THE WRIST

THE WRIST

Editors

H. KIRK WATSON, M.D.

Director
Connecticut Combined Hand Surgery Fellowship
Hartford Hospital
Connecticut Children's Medical Center
Hartford, Connecticut
Clinical Professor
Department of Orthopaedics
University of Connecticut School of Medicine
Farmington, Connecticut
Assistant Clinical Professor
Department of Orthopaedics, Rehabilitation, and Plastic Surgery
Yale University School of Medicine
New Haven, Connecticut

JEFFREY WEINZWEIG, M.D.

Assistant Professor
Division of Plastic Surgery
Department of Surgery
Brown University School of Medicine
Attending Plastic Surgeon
Department of Plastic Surgery
Rhode Island Hospital
Hasbro Children's Hospital
Providence, Rhode Island

with illustrations by Kate Sweeney

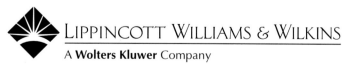

LIPPINCOTT WILLIAMS & WILKINS
A **Wolters Kluwer** Company
Philadelphia • Baltimore • New York • London
Buenos Aires • Hong Kong • Sydney • Tokyo

Acquisitions Editor: Robert Hurley
Developmental Editor: Keith Donnellan
Production Editor: Rosemary Palumbo
Manufacturing Manager: Tim Reynolds
Cover Designer: Co.Laborative Design
Compositor: Lippincott Williams & Wilkins Desktop Division

©2001 by LIPPINCOTT WILLIAMS & WILKINS
530 Walnut Street
Philadelphia, PA 19106 USA
LWW.com

All rights reserved. This book is protected by copyright. No part of this book may be reproduced in any form or by any means, including photocopying, or utilized by any information storage and retrieval system without written permission from the copyright owner, except for brief quotations embodied in critical articles and reviews. Materials appearing in this book prepared by individuals as part of their official duties as U.S. government employees are not covered by the above-mentioned copyright.

Printed and bound in China

Library of Congress Cataloging-in-Publication Data

The wrist /editors, H. Kirk Watson, Jeffrey Weinzweig.
   p. ; cm.
  Includes bibliographical references and index.
  ISBN 0-397-51726-2
  1. Wrist—Surgery. 2. Wrist—Wounds and injuries—Surgery. I. Watson, H. Kirk.
II. Weinzweig, Jeffrey, 1963– .
   [DNLM: 1. Wrist Joint. 2. Joint Diseases. 3. Wrist Injuries. WE 830 W95 2000]
RD559.W742 2000
617.5′74—dc21
                                           99-462327

Care has been taken to confirm the accuracy of the information presented and to describe generally accepted practices. However, the authors, editors, and publisher are not responsible for errors or omissions or for any consequences from application of the information in this book and make no warranty, expressed or implied, with respect to the currency, completeness, or accuracy of the contents of the publication. Application of this information in a particular situation remains the professional responsibility of the practitioner.

The authors, editors, and publisher have exerted every effort to ensure that drug selection and dosage set forth in this text are in accordance with current recommendations and practice at the time of publication. However, in view of ongoing research, changes in government regulations, and the constant flow of information relating to drug therapy and drug reactions, the reader is urged to check the package insert for each drug for any change in indications and dosage and for added warnings and precautions. This is particularly important when the recommended agent is a new or infrequently employed drug.

Some drugs and medical devices presented in this publication have Food and Drug Administration (FDA) clearance for limited use in restricted research settings. It is the responsibility of the health care provider to ascertain the FDA status of each drug or device planned for use in their clinical practice.

10 9 8 7 6 5 4 3 2 1

*For those without whom life would have no meaning,
Your forbearance—my thanks. For my Tracy, and
Hayes, Reid, Beecher, Aubrey, Drew, Jill, Lauren,
Monie and Beth.*

H.K.W.

*For my father and my mother,
Who taught me everything I know,
That really matters.*

J.W.

CONTENTS

Contributing Authors xi
Foreword by Julio Taleisnik xv
Preface xvii
Acknowledgments xix

SECTION I: INTRODUCTION TO THE WRIST

1. Evolution of the Wrist: The First 400 Million Years 1
   Jeffrey Weinzweig and H. Kirk Watson

2. Anatomy of the Wrist 7
   Marc Garcia-Elias

3. Kinematics of the Wrist 21
   Rita M. Patterson and Steven F. Viegas

4. Biomechanics of the Wrist 27
   Jaiyoung Ryu

SECTION II: EVALUATION OF WRIST SYMPTOMS

5. Examination of the Wrist 47
   Jeffrey Weinzweig and H. Kirk Watson

6. Imaging of the Symptomatic Wrist 61
   Yuming Yin and Louis A. Gilula

7. Wrist Arthroscopy 83
   Terry L. Whipple and Thomas A. Dwyer

8. Extraarticular Etiologies of Wrist Pain 95
   Martti Vastamäki

9. Carpal Tunnel Syndrome 107
   James C.Y. Chow

SECTION III: CONGENITAL AND PEDIATRIC ANOMALIES

10. Congenital Anomalies of the Wrist 123
    Dieter Buck-Gramcko

11. Pediatric Problems Involving the Wrist 149
    Jaiyoung Ryu and Bruce F. C. Gomberg

SECTION IV: CARPAL BONE FRACTURES

12. Carpal Bone Fractures (Excluding Scaphoid Fractures) 173
    Marc Garcia-Elias

13. Diagnosis and Management of Scaphoid Fractures 187
    David M. Kalainov and A. Lee Osterman

SECTION V: FRACTURE-DISLOCATIONS OF THE CARPUS

14. Carpal Dislocations and Instability 203
    Richard S. Idler

15. Open Reduction and Ligamentous Repair of Carpal Fracture-Dislocations 231
    Robert R. Slater, Jr. and Robert M. Szabo

16. Carpometacarpal Fractures and Fracture-Dislocations 255
    Marc Garcia-Elias

SECTION VI: WRIST AMPUTATION AND REPLANTATION

17. Transcarpal and Radiocarpal Wrist Amputation and Replantation 269
    David L. Cannon and James R. Urbaniak

SECTION VII: DISTAL RADIUS FRACTURES

18. Classification and Conservative Treatment of Distal Radius Fractures 277
    Diego L. Fernandez and Claude J. Martin

19. External Fixation of Distal Radius Fractures 299
    Michael E. Rettig, Keith B. Raskin, and Charles P. Melone, Jr.

20 Open Reduction and Internal Fixation of Distal Radius Fractures 311
Howard A. Lipton and Jesse B. Jupiter

21 Reconstruction of Secondary Carpal Problems Following Distal Radius Fracture 341
Brian Fingado and Scott W. Wolfe

SECTION VIII: THE DISTAL RADIOULNAR JOINT

22 Management of the Painful Distal Radioulnar Joint 369
Joseph E. Imbriglia and John W. Clifford

SECTION IX: KIENBÖCK'S DISEASE

23 Kienböck's Disease: Overview and Classification 395
Robert C. Kramer and David M. Lichtman

24 Theory and Etiology of Kienböck's Disease 411
H. Kirk Watson and Jeffrey Weinzweig

25 Lunate Revascularization 419
Hiroshi Yajima

SECTION X: CARPAL INSTABILITY

26 The Pathogenesis of Carpal Ligament Instability 431
Jack K. Mayfield

27 Dynamics of Carpal Instability 455
William B. Kleinman

28 Dorsal Wrist Syndrome: Predynamic Carpal Instability 483
Jeffrey Weinzweig and H. Kirk Watson

29 Ligamentous Repair for Scapholunate Instability and Dissociation 491
Mark S. Cohen and Julio Taleisnik

30 Lunotriquetral Joint Instability 501
Neal Hochwald and Martin A. Posner

31 Midcarpal Instability 511
Andrew E. Caputo, H. Kirk Watson, and Jeffrey Weinzweig

SECTION XI: OSTEOARTHRITIS OF THE WRIST

32 Limited Wrist Arthrodesis 521
Jeffrey Weinzweig and H. Kirk Watson

33 Proximal Row Carpectomy 545
Robert Lee Wilson and Douglas M. Hassan

34 Total Wrist Arthrodesis 555
Hill Hastings II and Martin I. Boyer

35 The Carpometacarpal Joint 567
N. George Kasparyan and Andrew J. Weiland

36 Crystalline Arthropathies of the Wrist 583
David B. Fulton and Peter J. Stern

SECTION XII: ULNAR WRIST PAIN

37 Overview of Ulnar Wrist Pain 591
James R. Skahen III and Andrew K. Palmer

38 Triangular Fibrocartilage Complex Injury and Repair 607
Scott D. Sagerman, Andrew K. Palmer, and Walter H. Short

39 Ulnar Impaction Syndrome 615
Andrew K. Palmer, Walter H. Short, and David A. Toivonen

40 Triquetral Impingement Ligament Tear Syndrome 633
H. Kirk Watson and Jeffrey Weinzweig

SECTION XIII: RHEUMATOID WRIST

41 Principles of Rheumatoid Arthritis 639
H. Kirk Watson and Jeffrey Weinzweig

42 Evaluation and Treatment of the Rheumatoid Wrist 645
Leonard K. Ruby and Charles Cassidy

43 Total Wrist Arthroplasty 659
Jay Menon

SECTION XIV: TUMORS OF THE WRIST

44 Benign Tumors of the Wrist 683
Michael J. Botte, Hoang N. Tran, Reid A. Abrams, Luke M. Vaughan, Richard A. Brown, Merlin L. Hamer, and Clifford W. Colwell

45 Malignant Tumors of the Wrist 723
Harold M. Dick and Robert J. Strauch

SECTION XV: REHABILITATION OF THE WRIST

46 Diagnosis and Management of Reflex Sympathetic Dystrophy (Complex Regional Pain Syndrome) 741
Lois Carlson and H. Kirk Watson

47 Therapeutic Management of the Wrist 757
Lois Carlson and Judy Stannard

SECTION XVI: ATLAS OF OPERATIVE TECHNIQUES IN WRIST RECONSTRUCTION

48 Casting for Limited Wrist Arthrodesis 777
Emmanuella Joseph, Richard J. DeRosa, Jr., and Lois Carlson

49 Capitate Shortening with Capitate-Hamate Fusion 785
Edward E. Almquist

50 Carpal Boss Repair 793
Jeffrey Weinzweig and H. Kirk Watson

51 Carpometacarpal Tendon Arthroplasty 797
H. Kirk Watson and Jeffrey Weinzweig

52 The Darrach Procedure 803
Charles Cassidy and Leonard K. Ruby

53 Distal Radioulnar Joint Dislocation Stabilization 811
H. Kirk Watson and Jeffrey Weinzweig

54 Distal Radius Bone Graft Harvest 815
Jeffrey Weinzweig and H. Kirk Watson

55 Dorsal Capsulodesis for Rotary Subluxation of the Scaphoid 819
Gerald Blatt

56 Dorsal Wrist Syndrome Repair 829
Jeffrey Weinzweig and H. Kirk Watson

57 Lunotriquetral Arthrodesis 833
H. Kirk Watson and Jeffrey Weinzweig

58 Matched Hemiresection–Interposition Arthroplasty 837
Robert S. Richards and James H. Roth

59 Matched Ulnar Arthroplasty 847
Jeffrey Weinzweig and H. Kirk Watson

60 Radial Shortening Osteotomy 855
Edward A. Stokel and Thomas E. Trumble

61 Radiocarpal Arthrodesis–Arthroplasty for Rheumatoid Arthritis 861
H. Kirk Watson and Jeffrey Weinzweig

62 Radiolunate Arthrodesis 867
Philippe Saffar

63 Radioulnar Arthrodesis 875
Joseph E. Imbriglia and John W. Clifford

64 Rotary Subluxation of the Scaphoid: Correction Using the Flexor Carpi Radialis 879
Giorgio A. Brunelli and Giovanni R. Brunelli

65 Reflex Sympathetic Dystrophy: Stress Loading Dystrophile Program 885
Lois Carlson and H. Kirk Watson

66 Sauvé-Kapandji Procedure 889
Peter J. Millroy

67 Scaphocapitate Arthrodesis 895
Vilijam Zdravkovic and Gontran R. Sennwald

68 Scaphoid Nonunion: Biconcave Bone Grafting 901
H. Kirk Watson and Jeffrey Weinzweig

69 Scaphoid Nonunion: Vascularized Bone Grafting 907
Alexander Y. Shin and Allen T. Bishop

70 Scapholunate Ligament Reconstruction Utilizing a Bone–Retinaculum–Bone Autograft 915
Michael T. LeGeyt and Arnold-Peter C. Weiss

71 Scapholunate Adavanced Collapse Wrist Reconstruction 921
Jeffrey Weinzweig and H. Kirk Watson

72 Trapezoidal Osteotomy of the Distal Radius 927
Jeffrey Weinzweig and H. Kirk Watson

73 Triscaphe Arthrodesis 931
H. Kirk Watson and Jeffrey Weinzweig

74 Ulnar Lengthening 939
Hermann Krimmer and Ulrich Lanz

75 Wrist Denervation 945
Guy Foucher and Allen T. Bishop

76 Wrist Stenosing Tenosynovitis: Cocompartment Release 953
H. Kirk Watson, James Michael Shenko, and Jeffrey Weinzweig

Subject Index 955

CONTRIBUTING AUTHORS

Reid A. Abrams, M.D. Associate Professor, Department of Orthopaedics, University of California, San Diego, 350 Dickinson Street, Mailcode 8894, San Diego, California 92103

Edward E. Almquist, M.D. Clinical Professor, Department of Orthopaedics, University of Washington School of Medicine, 600 Broadway, Suite 440, Seattle, Washington 98122

Allen T. Bishop, M.D. Professor, Department of Orthopaedic Surgery, Mayo Medical School; and Chief, Division of Hand Surgery, Department of Orthopaedic Surgery, Mayo Clinic, 200 First Street, SW, Rochester, Minnesota 55905

Gerald Blatt, M.D. Associate Clinical Professor, Department of Orthopedic Surgery, University of California at Los Angeles, 555 Westwood Plaza, Los Angeles, California 90024; and Senior Consultant, Department of Hand Surgery, Harbor–UCLA Medical Center, 1000 West Carson Street, Torrance, California 90509

Michael J. Botte, M.D. Clinical Professor, Department of Orthopaedic Surgery, University of California, San Diego, 200 West Arbor Drive, San Diego, California 92103; and Head, Section of Neuromuscular Reconstruction Surgery and Rehabilitation, Department of Orthopaedic Surgery, Scripps Clinic and Research Foundation, 10666 North Torrey Pines Road, La Jolla, California 92037

Martin I. Boyer, M.D. Assistant Professor, Department of Orthopaedic Surgery, Washington University School of Medicine, 1 Barnes Jewish Hospital Plaza, Suite 11300, West Pavillion, St. Louis, Missouri 63110

Richard A. Brown, M.D. Assistant Clinical Professor, Department of Orthopaedic Surgery, University of California, San Diego, 200 West Arbor Drive, San Diego, California 92103; and Department of Orthopaedic Surgery, Scripps Clinic and Research Foundation, 10666 North Torrey Pines Road, La Jolla, California 92037

Giorgio A. Brunelli, M.D. President, Foundation for Research in Spinal Cord Lesions, and Professor, Department of Orthopaedics, Clinica S. Rocco, Via Campiani 77, 25060 Cellatica, Italy

Giovanni R. Brunelli, M.D. Hand Surgery Service, Institute Ortopedico Galeazzi, Milan, Italy

Dieter Buck-Gramcko, M.D. Professor Emeritus, Department of Surgery, University of Hamburg, and Former Chief, Department of Hand Surgery, Wilhelmstift Children's Hospital, Liliencronstrasse 130, Hamburg D-22149, Germany

David L. Cannon, M.D. Assistant Professor, Department of Surgery, Uniformed Services University of Health Sciences, 4301 Jones Bridge Road, Bethesda, Maryland 20814; and Co-Director, Hand and Upper Extremity Division, Department of Orthopaedic Surgery, Navy Medical Center, 27 Effingham Street, Portsmouth, Virginia 23708

Andrew E. Caputo, M.D. Clinical Assistant Professor, Department of Orthopaedic Surgery, University of Connecticut Health Center, 10 Talcott Notch, Farmington, Connecticut 06032; and Co-director, Hand Surgery Service, Department of Orthopaedic Surgery, Hartford Hospital and Connecticut Children's Medical Center, Hartford, Connecticut 06106

Lois Carlson, O.T.R./L., C.H.T. Director, Connecticut Combined Hand Therapy (a division of Hartford Orthopaedic, Plastic, and Hand Surgeons, Inc.), 131 New London Turnpike, Suite 319, Glastonbury, Connecticut 06033

Charles Cassidy, M.D. Assistant Professor, Department of Orthopaedics, Tufts University School of Medicine and New England Medical Center, 750 Washington Street, Box 26, Boston, Massachusetts 02111

James C.Y. Chow, M.D. Clinical Assistant Professor, Department of Surgery, Southern Illinois University School of Medicine, Springfield, Illinois 62701; and President and Founder, Orthopaedic Center of Southern Illinois, P.O. Box 2064, 4121 Veterans Memorial Drive, Mount Vernon, Illinois 62864

John W. Clifford, M.D. Department of Orthopaedics, Kaiser Santa Teresa Community Hospital, 263 International Circle, Building 1, North, San Jose, California 95119

Mark S. Cohen, M.D. Assistant Professor, Hand and Elbow Program and Orthopaedic Education, Department of Orthopaedic Surgery, Rush-Presbyterian-St. Luke's Medical Center, Chicago, Illinois 60612

Clifford W. Colwell, M.D. Department of Orthopaedic Surgery, Scripps Clinic and Research Foundation, 10666 North Torrey Pines Road, La Jolla, California 92037

Richard J. DeRosa, Jr., O.T.C. Senior Orthopaedic Technologist, Casting Section, Orthopaedic Associates of Hartford, 85 Seymour Street, Suite 607, Hartford, Connecticut 06106

Harold M. Dick, M.D. Professor, Department of Orthopaedic Surgery, Columbia University, 622 West 168th Street; and Attending Physician, Department of Orthopaedics, New York Presbyterian Hospital, 622 West 168th Street, PH-1150, New York, New York 10032

Thomas A. Dwyer, M.D. 1226 West Landis Avenue, Pittsgrove, New Jersey 08318

Diego L. Fernandez, M.D., Ph.D. Associate Professor, Department of Orthopaedic Surgery, University of Berne, and Staff, Department of Orthopaedic Surgery, Lindenhof Hospital, Mittelstrasse 54, Berne CH-3010, Switzerland

Brian Fingado, M.D. Holy Cross Orthopaedics, 6000 North Federal Highway, Fort Lauderdale, Florida 33308

Guy Foucher, M.D. Ancien Chef de Clinique de la Faculté de Strasbourg, 4 Boulevard Edwards, Strasbourg 67000, France

David B. Fulton, M.D. Orthopaedic Surgeon, The Moore Orthopaedic Clinic, 1 Richland Medical Park, Suite 110, Columbia, South Carolina 29203

Marc Garcia-Elias, M.D, Ph.D. Staff, Hand & Upper Extremity Surgery, Institut Kaplan, Pg. Bonanova, 9, 2º, 2ª, Barcelona 08022, Spain

Louis A. Gilula, M.D. Professor, Mallinckrodt Institute of Radiology, Washington University School of Medicine, 510 South Kingshighway Boulevard; and Radiologist, Department of Radiology, Barnes Jewish Hospital, One Barnes Hospital Plaza, St. Louis, Missouri 63110

Bruce F.C. Gomberg, M.D., M.A. Resident, Department of Orthopedics, West Virginia University, 1 Hospital Drive, Box 9196, Morgantown, West Virginia 26506

Merlin L. Hamer, M.D. Department of Orthopaedic Surgery, Scripps Clinic and Research Foundation, 10666 North Torrey Pines Road, La Jolla, California 92037

Douglas M. Hassan, M.D. Attending Surgeon, Department of Surgery, St. Joseph's Medical Center, 1717 South J Street, Tacoma, Washington 98405

Hill Hastings II, M.D. Clinical Associate Professor, The Indiana Hand Center, Indiana University Medical School, 8501 Harcourt Road, Indianapolis, Indiana 46260

Neal Hochwald, M.D. Assistant Attending Surgeon, Department of Orthopeadics, Huntington Hospital, 270 Park Avenue, Huntington, New York 11743

Richard S. Idler, M.D. Clinical Associate Professor, Indiana Hand Center, Indiana University Medical School, 8501 Harcourt Road, P.O. Box 80434, Indianapolis, Indiana 46280

Joseph E. Imbriglia, M.D. Department of Orthopaedics, Western Pennsylvania Hand Center, 127 Anderson Street, #201, Pittsburgh, Pennsylvania 15212

Emmanuella Joseph, M.D. Fellow, Section of Plastic Surgery, Department of Surgery, Medical College of Ohio, 626 Pine Valley Lane, #203, Toledo, Ohio 43615

Jesse B. Jupiter, M.D. Professor, Department of Orthopaedic Surgery, Harvard Medical School, Shattock Street; and Chief, Department of Orthopaedics, Massachusetts General Hospital, 15 Parkman Street, ACC 527, Boston, Massachusetts 02114

David M. Kalainov, M.D. Instructor, Department of Orthopaedic Surgery, Northwestern University Medical School, 303 East Chicago Avenue; and Associate Attending, Department of Orthopaedic Surgery, Northwestern Memorial Hospital, 251 East Huron Street, Chicago, Illinois 60611

N. George Kasparyan, M.D., Ph.D. Staff Surgeon, Section of Hand Surgery, Department of Orthopaedic Surgery, Lahey Clinic, 41 Mall Road, Burlington, Massachusetts 01805

William B. Kleinman, M.D. Clinical Professor, Department of Orthopaedic Surgery, The Indiana Hand Center, Indiana University School of Medicine, 8501 Harcourt Road, Indianapolis, Indiana 46280

Robert C. Kramer, M.D. Hand Surgeon, Beaumont Bone and Joint Institute, 3650 Laurel Avenue, Beaumont, Texas 77707

Hermann Krimmer, M.D. University of Würzburg, Sanderring 2, Würzburg 97070, Germany; and Klinik fur Handchirurgie, Rhön Klinikum, Salzburger Liete 1, Bad Neustadt 97616, Germany

Ulrich Lanz, M.D. Professor, University of Würzburg, Sanderring 2, Würzburg 97070, Germany; and Chief, Klinik fur Handchirurgie, Rhön-Klinikum, Salzburger Liete 1, Bad Neustadt 97616, Germany

Michael T. LeGeyt, M.D. Staff Surgeon, Department of Orthopaedic Surgery, Bristol Hospital, 64 Brewster Road, Bristol, Connecticut 06010

David M. Lichtman, M.D. Adjunct Professor, Department of Surgery, Uniformed Services University of the Health Sciences, 4301 Jones Bridge Road, Bethesda, Maryland 20814; and Clinical Professor, Department of Orthopedic Surgery, The University of Texas Southwestern Medical Center at Dallas, 5323 Harry Hines Boulevard, Dallas, Texas 75235

Howard A. Lipton, M.D. Director, Hand Surgery Service, Department of Plastic and Reconstructive Surgery, Hadassah-University Hospital, Eiu Kerem, Jerusalem 91120, Israel

Claude J. Martin, M.D. Department of Medical Services, Commission of Health and Occupational Safety, 1199 DeBleury, Montreal, Quebec H3C4E1 Canada

Jack K. Mayfield, M.D. Adjunct Professor, Biological, Chemical, and Materials Engineering, Arizona State University; and Staff Surgeon, Department of Orthopaedic Surgery, St. Luke's Hospital, 525 N. 18th Street, #308, Phoenix, Arizona 85006

Charles P. Melone, Jr., M.D. Department of Orthopaedic Surgery, New York University Medical Center, 317 East 34th Street, New York, New York 10016

Jay Menon, M.D. (deceased) Consultant Hand Surgeon, Department of Orthopaedic Surgery, Southern California Permanente Medical Group, 9985 Sierra Avenue, Fontana, California 92335

Peter J. Millroy, M.D. Watkins Medical Center, 225 Wickham Terrace, Brisbane, Queensland 4000, Australia

A. Lee Osterman, M.D. Professor, Department of Orthopaedic Surgery, Thomas Jefferson University Hospital, Philadelphia, Pennsylvania, 19106, and Philadelphia Hand Center, 700 S. Henderson Road, #200, King of Prussia, Pennsylvania 19406

Andrew K. Palmer, M.D. Professor, Department of Orthopedic Surgery, State University of New York Health Science Center at Syracuse, 550 Harrison Center, Syracuse, New York 13202

Rita M. Patterson, Ph.D. Deputy Director, Biomechanical Research, and Associate Professor, Department of Orthopaedic Surgery and Rehabilitation, The University of Texas Medical Branch, 301 University Boulevard, Galveston, Texas 77555

Martin A. Posner, M.D. Clinical Professor, Department of Orthopaedics, New York University School of Medicine; and Hand Services, Hospital for Joint Diseases and Lenox Hill Hospital, 2 East 88th Street, New York, New York 10128

Keith B. Raskin, M.D. Clinical Associate Professor, Department of Orthopaedic Surgery, New York University Medical Center; and Attending Surgeon, New York University/ Hospital for Joint Diseases, 317 East 34th Street, 3rd Floor, New York, New York 10016

Michael E. Rettig, M.D. Assistant Professor, Department of Orthopaedic Surgery, New York University Medical Center, 317 East 34th Street, New York, New York 10016

Robert S. Richards, M.D., F.R.C.S.C. Associate Professor, Divisions of Orthopaedics and Plastic Surgery, Department of Surgery, University of Western Ontario, 1151 Richmond Street; and Attending Staff, Hand and Upper Limb Center, St. Joseph's Health Centre, 268 Grosvenor Street, London, Ontario N6A 4L6, Canada

James H. Roth, M.D., F.R.C.S.C. Professor, Department of Surgery, University of Western Ontario, 1151 Richmond Street; and Director, Hand and Upper Limb Centre, St. Joseph's Health Centre, 268 Grosvenor Street, London, Ontario, N6A 4L6, Canada

Leonard K. Ruby, M.D. Department of Orthopaedics, Tufts University School of Medicine and New England Medical Center, 750 Washington St., Box 26, Boston, Massachusetts 02111

Jaiyoung Ryu, M.D. Associate Professor, Department of Orthopedics, West Virginia University, 1 Hospital Drive, P.O. Box 9196, Morgantown, West Virginia 26506

Philippe Saffar, M.D. Surgeon, Department of Hand Surgery, Hospital Boucicaut, 78, rue de la Convention, 75730 Paris; and Head, Institut Francais de Chirurgie de la Main, 5 rue du Dome, Paris 92200, France

Scott D. Sagerman, M.D. Instructor, Department of Orthopaedics, Northwestern University Medical School, 303 East Chicago Avenue, Chicago, Illinois 60611; and Surgeon, Department of Orthopaedics, Northwest Community Hospital, 800 West Central Road, Arlington Heights, Illinois 60005

Gontran R. Sennwald, M.D. Chief Consultant, Hand Surgery Unit, Medical School of Geneva, CH1200 Geneva, Switzerland

James Michael Shenko, M.D. Department of Plastic Surgery, University of Massachusetts Memorial Health Care, 119 Belmont Street, Worcester, Massachusetts 01605

Alexander Y. Shin, M.D., U.S.N.R. Assistant Professor, Department of Othopaedic Surgery, University of California, San Diego, 350 Dickinson Street, Mailcode 8894, San Diego, California 92103; and Director, Hand & Microvascular Surgery, Department of Orthopaedic Surgery, Naval Medical Center San Diego, 34800 Bob Wilson Drive, San Diego, California 92134

Walter H. Short, M.D. Department of Orthopedic Surgery, State University of New York Health Science Center at Syracuse, 550 Harrison Center, Syracuse, New York 13202

James R. Skahen III, M.D. Director, Hand Surgery, Department of Orthopedic Surgery, Northeast Medical Center, Church Street, and Vice-President, Northeast Orthopedics, 354 Copperfield Boulevard, Concord, North Carolina 28025

Robert R. Slater, Jr., M.D. Assistant Professor, Department of Orthopaedic Surgery, University of California, Davis, 4860 Y Street, Suite 3800, Sacramento, California 95817

Judy Stannard, P.T. Connecticut Combined Hand Therapy, 131 New London Turnpike, Suite 319, Glastonbury, Connecticut 06033

Peter J. Stern, M.D. Professor and Chairman, Department of Orthopaedic Surgery, University of Cincinnati College of Medicine, 231 Bethesda, Cincinnati, Ohio 45267

Edward A. Stokel, M.D. Private Practice, 907 San Ramon Valley Boulevard, Suite 202, Danville, California 94526

Robert J. Strauch, M.D. Assistant Professor, Department of Orthopaedic Surgery, Columbia University, 622 West 168th Street; and Assistant Attending Surgeon, Department of Orthopaedic Surgery, New York-Presbyterian Hospital, 622 West 168th Street, PH11-1115, New York, New York 10032

Robert M. Szabo, M.D., M.P.H. Professor, Departments of Orthopaedic Surgery and Plastic Surgery, University of California, Davis, 4860 Y Street; and Chief, Hand and Upper Extremity, Department of Orthopaedic Surgery, University of California, Davis Health Care System, 2215 Stockton Boulevard, Sacramento, California 95817

Julio Taleisnik, M.D. Clinical Professor, Division of Orthopaedics, Department of Surgery, University of California, Irvine, School of Medicine, Irvine, California 92717

David A. Toivonen, M.D. Northeast Wisconsin Center for Surgery and Rehabililtation of the Hand, Ltd., 2555 Northern Road, Appleton, Wisconsin 54914

Hoang N. Tran, M.D. Resident, Department of Orthopaeddic Surgery, University of California, San Diego, 200 West Arbor Drive, San Diego, California, 92103; and Scripps Clinic and Research Foundation, 10666 North Torrey Pines Road, La Jolla, California 92037

Thomas E. Trumble, M.D. Chief, Division of Hand and Microvascular Surgery, and Professor, Department of Orthopaedics, University of Washington and Harborview Medical Center, 1959 NE Pacific Street, Box 356500, Seattle, Washington 98195

James R. Urbaniak, M.D. Virginia Flowers Baker Professor, Division of Orthopaedic Surgery, Department of Surgery, Duke University School of Medicine; and Vice-Chairman and Chief, Division of Orthopaedic Surgery, Department of Surgery, Duke University Medical Center, Trent Drive, Box 2912, Durham, North Carolina 27710

Martti Vastamäki, M.D., Ph.D. Associate Professor and Chief, Department of Hand Surgery, Orton Hospital, Tenholantie 10, Helsinki 00280, Finland

Luke M. Vaughan, M.D. Associate Clinical Professor, Department of Orthopaedic Surgery, University of California, San Diego/Thornton Hospital, San Diego, California 92103; and Head, Tumor Surgery, Department of Orthopaedics, Scripps Clinic and Research Foundation, 10666 North Torrey Pines Road, La Jolla, California 92037

Steven F. Viegas, M.D. Professor and Chief, Division of Hand Surgery, Department of Orthopaedics and Rehabilitation, The University of Texas Medical Branch, 301 University Boulevard, Galveston, Texas 77555

H. Kirk Watson, M.D. Director, Connecticut Combined Hand Surgery Fellowship, Hartford Hospital, Connecticut Children's Medical Center, Hartford, Connecticut; Clinical Professor, Department of Orthopaedics, University of Connecticut School of Medicine, Farmington, Connecticut; Assistant Clinical Professor, Department of Orthopaedics, Rehabilitation, and Plastic Surgery, Yale University School of Medicine, New Haven, Connecticut 06510; 85 Seymour Street, Suite 816, Hartford, Connecticut 06106

Andrew J. Weiland, M.D., Ph.D. Professor, Departments of Orthopaedic Surgery and Plastic Surgery, Cornell University Medical College, 535 East 70th Street, New York, New York 10021

Jeffrey Weinzweig, M.D. Assistant Professor, Division of Plastic Surgery, Department of Surgery, Brown University School of Medicine; Attending Plastic Surgeon, Department of Plastic Surgery, Rhode Island Hospital and Hasbro Children's Hospital, 2 Dudley Street, Suite 380, Providence, Rhode Island 02905

Arnold-Peter C. Weiss Professor, Department of Orthopaedics, Brown University School of Medicine, 2 Dudley Street, Suite 200, Providence, Rhode Island 02905

Terry L. Whipple, M.D. Clinical Assoiciate Professor, Department of Orthopaedics and Rehabilitation, University of Virginia School of Medicine, Charlottesville, Virginia 22908; and Director, Orthopaedic Research of Virginia, Health South Hospital, 7700 East Parham Road, Richmond, Virginia 23226

Robert Lee Wilson, M.D. Clinical Lecturer, Department of Surgery, University of Arizona, Tucson, Arizona 85719; and Hand Surgery Consultant, Phoenix Orthopedic Program, Maricopa Medical Center, 2601 E. Roosevelt Street, Phoenix, Arizona 85008

Scott W. Wolfe, M.D. Professor, Department of Orthopaedics, Yale University School of Medicine, 800 Howard Avenue, P.O. Box 208071; and Attending Surgeon, Department of Orthopaedics and Rehabilitation, Yale New Haven Hospital, 20 York Street, New Haven, Connecticut 06510

Hiroshi Yajima, M.D., Ph.D. Assistant Professor, Department of Orthopaedic Surgery, Nara Medical University, 840 Shijo-Cho, Kashihara, Nara 634-8522, Japan

Yuming Yin, M.D. Mallinckrodt Institute of Radiology, Washington University Medical Center, 510 South Kingshighway Boulevard, St. Louis, Missouri 63110

Vilijam Zdravkovic Kantonsspital Altsätten, Ch-9450 Altsätten, Switzerland

FOREWORD

"The game is afoot, Watson."
Sherlock Holmes

In 1994, Kirk Watson approached me with a question: Is there a place for yet another book dedicated to the wrist? He had been asked to edit such a text, but was concerned that the scientific literature was already saturated, and that any other publication on this subject would be at best redundant, at worst unnecessary. I knew, however, that a book containing Kirk's practical and commonsensical approach to the wrist, together with his vast experience, would be an important contribution. Over a period of at least twenty years, many of us, including Kirk, had managed to find answers to some of the many problems we faced in examining and treating patients with wrist problems. Much of our experience resulted from trial and error. Clearly, there was a need for a textbook which would describe this experience, and provide the practitioner with solutions to practical problems in a direct manner.

It was coincidental that this conversation took place exactly twenty years after Kirk and I first met and became aware of each other's interest in problems of the wrist. In 1974, we were both part of the delegation of the American Society for Surgery of the Hand, and attended the first combined meeting held with the Japanese Society for Surgery of the Hand. One day, after lunch, we found ourselves alone, and took a long walk, during which we shared our fascination with this complex and enigmatic joint. This was the first of many similar conversations, and the beginning of a respectful, challenging, and close friendship.

Indeed, during these encounters, we explored ideas which formed the foundation for subsequent research. Vivid in my mind is a period of three days in Paris, France, where Kirk and I participated in a symposium hosted by Professor Raoul Tubiana. Every day, at breakfast and during long taxi rides to and from the meeting, we would challenge each other with our ideas. By-products of our discussions included a consideration of carpal instability as dynamic or static, the relationship between the tilt of the distal radius and midcarpal alignment, and the difference in behavior of the carpus under kinetic and kinematic conditions. Throughout these very exciting exchanges, I learned to appreciate the wit, the intelligence, and the innovative thought process always at work in Kirk's mind, behind the droll, Gary Cooper-ish façade.

It is, therefore, not surprising that innovation and common sense are at the core of this book, edited by Dr. Watson and one of his former Hand Fellows, Dr. Jeffrey Weinzweig. They secured the cooperation of a superb group of contributors, and organized the text in a logical and readable fashion.

Editors' Comments are included at the end of many chapters whenever approaches or concepts would benefit. In addition, Drs. Watson and Weinzweig simplified the search for surgical techniques by placing step-by-step descriptions in single chapters within Section XVI, an Atlas of Operative Techniques in Wrist Reconstruction. I was honored by Dr. Watson's and Dr. Weinzweig's request that I provide a foreword to their book. This Dr. Watson is very much unlike the Dr. Watson of Sherlock Holmes fame. In Sir Arthur Conan Doyle's books, the brilliant mind belonged to Holmes, while Dr. Watson was merely his sidekick. Kirk Watson is, however, more like the Dr. Watson portrayed in the 1988 movie "Without a Clue." In that movie, Dr. Watson was in reality the mastermind detective, and Sherlock Holmes was a third-rate actor he hired to play the role of the master sleuth. Just like in the film, this Dr. Watson is the mastermind whose teachings and publications are behind many of our advances in understanding and treating the wrist.

Julio Taleisnik, M.D.

PREFACE

Four hundred million years of evolution have yielded the most complex human joint—*the wrist*. What originated as the pectoral fin of a primitive fish, a swimming appendage, has evolved into a weight-bearing joint and ultimately into an intricate structure capable of sophisticated multiplanar motion. Several carpal structures have emerged relatively recently, becoming more prominent and assuming crucial functional roles, while others have regressed, maintaining only vestigal roles. The past three decades have seen great strides in our understanding of wrist anatomy, function, and pathology, and in the development of solutions to complex clinical problems. Much has been learned concerning how, why, and under what conditions the wrist fails. These advances have been fueled by the fervor of both scientists and surgeons striving to better understand this fascinating joint.

This book is our attempt to portray the wrist as seen from the world's most expert eyes. Almost 100 authors from all over the world have contributed their thoughts, approaches, and clinical cases to produce this comprehensive volume. The assimilation of anatomy, theory, and technique is integral to the development of a three-dimensional conceptualization of the complexities of the wrist. The majority of chapters in Sections I through XV incorporate all of these elements in addressing a particular concept while others focus on each element specifically. Section XVI, the Atlas of Operative Techniques in Wrist Reconstruction, provides detailed, step-by-step demonstrations of dozens of reconstructive procedures while many other techniques are included in the body of the text. Complementing these clinical elements are over 500 color intraoperative photographs. Editors' Comments, which follow most chapters, provide additional perspectives, underscore crucial caveats, and elicit controversial issues from which the reader may benefit. As a result, there are discrepancies and disagreements throughout, as there should be in any unfinished work.

It will take many more decades of study before we have a complete understanding of the intricacies of the wrist. We feel very fortunate to have shared this journey with the numerous luminaries who have contributed to our current conceptualization of the wrist. To those who follow, enthusiastically seeking answers, we encourage you to search for new paths and explore novel concepts. *Carpe carpus!*

H. Kirk Watson, M.D
Jeffrey Weinzweig, M.D.

ACKNOWLEDGMENTS

The orchestration of almost 100 authors from a dozen countries was no easy task. The compilation of a comprehensive text demands attention to thousands of details and microdetails that could only be accomplished by a dedicated team of highly talented individuals committed to producing a book of the finest quality. We are extremely fortunate to have had just such a team involved in the gargantuan undertaking of producing *The Wrist*.

We are indebted to the scores of wrist aficionados who contributed their time and ingenuity to produce the 76 beautifully-crafted chapters that comprise *The Wrist*. Many of these chapters have been supplemented by the superb drawings of medical illustrator Kate Sweeney. These drawings provide additional clarity where complex anatomy and concepts need it most. The coordination of communications between artist and editors, editors and authors, editor and editor, and all sorts of other permutations and combinations, could only be accomplished by our gifted administrative assistant Barbara Smith, whom we have been fortunate enough to have had along for the roller coaster ride from day one. Her rare ability to grasp the only glimmer of light in the darkest storm, nurture it, then use it to burn off any remaining clouds, was instrumental in the completion of this text. Our appreciation transcends words.

Lippincott Williams & Wilkins provided us with an editorial and production staff with open minds and a willingness to allow us to digress now and then from convention. For that, and for our inclusion in virtually every decision and detail that contributed to the book's evolution, we are very grateful. Of course, we are not sure how wise it was to let us have our way, but we did enjoy the ride. We are especially grateful to our editors, Danette Knopp, Keith Donnellan, Rosemary Palumbo, and Robert Hurley, whose efforts in bringing this project to fruition have been extraordinary. In retrospect, each of those knock-down, drag-outs was certainly well worth the product that resulted.

THE WRIST

1

EVOLUTION OF THE WRIST
THE FIRST 400 MILLION YEARS

JEFFREY WEINZWEIG
H. KIRK WATSON

Inquiry into the origin of hands leads us down the animal phyla until we find the beginning of limbs in the primitive sharks. Here is the first sign—a lateral fold on each side, continuous from gill to anus, into which muscles grew in later development. The middle of each fold receded, but the two ends increased, so that it became the established order throughout all fishes to have two pectoral fins just behind the gills and two pelvic fins near the anus. Since then this tetrapod or four-limbed architecture has persisted through all consecutive classes—amphibians, reptiles, and mammals—up to man.

Sterling Bunnell, M.D.
Surgery of the Hand (1944)

The first paragraph of the original edition of Bunnell's classic treatise tersely traces the origin of the hand and deftly reinforces the concept of structural preservation through the evolutionary process (1). The present description of the evolution of the wrist represents not a compilation of evolutionary minutia reprocessed and conveyed as convoluted rhetoric, but rather an overview of this fascinating process presented as a concise discussion of a series of sequences that span almost half a billion years. In-depth treatises on this subject matter are alluded to, and their review, for the enthusiast, is encouraged.

The evolutionary development of the wrist joint began 400 million years ago, originating as the pectoral fin of *Crossopterygii*, a primitive fish (Fig. 1.1) (2). The *Crossopterygii* were the immediate predecessors of the lungfish *Dipnoi*, which possessed an articulated bony skeleton activated by muscles within the fins, analogous to intrinsic muscles. These fins, which were used for locomotion along shallow fresh waters, had a primitive carpus with multiple rays. This provided the basis for limb development (3). From these marginal rays the pisiform and prepollex ultimately developed, but there is no evidence to suggest they functioned as digits (2,4). Thus, the earliest form of the wrist was present in the pentadactyl limb.

This subclass of fish emerged from the water to become amphibians and developed lungs and limbs for terrestrial existence (1). As species became more terrestrial, the wrist evolved into a weight-bearing joint as the functional needs of the new environment dictated. The wrist evolved from a swimming appendage to a weight-bearing joint to a complex structure capable of fine movement in space as the evolutionary course progressed from amphibians to reptiles, mammals, primates, and, finally, humans.

Successful transition to terrestrial inhabitance was achieved by the *Eryops*, a land-dwelling amphibian approximately 3 m long that thrived 370 million years ago when amphibians were the dominant land animals. Further evolution of the crossopterygian pectoral fin, characterized by a shoulder girdle, humerus, radius, ulna, 11 or 12 carpal bones, and five phalanges, yielded the upper extremity of the *Eryops* (Fig. 1.2). The carpal bones of these primitive amphibians were arranged in a block-like mosaic pattern of three rows. The upper limb morphology of the *Eryops* persisted without significant change through the subsequent evolution of reptiles, which appeared 70 million years later (Fig. 1.3).

The reptilian wrist, a plantigrade structure, represented a reduction in the number of carpal bones, the result of either coalescence or elimination, in which 10 bones were arranged in two rows, the distal row of five carpal bones articulating with the metacarpals in pentadactylate fashion (Fig. 1.4). This primitive pentadactylate hand had two rows of carpal bones and, often, one to three carpal bones intercalated between the rows. The three bones of the proximal row—the radiale, intermedium, and ulnare—are named based on their relation to the forearm bones. The five carpal bones of the distal row are named, from radial to ulnar, I,

---

J. Weinzweig: Department of Plastic Surgery, Brown University School of Medicine, Rhode Island Hospital, and Hasbro Children's Hospital, Providence, Rhode Island 02905.

H. K. Watson: Connecticut Combined Hand Surgery Fellowship, Hartford Hospital, and Connecticut Children's Medical Center, Hartford, Connecticut 06106; Department of Orthopaedics, University of Connecticut School of Medicine, Farmington, Connecticut 06032; Department of Orthopedics, Rehabilitation, and Plastic Surgery, Yale University School of Medicine, New Haven, Connecticut 06520.

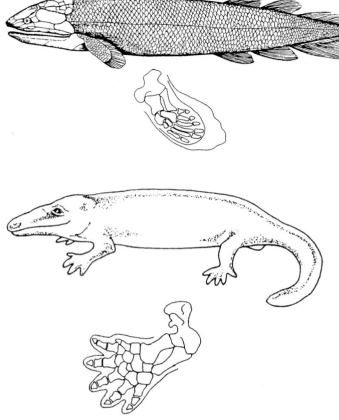

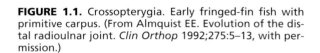

FIGURE 1.1. Crossopterygia. Early fringed-fin fish with primitive carpus. (From Almquist EE. Evolution of the distal radioulnar joint. *Clin Orthop* 1992;275:5–13, with permission.)

FIGURE 1.2. *Eryops.* Primitive amphibian with evolving carpus. (From Almquist EE. Evolution of the distal radioulnar joint. *Clin Orthop* 1992;275:5–13, with permission.)

II, III, IV, and V. From each of these distal row bones extended a number of phalanges. In modern amphibians, some of the carpal bones are fused or absent, and the digits are reduced in number (1). In the frog, the radius and ulna are fused, and only six of its original nine carpal bones remain. It is unknown whether the reduction in the number of carpal bones or digits occurred as a result of coalescence or elimination (4). However, some amphibian wrists, such as that of the alligator, do demonstrate evidence of carpal reduction by synostosis.

On the basis of temporal fenestrations, reptiles are divided into three classes: anapsids (turtles), diapsids (dinosaurs), and synapsids, which represent the basis for mammalian evolution (3). Seventy million years later, approximately 230 million years ago, during the Triassic period, the first mammals arose in the reptilian-dominated

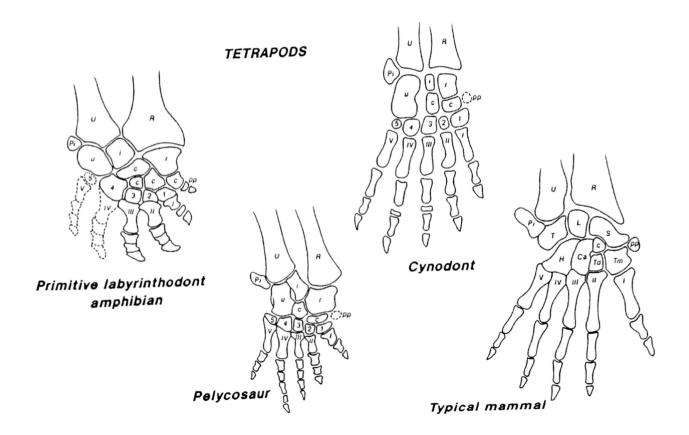

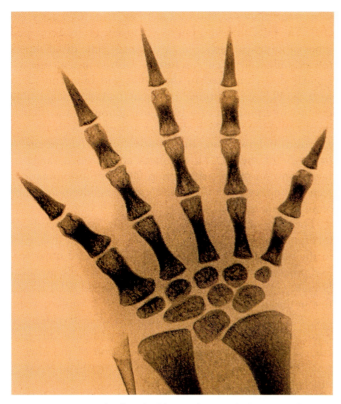

FIGURE 1.4. Hand of a Florida turtle, a primitive reptile. The radiale, intermedium, and ulnare, the three bones of the proximal carpal row, are seen distal to the os centrale. The phalangeal formula in this case is 2, 3, 3, 3, 2, which differs from the typical reptilian formula of 2, 3, 4, 5, 3. (From Bunnell S. *Surgery of the hand.* Philadelphia: JB Lippincott, 1944, with permission.).

world. The osseous morphology of the primitive mammalian wrist demonstrated remarkable similarity to that of the reptilian carpus; the phalangeal sequence revealed a reduction of the 2-3-4-5-3 pattern to 2-3-3-3-3.

One of the fundamental principles of Darwinism dictates that the most powerful force driving the machinery of evolutionary change is survival—the ability to adapt to the environment and compete for food (5). This is reflected in the metamorphosis of the carpus that occurs as functional demands, such as the need for increased strength, stability, or motion, dictate change. Therefore, it is not surprising that the carpus has undergone its most significant changes in species where the wrist is a weight-bearing joint. Carpal bones IV and V have fused in mammals, including man, to become the unciform (hamate). In primitive mammals there were three carpal bones and a pisiform in the proximal row and four bones in the distal row. Longitudinal weight-bearing through the carpus has resulted in addi-

tional carpal fusion or elimination. The scaphoid and lunate are supported by the radius, and the cuneiform (triquetrum) is supported by the ulna. The scaphoid articulates with the trapezium, trapezoid, and part of the os magnum (capitate); the lunate articulates with the os magnum and, usually, with the unciform as well, and the cuneiform articulates with the unciform (1).

In all carnivora, including seals and sea lions, the scaphoid and lunate are fused; in the hoofed animals, the trapezium is lost. In the primitive wrist, the trapezium, trapezoid, and os magnum each articulate with one metacarpal, and the unciform with the fourth and fifth; however, this arrangement has been modified with reductions in the number of metacarpal bones. The pisiform is not a true carpal bone, having developed as a sesamoid bone within a tendon at least as far back as the reptiles. In crocodiles and in most mammals it articulates with the ulna. In the carpus of most quadripeds and higher apes, the pisiform projects impressively from the volar aspect of the carpus. This and the tubercle of the scaphoid project for great muscle leverage in running, but the pisiform is rudimentary in man.

A change in the use of the hand for agility and quadrupedal gait in primitive species to its use for brachiation (the ability to swing progressively from hand to hand along a branch), manipulating rudimentary weapons, and, ultimately, handling tools is reflected in a number of evolutionary changes in the carpus (6). The primate wrist, although structurally similar to earlier forms of mammalian wrists, differs in three important respects: (a) recession or proximal migration of the distal ulna from its earlier direct articulation with the triquetrum and pisiform; (b) development of a synovially lined distal radioulnar joint (DRUJ) permitting pronation and supination of the wrist; and (c) appearance of the triangular fibrocartilage complex (TFCC) (2).

The first primate was a rodent-like creature, *Purgatorius ceratops,* after which prosimians appeared in the fossil record, 58 million years ago, during the Eocene epoch (5). The wrist of the prosimians strongly resembled that of the earlier primates: the distal radius and ulna are connected by an interosseous ligament, the radioulnar ligament (4), and the ulna articulates intimately with the triquetral and pisiform bones, assisting in weight transmission across the wrist (Fig. 1.5). The ulnocarpal and radiocarpal joints were completely separated from each other by a thick fibrous septum extending from the radioulnar ligament to the ulnar face of the lunate (7,8). To reinforce the plantigrade posture of the early mammals, two volar intracapsular ligaments, the palmar ulnocarpal ligament (PUCL), originating from the

FIGURE 1.3. Inferred transformation of the carpal architecture of the tetrapods based on descriptions and interpretations by various authors. **Left to right:** Primitive labyrinthodont amphibian; early mammal-like reptile pelycosaur; advanced mammal-like reptile cynodont; typical mammal. (From Lewis OJ. *Functional morphology of the evolving hand and foot.* Oxford: Clarendon Press, 1989, with permission.)

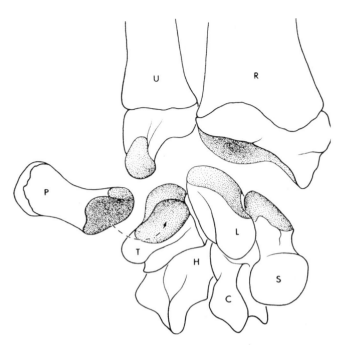

FIGURE 1.5. The palmar aspects of the carpal bones that participate in the radiocarpal articulation of *Procolbus verus* are shown; the articular surfaces of each participating bone are stippled in each case. C, capitate; H, hamate; T, triquetrum; L, lunate; S, scaphoid; P, pisiform; R, radius; U, ulna. Note the primitive articulations of the distal ulna with the pisiform and triquetrum as well as that of the pisiform with the triquetrum. (From Lewis OJ. Brachiation and the early evolution of the Hominoidea. *Nature* 1971;230:577–579, with permission.)

ulna, and the palmar radiocarpal ligament (PRCL), originating from the radius, evolved. The PUCL and PRCL, which shared a common insertion into the lunate, acted as a check to rein wrist extension during loading (2,9).

The wrist of the monkey differs only slightly from that of the prosimians. Proximal migration of the ulna is seen, although articulation with the pisiform and triquetral bones is maintained. The distal slip of the radioulnar interosseous ligament is expanded and forms an intermediate segment of the articular surface of the wrist joint, the precursor to the TFCC that evolved in later primates (10). Efficient swinging from branch to branch promoted the development of increased rotation at the wrist, and therefore, the syndesmosis of the DRUJ developed more motion. The DRUJ began to migrate proximally from the articulation of the triquetrum and pisiform to form a synovial joint (5). Brachiation required even more supination and pronation of the arm and further drove the development of the DRUJ (11). As the ulna retracted proximally, the meniscus became an articulating intercalation between the ulna and triquetrum. It ultimately fused into the triangular fibrocartilage in the later-developed *Hominidae*, as found in man (5).

A wrist demonstrating characteristics intermediate between those of monkeys and descendant hominoids is seen in the gibbons, which arose 18 to 22 million years ago (12). The DRUJ of the gibbons is, indeed, a fully developed synovial joint with articular cartilage (4). The distal slip of the radioulnar ligament has further evolved into a large triangular disc connected to the radius and ulna and fused with the PUCL. Additional proximal migration of the ulna permits interposition of a fibrocartilaginous, intraarticular meniscus through which the ulna articulates with the triquetrum and pisiform. Interposition of this meniscus, a precursor of the TFCC, facilitates an increased range of rotary motion of the carpus from 90° of pronosupination, seen in monkeys, to 150° to 180°, seen in gibbons and subsequent primates (12).

The rudimentary meniscal homolog is the result of incorporation of the meniscus into the triangular disc, seen in the wrist of the gorilla. The cartilage-covered ulnar styloid process articulates almost exclusively with the meniscal homolog in its own synovial cavity. A formal DRUJ is seen first in the chimpanzee, which arose 6.3 to 7.7 million years ago, the result of the distal radius and ulna developing a synovial articulation walled off by the triangular disc distally (2). With further proximal migration of the ulna, a small blind recess—the precursor to the prestyloid recess—developed (4).

The earliest undisputed hominid is *Australopithecus afarenesis*, a bipedal primate that arose 4 million years ago. The skeletal anatomy of this primate suggests its role as a link between living apes and humans (13). Evidence in the fossil record attributes an opposable thumb, a DRUJ that allowed pronosupination, and a relatively large brain to this species (14,15). The *Homo* species originated as *Homo habilis* 2 million years ago. With the exception of subtle intercarpal and carpometacarpal (CMC) changes especially adapted for tool handling, the wrist of modern *Homo sapiens* bears remarkable similarity to that of *Homo habilis*. The human wrist demonstrates significant withdrawl of the ulnar styloid beyond the confines of the prestyloid recess with subsequent loss of articular cartilage of the ulnar styloid (Fig. 1.6) (4). The DRUJ provides articulation for the articular cartilage-covered distal ulna (270° of its circumference) with the sigmoid notch of the distal radius. The TFCC is now comprised of the triangular disc, the meniscus, and the PUCL. The PRCL has split into two bands, which attach to the lunate, as the radiolunate ligament, and the capitate, as the radioscaphocapitate ligament. These structures contribute to the development of the volar wrist ligaments (2).

The characteristics of the carpus have changed relatively little over the last 4 million years. The most significant difference in hominid evolution during this period involved the size of the brain cavity and thus the ability to control and use this highly developed tool—the hand—with its remarkably mobile wrist (9,16). As a result, the *Homo habilis* are known to have used tools and weapons; they were thus more able to obtain food and defend themselves

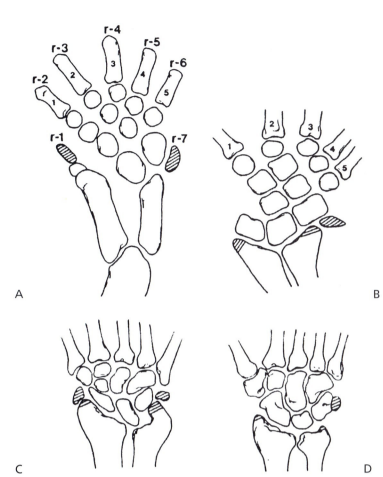

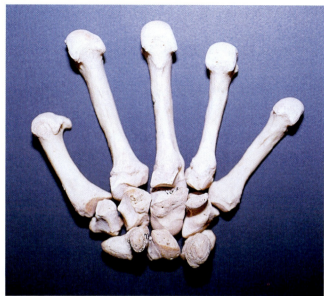

FIGURE 1.7. Peruvian *Homo sapiens* carpus and metacarpals approximately 5,000 years old. This relatively recent specimen no longer contains evidence of an articulation between the triquetrum and pisiform and the distal ulna which has long since migrated proximally. (Courtesy of Dr. Janet Monge and the Museum of Archeology and Anthropology of the University of Pennsylvania.)

FIGURE 1.6. Evolutionary scheme of the carpus. **A:** Primitive seven-rayed tetrapod. **B:** Early tetrapod. **C:** Embryonic human carpus. **D:** Adult human carpus. *r-1* and *r-7* of the primitive tetrapod persist as rudimentary elements in the human (represented as *shaded areas* in **B** and **C**). *r-2* is the first ray (thumb), *r-3* the second ray (index), etc., of the human tetrapod. The various carpal elements present in the primitive tetrapod ultimately formed specific parts of the present human carpus. The elementary *r-1* and *r-7* rays of the primitive tetrapod are represented in the human embryo as the radial styloid process and as a pisiform in the ulnar styloid process, as noted in **B**. (From Almquist EE. Evolution of the distal radioulnar joint. *Clin Orthop* 1992;275:5–13, with permission.)

as their ability to control their environment developed. The transition from *Homo habilis* to *Homo erectus* to *Homo sapiens* is reflected in increased height and brain size rather than notable changes in the carpus or DRUJ except for subtle intercarpal and CMC relationships, which provided additional adaptations to facilitate tool handling (Fig. 1.7) (16).

Philosopher-anthropologists have debated whether this extraordinary instrument encouraged the brain to evolve in an effort to put it to better use, or vice versa (5). Over 2,000 years ago, Galen addressed this question, providing his own insightful perspective:

> Thus, man is the most intelligent of the animals and so, also, hands are the instruments most suitable for an intelligent animal. For it is not because he has hands that he is the most intelligent, as Anaxagoras says, but because he is the most intelligent that he has hands, as Aristotle says, judging him most correctly. Indeed, not by his hands, but by his reason has man been instructed in the arts. Hands are an instrument, as the lyre is the instrument of the musician . . . (17).

REFERENCES

1. Bunnell S. *Surgery of the hand.* Philadelphia: JB Lippincott, 1944.
2. Russell GV, Stern PJ. The phylogeny of the wrist. *Am J Orthop* 1998;47:494–498.
3. Linscheid RL. Presidential address: The hand and evolution. *J Hand Surg [Am]* 1993;18:181–194.
4. Lewis OJ. *Functional morphology of the evolving hand and foot.* Oxford: Clarendon Press, 1989.
5. Almquist EE. Evolution of the distal radioulnar joint. *Clin Orthop* 1992;275:5–13.
6. Jenkins FA. Wrist rotation in primates: A critical adaptation for brachiators. *Symp Zool Soc Lond* 1981;48:429–451.
7. Lewis OJ. The hominoid wrist joint. *Am J Phys Anthrop* 1969;30:251–268.
8. Lewis OJ. Derived morphology of the wrist articulations and theories of hominoid evolution. Part II. The midcarpal joints of higher primates. *J Anat* 1985;142:151–172.
9. Marzke MW. Hominid hand use in the pliocene and pleistocene: Evidence from experimental archaeology and comparative morphology. *J Hum Evol* 1986;15:439–446.
10. Lewis OJ. Evolutionary change in the primate wrist and inferior radio-ulnar joints. *Anat Rec* 1965;151:275–286.

11. Cartmill M, Milton K. The lorisiform wrist joint and the evolution of "brachiating" adaptations in the hominoidea. *Am J Phys Anthrop* 1974;47:249–254.
12. Lewis OJ. The wrist articulations of the anthropoidea. In: Jenkins FA, ed. *Primate locomotion.* New York: Academic Press, 1974; 143–169.
13. Fleagle JG. *Primate adaptation and evolution.* San Diego: Academic Press, 1988.
14. Leakey R, Walker A. Homo erectus unearthed. *Natl Geogr* 1985; 168:624–631.
15. Weaver KF. The search for our ancestors. *Natl Geogr* 1985;168: 560–568.
16. Marzke MW. Origin of the human hand. *Am J Phys Anthrop* 1971;34:61–84.
17. Galen. *On the usefulness of the parts of the body.* Ithaca, NY: Cornell University Press, 1968. May MT, translator.

2

ANATOMY OF THE WRIST

MARC GARCIA-ELIAS

"Without anatomy, there is no surgery, no therapy, but only guessing and prejudices."

Gubarev, nineteenth century (1)

Despite the fact that the skeletal structures of the wrist were described by Vesalius in the sixteenth century (2), the anatomic and biomechanical complexity of its capsuloligamentous elements is still the subject of controversy (3–7). Only a thorough understanding of the spatial relationships among the different components of the wrist can permit adequate comprehension of its pathomechanics and direct appropriate treatment. In this chapter a review of the developmental anatomy, from a surgical perspective, is presented. The classical anatomic descriptions of the different structures are revisited, taking into account the findings of more recent investigations based on gross and microscopic dissections (8–11), specimen cross-sectional studies (12–15), histologic analysis of embryos (16), fetuses (17–19), and adult specimens (11,13), arthrotomography (20), arthroscopy (21–23), and magnetic resonance imaging of living subjects (24).

ONTOGENESIS OF THE CARPAL BONES

The first evidence of the trapezium, trapezoid, and capitate bones appears in the form of chondrifications of specific mesenchymal areas (called anlagen) within the wrist between the fourth and sixth weeks of embryonic development (16). The scaphoid originates from the fusion of two chondrified zones, called centralia (radiale distale and ulnare distale), a process that is not completed until the seventh week, when the embryo reaches 50 mm of crown–rump (CR) length. If these two elements do not fuse, a so-called os centrale (a supernumerary bone interposed between the distal part of the scaphoid and the neck of the capitate) may be found (1.5% of the population) (25).

The lunate evolves from a large nucleus of chondrification called *centralia intermedium,* which extends proximally between the two forearm bone primordia (16,26). The more proximal portion of this centralia, however, usually slows in growth and separates from the distal portion, joining the articular disc between the radius and ulna. By contrast, the distal portion chondrifies rapidly, becoming the definitive lunate. Occasionally, the proximal portion of the intermedium yields an accessory bone, called *os triangulare,* which is present between the triangular fibrocartilage and the lunate (0.7% of the population) (25).

The ulnar styloid process originates from a well-differentiated anlage, the chondrification of which results in the carpalia ulnare. At approximately the tenth week of ontogenesis, however, this carpalia tends to join the developing chondrified ulna. A similar evolution is found for the radial styloid process. It also evolves from an independent chondrification center (carpalia radiale), which fuses to the developing radius approximately during the seventh week of development. By the end of the eighth week, all carpal bones except the pisiform appear completely chondrified. The joint ligaments and capsule will not be completed until the third month. Further information about this complex ontogenic process can be found in the superb study by Čihác (16).

The timing of carpal bone ossification is also quite variable from one bone to another (27). The first ossified nuclei are those of the capitate and hamate, which appear during the first year of age. Ossification of the triquetrum occurs between the second and fourth years. The appearance of the lunate center of ossification ranges from 1 to 7 years of age. The scaphoid appears at the fifth year of age, and the pisiform ossifies between the eighth and the eleventh years of age. Double ossification centers for the lunate, scaphoid, and pisiform bones are not unusual They are often misinterpreted as fractures.

OSTEOLOGY OF THE ADULT WRIST

From an anatomic viewpoint, the carpus contains two rows of bones intercalated between the five metacarpals and the two forearm bones, the radius and ulna: the proximal row

---

M. Garcia-Elias: Department of Hand and Upper Extremity Surgery, Institut Kaplan, 08022 Barcelona, Spain.

Section I: Introduction to the Wrist

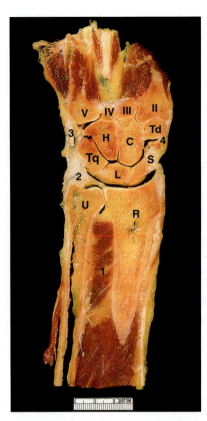

FIGURE 2.1. Frontal section of a human wrist demonstrating the articular relationship of the different bones of the carpus, with the exception of the trapezium, pisiform, and first metacarpal. *R*, radius; *U*, ulna; *S*, scaphoid; *L*, lunate, *Tq*, triquetrum; *Td*, trapezoid; *C*, capitate; *H*, hamate; *II–V*, bases of the metacarpals II to V; *1*, pronator quadratus muscle; *2*, triangular fibrocartilage complex; *3*, extensor carpi ulnaris tendon and sheath; *4*, dorsolateral scaphoid–trapezium ligament.

consists of the scaphoid, lunate, and triquetrum, and the distal row consists of the trapezium, trapezoid, capitate, and hamate (Fig. 2.1). Despite ontogenic evidence supporting the concept that the pisiform is a true carpal element (28), it is widely accepted that this bone functions as a sesamoid for the flexor carpi ulnaris tendon (9,29), and, therefore, it should not be considered a proximal carpal row bone. What follows is a brief description of the different bones involved in the wrist.

Distal Epiphysis of the Ulna

The distal end of the ulna (*os ulna*, also referred to as the ulnar head) is a rounded expansion that articulates with the ulnar-facing articular concavity of the distal radius (called the sigmoid notch). It has a conic shape and is covered with articular cartilage over three-quarters of its total circumference (3,6,30). The distal aspect of the head has three parts: (a) a lateral semilunar-shaped surface, slightly convex, covered by cartilage, for articulation with the undersurface of the triangular fibrocartilage; (b) a central rough depression, called the basistyloid fovea, for the attachment of different ligaments; and (c) a medial bony prominence, variable in length and size, called the ulnar styloid process. The dorsal nonarticular aspect of the ulnar head has a groove to accommodate the extensor carpi ulnaris.

Distal Epiphysis of the Radius

The carpal articular surface of the distal radius (*os radius*) is not flat and horizontally oriented but somewhat concave and tilted in two directions. In the sagittal plane, there is a slope of an average of 10.2° palmar tilt, and in the frontal plane, there is an ulnar inclination at an angle averaging 23.8° (31,32). To ensure articular congruency to the two articulating carpal bones, the radius has two facets (scaphoid and lunate fossae) separated by a cartilaginous sagittal ridge called the interfacet prominence (33,34) (Fig. 2.2). The biconcave scaphoid fossa is triangular or oval-shaped and has a smaller radius of curvature than that of the lunate fossa (32). The latter is more or less rectangular in shape, also biconcave although shallower, and less inclined toward the ulnar side than the scaphoid fossa.

Scaphoid Bone

The scaphoid (*os scaphoideum*) is the largest bone of the proximal carpal row and an important link between the

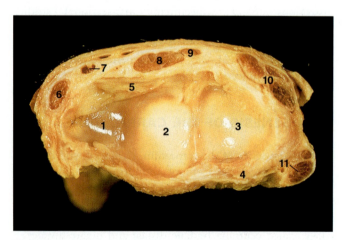

FIGURE 2.2. Distal articular surface of the radius with the attached *(1)* triangular fibrocartilage, *(2)* lunate fossa, *(3)* scaphoid fossa, *(4)* palmar radiocarpal ligaments (sectioned obliquely), *(5)* dorsal radiolunotriquetral ligament, *(6)* extensor carpi ulnaris tendon (sixth extensor compartment), *(7)* extensor digiti quinti proprius (fifth compartment), *(8)* extensor digitorum communis and indicis proprius (fourth compartment), *(9)* extensor pollicis longus (third compartment), *(10)* extensor carpi radialis brevis and longus (second compartment), and *(11)* extensor pollicis brevis and abductor pollicis longus (first compartment). **Editors' Notes:** *The lunate is thought of as the smaller of the two bones between the scaphoid and lunate; notice, however, the larger broad surface the lunate occupies on the distal radius. This is appropriate to the keystone bone of the wrist, which takes the greater load.*

proximal and distal carpal rows (4,35,36). Because of its peculiar shape, with a mediodistal concavity, anatomists have compared it to a boat (*scaphon* in Greek means "boat"). It has four articular facets covering approximately 80% of its entire surface: (a) a proximal surface, strongly convex, articulating with the scaphoid fossa of the radius; (b) an ulnar facet, semilunar in shape, that articulates with the lateral aspect of the lunate; (c) a distal ulnar concave facet facing the lateral aspect of the head of the capitate; and (d) a distal articular surface, convex and sometimes divided by a sagittal smooth ridge into two sectors, medial (that articulates with the trapezoid) and lateral (with the trapezium).

On the palmar aspect of the scaphoid, between the proximal and distal articular surfaces, there is a rough prominence, called the tubercle or tuberosity, that gives attachment to a number of strong ligaments while acting as a pivoting point for the flexor carpi radialis tendon. This nonarticular surface extends laterally, around the bone, forming the dorsolateral ridge or waist, an important area through which about 80% of the vascularity enters the bone (37,38). The proximal margin of the ulnar (lunate) articular surface contains a roughened edge giving attachment to the scapholunate interosseous membrane (11,34).

The long axis of the scaphoid is obliquely oriented in both the sagittal and coronal planes (4,36) (Fig. 2.3). Using computed tomography scans, Belsole et al. (39) found that the average three-dimensional scaphocapitate angle was 73°. This obliquity may explain the inherent instability of the bone when the ligaments to the adjacent structures have failed (40).

Lunate Bone

The lunate (*os lunatum*), considered by many to be the keystone of the carpus, has a sagittal moon-shaped configuration with four articular surfaces (proximal, distal, lateral, and medial) and two nonarticular sides (palmar and dorsal). The biconcave, distal articular surface of the lunate receives the head of the capitate and, in about a 65% of the population, the proximal pole of the hamate (41,42) (Fig. 2.4). The radial and ulnar articular surfaces that face the scaphoid and the triquetrum, respectively, are flat and semi-

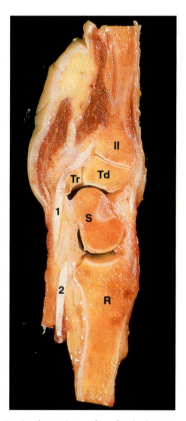

FIGURE 2.3. Sagittal section of a fresh human scaphoid *(S)*, demonstrating its oblique alignment relative to the long axis of the radius *(R)*. *Td*, Trapezoid; *Tr*, Trapezium; *II*, second metacarpal; *(1)* flexor carpi radialis tendon; *(2)* flexor pollicis longus. **Editors' Notes:** *The scaphoid exhibits poor mechanical advantage because the trapezium and trapezoid sit on the head, tending to drive it into flexion, and lie volar to the resistance of the proximal pole on the radius. There is always a significant flexion moment on the scaphoid.*

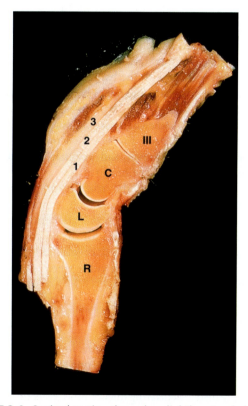

FIGURE 2.4. Sagittal section through a slightly extended lunate bone *(L)* and its relationship to the capitate *(C)*, radius *(R)*, and third metacarpal *(III)*. *1*, flexor digitorum; *2*, median nerve; *3*, flexor retinaculum. **Editors' Notes:** *Note that this lunate is thinner dorsally than volarly. Its neutral anatomy position, therefore, there will be volar translation and dorsal angulation or dorsal intercalated segment instability if all of the ligaments supporting the lunate were absent.*

lunar in shape, contain roughened proximal edges for insertion of the radioscapholunate and interosseous scapholunate and lunotriquetral membranes and ligaments.

The proximal articular surface is biconvex, with a radius of curvature larger than that of the corresponding scaphoid (4,40). In neutral position, approximately two thirds of this surface articulates with the radius, while the medial one third articulates with the central portion of the triangular fibrocartilage (31,32).

The overall shape of the lunate varies substantially from one individual to another. From a sagittal view, approximately 67% of lunates are thinner dorsally than volarly (type D lunates), although the opposite is found in 23% of the cases (43). From a frontal view, three different shapes have been described by Antuña-Zapico (44): type I (ulnar-based wedge shaped: 32% of the population), type II (parallel proximal and distal surfaces: 50%), and type III (V-shaped proximal articular surface: 18%). These anatomic characteristics have been regarded as important factors in the pathomechanics of Kienböck's disease (44) and carpal instabilities (36,40,43).

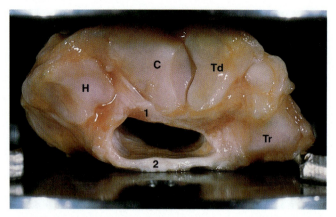

FIGURE 2.5. Transverse carpal arch, seen from distal to proximal. The bones fit together like stones in an arch, resisting high dorsopalmar compression loads without signs of failure. Such structural strength is provided by the stout transverse intercarpal ligaments *(1)* and flexor retinaculum *(2)*. *H*, hamate; *C*, capitate; *Td*, trapezoid; *Tr*, trapezium. **Editors' Notes:** *The flexor retinaculum is large and strong, and one would ascribe to it the job of maintaining the transverse carpal arch; however, Fisk and others have demonstrated that resecting the flexor retinaculum does not significantly change the arch and that carpal alignment is based on bone shape and ligament support.*

Triquetrum Bone

The triquetrum *(os triquetrum)* can also be compared to a boat with a moon-shaped base articulating with the ulnar aspect of the lunate. In addition, it has three other articular surfaces: distal, proximal, and anterior. The distal articular facet is in full contact with the hamate bone only when the wrist is ulnarly deviated. The radial half of its helicoid surface is horizontal and slightly biconcave, whereas the ulnar half is convex and somewhat dorsally oriented (45). The proximal articular surface, the so-called proximal pole, is small, triangular, and convex and in ulnar deviation is in contact with the triangular fibrocartilage.

The anterior aspect of the triquetrum contains two zones: a lateral rough surface, which contains vascular foramina and important ligamentous attachments, and an ulnar oval-shaped articular surface for the pisiform (9). The dorsal aspect of the triquetrum is divided into two rough areas by a transverse prominent ridge where strong dorsal ligaments attach.

Distal Carpal Row

Though anatomically independent, the four distal carpal row bones are functionally considered as one single unit. Indeed, a complex system of stout and strong interosseous (palmar, dorsal, and intraarticular) ligaments bind each to the other (15) so that intercarpal motion is minimal (Fig. 2.5).

Trapezium Bone

The trapezium *(os trapezium)* is the most mobile of the four distal carpal row bones and has four articular facets: (a) a distal articular surface for the first metacarpal, traditionally described as "saddle-shaped," concave in the flexion–extension plane and convex in the abduction–adduction plane (46); (b) a small ulnodistal triangular facet for articulation with the base of the second metacarpal; (c) a medial facet to the trapezoid; and (d) a somewhat concave, proximal surface that articulates with the scaphoid. Between the articular facet for the trapezoid and a palmar prominence (trapezial ridge), there is a vertical groove for the flexor carpi radialis tendon. The trapezial ridge is an important structure because it provides strong attachment to the transverse carpal ligament (12,47).

Trapezoid Bone

The smallest bone of the distal carpal row is the trapezoid *(os trapezoideum)*. It obviously has a trapezoidal shape, with four articular (superior, inferior, lateral, and medial) and two nonarticular (palmar and dorsal) surfaces. The distal articular surface of the trapezoid is wedge-shaped with a sagittal ridge fitting into a notch in the base of the second metacarpal. Its proximal articular surface has a shallow concavity, in continuity with that of the trapezium, for the scaphoid.

Capitate Bone

The capitate *(os capitatum)* is the largest carpal bone and the keystone of the transverse carpal arch (12) with a palmar surface, rough and somewhat prominent, constituting the floor of the carpal tunnel. This facet is important because it provides attachment to the crucial midcarpal crossing ligaments. The proximal one third of the bone (called the head of the capitate) is not perfectly spheroidal but contains three articular surfaces: one lateral for the scaphoid, another proximal for the lunate, and a medial, almost flat surface for the hamate bone (15,40). The distal articular surface of the bone is flat, articulating with the third metacarpal, except for its radial third, which is oblique and receives the ulnar prolongation (styloid process) of the second metacarpal (48). The medial articular aspect of the bone articulates with the hamate and has a roughened palmar depression where strong interosseous ligaments attach (15).

Hamate Bone

The hamate *(os hamati)* or unciform bone, named after its prominent palmar projection (the so-called hook of the hamate), constitutes the ulnar border of the carpal tunnel (46). It articulates distally with the fourth and fifth metacarpal bases through flat or slightly saddle-shaped articular surfaces (48). Proximally, the hamate has an ulnarly helicoid articulating surface matching that of the triquetrum (45). The palmar nonarticular surface of the hamate is characterized by the presence of the hook (also known as unciform process or *hamulus hamati*), a rounded apophysis, varying in size and shape, that gives attachment to important ligaments and muscles. The radial aspect of the hook constitutes the ulnar wall of the carpal tunnel and has a close relationship with the flexor tendons of the little finger (49).

ARTHROLOGY OF THE WRIST

The wrist is a complex composite joint composed of different articulations. The radius rotates around the ulnar head, constituting the distal radioulnar joint. The proximal carpal row moves on the radius and its ulnar prolongation, the triangular fibrocartilage, by means of the radiocarpal joint. There is motion between the proximal row bones at the scapholunate and lunotriquetral joints. Between the proximal and distal rows is a very mobile articulation, the midcarpal joint. Finally, the metacarpals articulate with the distal aspect of the distal carpal row through the carpometacarpal joints.

From a kinematic point of view, all these articulations can be grouped into three categories: (a) joints with significant mobility (distal radioulnar, radiocarpal, midcarpal, and pisotriquetral), (b) joints with less than 35° of maximum rotation (scapholunate, lunotriquetral), and (c) joints with minimal mobility (distal intercarpal joints). What follows is a brief description of the joints from the first group. The anatomy of the carpometacarpal joints is covered elsewhere in this book (see Chapters 16 and 35).

Distal Radioulnar Joint

The distal radioulnar joint has been defined as a diarthrodial trochoid articulation formed by the head of the ulna and the shallow sigmoid cavity of the lower end of the radius (50). The curvatures of the two articulating surfaces are not equal. The radius of the ulna is about two-thirds the length of the sigmoid notch concavity (30,51). This results in a relatively unstable articulation with reduced area of contact between the two bones (Fig. 2.6). To overcome this, different stabilizing structures exist: (a) the triangular fibrocartilage complex (TFCC), composed of the discus articularis, the palmar and dorsal radioulnar ligaments, the ulnocarpal ligaments, and the extensor carpi ulnaris (ECU) sheath; (b) the pronator quadratus muscle; and (c) the interosseous membrane (52,53). A description of the triangular fibrocartilage complex is presented below.

The central portion of the TFCC is a semicircular fibrocartilaginous structure interposed between the distal aspect of the ulna and the carpal bones. It is composed of two elements: the central disc and the peripheral radioulnar ligaments (17,51,54). The disc emerges from the ulnar edge of the distal radius and attaches medially to the basistyloid fovea of the ulna, preventing the ulnar dome

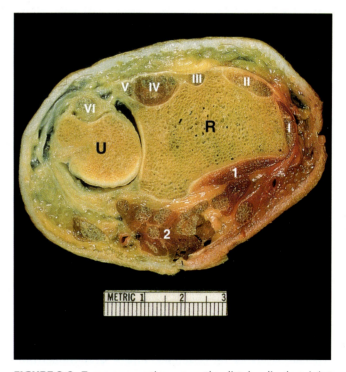

FIGURE 2.6. Transverse section across the distal radioulnar joint of a human wrist, demonstrating the asymmetric curvatures of the articular surfaces of the ulna *(U)* and radius *(R)*. *I–VI,* extensor compartments; *1,* pronator quadratus muscle; *2,* flexor digitorum. **Editors' Notes:** *Envision the dorsal and volar capsular structures of the radius–ulnar joint. From this view, they can become tight only at maximum supination or maximum pronation and, therefore, contribute poorly to stabilizing the ulna in other than those positions.*

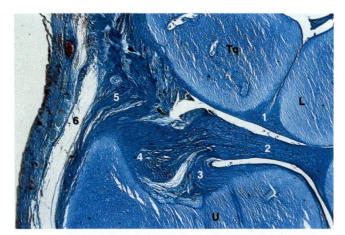

FIGURE 2.7. Frontal histologic section of the triangular fibrocartilage complex of a fetus, 105 mm CR. *Tq,* triquetrum; *L,* lunate; *U,* ulna; *1,* lunotriquetral ligament; *2,* discus articularis; *3,* insertion into the basistyloid fovea; *4,* insertion into the ulnar styloid process; *5,* meniscus homolog (well-vascularized synovial fold); *6,* sheath of the extensor carpi ulnaris. (Courtesy of Dr. Jordi Ardevol, Mataró, Spain.)

from direct contact with the ulnar part of the carpus (53). Nontraumatic perforations of the triangular fibrocartilage (TFC), caused by wear, are not unusual, and their prevalence increases with age from 7.6% in the third decade to 53% in the seventh decade (42,55).

The dorsal and palmar edges of the disc are thick, containing dense, longitudinally oriented collagen fibers (the palmar and dorsal radioulnar ligaments). These ligaments, often indistinguishable from the disc, have a double insertion into the basistyloid fovea and into the ulnar styloid process (17,54,56) (Fig. 2.7). Proximal to these two ligaments is the palmar and dorsal radioulnar capsule, which is lax, with no dense collagen fibers, in order to permit pronosupination. The ulnocarpal ligaments emerge from the anterior edge of the TFCC and consist of three fascicles that are further described below.

Radiocarpal Joint

The radiocarpal joint is a glenoid type of articulation consisting of two elements: (a) the antebrachial glenoid, formed by the distal articular surface of the radius and its ulnar prolongation, the articular disc of the triangular fibrocartilage, and (b) the carpal condyle, formed by the convex proximal articular facets of the scaphoid, lunate, and triquetrum. Within the joint capsule a number of palmar and dorsal ligaments exist, the inner sides of which appear resurfaced by synovial tissue (11,34). This tissue may form synovial recesses, commonly in front of the ulnar styloid (recessus prestyloideus) (17,56,57), and at the junction of the interfacet prominence and the palmar capsule (recessus prescaphoideus) (57).

Midcarpal Joint

The midcarpal joint combines three different types of articulations (6,41) (Fig. 2.8). Laterally, there is a glenoid joint in which the convex distal surface of the scaphoid articulates with the concavity formed by the trapezium, trapezoid, and lateral aspect of the capitate. The central part of the midcarpal joint is a ball-and-socket type of joint, concave proximally (scaphoid and lunate) and almost spherical distally (head of the capitate and sometimes the proximal pole of the hamate) (41,42). The ulnar part of the midcarpal joint (hamate–triquetral articulation) has a reciprocal helicoid or screw-shaped configuration on both sides (45). The midcarpal synovial cavity includes not only the space between the two rows but also the intervals between the bones of the proximal row.

In normal subjects there should be no communication between the midcarpal and radiocarpal joint cavities. When present, they are either traumatic or age-related perforations caused by wear (42,53,56). Mikic (57) found a high incidence of scapholunate (43%) and lunotriquetral (55%) perforations among 109 wrist specimens past the third decade.

Pisotriquetral Joint

The pisiform is a pea-shaped sesamoid bone enhancing the action of the flexor carpi ulnaris muscle (28). Distally, the pisiform is strongly connected to the hook of the hamate by the thick pisohamate ligament and to the base of the fifth

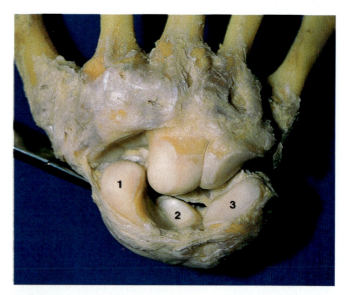

FIGURE 2.8. Opened midcarpal joint, viewed from the dorsum. Three articular structures are evident: *1,* scaphoid–trapezium–trapezoid (proximal condyle–distal glenoid); *2,* lunate–scaphoid–capitate (distal condyle–proximal glenoid); and *3,* triquetrum–hamate (helicoidal-shaped). **Editors' Notes:** *Picture this unit moving from a dorsal radial position to a volar ulnar position. This represents its maximum range. The midcarpal joint moves in limited fashion from dorsal ulnar to volar radial.*

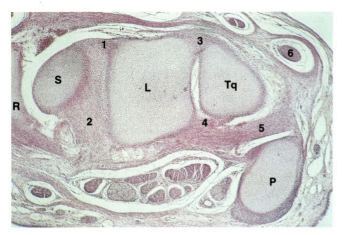

FIGURE 2.9. Transverse histologic section of the wrist of a 70-mm CR fetal specimen (Collection Domènech-Mateu, UAB, Bellaterra, Spain). *P*, pisiform; *Tq*, triquetrum; *L*, lunate; *S*, proximal pole of the scaphoid; *R*, radial styloid process; *1*, dorsal scapholunate ligament (transversely oriented); *2*, palmar scapholunate ligament (obliquely oriented, thus allowing rotational motion); *3*, dorsal lunotriquetral ligament; *4*, palmar lunotriquetral ligament; *5*, palmar–distal extension of the triangular–fibrocartilage complex (including the ulnocarpal ligaments); *6*, extensor carpi ulnaris tendon and sheath (sixth extensor compartment).

metacarpal by the pisometacarpal ligament (9). Other soft tissue attachments to the pisiform include the extensor retinaculum, the flexor retinaculum, and the abductor digiti minimi. The pisotriquetral joint has a very thin and loose capsule with no ligaments between the two articulating bones (Fig. 2.9). The synovial cavity is relatively large, bulging upward between the flexor carpi ulnaris tendon and the radiocarpal capsule. In approximately 30% of the population there is a comunication between this and the so-called recessus pretriquetralis of the radiocarpal joint (57).

LIGAMENTS OF THE WRIST

When surgically approaching the wrist, one should not expect to find a network of well-differentiated ligamentous structures with precise interligamentous spaces between them as portrayed in most textbooks. In fact, the majority of ligaments are intracapsular, contained within capsular sheaths of loose connective and fat tissue, making their recognition difficult (11). Furthermore, most carpal ligaments do not have distinct edges and demonstrate frequent anatomic variations in size and shape (Fig. 2.10). Not sur-

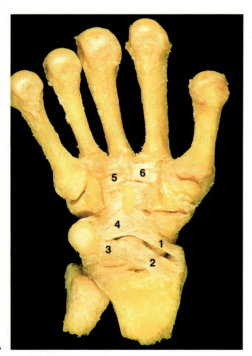 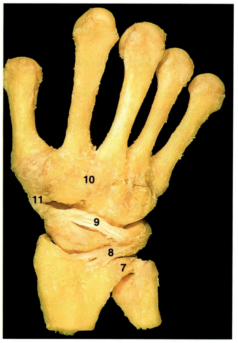

FIGURE 2.10. Anatomic dissection of the most significant ligaments of the wrist. **A:** Palmar view (ulnocarpal ligaments excluded) showing *1*, radioscaphocapitate ligament; *2*, long radiolunate ligament; *3*, palmar lunotriquetral interosseous ligament; *4*, palmar triquetrum–hamate–capitate ligamentous complex; *5*, palmar hamate–capitate interosseous ligament; and *6*, palmar capitate–trapezoid–trapezium interosseous ligament. **B:** Dorsal view, showing *7*, dorsal radioulnar ligament; *8*, dorsal radiolunotriquetral ligament; *9*, dorsal intercarpal ligament (distal fibers excluded); *10*, dorsal interosseous ligaments of the distal carpal row; and *11*, dorsolateral scaphoid–trapezium ligament. **Editors' Notes:** *Notice the predominantly upslope character of the ligaments and envision the sling of collagen running from dorsal to volar around the ulnar aspect of the wrist.*

TABLE 2.1. LIGAMENTS OF THE WRIST (CARPOMETACARPAL JOINTS EXCLUDED)

Extrinsic ligaments
  Palmar superficial
    Radioscaphocapitate
    Long radiolunate
      ulnocapitate
  Palmar deep
    Short radiolunate
    Ulnolunate
    Ulnotriquetral
    Radioscapholunate
  Dorsal
    Radiolunotriquetral
Intrinsic ligaments
  Proximal row
    Scapholunate[a]
    Lunotriquetral[a]
  Distal row
    Hamate–capitate[a]
    Capitate–trapezoid[a]
    Trapezoid–trapezium[a]
  Palmar midcarpal
    Triquetrum–hamate–capitate
    Scapho–capitate–trapezoid
  Dorsal midcarpal
    Dorsal intercarpal ligament
    Lateral scaphoid–trapezium–trapezoid

[a]Palmar and dorsal ligaments.

prisingly, descriptions of carpal ligaments in the literature are quite varied (3,6,35,36,58,59), with new additions recently reported (8,60).

Traditionally, wrist ligaments have been classified into two major categories: extrinsic and intrinsic (59) (Table 2.1). Extrinsic ligaments are those connecting the forearm bones and the carpus, whereas intrinsic ligaments have both attachments within the carpus. Intrinsic ligaments are short, stiff, and difficult to repair when ruptured; the extrinsic ligaments are longer, less stiff, and more easily repaired (14,61).

PALMAR EXTRINSIC LIGAMENTS

In most textbooks, palmar extrinsic ligaments have been described as two reversed V-shaped ligamentous bands, a proximal one connecting the two forearm bones to the triquetrum–lunate complex and a distal one linking the forearm to the capitate (59). Recent anatomic investigations, however, especially since the introduction of arthroscopy, have disclosed the need for further subdividing these ligaments into two subgroups: deep and superficial ligaments (21–23). Deep ligaments can be easily inspected from inside the joint under a thin synovial layer, whereas the superficial ligaments are hardly visible through the arthroscope. Furthermore, surgical exposure of the deep ligaments through an anterior approach is not possible unless the superficial ligaments are severed or retracted.

Palmar Superficial Extrinsic Ligaments

From lateral to medial, the first superficial ligament is the radioscaphocapitate (RSC) ligament. It originates from the rough palmar surface of the radial styloid process and has two components: radioscaphoid and radiocapitate (11,33,62). The radioscaphoid bundle (sometimes referred to as the radial collateral ligament) courses obliquely from the tip of the radial styloid to the proximal edge of tuberosity of the scaphoid, where it interconnects with the scaphocapitate ligament. The radiocapitate component of the RSC ligament courses around the palmar concavity of the scaphoid, proximal to the scaphoid tuberosity, forming a fulcrum over which the scaphoid rotates (63). Most of its distal fibers insert distally onto the palmar aspect of the body of the capitate. Its proximal fibers, however, do not insert on the capitate; they course around the distal margin of the palmar pole of the lunate, blending into the ulnocapitate ligament (8,35).

Medial to the RSC ligament is the long radiolunate ligament (long-RL), which connects the radius to the lunate. Its most superficial fibers frequently interconnect with the palmar lunotriquetral interosseous ligament (33). For this reason, some authors refer to this structure as the radiolunotriquetral ligament (58). Between the RSC and the long RL ligaments is an oblique interligamentous sulcus, well visualized from inside the joint (11,22,23).

Arising from the palmar edge of the triangular fibrocartilage is another superficial extrinsic ligament, called the ulnocapitate (UC) ligament (17,18,64). It also has two components, one for the capitate, another blending into the RSC ligament. The triangular sulcus between these latter fascicles and the distal edge of the long radiolunate ligament has been called the space of Poirier, a relatively weak area through which perilunar dislocations frequently occur (58,65).

Palmar Deep Extrinsic Ligaments

Under the most proximal fibers of the long-RL ligament is a flat sheet of short fibers, vertically oriented, originating from the anterior edge of the radius and inserting into the palmar aspect of the lunate (33)—the short radiolunate (short-RL) ligament, which plays an important role in preventing excessive extension of the lunate.

Adjacent to the short-RL ligament, under the fibers of the UC ligament, and frequently indistinguishable from these two structures, is the ulnolunate (UL) ligament. It arises from the anterior edge of the triangular fibrocartilage and courses vertically toward its distal insertion into the anterior aspect of the lunate (17,18,22). A similar structure, the ulnotriquetral (UTq) ligament, is found between the

TFC and the proximal pole of the triquetrum. These two ligaments, together with the superficial UC ligament, form the ulnocarpal ligamentous complex, an important structure in the stabilization of the distal radioulnar joint, and considered by many as an important part of the TFCC (50,52)

Frequently included as a deep extrinsic ligament is the radioscapholunate ligament of Kuenz-Testut (59). It originates from the anterior one-third of the interfacet prominence, and courses distally and dorsally until inserting at the base of the scapholunate joint. Recent anatomic studies, however, have demonstrated that this structure is not a true ligament but rather a neurovascular bundle supplying the scapholunate interosseous membrane (13,34).

DORSAL EXTRINSIC LIGAMENTS

There is only one dorsal extrinsic ligamentous complex, called the radiolunotriquetral (RLTq) ligament. It is formed by a thin, fan-shaped superficial radiotriquetral fascicle and a deep radiolunotriquetral fascicle (60). The superficial fascicle emerges partly from the ulnar half of the dorsal edge of the radius and partly from the dorsal border of the radial notch. It courses obliquely toward its distal insertion into a triangular rough facet located proximal to the dorsal tubercle (or ridge) of the triquetrum. Inseparable from this superficial band, the deep bundle arises from the medial third of the dorsal border of the radius and courses obliquely to insert into the distal part of the lunotriquetral articulation.

Despite having been described in many textbooks, no ulnar collateral ligament exists in the human wrist (3,17,66). The collagen tissue connecting the ulnar styloid process and the medial aspect of the triquetrum and pisiform does not have a histologic structure analogous to a true collateral ligament but is composed of a network of irregularly arranged loose connective tissue (17) (Fig. 2.7). In fact, because the wrist is not a true hinge joint, collateral ligaments are not expected to be present. Their absence is functionally compensated for by the extensor carpi ulnaris tendon and sheath (67,68).

INTRINSIC LIGAMENTS

Intrinsic ligaments are those that originate and insert into carpal bones (65). They can be classified into two categories: ligaments connecting bones of the same carpal row (interosseous ligaments), and ligaments crossing the midcarpal joint (midcarpal ligaments).

Proximal Row Interosseous Ligaments

Truly important from a biomechanical point of view are these collections of short fibers transversely binding the anterior and posterior aspects of the bones of the proximal row (19,64,69). The palmar scapholunate (SL) and lunotriquetral (LTq) interosseous ligaments are deep structures covered by the long-RL and UC ligaments, respectively, with which they interdigitate. The fibers of the dorsal scapholunate ligament are shorter and more transversely oriented than their palmar counterparts (19,68) (Fig. 2.9). As a result, the scaphoid has greater flexion–extension motion than the lunate, a rotation that occurs around a dorsally located hinge, which approximately coincides with the dorsal SL ligament. By contrast, the dorsal lunotriquetral ligament has fibers similarly oriented with those of the palmar side (11,64).

Connecting the palmar and dorsal SL and LTq ligaments, and following the proximal arc of the two joints, is the interosseous membrane, a fibrocartilage structure that prevents communication between the radiocarpal and midcarpal joint cavities (11,57). This structure has neither the histologic nor the mechanical properties of the true interosseous ligaments (19).

Distal Row Interosseous Ligaments

There are superficial interosseous ligaments on both palmar and dorsal aspects of the joints between the distal row bones (capitate–hamate, capitate–trapezoid, and trapezoid–trapezium joints). They are stout fibers, stiffer and stronger than those of the proximal carpal row (15,46). There are also deep interosseous ligaments within these joints, and in particular between the hamate and capitate (15,35). The assembly of ligaments converging on the palmar aspect of the capitate from the adjacent carpal and metacarpal bones has been called the radiate ligament (65).

Palmar Midcarpal Ligaments

Two groups of ligaments cross the palmar aspect of the midcarpal joint: one medial, another anterolateral. The medial complex, also known as the ulnar limb of the arcuate ligament or the triquetrum–hamate–capitate (TqHC) ligamentous complex, is formed by a group of fascicles connecting the anterolateral rough facet of the triquetrum to the anterior aspects of the hamate and capitate (70) (Fig. 2.11). It usually runs parallel to and often is indistinguishable from the UC ligament (35).

The anterolateral complex of ligaments crossing the midcarpal joint consists of a fan-shaped group of fascicles that emerge from the medial aspect of scaphoid tuberosity and diverge toward the palmar surface of the body of the capitate and the anteromedial aspect of the trapezoid (71,72). It is called the palmar scaphocapitate–trapezoid (SCTd) ligamentous complex and is covered by a synovial layer constituting the groove of the flexor carpi radialis tendon. In its oblique course, this ligamentous complex interconnects with the TqHC ligament proximally (9) and the

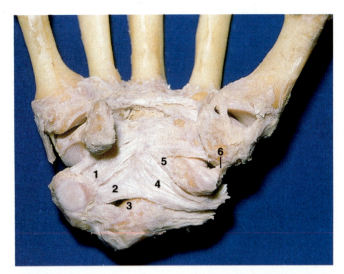

FIGURE 2.11. Palmar midcarpal crossing ligaments (radiocarpal joint disarticulated): *1*, triquetrum–hamate ligament; *2*, triquetrum–capitate ligament; *3*, space of Poirier; *4*, radioscaphocapitate ligament; *5*, scaphocapitate ligament; *6*, dorsolateral scaphotrapezium ligament.

capitate–trapezoid and trapezoid–trapezium palmar interosseous ligaments distally. As shown in recent investigations, this ligament probably plays an important role as a major distal stabilizer of the scaphoid (9,69).

Dorsal Midcarpal Ligaments

Two consistent ligamentous structures cross the dorsal aspect of the midcarpal joint: the dorsal intercarpal (DI) ligament (60) and the dorsolateral scaphoid–trapezium–trapezoid (STT) ligament (69).

The DI ligament arises from the dorsal rim of the triquetrum, where it blends with the distal insertions of the dorsal radiocarpal ligament (60). In its medial-to-lateral course it crosses, but does not insert on, the dorsum of the head of the capitate. At the level of the scaphocapitate–trapezoid corner, this band fans out toward its distal insertions to the dorsal surface of the trapezoid and dorsolateral side of the trapezium (35). The more proximal fibers of this ligament (called by some authors the dorsal scaphotriquetral ligament) are somewhat thicker and stiffer than the distal ones and follow the distal edge of the lunate, interconnecting with the more distal fascicles of the dorsal LTq interosseous ligament first and the dorsal SL interosseous ligament later, until inserting along the dorsolateral ridge of the scaphoid.

The dorsolateral STT ligament has not been well defined until recently (69) and probably has an important stabilizing effect on the scaphoid–trapezium joint (Fig. 2.12). Proximally, it originates on a rough area located on the lateral aspect of the scaphoid tuberosity and fans out to insert distally into the lateral tubercle of the trapezium and

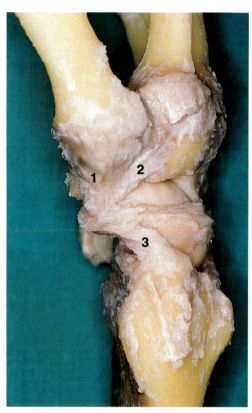

FIGURE 2.12. Lateral view of the wrist demonstrating the fan-shaped dorsolateral scaphoid–trapezium–trapezoid ligamentous complex. *1*, scaphoid–trapezium fascicle (vertical fibers); *2*, scaphoid–trapezoid fascicle (oblique fibers); *3*, radioscaphoid fascicle, portion of the radioscaphocapitate ligament (also referred to as the radial collateral ligament). **Editors' Notes:** *The oblique line on the distal pole of the scaphoid represents the restricted plane of motion of the trapezium–trapezoid from dorsal radial to volar ulnar across the distal scaphoid.*

dorsal aspect of the trapezoid. These latter fascicles are covered by the distalmost fibers of the dorsal intercarpal ligament.

RETINACULAR SYSTEM OF THE WRIST

The flexor carpi ulnaris (FCU) is the only forearm muscle with a major distal insertion on the carpus. It attaches to the pisiform, which, in turn, is connected to the hook of the hamate via the pisihamatum ligament and to the fifth metacarpal by means of the pisometacarpicum ligament (9). The flexor carpi radialis (FCR) tendon inserts on the anterior aspect of the base of the second metacarpal. The wrist extensors—extensor carpi radialis longus (ECRL), extensor carpi radialis brevis (ECRB), and extensor carpi ulnaris (ECU)—insert on the dorsal surface of the bases of the second, third, and fifth metacarpal bones, respectively. Other tendons crossing the wrist joint are the abductor pollicis longus (APL) and the extensor pollicis brevis

(EPB) laterally, the extensor pollicis longus (EPL), the extensor digitorum communis (EDC), the extensor indicis proprius (EIP), and the extensor propius digiti quinti (EPDQ) dorsally, and the flexor digitorum sublimis (FDS) and profundus (FDP) and the flexor pollicis longus (FPL) palmarly (66).

A complex retinacular system derived from the deep sheath of the antebrachial fascia and consisting of the flexor and extensor retinaculum establishes a relationship between these tendons and the multiple wrist capsular structures.

Flexor Retinaculum

The forearm fascia becomes thicker at the distal forearm, where it receives arcuate tendinous expansions emerging from the FCU, FCR, and palmaris longus tendons. At the proximal carpal row level, the thickness of the flexor retinaculum is very significant, its deepest fibers [called the transverse carpal (TC) ligament] having a transverse orientation, attaching laterally on the scaphoid tuberosity and medially on the pisiform (49). More distally, at the level of the distal carpal row, the fibers of the flexor retinaculum grow thicker and connect the hook of the hamate to the palmar ridge of the trapezium. Medially and laterally, the TC ligament blends with the transverse intercarpal ligaments, thus closing the carpal tunnel, the oval compartment that contains the nine flexor digitorum tendons and the median nerve. The floor of the carpal tunnel is formed by the fibrous layer covering the palmar carpal ligaments. The FCR tendon is not contained in the carpal tunnel but within a separate tunnel defined by a fibrous sagittal septum that arises from the palmar aspect of the trapezoid and joins the inner fibers of the TC ligament near its lateral insertion on the trapezium ridge.

Extensor Retinaculum

The dorsal retinaculum of the wrist also originates from the deep forearm fascia and consists of two layers: the supratendinous and the infratendinous layers (66) (Fig. 2.6). Between the supratendinous layer and the radius are six longitudinal fibrous septa that create six compartments for the different tendons crossing the wrist (Fig. 2.13).

The first compartment, on the lateral border of the wrist, contains the APL and EPB tendons. The second compartment holds the ECRL and ECRB tendons. The third compartment, which lies ulnar to Lister's tubercle, contains the EPL tendon. The floor of the fourth and fifth compartments, which contain the EDC and EIP in the former and the EPDQ in the latter, is formed by the infratendinous retinaculum, a sheet of parallel fibers, narrower and shorter than those of the supratendinous retinaculum, that blend with the dorsal wrist capsule and the corresponding sagittal septa. The sixth compartment, for the ECU tendon, is an independent fibrous tunnel formed entirely by the

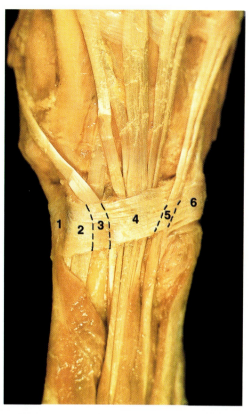

FIGURE 2.13. Extensor retinaculum forming the sixth extensor compartment: *1*, extensor pollicis brevis and abductor pollicis longus (first compartment); *2*, extensor carpi radialis brevis and longus (second compartment); *3*, extensor pollicis longus (third compartment); *4*, extensor digitorum communis and indicis propius (fourth compartment); *5*, extensor propius digiti quinti (fifth compartment); *6*, extensor carpi ulnaris tendon (sixth extensor compartment). **Editors' Notes:** *The extensor retinaculum is actually proximal to the radial carpal joint, and a transverse incision allows exposure throughout the wrist whether radial sided or ulnar sided surgery is necessary. The transverse incision allows one to work on the distal radius proximal to the extensor retinaculum as well as within the joint, say, for example, treating radius fractures. The extensor retinaculum may be narrowed without interfering with its functional capacity.*

infratendinous retinaculum, separated from the supratendinous layer by loose connective tissue (66,67).

The thickest fibers of the extensor retinaculum insert laterally into the radius, forming the lateral septum for the first compartment. These fascicles run obliquely from lateral to medial and from proximal to distal, over the extensor tendons, until attaching to the ulnar side of the triquetrum and the pisiform, where they blend with expansions of the FCU tendon and the origins of the abductor digiti quinti.

ACKNOWLEDGMENT

I wish to acknowledge the support provided for my anatomic research by Professor Josep Mª Domènech-

Mateu, Chief of the Department of Morphological Sciences of the Faculty of Medicine of the Universitat Autònoma de Barcelona. I am also grateful to Drs. Ronald Linscheid and William P. Cooney for their continuous encouragement and help during the last decade, and also for allowing publication of the cross-sectioned cadaver wrists that appear in this chapter.

EDITORS' COMMENTS

The wrist has two primary functions: the first and foremost is to transfer load from the digits to the forearm and on to the axial skeleton; the second is to allow finite positioning of the fingers and fist for function. It is the combination of the motion requirements and the load transference requirements that are the basis for most of the problems in the wrist. These problems statistically resolve to the scaphoid. The scaphoid and lunate are the main load transference bones. They perform well in the in-line or neutral position but are extremely susceptible to injury, particularly at the limits of the motion range. Once loads have left the wrist on their proximal trek, they are primarily the responsibility of the radius. The ulna carries little or no load in terms of in-line transmission from the hand. In full pronation, the ulna is mostly uncovered, and its end can be palpated in the fully pronated position. The planes of motion of the ulnar carpals lie more in line with the long axis of the forearm and are not adapted for load transference despite anatomic studies that demonstrate 20% of the load on the end of the ulna in certain conditions. As the loads increase, they will migrate to the perpendicularly aligned joints and transfer to the scaphoid, lunate, and radius. The human ulna is a phylogenetic requirement for the wrist but is not necessary for the wrist or its function. The distal ulna must be accounted for, stabilized, and protected by the wrist. The ulna needs the wrist. The wrist does not need the ulna. The main in-line loads traveling up the radius are transmitted to the ulna by the interosseous membrane and to the humerus across the radial capitellar joint. The elbow, of course, is primarily comprised of the ulna. The importance of the radial head to the functioning arm can not be overestimated.

The wrist is inherently unstable to the extent that the bones are held in positions that they would not assume based entirely on their shape. The position a bone would assume based on its shape is called its *neutral* anatomy position, as opposed to its *normal* anatomy position.

The distal end of the radius slopes volarly and ulnarly. The neutral anatomy position of the carpals is, therefore, volar–ulnar dislocation. The neutral anatomy position of the scaphoid is to flex and supinate, with the proximal pole escaping from beneath and riding up on the dorsum of the capitate. The neutral anatomy position of the lunate is actually twofold, based on whether the lunate is thinner dorsally or thinner volarly. Sixty-seven percent or just under three-quarters of lunates are thinner dorsally and will angle dorsally and migrate volarly (DISI) in their neutral anatomy position. Nearly a quarter of lunates are thinner volarly and will angle volarly and migrate dorsally (VISI) in their neutral anatomy position. An intact ligamentous system is, therefore, integral to the function of the wrist.

The wrist, therefore, is totally dependent on its ligamentous system for support. There are three main categories of ligaments. First are the short interosseous ligaments that are highly restrictive to the motion of their associated bones. Second are long wrist ligaments that may be favorably compared to springlines on a boat tied up into dock. Springlines are long lines that run from the dock at one end of the boat to the other end of the boat. This prevents displacement along the long axis of the line but allows the boat to move up and down in its slip with tide and wind changes. The long ligaments of the wrist are similar in that they restrain a specific shift direction of the carpals without limiting motion between carpals. The third type of ligament is probably best represented by the volar radial–scapholunate ligament, which is a recruitment-type ligament filled with stretch and pressure sensors. Vessels are coiled, similar to a phone cord, allowing significant stretching, and this third type of ligament probably calls for or recruits additional muscle power as it is stretched. The speed of stretch as well as the extent of stretch may both play a role in calling for additional muscle power support for the wrist.

The scaphoid is unique in the skeleton because of its propensity to produce clinical problems. The scaphoid is so mechanically disadvantaged as to be far and away the most common cause of wrist symptoms. Without the scaphoid's peculiar anatomy, the wrist would offer only slightly more challenge than the elbow. Ninety percent of all ganglia occur as scaphoid problems, either from the dorsal scapholunate joint, the volar scaphoradial joint, or from the triscaphe joint. The common patterns of degenerative arthritis of the wrist begin with periscaphoid joints. The clinical diagnosis of dorsal wrist syndrome, which is scaphoid in origin, is the most common wrist disorder (see Chapter 28). Understanding carpal anatomy is integral to understanding carpal pathology.

REFERENCES

1. Zhdanov DA. Anatomy and medicine. *Acta Anat* 1975;93: 496–505.
2. Dobyns JH, Linscheid RL. A short history of the wrist joint. *Hand Clinics* 1997;13:1–12.

3. Lewis OJ, Hamshere RJ, Bucknill TM. The anatomy of the wrist joint. *J Anat* 1970;106:539–552.
4. Kauer JMG. The interdependence of carpal articulation chains. *Acta Anat* 1974;88:481–501.
5. Landsmeer JMF. *Atlas of anatomy of the hand.* New York: Churchill Livingstone, 1976.
6. Bonnel F, Allieu Y. Les articulations radio-cubito-carpienne et médiocarpienne. *Ann Chir Main* 1984;3:287–296.
7. Berger RA, Blair WF. The radioscapholunate ligament: A gross and histologic description. *Anat Rec* 1984;210:393–405.
8. Sennwald G, Zdravkovic V, Oberlin C. The anatomy of the palmar scaphotriquetral ligament. *J Bone Joint Surg Br* 1994;76: 146–149.
9. Pevny T, Rayan GM, Egle D. Ligamentous and tendinous support of the pisiform. Anatomic and biomechanic study. *J Hand Surg [Am]* 1995;20:299–304.
10. Apergis EP. The unstable capitolunate and radiolunate joints as a source of wrist pain in young women. *J Hand Surg [Br]* 1996;21: 501–506.
11. Berger RA. The ligaments of the wrist: A current overview of anatomy with considerations of their potential functions. *Hand Clin* 1997;13:63–82.
12. Garcia-Elias M, An K, Cooney WP, et al. Transverse stability of the carpus. An analytical study. *J Orthop Res* 1989;7:738–743.
13. Hixson ML, Stewart C. Microvascular anatomy of the radioscapholunate ligament of the wrist. *J Hand Surg [Am]* 1990;15: 279–282.
14. Johnston RB, Seiler JG, Miller EJ, et al. The intrinsic and extrinsic ligaments of the wrist. A correlation of collagen typing and histologic appearance. *J Hand Surg [Br]* 1995;20:750–754.
15. Ritt MJ, Berger RA, Bishop AT. The capitohamate ligaments: A comparison of biomechanical properties. *J Hand Surg [Br]* 1996; 21:451–454.
16. Cihác R. Ontogenesis of the skeleton and intrinsic muscles of the human hand and foot. *Ergeb Anat Entwickl Ges* 1972;46:1–189.
17. Garcia-Elias M, Domènech-Mateu JM. The articular disc of the wrist. Limits and relations. *Acta Anat* 1987;128:51–54.
18. Hogikyan JV, Louis DS. Embryologic development and variations in the anatomy of the ulnocarpal ligamentous complex. *J Hand Surg [Am]* 1992;17:719–723.
19. Berger RA. The gross and histologic anatomy of the scapholunate interosseous ligament. *J Hand Surg [Am]* 1996;21:170–178.
20. Berger RA, Blair WF, El-Khoury GY. Arthrotomography of the wrist: The palmar radiocarpal ligaments. *Clin Orthop* 1984;186: 224–229.
21. North ER, Thomas S. An anatomic guide for arthroscopic visualization of the wrist capsular ligaments. *J Hand Surg [Am]* 1988; 13:815–822.
22. Cooney WP, Dobyns JH, Linscheid RL. Arthroscopy of the wrist: anatomy and classification of carpal instability. *J Arthrosc Rel Surg* 1990;6:133–140.
23. Sennwald G, Fischer M, Jacob HAC. Arthroscopie radio-carpienne et médio-carpienne dans les instabilités du carpe. *Ann Chir Main* 1993;12:26–38.
24. Skahen JR III, Palmer AK, Levinsohn EM, et al. Magnetic resonance imaging of the triangular fibrocartilage complex. *J Hand Surg [Am]* 1990;15:552–557.
25. Ebri B, Ros R, Monzon A, et al. Contribución al estudio de los huesos accesorios de la mano. *Rev Esp Cir Mano* 1982;24:65–76.
26. Beatty E. Upper limb tissue differentiation in the human embryo. *Hand Clin* 1985;1:391–403.
27. Hugues PCR, Tanner JM. The development of carpal bone fusion as seen in serial radiographs. *Br J Radiol* 1966;39:943–949.
28. May O. Le pisiforme: sésamoïde ou os carpien. *Ann Chir Main* 1996;4:265–271.
29. Harris HA. The pisiform bone. *Nature* 1944;153:715.
30. Hagert C. The distal radioulnar joint. *Hand Clin* 1987;3:41–50.
31. Schuind F, Linscheid RL, An KN, et al. A normal data base of posteroanterior roentgenographic measurements of the wrist. *J Bone Joint Surg Am* 1992;14:1418–1429.
32. Boabighi A, Kuhlmann JN, Guérin-Surville H. Nouvelle approche radiologique de l'articulation radiocarpienne. *J Radiol* 1988;69:465–467.
33. Berger RA, Landsmeer JMF. The palmar radiocarpal ligaments: a study of adult and fetal human wrist joints. *J Hand Surg [Am]* 1990;15:847–854.
34. Berger RA, Kauer JMG, Landsmeer JMF. Radioscapholunate ligament. A gross anatomic and histologic study of fetal and adult wrists. *J Hand Surg [Am]* 1991;16:350–355.
35. Berger RA, Garcia-Elias M. General anatomy of the wrist. In: An KN, Berger RA, Cooney WP, eds. *Biomechanics of the wrist joint.* New York: Springer-Verlag, 1991;1–21.
36. Cooney WP, Garcia-Elias M, Dobyns JH, et al. Anatomy and mechanics of carpal instability. *Surg Rounds Orthop* 1989;3:15–25.
37. Taleisnik J, Kelly PJ. The extraosseous and intraosseous blood supply of the scaphoid bone. *J Bone Joint Surg Am* 1966;48: 1125–1137.
38. Gelberman RH, Gross M. The vascularity of the wrist. Identification of arterial patterns at risk. *Clin Orthop* 1986;202:40–49.
39. Belsole RJ, Hilbelink DR, Llewellyn JA, et al. Carpal orientation from computed reference axes. *J Hand Surg [Am]* 1991;16: 82–90.
40. Kauer JMG. The mechanism of the carpal joint. *Clin Orthop* 1986;202:16–26
41. Burgess RC. Anatomic variations of the midcarpal joint. *J Hand Surg [Am]* 1990;15:129–131.
42. Viegas SF, Patterson RM, Hokanson JA, et al. Wrist anatomy: incidence, distribution, and correlation of anatomic variations, tears, and arthrosis. *J Hand Surg [Am]* 1993;18:463–475.
43. Watson HK, Yasuda M, Guidera PM. Lateral lunate morphology: An x-ray study. *J Hand Surg [Am]* 1996;21:759–763.
44. Antuña-Zapico JM. *Malacia del semilunar.* Valladolid: Secretariado de publicaciones de la Universidad de Valladolid, 1966.
45. Weber ER. Concepts governing the rotational shift of the intercalated segment of the carpus. *Orthop Clin North Am* 1984;15: 193–207.
46. Garcia-Elias M, An KN, Cooney WP, et al. Stability of the transverse carpal arch: An experimental study. *J Hand Surg [Am]* 1989; 14:277–281.
47. Cooney WP, Lucca MJ, Chao EYS, et al. The kinesiology of the thumb trapeziometacarpal joint. *J Bone Joint Surg Am* 1981;63: 1371–1381.
48. El Bacha A. Les articulations carpo-métacarpiennes a l'exception de la trapézo-métacarpienne. In: Tubiana R, ed. *Traité de Chirurgie de la Main.* Paris: Masson, 1980:193–205.
49. Jessurun W, Hillen B, Zonneveld F, et al. Anatomical relations in the carpal tunnel: A computed tomographic study. *J Hand Surg [Br]* 1987;12:64–67.
50. Bowers WH. Instability of the distal radioulnar articulation. *Hand Clin* 1991;7:311–327.
51. af Ekenstam FW, Hagert CG. Anatomical studies on the geometry and stability of the distal radioulnar joint. *Scand J Plast Reconstr Surg* 1985;19:17–25.
52. Garcia-Elias M, Lluch AL, Vidal AM. Surgical treatment of acute dislocations of the distal radio-ulnar joint. *J Orthop Surg Tech* 1995;9:33–43.
53. Palmer AK. The triangular fibrocartilage complex of the wrist—anatomy and function. *J Hand Surg [Am]* 1981;6:153–165.
54. Mikic ZD. Detailed anatomy of the articular disc of the distal radioulnar joint. *Clin Orthop* 1989;245:123–132.
55. Mikic ZD. Age changes in the triangular fibrocartilage of the wrist joint. *J Anat* 1978;126:367–384.

56. Kauer JMG. The articular disc of the hand. *Acta Anat* 1975;93:590–611.
57. Mikic ZD. Arthrography of the wrist joint. *J Bone Joint Surg Am* 1984;66:371–378.
58. Mayfield JK, Johnson RP, Kilcoyne RF. The ligaments of the human wrist and their functional significance. *Anat Rec* 1976;186:417–428.
59. Taleisnik J. The ligaments of the wrist. *J Hand Surg [Am]* 1976;1:110–118.
60. Mizuseki T, Ikuta Y. The dorsal carpal ligaments: their anatomy and function. *J Hand Surg [Br]* 1989;14:91–98.
61. Mayfield JK, Williams WJ, Erdman AG, et al. Biomechanical properties of human carpal ligaments. *Orthop Trans* 1979;3:143–144.
62. Siegel DB, Gelberman RH. Radial styloidectomy: An anatomical study with special reference to radiocarpal intracapsular ligamentous morphology. *J Hand Surg [Am]* 1991;16:40–44.
63. Linscheid RL. Kinematic considerations of the wrist. *Clin Orthop* 1986;202:27–39.
64. Ambrose L, Posner MA. Lunate–triquetral and midcarpal joint instability. *Hand Clin* 1992;8:653–668.
65. Taleisnik J. Wrist: anatomy, function, and injury. In: *AAOS instructional course lectures*. St Louis: CV Mosby, 1978;61–87.
66. Taleisnik J, Gelberman RH, Miller BW, et al. The extensor retinaculum of the wrist. *J Hand Surg [Am]* 1984;9:495–501.
67. Spinner M, Kaplan EB. Extensor carpi ulnaris. Its relationship to the stability of the distal radioulnar joint. *Clin Orthop* 1970;68:124–129.
68. Kauer JMG. Functional anatomy of the wrist. *Clin Orthop* 1980;149:9–20.
69. Garcia-Elias M. Kinetic analysis of carpal stability during grip. *Hand Clin* 1997;13:151–158.
70. Lichtman DM, Shneider JR, Swafford AR, et al. Ulnar midcarpal instability: Clinical and laboratory analysis. *J Hand Surg [Am]* 1981;6:515–523.
71. Drewniany JJ, Palmer AK, Flatt AE. The scaphotrapezial ligament complex: An anatomic and biomechanical study. *J Hand Surg [Am]* 1985;10:492–498
72. Masquelet AC, Strube F, Nordin JY. The isolated scapho-trapezio-trapezoid ligament injury. Diagnosis and surgical treatment in four cases. *J Hand Surg [Br]* 1993;18:730–735.

3

KINEMATICS OF THE WRIST

RITA M. PATTERSON
STEVEN F. VIEGAS

Investigations of normal wrist kinematics date back to the late nineteenth century. These studies utilized planar x-rays to study both cadaver specimens and living subjects and were highly qualitative in nature (1–6). Sparked specifically by the need for treatment modalities for patients with advanced rheumatoid arthritis and posttraumatic instabilities, investigators searched for a more accurate and quantitative description of wrist kinematics. Recognizing the limitations of planar x-rays, investigators later used stereoscopic x-rays to attempt to analyze the three-dimensional (3-D) properties of wrist kinematics (7,8). Other investigators have used 3-D techniques such as sonic digitizers (9–13), instrumented electromechanical linkages (14,15), radiostereophotogrammetric techniques (16–19), or 3-D computer imaging (20). These studies gave the first insight into carpal bone kinematics; however, their methods were based on static analyses. The musculoskeletal control necessary to perform these static positions is significantly different from that needed to produce dynamic motion. The kinematic results also differ between static and dynamic motion.

There are many methods to measure joint kinematics, and the precision of the kinematic measurements needed is dependent on the specific goals of the study and the way the measurements were conducted. Radiographic measurements, including planar x-rays, biplanar x-rays, CT scans, and MRI scans, are limited to static or quasistatic studies. The relatively slow capture time for even the fastest imaging technology currently available on standard machines requires that the subject be perfectly stationary while the scan is being conducted. For a static, cadaveric specimen, this is not a problem. In dynamic studies or live-subject studies, however, because the musculoskeletal control necessary to perform such fixed (static) positions is significantly different from that used in a continuously moving action, the kinematic results also differ. In addition, for the live subject, scans of the bones made for each of many small postural changes over an entire range of motion (ROM) would constitute excessive x-ray exposure. Thus, *in vivo* radiographic studies are limited to larger-angle samples (5–10°) (21,22), and all radiographic studies are limited to the gross approximation of dynamic motion by repeated static positioning (3–8,16–19,23–28). Other means of studying human joint motion include the use of attached active or passive markers or transmitters, the positions of which are recorded by multiple sensors. Combined, these sensor arrays produce a 3-D path and marker site orientation for the motion of interest.

FLEXION–EXTENSION

Third Metacarpal Capitate Joint Motion

There is little motion in the distal carpal row between the third metacarpal and the capitate (29), implying that global wrist motion can be measured using either the third metacarpal or the capitate's angle with respect to the radius. Figure 3.1 displays third metacarpal–radius and capitate–radius angles. The average difference in capitate–radius and third metacarpal–radius angles at each respective flexion–extension wrist angle for all wrists was 1.1° ± 1.6°.

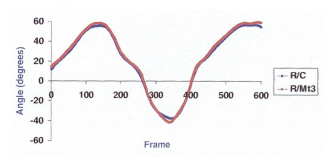

FIGURE 3.1. Normal flexion-extension angles of the capitate and third metacarpal with respect to the radius.

R. M. Patterson and S. F. Viegas: Department of Orthopaedic Surgery and Rehabilitation, The University of Texas Medical Branch, Galveston, Texas 77555.

TABLE 3.1. REPORTED CONTRIBUTIONS OF THE PROXIMAL AND MIDCARPAL JOINTS TO FLEXION–EXTENSION OF THE WRIST

Author	Flexion		Extension	
	RC	MC	RC	MC
Fick (33)	45–50	30–35	35	50
Kapandji (34)	50	35	35	50
Kaplan (23)	65–75	25–35	15–25	79–85
Steindler (35)	RC > MC		RC < MC	
Patterson (29)	RC > MC		RC < MC	
Garcia-Elias et al. (30)	49.7%	50.3%	62.1%	37.9%
Wright (25)	30	50	28	16
Sarrafian et al. (6)	40%	60%	66.5%	33.5%
Ruby et al. (18)	MC > RC		MC > RC	
Jackson et al. (15)	19.0	24.3	18.6	49.5
DeLange et al. (16)	40	82	18	66
Smith (17)	37	69	17	40
Brumfield et al. (28)	RC < MC		RC ≠ MC	
Horwitz (26)	18	67	24	33
Fisk (4)	RC = MC		RC = MC	
Bunnell (3)	22	22	44	34
Serage et al. (19)	RC > MC		RC = MC	
Sennwald (36)	RC > MC		RC > MC	
Berger et al. (9)	RC > MC		RC > MC	

MC, midcarpal; RC, radiocarpal.
Numbers given in degrees unless otherwise marked.

Radiocarpal and Midcarpal Motion

There have been several studies investigating the relative angles between carpal bones. There are conflicting reports of the contribution of the radiocarpal and midcarpal joints to the flexion and extension of the wrist (Table 3.1). Several authors have reported that the radiolunate joint contributes more to extension, and the midcarpal joint contributes more to flexion (6,15,25–28). Others (3,4,30) have reported that there is an equal contribution of the radiocarpal and midcarpal joints to flexion and that the radiocarpal joint contributes more to extension. Several other authors state that the radiocarpal joint contributes more to flexion and that the midcarpal joint contributes more to extension (16,17,19,23,24). The confusing results may be related to the way each author reports the results. Carpal angles can be reported as the relative angle with respect to another bone (as in the data reported here) or as an angle relative to a starting position. Relative angles give intermediate information throughout the ROM about the path that the objects move through, whereas angles relative to a starting position give information about the endpoints of the motion.

There is relatively little out-of-plane (pronation–supination and radioulnar deviation) motion of the carpal bones during flexion and extension of the wrist. The amount of angulation each joint contributes to the ROM, however, in a normal wrist is not constant during all phases of motion. During global wrist motion, the radiolunate joint contributes more motion in flexion (Fig. 3.2) than the capitolunate joint, and the capitolunate joint contributes more motion in extension than the radiolunate joint (Fig. 3.3). Capitolunate angles ranged from 16.9° extension to 29.5° flexion with a total ROM of 46.4°. Radiolunate angles ranged from 12.2° extension to 58.3° flexion with a total ROM of 70.5°.

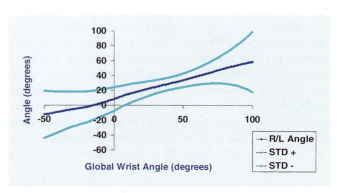

FIGURE 3.2. Graph displaying average radiolunate angles for each condition. Flexion is indicated by positive angles, and extension by negative angles.

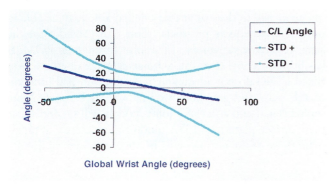

FIGURE 3.3. Graph displaying average capitolunate angles for each condition. Flexion is indicated by positive angles, and extension by negative angles.

TABLE 3.2. REPORTED AXIS OF ROTATION FOR FLEXION–EXTENSION OF THE WRIST

Author	Flexion–Extension axis of rotation
Fick (33)	Two parallel axes in the RC and MC joints
Wright (25)	Flexion: head of the capitate
	Extension: intercarpal joint
Kapandji (34)	Two parallel axes in the RC and MC joints
MacConaill (37)	Head of the capitate
Volt (32)	Head of the capitate
Youm (12)	Head of the capitate
Andrews (10)	Head of the capitate
Brumbaugh (11)	Head of the capitate
Jackson (15)	Head of the capitate
Patterson (29)	ISA calculated in head of the capitate and beyond

MC, midcarpal; RC, radiocarpal.

RADIOULNAR DEVIATION

In radioulnar (RU) deviation, the deviation excursions of the distal carpal bones exceed those of the proximal ones. The out-of-plane rotations during RU deviation are of the same order of magnitude as the principal (RU deviation) rotations, in contrast to the relatively small out-of-plane rotations of the carpal bones during wrist flexion and extension.

During ulnar deviation, there is a gliding movement of the proximal row on the radial and triangular ligament surfaces (25). The scaphoid rotates most in the dorsal direction, creating a greater proximal-to-distal height of the scaphoid on x-ray. The carpal bones supinate, and the triquetrum migrates distally along the hamate, assuming a lower position, and becomes dorsiflexed (16). The hamate "engages" against the triquetrum at the helicoidal triquetrohamate joint, causing the triquetrum and hamate to overlap on x-ray.

During radial deviation the movement takes place at the midcarpal row entirely. There is no movement of the proximal row relative to the radius (25). The scaphoid and lunate rotate in the palmar direction (volarflex), the carpal bones pronate, and the trapezoid and trapezium ride dorsally on the distal neck of the scaphoid (16). The hamate disengages from the triquetrum, and the two bones separate, causing them not to overlap on x-ray.

INSTANTANEOUS SCREW AXIS

The instantaneous screw axis (ISA) is another measurement that can be calculated. Investigators have reported on the center of rotation (COR) for a specific wrist motion. The COR is a geometric calculation based on strictly planar motion. It is typically a gross estimate of the rotation center using large angular changes (>5°). Wright (25) reported that the COR was in the head of the capitate for flexion of the wrist and in the intercarpal joint during extension of the wrist. Several other authors have stated that the COR for flexion and extension of the wrist is located in and confined to the head of the capitate (10,11,13,15,31,32). Others believe that there are two parallel and closely spaced axes of rotation located in the radiocarpal and midcarpal joints (32, 33) (Table 3.2).

The data presented here differ in that a high-speed ISA was calculated for each rotation and displacement at each time interval. The ISA surface of vectors (ISA axode) constitutes the signature surface characteristic for each bone and gives insight into the instantaneous motion (kinematics) of that joint during a specific global wrist motion (Fig. 3.4).

The distancing of the ISA from the previously reported COR of the wrist in the head of the capitate results in part

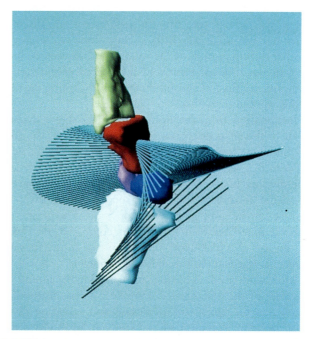

FIGURE 3.4. Lateral view of an instantaneous screw axis surface for flexion and extension of a normal wrist.

from the translational motion that occurs between the bones during motion of the carpus. The instantaneous axis of rotation of pure sliding motion is at infinity. Thus, it is expected that limited gliding or slippage between curved articular surfaces would produce a distantly placed ISA, as seen in this case. The problem is to relate the ISA with historical COR results. Fundamentally, ISA and COR measurements can not be compared directly because of the difference in constraints imposed in each case. The COR calculations reported in previous studies have been made from wrists that were constrained to move in a plane. This forces the COR to be normal to that plane of motion. This constrained motion does not represent the true multiplanar motion of the carpus and thus does not offer insight into its relative kinematics. External constraints (i.e., external forces) are necessary to produce planar motion and will influence the location of the COR. It provides no information about the path taken by the multiple-link joint to provide that gross motion. The ISA method provides the detail. The use of COR calculations for the wrist is like saying the trip from Los Angeles to San Francisco via the Pacific Coast Highway takes 8 hours, is south–north, and traverses an average elevation of 500 feet. The actual drive is, like ISA calculations, a thrilling and at times terrifying, twisting, turning road filled with incredible vistas of the Pacific coast. Both COR and ISA methods are valuable, but the latter provides a great deal more information. It represents the continuously changing relationship between carpal bones during continuous motion.

Thus, there is a dilemma in adequately comparing results from this study with most past work (i.e., they are really not comparable). The ISA vector surfaces (axodes) generated for normal wrists (third metacarpal motion relative to the radius) were smooth surfaces without discontinuity because there was little change from one vector to another during motion of the wrist. The ISA vectors, however, are not located exclusively in the head of the capitate but travel within and around the carpus, including the head of the capitate (Fig. 3.4).

Information from the normal ISA data shows that the COR of the wrist does pass through the head of the capitate but is not limited to the capitate. In addition, the angle between ISA vectors indicates a directional shift in the ISA. The distance between ISA vectors indicates a difference in calculated relative sliding of the bones during the wrist motion for the same global wrist position. The greater the distance noted between ISA vectors compared to normal, the greater the likelihood that abnormal kinematics has occurred, especially in the sliding component.

More work needs to be done in explaining the clinical significance of the ISA surface. However, it has clearly illustrated that the kinematics of flexion and extension of the wrist are more complicated and can not be modeled as a fixed hinge or ball joint. The real value of using the ISA method of analysis is to understand the continuously changing geometry to the extent that one day one may be able to provide an adequate prosthetic joint that provides for the same geometric variability of the joint through its ROM. It has been observed that simple hinge-type prosthetic devices (fixed COR) do not adequately reproduce normal junction of the wrist and are short-lived *in vivo* as a result. More sophisticated and successful joint models will be derived as their surface pattern and ISA motion more closely approximate those of the normal wrist in unconstrained motion.

SUMMARY

- There is little motion in the distal carpal row between the third metacarpal and the capitate, which implies that global wrist motion can be measured using either the third metacarpal or the capitate's angle with respect to the radius.
- Normal carpal motion during wrist flexion and extension does not have an ISA fixed in or limited to the capitate. This changes the understanding of carpal kinematics from that previously based on studies suggesting that the COR was fixed in the capitate.
- During global wrist motion, the radiolunate joint contributes more motion in flexion than the capitolunate joint, and the capitolunate joint contributes more motion in extension than the radiolunate joint.
- Translational motion is a real and measurable component of normal carpal kinematics.
- During ulnar deviation, the scaphoid dorsiflexes, the carpal bones supinate, and the triquetrum migrates distally along the hamate.
- During radial deviation, the scaphoid and lunate volarflex, the carpal bones pronate, the trapezoid and trapezium ride dorsally on the distal neck of the scaphoid, and the hamate disengages from the triquetrum.

EDITORS' COMMENTS

One problem with wrist kinematics is that history has constrained wrist evaluation to dorsiflexion, volarflexion, radial deviation, and ulnar deviation determined by the plane of the metacarpals. The wrist has little regard for the plane of the metacarpals and functions through a long range of dorsoradial angulation to volar–ulnar angulation and a very short restricted range between volar–radial angulation and dorsal–ulnar angulation. Seen end on, the maximal deviation of the wrist in any direction describes an oval plane. The metacarpals form a very arbitrary set of axes within this oval. Meaningful wrist kinematics must be done relative to the functional motion of the wrist and not the plane of the metacarpals.

From the clinician's point of view, the basic principle is to define any adequate cartilage surfaces in a damaged wrist and rebuild the wrist around that joint, accepting concomitant limitations of motion. Minimal motion established at the center of an axis can demonstrate significantly greater motion at a distance along that axis. Cadaveric studies demonstrate little motion difference between STT and capitate–scaphoid fusions. With STT fusion, the trapezoid–capitate joint develops some motion over time, probably with ligament attenuation. This minimal motion between trapezoid and capitate following STT arthrodesis produces the significant total wrist motion difference seen *in vivo* with STT over capitate–scaphoid fusion.

Other than load transference, motion is what the wrist is all about. Wrist arthrodesis is to be avoided. Even small amounts of motion make a big difference in functional capacity. Time is part of the equation. If an asymptomatic wrist with some motion and an expected life span of 10 years can be achieved, this represents many thousands of man-hour activities in a significant portion of the patient's life. Salvage procedures are available when needed. A patient may tell the surgeon that he wants "one procedure and never wants to worry about the wrist again." The patient is better advised to go for a painless functional wrist, even with an expected time limit.

As the wrist ulnar deviates into power position, the entire proximal row dorsiflexes. This tends to move the capitate and hand dorsally, but the downslope movement of the lunate maintains a collinear axis between the capitate and radius. In radial deviation, the scaphoid must lie more perpendicular to the axis of the wrist and, in flexing, carries the lunate and triquetrum into the volarflexed position of radial deviation. The symptom-producing problem of a dorsiflexed Colles' fracture is the dorsiflexion of the proximal row in ulnar deviation, but downslope volarly has now become upslope, and the translation component does not occur, so the entire hand is displaced dorsally in power grip, creating a cantilever and overloading the ligament support. This is the symptomatic wrist that will develop in an active person 6 months or so following a Colles' fracture that has been left in dorsiflexion.

Picturing the scaphoid from a lateral view serves as a mnemonic for these kinematics, as the scaphoid in radial deviation must get out of the way of the radial deviating wrist, taking the proximal row into flexion with it, and, in ulnar deviation, it lines up more with the long axis of the radius, carrying the proximal row into dorsiflexion.

Table 3.1 reports contributions of the proximal and midcarpal joints to flexion–extension of the wrist.

REFERENCES

1. Gilford WW, Bolton RH, Lambrinundri C. The mechanism of the wrist joint with special reference to fractures of the scaphoid. *Guys Hosp Rep* 1943;92:52–59.
2. Henke W. Die bewegungen der wandwurzel. *Z Rad Med* 1859; III:27–42.
3. Bunnell S. *Surgery of the hand, the normal hand, 3rd ed.* Philadelphia: JB Lippincott, 1956;34–37.
4. Fisk GR. Carpal instability and the fractured scaphoid. *R Coll Surg Engl* 1970;46:63–76.
5. Bryce TH. On certain points in the anatomy and mechanism of the wrist-joint reviewed in light of a series of Roentgen ray photographs of the living hand. *J Anat Physiol* 1896;31:59–79.
6. Sarrafian SK, Melamed JL, Goshgarian GM. Study of wrist, motion in flexion and extension, *Clin Orthop* 1977;126:153–159.
7. Von Bonin G. A note on the kinematics of the wrist-joint, *J Anat* 1929;63:259–262.
8. Savelberg H, Otten JDM, Kooloos JGM, et al. Carpal bone kinematics and ligament lengthening studied for the full range of joint movement. *J Biomech* 1993;26:1389–1402.
9. Berger RA, Crowninshield RD, Flatt AE. The three-dimensional rotational behavior of the carpal bones. *Clin Orthop* 1982;167: 303–310.
10. Andrews JG, Youm YA. A biomechanical investigation of wrist kinematics. *J Biomech* 1979;12:83–93.
11. Brumbaugh RB, Crowninshield RD, Blair WF, et al. An *in-vivo* study of normal wrist kinematics. *J Biomech Eng* 1982;104: 176–181.
12. Youm Y, McMurtry RY, Flatt AE, et al. Kinematics of the Wrist. *J Bone Joint Surg Am* 1978;60:423–431.
13. Youm Y, Flatt AE. Kinematics of the wrist. *Clin Orthop* 1980; 149:21–32.
14. Sommer HG III, Miller NR. A technique for kinematic modeling of anatomical joints. *J Biomech Eng* 1980;102:311–317.
15. Jackson WT, Hefzy MS, Guo H. Determination of wrist kinematics using a magnetic tracking device. *Med Eng Phys* 1994;16: 123–133.
16. deLange A, Kauer JMG, Huiskes R. Kinematic behavior of the human wrist joint: A Roentgen-stereophotogrammetric analysis. *J Orthop Res* 1985;3:56–64.
17. Smith DK, Cooney WP, Linscheid RL, et al. Effects of a scaphoid waist osteotomy on carpal kinematics. *J Orthop Res* 1989;7: 590–598.
18. Ruby LK, Cooney WP III, An KN, et al. Relative motion of selected carpal bones: A kinematic analysis of the normal wrist. *J Hand Surg [Am]* 1988;13:1–10.
19. Seradge H, Owens W, Seradge E. The effect of intercarpal joint motion on wrist motion: Are there key joints? An *in vitro* study. *Orthopedics* 1995;18:727–732.
20. Belsole RJ, Hilbelink D, Llewellyn JA, et al. Scaphoid orientation and location for computed three dimensional carpal models. *Orthop Clin North Am* 1986;173:505–510.
21. Woltring HJ, Huiskes R, DeLange D. Finite centroid and helical axis estimation from noisy landmark measurements in the study of human joint kinematics. *J Biomech* 1985;18:379–389.
22. Spoor CW. Explanation, verification and application of helical-axis error propagation formulas. *Hum Movement Sci* 1984;3: 95–117.
23. Kaplan E. *Functional and surgical anatomy of the hand, 2nd ed.* Philadelphia: JB Lippincott, 1965;248.
24. *Cunningham's textbook of anatomy.* New York: Oxford University Press, 1953;370.
25. Wright DR. A detailed study of movement of the wrist joint. *J Anat* 1935;70:137–143.
26. Horwitz T. An anatomic and roentgenologic study of the wrist joint. *Surgery* 1940;7:773–783.
27. *Gray's anatomy, 35th Br ed.* London: Warwick and Williams, 1973;438.
28. Brumfield RH Jr, Nickel VL, Nickel E. Joint motion in wrist flexion and extension. *South Med J* 1966;59:909–910.

29. Patterson RM, Nicodemus CL, Viegas SF, et al. Normal wrist kinematics and the analysis of the effect of various dynamic external fixators for treatment of distal radius fractures. *Hand Clin* 1997;13:129–142.
30. Garcia-Elias M, Cooney WP, An KN, et al. Wrist kinematics after limited intercarpal arthrodesis. *J Hand Surg [Am]* 1989;14:791–799.
31. Youm Y, Flatt AE. Design of a total wrist prosthesis. *Ann Biomed Eng* 1984;12:247–262.
32. Voltz RG. The development of a total wrist arthroplasty. *Clin Orthop* 1976;116:209–214.
33. Fick R. *Anatomie und Mechanik der Gelenke.* Jena: Gustav Fisher, 1911;357.
34. Kapandji IA. *The physiology of the joints, vol. 1: Upper limb,* 5th ed. New York: Churchill Livingston, 1982:138–149.
35. Steindler A. *Kinesiology of the human body under normal and pathologic conditions.* Springfield, IL: Charles C. Thomas, 1955.
36. Sennwald GR, Zdradovic V, Kern HP, et al. Kinematics of the wrist and its ligaments. *J Hand Surg [Am]* 1993;8:805–814.
37. MacConaill MA. The mechanical anatomy of the carpus and its bearings on some surgical problems. *J Anat* 1941;75:166–175.

4

BIOMECHANICS OF THE WRIST

JAIYOUNG RYU

To position the hand optimally in space for specific tasks, the wrist must strike a crucial balance between mobility and stability. A ball-and-socket joint, the basic design for the hip and shoulder joints, provides a large arc of motion but is a poor precursor for the wrist, as its inherent instability is checked mainly by bulky surrounding muscles. The wrist cannot afford such bulk, else its performance would be hindered greatly. Thus, the wrist developed in another way to maintain both mobility and stability: multilinked rows. Each link has a small degree of motion but good stability. When assembled, the wrist combines the motions of the multiple links. The links, despite their advantages, do decrease wrist stability somewhat. To compensate, the wrist includes not only multilinked rows, but columns of these rows as well. An et al. compared the wrist with a Rubik's cube, with its comparable arrangement of rows and columns (1). The traditional row theory (Fig. 4.1) and the columnar theory (2–5), which was first proposed by Navarro (6,7) and then modified by Taleisnik (8–10) (Fig. 4.2), were developed to explain how the columns and rows affect wrist motion and stability.

The scaphoid, which connects the proximal and distal rows, makes carpal kinematics and kinetics more complex. Linscheid and Dobyns introduced the slider–crank mechanism of the scaphoid to explain its role (11). Lichtman et al. later proposed the ring concept in which the proximal and distal rows are connected with radial mobile and ulnar rotatory links (12). Craigen and Stanley (13) observed that there are two kinds of people: those whose scaphoid stays vertical and translates through radioulnar deviation (RUD) and those whose scaphoid flexes with ulnar deviation. Thus, they felt that carpal kinematics covered a spectrum from the row theory to the column theory that is normally distributed. They reported that women were more likely to have column-type wrists.

Each theory has merit in explaining certain motions or certain stability/instability patterns. However, none explains wrist joint mechanics as a whole. A four-unit concept (Fig. 4.3) is proposed later in this chapter.

Many advances have been made toward understanding the biomechanics of this intriguing joint during the last two to three decades. Yet, we still do not have a reasonable or accurate model for the wrist. Biomechanics of the wrist is a science that certainly has a long way to evolve in the future. I have tried to make this chapter as comprehensive as the given space allows. The reader is encouraged to explore the subject in greater detail through the references.

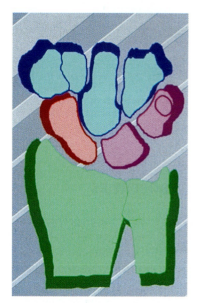

FIGURE 4.1. Classical row theory of the wrist. Note that the scaphoid bridges the proximal and distal rows rather than functioning as just one of the proximal row bones. Also note that the lunocapitate and the scaphotrapeziotrapezoid joints, together called the midcarpal joint, are located at two different levels with obviously different axes of rotations. Thus, the row theory cannot explain carpal kinematics.

J. Ryu: Department of Orthopedics, West Virginia University, Morgantown, West Virginia 26506.

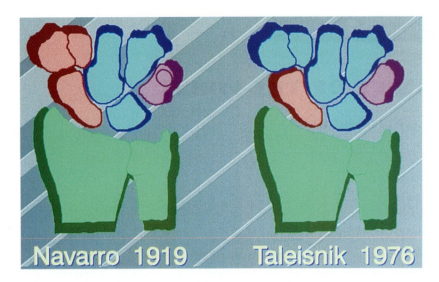

FIGURE 4.2. The columnar theory was first proposed by Navarro, then modified by Taleisnik. Taleisnik's modification, including the trapezium and trapezoid in the central column, makes a lot of biomechanical sense because there is almost no motion among distal row carpal bones. Eliminating the pisiform also makes sense because it does not contriburte to load bearing in the wrist. However, when one thinks about how much motion is present at the lunocapitate joint, it becomes clear that we cannot explain kinematics of the carpal bones with a theory that puts these two mobile bones into a single group.

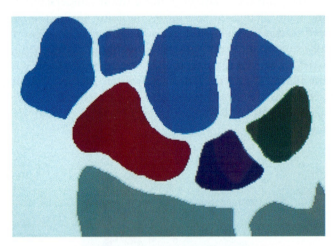

FIGURE 4.3. The "four-unit concept" was derived from a recent carpal kinematic study (58) that showed the distal carpal bones moved as a single unit while the scaphoid, lunate, and triquetrum moved independently. It is proposed that this concept be used in describing normal or pathokinematics of the wrist as well as stability and instability of the wrist.

MATERIAL PROPERTIES

The material properties of the carpal ligaments are generally agreed on by several investigators (14–16). The intrinsic ligaments, such as the scapholunate (SL) or lunotriquetral (LT) interosseous ligaments, are much stronger (ultimate strength of up to 300 N) than the extrinsic ligaments, such as the radioscaphocapitate or the long radiolunate ligaments (approximately 100 N). The former also have much greater strain at failure (over 50%) because they are more elastic than the latter, which have 10% to 35% strain at failure. Berger (17) recently studied the material properties of the subregions of the SL and LT ligaments. The dorsal region of the SL ligament was the strongest, requiring more than 250 N to fail, followed by the palmar region, failing at about 125 N. A reversed pattern was observed in the LT ligament. In both SL and LT ligaments, the fibrocartilaginous proximal region was quite weak, failing at approximately 25 N. Kim et al. developed a cross-sectional area measurement technique for intrinsic and extrinsic wrist ligaments using MRI (18,19). A method to represent articular surfaces of the carpal bones has also been developed (20).

NORMAL WRIST STRENGTH

Ryu et al. measured wrist strength in 100 (50 male and 50 female) normal subjects (21). They used custom-built torque cell dynamometers for wrist flexion, extension, and radial and ulnar deviations (Fig. 4.4A), forearm pronosupination (Fig. 4.4B), and a strain gauge for grip strength (Fig. 4.4C).

Men were 40.5% stronger than women in grip strength and 47.5% (44.1% to 51.6%) stronger for other measured strengths (Fig. 4.5). Dominant sides were 7% stronger than nondominant sides. Extension had only 45% of flexion strength while radial deviation accounted for 92% of ulnar deviation and pronation for 82% of supination.

WRIST MOTION (AS A WHOLE)

In general, the wrist is known to have three degrees of freedom: flexion–extension (FE) of 140°, RUD of 65°, and some pronosupination (PR).

Functional Range of Motion of the Wrist

Ryu et al. examined 40 normal subjects (20 men and 20 women) to determine the ideal range of motion required

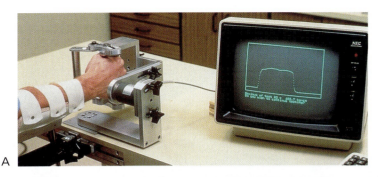

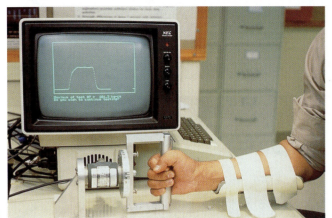
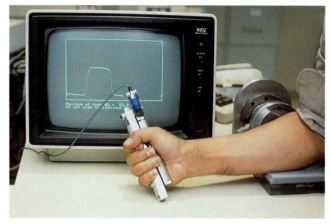

FIGURE 4.4. Custom-built torque cell dynamometers for measuring wrist flexion and radial and ulnar deviations **(A)**, for arm pronosupination **(B)**, and a strain gauge for grip strength **(C)**.

FIGURE 4.5. Functional evaluation of normal wrist strength. Men were 40.5% stronger than women in grip strength and 47.5% (44.1%–51.6%) stronger for other measured strengths. Dominant sides were 7% stronger than nondominant sides. Extension demonstrated only 45% of flexion strength, radial deviation (*RD*) accounted for 92% of ulnar deviation (*UD*), and pronation demonstrated 82% the strength of supination.

to perform activities of daily living (22) (Fig. 4.6). Wrist flexion and extension, as well as radial and ulnar deviation, were measured simultaneously with a biaxial wrist electrogoniometer. The entire battery of evaluated tasks could be achieved with 60° of extension, 54° of flexion, 40° of ulnar deviation, and 17° of radial deviation. These data reflected the maximum wrist motion required for the daily activities. The majority of the hand placement and range-of-motion tasks studied in this project could be accomplished with 70% of the maximal range of wrist motion (Fig. 4.7). This converts to 40° each of wrist flexion and extension and 40° of combined RUD (Fig. 4.8).

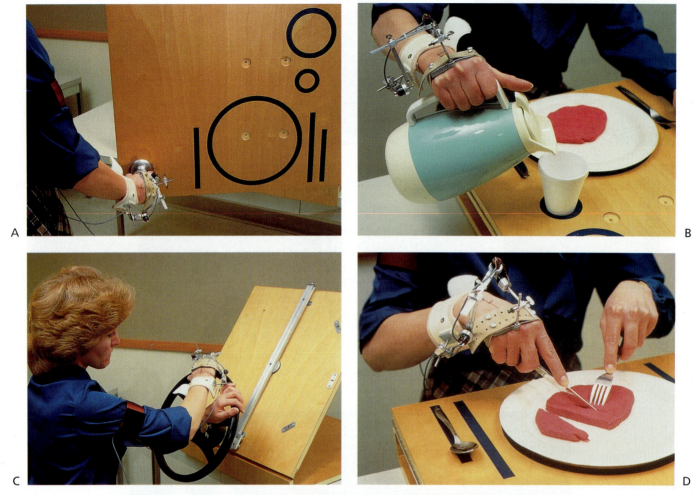

FIGURE 4.6. Forty normal subjects' wrist motions were examined with a custom-built electrogoniometer while they performed 24 different activities of daily living, including opening/closing a door **(A)**, pouring water into a cup **(B)**, turning a steering wheel **(C)**, and holding and cutting a steak **(D)**.

This study set the normal standards for the functional range of wrist motion.

Palmer et al. (23) investigated the same subject using a similar mechanical electrogoniometer. The raw data were very similar to those of Ryu et al. However, Palmer et al. associated much less motion (5° of flexion, 30° of extension, 10° of radial deviation, and 15° of ulnar deviation) with functional wrist motion. The difference between the studies rests almost purely on the disparity between the two statistical analyses. Palmer et al. averaged the ranges of motion required for all tested activities, which may not satisfy the majority of the daily activities in a normal fashion.

Nelson (24) used a custom-modified DonJoy wrist splint that limited wrist motion to 5° of flexion, 6° of extension, 7° of radial deviation, and 6° of ulnar deviation on 12 volunteers. He found that the subjects were able to perform a majority of their activities of daily living with a minimal degree of difficulty or frustration and with satisfactory outcome. Therefore, Nelson concluded that the functional range of motion of the wrist was much smaller (same as the limits created by the splint) than reported by others. Other investigators (25–27) have also studied the subject.

The major difference among investigators on this issue seems to be the definition of "functional" range of motion,

FIGURE 4.8. Although other investigators (23,24) claimed the functional range of wrist motion to be much smaller, Ryu et al. (22) believe that 40° each of wrist flexion and extension, 10° of radial deviation, and 30° of ulnar deviation is the functional range of wrist motion. This is defined as the capability to perform most activities of daily living in a normal fashion within the same range of motion.

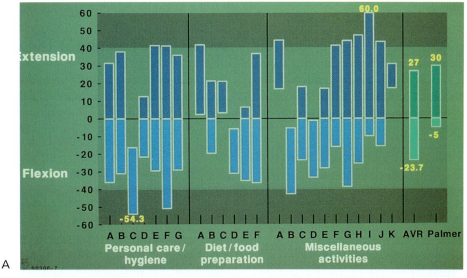
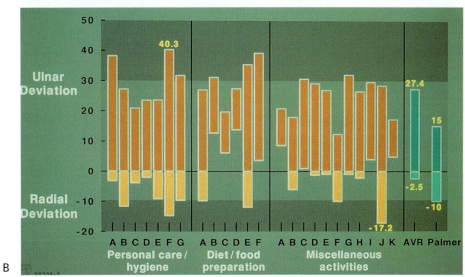

FIGURE 4.7. Functional evaluation of normal wrist motion. Flexion–extension **(A)** and radioulnar deviation (RUD) **(B)** were needed to fulfill the 24 activities of daily living. With 40° each of flexion and extension, and 40° of combined RUD, most activities could be performed in a normal fashion.

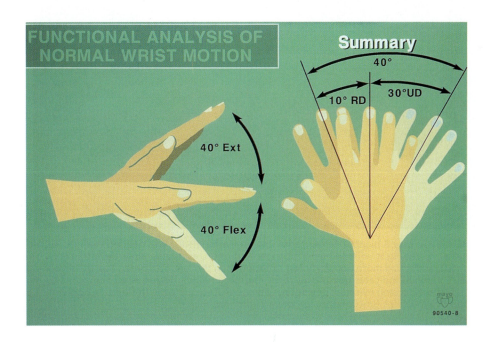

which differs from person to person depending on his or her vocational and avocational activities. Perhaps the term "functional" is viewed too generally. Health professionals treating wrist pathologies must first ascertain the individual patient's needs and then devise a plan to regain that specific "functional" range of motion.

Physiologic Motion of the Wrist

Bagg et al. carried out a study to delimit the global motion of the wrist, that is, the contribution of RUD to FE and of FE to RUD (Bagg MR, Ryu J, Kato H, et al., unpublished data.). With a biaxial goniometer, both RUD and FE were measured

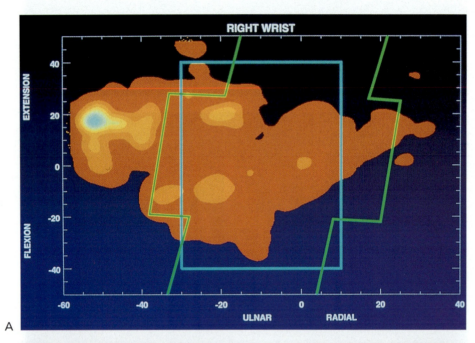

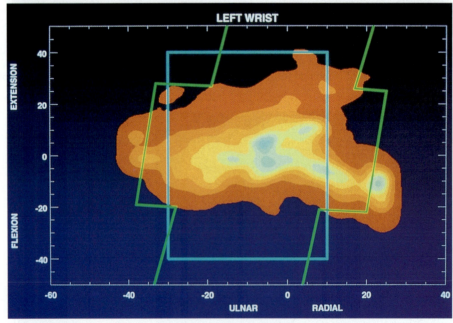

FIGURE 4.9. To play a piano, a larger radioulnar deviation (RUD) was needed than for activities of daily living. The right wrist **(A)** used much more motion, especially ulnar deviation (UD), than the left **(B)**, and it had more nonphysiologic motion than the left. The *green box* (resembling the Chevrolet insignia) indicates physiologic wrist motion in which flexion is accompanied by ulnar deviation and extension by radial deviation, whereas RUD occurred with slight flexion-extension. The *cyan box* indicates functional range of wrist motion.

simultaneously in 41 adult subjects with no history of upper extremity trauma or pathology. Measurements were recorded with the forearm in both neutral and pronated positions. Volunteer subjects were asked to move their wrists in what they perceived to be normal up-and-down and side-to-side motion. The mean slope for each motion was identified by combining the slopes of the individual motion curves. The "physiologic" axis for each motion was determined by converting slope to degrees and measuring from the RUD axis. The wrist radially deviated when it extended and ulnarly deviated when it flexed, as in a dart-throwing motion. As the wrist radially deviated, it flexed slightly, and vice versa (Fig. 4.9).

Range of Motion of the Wrist for Specific Activities

Unlike gait in the lower extremities, the wrist does not have a set motion. It must accommodate for the widely varying tasks the hand performs at certain times. Health professionals dealing with wrist injuries should aim for an optimal range of motion for each patient after considering the patient's occupation, avocational activities, age, hand dominance, etc. Only with this information can hand surgeons weigh the importance of motion and stability for the individual patient and choose an appropriate treatment modality for him or her.

To meet this basic goal, Ryu and his colleagues studied the wrist range of motion required in several specific activities, such as piano, violin, basketball, tennis, baseball, bowling, table tennis, golf, and typing (29–36). Either a custom-built biaxial electrogoniometer or a biaxial flexible electrogoniometer (Penny and Giles, Blackwood, UK) was used to measure motion in these studies (Table 4.1).

To play piano, a larger RUD was needed than for activities of daily living. The right wrist used much more motion than the left, particularly in ulnar deviation (UD); it also relied substantially more on nonphysiologic motion (Fig. 4.9). This may explain the glut of overuse syndromes in the right wrists of pianists as compared to the left. Trills and arpeggios required wider wrist motion than octaves or broken octaves. The amount of wrist motion used by weight-playing pianists was smaller than that used by pianists using the traditional method, although weight players showed greater FE activity in arpeggios and trills.

Violinists used more motion in the right wrist than the left, but the left wrist had more nonphysiologic motion, a combination of extreme flexion and radial deviation.

During keyboard typing, the range of wrist motion was about 40° of the wrist-flexed position in FE and 30° of the wrist ulnarly deviated position in RUD in both wrists. Standard posture did not reduce the range of motion of typists' wrists when compared to their own typing postures. Range of wrist motion was significantly reduced by a wrist or arm support device, which suggests that use of these support devices could help typists lessen overuse injuries.

Golfers frequently used their left wrist beyond the functional range of motion. The right wrist, however, remained

TABLE 4.1. RANGE OF MOTION OF THE WRIST IN DIFFERENT ACTIVITIES

	Right				Left			
	F	E	RD	UD	F	E	RD	UD
Functional ROM (for ADL) (77)	40	40	10	30	40	40	10	30
Piano								
Classical music	18	29	28	54	23	20	17	33
Practice exercise	16	26	28	53	19	16	12	29
Violin[a]	34	40	25	8	36	12	12	9
Keyboard typing	−8	47	−5	36	−7	46	−6	33
Golf[b]	0	53	21	23	−7	52	24	27
Baseball								
Batting[c]	14	68	23	39	4	58	19	33
Straight pitching[d]	28	55	16	20				
Curved pitching[e]	28	50	12	24				
Basketball[f]	70	50	12	10				
Bowling[g]	31	24	15	11				

[a]All violinists were right-hand dominant.
[b]All golfers were right-hand dominant.
[c]Right wrist is the top wrist, and the left wrist is the bottom wrist.
[d]Only pitching wrist was measured.
[e]Only pitching wrist was measured.
[f]Data for dominant shooting wrist was recorded as right wrist. Nondominant wrist needed minimal range of motion (32° of flexion–extension and 16° of radioulnar deviation).
[g]Data for dominant throwing wrist was recorded as right wrist.
ADL, activities of daily living; F, flexion; E, extension; RD, radial deviation; UD, ulnar deviation; ROM, range of motion.
Data from Ryu J, Cooney WP, Askew LJ, et al. Functional ranges of motion of the wrist joint. J Hand Surg [Am] 1991;16:409–419.

within range. Advanced golfers used less left wrist motion but more right wrist motion than intermediate-level golfers.

Bowlers used more motion (58° of FE and 32° of RUD) for their curved deliveries than for straight deliveries (50° of FE and 21° of RUD). In the advanced bowler's group, the wrist was more flexed and ulnarly deviated during forward swing, as opposed to extension and radial deviation during release and follow through of curved delivery. Some advanced bowlers showed a decrease in wrist flexion and a significant increase in ulnar deviation during curved delivery.

Baseball players used a large amount of extension and RUD for both pitching and batting. However, the requirement for flexion in baseball was extremely small, particularly for batting. During batting, the top wrist required more FE and RUD than the bottom wrist.

In basketball free throw shooting, the dominant shooting wrist required large FE but small RUD. The nondominant wrist needed minimal motion in both axes. Players who had more consistent wrist motion with less standard deviation had a better shooting success rate.

In general, the flexible or rigid electrogoniometer seems to provide a reliable and reproducible tool for evaluation of wrist motion. The insight these evaluations provide into the functional assessment of wrist pathology and potential treatment outcomes offers hand surgeons invaluable help in selecting therapeutic techniques to aid patients suffering from wrist impairment. If the selection can be tailored to meet occupational and avocational wrist motion requirements, hand surgeons will be that much further inclined toward meeting patients' needs and returning them to the activities their former dexterity had led them to expect.

CARPAL KINEMATICS

Normal Carpal Kinematics: The Four-Unit Concept

Wrist motion is produced by the interaction and accumulation of individual three-dimensional motions among carpal bones. Since the late 1800s, many investigators have attempted to learn about individual carpal motions through anatomic dissection (37,38), plain x-rays (37,39–45), stereoscopic x-rays (46), and cineradiography (45,47).

In 1972, Linscheid, Dobyns, and their colleagues (11) established the concept of carpal instability, which attracted many hand surgeons to the study of carpal kinematics. Many new techniques have been developed for more precise three-dimensional measurement of carpal motion. Researchers have used cadaveric models with each carpal bone labeled with special markers—light-emitting diodes (48,49), sonic pulsation markers (50), metal staples (51), radiopaque pellets (52–55)—then measuring the spatial position of carpal markers with a computer-controlled digitizer. Other techniques such as electrogoniometers (56), radiostereophotogrammetric techniques (52), and three-dimensional computer imaging (57) have also been utilized. The resultant data differ from one study to another.

Carpal motion results from the intercalation of carpal bone geometry, the restraining forces of ligament and capsular structures, and loading force. Therefore, in studying kinematics using cadaver specimens, it is important to standardize these factors in accordance with physiologic conditions. In most previous studies, the wrist was not actively loaded (50), or the number of loading tendons was limited (51–55). In all studies, wrist specimens were forced to FE and RUD in an orthogonal plane rather than allowing physiologic motion with a combination of FE and RUD. No study applied force to the wrist from all the finger and wrist extrinsic tendons that cross the wrist joint. Furthermore, most studies dissected the dorsal capsule and ligament to place carpal markers on or in the carpal bones, thus damaging the integral structures (51–55).

To obtain accurate measurements of carpal motion and rotation angles that would be of value in diagnosing carpal instabilities, understanding various wrist pathologies, presaging appropriate treatments, and designing kinematically compatible prostheses, Kato et al. studied three-dimensional carpal rotation angles during normal wrist motion under physiologic conditions (58,59).

Two K-wires were inserted into each of the carpal bones of 12 fresh-frozen human cadaveric upper extremities amputated at the midhumeral level. Custom-designed markers with four reference points were attached to the K-wires. All finger and wrist flexor and extensor tendon groups were incised proximal to the wrist and loaded according to the ratio of physiologic muscle cross-sectional areas. Wrist capsular structures and soft tissue were kept intact. Tendon loading of the wrist was the sole source of power; the wrist was allowed to move without any external restraints (Fig. 4.10). The resultant motion of the wrist was surprisingly similar to that in the "physiologic wrist motion" study (28), previously noted in this chapter (Fig. 4.11).

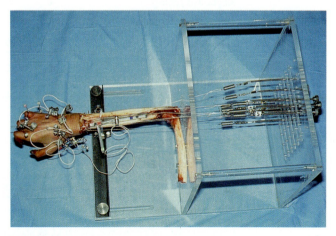

FIGURE 4.10. Static wrist simulator with a specimen mounted.

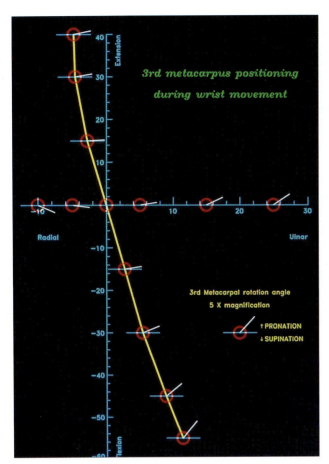

FIGURE 4.11. The wrist cadaver model generated motion almost identical to the physiologic motion noted in an *in vivo* study.

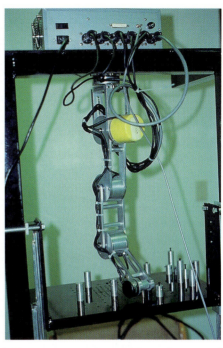

FIGURE 4.12. A custom-designed three-dimensional digitizer, with six optical encoders, that was used to track the carpal marker positions with accuracy.

In studying FE, the wrist was positioned from 40°, 30°, and 15° of extension, neutral, to 15°, 30°, 45°, and 55° of flexion. In studying RUD, the wrist was positioned 10° and 5° radially, neutral, and 5°, 15°, and 25° ulnarly. The markers allowed carpal motion to be tracked by a custom-designed three-dimensional digitizer with six optical encoders (Fig. 4.12) and computer software. Data were analyzed using Scheffe's analysis of variance; the reproducibility of measured rotation angles was determined via checks for inherent error in the digitizing system and repetitive examination of a single specimen to calculate standard error.

In wrist extension positions, there was no significant difference in the carpal extension angle between the scaphoid and distal carpus. In all wrist positions, the absolute scaphoid angle was greater than that of the lunate. As the wrist moved from 40° extension to 55° flexion, the total range of flexion motion was 73° (77%) in the scaphoid, 46.3° (49%) in the lunate, and 57.8° (61%) in the triquetrum. The total range of scaphoid extension-flexion was significantly greater than that of wrist extension motion (Fig. 4.13). Fifty-nine percent of wrist extension occurred at the radiocarpal joint, and 41% at the midcarpal joint, which was similar to the results reported by Sarrafian et al. (45).

In analyses of extension–flexion angles during wrist deviation, no significant extension–flexion motion was noted in the distal carpal bones. Conversely, all proximal carpal bones extended as the wrist moved from radial to ulnar deviation. In the proximal carpal bones, extension–flexion angles were almost equal. As the wrist shifted from 10° radial to 25° ulnar deviation, the total extension angle range was 20.7° in the scaphoid, 22.4° in the lunate, and 16.9° in the triquetrum. Midcarpal joint motion contributed 78% of radial deviation and 60% of ulnar deviation of the wrist. The RUD angles in carpal bones during wrist deviation showed that the proximal and distal carpal rows angulated in the same direction. Deviation excursion of the proximal carpal row was less than one-half that of the wrist, especially during radial deviation. No significant difference existed in deviation angles among the distal carpal bones.

The three-dimensional range of carpal motion during 40° extension to 55° flexion and during deviation 10° radially to 25° ulnarly revealed that the distal carpal bones move as a single kinematic unit. Kobayashi et al. (60) recently verified this in their study using a three-dimensional biplanar x-ray technique. The proximal carpal bones moved independently. Thus, wrist motion seems to be comprised of four kinematic units: the scaphoid, lunate, triquetrum, and the distal carpal row (Fig. 4.3). I propose this "four-unit concept" to describe carpal kinematics instead of rows, columns, or a ring.

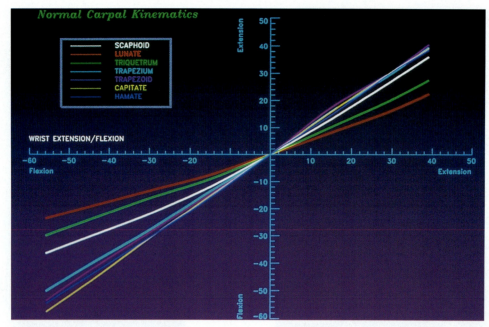

FIGURE 4.13. A sample graph demonstrating flexion–extension motion of individual carpal bones while the wrist moved from flexion to extension. Note that the four distal bones moved as a unit.

One of the pitfalls of this study and all others is that measurements are done in a static condition, which may differ from the way we use our wrists dynamically. To solve this problem, researchers are building "dynamic wrist simulators" (61–65). To eliminate the inconvenience and limitations of using cadaveric specimens, finite element modeling of the wrist is being studied (18,66).

Carpal Kinematics in Rotary Subluxation of the Scaphoid

Using techniques fairly similar to those that revealed normal human carpal kinematics, Tokunaga et al. investigated the altered kinematics produced by rotary subluxation of the scaphoid (RSS) in 12 cadaver specimens (67). Physiologic conditions were maintained in all specimens. Serial sectioning of the SL interosseous, radioscaphocapitate, and radioscapholunate ligaments was performed arthroscopically, leaving the other capsular structures of the wrist intact. Complete sets of data were collected and digitized using custom-designed computer software before and after each sectioning in eight wrist FE and six RUD positions.

After sectioning of the SL interosseous ligament, the scaphoid flexed while the lunate and triquetrum extended significantly during movement of the wrist from neutral to flexion positioning when compared to normal wrist kinematics ($p < 0.05$). No significant changes occurred during wrist extension. As the wrist moved from neutral to flexion position, the SL angle increased by 27.8°. The stability of the scaphoid and lunate was not significantly changed by sectioning of either the radioscaphocapitate or radioscapholunate ligament with the SL interosseous ligament. Sectioning all three ligaments resulted in the greatest displacement of the proximal carpal bones. From extension to 20° of wrist flexion, the scaphoid moved in unison with the distal carpal row. The lunate tended to maintain extension, and the SL angle increased by 33.5°. In RSS, when compared to normal wrist, the scaphoid flexed and pronated, the lunate extended and radially deviated, and the triquetrum radially deviated (Fig. 4.14). This finding was recently supported by Short et al. (64).

According to clinical reports, increased radiolunate angles are to be expected on radiographs in SL dissociations. This is probably because the patients had suffered the condition for an extended period of time before proper diagnosis was made, thereby altering soft tissues and producing ligamentous stress and possibly even bony structures. The early stages of acute scaphoid subluxation may not exhibit alteration radiographically. In general, this study produced smaller changes in carpal kinematics subsequent to RSS than in the findings of Ruby et al. (68). This may result either from the preservation of all surrounding capsular structures by Tokunaga et al., thereby curtailing wrist instability, or from the loading of all tendons crossing the wrist, which then functioned as dynamic carpal stabilizers.

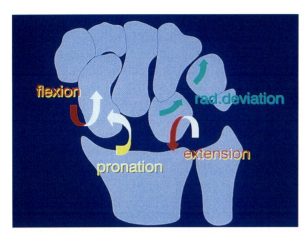

FIGURE 4.14. Rotary subluxation of the scaphoid. In scapholunate dissociation, when compared to normal wrists, the scaphoid flexed and pronated, the lunate extended and radially deviated, and the triquetrum radially deviated.

Carpal Kinematics in Lunotriquetral Dissociation

Li et al. investigated LT dissociation (69) in six cadaveric wrists. They performed three sets of digitization: on the intact wrist, after arthroscopic sectioning of the LT interosseous ligament, and then after further sectioning of the volar radiolunotriquetral ligament. During 10° radial and 25° ulnar deviation in intact wrists, the lunate expressed little motion (12°, 33%), the scaphoid showed comparatively more (14°, 40%), and the triquetrum exhibited the most proximal row motion (18°, 52%). In the distal row, the capitate (33°, 94%) and the hamate (32°, 92%) moved as a single unit. Traveling from 45° flexion to 55° flexion, there were varying degrees of proximal carpal bone motion. The capitate and hamate again moved as one. In the proximal row, the scaphoid exhibited the greatest amount of motion (74°), the lunate moved 51°, and the triquetrum 58°. Hypermobility of the LT joint was noted after sectioning of the LT interosseous ligament. Lunate and scaphoid RUD motions were virtually unchanged when compared with those in the intact wrists. Triquetrum motion significantly increased during ulnar deviation but increased only slightly throughout wrist FE. Further sectioning of the radiolunotriquetral ligament significantly increased LT joint motion in extension, mainly to a 4° decrease in lunate motion and a 3° increase in triquetrum motion from those values observed in intact wrists. This study suggested that the volar interosseous ligament stabilizes the LT joint during ulnar deviation, whereas the volar radiolunotriquetral ligament stabilizes the LT joint during wrist flexion. These results were similar to those reported by Horii et al. (70), although the alteration of carpal kinematics was smaller in the study by Li et al.

Carpal Kinematics in Ulnar Variance

In a study of ulnar variant kinematics (70), the ulnas of six specimens were osteotomized, and the impact on carpal motion of neutral, 5 mm ulnar lengthening, and 5 mm shortening during FE and RUD was quantified. Ulnar lengthening caused significant reduction in extension motion of the lunate and scaphoid during ulnar deviation. During FE motion, the proximal carpal bones, especially the lunate, locked at 20° flexion in some specimens after ulnar lengthening but were suddenly released as the wrist moved to neutral position. During flexion, ulnar deviation of all bones was significantly limited. During ulnar deviation, all carpal bones showed significant pronation, but radial deviation caused no significant alteration in motion.

Ulnar shortening yielded a significantly decreased flexion range for all proximal carpal bones, but rotation and deviation caused no significant decreases in flexion. During ulnar deviation, extension of the scaphoid and triquetrum increased significantly, but the lunate underwent no changes.

This study showed that, from a kinematic point of view, 5 mm of ulnar lengthening limited carpal motion by pushing the lunate into the scaphoid, thus narrowing the space between the radius and the scaphoid, whereas 5 mm of ulnar shortening had little impact on wrist dexterity.

Carpal Kinematics in Other Conditions

Carpal kinematic changes in other wrist conditions have been studied: different treatments of RSS [scaphotrapeziotrapezoid (STT) fusion, scaphocapitate (SC) fusion, Blatt procedure, SL fusion] (71), comparison of LT and CLTH fusion in LT dissociation (72), effects of scaphoid angle in STT fusion (73), malunion of Colles' fracture (55,74–76), effects of resection of the distal pole of the scaphoid (77), and effects of excision of the volar tubercle of the trapezium during scaphoid fixation (78).

FORCE, CONTACT AREA, AND PRESSURE ANALYSIS ON THE WRIST

Forces on the wrist can be either extrinsic or intrinsic. Extrinsic forces on the wrist are those externally applied and can be either positive (compressive) or negative (distractive), vary greatly (e.g., force from a floor during push-ups and that from a heavy fall), and have unlimited combinations. Intrinsic forces are those exerted by muscle–tendon units that cross the wrist, including all thumb, finger, and wrist motors.

Forces are distributed throughout carpometacarpal, intercarpal, and radioulnar–carpal joints. Force distribution is controlled by many factors, including complex bony geometry with anatomic variances, different load-bearing surface characteristics (e.g., cartilage to cartilage vs. cartilage to triangular fibrocartilage), contact area, constraints of varying ligamentous and capsular structures (e.g., mechanical differences between extrinsic and intrinsic ligaments), and infinite positions and motions of the wrist. These numerous factors, along with lack of a physiologic model of the human wrist, make force analysis of the wrist very difficult, demanding development of new theoretical solutions and experimental methods. We need to know the force and contact area to measure pressure. The problem is further complicated because the contact area increases as the force increases to a point (maximum contact area). In addition, a part of the contact area can have higher or lower pressure than another part of the same contact area.

During the last two to three decades, force analysis of the wrist has been studied through free-body diagrams, strain gauges, force and pressure transducers, pressure-sensitive film, a rigid-body spring model, and a finite element model.

Normal Force, Contact Area, and Pressure in the Wrist

Normal force distribution data have been gathered by various investigators (79–86) utilizing different techniques (Table 4.2). The data vary from one investigator to another and are even more varied if force distribution is measured when the wrist and forearm are not in neutral position. However, most investigators seem to agree that approximately 20% of force is transmitted by the distal ulna through the triangular fibrocartilage complex (TFCC), and the remaining 80% runs through the radius in the neutral position. Sixty percent of the radiocarpal load is reported to go through the radioscaphoid joint, and the other 40% through the radiolunate joint (87).

Wrist position and forearm rotation do not seem to change force transmission significantly. However, Hara et al. (79) reported decreased load transmission through the TFCC (8% from 15% in neutral position) with the wrist in ulnar deviation, while the load through the lunate fossa increased (50% from 35% in neutral) and the load through the radioscaphoid fossa decreased (42% from 50% in neutral). Werner et al. (86) reported increased load through the TFCC (37%) with the forearm in pronation. They explained the increased load to be the result of relative ulnar positive variance. In contrast, Trumble et al. (85) reported slightly decreased load transfer through the TFCC (15%) with the forearm in pronation.

As for the midcarpal joint, the load is distributed approximately 23% through the STT joint, 28% through the SC joint, 29% through the lunocapitate (LC) joint, and 20% through the triquetrohamate (TH) joint (88).

Viegas et al. (87) reported that the amount of contact in the proximal wrist joint accounts for only 20% of the available joint surface. This report was challenged by Hara et al. (79) because they consistently observed a relatively low articular pressure of about 0.5 MPa.

As load increases, cartilage compresses, resulting in an increasingly larger contact area until the cartilage cannot

TABLE 4.2. FORCE ANALYSIS OF THE NORMAL WRIST

Wrist Position	Investigators	Radiocarpal (%)		Ulnocarpal (%)	
		RS	RL	UL	UT
Neutral	Palmer & Werner (81)	82		18	
	Trumble et al. (85)	83		17	
	Horii et al. (80)	46	32	14	8
	Patterson et al. (82)	62		38	
	Hara et al. (79)	50	35		15
	Short et al.(84)	77		23	
	Schuing et al.(83)	55	35		10
Flexion	Trumble et al.(85)	85		15	
	Hara et al.(79)	37	50		13
Extension	Trumble et al.(85)	76		24	
	Hara et al.(79)	40	50		10
Radial deviation	Trumble et al.(85)	88		12	
	Hara et al.(79)	52	30		18
	Werner et al.(86)	87		13	
Ulnar deviation	Trumble et al.(85)	80		20	
	Hara et al.(79)	42	50		8
	Werner et al.(86)	72		28	
Pronation	Trumble et al.(85)	85		15	
	Werner et al.(86)	63		37	
Supination	Trumble et al.(99)	81		19	
	Werner et al.(86)	86		14	

RS, radioscaphoid; RL, radiolunate; UL, ulnolunate; UT, ulnotriquetral.

compress any further. That point is the maximum contact area, with the load reported to be in the range of 45 to 50 lb (87). Additional load does not result in increased contact area. As load increases, pressures measured in the contact areas increase. As the wrist flexes, the contact area moves to the dorsal aspect of the articular surface of the distal radius, and the contact area moves palmarward as the wrist extends.

In a study by Viegas et al., average high contact pressures within the scaphoid and lunate fossae varied with joint position; however, they were fairly low—in the range of 4 to 30 MPa (87). Palmer and Werner (81) found three distinct contact areas when 20 lb was loaded through the prime wrist movers. The peak pressures in the ulnolunate, radiolunate, and radioscaphoid joints were 1.4, 3.0, and 3.3 MPa, respectively. The peak pressure of the lunate decreased with radial deviation and increased with ulnar deviation, flexion, and extension (79).

CONTACT AREA AND PRESSURE ANALYSIS OF THE WRIST

Forces and Pressure on the Wrist in Scapholunate Dissociation

Viegas et al. (89) found an overall decrease in load in the lunate fossa and a significant increase in load in the scaphoid fossa with stage III perilunate instability. Both STT and SC fusions transmitted almost the entire load through the scaphoid fossa; SL, SLC, and LC fusions all distributed load more proportionately through both the scaphoid and lunate fossae. Other studies regarding force changes after various intercarpal fusions are noted in the following section on Kienböck's disease.

Forces and Pressure on the Wrist after Surgical Treatment Modalities for Kienböck's Disease

Many investigators have analyzed pressure of the wrist after various treatment modalities for Kienböck's disease.

Palmer and Werner and their colleagues (81,90) studied the effect of ulnar lengthening and shortening on force transmission through the radioulnar carpal joint. Lengthening the ulna by 2.5 mm in the intact wrist increased the force on the ulna from 18.4% to 41.9% of the total axial load. Shortening the ulna by 2.5 mm decreased axial load from 18.4% to 6.2%.

The same research group studied load changes to the distal radioulnar joint (DRUJ) after leveling procedures (91,92). They found radial shortening and ulnar lengthening led to increased pressure at the DRUJ and caused shifting of the location of the center of pressure distally within the sigmoid notch. Radial displacement of the distal radial fragment at the time of radial shortening, however, decreased the peak pressures.

Trumble and his colleagues (93,94) measured lunate strain with electronic strain gauges and found that STT fusion and joint leveling procedures were successful in relieving lunate loading throughout a functional range of wrist motion and forearm rotation, but that capitohamate (CH) fusion was ineffective.

Masear et al. (95) used strain gauges to compare the effectiveness of three procedures used to unload the lunate. Ulnar lengthening of 3 mm was the most effective method of lunate strain reduction; CH fusion decreased compressive strain but increased shear strain, and STT fusion significantly increased both compressive and shear strain in the lunate.

An, Horii, and their colleagues (96,80), using their two-dimensional rigid body spring model of the wrist, found that limited intercarpal fusions (STT, SC, and CH fusions) reduced compressive loading at the radiolunate joint by no more than 15% of the original load. Although CH fusion combined with capitate shortening was successful in relieving radiolunate forces, it dramatically overloaded the adjacent scaphotrapezial and TH forces. In contrast, a 4-mm lengthening of the ulna or shortening of the radius resulted in a 45% reduction of radiolunate load with only moderate changes in force at the midcarpal and radioscaphoid joints.

Using a two-dimensional mathematical model, Watanabe et al. (97) studied patients after radial wedge osteotomy for Kienböck's disease. They found that total force through the LC, radiolunate, and ulnolunate joints decreased by 23%, 10%, and 36%, respectively.

Short et al. (84) found that STT fusion with the scaphoid in neutral or extended positions unloaded the lunate fossa. However, STT fusion with the scaphoid in flexion did not affect lunate load.

Forces and Pressure on the Wrist in Fracture/Malunion of the Distal Radius

Distal radius fracture is another wrist pathology extensively studied for its effect on contact area and pressure to the joint.

Short et al. (98), through their study using pressure-sensitive film, found that the load through the ulna increased from 21% to 67% of the total load as the angulation of the distal radial fragment increased from 10° of palmar tilt to 45° of dorsal tilt. The pressure distribution on the ulnar and radial articular surfaces changed in position and became more concentrated as dorsal angulation increased.

In a simulated malunion of the distal radius, Pogue et al. (99) observed that radial shortening to any degree slightly increased the total contact area in the lunate fossa but was significant at 2 mm of shortening. Angulating the distal radius more than 20°, either palmarly or dorsally, caused a dorsal shift in the scaphoid and lunate high-pressure areas. The loads were more concentrated, but there was no change in the load distribution between the scaphoid and lunate. Decreasing the radial inclination shifted the load distribution from the scaphoid fossa to the lunate fossa.

Miyake et al. (100) noted that the stress area in the volar regions of the radiolunate joint under normal pressure in neutral position shifted to dorsal regions and decreased in size at 30° of dorsal angulation. Their results agreed with those from a study by Kazuki et al. (101), who found a 27% increase in pressure to the radiolunate joint with 2.5 mm ulnar minus variance and a 22% increase in radiolunate joint pressure with 2.5 mm ulnar plus variance.

Using pressure sensitive film, Baratz et al. (102) found that mean contact stresses were significantly increased with stepoffs of 1 mm or more on the lunate fossa. Maximum stresses and overloaded areas were significantly increased with stepoffs of 2 mm or more. However, using a similar technique, Wagner et al. (103) found that the only statistically significant effect of a lunate fossa depression was an increase in scaphoid fossa pressure with a 3-mm stepoff and the hand in neutral position. Scaphoid fossa depression had more significant effects. With a 1-mm scaphoid fossa depression, lunate fossa pressures increased in neutral position and in radial deviation.

Forces and Pressure on the Wrist in Surgical Treatments for Ulnar Impaction Syndrome

Trumble et al. (40), using load cells in axially loaded cadaver arms, found that the load through the ulna decreased after silicone arthroplasty, hemiresection arthroplasty, and Darrach procedure to 3.6%, 2.4%, and 1.0%, respectively, all from the preoperative 17%.

MOMENT ARM AND TENDON EXCURSION

Quantifying the moment arms (MA) of tendons crossing a joint is crucial to understanding joint kinetics, obtaining balance after tendon transfers, creating sensible research models, and designing joint prostheses. Joints are moved by the summation of muscle forces applied through tendons across the joint surface. Many investigators (5,49,104–109) have worked on MA and/or tendon excursion around the wrist.

Normal Moment Arm and Tendon Excursion

Ohnishi et al. studied the effective MAs of all tendons crossing the wrist (110), using the joint–tendon excursion technique, with which MAs are accurately measured without identifying the axis of joint rotation (111). An eight-channel digital data acquisition and storage system was employed to monitor wrist position and excursion of six tendons simultaneously in five fresh-frozen cadaveric upper extremities. A custom electrogoniometer utilizing two rotary potentiometers monitored angular displacement of the wrist into FE and RUD (Fig. 4.15). Data for each measurement proved repeatable and consistent. Figure 4.16 is an example of the raw data obtained for one tendon in a fixed wrist position with the least-squares polynomial fit applied. Figure 4.17 represents a "cross-sectional" view of the MAs for each tendon group held in a neutral wrist and forearm position.

The study showed that each tendon's MA varied depending on forearm and wrist position. This finding indicated that changing the position of the forearm and wrist results in changing the direction of pull for each of the tendons with respect to wrist structure (43). Because the radius and carpal bones are so strongly linked by tight ligamentous systems—especially the extrinsic volar ligaments—it would appear that the greatest MA change for the tendon–joint mechanism occurs when the tendon's locating mechanism is shifted between bony structures and the skin surface. The flexor carpi radialis (FCR) originates at the medial epicondyle and inserts at the bases of the second and third metacarpals. It runs more centrally through the wrist when the forearm is held in supination than it does in neutral or pronated positioning. This explains why the FCR has a greater MA in FE and a smaller MA in RUD for neutral versus pronated forearm positions (Fig. 4.18). A reverse process affects extensor groups originating at the lateral epicondyle. In the pronated forearm position, extensors, especially radially located tendons, tend to displace more centrally, creating greater MAs in FE than RUD. Pronation also causes the extensor digitis minimi (EDM) and EDC-3,4, located more

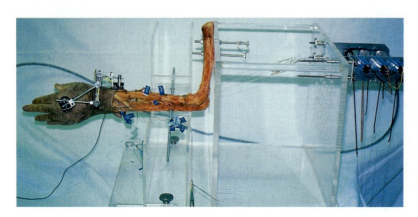

FIGURE 4.15. The setup used to examine the tendon excursion and moment arm of all tendons that cross the wrist.

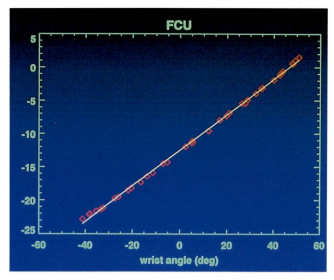

FIGURE 4.16. A sample graph of extensor carpi ulnaris (ECU) tendon excursion versus wrist angular change. The slope of this line is defined as the moment arm of the ECU.

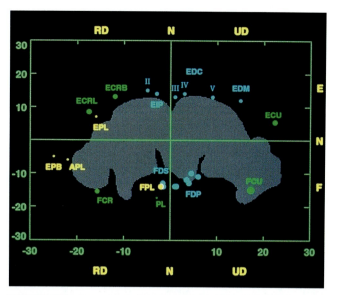

FIGURE 4.17. Cross-sectional view of the moment arms for each tendon held in neutral wrist and forearm rotation. Note that the outline of dots, each of which represents a tendon unit, is similar to the bony geometry of the wrist. *N*, neutral; *RD*, radial deviation; *UD*, ulnar deviation; *ECRL*, extensor carpi radialis longus; *ECRB*, extensor carpi radialis brevis; *EPL*, extensor pollicis longus; *EPB*, extensor pollicis brevis; *FCR*, flexor carpi radialis; *FPL*, flexor pollicis longus; *ECU*, extensor carpi ulnaris; *FCU*, flexor carpi ulnaris; *EDM*, extensor digitis minimi; *APL*, abductor pollicis longus.

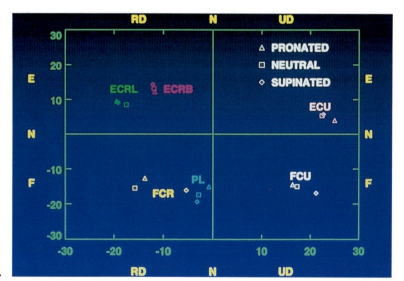

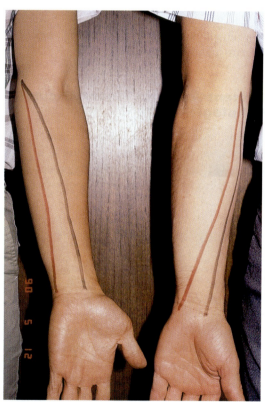

FIGURE 4.18. A: The flexor carpi radialis (FCR) functioned as a much stronger radial deviator when the forearm was in pronation, compared to when it was in supination, and the flexor carpi ulnaris (FCU) functioned as a much stronger ulnar deviator when the forearm was in supination. *RD*, radial deviation; *UD*, ulnar deviation. **B:** The man on the left is facing the reader with his forearm supinated; the man on the right is facing the wall with his forearm pronated. The *black line* is drawn over the course of the FCR, and the *red line* over the FCU. It becomes clear how the FCR becomes a stronger radial deviator with the forearm pronated, and how the FCU becomes a stronger ulnar deviator with the forearm supinated.

ulnarly to the center of rotation, to have smaller MAs in FE and greater MAs in RUD. The extensor pollicus longus (EPU) and extensor pollicus brevis (EPB), acting as wrist flexors, are displaced dorsally in the forearm pronated position, resulting in smaller MAs in FE. The amount of change in MA caused by forearm rotation demonstrates the degree of mobility of each tendon within its sheath. The directions of the extensor carpi ulnaris (ECU) and flexor carpi ulnaris (FCU), which lie parallel to the ulna, are less affected by forearm position. The ECU has greater MAs in FE with a supinated versus pronated forearm. The change results from the relationship between the radius and ulna.

During forearm rotation, the ECU is tightly coupled to the ulna by the fibroosseous tunnel and changes its geometry with respect to the radius and carpus, thus placing the ECU more dorsal to the FE axis in supination than in pronation. This gives the ECU a larger MA in supination. The ulnar head also displaces volarly in supination, resulting in a greater MA of the FCU. As the wrist deviates radially, the scaphoid pole flexes. Ulnar deviation causes the scaphoid to extend, the triquetrum to move volarly, and the hamate to flex. These carpal movements affect the positions of tendons running on or near the carpus and explain why the FCR and ECU have greater MAs in FE with the wrist radially deviated, whereas the FCU has a greater MA with the wrist ulnarly deviated. Tendons with greater MAs at a joint generate higher forces on that joint.

Moment Arm and Tendon Excursion in Pathologic Wrists

Recently, researchers have studied changes of MA and tendon excursion after scaphoid fracture (112), distal radius fracture (113), and radial shortening procedures (114). The interested reader is directed to the references.

EDITORS' COMMENTS

There is a poorly understood adaptive process in the wrist where ligament length can change with demand. For the most part, this is a healthy process that allows a professional musician, athlete, or employee to steadily improve his or her technical proficiency. There is, unfortunately, a fine line between the adaptive ligament stretch/attenuation and certain pathologic conditions. The gamekeeper's thumb is most probably an example of that attenuation carried to extreme. The ongoing activity of snapping the neck of rabbits over the thumb stretches and attenuates the metacarpophalangeal (MP) joint ulnar collateral ligament, eventually achieving total instability. It is probable that many wrist ligament injuries are accumulations of chronic overload and multiple subclinical traumatic events.

The human wrist has a wide variation of normal, with different individuals sharing carpal loads in different ways and major changes in ligament stability between individuals. Some wrists with complete SL dissociation may function normally because in that patient, all ligaments are strong and tight. This type of patient cannot hyperextend the MP joints and cannot forwardflex their bodies enough to touch below midtibia. This is the type of patient who does well with fibrous stability of a scaphoid nonunion.

Contrarily, loose-jointed hypermobile wrists may allow better function as a musician but deny that individual certain athletic prowess with even minor tears of the volar SL interosseous ligaments. The collagen elastic fiber content will determine whether the same injury will cause fracture or ligament tear. There is a difference between individuals, and there is an age-dependent change between the ligamentous mobility of a 10-year-old girl and the kinematics of that wrist at age 40.

Phylogenetically, the ulna is present, and the wrist must deal with it. Evolution has gradually backed the ulna off from the wrist, and the wrist now stands as an independent structure free of the ulna. However, the existence of the ulna must be dealt with by the wrist, and the anatomic relationships between the two should be seen in this light. The ulna needs the wrist. The wrist does not need the ulna. The wrist is a functional entity unto itself. The ulna can be genetically very short or surgically removed and not affect the function of the wrist. Load has been demonstrated on the distal ulna. If the ulna is long enough, some loads will traverse the triangular fibrocartilage. As the loads increase, this collagen compresses, transferring load to cartilage, which then compresses, transferring load to bone. At the highest possible loads, 100% will pass from bone to bone, that is from scaphoid and lunate to the radius.

The triangular fibrocartilage has received far more attention than it deserves, in part because it carries a complex name. Basically, this structure consists of two ligaments running from the radius volarly to the ulna and from the radius dorsally to the ulna. These are the main stabilizers of the distal ulna. Other than instability of the distal ulna, problems of the triangular fibrocartilage are significantly overdiagnosed. Statistically, this structure plays only a very minor role in the production of symptoms in the human wrist. The ligaments that arise from the triangular fibrocartilage run volarly to the lunate and triquetrum and are part of the ulnar sling mechanism. The ulnar sling mechanism may be thought of as two loafers, placed heel to heel, where the two heels represent the triangular fibrocartilage. The carpals would be represented by the heel of the wearer. They are surrounded by a cuff of collagen that incorporates the fourth, fifth, and sixth extensor tendon tunnels dorsally, swings around the ulnar side of the triquetrum, and includes the ulnolunate and ulnotriquetral ligaments volarly. The second shoe proximally forms a similar sling around the DRUJ, comprising the tendon tunnels and capsule of the joint. Because the entire complex is interconnected, and because there is almost always adequate stability within the structure, there is rarely a need to repair ligament tears of the triangular fibrocartilage. There are problems that arise and produce symptoms. These are discussed in the chapters on ulnar wrist pain.

REFERENCES

1. An KN, Berger RA, Cooney WP. *Biomechanics of the wrist joint.* New York: Springer-Verlag, 1991;ix–x.
2. Brash JC, Jamieson EB. *Cunningham's text-book of anatomy, 8th ed.* New York: Oxford University Press, 1943.
3. Destot E. *Injuries of the wrist. A radiological study.* London: Earnest Benn, 1925.
4. Hollingshead WH. *Anatomy for surgeons, 2nd ed, vol 3.* New York: Harper & Row, 1969.
5. Kaplan EB. *Functional and surgical anatomy of the hand, 2nd ed.* Philadelphia: JB Lippincott, 1965.
6. Navarro A. Luxaciones del carpo. *An Fac Med (Montevideo)* 1921;6:113.
7. Navarro A. Anatomia y fisiologia del carpo. *An Inst Clin Quir Cir Exp Montevideo* 1935.
8. Taleisnik J. The ligaments of the wrist. *J Hand Surg [Am]* 1976;1:110–118.
9. Taleisnik J. Wrist: Anatomy, function and injury. *AAOS Instruct Course Lect* 1978;27:61.
10. Taleisnik J. Post-traumatic carpal instability. *Clin Orthop* 1980;149:73–82.
11. Linscheid RL, Dobyns JH, Beabout JW, et al. Traumatic instability of the wrist. Diagnosis, classification, and pathomechanics. *J Bone Joint Surg Am* 1972;54:1612–1632.
12. Lichtman DM, Swafford AR, Schneider JR. *Midcarpal instability.* Paper presented at the 34th annual meeting of the American Society for Surgery of the Hand, Atlanta, GA, February 1980.
13. Craigen MA, Stanley J. Wrist kinematics. Row, column or both? *J Hand Surg [Br]* 1995;20:165–170.
14. Mayfield JK, Williams WJ, Erdman AG, et al. Biomechanical properties of human carpal ligaments. *Orthop Trans* 1979;3:143–144.
15. Nowak MD, Logan SE. Strain-rate-dependent permanent deformation of human wrist ligaments. *Biomed Sci Instrum* 1988;24:61–65.
16. Schuind F, An KN, Berglund L, et al. The distal radio-ulnar ligaments: A biomechanical study. *J Hand Surg [Am]* 1991;16:1106–1114.
17. Berger RA. The gross and histologic anatomy of the scapholunate interosseous ligament. *J Hand Surg [Am]* 1996;21:170–178.
18. Han JS, Nieman JC, Ryu J. *Finite element analysis of the human wrist.* Paper presented at the American Association for Hand Surgery 26th Annual Meeting, Palm Springs, California, January 1996.
19. Kim HK, Ryu J, Han JS, et al. *A new cross-sectional area measurement technique for intrinsic and extrinsic human wrist ligaments: in-situ MRI study.* Paper presented at the Second World Congress of Biomechanics, Amsterdam, The Netherlands, July 1994.
20. Wang H, Ryu J, Han J, et al. *A new method for the representation of articular surfaces.* Paper presented in the Transactions of ASME, Anaheim, California, November 1992.
21. Ryu J, Askew LJ, Chao EYS, et al. *Biomechanical measurements of human wrist joint strength.* Paper presented at the Orthopaedic Research Society 1986 Annual Meeting, vol 11, New Orleans, Louisiana, February 1986.
22. Ryu J, Cooney WP, Askew LJ, et al. Functional ranges of motion of the wrist joint. *J Hand Surg [Am]* 1991;16:409–419.
23. Palmer AK, Werner FW, Murphy D, et al. Functional wrist motion: a biomechanical study. *J Hand Surg [Am]* 1985;10:39–46.
24. Nelson DL. Functional wrist motion. *Hand Clin* 1997;13:83–92.
25. Brumfield RH, Champoux JA. A biomechanical study of normal functional wrist motion. *Clin Orthop* 1984;187:23–25.
26. Mann KA, Werner FW, Palmer AK. Frequency spectrum analysis of wrist motion for activities of daily living. *J Orthop Res* 1989;7:304–306.
27. Sugimoto A, Hara Y, Findley TW, et al. A useful method for measuring daily physical activity by a three-direction monitor. *Scand J Rehabil Med* 1977;29:37–42.
28. Deleted in proof.
29. Azuma T, Ryu J, Li G, et al. *Wrist motion study in typing.* Paper presented at the American Society for Surgery of the Hand 48th Annual Meeting, Kansas City, Missouri, September–October 1993.
30. Chung I, Ryu J, Ohnishi N, et al. Wrist motion analysis in pianists. *Med Problems Perform Artists* 1992;7:1–52.
31. Kihira M, Ryu J, Han JS, et al. *Kinematic study of the wrist during golf swing.* Paper presented at the American Society for Surgery of the Hand 47th Annual Meeting, Phoenix, Arizona, November 1992.
32. Li G, Ryu J, Han JS, et al. *Wrist motion analysis during bowling.* Paper presented at the American Society for Surgery of the Hand 47th Annual Meeting, Phoenix, Arizona, November 1992.
33. Li G, Ryu J, Hawkins D, et al. *Analysis of wrist motion in baseball.* Paper presented at the American Society for Surgery of the Hand 48th Annual Meeting, Kansas City, Missouri, September–October 1993.
34. Ohnishi N, Ryu J, Chung I, et al. Analysis of wrist motion during basketball shooting. In: Nakamura R, Linscheid RL, Miura T, eds. *Wrist disorders.* Tokyo: Springer-Verlag, 1992;49–55.
35. Ryu J, Han JS, Li G. *Range of wrist motion expressed in selected sports endeavors.* Paper presented at the Société Internationale de Recherche Orthopédique et de Traumatologie (SIROT) VI World Congress, Seoul, Korea, August 1993.
36. Tokunaga D, Ryu J, Kihira M, et al. *The biomechanics of wrist motion in tennis players.* Paper presented at the American Society for Surgery of the Hand 47th Annual Meeting, Phoenix, Arizona, November 1992.
37. Bryce TH. On certain points in the anatomy and mechanism of the wrist joint reviewed in the light of a series of roentgen ray photographs of the living hand. *J Anat* 1896;31:59–79.
38. Johnson HM. Varying positions of the carpal bones in the different movements at the wrist. *J Anat Physiol* 1907;41:109–122.
39. Brumfield RH, Nickel VL, Nickel E. Joint motion in wrist flexion and extension. *South Med J* 1966;59:909–910.
40. Cyriax EF. On the rotary movements of the wrist. *J Anat* 1925;60:199–201.
41. Gilford WW, Bolton RH, Lambrinundri C. The mechanism of the wrist joint with special reference to fractures of the scaphoid. *Guys Hosp Rep* 1943;92:52–59.
42. Henke W. Die Bewegungen der Wandwurzel. *Z Radiol Med* 1859;III:27–42.

43. Kauer JMB. The independence of the carpal articulation chains. *Acta Anat (Basel)* 1974;88:481–501.
44. MacConaill MA. The mechanical anatomy of the carpus and its bearing on some surgical problems. *J Anat* 1941;75:1166–1175.
45. Sarrafian SK, Melamed JL, Goshgarian GM. Study of wrist motion in flexion and extension. *Clin Orthop* 1977;126:153–159.
46. Wright RD. A detailed study of movement of the wrist joint. *J Anat* 1935;70:137–142.
47. Arkless R. Cineradiography in normal and abnormal wrists. *Am J Roentgenol* 1966;96:837–844.
48. Andrew JG, Youm YA. A biomechanical investigation of wrist kinematics. *J Biomech* 1979;12:83–93.
49. Youm Y, McMurtry RY, Flatt AE, et al. Kinematics of the wrist. *J Bone Joint Surg Am* 1978;60:423–431.
50. Berger RA, Crowninshield RD, Flatt AE. The three-dimensional rotational behavior of the carpal bones. *Clin Orthop* 1982;167:303–310.
51. Ruby LK, Cooney WP, An KN, et al. Relative motion of selected carpal bones. A kinematic analysis of the normal wrist. *J Hand Surg [Am]* 1988;13:1–10.
52. deLange A, Kauer JMG, Huiskes R. Kinematic behavior of the human wrist joint: a roentgen-stereophotogrammetric analysis. *J Orthop Res* 1985;3:56–64.
53. Garcia-Elias M, Cooney WP, An KN, et al. Wrist kinematics after limited intercarpal arthrodesis. *J Hand Surg [Am]* 1989;14:791–799.
54. Horii E, Garcia-Elias M, An KN, et al. A kinematic study of luno-triquetral dissociations. *J Hand Surg [Am]* 1991;16:355–362.
55. Smith DK, An KN, Cooney WP, et al. Effects of a scaphoid waist osteotomy on carpal kinematics. *J Orthop Res* 1989;7:590–598.
56. Sommer HG III, Miller NR. A technique for kinematic modeling of anatomical joints. *J Biomech Eng* 1980;102:311–317.
57. Belsole RJ, Hilbelink D, Llewellyn JA, et al. Scaphoid orientation and location for computed three dimensional carpal models. *Orthop Clin North Am* 1986;173:505–510.
58. Kato H, Ryu J, Tokunaga D. *Normal human carpal kinematics.* Paper presented at the Vth World Congress, International Federation of Societies for Surgery of the Hand (IFSSH), Paris, France, May 1992.
59. Kato H, Ryu J, Tokunaga D, et al. *Carpal kinematics: normal and in rotary subluxation of the scaphoid.* Paper presented at the American Society for Surgery of the Hand 46th Annual Meeting, Orlando, Florida, October 1991.
60. Kobayashi M, Berger RA, Linscheid RL, et al. Intercarpal kinematics during wrist motion. *Hand Clin* 1997;13(1):143–149.
61. Chang C, Kish V, Ryu J, et al. *Development of passive dynamic wrist simulator.* Paper presented at the IASTED (International Association of Science and Technology for Development) International Conference on Modeling and Simulation, Pittsburgh, Pennsylvania, May 1993.
62. Colbaugh R, Glass K, Ryu J. Adaptive control of a human wrist motion simulator. *Int J Model Simulat* 1991;11:93–103.
63. Han JS, Ryu J. Force transmission through the distal radius and ulna during dynamic loading. *J Bone Joint Surg Br* 1993;75[Suppl III]:203.
64. Short WH, Werner FW, Fortino MD, et al. A dynamic biomechanical study of scapholunate ligament sectioning. *J Hand Surg [Am]* 1995;20:986–999.
65. Werner FW, Palmer AK, Somerset JH, et al. Wrist joint motion simulator. *J Orthop Res* 1996;14:639–646.
66. Nieman JC, Han JS, Ryu J. *Finite element analysis of the human wrist.* Paper presented at Annual Meeting, Bioengineering Division, American Society of Mechanical Engineering (ASME), San Francisco, California, November 1995.
67. Tokunaga D, Ryu J, Kato H, et al. *Carpal kinematics in rotary subluxation of the scaphoid.* Paper presented at the Vth World Congress, International Federation of Societies for Surgery of the Hand (IFSSH), Paris, France, May 1992.
68. Ruby LK, An KN, Linscheid RL, et al. The effects of scapholunate ligament section on scapholunate motion. *J Hand Surg [Am]* 1987;12:767–771.
69. Li G, Rowen B, Tokunaga D, et al. Carpal kinematics of lunotriquetral dissociations. *Biomed Sci Instrum* 1991;27:273–281.
70. Kihira M, Ryu J, Rowen B. *Carpal kinematics in ulnar variance.* Paper presented at the Vth World Congress, International Federation of Societies for Surgery of the Hand (IFSSH), Paris, France, May 1992.
71. Azuma T, Ryu J, Han JS, et al. Carpal kinematic changes due to the different treatment of rotary subluxation of the scaphoid. *J Bone Joint Surg Br* 1993;75[Suppl III]:203.
72. Yang SB, Ryu J, Han JS, et al. *Comparison of LT and CLTH arthrodesis in lunotriquetral dissociation.* Paper presented at the Third Inter-meeting, Société Internationale de Recherche Orthopédique et de Traumatologie (SIROT), Boston, Massachusetts, October 1994.
73. Azuma T, Ryu J, Han JS, et al. Effect of scaphoid angle for STT fusion on carpal kinematics. *J Bone Joint Surg Am* 1994;18:554–555.
74. Burgess RC. The effect of a simulated scaphoid malunion on wrist motion. *J Hand Surg [Am]* 1987;12:774–776.
75. Li G, Ryu J, Han JS. *Quantitative analysis of carpal kinematics in malunion of Colles' fracture.* Paper presented at the American Society for Surgery of the Hand 50th Annual Meeting, San Francisco, California, September 1995.
76. Smith DK, Cooney WP, An KN, et al. The effects of simulated unstable scaphoid fractures on carpal motion. *J Hand Surg [Am]* 1989;14:283–291.
77. Kim HK, Whipple TL, Ryu J, et al. *Effects of resection of the distal pole of the scaphoid on carpal kinematics.* Paper presented at the Third Inter-meeting, SIROT, Boston, Massachusetts, October 1994.
78. Kim H, Whipple TL, Ryu J, et al. Effect on carpal kinematics of excision of the volar tubercle of the trapezium during scaphoid fracture fixation. *J Bone Joint Surg Am* 1995;19:558–559.
79. Hara T, Horii E, An KN, et al. Force distribution across wrist joint: application of pressure-sensitive conductive rubber. *J Hand Surg [Am]* 1992;17:339–347.
80. Horii E, Garcia-Elias M, Bishop AT, et al. Effect on force transmission across the carpus in procedures used to treat Kienböck's disease. *J Hand Surg [Am]* 1990;15:393–400.
81. Palmer AK, Werner FW. Biomechanics of the distal radioulnar joint. *Clin Orthop* 1984;187:26–35.
82. Patterson RM, Todd P, Viegas SF, et al. *Forearm load distribution.* Paper presented at the Ninth Annual Conference on Biomedical Engineering Research, Houston, Texas, 1991.
83. Schuing F, Cooney WP, Linscheid RL, et al. Force and pressure transmission through the normal wrist: A theoretical two-dimensional study in the posteroanterior plane. *J Biomech* 1995;28:587–601.
84. Short WH, Werner FW, Fortino MD, et al. Distribution of pressures and forces on the wrist after simulated intercarpal fusion and Kienböck's disease. *J Hand Surg [Am]* 1992;17:443–449.
85. Trumble TE, Glisson RR, Seaber AV, et al. Forearm force transmission after surgical treatment of distal radioulnar joint disorders. *J Hand Surg [Am]* 1987;12:196–202.

86. Werner FW, Glisson RR, Murphy D, et al. Force transmission through the distal radioulnar carpal joint: Effect of ulnar lengthening and shortening. *Handchirurgie* 1986;18:304–308.
87. Viegas SF, Tencer AF, Cantrell J, et al. Load transfer characteristics of the wrist. Part I. The normal joint. *J Hand Surg [Am]* 1987;12:971–978.
88. Viegas SF, Patterson RM, Peterson PD, et al. Load mechanics in the midcarpal joint. *J Hand Surg [Am]* 1993;18:14–18.
89. Viegas SF, Patterson RM, Peterson PD, et al. Evaluation of the biomechanical efficacy of limited intercarpal fusions for the treatment of scapho-lunate dissociation. *J Hand Surg [Am]* 1990;15:120–128.
90. Werner FW, Glisson RR, Murphy DJ, et al. Force transmission through the distal radioulnar carpal joint: effect of ulnar lengthening and shortening. *Handchir Mikrochir Plast Chir* 1986;18:304–308.
91. Werner FW, Murphy DJ, Palmer AK. Pressures in the distal radioulnar joint: effect of surgical procedures used for Kienböck's disease. *J Orthop Res* 1989;7:445–450.
92. Werner FW, Palmer AK. Biomechanical evaluation of operative procedures to treat Kienböck's disease. *Hand Clin* 1993;9:431–443.
93. Coe MR, Trumble TE. Biomechanical comparison of methods used to treat Kienböck's disease. *Hand Clin* 1993;9:417–429.
94. Trumble T, Glisson RR, Seaber AV, et al. A biomechanical comparison of the methods for treating Kienböck's disease. *J Hand Surg [Am]* 1986;11:88–93.
95. Masear VR, Zook EG, Pichora DR, et al. Strain-gauge evaluation of lunate unloading procedures. *J Hand Surg [Am]* 1992;17:437–443.
96. An KN. The effect of force transmission on the carpus after procedures used to treat Kienböck's disease. *Hand Clin* 1993;9:445–454.
97. Watanabe K, Nakamura R, Horii E, et al. Biomechanical analysis of radial wedge osteotomy for the treatment of Kienböck's disease. *J Hand Surg [Am]* 1993;18:686–690.
98. Short WH, Palmer AK, Werner FW, et al. A biomechanical study of distal radial fractures. *J Hand Surg [Am]* 1987;12:529–534.
99. Pogue DJ, Viegas ST, Patterson RM, et al. Effects of distal radius fracture malunion on wrist joint mechanics. *J Hand Surg [Am]* 1990;15:721–727.
100. Miyake T, Hashizume H, Inoue H, et al. Malunited Colles' fracture. Analysis of stress distribution. *J Hand Surg [Am]* 1994;19:737–742.
101. Kazuki K, Kusunoki M, Shimazu A. Pressure distribution in the radiocarpal joint measured with a densitometer designed for pressure-sensitive film. *J Hand Surg [Am]* 1991;16:401–408.
102. Baratz ME, Des Jardins JD, Anderson DD, et al. Displaced intra-articular fractures of the distal radius: the effect of fracture displacement on contact stresses in a cadaver model. *J Hand Surg [Am]* 1996;21:183–188.
103. Wagner WF, Tencer AF, Kiser P, et al. Effects of intra-articular radius depression on wrist joint contact characteristics. *J Hand Surg [Am]* 1996;21:554–560.
104. Boyes JH. *Bunnell's surgery of the hand, 5th ed.* Philadelphia: JB Lippincott, 1970.
105. Brand PW. Biomechanics of tendon transfer. *Orthop Clin North Am* 1974;5:205–230.
106. Brand PW. *Clinical mechanics of the hand.* St Louis: CV Mosby, 1985.
107. Ketchum LD, Brand PW, Thompson D, et al. The determination of the moments for extension of the wrist generated by muscles of the forearm. *J Hand Surg [Am]* 1978;3:205–211.
108. Tolbert JR, Blair WF, Andrews JG, et al. The kinetics of normal and prosthetic wrists. *J Biomech* 1985;18:887–897.
109. Youm Y, Thambyrajah K, Flatt AE. Tendon excursion of the wrist movers. *J Hand Surg [Am]* 1984;9:202–209.
110. Ohnishi N, Ryu J, Colbaugh R, et al. *Tendon excursion and moment arm of wrist motors and extrinsic finger motors at the wrist.* Paper presented at the American Society for Surgery of the Hand 45th Annual Meeting, Toronto, Canada, September 1990.
111. An KN, Takahashi K, Harrigan TP, et al. Determination of muscle orientation and moment arms. *J Biomech Eng* 1984;1:280–282.
112. Tang JB, Ryu J, Han JS, et al. Biomechanical changes in wrist flexor and extensor tendons following loss of scaphoid integrity. *J Orthop Res* 1997;15:69–75.
113. Tang JB, Ryu J, Han JS, et al. *Biomechanical changes in wrist motor tendons following fractures of the distal radius.* Paper presented at the Orthopaedic Research Society 43rd Annual Meeting, San Francisco, California, February 1997.
114. Tang JB, Ryu J, Kish V. *Effect of distal radial shortening on muscle length and moment arms of the wrist flexors and extensors.* Paper presented at the Orthopaedic Research Society 43rd Annual Meeting, San Francisco, California, February 1997.

5

EXAMINATION OF THE WRIST

JEFFREY WEINZWEIG
H. KIRK WATSON

The carpus represents a highly complex anatomic structure encompassing more than 20 radiocarpal, intercarpal, and carpometacarpal (CMC) joints in addition to the distal radioulnar joint (DRUJ), which collectively link the forearm to the hand. This amalgamation of bony interconnections that forms the wrist joint provides structural stability for the hand, enabling it to endure loading while facilitating the multiplanar motion required.

It would be incomplete, if not unfair, to refer to the wrist solely in terms of its bony composition, for, in addition to the eight bones that comprise its core structure, a number of important soft tissue structures warrant discussion, as it is often these elements from which carpal bone pathology must be differentiated. Specific maneuvers during a thorough physical examination must address both intra- and extraarticular soft tissue etiologies for wrist symptomatology. Indeed, a number of such maneuvers have been developed to assess instability among the 26 named intercarpal ligaments and the triangular fibrocartilage complex (TFCC) (intraarticular sources of wrist pathology), as well as symptomatology emanating from among the 24 tendons that cross the carpus to insert distally. Such extraarticular causes of wrist pain include stenosing tenosynovitis of the first dorsal compartment, or de Quervain's disease, and synovitis of the sheath of the extensor carpi ulnaris (ECU) tendon within the sixth dorsal compartment, commonly referred to as ECU tendonitis. A discussion of our approach to the physical examination of the wrist, as well as a number of diagnostic maneuvers commonly performed by others, is presented.

J. Weinzweig: Department of Plastic Surgery, Brown University School of Medicine, Rhode Island Hospital, and Hasbro Children's Hospital, Providence, Rhode Island 02905.

H. K. Watson: Connecticut Combined Hand Surgery Fellowship, Hartford Hospital, and Connecticut Children's Medical Center, Hartford, Connecticut 06106; Department of Orthopaedics, University of Connecticut School of Medicine, Farmington, Connecticut 06032; Department of Orthopedics, Rehabilitation, and Plastic Surgery, Yale University School of Medicine, New Haven, Connecticut 06520.

HISTORY

A physical examination can be considered complete, and the information obtained adequate to either make a specific diagnosis or formulate a focused differential, only if accompanied by a thorough history. Information regarding the patient's (a) age, (b) handedness, (c) chief complaint (the patient must be specifically asked to identify the single most bothersome problem which he or she would prefer to have eliminated if only one could be addressed), (d) occupation, (e) avocational activities, (f) any previous wrist injury and/or surgery, (g) the exact onset of symptoms and their relation to specific activities, (h) factors that exacerbate or improve them, (i) the frequency and duration of postactivity ache, (j) any subjective loss of wrist motion, (k) current work status, and, certainly, (l) whether a worker's compensation claim is involved will always complement findings noted during physical examination.

Suspicions of secondary gain must be perceived by the clinician as early as possible, for these can dramatically alter the accuracy of the physical examination and require modifications of physical exam techniques. A number of distraction or substitution maneuvers have been developed to aid in distinguishing between real and contrived symptoms and findings, and these are also presented.

PHYSICAL EXAMINATION

Obtaining a thorough history from a given patient permits the clinician to proceed with a focused examination. Radial wrist pain following a fall on an outstretched hyperextended hand certainly suggests a different diagnosis than does ulnar wrist pain without a history of injury. A clinician's degree of comfort with a certain diagnosis based on a physical examination that is consistent with the patient's history can only come with experience. Just looking at the hand may provide significant information. Scapholunate advanced collapse (SLAC) almost always has an oblique dorsal swelling extending from distal radially over the scaphoid to proximal ulnarly over the lunate. A carpal boss may demonstrate a bony prominence. Disuse trophic changes will indicate a longstanding difficult problem. Trophic changes can be accurately described with the following observations: (a) flattening of the cuticle base—seen in lateral silhouette, the bump of skin at the nail base will be flat and in the plane of the nail; (b) decrease in pulp bulk—seen laterally and volarly compared to the same finger on the opposite hand, there will be a decrease in overall size; (c) increased nail curvature—seen from laterally and end on, the nail will demonstrate an increased radius of curvature; (d) fingerprint changes—the fingerprints will be smoother and often drier than the opposite side.

WRIST MOTION

The examination should commence with an evaluation of passive and active range of motion of both wrists. With the physician and patient seated across from each other, and the patient's upper arms fully adducted with elbows resting on the exam table, an assessment of flexion and extension is performed. Any loss of motion compared with the contralateral asymptomatic wrist should be noted. In our experience, any loss of passive flexion has consistently represented a sign of underlying organic carpal pathology. For instance, it is rare that a patient with Kienböck's disease, even stage I, will not present with some degree of loss of passive flexion.

With the patient's upper arms still adducted, a bilateral assessment of pronation and supination is made with the examiner's hands rotating the patient's wrists from the midforearm level. Full forced pronosupination without pain will eliminate the DRUJ and TFCC as potential sources of the patient's symptomatology. Any degenerative disease or dislocation of the DRUJ, triquetral impaction ligament tear (TILT) syndrome, or substantial tear of the TFCC will result in pain and/or diminished pronosupination. Compression of the distal radius and ulna against each other will also elicit pain in the presence of DRUJ instability or degenerative joint disease (DJD).

RADIAL WRIST EXAM

The vast majority of carpal pathology originates on the radial aspect of the wrist. In fact, approximately 95% of all DJD of the wrist occurs as a periscaphoid problem, with arthritic changes involving the SLAC pattern in 55%, the triscaphe joint in 26%, and a combination of these in 14%. With this in mind, a systematic clinical examination consisting of five maneuvers has evolved (1,2). Each of these maneuvers is not necessarily diagnostic by itself, nor intended to be. However, a diagnosis can almost always be derived by coupling the entire picture of the patient's wrist mechanics and pathomechanics with the history, symptomatology, and radiographic examination.

Dorsal Wrist Syndrome: Scapholunate Joint

Identification of the scapholunate (SL) joint is facilitated by following the course of the third metacarpal proximally until the examiner's thumb falls into a recess (Fig. 5.1). That recess lies over the capitate with the wrist in flexion. The SL articulation is readily palpable just proximal between the extensor carpi radialis brevis and the extensors of the fourth compartment. A normal joint will produce no pain with palpation; SL dissociation, Kienböck's disease, dorsal wrist syndrome (DWS), or other pathology involving the SL or radiolunate joints, or the lunate itself, will elicit pain with direct palpation.

Finger Extension Test

The increased mechanical advantage of carpal loading during the finger extension test (FET) produces a reliable indicator of carpal pathology. With the patient's wrist held passively in flexion, the examiner resists active finger extension (Fig. 5.2). In patients with significant periscaphoid inflam-

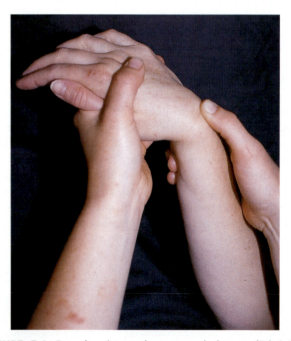

FIGURE 5.1. Dorsal wrist syndrome: scapholunate (SL) joint. Identification of the SL joint is facilitated by following the course of the third metacarpal proximally until the examiner's thumb falls into a recess. The SL articulation is readily palpable between the extensor carpi radialis brevis and the extensors of the fourth compartment.

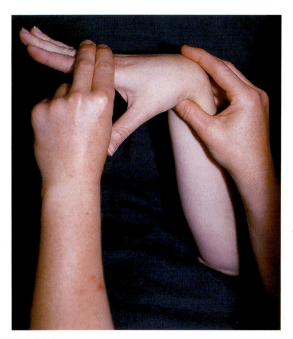

FIGURE 5.2. Finger extension test. With the patient's wrist held passively in flexion, the examiner resists active finger extension.

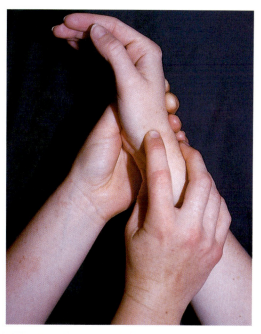

FIGURE 5.3. Articular–nonarticular (ANA) junction of scaphoid. With the wrist in ulnar deviation, the ANA junction is easily palpated just distal to the radial styloid. The ANA maneuver is performed with the examiner's index finger firmly palpating the radial aspect of the patient's wrist just distal to the radial styloid with the wrist initially in radial deviation. Pressure is maintained as the patient's wrist is brought into ulnar deviation with the examiner's other hand.

matory change, radiocarpal or midcarpal instability, symptomatic rotary subluxation of the scaphoid (RSS), or Kienböck's disease, the combined radiocarpal loading and pressure of the extensor tendons will cause considerable discomfort. In our experience, patients with these carpal disorders always demonstrate a positive FET. The FET has become a very reliable indicator of problems at the SL joint. Full-power finger extension against resistance (i.e., a negative FET) almost always eliminates DWS, RSS, Kienböck's disease, midcarpal instability, SLAC, and carpal disease in general involving scaphocapitate, lunate, and radius articulations (see Substitution Maneuvers below).

Articular–Nonarticular Junction of Scaphoid

The proximal pole of the scaphoid articulates with the radius within the radiocarpal joint. The articular surface of the proximal scaphoid continues distally toward a junctional point along the radial aspect, where the cartilage changes from articular to nonarticular. With the wrist in radial deviation, that articular–nonarticular (ANA) junction is obscured by the radial styloid. With the wrist in ulnar deviation, the ANA junction is easily palpated just distal to the radial styloid. The ANA maneuver is performed with the examiner's index finger firmly palpating the radial aspect of the patient's wrist just distal to the radial styloid with the wrist initially in radial deviation and then in ulnar deviation (Fig. 5.3). The normal asymptomatic wrist will demonstrate mild to moderate tenderness and discomfort at the ANA junction with direct palpation in almost every individual. However, the patient with periscaphoid synovitis, scaphoid instability, nonunion, or SLAC changes will experience severe pain with this maneuver. For purposes of comparison, it is useful to perform this maneuver as a bilateral examination.

Scaphotrapeziotrapezoid or Triscaphe Joint

Identification of the scaphotrapeziotrapezoid (STT) or triscaphe joint is facilitated by following the course of the second metacarpal proximally until the examiner's thumb falls into a recess (Fig. 5.4). That recess is the triscaphe joint. A normal joint will produce no pain with palpation. Any triscaphe synovitis, degenerative disease, or other pathology involving the joint or scaphoid will elicit pain with direct palpation.

Scaphoid Shift Maneuver

The scaphoid shift (SS) maneuver provides a qualitative assessment of scaphoid stability and periscaphoid synovitis

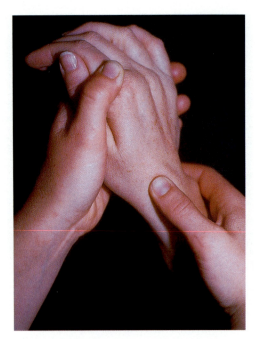

FIGURE 5.4. Scaphotrapeziotrapezoid or triscaphe joint. Identification of the triscaphe joint is facilitated by following the course of the second metacarpal proximally until the examiner's thumb falls into a recess, just radial to the anatomic snuff box. (From Watson HK, Weinzweig J. Physical examination of the wrist. *Hand Clin* 1997;13:17–34, with permission.)

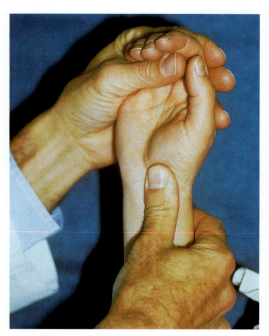

FIGURE 5.5. Scaphoid shift maneuver. The examiner grasps the wrist from the radial side, placing his thumb on the palmar prominence of the scaphoid while wrapping his fingers around the distal radius. This enables the thumb to push on the scaphoid with counterpressure provided by the fingers. The examiner's other hand grasps the patient's hand at the metacarpal level to control wrist position. Starting in ulnar deviation and slight extension, the wrist is moved radially and slightly flexed with constant thumb pressure on the scaphoid. (From Watson HK, Weinzweig J. Physical examination of the wrist. *Hand Clin* 1997;13:17–34, with permission.)

when compared with the contralateral asymptomatic wrist (1). This exam, therefore, is meaningful only when performed bilaterally.

With the patient's forearm slightly pronated, the examiner grasps the wrist from the radial side, placing a thumb on the palmar prominence of the scaphoid while wrapping fingers around the distal radius. This enables the thumb to push on the scaphoid with counterpressure provided by the fingers (Fig. 5.5). The examiner's right thumb is used to examine the patient's right scaphoid; the left thumb is used to examine the left scaphoid. The examiner's other hand grasps the patient's hand at the metacarpal level to control wrist position. Starting in ulnar deviation and slight extension, the wrist is moved radially and slightly flexed with constant thumb pressure on the scaphoid.

When the wrist is in ulnar deviation, the scaphoid axis is extended and lies nearly in line with the long axis of the forearm (Fig. 5.6A). As the wrist deviates radially and flexes, the scaphoid also flexes and rotates to an orientation more nearly perpendicular to the forearm, and its distal pole becomes prominent on the palmar side of the wrist (Fig. 5.6B). The examiner's thumb pressure opposes this normal rotation and creates a subluxation stress, causing the scaphoid to shift in relation to the other bones of the carpus (Fig. 5.6C). With experience, the wrist can be placed in the position of maximum scaphoid mobility (slight ulnar deviation and wrist flexion), and the scaphoid pistoned dorsally and volarly. This "scaphoid shift" may be subtle or dramatic. In a patient with rigid periscaphoid ligamentous support, only minimal shift is tolerated before the scaphoid continues to rotate normally, pushing the examiner's thumb out of the way. In patients with ligamentous laxity, the combined stresses of thumb pressure and normal motion of the adjacent carpus may be sufficient to force the scaphoid out of its elliptical fossa and up onto the dorsal rim of the radius (Fig. 5.7). As thumb pressure is withdrawn, the scaphoid returns abruptly to its normal position, sometimes with a resounding "thunk."

The scaphoid may shift smoothly and painlessly or with a gritty sensation, or clicking, accompanied by pain. Grittiness suggests chondromalacia or loss of articular cartilage, and clicking or catching may indicate bony change sufficient to produce impingement. Pain is a significant finding, especially when it reproduces the patient's symptoms. Pain associated with unilateral hypermobility of the scaphoid is virtually diagnostic of rotary subluxation or scaphoid nonunion. A less well localized pain associated with normal or decreased mobility is encountered in patients with periscaphoid arthritis, whether of triscaphe or SLAC pattern.

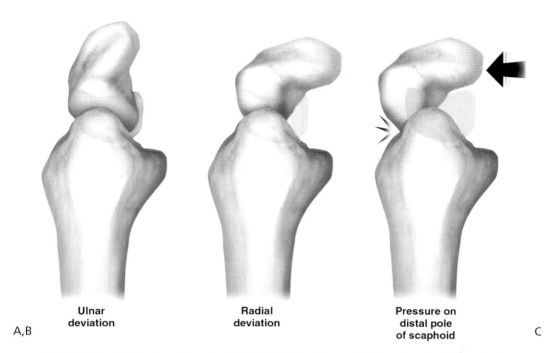

FIGURE 5.6. Mechanism of scaphoid shift. **A:** When the wrist is in ulnar deviation, the long axis of the scaphoid is nearly in line with the axis of the radius. **B:** In radial deviation, the axis of the scaphoid is nearly perpendicular to the axis of the wrist, and its distal pole becomes prominent on the palmar side of the wrist. **C:** The examiner's thumb prevents the normal palmar tilt of the scaphoid, and, in a patient with ligamentous laxity, the scaphoid can be forced out of its elliptical fossa and up onto the dorsal rim of the radius.

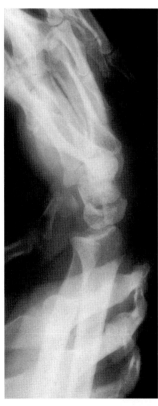

FIGURE 5.7. Scaphoid shift dynamics. On this lateral x-ray, the examiner's thumb is displacing the proximal pole of the scaphoid up onto the dorsal rim of the radial fossa. Scaphoid shift accurately evaluates the comparative scaphoid mobility. (From Watson HK, Weinzweig J. Physical examination of the wrist. *Hand Clin* 1997;13:17–34, with permission.)

Experience performing the SS maneuver is essential to obtaining useful diagnostic information and distinguishing the normal wrist from the pathologic one. Two hundred nine of 1,000 normal asymptomatic subjects examined demonstrated a unilateral abnormal SS maneuver with hypermobility of the scaphoid and/or pain (3). This represents 21% of examined subjects and 10% of examined wrists and makes the point that some degree of periscaphoid ligamentous injury is extremely common. Bilateral positive SS maneuvers were excluded. Therefore, it is probable that nearly 25% (or more) of normal adults have sustained some attenuation or ligament rupture involving the scaphoid.

ULNAR WRIST EXAM

Ulnar wrist pain is a complex problem requiring a keen understanding of both the intraarticular and extraarticular anatomy of the region. Distinguishing among abnormalities involving the DRUJ, the TFCC, and the ulnar carpus necessitates discerning soft tissue problems from bony ones.

The Distal Radioulnar Joint

An abnormality of the DRUJ, such as degenerative disease or subluxation, should be immediately suspected on the basis of decreased or painful pronosupination. With the patient's hand in full ulnar deviation, significant pain

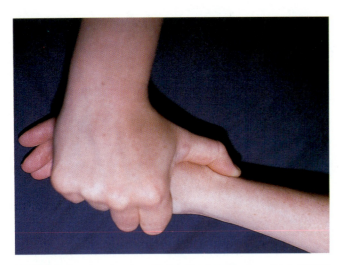

FIGURE 5.8. Examination of the distal radioulnar joint (DRUJ). With the patient's hand in full ulnar deviation, significant pain elicited by pressing on the ulnar head by the examiner's thumb is suggestive of DRUJ pathology.

elicited by pressing on the ulnar head by the examiner's thumb (Fig. 5.8) is suggestive of DRUJ pathology. Pain produced during pronosupination while the ulnar head is pressed volarward and the pisiform is pressed dorsally is often indicative of an ulnar impingement or impaction syndrome (4).

The Triangular Fibrocartilage Complex

The diagnosis of a TFCC tear or injury is one of exclusion, as it is difficult, if not impossible, to confirm the diagnosis on the basis of physical examination alone. Other more common causes of ulnar wrist pain, such as DJD and carpal instability, must first be excluded. Examination may demonstrate loss of forearm pronosupination and wrist motion, tenderness over the TFCC dorsally, and a palpable and/or audible click with forearm rotation or radioulnar deviation of the wrist (5). Pathology of the TFCC may demonstrate changes on three-compartment wrist arthrography (6). The presence of a radiocarpal–DRUJ arthrographic communication is pathognomonic of a TFCC perforation. However, perforations are common and do not in themselves indicate pathology.

The significant pathology of the TFCC is rupture of either the dorsal or volar ligaments that run from the radius to the ulna. The collagenous fill material that lies between these ligaments is frequently frayed or perforated with no clinical effect. It is not uncommon for patients whose major wrist pathology is radial, involving the scaphoid, lunate, and/or radius having undergone prolonged immobilization and disuse, that they will present with complaints on the ulnar side of the wrist with little or no complaint radially. If these patients are placed on 5 hours of heavy loading on a BTE machine or other artificial activity program, the symptoms will shift to the real source of the problem on the radial side of the wrist. Evaluation at the end of this 5-hour period will verify the radial-sided synovitis and pathology.

The Lunotriquetral Joint

Manipulation of the lunotriquetral (LT) articulation to localize pathology to this joint can be done in several ways.

The LT *compression test* directs load across the LT joint along an ulnoradial axis by palpating immediately beyond the ulnar styloid within the "ulnar snuff box." This space is circumscribed by the ECU and flexor carpi ulnaris (FCU) tendons running posteriorly and anteriorly over the ulna at the wrist. In radial deviation, the floor of this depression is formed by the triquetrum; in ulnar deviation, by the joint between the triquetrum and hamate (4). Direct pressure in this area will elicit pain from a patient with LT joint instability, degenerative disease, or partial synchondrosis.

Ballottement tests, or shear tests, demonstrate joint instability by exerting pressure in opposite directions on adjacent carpal bones.

Instability of the SL joint can be elicited by applying palmar pressure on the volar tubercle of the scaphoid with the examiner's index finger and dorsal pressure on the lunate with the examiner's thumb. Ligamentous injury is demonstrated by painful shearing of the SL joint (4).

Instability of the LT joint can be demonstrated in a similar fashion by *Reagan's test* (7). The examiner's thumb is used to apply pressure on the patient's lunate dorsally while his index finger applies pressure on the triquetrum volarly (Fig. 5.9). *Masquelet's test* (8) is another ballottement test of the LT joint in which the examiner uses both hands to apply shear force across the articulation (Fig. 5.10). The examiner's thumbs are used to apply dorsal

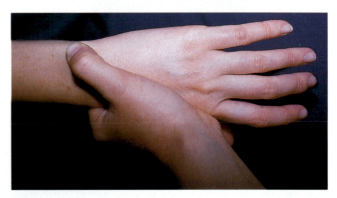

FIGURE 5.9. Reagan's test of lunotriquetral instability. The examiner's thumb is used to apply pressure on the patient's lunate dorsally while his index finger applies pressure on the triquetrum volarly.

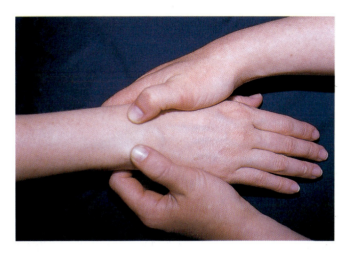

FIGURE 5.10. Masquelet's test of lunotriquetral (LT) instability. The examiner uses both hands to apply shear force across the LT joint. The examiner's thumbs are used to apply dorsal pressure to the lunate and triquetrum while counterpressure is applied to these bones volarly by the examiner's index fingers.

pressure to the lunate and triquetrum while counterpressure is applied to these bones volarly by the examiner's index fingers.

Triquetral Impingement Ligament Tear

We have recently described a new etiology for ulnar wrist pain that specifically involves the triquetrum (9) (see Chapter 40). The triad of localized triquetral pain along the proximal ulnar slope of the bone, a history of a hyperflexion injury, and normal radiographs is diagnostic of TILT. The mechanism of this syndrome involves a cuff of fibrous tissue that has become detached from the ulnar sling mechanism and chronically impinges on the triquetrum, resulting in synovitis, bony eburnation, and pain. The TILT syndrome is also produced by ulnar carpal translation against the ulnar sling mechanism. Point tenderness can be appreciated by palpating the ulnar aspect of the triquetrum just distal to the ulnar styloid (Fig. 5.11).

THE RADIOCARPAL AND MIDCARPAL JOINTS

The *anteroposterior drawer test* can be used to evaluate instability of either the radiocarpal or midcarpal joints (4). One of the examiner's hands holds the patient's hand by the metacarpals to apply axial traction while the other hand stabilizes the patient's forearm. While traction is maintained, anteroposterior force is applied, and a drawer is elicited at the radiocarpal, and then the midcarpal, joint (Fig. 5.12).

The *"pivot shift"* test of the midcarpal joint consists of supinating and volar subluxing the distal row of the carpus (10). With the patient's elbow at 90°, the hand is placed in a fully supinated position while the distal forearm is held firmly. The wrist is maintained in a neutral position while the hand is moved into full radial deviation. The ulnar side of the carpus is forced into further supination and a volar subluxed position. At this point, the hand is moved from radial to full ulnar deviation (Fig. 5.13). Instability secondary to excessive ligamentous laxity or rupture will allow the capitate to volarly sublux from the lunocapitate fossa during this maneuver.

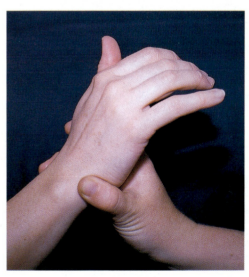

FIGURE 5.11. Triquetral impingement ligament tear. Point tenderness can be appreciated by palpating the ulnar aspect of the triquetrum just distal to the ulnar styloid.

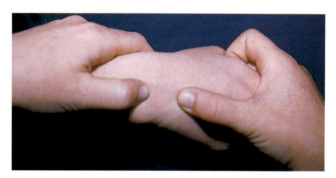

FIGURE 5.12. The anteroposterior drawer test of radiocarpal or midcarpal instability. One of the examiner's hands holds the patient's hand by the metacarpals to apply axial traction while the other hand stabilizes the patient's forearm. While traction is maintained, anteroposterior force is applied, and a drawer is elicited at the radiocarpal and then the midcarpal joint.

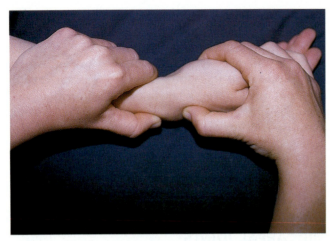

FIGURE 5.13. The "pivot shift" test of midcarpal instability. This maneuver consists of supinating and volar subluxing the distal row of the carpus. With the patient's elbow at 90°, the hand is placed in a fully supinated position while the distal forearm is held firmly. The wrist is maintained in a neutral position while the hand is moved into full radial deviation. The ulnar side of the carpus is forced into further supination and a volar subluxed position.

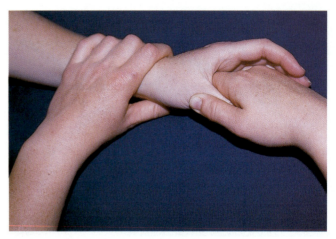

FIGURE 5.14. The grind test. The patient's thumb is gently rotated while axial loading is applied to the basal joint.

THE CARPOMETACARPAL JOINT

The CMC joints link the digital rays with the carpus. Normally, there is no clinically detectable mobility at the second and third CMC joints, and only several degrees of motion at the fourth CMC joint, which is functionally negligible. The fifth CMC joint has approximately 20° of motion, which permits functional adaptation to the transverse arch of the palm (4).

The first CMC (trapeziometacarpal) joint is functionally the most important, as it allows movement of the entire column of the thumb. Movements of this joint are quite complex, involving multiplanar motion that includes anteposition, retroposition, adduction, and abduction. In fact, Kapandji has described a method of evaluation of thumb opposition that defines 11 stages (11).

Trapeziometacarpal Joint DJD

Although degenerative disease can involve any of the five CMC joints secondary to arthritis or trauma, the first CMC joint is most commonly involved. Four maneuvers permit complete evaluation of this complex joint. A patient with pronounced DJD of the first CMC joint will experience moderate to severe discomfort or pain with each of these maneuvers.

Grind Test

The examiner produces in-line compression on the metacarpal, forcing it toward the trapezium. The index and thumb of the examiner's opposite hand then move the base of the metacarpal volarly and dorsally (Fig. 5.14). Areas of eburnated bone and chondromalacia are easily elicited. The position of the metacarpal may be changed, the shear motion at the base of the metacarpal recreated, and other areas of the joint evaluated. Aside from the objective evidence elicited, the maneuver will be painful.

Adduction or Compression Test

The examiner's thumb is placed on the midportion of the patient's first metacarpal while his fingers are placed along the length of the fifth metacarpal. The first and fifth metacarpals are then compressed toward each other with gentle pressure (Fig. 5.15).

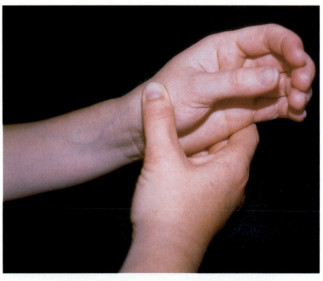

FIGURE 5.15. The compression test. The first and fifth metacarpals are compressed toward each other with gentle pressure. (From Watson HK, Weinzweig J. Physical examination of the wrist. *Hand Clin* 1997;13:17–34, with permission.)

Abduction Test

The examiner brings the thumb dorsally into the plane of the fingers with pressure on the volar head of the metacarpal.

Resisted Opposition Maneuver

The patient's hand is positioned flat with the palm facing upward. The examiner's index and middle fingers are placed on the volar radial aspect of the distal phalanx of the patient's thumb, and active opposition is resisted (Fig. 5.16).

The Carpal Boss

The carpal boss represents a partial or complete coalition or synchondrosis of the second and third CMC joints. This anomaly is often asymptomatic but may result in pain secondary to degenerative change or trauma. Examination involves ballottement or malalignment of these joints by grasping the heads of the second and third metacarpals with the examiner's thumb and index fingers of each hand and shifting one metacarpal head volarly and the other dorsally simultaneously (12) (Fig. 5.17). The secondary maneuver is to flex the metacarpo-phalangeal (MP) joints of the index and middle rays completely and abduct and adduct the proximal phalanges, rotating the metacarpals.

EXTRAARTICULAR ETIOLOGIES OF WRIST PAIN

De Quervain's Disease

Stenosing tenosynovitis of the first dorsal compartment is a common cause of wrist and hand pain involving the abductor pollicis longus (APL) and extensor pollicis brevis (EPB) sheaths at the radial styloid process (12). The diagnosis is easily made after eliciting the complaint of several weeks or months of pain localized to the radial side of the wrist, aggravated by movement of the thumb, with a history of chronic overuse of the wrist and hand. The findings of local tenderness and moderate swelling of the extensor retinaculum of the wrist over the first dorsal compartment and a positive *Finklestein's test* (14) confirm the diagnosis. This test is performed by having the patient grasp his own thumb within his ipsilateral palm. Moderate to severe pain is elicited as the patient's wrist is brought from radial deviation into extreme ulnar deviation. An asymptomatic patient without de Quervain's disease will also experience mild discomfort with this maneuver. A "wet leather sign," or crepitus with movement of the involved tendons, may also be observed.

Extensor Carpi Ulnaris Disorders

In addition to the triangular fibrocartilage and ulnocarpal ligaments (the TFCC), stability of the radioulnar–carpal unit is also influenced by the conformation of the sigmoid notch, the interosseous membrane, the extensor retinaculum, the pronator quadratus, and the ECU (15). The ECU sheath extends from the ECU groove on the ulnar head to the dorsal base of the fifth metacarpal. Conditions such as ECU synovitis or tendinitis, subluxation, stenosis, and partial rupture will each result in pain on direct palpation of the tendon at the level of, or just distal to, the ulnar head with the wrist in ulnar deviation.

Pisiform Fracture and Subpisiform DJD

Pisiform fractures occur uncommonly, representing approximately 1% of all carpal bone fractures (16). Diagnosis is often overlooked because roughly 50% of all pisiform

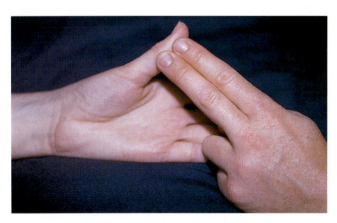

FIGURE 5.16. The resisted opposition maneuver. The examiner's index and middle fingers are placed on the volar radial aspect of the distal phalanx of the patient's thumb, and active opposition is resisted.

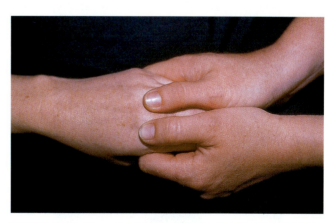

FIGURE 5.17. The carpal boss. Examination involves ballottement or malalignment of these joints by grasping the heads of the second and third metacarpals with the examiner's thumb and index fingers of each hand and shifting one metacarpal head volarly and the other dorsally simultaneously. (From Watson HK, Weinzweig J. Physical examination of the wrist. *Hand Clin* 1997;13:17–34, with permission.)

fractures are associated with more severe upper extremity injuries (17). In addition, pisiform fractures are missed because they are difficult to see on routine radiographs of the wrist. Subpisiform DJD, usually secondary to delayed diagnosis of pisiform fractures or untreated injuries, is another infrequent etiology of ulnar wrist pain. Examination is performed quite easily, with gentle thumb pressure applied directly over the volar surface of the pisiform (Fig. 5.18).

Hook of the Hamate

Pain secondary to an acute fracture or nonunion of the hook of the hamate can be an elusive cause of wrist pain (18). Examination of the hook of the hamate is performed by deep palpation over the tip of the hamular process in the palm by the examiner's thumb and by pressure on the dorsal ulnar aspect of this bone with the examiner's index and middle fingers (19) (Fig. 5.19). The hook can easily be located by first placing one's thumb on the volar pisiform. Movement approximately 2 cm along a line connecting the pisiform to the head of the second metacarpal (45° angle) will locate the hamular process.

Intersection Syndrome

Pain and swelling of the muscle bellies of the APL and EPB in the area where they cross the common radial wrist extensors are characteristic of intersection syndrome. This area is approximately 4 cm proximal to the radiocarpal joint (Fig. 5.20).

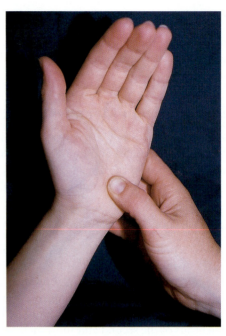

FIGURE 5.19. Examination of the hook of the hamate. Deep palpation over the tip of the hamular process in the palm is applied by the examiner's thumb, with simultaneous pressure applied on the dorsal ulnar aspect of this bone with the examiner's index and middle fingers.

With severe cases, swelling, redness, and crepitus may be found. Examination of this region with gentle palpation will elicit marked tenderness. Tenosynovitis of the second dorsal compartment is the etiology of this disorder (20), which occurs less commonly than de Quervain's disease and must be differentiated from it.

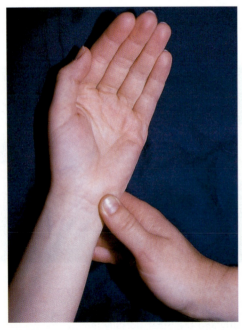

FIGURE 5.18. Examination of the pisiform. Gentle thumb pressue is applied directly over the volar surface of the pisiform.

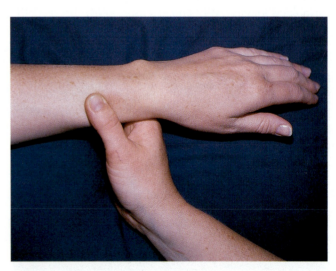

FIGURE 5.20. Intersection syndrome. The area where the abductor pollicis longus and extensor pollicis brevis cross the common wrist extensors is located approximately 4 cm proximal to the radiocarpal joint. Examination of this region with gentle palpation will elicit marked tenderness.

Flexor Carpi Radialis Tendinitis

Flexor carpi radialis (FCR) tendinitis, often seen in laborers who perform repetitive wrist motions, can cause pain over the flexor aspect of the wrist. On examination, pain is elicited by palpating over the osteofibrous FCR tunnel, which begins approximately 3 cm proximal to the wrist and extends to the main insertion of the FCR on the base of the second metacarpal. There is usually increased pain with resisted wrist flexion and resisted radial deviation of the wrist. Frequently, redness is noted along the FCR.

SUBSTITUTION MANEUVERS

Ficticious complaints presented for secondary gain can be difficult to distinguish from actual symptomatology. In order to do so, it is necessary to incorporate within the physical examination a number of substitution or distraction maneuvers. These maneuvers take advantage of the clinician's knowlege of wrist anatomy and biomechanics as well as the patient's ignorance in these areas. It is not unusual that secondary gain will govern the patient's complaint and clinical picture. Secondary gain may be seen most commonly as financial but may also exist in terms of attention from a relative or an avenue for escape from unwanted activities, be they work or sport. The following are comments and techniques to elicit the truth in the face of obfuscation.

Teeth Suck

This is an interesting phenomenon in which the patient will suck air across closed teeth. We have found this to be almost universally a sign of overplay, usually employed by those with less than sophisticated intellect. Teeth suck may be interpreted as "I'd like to make you believe you are killing me, but it really doesn't hurt very much."

Overprotection

Patient will be seen with an overprotection of the extremity where gentle skin touching and gentle passive range of motion produces a major withdrawal and complaint of severe pain. Barring reflex sympathetic dystrophy and certain neurologic conditions, there is nothing that will produce severe pain from both very gentle passive motion of a joint and the examiner's contact with the skin. This major overprotection picture is not infrequently associated with professed total inability to move any joints actively, and the passive fist evaluation is useful.

Passive Fist

In this case, the patient will refuse any active closure of the fingers, and attempted passive flexion of the fingers will activate the finger extensors to hold them open. The approach here is to passively fully flex the fingers into a fist and maintain them in that position until the active extensors relax. With some distraction such as examining the opposite hand simultaneously, a finger that is released from passive flexion will remain fully flexed. Often, if the entire hand is released, the fingers will momentarily remain completely flexed, which indicates that the sublimus and profundus are actively maintaining flexion. Then, one can often have the patient extend a finger a few degrees, perhaps a pulp-to-palm distance of 2 cm, and then draw the finger back in; they will frequently abandon the position that they cannot close the fingers.

Shoulder Abduction

Patients with major overprotection frequently will maintain the shoulder in an adducted, internally rotated position and complain of severe pain and inability to abduct the shoulder, either actively or passively. If one has the patient stand and then bend forward, supporting the weight on the seat of a chair with the opposite arm, the involved shoulder will be relaxed, and the arm will hang toward the floor. By flexing the neck, the patient's ear can be placed along the humerus of the involved extremity. Have the patient stand up, maintaining the humerus alongside the ear. As the patient stands, the arm, of course, is in the fully abducted position, and the patient is obviously holding it there at that point.

Spurious Flexor Pollicis Longus Power

If one suspects the overprotection mechanism is going to play a role in a patient who is generally cooperative, then early examination of the flexor pollicis longus will help. The power of the flexor pollicis longus cannot be broken by the examiner's hand. The patient who does not realize this significant power will allow the distal joint of the thumb to be opened too easily. The thumb flexion will be matched to the power of much smaller muscles. Even with major wrist problems, a supported wrist with supported CMC and MP joints will allow significant power to be transmitted to the distal joint of the thumb. If the examiner can open the distal joint of the thumb, the patient is overplaying the symptoms.

Volar Plate Test

Reflex sympathetic dystrophy can produce a major pain component throughout the extremity, and even minor motions can be painful, but reflex sympathetic dystrophy will be associated with positive volar plate tests. This is accomplished by passively flexing the proximal interphalangeal (PIP) joint and can be done with distraction maneuvers, where one is examining both hands and directing attention to the normal side while passively flexing the PIP joint in one of the fingers on the involved side. A negative volar plate test, that is, no significant withdrawal or pain response to forced passive flexion of the middle joint, means there is no active reflex sympathetic dystrophy. A specific joint volar plate test may be positive in an injured finger with chronic symptoms following volar plate avulsion of the PIP joint.

Finger Extension Test

This is a useful substitution maneuver for the wrist in that it is performed away from the wrist. The examiner finishes the examination of the wrist, makes this known and proceeds to examine the thumb and fingers. The wrist is held in passive flexion. The patient is requested to maintain full extension of all MP and interphalangeal (IP) joints, and the examiner attempts to passively flex the fingers. If this can be done with good power and without producing significant pain, there is no radial wrist disease. This includes all of the phenomena involving the distal radius, scaphoid, lunate, capitate, trapezium, and trapezoid. This does not test CMC disease of the first ray and does not impact on triquetral–lunate or ulnar-sided problems. The positive FET tells you only that you have radial-sided wrist problems, but the negative FET is probably more valuable in that it means there is no significant radial-sided wrist disease.

Two-Point Substitution

Wrist disease may or may not involve the median or ulnar nerves, but sensory abnormalities are frequently claimed where none exist. Utilizing a moving two-point stimulus, normally with a 4-mm distance between points, a subjective exam can be turned into an objective one by paying attention to the patient response. The principle here lies in obtaining a different response between the one- and two-point applications. At one end of the intellectual spectrum, the response will be "two" when one is applied and "one" when two are applied. This, of course, means that they are easily telling the difference between two and one, which is all that is required. At a more normally sophisticated level, one requests the patient to respond with a "one" or a "two" on each application, even when they claim they can tell no difference between one and two. This will frequently produce a pattern demonstrating that they can tell the difference. If one rapidly applies one or two pins to various pulps of the fingers, a not uncommon substitution response will be a patient stating "one" when two are applied and saying nothing when one is applied. This pattern is recognizable in just four or five applications of the two point. Another maneuver is useful when one nerve is claimed to be numb but other areas are normal. One rapidly applies one or two pins, alternating on the normal areas in a consistent pattern, eliciting a "one," then "two," then "one," then "two"

response from the patient over and over, then moving to the purported numb areas where a patient with no sensation would still tend to reply "one" and "two," as you have established the pattern of alternating responses. A patient who is substituting will be sure to break the pattern in some fashion so as not to give an accurate response. The alternating one and two pins must be done fairly rapidly to establish a pattern.

Finger Extension and Intrinsics

If a patient is claiming an inability to open the fingers, he is asked to abduct the fingers or adduct the fingers; one can visualize or palpate the extensor digitorum communis acting to maintain the position of the MP joints, whereas intrinsics fired in the absence of any extrinsic extensor will produce full MP flexion.

Handling the Malingering Patient

An example may be suggestive: A 13-year-old girl would wake in the middle of the night screaming in pain with a right middle finger locked in a swan-neck position. The entire family would make their way to the emergency room. This patient was taken to the operating rooms of two different hospitals, but when she was put to sleep, the finger became normal, and no surgery was carried out. On examination, of course, she was producing a physiologic swan-neck. We used x-ray examination to separate the patient from her family and then looked the patient in the eye and made sure she understood the game was up without saying so. She was told, "We will teach you how to unlock this, and we do not ever expect to hear that it needs medical attention again." The family was then brought in and we explained that we had taught her how to unlock the finger, and should this recur in the middle of the night, we expect that this knowledge would solve the problem. Three months later, the child had had one or two episodes of locking, which she had unlocked herself, disturbing no one, for which the sizable family was eternally grateful.

CONCLUSION

A complete examination of the wrist necessitates both an accurate history and a thorough understanding of carpal anatomy, biomechanics, and pathology. A thorough examination may necessitate evaluation of the radial and ulnar aspects of the carpus as well as potential extraarticular etiologies of wrist pain. A carefully obtained history can assist in focusing the examination. Because the majority of carpal disorders involve the radial wrist, our standard approach to the examination consists of five maneuvers: (a) ANA, (b) STT, (c) DWS, (d) SS, and (e) FET. Additional diagnostic tests, as described, are indicated by ulnar wrist or extraarticular symptomatology. Substitution maneuvers serve to distinguish between actual and fictitious findings on examination.

REFERENCES

1. Watson HK, Weinzweig J. Physical examination of the wrist. *Hand Clin* 1997;13:17–34.
2. Watson HK, Weinzweig J. Intercarpal arthrodesis. In: Green DP, Hotchkiss RN, Pederson WC, eds. *Operative hand surgery, 4th ed.* New York: Churchill Livingstone, 1999;108–130.
3. Watson HK, Ashmead D, Makhlouf MV. Examination of the scaphoid. *J Hand Surg [Am]* 1988;13:657–660.
4. Tubiana R, Thomine JM, Mackin E. *Examination of the hand and wrist.* Philadelphia: CV Mosby, 1995;197–218.
5. Palmer AK. Partial excision of the triangular fibrocartilage complex. In: Gelberman RH, ed. *Master techniques in orthopaedic surgery: the wrist.* New York: Raven Press, 1994;207–218.
6. Levinsohn EM, Palmer AK, Coren AB, et al. Wrist arthrography: the value of the three-compartment injection technique. *Skel Radiol* 1987;16:539–544.
7. Reagan DS, Linscheid RL, Dobyns JH. Lunotriquetral sprains. *J Hand Surg [Am]* 1984;9:502–514.
8. Masquelet AC. L'examen clinique du poignet. *Ann Chir Main* 1989;8:159–167.
9. Watson HK, Weinzweig J. Triquetral impaction ligament tear (TILT) syndrome. *J Hand Surg [Br]* 1999;24:350–358.
10. Stanley J, Saffar P. *Wrist arthroscopy.* Philadelphia: WB Saunders, 1994.
11. Kapandji AI. Cotation clinique de l'opposition et de la contreopposition du pouce. *Ann Chir Main Memb Super* 1986;5:67–73.
12. Cuono CB, Watson HK, Masquelet AC. The carpal boss: Surgical treatment and etiological considerations. *Plast Reconstr Surg* 1979;63:88–93.
13. Leao L. De Quervain's disease: A clinical and anatomical study. *J Bone Joint Surg Am* 1958;40:1063–1070.
14. Finkelstein H. Stenosing tendovaginitis at the radial styloid process. *J Bone Joint Surg* 1930;12:509–540.
15. Bowers WH. The distal radioulnar joint. In: Green DP, ed. *Operative hand surgery.* New York: Churchill Livingstone, 1993: 973–1019.
16. Vasilas A, Grieco RV, Bartone NF. Roentgen aspects of injuries to the pisiform and pisotriquetral joint. *J Bone Joint Surg Am* 1960; 42:1317–1328.
17. Failla JM, Amadio PC. Recognition and treatment of uncommon carpal fractures. *Hand Clin* 1988;4:469–476.
18. Watson HK, Rogers WD. Nonunion of the hook of the hamate: An argument for bone grafting the nonunion. *J Hand Surg [Am]* 1989;14:486–490.
19. Stark HH, Jobe FW, Boyes JH, et al. Fracture of the hook of the hamate in athletes. *J Bone Joint Surg Am* 1977;59:575–582.
20. Grundberg AB, Reagan DS. Pathologic anatomy of the forearm: Intersection syndrome. *J Hand Surg [Am]* 1985;10:299–302.

6

IMAGING OF THE SYMPTOMATIC WRIST

**YUMING YIN
LOUIS A. GILULA**

The most common symptom leading a patient who has a wrist disorder to seek medical assistance is wrist pain. Wrist pain has many causes and may have a wide variety of clinical histories and presentations. However, these disparate clinical presentations can be generally classified into three categories: (a) acute wrist pain after traumatic injury, (b) chronic wrist pain with a history of remote traumatic injury, or (c) atraumatic continuous or intermittent wrist pain (1).

Diagnostic imaging is usually necessary to identify the causes of wrist pain in clinical practice. The introduction of many new imaging modalities has expanded the use of diagnostic imaging. Many imaging techniques available to evaluate the underlying causes of wrist pain include plain radiography, conventional tomography, computed tomography (CT), ultrasound, scintigraphy (bone scan), arthrography, and magnetic resonance imaging (MRI). However, on the other hand, these readily available imaging techniques are easily abused or overused, and use of many unnecessary imaging studies can significantly increase the cost of medical care. Clearly understanding the indications for the different imaging modalities for specific pathologic conditions and the basic imaging appearances for various conditions becomes essential to correctly select the proper imaging study. The imaging approach for each different clinical presentation is commonly different. A tailored algorithmic approach using different imaging techniques for different clinical presentations is useful (1–7).

CONVENTIONAL RADIOGRAPHY

For musculoskeletal disorders, conventional radiography is the single most important imaging examination when an imaging study is deemed to be necessary (8–11). In most cases, conventional radiography can provide enough information for management (7,12,13). The number and types of exposures for a routine examination vary in different institutions. However, some general rules should be followed. In general, a minimum of frontal and lateral views of the joint or bone in question should be obtained. It is important to remember to tailor the number and specific projections of radiographic exposures to the clinical problem. Our routine examination is composed of four radiographic exposures: posteroanterior (PA), 45° pronated oblique, PA obtained in ulnar deviation, and a neutral lateral position (Fig. 6.1) (14). This series is designed to survey the wrist for gross abnormalities. Although, in general, at least two views perpendicular to each other are considered to provide the essential images for most joint and long bone studies, because of the anatomic complexity of the wrist joint, we consider the four-view wrist series to be necessary and important both for diagnosis and for selecting further imaging studies (7,11,12,15). There are some exceptions: for example, patients with possible arthritis, either rheumatoid arthritis or osteoarthritis, who are being surveyed for presence of anatomic abnormalities may require only a PA view. In some follow-up studies, as for fracture follow-up, only two views, PA and lateral, may provide most of the information. However, often an oblique view in fracture follow-up may be very valuable. The PA wrist view is particularly useful and important to survey the carpus. The 45° PA oblique view is the only view of this series that profiles the trapeziotrapezoidal joint (Fig. 6.1B). This view also provides an oblique view of the scaphoid that often profiles the scaphoid waist clearly. The PA ulnar deviation view elongates the scaphoid to more full profile in addition to providing an additional view of the carpal bones (Fig. 6.1C). The routine four-view wrist series potentially can establish or confirm many incidental conditions, such as a congenital anomaly, or painful conditions such as fractures, dislocations, arthritis including osteoarthritis, Kienböck's disease,

---

Y. Yin: Mallinckrodt Institute of Radiology, Washington University Medical Center, St. Louis, Missouri 63110.

L. A. Gilula: Mallinckrodt Institute of Radiology, Washington University Medical Center; Department of Radiology, Barnes-Jewish Hospital, St. Louis, Missouri 63110.

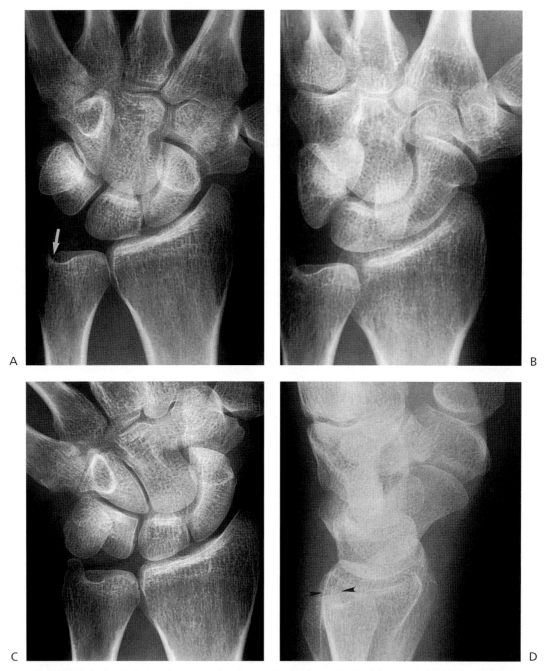

FIGURE 6.1. Four views of a normal wrist. **A:** Posteroanterior (PA) in neutral position. **B:** 45° pronated oblique. **C:** PA with ulnar deviation. **D:** Lateral view of the left wrist in neutral position. Recognition that the ulnar styloid is profiled differently on the PA and lateral views, as shown here (extensor carpi ulnaris groove, *arrow* in **A**, is radial to the base of the ulnar styloid on the PA view; and the ulnar styloid, between *arrowheads* in **D**, projects in the dorsal or middle third of the ulna in the lateral view), supports correct positioning of the wrist.

or ulnar impaction syndrome (Fig. 6.2). Sometimes, an additional view may be needed to profile a specific location or structure, such as the carpal boss view to evaluate the cause of a clinical carpal boss (Fig. 6.3). These are only some of the conditions that cause dorsal wrist pain. Fluoroscopic "spot" films allow optimal profiling of symptomatic sites for evaluation of a possible abnormality. Sometimes, without fluoroscopy, multiple exposures may be taken every 5° to 10° tangent to a surface in question by rotating either the wrist or x-ray tube to profile a specific anatomic structure. When a probable fracture is not demonstrated but is highly suspected, a repeat four-view exam of the wrist 2 to 3 weeks posttrauma is the most economical imaging method to detect subtle fractures (16). However, if demonstration that no fracture line exists would return a patient to function (work) faster, then MRI performed immediately may be more cost effective by preventing loss of work by the patient.

Plain radiography is a more straightforward imaging method for bone structures; however, it projects the three-dimensional structure of the body into a two-dimensional image, which creates overlapping or superimposed structures along the projected direction. Such overlapping sometimes obscures the abnormality, leading to a missed diagnosis. To overcome this problem, tomographic techniques were developed.

CONVENTIONAL TOMOGRAPHY

Conventional tomography is a technique whereby an anatomic structure is demonstrated by blurring structures above and below the x-ray focus plane. Conventional tomography achieves its effect by moving the x-ray tube and film cassette in opposite directions on either side of the patient during the radiographic exposure so that the structure of interest in the topographic plane remains

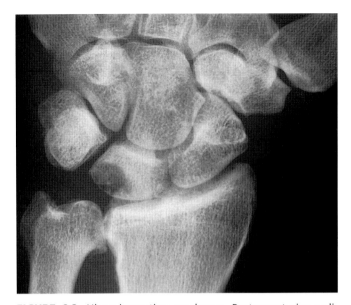

FIGURE 6.2. Ulnar impaction syndrome. Posteroanterior radiograph of the left wrist demonstrates focal decreased bone density involving the proximal ulnar corner of the lunate. The ulna has positive variance and an osteophyte at the distal radioulnar joint. **Editors' Notes:** *This x-ray demonstrates significant degenerative arthritis of the distal radioulnar joint as well as the changes of ulnar impaction syndrome. Typically, ulnar impaction syndrome demonstrates less dramatic lunate changes and no degenerative arthritis of the distal radioulnar joint.*

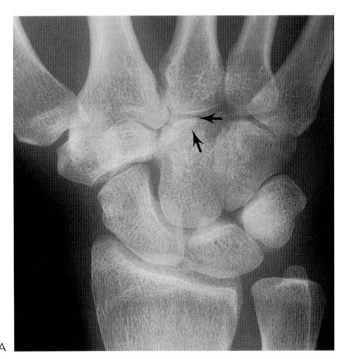
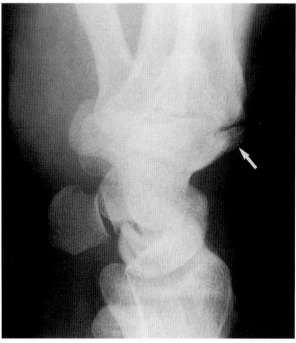

FIGURE 6.3. Carpal boss view. **A:** Posteroanterior radiograph demonstrates an extra small bone density *(arrows)* overlapping the third carpometacarpal joint. **B:** The carpal boss view demonstrates a separate ossicle *(arrow)*, the os styloideum, as a cause for the carpal boss. (From Gilula L, Yin Y, eds. *Imaging of the wrist and hand.* Philadelphia: WB Saunders, 1996, with permission.) **Editors' Notes:** *This os styloidium lies dorsal and is responsible for the clinical entity carpal boss. Carpal boss represents a highly localized degenerative change in the dorsalmost aspect of the capitate, trapezoid, index metacarpal, middle metacarpal unit. Similar phenomena are rare in the other carpals. Treatment is to resect the dorsal degenerative change, being sure to radically cut back to normal joint surfaces.*

sharp. At the same time those structures above and below the imaging plane are blurred because their positions are out of focus. Conventional tomography was a very useful technique before computerized tomography was invented. However, conventional tomography has been largely replaced by CT and MRI. Conventional tomography is well suited for evaluation of bone but is generally not useful for the soft tissue in the hand and wrist (17). Because conventional tomography offers easy access to multiplanar imaging in the wrist and is less expensive than CT and MRI, it may still be used in some places (18), but because of the blurring effect associated with conventional tomography, conventional tomographic images are not always as definitive as images produced by computerized tomography. Conventional tomography of the hand and wrist has been most often used in the evaluation and follow-up of traumatic carpal bone injuries, but it can also be used in assessment of Kienböck's disease (Fig. 6.4), premature physeal fusion, and congenital anomalies.

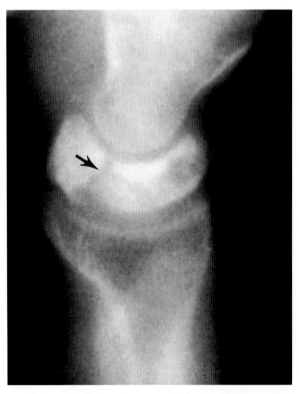

FIGURE 6.4. Kienböck's disease with lunate fracture. Sagittal conventional tomography demonstrates a vertical linear fracture radiolucency *(arrow)* in the middle of the lunate with diffuse increased density of the lunate underneath the *arrow*. **Editors' Notes:** *Kienböck's disease is a disease of the cancellous bone. Cartilage remains normal, the cortex collapses, and fractures are terminal events to the cancellous bone death.*

COMPUTED TOMOGRAPHY

Computed tomography is a technique using computer technology to create cross-sectional images. The major advantages of CT over conventional radiography relate to the ability of CT to directly display a cross-sectional anatomic image without obscuration by surrounding tissue. It provides excellent contrast resolution between tissues and has the capability of image manipulation and the ability to simultaneously compare both sides of the body. CT can accurately measure tissue attenuation coefficients. Iodinated contrast agents may be used intravenously to enhance the CT images, increasing the x-ray attenuation of tissues holding the contrast material and demonstrating the local blood flow.

With high resolution and fast scan capabilities, CT has become more and more popular in the diagnosis of wrist problems. Because of the anatomic configuration and placement of the wrist in the body, direct multiple-plane imaging can be acquired at the wrist joint including sagittal, axial, coronal, and other oblique planes (5,19–21). Reports have shown that CT scanning is a useful tool in evaluating many wrist disorders, such as subtle traumatic injury (Fig. 6.5) or complex wrist trauma (21) (Fig. 6.6) and in diagnosing and localizing intraarticular bodies (22–27), loss of articular cartilage, intraosseous lucent defects or "cysts," bone irregularities, and soft tissue abnormalities (22). CT is very useful to evaluate bony union after traumatic injury or operations with or without bone graft (23) (Fig. 6.7). It is particularly advantageous in its ability to obtain diagnostic information in the presence of metal fixation or cast immobilization (5,24), even in the presence of multiple internal fixation pins. Axial CT scan is very useful to evaluate distal radioulnar joint (DRUJ) subluxation (Fig. 6.8) and incongruity (26–28) and has also been used for carpal tunnel syndrome (29–34).

When a traumatic injury involves the epiphyseal plate, it is important to know whether this injury will damage the growth cartilage and cause early fusion of the growth cartilage. CT is a very useful tool to evaluate early growth plate closure after trauma (Fig. 6.9). In addition, it can be very helpful to identify articular fractures and intraarticular fragments, which may be difficult to discern on plain films (Fig. 6.6). In cases where the fracture involves the articular surface, it is very important to assess the displacement of fracture fragments. Any stepoff of more than 1 or 2 mm of the articular surface should be considered for surgical reduction and fixation (12). This makes CT examination extremely valuable because CT allows more accurate assessment of fragment displacement than any other imaging modality (35).

Three-dimensional CT of the wrist has demonstrated carpal volume, contour, and spatial position (36–38). Three-dimensional surface reconstruction has demonstrated the vascular anatomy of the carpus (39). Three-dimensional reconstruction of CT scan data has been used

text continues on p. 69

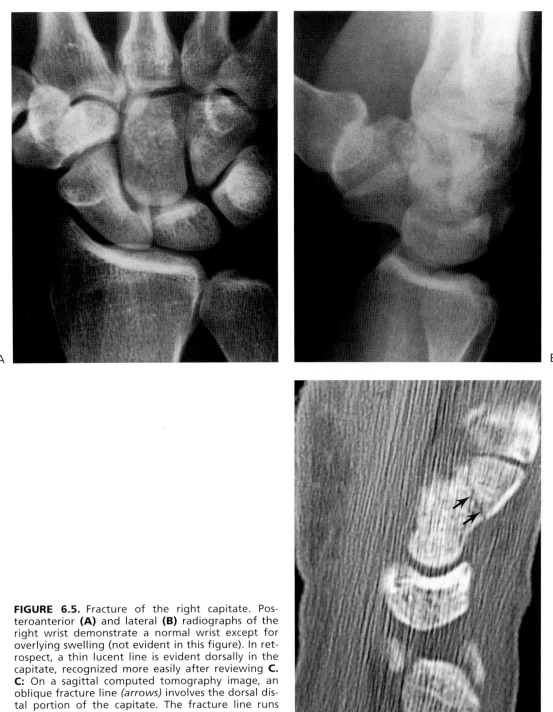

FIGURE 6.5. Fracture of the right capitate. Posteroanterior **(A)** and lateral **(B)** radiographs of the right wrist demonstrate a normal wrist except for overlying swelling (not evident in this figure). In retrospect, a thin lucent line is evident dorsally in the capitate, recognized more easily after reviewing **C**. **C:** On a sagittal computed tomography image, an oblique fracture line *(arrows)* involves the dorsal distal portion of the capitate. The fracture line runs from proximal dorsal to distal ventral with 0.5-mm separation of the fracture fragments.

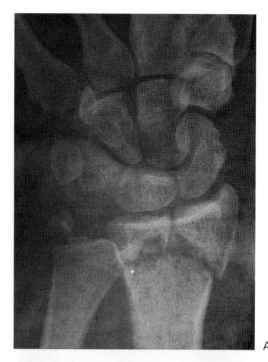

FIGURE 6.6. Distal radius fracture. **A:** Posteroanterior radiograph of the left wrist demonstrates comminuted intraarticular distal radius and base of ulnar styloid fractures. **B:** Axial computed tomography (CT) image of the same wrist shows a distal radius fracture. A cortical fracture is located in the radius fracture gap *(arrow)*. (Dorsal is toward the bottom of the figure.) **C:** An oblique sagittal CT image demonstrates the fracture fragment in **B** *(arrow)* located between the two distal radius fragments projecting into the radiocarpal joint space. (From Gilula L, Yin Y, eds. *Imaging of the wrist and hand.* Philadelphia: WB Saunders, 1996, with permission.) **Editors' Notes:** *The x-ray seen in* **A** *should alone be sufficient to send the hand surgeon to the operating room. One can demonstrate a segment of cortex that is rotated in a 90° malalignment. Direct visualization of the joint is indicated in this type of injury, and CT scans are usually not necessary, as the surgeon should be directly viewing the fragments.*

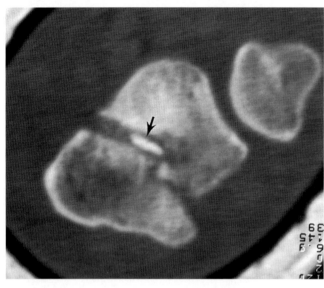
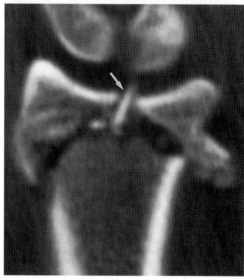

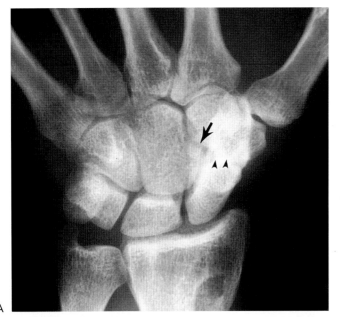
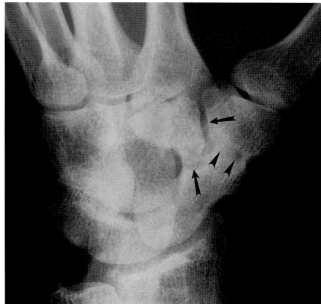
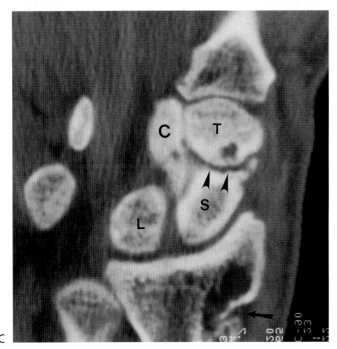

FIGURE 6.7. Left wrist pain following scaphotrapeziotrapezoidal arthrodesis. Posteroanterior **(A)** and 45° oblique **(B)** radiographs of the left wrist demonstrate apparent bony bridging across the scaphotrapezial joint *(arrowheads)*. A radiolucent space is visible at the scaphotrapezoidal joint and trapeziotrapezoidal joints *(arrows);* however, there is still questionable fusion at the scaphotrapezoidal joint. **C:** Coronal computed tomography image demonstrates no union between the scaphoid and trapezoid *(arrowheads)*. This was also true on all other sections. The distal radius lucency is a bone graft donor site *(arrow)*. T, trapezoid; S, scaphoid; C, capitate; L, lunate. (From Gilula L, Yin Y, eds. *Imaging of the wrist and hand*. Philadelphia: WB Saunders, 1996, with permission.)

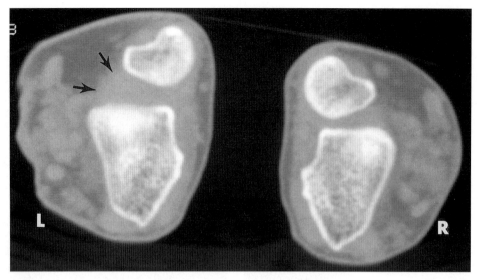

FIGURE 6.8. Axial images of both overpronated wrists show left distal radioulnar joint widening and soft tissue swelling *(arrows)*. R, right; L, left. (From Gilula L, Yin Y, eds. *Imaging of the wrist and hand.* Philadelphia: WB Saunders, 1996, with permission.)

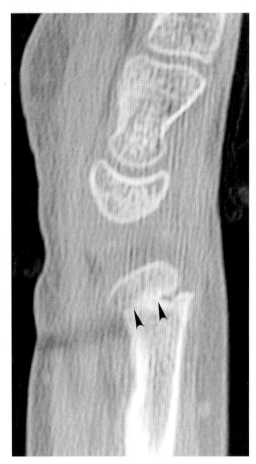

FIGURE 6.9. An 11-year-old boy with a history of fractures of the right distal radius and ulna. Sagittal computed tomography image shows bony fusion *(arrowheads)* at the palmar two-thirds of the distal ulnar growth plate, and the epiphysis is tilted palmarly from continued epiphyseal plate growth dorsally. (Courtesy of Harvey Mirly, M.D., Belleville Orthopedics, Belleville, IL.)

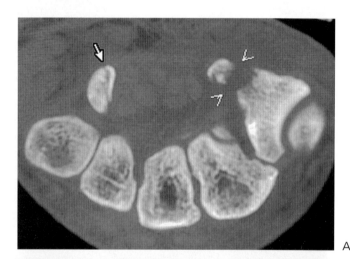

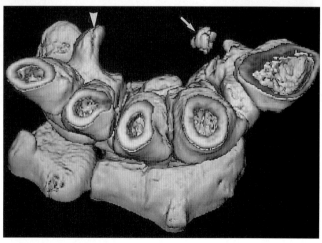

FIGURE 6.10. A: Axial image demonstrates trapezial *(arrowheads)* and hook of the hamate *(arrow)* fractures. **B:** A three-dimensional image of the same wrist demonstrates a small trapezial fracture fragment *(arrow)* and a fracture line *(arrowhead)* in the hook of the hamate. (Courtesy of Ken L. Schreibman, M.D., Ph.D., Department of Radiology, University of Wisconsin Medical Center, Madison, WI.)

for surgical planning (Fig. 6.10) (40). Spiral CT has shown the advantages of faster scans and multiple-plane reconstruction with good resolution (41–43).

CT does have disadvantages. These include partial volume effects, movement and metal artifacts, higher radiation dose during some examinations, and poor characterization of some types of tissue. However, CT is useful in determining fatty tissue and the presence of fluid and air.

ARTHROGRAPHY

Arthrography is performed by injecting contrast agents into a synovial joint to outline the internal contour of the synovial compartment or envelope (Fig. 6.11). This procedure is ideally monitored under fluoroscopy and is an invasive procedure in that a needle must be inserted into the joint for injection. In spite of introduction of new imaging modalities such as CT and MRI, arthrography retains its importance in assessment of abnormalities of the articular cartilage, synovium, capsular, interosseous ligaments, and intraarticular cartilaginous and osseous bodies (44–46). Currently, arthrography remains the best imaging technique to demonstrate communicating defects in intrinsic ligaments of the carpal bones, capsular abnormalities, and the triangular fibrocartilage complex (47,48) (Fig. 6.12). Arthrographically demonstrable ligament or

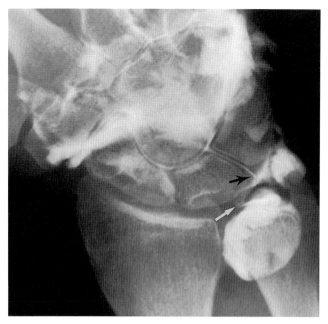

FIGURE 6.12. A posteroanterior view of a right wrist in another patient demonstrates communicating defects of the lunotriquetral ligament *(black arrow)* and the midportion of the triangular fibrocartilage *(white arrow)* during midcarpal joint arthrography. **Editors' Notes:** *The use of arthrograms has steadily declined. Dye passing between surfaces of any particular joint should not dictate the area for surgery. The synovium can seal over a joint, preventing dye from passing through injured interosseous ligaments, making the arthrogram an occasional confirmatory study but generally not indicated. The clinical exam holds sway.*

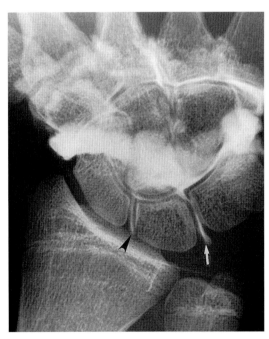

FIGURE 6.11. An anteroposterior view of a left wrist with radial deviation demonstrates a normal midcarpal joint wrist arthrogram. The distal surfaces of normal scapholunate *(arrowhead)* and lunotriquetral *(arrow)* ligaments are clearly seen.

capsule defects, however, do not always correlate with patient symptoms and signs (49). So it is better to use the words "communicating defect" or "perforation" to describe the communication between adjacent compartments because we do not know whether the communication resulted from a true "tear" of tissue or just a gradually developing hole. Bilateral symmetric defects infrequently correlate with the clinical picture and are probably degenerative or old posttraumatic in nature. Thus, if an abnormal finding is found on an arthrogram of the symptomatic wrist, the asymptomatic wrist should also undergo arthrography to exclude fortuitous association of symptoms with either developmental, old posttraumatic, or degenerative changes. Although it is unproven, potentially the asymmetric arthrographic defects that correlate with the patient's history and physical findings are likely to be the cause of wrist pain (50).

BONE SCINTIGRAPHY (BONE SCAN)

Bone scintigraphy is a study of bone metabolism depending on two factors: bone turnover with osteoblastic activity and local blood supply. It is performed by injecting a radioactive

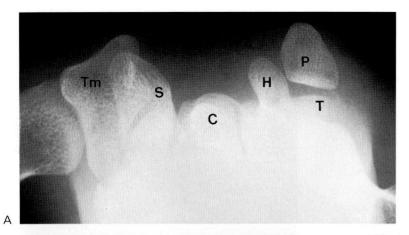
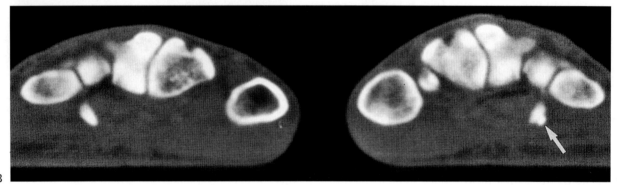

FIGURE 6.13. A: A carpal tunnel view of a normal right wrist. *C,* capitate; *H,* hamate; *P,* pisiform; *S,* scaphoid; *T,* triquetrum; *Tm,* trapezium. **B:** An axial computed tomography scan image of both wrists shows a small high-density calcification, which was hot on bone scintigram, near the hook of the hamate *(arrow),* most consistent with calcific tendonitis. (From Gilula L, Yin Y, eds. *Imaging of the wrist and hand.* Philadelphia: WB Saunders, 1996, with permission.)

agent into the body and detecting its distribution by a γ-camera. A three-phase bone scan may be performed. Phase I—the radionuclide angiogram or intravascular phase—demonstrates the vascular flow of the area examined. Phase II—blood pool, tissue phase, or extracellular space imaging immediately following the angiogram image—reflects the relative vascularity and extracellular radioactive agent uptake of the area of interest. Phase III—delayed or metabolic imaging—usually is obtained about 3 to 4 hours after injection of the radioactive agent. The delayed images reflect the bone turnover with osteoblastic activity in a particular anatomic area (51–53).

The major advantage of a bone scan is to image the entire or a selected area of the skeleton at one time. Currently, no other imaging method can perform a similar function. This unique feature makes it valuable in searching for metastatic bone disease. It is also good for localizing other wrist pathology such as degenerative joint disease, subtle fractures, avascular necrosis (AVN) of the carpal bones, radioulnar arthritis, septic or inflammatory arthritis, ulnocarpal or radioulnar impingement, and reflex sympathetic dystrophy syndrome (54,55). The abnormal bone scan may show either a "hot" area, which is increased uptake of the radioactive agent, such as in most tumors, trauma, or osteomyelitis, or a "cold" area, which is decreased uptake of the radioactive agent, for example, in the early stage of osteonecrosis (56).

Bone scintigraphy is valuable to exclude metabolically active osseous abnormalities that are not evident on plain radiographs (11,15). In general, if the bone scan is "hot" diffusely, synovitis, reflex dystrophy, or disuse osteoporosis should be considered. If there is a very hot focal abnormality corresponding to the location of the patient's symptoms, additional imaging techniques should be performed to define osteochondral and soft tissue pathology. Depending on the preference of the imager and the available technique, conventional tomography, CT (Fig. 6.13), or MRI may be the next modality of choice (Fig. 6.14). Bone scan has been used to detect subtle bone fracture; however, it cannot make the definite diagnosis unless proved by another imaging modality such as delayed plain radiographs, CT, or MRI. Currently, most authors agree that MRI is by far the most sensitive technique to detect subtle fractures (57,58). However, one comparison study did not demonstrate that MRI is superior to three-phase bone scintigraphy in the diagnosis of the subtle scaphoid fracture, which was normal on plain radiographs (51).

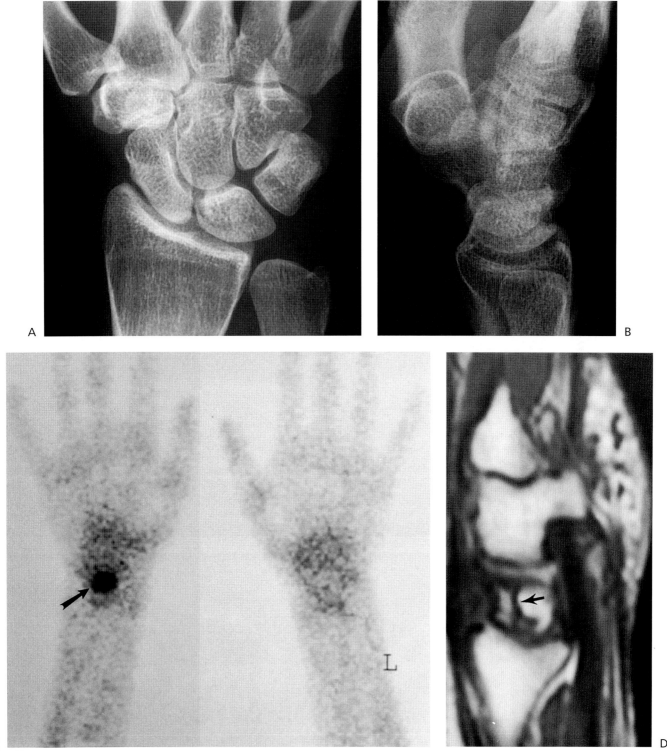

FIGURE 6.14. A 41-year-old woman had persistent right wrist pain after mild trauma. Posteroanterior **(A)** and lateral **(B)** views of the right wrist are normal. **C:** On the palmar bone scan of both wrists, a very hot spot (increased uptake of ^{99m}Tc) involves the right lunate area *(arrow)*. **D:** Sagittal T1 (266/17)-weighted image demonstrates a vertical linear decreased signal in the lunate *(arrow)*, consistent with a vertical fracture of the lunate.

DIAGNOSTIC ULTRASOUND

Diagnostic ultrasound is a well-developed technique; however, it is a relatively new application for the musculoskeletal system in some places in the world. Some of the recent improvements in equipment make it possible to apply this technique to the hand and wrist. Two major advantages of diagnostic ultrasound are the absence of ionizing radiation and relatively lower cost than some imaging modalities. In addition, it is easy to compare the abnormal with the normal side and can be performed at the bedside or in the operating room. The equipment is relatively small and light, which allows it to be transported relatively easily. These features make the examining technique easily accepted and potentially readily available. However, the ability to see all structures is limited, and the image quality of diagnostic ultrasound may be limited. It is also important to realize that the diagnostic ultrasound is operator dependent, and it is relatively difficult to interpret the image in isolation. Usually a radiologist specialized in ultrasound is needed. Applications of ultrasound in musculoskeletal lesions include evaluations of ligaments and tendons (59), evaluation of soft tissue masses, and evaluation of intraarticular and periarticular fluid collection (60). It is extremely useful to demonstrate fluid collections such as ganglion cysts (61–63) (Fig. 6.15). It also helps to locate foreign bodies, and ultrasound-guided needle aspiration and injection has become more and more popular (64).

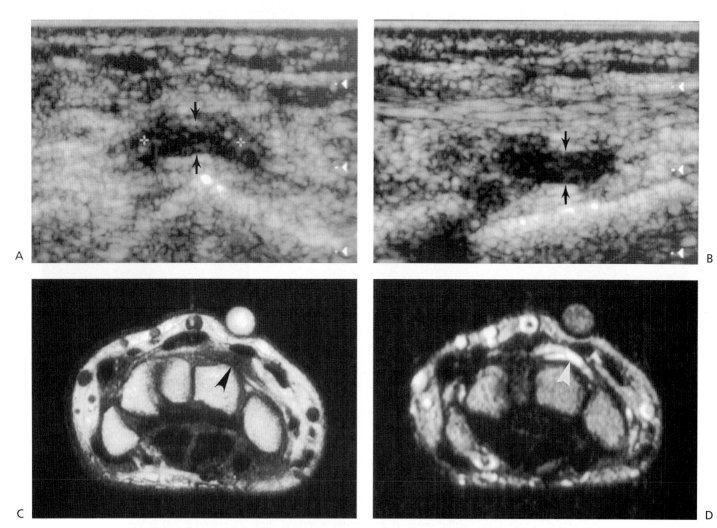

FIGURE 6.15. A patient with chronic dorsal left wrist pain. Transverse **(A)** and longitudinal **(B)** ultrasound images of the left wrist demonstrate an ovoid hypoechoic area *(between arrows)*. Axial magnetic resonance images of the same region demonstrate a ganglion *(arrowheads)*, which is a region of low signal on T1 (577/20) **(C)** and high signal on T2 (2,500/90) **(D)**. (Courtesy of Ken L. Schreibman, M.D., Ph.D., Department of Radiology, University of Wisconsin Medical Center, Madison, WI.)

MAGNETIC RESONANCE IMAGING

Magnetic resonance imaging is a study of human tissue characteristics, specifically hydrogen protons within the human body. The hydrogen proton mainly exists in the water content and also fatty tissues; therefore, the MRI image represents the distribution of water or fat within the human body. Many factors influence the quality of MRI images, including the type of machine, strength of magnet, quality and type of coil, specific imaging plane, proper slice thickness, optimal pulse sequences, and number of excitations averaged. Many pulse sequences have been developed to display pathology and decrease the imaging time. However, the traditional spin-echo sequences remain the mainstream of most clinical practices. Manipulating the different MRI parameters can produce different levels of tissue contrast and signal intensity, which, on the other hand, can be confusing to clinicians and even to some radiologists. For simplification purposes, the image contrast obtained in the standard spin-echo sequence can be divided into three general categories based on the combination of repetition time (TR) and echo time (TE). They are T1-weighted images, proton density (PD)-weighted images, and T2-weighted images. Generally, T1-weighted and PD-weighted images can provide the best anatomic detail, whereas T2-weighted images best demonstrate edema, inflammation, and neoplasm. Compared with normal, abnormal tissue generally presents low signal intensity on T1-weighted SE images, which is significantly lower than that of fat and lower than or equal to that of muscle. Contrary to T1-weighted images, on T2-weighted SE images, the abnormal tissue often has increased signal intensity. Not all abnormal tissue has the same appearance, with the exception that abnormal tissue containing fat, fibrotic tissue, or hemorrhage may look different, depending on the composition of the tissues.

With general knowledge about the imaging characteristics of abnormal tissue, it is generally accepted that the T1-weighted sequence is the most useful to evaluate bone marrow changes, while the T2-weighted sequence is the most useful to evaluate change in muscle, emphasizing the water content of tissues. Intravenous injection of gadopentate dimeglumine (Gd-DTPA), known as gadolinium, can increase signal intensity on T1-weighted imaging sequences to provide enhanced MR images. Because Gd-DTPA passes through the vascular system, Gd-DTPA reflects the blood supply and vascularity of the region. Many advantages of MRI make it a very useful diagnostic tool in the musculoskeletal system (65–67). Because it is very sensitive to bone marrow changes, MRI is very valuable in detecting any pathologic process that involves bone marrow, such as infection, bone trauma, and neoplasm. MRI is also an excellent way to demonstrate soft tissue abnormalities.

Many studies have demonstrated that MRI is an effective method to help determine the cause of wrist pain by demonstrating a broad spectrum of abnormalities, including those of bone, cartilage, ligaments, and tendons (68–70). MRI is useful in the detection, characterization, and staging of osseous injury and disease, although currently CT usually provides superior detail in the depiction of bone cortex. MRI may demonstrate cartilage loss in inflammatory or noninflammatory arthropathies, and its superior soft tissue contrast makes it the method of choice for evaluating synovial processes. MRI is an excellent tool to demonstrate fluid collections (71) (Fig. 6.16). Lesions of ligaments and tendons are readily demonstrated by MRI. One unique value is that MRI can demonstrate extrinsic ligamentous anatomy,

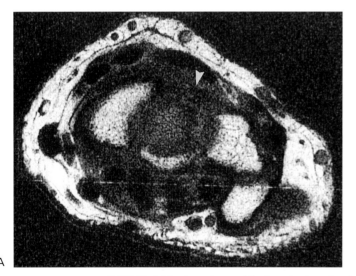
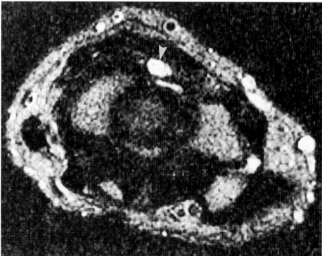

FIGURE 6.16. A patient with chronic dorsal wrist pain after surgical resection of a right wrist ganglion. Axial magnetic resonance images of the same region demonstrate a fluid collection *(arrowheads)* that has low signal on T1 (798/20) **(A)** and high signal on T2 (2,500/90) **(B)**. This is consistent with a recurrent ganglion.

which is difficult to demonstrate by any other means (72,73). It is also helpful to evaluate the viability of bone by demonstrating normal bone marrow signal. Although arthrography remains the standard of reference in the detection of perforations of the intrinsic ligaments of the wrist, MRI has shown promise in depicting the small interosseous ligaments. Dynamic MRI examination has been shown to be valuable in evaluating stability of the triangular fibrocartilage (TFC) and ulnocarpal impaction (74). By means of dynamic MRI, it is possible to make a preoperative diagnosis of an ulnocarpal impingement caused by instability of the ulnar attachment of the TFC. This kind of impingement could not be ascertained arthroscopically (75). Even a small tendon dislocation can be demonstrated by dynamic MRI. Tendinitis and tenosynovitis can be diagnosed and accurately assessed with MR imaging (76).

Musculoskeletal tumors of the hand and wrist are relatively uncommon. MRI is helpful in defining the extent of the lesion and some of the histologic characteristics (77). Radiologists need to be aware of the full spectrum of wrist abnormalities and their characteristic accompanying MRI findings (66).

However, there are limitations of MR imaging. First of all, MRI can not provide a specific histologic diagnosis under most situations. It is insensitive to gas and small calcifications and is unable to display bone cortex with fine detail. Some patients who are medically unstable, such as those with claustrophobia, cardiac pacemakers, cerebral aneurysm clips, or metallic foreign bodies (especially those in the eye) can not undergo MRI examination. The strong magnetic field may cause deflection of metallic objects and malfunction of an electronic device. The presence of metallic objects may cause focal loss of signal with regional distortion called artifacts. However, the artifacts produced by metallic objects are more localized in MRI than CT. Currently, MRI is an expensive examination. Newer dedicated low-field MRI systems have been developed and may prove to be more cost-effective for the diagnosis of some problems in the extremities (78). Despite the cost of MRI, studies have shown that when used properly, MRI is a cost-effective technique for avoiding unnecessary surgery and affects patient outcome by improving surgical decision making (79–81).

After review of each individual imaging modality, a decision about how to select an adequate technique for an individual patient becomes an important issue. To select an adequate imaging technique, the examiner needs not only to be familiar with the characteristics of each individual imaging technique but also needs to understand the clinical problem. The following algorithms are not meant to be clinically exhaustive but are designed to give a perspective for imaging the painful wrist. In any event, a careful clinical history and physical examination provide the foundation for requesting an imaging study. Plain radiography is the single most important and fruitful imaging exam and is certainly necessary before any other imaging study when an imaging study is deemed to be necessary (82,83). The major goals of a physical

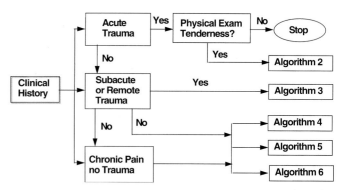

FIGURE 6.17. Algorithm 1: Imaging algorithm for differing presentations. (Modified from Gilula L, Yin Y, eds. *Imaging of the wrist and hand.* Philadelphia: WB Saunders, 1996, with permission.)

examination are to localize the site(s) of maximum tenderness, produce stresses that cause the presenting symptoms, and detect any association with underlying anatomic structures. Once a painful and/or symptomatic spot is found, the next step is to evaluate its anatomic and physiologic character (1).

ALGORITHMIC APPROACH TO IMAGING

As described above, before any kind of imaging study is begun, a clinical history and physical examination are extremely important to determine the kind of imaging approach to be used (Fig. 6.17). An algorithmic approach is intended to provide a systematic and economic way to determine the final diagnosis for certain clinical presentations. When a patient presents with a history of acute trauma, a traumatic injury to bone or soft tissue should be the major consideration. If the patient presents with a history of a subacute or remote trauma with wrist pain, a subtle fracture, TFC injury, or carpal instability secondary to ligament injury are some of the major concerns. The algorithm for subacute or remote trauma is designed to approach the above abnormalities. If the patient presents with chronic pain without a history of trauma, then infection, synovitis, AVN, tumor, chondromalacia, osteoarthritis, and other nontraumatic causes should be considered.

ALGORITHM FOR ACUTE TRAUMA TO THE WRIST

When a history of acute trauma is present, careful physical examination is usually very important to determine whether an imaging study is necessary (Fig. 6.18). One most important sign is to find the precise site of tenderness. A focal traumatic tissue injury is nearly always accompanied by tenderness. When there is no area of tenderness and/or pain, in general no imaging examination is necessary. However, a careful search for tenderness must be made before it is possible to say that tenderness is absent. When there are identifi-

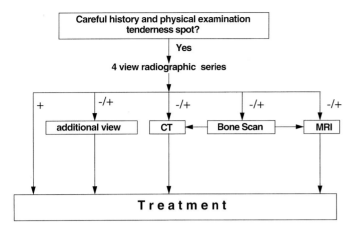

FIGURE 6.18. Algorithm 2: Algorithm for acute trauma to the wrist. +, definitive diagnosis; –, normal; ±, indeterminate/equivocal.

able symptoms, especially with focal tenderness and/or deformity with history of trauma, an injury to bone and/or soft tissue is the major entity to exclude. The algorithm for acute wrist trauma is designed to exclude bone fracture and joint dislocation first by using four roentgenographic plain film views. If the plain films clearly demonstrate a fracture and/or dislocation, the patient may be treated without additional imaging studies. If the plain films show a complex abnormality or a subtle fracture, but something needs to be further clarified, additional radiographic views commonly may suffice. In addition, if a radiographic abnormality correlating with the patient's signs and symptoms cannot be seen, especially if the patient has focal tenderness, additional radiographic views should be the first choice to profile a subtle fracture as well as a subtle subluxation or dynamic subluxation and dislocation. These additional views should usually be performed under the direction of a radiologist or someone who is specially trained to tailor the views for the specific site of tenderness with additional films. Fluoroscopic spot films can be extremely helpful to precisely profile bone surfaces to show subtle cortical abnormalities and evaluate dynamic changes between bones. If these additional views do not show an abnormality to explain the pain, further additional imaging studies may be considered. For bone and joint trauma, a routine four-view wrist series (Fig. 6.1) will display most of the abnormalities such as fracture or dislocation. This examination may lead to prompt treatment for those patients.

For more subtle fracture or soft tissue injury, bone scan (scintigraphy), CT, MRI, or arthrography may be of value. Bone scintigraphy is a sensitive survey tool for finding an osteochondral abnormality; however, it is not specific. Many conditions may display increased uptake of the radioactive agent. When a very "hot" spot exists, it is usually correlated with pathology, and further exams should be performed to explain this abnormality. But, because either subtle fractures or soft tissue injury may cause the increased uptake, CT and/or MRI of the wrist may help define the abnormal "hot"

spot. Because no objectively proven algorithmic approach for evaluation of various wrist problems has been reported, the preferences of the examiner play an important role in deciding which imaging method will be the next examination. Choice of the next examination also depends on what further information is desired and the availability of various imaging modalities. If both MRI and CT are available, the choice may be somewhat arbitrary; however, important differences exist. CT may better define cortical defects and is also better at demonstrating the presence of small fracture fragments than MRI. If CT shows a fracture that corresponds to the site of clinical suspicion, then the patient may proceed for treatment. If the CT is normal, the imaging evaluation may be stopped, and treatment may be expectant with appropriate follow-up. If there is a strong suspicion of fracture or other traumatic abnormalities, MRI may be helpful. The MRI shows marrow abnormalities much better than CT and is more sensitive to showing fractures or other trauma such as bone bruise involving the marrow space in any plane than is CT. The MRI is also the best imaging technique to demonstrate soft tissue edema.

When bone injury has been completely excluded, demonstration of soft tissue injury, especially ligament injury, may have important clinical significance. Demonstrable wrist instability may or may not present after ligament injury. An instability series is designed to demonstrate different patterns of wrist instabilities. However, many wrist instabilities may not be evident clinically. Wrist arthrography remains the best way to demonstrate intrinsic ligament (scapholunate, lunotriquetral) and TFC defects. Those defects may or may not correlate with clinical symptoms. MRI is becoming useful in evaluating injuries to the interosseous ligaments and ventral and dorsal radiocarpal and ulnocarpal ligaments, TFC abnormalities, and DRUJ instability. In our opinion, despite the increasing value of MRI for ligament and cartilage abnormalities, MRI should not be routinely used for these problems until its accuracy in each institution is established.

ALGORITHM FOR SUBACUTE AND REMOTE WRIST TRAUMA

With the patient who presents with persistent pain of a subacute (4–36 weeks) or chronic (longer than 36 weeks) duration, a slight variation of the approach to the acute patient may be used (Fig. 6.19). In this situation, excluding the trauma-related injury is the major task. Other causes of the symptoms should also be considered. After the history and physical exam have been performed, whether there is focal tenderness or not, a routine four-view radiographic examination remains the most valuable initial imaging study. If there is an abnormality, such as a previously undiagnosed fracture, imaging studies could stop at this point, and the treatment could be instituted. If there is a questionable fracture that is not clearly profiled, additional films, especially fluoroscopic

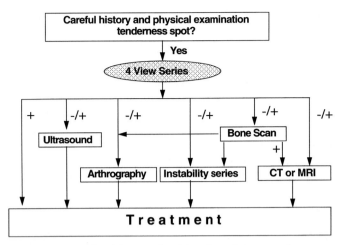

FIGURE 6.19. Algorithm 3: Algorithm for subacute and remote wrist trauma. +, definitive diagnosis; −, normal; ±, indeterminate/equivocal.

spot films, may demonstrate a subtle fracture or subluxation. If there is abnormal intercarpal alignment, such as abnormal lunate tilting, a tailored instability series would be the next appropriate test to see if there is associated abnormal intercarpal movement during wrist motion or under stress (84). Abnormal carpal alignment in association with abnormal intercarpal motion is evidence of a "carpal instability." The carpal instability may be static or dynamic. A static carpal instability is defined as an abnormal alignment or angulation that can be demonstrated on regular radiographs. A dynamic carpal instability is defined as abnormal alignment, angulation, or movement that can be demonstrated only by study with motion or under stress. The instability series films are designed to demonstrate such abnormalities as an abnormal gap or motion within the carpal joints. Integrity of the intrinsic ligaments (e.g., scapholunate, lunotriquetral) and the TFC are most accurately assessed by wrist arthrography. An abnormal arthrogram may allow subclassification of instabilities into various types of instability patterns, such as carpal instability dissociated (CID), to support the clinical diagnosis and lead to treatment.

If additional studies are normal, bone scintigraphy may be used as a survey tool to find an abnormal osteochondral site. Again, if the abnormal increased uptake is centered in a bone, CT or MRI has to be used to demonstrate the abnormal bone pathology. To confirm a subtle fracture, MRI is extremely sensitive to bone bruise and edema. CT may also demonstrate a subtle cortical break.

Further, if an intracarpal abnormality, such as an intraosseous lucency associated with focal tenderness, is identified on plain film, the instability series, or an arthrogram, an MRI may be of value to determine the nature and content of the lesion. In other words, if the lesion is fluid in nature, it could be consistent with a ganglion or synovial cyst. Both MRI and CT can be equally useful in localizing the lesion palmarly or dorsally and characterizing the margins of the lesion. This information may be useful in deciding the route of the operative approach (22,85). CT may be of value when additional information is desired about cortical and trabecular detail. When an intracarpal lesion is identified, bone scintigraphy is of value to see if the lesion is physiologically active. Bone scintigraphy can be used to survey the wrist at any stage in this algorithm to detect evidence of an active osteochondral abnormality not shown on routine radiographs. It is also valuable to assess the physiologic activity of a previously documented osseous abnormality. Finally, bone scintigraphy can be used to see if there is a diffuse abnormality present, such as from synovitis or reflex sympathetic dystrophy. If focal increased uptake is centered around a joint, a ligamentous abnormality may be suspect, and this could be confirmed or rejected by an arthrogram. However, it may be difficult to separate activity over a solitary bone or about a joint. It has been our experience that a focally moderately hot or very hot spot on scintigraphy suggests clinically relevant pathology, which may be demonstrated on additional imaging studies (e.g., MRI or CT). In any event, bone scintigraphy is useful to demonstrate abnormal uptake of the radioactive agents. Both MRI and CT have the ability to clarify the abnormality.

ALGORITHM FOR OSTEONECROSIS

Many entities other than trauma can cause a painful wrist. These may or may not be suspect clinically and at times can be detected on plain radiographs (Fig. 6.20). One of these is osteonecrosis or avascular necrosis (AVN), which can be either traumatic or idiopathic. The traumatic form is most common to occur in the proximal pole of the scaphoid after

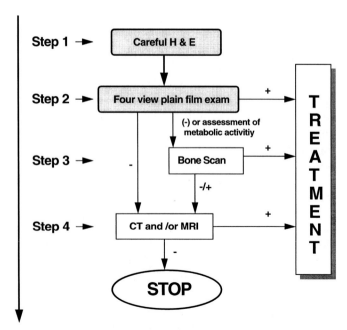

FIGURE 6.20. Algorithm 4: Algorithm for osteonecrosis. +, definitive diagnosis; −, normal; ±, indeterminate/equivocal. (From Gilula L, Yin Y, eds. *Imaging of the wrist and hand.* Philadelphia: WB Saunders, 1996, with permission.)

a fracture (Fig. 6.21) (86,87). Avascular necrosis in bones such as the capitate and hamate have also been reported after fracture (88–91). The idiopathic form of AVN in the carpus most commonly involves the lunate and is called Kienböck's disease, lunate malacia, or lunatomalacia (92,93). The idiopathic form of AVN can also involve the scaphoid (94–97) and capitate (98–100). Other rare causes such as gout have also been reported to cause capitate osteonecrosis (101). Again, the standard four-view plain film series is the first imaging exam to perform. If that is positive (shows AVN), treatment can be instituted. If the plain film exam is normal or questionable, then scintigraphy, CT, or MRI can be utilized. Controversy exists about which of these three procedures should be used next. Bone scintigraphy has the advantage of surveying the entire carpus for physiologically abnormal activity and may demonstrate early avascular changes (102,103). If this exam is normal, CT would usually not be of any value. However, MRI could potentially still be of value. In rare cases where the amount of healing and dead bone is in balance, the scintigram can be normal, and the MRI can show an abnormality. If the bone scintigram is abnormal, it is debated if treatment should be instituted at this time as various conditions can cause a carpal bone to be abnormal on scintigraphy. In general, the abnormal scintigram is not specific enough to differentiate among such diverse conditions as fracture, AVN, bone marrow edema, painful focal intracarpal defects, etc., MR imaging is extremely useful to detect early phases of AVN, permitting diagnosis before collapse of the carpal bones has occurred. The sensitivity of MRI allows differentiation of subtle changes in the bone marrow signal. The prognosis of scaphoid fractures and estimation of likelihood of AVN of the proximal fragment can be inferred by using gadolinium enhancement to evaluate bone marrow vascularity (104). If both the MRI and the bone scintigram are normal, then for practical purposes AVN has been excluded (105).

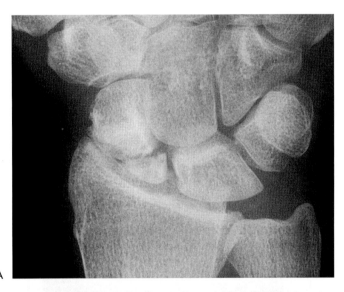

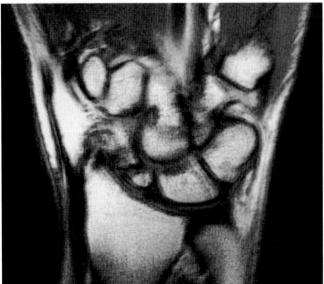

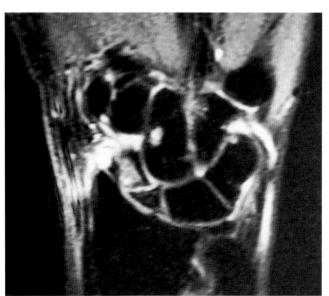

FIGURE 6.21. A 41-year-old woman with a scaphoid fracture evaluated for possible avascular necrosis. **A:** A posteroanterior radiograph demonstrates a proximal one-third scaphoid fracture with slightly increased bone density of the proximal fragment. Coronal T1 **(B)** and short T1 inversion recovery (STIR) images **(C)** demonstrate that the proximal fragment has a normal bone marrow signal that is bright on T1 and dark on STIR images. The signal is isointense with other carpal bones on T1 **(B)** and slightly hyperintense to other carpal bones on STIR, which supports a minimal amount of edema. The magnetic resonance imaging study demonstrates no evidence of avascular necrosis. Much edema involves the distal scaphoid fracture fragment, and a cyst involves the waist of the capitate.

ALGORITHM FOR FOCAL BONE LESIONS

In evaluating the plain radiographs of a patient with a painful wrist, a focal bone lesion may be found. The question then arises if this lesion is causing the patient's pain, or if it is an incidental finding of no clinical significance (Fig. 6.22). A focal defect or abnormality in a bone can be present from a variety of causes, including infection, synovitis, metastatic disease, trauma (vibration injury), particulate synovitis, infection, etc., as well as a congenital or developmental defect. When a lesion is found, additional plain radiographic views may be of value to further characterize the lesion. If it has a benign appearance such as with sclerotic, sharp, or regular margins, no further evaluation is needed. Alternatively, if it is indeterminate, further evaluation is indicated. If a lesion cannot be defined as active or quiescent, bone scintigraphy is valuable to demonstrate whether the lesion is metabolically active. If the lesion is demonstrated to be metabolically active and shows a prominent increased uptake of radioisotope, this strongly supports the need for further imaging. As mentioned in the above algorithms, to clarify the abnormal scintigram, MRI and/or CT may be necessary. These two modalities are useful to demonstrate anatomic detail as well as to show the extent of a lesion. MRI is the best technique available to show bone marrow changes and the associated soft tissue component of a lesion (Fig. 6.23). The CT can be valuable to assess the bone cortex detail in the following conditions: when MRI may not be available, when more subtle cortical or trabecular detail is desired, or when the lesion is sclerotic.

ALGORITHM FOR INFECTION

Pyarthrosis, osteomyelitis, septic tenosynovitis, and superficial soft tissue infections can all present as wrist pain. In most situations, infection may be suspected on the basis of clinical presentation and physical examination findings (Fig. 6.24). However, noninfectious synovitis may have the same clinical appearance as infection. Plain films provide the easiest and least expensive survey of the wrist. A plain film exam may show bone destruction and soft tissue swelling. In the patient with acute symptoms and history, additional views may be necessary to profile symptomatic sites to demonstrate any subtle bone abnormality. It is advisable to perform any additional views under the direction of a radiologist or a person experienced with the technique of profiling cortical surfaces. Alternatively, fluoroscopy with a small focal spot technique may allow precise profiling of a cortical lesion.

If such views still do not demonstrate an abnormality, bone scintigraphy can be performed. As stated before, bone scintigraphy is very good at localizing an abnormality. If bone scintigraphy is negative, practically speaking the workup can stop. If bone scintigraphy is moderately or strongly positive, further studies should be performed to clarify causes of the abnormal scintigram. In the patient with the clinical picture of chronic infection or synovitis and no plain film abnormality, additional views could be of value. The CT could be of value to look for subtle cortical abnormalities and adjacent soft tissue abnormalities; however, MRI provides the best means to look for a soft tissue or intraosseous marrow abnormality to support the diagno-

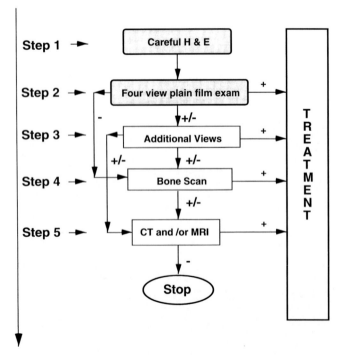

FIGURE 6.22. Algorithm 5: Algorithm for focal bone lesions. +, definitive diagnosis; −, normal; ±, indeterminate/equivocal. (From Gilula L, Yin Y, eds. *Imaging of the wrist and hand.* Philadelphia: WB Saunders, 1996, with permission.)

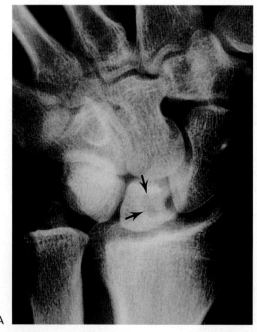

FIGURE 6.23. Painful carpal hole consistent with a cyst or intraosseous ganglion and not avascular necrosis. **A:** A posteroanterior view of the wrist shows a well-defined subarticular defect in the radial side of the lunate (*arrows*).

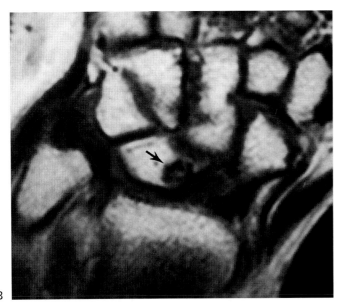
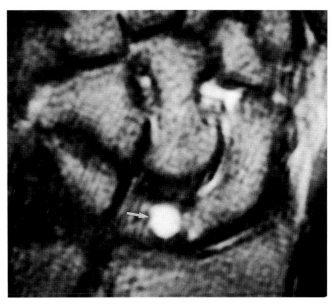

FIGURE 6.23. *(continued)* **B:** T1 (300/17)-weighted magnetic resonance image in the coronal plane demonstrates decreased signal on the radial side of the lunate *(arrow)*. The ulnar side of the lunate is normal. **C:** Coronal T2 (3,000/90)-weighted image demonstrates increased signal in the same region compatible with fluid *(arrow)*. (From Gilula L, Yin Y, eds. *Imaging of the wrist and hand.* Philadelphia: WB Saunders, 1996, with permission.)

sis of infection or synovitis. If MRI is normal, for practical purposes an imaging workup can stop. If MRI is positive, treatment can be instituted. Depending on the clinical situation, biopsy or culture, possibly under radiologic control, may be indicated before treatment with antibiotics.

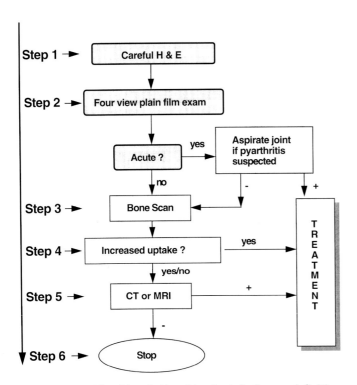

FIGURE 6.24. Algorithm 6: Algorithm for infection. +, definitive diagnosis; –, normal; ±, indeterminate/equivocal. (From Gilula L, Yin Y, eds. *Imaging of the wrist and hand.* Philadelphia: WB Saunders, 1996, with permission.)

EDITORS' COMMENTS

It is a wonderful advantage to be able to "see" inside the wrist. All too often, however, when the diagnosis is obvious, the imaging is obvious and when the diagnosis is obscure, the imaging is obscure. *The clinical exam is everything.* We can't emphasize strongly enough that the clinician must find his way without an imaging lamp. There is no question that plain x-rays, obliques, and multiple views are all of the highest value in determining a treatment plan for fractures, but recognize that the clinical exam and the degree of tissue response indicate a fracture or major ligamentous interruption, even without plain x-rays. Similarly, a pansynovial problem puts you in the categories of infection or inflammatory arthritis. Severe pain and significant loss of range of motion without trauma leads you toward avascular necrosis, whereas a milder set of similar symptoms lead you toward ligamentous injury.

The authors have outlined an approach to the wrist based on injury and presumptive diagnosis. We have used their algorithm pattern.

Algorithm for acute trauma to the wrist: Relate the time since injury to the degree of soft tissue response. If major soft tissue response is noted, one would proceed directly to plain films, as there is an inability to examine and isolate structures clinically. With less serious trauma, or longer duration from injury, a more precise exam would call for oblique or special films as part of the initial imaging. Fluoroscopic evaluation is not necessary in the usual clinical setting. Scintigraphy is also not indicated as the trauma will produce increased uptake and the clinical exam will tell you as much. CT, MRI and arthroscopy also have little place in the acute injury. The body has a manifestly beautiful system for dealing with trauma; as long as circulatory compromise, soft tissue injury, or skeletal damage does not require surgery, then immobilization may be instituted without further esoteric imaging. Suspicion of scaphoid fracture requires another x-ray with a Stetcher or elongation scaphoid view at 10 to 14 days. Acute major scapholunate interosseous ligament rupture may require open repair, preferably within the first two weeks following injury. A clinical examination at 7 to 10 days is important in the face of obvious, significant wrist injury and negative x-rays.

Algorithm for subacute wrist trauma: The authors have described subacute trauma as 4 to 36 weeks and chronic as longer than 36 weeks; our comments will apply within this time frame. The clinical exam now takes on a more definitive role in making the diagnosis. Plain films along with any localizing views that correspond to the clinical exam are indicated in all cases.

By four weeks or more, highly accurate localization of the injured structures should be clinically possible. For the sake of this algorithm, we're assuming that the plain films and localizing films of the symptomatic area are negative. This would include x-rays of the opposite wrist, particularly if there is an unwarranted amount of volar or dorsal intercalated segment instability (VISI or DISI) on lateral views, a fluted champagne glass appearance of the triquetral-lunate joint, or carpal alignment problems. There are centers where extensive experience allows some intelligent interpretation of arthrography, but in general wrist arthrography is not indicated. No surgical repair decision should be based on dye passing between normally closed off joint spaces.

The clinical exam should preclude the need for scintigraphy, with the exception of some highly specialized circumstances, such as suspected metastatic bone disease. On rare occasions, scintigraphy is used in a negative fashion; for example, in a patient with an entirely normal clinical exam and positive substitution maneuvers, negative scintigraphy can be used to "prove" to the patient that there is no structural abnormality preventing his or her full work and functional activities.

Ultrasound should probably be limited to the localization of foreign bodies, although recent work has demonstrated the ability to ascertain traumatic interosseous membrane injury. MRI deserves somewhat more attention in a changing world. Clearly, MRI is a work in progress. At this time its main advantage to the clinician is for evaluation of a wrist that has significant symptoms and a major limitation of passive wrist flexion, negative x-rays, and a high index of suspicion of early Kienböck's Disease. For many years, the number of MRIs of the wrist performed on patients with ongoing, undiagnosed problems has been increasing. MRI has contributed little to these cases. There are centers where small coils and trained interpreters are pushing the frontier of what MRI is capable of determining. At this time, it is not possible to accurately determine definitive ligamentous interpretation on MRI when this interpretation is not clinically diagnosable. For ligament rupture, an MRI alone is not yet able to send the surgeon to the operating room.

Tomograms and CT scans also require special comment. Depending on the setting in which the clinician functions, one or the other of these studies is often indicated once a high degree of localization of the lesion has been achieved clinically and/or plain films demonstrate a bone/articular lesion which requires more accurate localization and definition for a treatment plan. These studies are indicated for delineation and added definition and are not indicated without a presumptive clinical and/or x-ray diagnosis.

Algorithm for osteonecrosis: Here MRI can demonstrate changes not available from any other modality.

Algorithm for focal bone lesions: If the bone lesion has been identified and a presumptive diagnosis made, clarification of its nature may require MRI and/or CT scan. These studies are not indicated for evaluation of an enchondroma where characteristics on plain film are sufficient.

Algorithm for suspected infection: If the clinical exam and plain films do not sufficiently delineate the problem, and it remains a clinically presumptive diagnosis, as with mycobacterium marinum, MRI may contribute to the diagnosis and a treatment plan.

Clearly, we have taken a position on imaging that might not apply in certain institutions, or where an individual has special training with an imaging technique. Clinical diagnosis is everything, corroborated by plain x-rays, and turns to more esoteric imaging studies not for diagnosis, but as tools of expansion, clarification, and planning.

REFERENCES

1. Yin YM, Mann FA, Gilula LA. Algorithmic approach to wrist pain. In: Gilula LA, Yin YM, eds. *Imaging of the wrist and hand.* Philadelphia: WB Saunders, 1996;587–599.
2. Hodgson SP, Royle SG, Stanley JK. An approach to the diagnosis of chronic wrist pain. *J R Coll Surg Edinb* 1995;40:407–410.
3. Stanley JK, Hodgson SP, Royle SG. An approach to the diagnosis of chronic wrist pain. *Ann Chir Main Memb Super* 1994;13:202–205.
4. Larsen CF, Brondum V, Wienholtz G, et al. An algorithm for acute wrist trauma. A systematic approach to diagnosis. *J Hand Surg [Br]* 1993;18:207–212.
5. Stewart NR, Gilula LA. CT of the wrist: A tailored approach. *Radiology* 1992;183:13–20.
6. Pin PG, Young VL, Gilula LA, et al. Wrist pain: a systematic approach to diagnosis. *Plast Reconstr Surg* 1990;85:42–46.

7. Gilula LA, Destouet JM, Weeks PM, et al. Roentgenographic diagnosis of the painful wrist. *Clin Orthop* 1984;187:52–64.
8. Belhobek GH, Richmond BJ, Piraino DW, et al. Special diagnostic procedures in sports medicine. *Clin Sports Med* 1989;8:517–540.
9. Berquist TH. Wrist disorders: what should we be looking for with imaging techniques? *J Hand Ther* 1996;9:108–113.
10. Skirven T. Clinical examination of the wrist. *J Hand Ther* 1996;9:96–107.
11. Wilson AJ, Mann FA, Gilula LA. Imaging the hand and wrist. *J Hand Surg [Br]* 1990;15:153–167.
12. Young VL, Higgs PE. Evaluation of the patient presenting with a painful wrist. *Clin Plast Surg* 1996;23:361–368.
13. Metz VM, Wunderbaldinger P, Gilula LA. Update on imaging techniques of the wrist and hand. *Clin Plast Surg* 1996;23:369–384.
14. Yin YM, Mann FA, Gilula LA. Positions and techniques. In: Gilula LA, Yin YM, eds. *Imaging of the wrist and hand.* Philadelphia: WB Saunders, 1996;93–158.
15. Totty WG, Gilula LA. Imaging of the hand and wrist. In: Gilula LA, ed. *The traumatized hand and wrist.* Philadelphia: WB Saunders, 1992;1–12.
16. Doczi J, Springer G, Renner A, et al. Occult distal radial fractures. *J Hand Surg [Br]* 1995;20:614–617.
17. Whitten CG, El-Khoury GY. Conventional tomography of the wrist and hand. In: Gilula LA, ed. *Imaging of the wrist and hand.* Philadelphia: WB Saunders, 1996;351–366.
18. Smith DK, Linscheid RL, Amadio PC, et al. Scaphoid anatomy: evaluation with complex motion tomography. *Radiology* 1989;173:177–180.
19. Biondetti PR, Vannier MW, Gilula LA, et al. Wrist: coronal and transaxial CT scanning. *Radiology* 1987;163:149–151.
20. Aaron JO. A practical guide to diagnostic imaging of the upper extremity. *Hand Clin* 1993;9:347–358.
21. Patel RB. Evaluation of complex carpal trauma: thin-section direct longitudinal computed tomography scanning through a plaster cast. *J Comput Assist Tomogr* 1985;9:107–109.
22. Quinn SF, Belsole RJ, Greene TL, et al. Advanced imaging of the wrist. *Radiographics* 1989;9:229–246.
23. Quinn SF, Murray W, Watkins T, et al. CT for determining the results of treatment of fractures of the wrist. *Am J Roentgenol* 1987;149:109–111.
24. Quinn SF, Belsole RJ, Greene TL, et al. CT of the wrist for the evaluation of the traumatic injuries. *Crit Rev Diag Imag* 1989;29:357–380.
25. Scheffler R, Armstrong D, Hutton L. Computed tomographic diagnosis of distal radio-ulnar joint disruption. *J Can Assoc Radiol* 1984;35:212–213.
26. McNiesh LM. Unique musculoskeletal trauma. *Radiol Clin North Am* 1987;25:1107–1132.
27. Sclafani SJA. Dislocation of the distal radioulnar joint. *J Comput Assist Tomogr* 1981;5:450.
28. Mino DE, Palmer AK, Levinsohn EM. Radiography and computerized tomography in the diagnosis of incongruity of the distal radio-ulnar joint. A prospective study. *J Bone Joint Surg Am* 1985;67:247–252.
29. Dekel S, Papaioannou T, Rushworth G, et al. Idiopathic carpal tunnel syndrome caused by carpal stenosis. *BMJ* 1980;31:1297–1299.
30. Jessurun W, Hillen B, Zonneveld F, et al. Anatomical relations in the carpal tunnel: A computed tomographic study. *J Hand Surg [Br]* 1987;12:64–67.
31. Jetzer T, Erickson D, Webb A, et al. Computed tomography of the carpal tunnel with clinical and surgical correlation. *CT Clin Symp* 1984;7:2–7.
32. Hindman BW, Avolio RE. High resolution scanning of the hand and wrist. *CT Clin Symp* 1985;8:2–11.
33. Hauser H, Rheiner P. Computed tomography of the hand. Part II: Pathological conditions. *Medicamundi* 1983;28:129–135.
34. Merhar GL, Clark RA, Schneider HJ, et al. High-resolution computed tomography of the wrist in patients with carpal tunnel syndrome. *Skel Radiol* 1986;15:549–552.
35. Pruitt DL, Gilula LA, Manske PR, et al. Computed tomography scanning with image reconstruction in evaluation of distal radius fractures. *J Hand Surg [Am]* 1994;19:720–727.
36. Biondetti PR, Vannier MW, Gilula LA, et al. Three-dimensional surface reconstruction of the carpal bones from CT scans: transaxial versus coronal technique. *Comput Med Imag Graphics* 1988;12:67–73.
37. Offutt CJ, Vannier MW, Gilula LA, et al. Volumetric 3-D imaging of computerized tomography scans. *Radiol Technol* 1990;61:212–219.
38. Tamai K, Ryu J, An KN, et al. Three-dimensional geometric analysis of the metacarpophalangeal joint. *J Hand Surg [Am]* 1988;13:521–529.
39. Oberlin C, Salon A, Pigeau I, et al. Three-dimensional reconstruction of the carpus and its vasculature: An anatomic study. *J Hand Surg [Am]* 1992;17:767–772.
40. Weeks PM, Vannier MW, Stevens WG, et al. Three dimensional imaging of the wrist. *J Hand Surg* 1985;10:32–39.
41. Zeman RK, Fox SH, Silverman PM, et al. Helical (spiral) CT of the abdomen. *Am J Roentgenol* 1993;160:719–725.
42. Fishman EK, Wyatt SH, Bluemke DA, et al. Spiral CT of musculoskeletal pathology: preliminary observations. *Skel Radiol* 1993;22:253–256.
43. McEnery KW, Wilson AW, Murphy WA. *Spiral CT evaluation of wrist trauma.* Exhibit presented at ARRS meeting, San Francisco, April 1993.
44. Manaster BJ. Digital wrist arthrography: precision in determining the site of radiocarpal–midcarpal communication. *Am J Roentgenol* 1986;147:563–566.
45. Manaster BJ. The clinical efficacy of triple-injection wrist arthrography. *Radiology* 1991;178:267–270.
46. Levinsohn EM, Rosen ID, Palmer AK. Wrist arthrography: value of the three-compartment injection method. *Radiology* 1991;179:231–239.
47. Gundry CR, Kursunoglu-Brahme S, Schwaighofer B, et al. Is MR better than arthrography for evaluating the ligaments of the wrist? *In vitro* study. *Am J Roentgenol* 1990;154:337–341.
48. Frahm R, Saul O, Mannerfelt L. Diagnostic applications of wrist arthrography. *Arch Orthop Trauma Surg* 1990;109:39–42.
49. Cantor RM, Stern PJ, Wyrick JD, et al. The relevance of ligament tears or perforations in the diagnosis of wrist pain: an arthrographic study. *J Hand Surg [Am]* 1994;19:945–953.
50. Yin Y, Evanoff BA, Gilula LA, et al. Surgeons' decision making in patients with chronic wrist pain: role of bilateral three-compartment wrist arthrography—prospective study. *Radiology* 1996;200:829–832.
51. Tiel-van Buul MMC, Roolker W, Verbeeten BWB Jr, et al. Magnetic resonance imaging versus bone scintigraphy in suspected scaphoid fracture. *Eur J Nucl Med* 1996;23:971–975.
52. Maurer AH. Nuclear medicine in evaluation of the hand and wrist. *Hand Clin* 1991;7:183–200.
53. Holder LE. Bone scintigraphy. In: Gilula LA, Yin YM, eds. *Imaging of the wrist and hand.* Philadelphia: WB Saunders, 1996;319–350.
54. Patel N, Collier BD, Carrera GF, et al. High-resolution bone scintigraphy of the adult wrist. *Clin Nucl Med* 1992;17:449–453.
55. van Beek EJ, van Buul MM, Broekhuizen AH. Diagnostic problems of scaphoid fractures: the value of radionuclide bone scintigraphy. *Neth J Surg* 1990;42:50–52.
56. Makino N, Ishigaki T, Sakuma S, et al. [Three-phase bone scintigraphy of Kienböck disease] (Jpn). *Kaku Igaku* 1992;29:1419–1427.

57. Gaebler C, Kukla C, Breitenseher M, et al. Magnetic resonance imaging of occult scaphoid fractures. *J Trauma* 1996; 41:73–76.
58. Peh WC, Gilula LA, Wilson AJ. Detection of occult wrist fractures by magnetic resonance imaging. *Clin Radiol* 1996;51:285–292.
59. Buyruk HM, Stam HJ, Lameris JS, et al. Colour Doppler ultrasound examination of hand tendon pathologies. A preliminary report. *J Hand Surg [Br]* 1996;21:469–473.
60. Read JW, Conolly WB, Lanzetta M, et al. Diagnostic ultrasound of the hand and wrist. *J Hand Surg [Am]* 1996;6:1004–1010.
61. Bianchi S, Abdelwahab IF, Zwass A, et al. Ultrasonographic evaluation of wrist ganglia. *Skel Radiol* 1994;23:201–203.
62. Berghoff RA Jr, Amadio PC. [Dorsal wrist ganglion. Cause of dorsal wrist pain] (Ger). *Orthopade* 1993;22:30–35.
63. Steiner E, Steinbach LS, Schnarkowski P, et al. Ganglia and cysts around joints. *Radiol Clin North Am* 1996;34:395–425.
64. Breidahl WH, Adler RS. Ultrasound-guided injection of ganglia with corticosteroids. *Skel Radiol* 1996;25:635–638.
65. Pretorius ES, Epstein RE, Dalinka MK. MR imaging of the wrist. *Radiol Clin North Am* 1997;35:145–161.
66. Oneson SR, Scales LM, Erickson SJ, et al. MR imaging of the painful wrist. *Radiographics* 1996;16:997–1008.
67. Siegel S, White LM, Brahme S. Magnetic resonance imaging of the musculoskeletal system. Part 5. The wrist. *Clin Orthop* 1996; 332:281–300.
68. Yu JS. Magnetic resonance imaging of the wrist. *Orthopedics* 1994;17:1041–1048.
69. Smith DK. MR imaging of normal and injured wrist ligaments. *Magn Reson Imag Clin North Am* 1995;3:229–248.
70. Rettig ME, Raskin KB, Melone CP Jr. Clinical applications of MR imaging in hand and wrist surgery. *Magn Reson Imag Clin North Am* 1995;3:361–368.
71. Vo P, Wright T, Hayden F, et al. Evaluating dorsal wrist pain: MRI diagnosis of occult dorsal wrist ganglion. *J Hand Surg [Am]* 1995;20:667–670.
72. Adler BD, Logan PM, Janzen DL, et al. Extrinsic radiocarpal ligaments: magnetic resonance imaging of normal wrists and scapholunate dissociation. *Can Assoc Radiol J* 1996;47:417–422.
73. Timins ME, Jahnke JP, Krah SF, et al. MR imaging of the major carpal stabilizing ligaments: normal anatomy and clinical examples. *Radiographics* 1995;15:575–587.
74. Escobedo EM, Bergman AG, Hunter JC. MR imaging of ulnar impaction. *Skel Radiol* 1995;24:85–90.
75. Gabl M, Lener M, Pechlaner S, et al. The role of dynamic magnetic resonance imaging in the detection of lesions of the ulnocarpal complex. *J Hand Surg [Br]* 1996;21:311–314.
76. Klug JD. MR diagnosis of tenosynovitis about the wrist. *Magn Reson Imag Clin North Am* 1995;3:305–312.
77. Kransdorf MJ, Murphey MD. MR imaging of musculoskeletal tumors of the hand and wrist. *Magn Reson Imag Clin North Am* 1995;3:327–344.
78. Kersting-Sommerhoff B, Hof N, Lenz M, et al. MRI of peripheral joints with a low-field dedicated system: a reliable and cost-effective alternative to high-field units? *Eur Radiol* 1996;6: 561–565.
79. Trieshmann HW Jr, Mosure JC. The impact of magnetic resonance imaging of the knee on surgical decision making. *Arthroscopy* 1996;12:550–555.
80. Williams RL, Williams LA, Watura R, et al. Impact of MRI on a knee arthroscopy waiting list. *Ann R Coll Surg Engl* 1996;78: 450–452.
81. Song SJ. Aspects of musculoskeletal magnetic resonance imaging. *Aust Fam Physician* 1995;24:550–551.
82. Brown DE, Lichtman DM. The evaluation of chronic wrist pain. *Orthop Clin North Am* 1984;15:183–192.
83. Beckenbaugh RD. Accurate evaluation and management of the painful wrist following injury. An approach to carpal instability. *Orthop Clin North Am* 1984;15:289–306.
84. Truong NP, Mann FA, Gilula LA, et al. Wrist instability series: Increased yield with clinical radiologic screening criteria. *Radiology* 1994;192:481–484.
85. Hollister AM, Sanders RA, McCann S. The use of MRI in the diagnosis of an occult wrist ganglion cyst. *Orthop Rev* 1989;18: 1201–1202.
86. Cooney WP, Linscheid RL, Dobyns JH. Scaphoid fractures. Problems associated with nonunion and avascular necrosis. *Orthop Clin North Am* 1984;15:381–391.
87. Filan SL, Herbert TJ. Avascular necrosis of the proximal scaphoid after fracture union. *J Hand Surg [Br]* 1995;20:551–556.
88. Failla JM. Osteonecrosis associated with nonunion of the hook of the hamate. *Orthopedics* 1993;16:217–218.
89. Failla JM. Hook of hamate vascularity: vulnerability to osteonecrosis and nonunion. *J Hand Surg [Am]* 1993;18: 1075–1079.
90. Telfer JR, Evans DM, Bingham JB. Avascular necrosis of the hamate. *J Hand Surg [Br]* 1994;19:389–392.
91. Lowry WE Jr, Cord SA. Traumatic avascular necrosis of the capitate bone-case report. *J Hand Surg [Am]* 1981;6:245–248.
92. Linscheid RL. Kienböck's disease. *Instr Course Lect* 1992;41: 45–53.
93. Almquist EE. Kienböck's disease. *Clin Orthop* 1986;202:68–78.
94. Herbert TJ, Lanzetta M. Idiopathic avascular necrosis of the scaphoid. *J Hand Surg [Br]* 1994;19:174–182.
95. Jensen CH, Leicht P. Idiopathic avascular necrosis of the scaphoid in a child. *Scand J Plast Reconstr Surg Hand Surg* 1995; 29:359–360.
96. Dossing K, Boe S. Idiopathic avascular necrosis of the scaphoid. Case report. *Scand J Plast Reconstr Surg Hand Surg* 1994;28: 155–156.
97. Martini G, Valenti R, Giovani S, et al. Idiopathic avascular necrosis of the scaphoid. A case report. *Recent Prog Med* 1995; 86:238–240.
98. Millez PY, Kinh Kha H, Allieu Y, et al. Idiopathic aseptic osteonecrosis of the capitate bone. Literature review apropos of 3 new cases. *Int Orthop* 1991;15:85–94.
99. Arcalis Arce A, Pedemonte Jansana JP, Massons Albareda JM. Idiopathic necrosis of the capitate. *Acta Orthop Belg* 1996;62: 46–48.
100. Kutty S, Curtin J. Idiopathic avascular necrosis of the capitate. *J Hand Surg [Br]* 1995;20:402–404.
101. De Smet L, Willemen D, Kimpe E, et al. Nontraumatic osteonecrosis of the capitate bone associated with gout. *Ann Chir Main Memb Super* 1993;12:210–212.
102. Pin PG, Semenkovich JW, Young VL, et al. Role of radionuclide imaging in the evaluation of wrist pain. *J Hand Surg [Am]* 1988;13:810–814.
103. Reinus WR, Conway WF, Totty WG, et al. Carpal avascular necrosis: MR imaging. *Radiology* 1986;160:689–693.
104. Golimbu CN, Firooznia H, Rafii M. Avascular necrosis of carpal bones. *Magn Reson Imag Clin North Am* 1995;3:281–303.
105. Imaeda T, Nakamura R, Miura T, et al. Magnetic resonance imaging in Kienböck's disease. *J Hand Surg [Br]* 1992;17: 12–19.
106. Metz VM, Schimmerl SM, Gilula LA, et al. Wide scapholunate joint space in lunotriquetral coalition: a normal variant? *Radiology* 1993;188:557–559.

7

WRIST ARTHROSCOPY

TERRY L. WHIPPLE
THOMAS A. DWYER

Arthroscopy has clearly revolutionized the practice of orthopedic surgery. In 1918, Takagi initiated endoscopic examination of the knee using a #22 French cystoscope (1). However, it was not until 1931 that he compiled unprecedented clinical experience in endoscopic knee examination after developing a 3.5-mm arthroscope that incorporated a lamp and magnifying optics that provided a clear visual field. Wantanabe, a protégé of Takagi, published his *Atlas of Arthroscopy* in 1969, which convincingly demonstrated endoscopic photography of the knee (1). Only then did the technique gain clinical credibility and acceptance. Using the improved #21 arthroscope developed by Wantanabe in 1958, several North American surgeons established the application of Wantanabe's techniques in the United States and Canada. The subsequent development of fiberoptic technology led to further improvement in arthroscope designs, and orthopedic surgeons around the world began to incorporate arthroscopy into their practice of orthopedic surgery. The improved precision and reduced morbidity afforded by arthroscopic techniques truly heralded a new era in orthopedic surgery.

The development of the Wantanabe #24 arthroscope in 1970 paved the way for the earliest reported experiences with wrist arthroscopy. Wantanabe reported his experience with 21 wrist arthroscopies between 1970 and 1972, and Chen published his results of 34 clinical arthroscopies of the wrist and finger joints. These pioneer attempts afforded limited viewing of the articular surface anatomy of the wrist, prompting Chen to conclude that "there were still many problems" (2).

The birth of modern-day wrist arthroscopy occurred in 1985, when Whipple described precisely located wrist portals based on anatomic landmarks and developed standardized methods for reviewing wrist anatomy. In 1986, Whipple introduced the use of joint distraction as a technique for gaining additional instrumentation working space and providing adequate exposure to the radiocarpal and midcarpal spaces (3). The development of small 2- to 3-mm instruments designed specifically for use in the wrist followed shortly thereafter. In a decade, wrist arthroscopy as a diagnostic and therapeutic tool has evolved into a reliable means of treating disorders of the wrist.

The complexity of the wrist frequently makes localization of pain difficult. The wrist consists of three joints (distal radioulnar, radiocarpal, and midcarpal), the radius and ulna, eight carpal bones, the triangular fibrocartilage complex (TFCC), and 27 ligaments, both extrinsic and intrinsic. A multitude of complex static and dynamic injury patterns exist, which frequently make diagnosis difficult.

The normal wrist complex moves in a synchronous and coordinated manner as a result of musculotendinous units working in conjunction with a multitude of ligamentous attachments. Wrist injury results in a disruption of this pattern and the development of wrist discomfort.

The foundation for the successful diagnostic evaluation of the wrist is a thorough history and physical examination. Physical examination should include a systematic palpation of each anatomic landmark, provocative maneuvers, strength testing, and selective anesthetic injections. Standardized x-ray evaluation of the wrist is a useful adjunct, and additional diagnostic tests such as tomograms, CT scans, and technetium-99 bone scans may be obtained on a selective basis. Arthrograms and magnetic resonance images can provide indirect evidence of soft tissue defects and ligaments and tendons. Despite the excellent specificity of triple-injection cinearthrography in defining injuries of the wrist, the fact that this particular procedure is not exceptionally sensitive is a concern, especially if its use is exclusionary in nature (4,5). For MRI to be effective in detecting wrist injuries, a strong magnet is required as well as specific surface coils to improve resolution (6). Standard MR imaging effectively evaluates the TFCC, although imaging of the intrinsic and extrinsic ligaments is not consistent (7). Neither arthrograms nor MRI is a reliable means of evaluating synovium or articular cartilage defects.

Wrist arthroscopy, which allows for visual inspection and palpation of all intraarticular structures, is an unparalleled means of examining the soft tissues and articular surfaces of

---

T. L. Whipple: Department of Orthopaedics and Rehabilitation, University of Virginia School of Medicine, Charlottesville, Virginia 22908; and Orthopaedic Research of Virginia, Health South Hospital, Richmond, Virginia 23226.

T. A. Dwyer: Pittsgrove, New Jersey 08318.

the wrist. Moreover, arthroscopy is the only modality that allows a detailed determination of both the size and extent of intraarticular pathology.

The clinical utility of wrist arthroscopy has been the focus of a number of recent articles. Wrist arthroscopy has been advocated as a beneficial diagnostic tool, a method of staging a known diagnosis, and as a means of definitive treatment for wrist pathology (8). Nagle and Benson reported that diagnostic arthroscopy was 98% effective in the accurate establishment of suspected wrist diagnoses (8). Adolfson reported success in establishing a previously unknown diagnosis in 21 of 30 patients (9). Similarly, Bleton et al. reported success in 22 of 33 patients (10). Sennwald et al. have particularly emphasized the benefits of arthroscopy in identifying multiple partial injuries in the wrist not readily apparent on arthrography (11).

Wrist arthroscopy has also been advocated as a means of staging wrist pathology, thereby guiding future clinical management. Specifically, intraarticular fractures, ligamentous disruptions, degenerative arthritis, and Kienböck's disease are amenable to arthroscopic evaluation, with future treatment dictated by arthroscopic findings (8,12). Wrist arthroscopy has been reported as a useful tool for evaluating the patient with undiagnosed wrist pain of longer than 3 months' duration (13) and in the management of cartilaginous lesions of the wrist (14,15).

Perhaps the most rapidly expanding indication for wrist arthroscopy is the definitive arthroscopic management of numerous wrist afflictions. The therapeutic indications for wrist arthroscopy have evolved to include the repair of peripheral TFCC lesions, debridement of central TFCC lesions, debridement of chondral lesions, synovectomy, irrigation and debridement of septic arthritis, arthroscopic reduction and internal fixation of intraarticular distal radius fractures and carpal fractures, radial styloidectomy, lysis of adhesions, removal of loose bodies, ganglionotomy, and arthroscopic excision of the distal ulna (8,14–28).

SURGICAL TECHNIQUE

Wrist arthroscopy is a minimally invasive surgical procedure that usually can be performed on an outpatient basis. The space required to manipulate instruments within the radiocarpal and midcarpal joints is obtained by placing traction across the wrist. The traction is applied through finger traps placed on two or three digits. Soft, flexible nylon finger traps are ideally suited for this purpose, as they are less traumatic and provide for more surface area for traction force distribution than metal finger traps. Joint traction may be supplied through a system of weights and pulleys. Alternatively, the Traction Tower (Linvatec Corp., Largo, FL) is ideally suited and specifically designed for wrist arthroscopy. It can be completely sterilized and allows for universal positioning of the wrist at surgery while avoiding cumbersome, unsterile traction and countertraction arrangements. Wrist arthroscopy requires video magnification because of the smaller-diameter arthroscopes used for the procedure. The standard 2.7-mm telescope with a 30° angled field of vision will usually suffice, though smaller arthroscopes are available. As with other joints, lactated Ringer's solution is well suited for arthroscopy of the wrist. With a patent inflow cannula with at least a 16-gauge bore, gravity-fed inflow is sufficient in almost all cases. Irrigation lines equipped with a small pinch chamber allow additional fluid to be pumped into the joint quickly and conveniently when required. The probe is perhaps the most useful diagnostic tool in arthroscopy and is an essential component of any instrument tray. A dissector, grasper, and several cutting instruments (baskets, arthroscopy knives, suction punch) round out the necessary manual instruments. For many cutting tasks, power instruments are advantageous because of their rapidly repeating cutting action and should be available to the wrist arthroscopist.

The operating room should be large enough to accommodate the necessary equipment. The room should be arranged to provide ample room for the surgeon to sit adjacent to the head of the table, facing the dorsum of the wrist. The patient is positioned supine with the shoulder abducted 60° to 90° on a narrow hand table or two arm boards affixed to the side of the table. A pneumatic tourniquet should be placed on the arm and utilized according to the surgeon's preference. The wrist should be circumferentially shaved from the midmetacarpals to 1 in. proximal to the radial styloid. The extremity is prepped and draped in routine sterile fashion. Sterile finger traps are applied to two or three digits.

The assistant, who generally sits next to the surgeon, is crucial for successful and efficient execution of arthroscopic wrist procedures. The assistant may be called on to stabilize the arthroscope at times and thus should have a clear view of the video monitor. In addition, the assistant should be familiar with the operation of all instrumentation and is responsible for the maintenance of an adequate irrigation system.

Our preferred method of applying traction across the wrist utilizes the Traction Tower. The base of the tower rests on the hand table with a circumferential strap about the patient's arm and hand table. Finger traps are attached to the spreader bar and traction is applied by raising the height of the tower. A spring scale allows the surgeon to calibrate the amount of applied traction. Usually 7 to 10 lb of traction will suffice. The tower is equipped with a universal joint, which allows the surgeon to adjust the wrist to the most appropriate position at surgery, facilitating the surgical procedure.

LANDMARKS

An intimate knowledge of the topographic anatomy of the wrist is necessary to safely and effectively perform the technique of wrist arthroscopy. Several surface landmarks can be identified by palpation and are sufficient to allow direct surgical approaches to most intraarticular structures in the wrist with precision and confidence. Bony landmarks include the radial styloid, which is easily palpated with the wrist in passive extension; most of the dorsal margin of the distal radius, including Lister's tubercle, is identifiable. The interval between the radius and the head of the ulna is best identified with the wrist in supination. Distally, the prominent base of the first metacarpal can be palpated, as are the bases of the second and third metacarpals. Midway between the base of the second metacarpal and Lister's tubercle is a soft spot, which marks the midcarpal space. The midcarpal space is located 8 to 10 mm distal to the dorsal margin of the radius and essentially follows the same contour as the distal radius.

The dorsal extensor retinaculum is oriented obliquely across the distal radius and ulna. It overlies and compartmentalizes all of the wrist extensor tendons. Tendon landmarks on the dorsal wrist are readily identifiable. Palpate the point of intersection of the second and third extensor compartments, the extensor carpi radialis longus (ECRL) and extensor pollicis longus (EPL), respectively. A straight line drawn from this intersection to Lister's tubercle marks the course of the EPL tendon. Ulnar to the EPL, it is possible to feel the radial margin of the fourth extensor compartment. The ulnar margin of the fourth compartment is found immediately distal to the interval between the radius and ulna. Coursing distally from the radial aspect of the ulnar styloid, the prominent extensor carpi ulnaris (ECU) tendon (sixth extensor compartment) should be identified (29).

The dorsum of the wrist contains arborizations of the dorsal cutaneous branches of the radial and ulnar nerves. Although variable in location, the radial cutaneous nerve is usually located in close approximation to the intersection of the second and third extensor compartments. This nerve arborizes immediately proximal to this point and commonly has three main branches. The dorsal cutaneous branch of the ulnar nerve courses superficially around the ulna from the volar to the dorsal surface. Last, the location of the radial artery must be remembered at the volar and radialmost aspect of the anatomic snuffbox.

PORTALS

Portal placement for reproducible wrist arthroscopy techniques was developed and described by Whipple et al. in 1986 (30). The technique requires precise identification of the aforementioned intersecting landmarks. Once located, these landmarks should be drawn precisely on the dorsum of the wrist before surgical incisions are made. As discussed, bony landmarks to be detailed preoperatively include the radial styloid, dorsal margin of the radius, Lister's tubercle, ulnar styloid, ulnar head, and the bases of the second and third metacarpals. Tendon landmarks to be identified include the ECRL (II), EPL (III), extensor digitorum communis (EDC) (IV), and the ECU (VI). For radiocarpal space arthroscopy, the portals are identified between the respective extensor tendons (Fig. 7.1). The 1–2 portal, located between the compartments for the abductor pollicis longus (APL) and the extensor pollicis brevis (EPB), and the ECRL and extensor carpi radialis brevis (ECRB) tendons, should be made as dorsal as possible to avoid injury to the radial artery (Fig. 7.2). This portal is useful for visualizing intraarticular dorsal anatomy, such as ganglia, as an inflow portal for ulnar pathology or for instrumentation for radial styloidectomy. The 3–4 portal, located between the EPL and EDC tendons distal to Lister's tubercle, is the primary entry portal for the arthroscopy (Fig. 7.3). The 4–5 portal, located between the EDC and EDQ tendons, is the primary accessory portal for instrumentation. The portal is located immediately above the TFCC attachment to the radius. The 6R portal is located just radial to the ECU tendon and is useful for arthroscopic viewing of the lunotriquetral ligament and as an accessory portal for TFCC procedures. Entry into this portal is through the dorsal

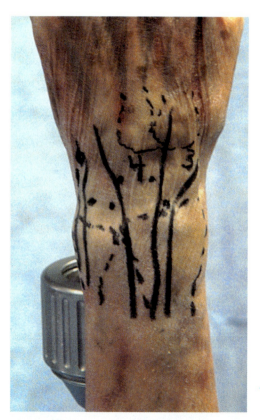

FIGURE 7.1. Arthroscopic landmarks and portals: *3*, extensor pollicis longus (EPL); *4*, extensor digitorum longus (EDC); *6*, extensor carpi ulnaris (ECU). The base of the second and third metacarpals and the distal radius and ulna are marked in *dashed lines*.

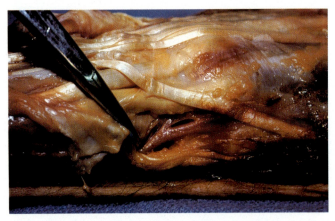

FIGURE 7.2. Dissection of the anatomic snuffbox of a right wrist. *Hemostat* points to the radial artery in the volar aspect of the snuffbox between the first and second extensor compartments. Arthroscopic entry through the 1–2 portal should stay in the dorsal safe zone of the snuffbox.

ligamentous portion of the TFCC immediately beneath the lunotriquetral ligament. The 6U portal, located ulnar to the ECU tendon, enters the radiocarpal joint through the prestyloid recess, just over the TFCC articular disc. One must be careful to avoid injury to the dorsal sensory branch of the ulnar nerve when establishing this portal. This is the

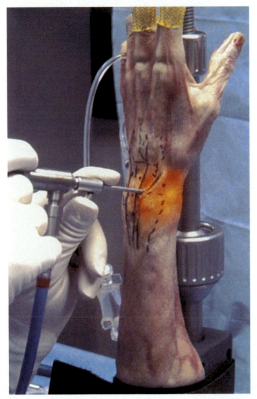

FIGURE 7.3. Arthroscope insertion through the 3–4 portal of a left wrist, the primary portal for diagnostic and surgical procedures in the radiocarpal space.

primary portal for the inflow–outflow cannula and affords the best arthroscopic view of the ulnocarpal ligaments (29,31).

Midcarpal joint arthroscopy allows visualization of intercarpal pathology through four portals. The most commonly utilized portal is the radial midcarpal portal (RMC), located approximately 1 cm distal to the 3–4 portal in line with the radial border of the third metacarpal. This is the primary portal for introduction of the arthroscope and enters the midcarpal space at the scaphocapitate interval. The ulnar midcarpal portal (UMC) is located at the same level as the RMC but in the midaxial line of the fourth metacarpal. This is the primary accessory portal for instrumentation in midcarpal arthroscopy. The portal enters the joint at the four-corner intersection of the capitate, hamate, triquetrum, and lunate.

Two accessory portals have been described. On the radial side of the wrist, the scaphotrapeziotrapezoid (STT) portal allows instrumentation of the STT joint. The portal is located ulnar to the EPL tendon in line with the radial margin of the second metacarpal. One must be careful not to displace the EPL tendon radially while establishing the STT portal to avoid possible injury to the radial artery (32). The ulnar accessory portal enters the triquetrohamate (TH) joint just ulnar to the ECU tendon. This portal is useful for inflow–outflow or for instrumentation of the TH joint.

Several technical points should be adhered to while establishing arthroscopic wrist portals. Initial localization of a portal and the projected angle of entry should begin with placement of a hypodermic needle percutaneously to the location desired. One must remember to take into account the 11° volar slope and 22° radioulnar inclination of the distal radius when entering the radiocarpal joint. After the appropriate location and angle of entry is confirmed with a hypodermic needle, the skin overlying the portal is incised with a #11 blade. This is accomplished by holding the scalpel stationary and drawing the underlying skin into the blade. The incision should be made through the dermis only. A mosquito hemostat is then utilized to spread the subcutaneous tissues and sensory nerves away down to the dorsal capsule of the wrist. A tapered, blunt trocar and sheath is then utilized to penetrate the capsule with a twisting motion. The surgeon's index finger should be positioned on the shaft of the trocar just proximal to the distal tip to avoid inadvertent plunging into the joint.

SYSTEMATIC ARTHROSCOPIC EXAMINATION

Wrist arthroscopy requires a systematic evaluation of each identifiable intraarticular structure. As mentioned previously, the 3–4 portal is the workhorse portal for radiocarpal joint arthroscopy. On penetration of the joint, the radioscapholunate ligament (RSL) is usually the first identifiable structure. It appears deep to a synovial tuft, which covers the ligament and serves as a useful reference point when first entering the radiocarpal joint. This synovial tuft consistently serves as a marker for the distal scapholunate ligament and proximal sagittal ridge of the radius. The arthroscope is maneuvered up the slope of the radius to the radial styloid with its capsular tissue attachment, the radial collateral ligament (33). As the arthroscope is directed further radially, one falls into the radial recess. Turning the arthroscope dorsally allows the surgeon to view the dorsal capsule of the wrist joint as it attaches to the dorsal lip of the radius. As the arthroscope is drawn into the scaphoid fossa of the radius, the volar ligamentous supports are inspected. Beginning radialward, the stout radioscaphocapitate ligament (RSCL) is viewed. This ligament provides stability to the scaphoid and maintains its proper alignment. The articular surface of the scaphoid and the scaphoid fossa are assessed and probed with the heel of the instrument. Progressing ulnarward, the radiolunate ligament is seen as an oblique structure distinct from the RSCL. Following the smooth convexity of the scaphoid brings the scapholunate ligament into view. The scapholunate ligament may be difficult to distinguish from articular cartilage in the normal wrist. It may appear as an indentation of dimple but is most easily appreciated on blunt palpation with the heel of a probe as a ligamentous structure. The probe is extremely useful for identifying the ligament margins and assessing for tears. In cases of suspected pathology, provocative stress testing should be performed while viewing the ligament to access for instability.

Wrist extension allows improved visualization of the dorsal surface of the scaphoid and lunate, whereas flexion of the wrist allows improved visualization of the volar surfaces. Ulnar to the scapholunate ligament is the articular surface of the lunate. The triangular fibrocartilage (TFC), one component of the TFCC, is an articular disc that is generally thin centrally and thick peripherally. On probing, the intact disc feels semirigid, and a "trampoline test" should be performed to evaluate its integrity (34). After systematic evaluation of the TFCL, the arthroscope should be advanced ulnarly and volarly into the prestyloid recess, which communicates with the radiocarpal space through a normal hiatus in the ulnar TFC.

The ulnocarpal ligaments include the ulnolunate and ulnotriquetral ligaments, which arise from a common origin at the TFC and ulna and bifurcate just distal to the TFC. These ligaments, in addition to the triquetral articular surface and the lunotriquetral (LT) ligament, are best visualized from the 6R portal. Pronation and supination of the wrist under arthroscopic control enhances visualization of the ulnar radiocarpal structures.

A complete arthroscopic examination of the wrist requires visualization of the midcarpal space. Because there is no normal communication between the radiocarpal and midcarpal spaces, irrigation is usually delivered through the arthroscope sheath. As with assessment of the radiocarpal space, the midcarpal space should be examined systematically, looking first for suspected pathology.

The RMC is the workhorse for examination of the midcarpal joint. Through the RMC portal, the arthroscope enters the joint between the scaphoid and the capitate. Generally, examination begins radially by following the smooth concave surface of the scaphoid. The first joint encountered is the capitate–trapezoid joint. Viewing distally, the trapezium can be seen in the background, and the trapezoid in the foreground. Degenerative changes are frequently encountered in the STT articulation, and it is not unusual to find the distal pole of the scaphoid entirely devoid of hyaline cartilage (29). Bubbles frequently collect in this region and are easily evacuated when touched with a percutaneous hypodermic needle. Examination continues as the arthroscope is maneuvered back down the concave surface of the scaphoid to the scapholunate interval. There are no intrinsic intercarpal ligaments in the midcarpal space, which allows easy recognition of this interval. Marginal fraying of the articular cartilage in this region may be a subtle but significant sign of rotary subluxation of the scaphoid (29). Provocative stress testing should be utilized to dynamically assess the joint. The articular surface of the lunate should be inspected. The lunate may contain one or two distal articular facets (Fig. 7.4). One facet accommodates the head of the capitate, and a smaller facet may exist to accommodate the proximal pole of the hamate (35). The lunotriquetral interval should be examined during application of dorsal and volar pressure to the triquetrum. Under normal circumstances, no anterior or posterior translation

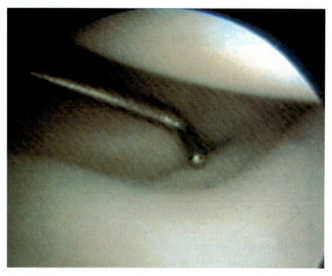

FIGURE 7.4. Arthroscopic view of the midcarpal space of a left wrist viewed from the radial midcarpal portal. A 1-mm hook probe is inserted through the ulnar midcarpal portal. The probe overlies the lunotriquetral space; the tip of the probe indicates a second facet on the lunate that accommodates the proximal pole of the hamate.

should exist between the carpal bones (29). The triquetrohamate joint is a saddle-shaped joint that is normally very tight. If manipulation of the joint produces distraction, midcarpal instability (MCI) may be present. Another sign of MCI is the presence of an articular defect on the proximal pole of the hamate. Withdrawal of the arthroscope slightly allows the surgeon to view the capitohamate joint. This is a planar joint with its articulating surface only partially covered by articular cartilage. Extend the wrist and view dorsalulnar to view the dorsal capsule of the distal carpal row and assess whether the dorsal capsule has avulsed from the hamate, from the capitate, or both (32). Finally, look for articular degeneration on the head of the capitate. If necessary, the ulnar midcarpal portal is easily established if accessory instrumentation of the midcarpal space is desired.

TRIANGULAR FIBROCARTILAGE COMPLEX

Ulnar-sided wrist pain is a diagnostic problem often encountered by the orthopedic surgeon. Disorders of the TFCC are being increasingly recognized as a significant source of ulnar wrist dysfunction, and the diagnosis of a TFCC lesion should be entertained in any patient who presents with ulnar-sided wrist complaints. The TFCC is a cartilaginous and ligamentous structure with several biomechanical functions. The TFCC transmits 20% of axial load from the ulnar carpus to the distal ulna and is a major stabilizer of both the distal radioulnar joint (DRUJ) and the ulnar carpus (36–41). However, studies have confirmed that the central two thirds of the disc can be excised with no change in its load-bearing status or stability (41). The TFCC arises from the distal sigmoid notch of the radius and inserts into the base of the ulnar styloid and ulnocarpal complex. The central portion of the TFCC is thin, mechanically weak, and composed of interwoven, obliquely oriented collagen fibers (42). Vascular studies have shown it to be relatively avascular with a poor potential for healing (43). The peripheral TFCC, on the other hand, is ligamentous and highly vascularized (44). The blood supply of the TFCC originates from the palmar and dorsal branches of the anterior interosseous artery (44,45). This vascular organization provides foundation for the belief that the periphery of the TFCC has an intrinsic capacity for healing, making repair of peripheral lesions a preferred treatment to debridement. Historically, both the central and radial TFCC were thought to be poorly vascularized. However, recent morphologic studies provide evidence for vascularity of the dorsal volar radial insertion of the TFCC, making repair of some radial lesions a rational treatment alternative (42).

In 1988 a classification system for describing TFCC injuries was introduced by Palmer (46); it provided a common frame of reference for discussion of the TFCC. Palmer classified TFCC tears as traumatic (class I) or degenerative (class II). Traumatic lesions are further subdivided by their location: I-A, central; I-B, peripheral; I-C, distal; I-D, radial. Class II (degenerative) lesions, in contrast to class I lesions, are all centrally located and frequently associated with ulnar positive variance.

The integrity of the TFCC may be investigated by a number of diagnostic techniques, but arthroscopy is considered the gold standard for the diagnosis of TFCC lesions (47). Previously, the diagnosis of a repairable TFCC lesion resulted in an arthrotomy for definitive surgical treatment. Today, TFCC lesions can be definitively treated arthroscopically as a result of the advantages of magnification and illumination. The arthroscopic appearance of a torn TFCC will vary depending on its thickness and the degree of degenerative changes present in the joint. Tears in thin discs tend to gap open, allowing easy recognition, whereas tears in thicker discs may lie closed and obscured unless probed and retracted (29). Diagnosis of a TFCC tear is facilitated by squeezing the dorsal and volar aspect of the DRUJ capsule, which will evert the edges of a subtle tear of the TFCC. These tears should be distinguished from the prestyloid recess and the occasionally present capsular opening into the pisiform–triquetral space.

The goals of surgical treatment of TFCC lesions are to eliminate unstable tissue by excision or repair and to minimize tear propagation. Instrumentation for arthroscopic treatment of the TFCC should include a traction mechanism, miniaturized arthroscopic knives, a suction punch, angled basket forceps, and a small motorized shaver system. An inflow cannula established in the 1–2 portal would be effective and out of the way of surgical manipulation of the TFCC. A 30° angled arthroscope introduced through the 3–4 portal will provide a detailed view of the TFCC disc. Visualization of the volar ulnocarpal ligaments is best accomplished through the 6R or 6U portal. Accessory instrumentation may be placed in the 4–5 or 6R portals.

Class I-A tears are isolated central lesions of the TFCC without instability of the DRUJ. For those patients who fail conservative treatment, limited arthroscopic debridement of the unstable portion of the tear will provide excellent palliation of symptoms by relieving mechanical ulnocarpal impingement. Irregular fibrocartilage may be readily excised with a suction punch, angled basket forceps, or arthroscopic knife. Thin, friable tissue is most easily debrided with a small powered shaver.

On occasion, it may be necessary to exchange portals with the arthroscope and accessory instruments if a more radial approach to the lesion is deemed more effective. If a prominent ulnar head exists because of positive ulnar variance or fracture shortening of the radius, especially in a wrist with chondromalacia of the lunate or ulnar head, consideration should be given to a leveling procedure on the ulna. These cases are best treated by arthroscopic wafer resection or formal ulnar shortening osteotomy. Osterman et al. (48), Wnorowski et al. (28), and Whipple (29) have all described their technique for arthroscopic wafer resection. The presence of lunotriquetral instability would mitigate in favor of a formal ulnar shortening to unload the ulnar head and tighten the ulnocarpal ligaments, stabilizing the lunotriquetral joint. If no significant lunotriquetral instability is noted, the central TFCC tear is debrided as previously described. Initial ulnar head debridement is accomplished with a small osteotome through the 4–5 or 6R portal. Slivers of ulnar head are removed while the wrist is gradually rotated from full supination to full pronation. Complete resection of the dorsal ulnar head may require instrumentation through the 6U portal. Resection of the palmar ulnar head can be achieved by leaving the arthroscope in the 6R portal, passing the osteotome through the 3–4 portal, and pronating the wrist. The residual ulnar head is finely contoured with small arthroscopic burrs through the portals that provide necessary access. Confirm the amount of ulnar resection by radiographs at the termination of the procedure. On completion of a simple debridement procedure, the portals may be closed or left open at the surgeon's preference, and the wrist is placed in a light sterile dressing incorporating a volar split for 3 to 5 days. Thereafter, early motion and return to function are permitted, with activity governed by the patient's comfort (18). Following arthroscopic wafer resection, the same dressing is used for seven days. Pronation and supination are permitted immediately.

Peripheral TFCC lesions (class I-B) may occur in conjunction with Smith's fractures of the distal radius, volar Barton's fractures, or hyperrotation injuries. These lesions can be repaired arthroscopically with superb results (49). A TFCC repair kit has been designed to facilitate this procedure (Linvatec Corp., Largo, FL). A diagnostic arthroscopy is initiated with the arthroscope in the 3–4 portal, and 6R and 6U portals are established once a peripheral tear is identified. Initially, the torn peripheral edge of the TFCC is debrided with a shaver or suction punch through the 6R portal. Next a longitudinal incision is created proximally from the 6R portal over the sixth extensor compartment. The retinacula over the common extensor and ECU tendon are incised, and the ECU tendon is retracted radially or ulnarward for suture placement.

The TFCC repair kit consists of a cannulated needle through which sutures are introduced and a suture retriever. The central disc is sutured to the floor of the ECU tendon sheath by inserting the curved cannulated needle through the floor of the ECU tendon sheath over the DRUJ, directing it upward through the edge of the TFC central disc. Through a more distal site in the floor of the ECU tendon sheath, the suture retriever is introduced, and the wire loop is deployed. The wire loop is then placed over the tip of the cannulated needle at the dorsal edge of the TFC disc, and 2 to 3 cm of 2-0 PDS suture is deployed. Withdrawal of both instruments brings the two arms of the suture out the ECU tendon sheath (Fig. 7.5). This step is then repeated two to four times, depending on the size of the peripheral tear. The forearm is then placed in neutral rotation, and the sutures are tied down over the floor of the ECU compartment. The extensor retinaculum is closed with interrupted sutures, and the skin is closed in subcuticular fashion. Postoperatively, the patient is placed in a sugar-tongs splint or long-arm cast for 3 to 4 weeks and then gradually mobilized. Impact loading of the wrist is not permitted for three months. Arthroscopic repair of peripheral TFCC injuries has yielded good to excellent results and return to previous occupation in 80% to 85% of patients (50).

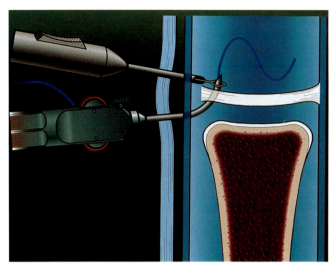

FIGURE 7.5. Artist rendering of technique to repair peripheral detachment of the triangular fibrocartilage complex with an Inteq repair kit.

Class I-C lesions involve disruption of the ulnocarpal ligament complex. Arthroscopically, one may fully visualize the pisotriquetral joint, indicating pathology involving the ulnar extrinsic ligaments. Those tears that do not heal with conservative treatment require open operative treatment. The type of open repair is controversial.

Class I-D lesions involve radial detachment of the TFCC from the sigmoid notch of the radius. These detachments may be repaired back to the radius using 0.035 Kirschner wires (51) or arthroscopically with small suture anchors (Micro Statak or Mitek). With the arthroscope in the 6U or 3–4 portal, a small curette or shaver is introduced through the 4–5 portal, and the dorsal ulnar rim of the radius adjacent to the sigmoid notch is debrided. With the wrist in flexion, a small dorsal arthrotomy is created by extending the 4–5 portal. The suture anchor is placed into subchondral bone at the dorsal edge of the sigmoid notch. Suture tails are then placed through the bony avulsion or the dorsal edge of the TFC and tied securely. Postoperatively, the wrist is immobilized in slight pronation and extension for 4 weeks, after which gradual mobilization is allowed.

Class II degenerative lesions are all centrally located and appear to be strongly correlated with positive ulnar variance.

Palmer proposed that degenerative lesions of the TFCC result from longstanding repetitive loading as a consequence of repetitive forearm rotation in an ulnar-positive wrist (46).

These lesions begin with TFCC wear and progress to chondromalacia of the lunate or ulna, subsequent TFCC perforation, lunotriquetral ligament perforation, and ultimately to degenerative arthritis of the ulnocarpal complex. Arthroscopic treatment for degenerative lesions of the central TFCC tear have been previously described. In addition, complete treatment of class I lesions requires an ulnar leveling procedure. In early lesions (class II-A and II-B), an open wafer procedure is indicated. In class II-C lesions, an arthroscopic wafer procedure is a reasonable treatment plan (52). In the final stages of degenerative lesions (class II-D and II-E) of the TFCC, salvage procedures or limited carpal fusions seem appropriate.

ARTICULAR FRACTURES OF THE RADIUS

Intraarticular fractures of the distal radius can be problematic. They disrupt the articular surface, producing intraarticular bleeding, which evokes a potent inflammatory response and may produce fibrous adhesions. The primary goal in the treatment of intraarticular fractures is the restoration of the articular surface in order to promote ideal long-term wrist function. External fixation of distal radius fractures corrects radial shortening and metaphyseal angulation but does not usually restore articular congruity with impacted fragments (53,54). Percutaneous and limited open reduction under fluoroscopic imaging reduces articular incongruities but does not address associated carpal ligament injuries that may go undetected (55,56).

Arthroscopically assisted reduction and internal fixation of articular fractures of the distal radius was first attempted in 1986 (29). The technique offers the advantages of anatomic restoration of articular incongruities, joint cleansing, greatly reduced surgical trauma, evaluation and concurrent treatment of associated intraarticular injuries, and earlier mobilization when compared to other methods of treatment. The technique is indicated when an articular stepoff of 2 mm or more exists in the radiocarpal joint or DRUJ after closed reduction or when an associated carpal ligamentous injury of DRUJ instability is suspected. Arthroscopic reduction and internal fixation of the distal radius is contraindicated in cases of suspected compartment syndrome or in an open joint with significant soft tissue injury.

Quality radiographs in multiple planes should be obtained after closed reduction of a distal radius fracture. A CT scan is the best method of assessing the articular surface if articular extension of a fracture is suspected. The CT scan cuts should parallel the slope of the distal radius, inclined volarly and ulnarward from the transverse plane. Arthroscopic reduction and internal fixation (ARIF) should be considered if the fracture lines are not uniform, are angulated, or if sagittal and coronal measurements are enlarged compared with the contralateral wrist on plain radiographs (21).

The ideal timing for this technique is 48 to 72 hours after injury. Earlier intervention will usually encounter too much bleeding from the fracture site to maintain a clear visual field. Longer delays result in tenacious fibrin precipitate formation, which obscures vision and is difficult to remove from the joint. A Traction Tower is useful for this procedure because it allows fracture manipulation under constant tension. The forearm is prepped and sterilely draped, and a compressive elastic bandage or Coban (3M, Minneapolis, MN) is wrapped about the forearm to restrict fluid extravasation into muscle compartments through fracture planes. The tower is angulated in the direction opposite the mechanism of injury. The 2.7-mm arthroscope is introduced through the 3–4 portal, and accessory instrumentation through the 4–5 and/or 1–2 portal. The joint is lavaged, and all clot, fibrin cartilage, and bone debris are removed. The articular surface of the radius is then explored arthroscopically, and all fracture planes are identified. Some fracture fragments may be nondisplaced with no separation of the fracture lines. These fragment relationships should not be disturbed. It may be necessary to transfer the arthroscope to the 1–2 portal to evaluate dorsal rim fractures, which are easily overlooked from the 3–4 portal. Importantly, a thorough examination is conducted to identify concomitant injuries to ligamentous structures or the TFCC.

A number of studies have detailed an extremely high incidence of associated intraarticular injuries when intraarticular distal radius fractures are arthroscopically investigated. The TFCC, in particular, is highly prone to injury (26,56–58). These lesions should be addressed in routine fashion after arthroscopic reduction of the distal radius fracture.

Once the complete fracture pattern has been identified, fragments are disimpacted with a dissecting probe by prying between fracture lines. A location near the midpoint of each fragment and between dorsal tendons is selected, and hypodermic needles are inserted perpendicular to the fracture lines in percutaneous fashion into each fragment. Using the needle as a guide to avoid injury to subcutaneous nerves or tendons, 0.45 Kirschner wires are then drilled into each major fragment, stopping short of the fracture plane. Beginning first with the largest fragments, individual pieces of the articular cartilage are reduced by pin manipulation and manual external compression. (Fig. 7.6). A bone tenaculum is often useful to aid in reduction. Once the fracture fragments are anatomically reduced, the K-wires are advanced across the fracture planes into the adjacent fragments to reestablish the articular surface. Fracture reduction should begin with the largest fragments and proceed sequentially to the smaller fragments (29). Some authors

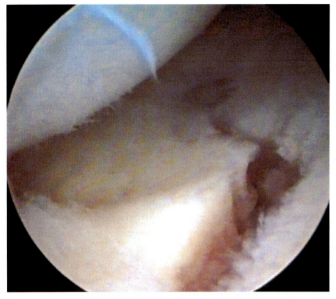 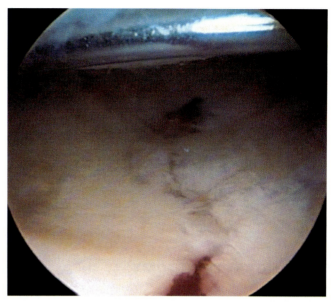

FIGURE 7.6. A: Arthroscopic view of intraarticular distal radius fracture line, left wrist, extending ulnarward toward a small central defect in the triangular fibrocartilage complex. **B:** Arthroscopic view of the same fracture after reduction and cross pinning. Pins are inserted parallel to the 18-gauge needle seen at the top of the image.

advocate reduction of the radial styloid first to provide a landmark to which other fragments are reduced (22,26). Numerous K-wires may be necessary. The hand is pronated and supinated to confirm that the K-wires do not cross the DRUJ.

The technique is somewhat tedious and requires patience but yields a nice articular reconstruction. Intraoperative radiographs or fluoroscopy is utilized to confirm satisfactory fracture reduction of the articular surfaces and to adjust the depth of K-wire penetration. Additional fixation may be required to maintain the normal palmar tilt of the articular surface. This is accomplished with a radial styloid pin across the metaphysis. Significant cortical comminution may be present in Smith's or Colles' fractures and should be addressed with the addition of a volar or dorsal buttress plate, respectively. External fixation should be considered when significant metaphyseal comminution is present. Generally, the external fixator is easier to apply after the articular surface has been reconstructed so that the frame does not interfere with the surgical manipulation of the articular surfaces. If deemed necessary, cancellous bone grafting may be performed through a small incision between the fourth and fifth dorsal compartments (22).

Postoperatively, the pins are bent and cut external to the skin. A short-arm cast or plaster splints are applied and are removed at 2 weeks in most cases. Controlled, gentle passive range-of-motion exercises are then permitted. Early motion with manual traction applied to the fingers prevents joint compression and arthrofibrosis. A functional range splint is used for protection until fracture healing has occurred. Pins are generally removed 3 to 4 weeks postoperatively in the office without anesthesia. In most cases, improved reduction of the articular surface is obtained after ARIF of the distal radius. Reports suggest that 80% good to excellent results can be expected with minimal significant complications (26).

RADIAL STYLOIDECTOMY

A characteristic pattern of arthritis develops following chronic scapholunate dissociation or scaphoid nonunion, both of which dissociate the lunate from the distal carpal row. The capitate migrates proximally, creating shear forces and ultimately degenerative changes at the distal pole of the lunate. The distal pole of the scaphoid is also compressed against the radial styloid, causing concentrated articular degeneration. In response, the radial styloid may elongate from osteophyte formation. This pattern of radioscaphoid and capitolunate degeneration is characterized as scapholunate advanced collapse—a SLAC wrist. In cases of SLAC wrist where radioscaphoid pain is the primary problem and the patient is concerned with expedient pain relief rather than a more definitive treatment plan, an arthroscopic radial styloidectomy is an option. The technique is minimally invasive and requires virtually no recuperation. In many cases, this procedure proves to be extremely effective in reducing SLAC wrist pain and forestalling ultimate intercarpal or complete wrist fusion (59). Arthroscopic radial styloidectomy is performed using the same basic wrist arthroscopy setup as previously described. An inflow cannula is placed in the 6U portal, and a 2.7-mm arthroscope is introduced through the 3–4 portal. A 1–2 arthroscopic portal is created through which a powered burr is manipulated for the radial styloid resection. The burr is utilized to create a sagittal line on the articular surface of the radius midway between the sagittal ridge and the tip of the radial styloid. The burr is then utilized to resect all bone radial to the sagittal line, creating a surface perfectly horizontal to the long access of the radius. Intraoperative radiographs or fluoroscopy is utilized to confirm adequate resection in the appropriate plane. Postoperatively, a sterile compressive dressing is applied for 3 to 5 days, after which range of motion is permitted as comfort allows (59).

DORSAL GANGLIONOTOMY

Dorsal wrist ganglia represent the majority of soft tissue tumors of the hand. Failing conservative treatment, symptomatic dorsal ganglia are generally excised. Open ganglionectomy, however, trades a bump for a scar, and recurrence rates have been reported to be as high as 40% (60). This high failure rate is thought to be the result of inadequate resection of the dorsal ganglion stalk, which is based at the scapholunate ligament and its dorsal capsular attachments. This stalk can be well visualized arthroscopically, appearing as a pearl-like structure emanating dorsal to the scapholunate ligament.

The wrist is positioned in the standard fashion for diagnostic wrist arthroscopy. The arthroscope is introduced through the ulnarly located portals (4–5 or 6R), preserving the 3–4 portal for ganglion wall excision. The 3–4 portal is established directly through the ganglion, and the powered shaver is inserted. The cystic defect and ganglion stalk are excised, and their origin at the lunate and the scaphoid is abraded. Care is taken not to disrupt any more of the scapholunate interosseous ligament than is directly involved in the ganglion. The shaver is slowly withdrawn while the complete ganglion stalk is excised in addition to a small portion of the dorsal wrist capsule. Resection is completed when the overlying extensor tendons are visualized. Care must be taken not to injure the overlying extensor tendons. Postoperatively, a soft compressive dressing is applied, and the patient is allowed immediate use of the hand. Normal activities are allowed within 2 to 3 days of cyst excision (19).

Arthroscopic ganglion resection is a safe and effective procedure. The technique minimizes surgical scarring and results in a lower recurrence rate than open ganglionectomy (27). The procedure results in complete removal of the dorsal wrist ganglion stalk. Failure to excise this stalk in open ganglionectomy procedures is thought to be responsible for their higher recurrence rate. Moreover, the procedure allows for definitive treatment of both the ganglion and all other associated intraarticular pathology.

Although arthroscopic ganglionectomy is considered to be a safe procedure, the small number of wrist arthroscopy cases in the literature precludes an accurate assessment of the true incidence of complications. However, wrist arthroscopy is a safe procedure with overall complication rates reported to be approximately 2% (61). Complications are best avoided by strict adherence to arthroscopic technique and periodic evaluation of the applied traction force across the wrist and the soft tissue compartments of the forearm. Most of the potential complications inherent in wrist arthroscopy are related to the establishment of arthroscopic portals. A thorough knowledge of the anatomy of the dorsal wrist is critical if iatrogenic injury to the sensory nerves, radial artery, and extensor tendons is to be avoided. The principles of arthroscopic wrist portal establishment and the technique of introducing instrumentation into the wrist joint have been thoroughly described. Attention to detail should eliminate most pitfalls related to this procedure.

Wrist arthroscopy is a safe and effective means of diagnosing, staging, and definitively treating a number of afflictions involving the wrist. The technique is unparalleled for examination of the soft tissues and articular structures of the wrist joint. Wrist arthroscopy uniquely allows determination of both the size and extent of all intraarticular wrist pathology. The therapeutic indications for the procedure continue to expand rapidly. The new world of wrist arthroscopy has emerged, permanently changing the past and providing the necessary structure for a stimulating and exciting new future.

EDITORS' COMMENTS

Wrist arthroscopy stormed into the arena on the heels of knee and shoulder arthroscopy in the 1980s. It gave us our first opportunity to directly visualize the surfaces of most of the internal structures of the wrist. We were not prepared for the number and degree of surface abnormalities, synovial fraying, small cartilage defects, tears, flaps, and multiple minor ligament abnormalities. Looming large are the changes on the surface of the triangular fibrocartilage. These are now recognized for their commonness in totally asymptomatic wrists. The decision to operate on a wrist is not based on a diagnosis. The actual decision for surgery is based on the degree of a patient's symptoms, interference with the quality of life, the inability to function at employment, or the intensity of pain. These are the factors that determine surgery, not the diagnosis. There are exceptions such as an asymptomatic scaphoid nonunion in a young individual because of the known propensity for degenerative change. For the most part, we operate to solve a patient's problem. Having first made the decision that repair is indicated, one must then determine what to do about what is causing the problem. With an adequate knowledge of the wrist, it is not necessary to arthroscope and see the pathology before surgery. It is not necessary to know the degree of tear of a triquetral–lunate interosseous ligament rupture. At surgery, if the tear is central and not complete, the problem can be solved with a step-cut shortening of the ulna. If the tear is total, with significant abnormal motion between the triquetrum and lunate, then limited wrist arthrodesis is indicated. An accurate determination of this degree of tear is better done under direct visualization. The wrist surgeon requires the ability to shift gears.

If the diagnosis is dorsal wrist syndrome, and the examiner suspects major tearing of the scapholunate interosseous system in spite of negative x-rays, then the patient and surgeon agree to an option approach. The surgeon carries the option to the operating room of either a dorsal wrist repair and 2 days in a dressing or triscaphe arthrodesis or major ligament reconstruction and 6 weeks in a cast. The degree of tear is better determined at open surgery with the ability to significantly load the interosseous ligament and separate the nonstructural synovial attachments.

Every 30 seconds of surgery may represent a year of patient activity, and it is far more important to see it all and get it right than to be under arthroscopic restrictions for the sake of minimal morbidity variance. This is not to discourage certain surgeons from perfecting arthroscopic techniques that will in time allow some definitive procedures through the arthroscope. From the view of a reconstructive wrist surgeon, arthroscopy is seldom indicated and never necessary.

REFERENCES

1. Wantanabe M, Takeda S, Ikeuchi H. *Atlas of arthroscopy*, 2nd ed. Tokyo: Igaku Shoin, 1969
2. Chen YC. Arthroscopy of the wrist and finger joints. *Orthop Clin North Am* 1979;10:723–733.
3. Whipple TL, Marotta J, Powell JH III. Techniques of wrist arthroscopy. *Arthroscopy* 1986;2:244–252.
4. Weiss AC, Akelman E, Lambiase R. Comparison of the findings of triple-injection cinearthrography of the wrist and those of arthroscopy. *J Bone Joint Surg Am* 1996;78:348–356.
5. Cooney WP. Evaluation of chronic wrist pain by arthrography, arthroscopy, and arthrotomy. *J Hand Surg [Am]* 1993;18: 815–822.
6. Totterman SM, Heberger R, Miller R, et al. Two piece wrist surface coil. *Am J Roentgenol* 1991;156:343–344.
7. Golimbu CN, Firoozania H, Melone CP Jr, et al. Tears of the triangular fibrocartilage complex of the wrist: MR imaging. *Radiology* 1989;173:731–733.
8. Nagle DJ, Benson LS. Wrist arthroscopy: indications and results. *Arthroscopy* 1992;8:198–203.
9. Adolfsson L. Arthroscopy for the diagnosis of post-traumatic wrist pain. *J Hand Surg [Br]* 1992;17:46–50.
10. Bleton R, Alnot JY, Levame JH. Therapeutic possibilities of arthroscopy in chronic painful wrists. Apropos of 27 cases with 55 arthoscopies [French]. *Ann Chir Main Memb Super* 1993;12: 313–325.
11. Sennwald G, Fischer M, Jacob HAC. Radio-carpal and medio-carpal arthroscopy in instability of the wrist [French]. *Ann Chir Main Memb Super* 1993;12:26–38.
12. Wantanabe K, et al. Arthroscopic assessment of Kienböck's disease. *Arthroscopy* 1995;11:257–262.
13. Koman LA, Poehling GG, Toby EB, et al. Chronic wrist pain: indications for wrist arthroscopy. *Arthroscopy* 1990;6:116–119.
14. Savoie F. The role of arthroscopy and the diagnosis and management of cartilaginous lesions of the wrist. *Hand Clin* 1995;11:1–5.
15. Bain G, Roth J. The role of arthroscopy in arthritis. *Hand Clin* 1995;11:51–58.
16. Whipple TL, Cooney WP, Osterman AL, et al. *Wrist arthroscopy* Chapter 10.
17. Rettig ME, Amadio PC. Wrist arthroscopy: indications and clinical applications. *J Hand Surg [Br]* 1994;19:774–777.
18. Whipple TL, Geissler WB. Arthroscopic management of wrist triangular fibrocartilage complex injuries in the athlete. *Orthopedics* 1993;16:1061–1067.
19. Savoie FH, Whipple TL. The role of arthroscopy in athletic injuries of the wrist. *Clin Sports Med* 1996;15:219–233.
20. Whipple TL. The role of arthroscopy in the treatment of wrist injuries in the athlete. *Clin Sports Med* 1992;11:227–238.
21. Whipple TL. The role of arthroscopy in the treatment of intra-articular wrist fractures. *Hand Clin* 1995;11:13–18.
22. Geissler W. Arthroscopically assisted reduction intra-articular fractures of the distal radius. *Hand Clin* 1995;11:19–29.
23. Wolfe S, Easterling K, Yoo H. Arthroscopic-assisted reduction of distal radius fractures. *Arthroscopy* 1995;11:706–714.
24. Leibovic S, Geissler W. Treatment of complex intra-articular distal radius fractures. *Orthop Clin North Am* 1994;25:685–706.
25. Geissler W, Freeland A. Arthroscopically assisted reduction of intra-articular distal radial fractures. *Clin Orthop* 1996;327: 125–134.
26. Culp R, Osterman A. Arthroscopic reduction and internal fixation of distal radius fractures. *Orthop Clin North Am* 1995;26: 739–748.
27. Osterman A, Raphael J. Arthroscopic resection of dorsal ganglion of the wrist. *Hand Clin* 1995;11:7–12.
28. Wnorowski D, Palmer AK, Werner FW, et al. Anatomic and biomechanical analysis of the arthroscopic wafer procedure. *Arthroscopy* 1992;8:204–212.
29. Whipple TL. *Arthroscopic surgery: the wrist*. Philadelphia: JB Lippincott, 1993.
30. Whipple TL, Marotta JJ, Powell JH 3rd. Techniques of wrist arthroscopy. *Arthroscopy* 1986;2:244–252.
31. Bettinger PC, Cooney WP, Borger RA. Arthroscopic anatomy of the wrist. *Orthop Clin North Am* 1995;26:707–719.
32. Viegas SF. Midcarpal arthroscopy: anatomy and portals. *Hand Clin* 1994;10:577–587.
33. Buterbaugh GA. Radiocarpal arthroscopy portals in normal anatomy. *Hand Clin* 1994;10:567–576.
34. Hermansdorfer JC, Kleinman WB. Management of chronic peripheral tears of the triangular fibrocartilage complex. *J Hand Surg [Am]* 1991;16:340–346.
35. Viegas SF. Intraarticular ganglion of the dorsal interosseous scapholunate ligament: a case for arthroscopy. *Arthroscopy* 1986; 2:93–95.
36. Ekenstam FW, Palmer AK, Glisson RR. The load on the radius and ulna in different positions of the wrist and forearm. A cadaver study. *Acta Orthop Scand* 1984;55:363–365.
37. Palmer AK. The distal radioulnar joint. *Hand Clin* 1987;3: 31–40.

38. Palmer AK, Glisson RR, Werner FW. Relationship between ulnar variance and TFCC thickness. *J Hand Surg [Am]* 1984;9:681–683.
39. Palmer AK, Werner FW. The triangular fibrocartilage complex of the wrist—anatomy and function. *J Hand Surg* 1981;6:153–162.
40. Palmer AK, Werner FW. Biomechanics of the distal radioulnar joint. *Clin Orthop* 1984;187:26–31.
41. Palmer AK, Werner FW, Glisson RR, et al. Partial excision of the triangular fibrocartilage complex. *J Hand Surg [Am]* 1988;12:391–394.
42. Chidgey LK. Histologic anatomy of the triangular fibrocartilage. *Hand Clin* 1991;7:249–262.
43. Bednar MS, Arnoczky SP, Weiland AJ. The microvasculature of the triangular fibrocartilage complex: its clinical significance. *J Hand Surg [Am]* 1991;16:1101–1105.
44. Thiru-Pathi RG, Ferlic DC, Clayton ML, et al. Arterial anatomy of the triangular fibrocartilage of the wrist and surgical significance. *J Hand Surg [Am]* 1986;11:258–263.
45. Schmidt HM, Lanz U. *Chirurgische Anatomie der Hand.* Stuttgart: Hippokrates Verlag, 1992.
46. Palmer AK. Triangular fibrocartilage complex lesions: a classification. *J Hand Surg [Am]* 1989;14:594–606.
47. Nagle DJ. Arthroscopic treatment of degenerative tears of the triangular fibrocartilage. *Hand Clin* 1994;10:615–624.
48. Osterman AL, Bori FW, Maitin E. Arthroscopic debridement of triangular fibrocartilage complex tears. *Arthroscopy* 1990;6:120–124.
49. Corso S, Whipple T, Savoie FH, et al. *Arthroscopic repair of triangular fibrocartilage complex lesions of the wrist: a multicenter study.* Paper presented at the annual meeting of the Arthroscopy Association of North America, Orlando, FL, 1994.
50. DeAriv DW, Poehling GG, et al. *Toughy needle technique for peripheral TFCC repair.* Paper presented at the American Society for Surgery of the Hand Annual Meeting, Cincinnati, OH, 1994.
51. Bednar JM, Osterman AL. The role of arthroscopy in the treatment of traumatic triangular fibrocartilage injuries. *Hand Clin* 1994;10:605–614.
52. Palmer AK. Triangular fibrocartilage disorders: injury patterns and treatment. *Arthroscopy* 1990;6:125–132.
53. Jenkins NH, Jones DG, Johnson SR, et al. External fixation of Colles' fractures. *J Bone Joint Surg Br* 1987;69:207–211.
54. Weber SC, Szabo RM. Severely comminuted distal radial fracture as an unsolved problem: complications associated with external fixation and pins and plaster techniques. *J Hand Surg [Am]* 1986;11:157–167.
55. Fernandez DL, Geissler WB. Treatment of displaced articular fractures of the radius. *J Hand Surg [Am]* 1991;16:375–384.
56. Geissler WB, Fernandez DL. Percutaneous and limited open reduction of the articular surface of the distal radius. *J Orthop Trauma* 1991;5:255–267.
57. Hanker GJ. *Wrist arthroscopy and distal radius fractures.* Paper presented in proceedings of the American Academy Orthopedic Surgeons Annual Meeting, Washington, DC, 1992.
58. Richards RS, Roth JH, Bennett JD, et al. *Arthroscopy and distal radius fractures.* Paper presented in proceedings of the American Society For Surgery of the Hand, Cincinnati, OH, 1994.
59. Whipple TL. Advanced wrist arthroscopy procedures. *AAOS Instruct Course Lect* 1996.
60. McEvedy BV. Simple ganglia: a review of modes of treatment and an explanation for the frequent failures of surgery. *Lancet* 1965;266:135.
61. Small NC. Complications in arthroscopy: the knee and other joints. *Arthroscopy* 1986;2:253–258.

8

EXTRAARTICULAR ETIOLOGIES OF WRIST PAIN

MARTTI VASTAMÄKI

Extraarticular wrist pain may result from cutaneous, tenosynovial, neural, vascular, or muscular lesions. In most cases, pain is caused by tenosynovial or neural disorders such as tendinitis/tenosynovitis or nerve entrapment.

Painful cutaneous or subcutaneous lesions such as glomus tumors are very rare in the wrist, as are vascular or muscular lesions. In fact, the only muscles existing in the region of the wrist are hypertrophied extensions of the normal muscles of the wrist tendons (Fig. 8.1) or actual anomalous muscles. The only relevant painful vascular disorders existing at the wrist level are uncommon arteriovenous fistulas or hemangiomas and the hypothenar hammer syndrome.

The purpose of this chapter is to acquaint the reader with the most current knowledge on extraarticular painful disorders involving the wrist.

TENDINOPATHIES

Tendinopathies are, in most cases, related to some kind of tendon overuse. Overuse is defined as a level of repetitive microtrauma sufficient to overwhelm the tissues' ability to adapt. Key risk factors for developing tendinopathies include repetition, high force, awkward joint posture, direct pressure, vibration, and prolonged constrained posture. Some kind of tendinopathy is always present in an overuse syndrome, which may also be called repetitive strain injury or cumulative trauma disorder. Repetitive strain injuries account for the major portion of all occupational illnesses. Tendinopathies are also common in athletes.

At the wrist level, numerous tendons may be affected. Diagnosis of tendinitis or tenosynovitis may be evident, as in de Quervain's disease, or more complicated, as in intersection syndrome. Symptoms and clinical findings may simulate those of tendinitis, but the etiology of various disorders may be of neural origin, even emanating from the brachial plexus as in thoracic outlet syndrome (TOS). In young people under the age of 25 years, tendinopathies are not common without very excessive overuse. A hand surgeon should consider nerve disorders, especially TOS, when faced with a young patient with one or two tenolysis scars in the wrist who is still complaining of persistent pain.

The course and prognosis of tendinopathies, especially overuse syndromes, are understood best by reviewing the pathologic stages of the inflammatory response (1):

1. The inflammatory stage starts immediately after injury, lasting 2 days to 2 weeks unless there is further injury. Clinical symptoms include pain, swelling, erythema, warmth, and tenderness.
2. The proliferative stage lasts 1 to 2 weeks and is a time when collagen and ground substances are produced. The area is highly susceptible to injury during this stage. Only low-level activity is encouraged, and movement should be limited to a pain-free range.
3. During the maturation stage, further healing is completed over 6 to 12 weeks. Full unrestricted activity should be avoided until this process is complete.

A major goal of treatment is to prevent fibrosis. Immobilization of the wrist is important. Most tendinopathies respond well to conservative treatment involving appropriate work and leisure restrictions, immobilization, therapy, nonsteroidal antiinflammatory medication, and occasional steroid injections. Early recognition and appropriate treatment can usually avoid the chronic longstanding problem and the need for surgery.

Overuse Syndromes of the Wrist

The wrist is the most frequent site of tendinitis and overuse syndromes. Tendons are most frequently affected where they pass through a fibroosseus tunnel. Overuse syndromes of the wrist include tenosynovitis of the dorsal wrist exten-

---

M. Vastamäki: Department of Hand Surgery, Orton Hospital, 00280 Helsinki, Finland.

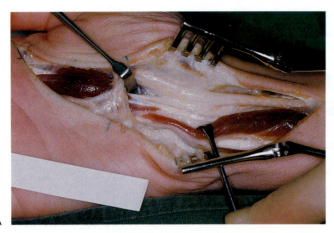 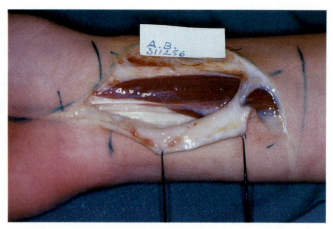

FIGURE 8.1. Hypertrophied extensions of normal muscles of wrist tendons causing symptoms. **A:** Flexor superficialis. **B:** Palmaris longus.

sor compartments and tenosynovitis of the flexor tendons of the wrist. Extensor tenosynovitis can involve any of the extensor tendons found in any of the six dorsal compartments (Table 8.1).

Extensor Compartment Tendinopathies

De Quervain's Disease

The first dorsal compartment contains the abductor pollicis longus (APL) and the extensor pollicis brevis (EPB) confined by the radial styloid and covered by a synovial-lined ligament of 4 cm. The tendons deviate as they pass through the tunnel, and this angle increases with ulnar deviation of the wrist. Anatomic variability is very common. The APL usually has two or more, even four or five, tendon slips (2). The APL and EPB are located within separate compartments in a third of normal individuals (3,4), but patients with de Quervain's disease have this anatomic variation more frequently (5).

De Quervain is credited with first describing stenosing tenosynovitis of the APL and EPB in 1895 (6). It is associated with activities requiring forceful grasp coupled with ulnar deviation or repetitive use of the thumb. Those at risk include knitters, laboratory technicians, carpenters, filing clerks, and mail sorters. Sports, such as racquet sports, golf, fly fishing, javelin, and discus throwing, may also produce the disease. A number of case reports have described rare causes of de Quervain's disease or other conditions resembling it. Weinzweig et al. (7) reported a bilateral case of de Quervain's disease caused by cavernous hemangiomas. Gillet et al. (8) reported a patient with fluoroquinoline-induced tenosynovitis of the first compartment of the wrist mimicking de Quervain's disease. Fromm et al. (9) published a case of an osteoid osteoma of the radial styloid resembling de Quervain's disease.

The presenting symptom of de Quervain's disease is pain on the radial aspect of the wrist and thumb, especially over the radial styloid, intensified by movement of the wrist and thumb. Physical examination reveals tenderness over the radial styloid and often also 1.5 to 2.5 cm distal and/or proximal to it. Swelling of the same area is typical; crepitus and triggering are more rarely seen. In chronic cases, fibrous thickening of the compartment sheath can be palpated.

A positive Finkelstein's test, (i.e., reproduction of pain with ulnar deviation of the wrist while the thumb is adducted causing maximum excursion of the APL and EPB) is typical but not pathognomonic of de Quervain's disease (10). This test must be interpreted with caution. It may also be positive in Wartenberg's syndrome, basilar thumb arthrosis, or intersection syndrome. Deviating the wrist using pressure over the index–metacarpal avoids confusion with thumb conditions. Symptoms can also be produced by resisted thumb extension with the wrist in maximum radial deviation. The differential diagnosis of pain in this region also includes scaphoid fracture and scapho-trapezial arthrosis.

A variation of Finkelstein's test can be useful to rule out incomplete release of previous de Qurevain's disease (11). If the usual Finkelstein's test is positive, full abduction of the APL followed by flexion of the thumb metacarpophalangeal joint will isolate the action of the EPB. Pain will occur if the EPB lies in a separate sheath and was not released.

TABLE 8.1. EXTENSOR COMPARTMENT TENDINITIS

Compartment	Disorder
First	De Quervain's disease
Second	Intersection syndrome
Third	Extensor pollicis longus tendinitis
Fourth	Extensor indicis proprius syndrome
Fifth	Extensor digiti minimi tendinitis
Sixth	Extensor carpi ulnaris tendinitis

Treatment of de Quervain's disease follows the standard protocol for overuse syndromes. Numerous nonoperative and operative treatment modalities have been advocated for this disorder. Nonoperative techniques have centered on the use of steroid and local anesthetic injections into the first dorsal compartment, immobilization of the wrist and thumb in a splint, and a combination of these two methods.

Harvey et al. (12) stressed an accurate injection technique. First, place the needle in the distal end of the compartment while injecting local anesthetic. Swelling at the proximal margin of the extensor retinaculum then confirms correct needle position, and the corticosteroid is delivered into the compartment. They reported that simple injection, without splinting, resolved 80% of de Quervain's disease. Witt et al. (13) reported, in a prospective study, a satisfactory outcome in 62% with simple injection. Weiss et al. (14) compared the use of a mixed steroid/lidocaine injection alone, an immobilization splint alone, and the simultaneous use of both. They recommended the use of a mixed steroid/lidocaine injection alone. No additional benefit was produced by the addition of splint immobilization.

A total lack of progress after 6 to 8 weeks of conservative treatment is an indication that surgical release may be necessary. Surgery involves decompression of the first dorsal compartment with care taken to divide any septation present in the compartment. The compartment for the EPB can be deceptively hidden under or dorsal to the fibrous APL sheath. Because the APL usually has two or more tendon slips, the surgeon may perform an insufficient release. A transverse incision creates a minimal scar, but most authors advocate a longitudinal one, especially because of the risk of injury to the radial sensory nerves (15–18) (Fig. 8.2).

Recognized complications of surgical release include injury to the superficial radial nerves, inadequate decompression, volar tendon subluxation, hypertrophic scarring, tendinous adhesions, and persistent symptoms.

Intersection Syndrome

Intersection syndrome is an inflammatory condition of the second dorsal compartment of the wrist located at the site of intersection of the APL and EPB muscles and the radial wrist extensors, extensor carpi radialis longus (ECRL) and extensor carpi radialis brevis (ECRB) (19). It occurs in active people such as rowers (oarsman's wrist), canoeists, weight lifters, recreational tennis enthusiasts, and industrial workers with repetitive wrist motion.

Pain and swelling over the radiodorsal portion of the distal forearm, 5 cm to 7 cm proximal to Lister's tubercle, differentiates intersection syndrome from the more distal de Quervain's disease. In severe cases, palpable crepitus is noted with wrist or thumb motion (peritendinitis crepitans) (20). An exertional compartment syndrome of the APL and EPB, inflammation or adventitial bursa formation of the intersection of the APL and EPB and ECRL and ECRB, and stenosing tenosynovitis of the ECRL and ECRB have been postulated to be the pathophysiologic etiology of intersection syndrome (21–23).

Initial treatment includes rest, splinting in 20° of wrist extension, antiinflammatory medication, and a corticosteroid injection. Phonophoresis and deep friction massage followed by exercises for stretching and strengthening may be useful (24). Surgical treatment is seldom necessary; it consists of release and tenosynovectomy of the second dorsal compartment, exploration of the intersection zone with debridement of any inflammatory or bursal tissue, and release of the fascial sheaths of the APL and EPB.

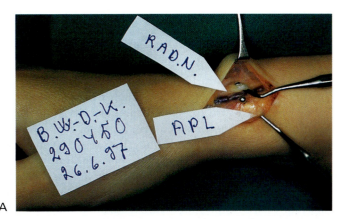 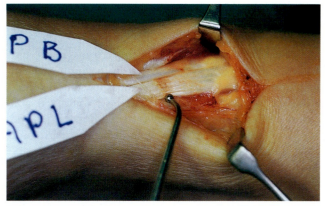

FIGURE 8.2. Author's approach to de Quervain's disease. **A:** One of three or four branches of the radial sensory nerve lies very close to the tendons. *APL,* abductor pollicis longus; *RAD.N.,* radial sensory nerve. **B:** Extensor pollicis brevis and abductor pollicis longus tendons are released from their separate sheaths. *PB,* extensor pollicis brevis. **Editors' Notes:** *A transverse incision with blunt spreading dissection protects the superficial radial nerves and allows excellent visualization of the entire first dorsal compartment. Cosmesis in this very noticeable area is significantly better than with a longitudinal incision.*

Extensor Pollicis Longus Tendinitis

Extensor pollicis longus (EPL) tendinitis rarely occurs as an isolated condition, although it can develop with activities that require repetitive thumb and wrist motion. Predisposing factors include rheumatoid arthritis, direct trauma, and distal radius fracture. The EPL is at risk of developing tenosynovitis as it passes around Lister's tubercle (25). Pain aggravated by motion of the thumb is located on the ulnar edge of the anatomic snuff box. Tenosynovitis of the EPL and subsequent rupture of the tendon were first reported in Prussian drummers (drummer boy's palsy) (26). Stenosing tenosynovitis occurs when the EPL muscle extends into a tight third compartment, constricting normal thumb flexion.

The EPL tendon attrition and rupture are more likely to occur after a nondisplaced, rather than a displaced, distal radius fracture (27,28). Overall, overuse is an unusual cause of rupture. It usually occurs after a Colles' fracture or in patients with rheumatoid arthritis.

Treatment of EPL tenosynovitis is the same as that for de Quervain's disease except injections are not proposed because of the possibility of circulatory compromise of the tendon. Surgical treatment consists of release of the third dorsal compartment and transposition of the EPL dorsal to the extensor retinaculum.

Extensor Indicis Proprius Syndrome

Tenosynovitis of the fourth dorsal compartment presents as pain, tenderness, and swelling over the dorsum of the hand and wrist. Tenosynovitis of the common digital extensors is uncommon except in rheumatoid arthritis.

Ritter and Inglis described the extensor indicis proprius (EIP) syndrome in 1969 (29). The musculotendinous junction of the EIP enters the fourth dorsal compartment in 75% of patients (30). The cause of discomfort is thought to be muscular hypertrophy following exercise or synovitis from repetitive motion.

Spinner and Olshansky (31) described a diagnostic test in which the patient's wrist is placed in maximum flexion and the index finger is extended against resistance, reproducing the patient's pain in a positive test. Weinzweig and Watson refer to a similar maneuver as the finger extension test (FET) (see Chapter 5). Swelling distal to the extensor retinaculum may also be the result of a dorsal carpal ganglion or, in rare cases, hypertrophy of an extensor digitorum brevis muscle.

In addition to standard treatment, a forearm-based splint extending over the metacarpophalangeal joints can be employed. As symptoms may be slow to resolve, at least 3 to 4 months of conservative treatment should be allowed before considering surgery (i.e., decompression/release of the fourth compartment and tenosynovectomy).

Extensor Digiti Minimi Tendinitis

Extensor digiti minimi (EDM) tendinitis of the fifth dorsal compartment is occasionally reported after wrist trauma and overuse (32–34). Pain and swelling on the dorsum of the wrist, just distal to the ulnar head, may be found on examination. The EDM tenosynovitis can be associated with the inability to extend the little finger at the metacarpophalangeal joint. Treatment involves the use of an ulnar gutter splint, antiinflammatory medication, and corticosteroid injection into the fifth dorsal compartment. If decompression becomes necessary, care must be taken to avoid damage to the dorsal sensory branch of the ulnar nerve. Surgical exploration may reveal multiple tendon slips of the EDM (34).

Extensor Carpi Ulnaris Tendinitis

Extensor carpi ulnaris (ECU) tendinitis is the second most common stenosing tenosynovitis of the wrist. It is one of many pathologic entities that produce pain and swelling along the dorsal ulnar aspect of the wrist, and therefore, this diagnosis may be overlooked. An ECU tendinidis may occur secondary to posttraumatic ECU subluxation as well as in athletes participating in sports that require repetitive wrist motion, such as rowing, baseball, golf, and racquet sports. Often the patient can recall a specific insult, usually a direct blow or a twisting injury of the wrist (35). A predisposing cause may be recurrent subluxation of the ECU tendon following a tear in the ulnar side of the compartment.

The ECU is unique among the extensor tendons because it passes through its own fibroosseous tunnel, separate from the overlying extensor retinaculum (36). The fibrous sheath overlying the ECU may be ruptured in forced supination, flexion, and ulnar deviation of the wrist (1). This rupture may occur even with an intact extensor retinaculum resulting in subluxation of the ECU and tenosynovitis (37).

On examination, tenderness along the ECU tendon is increased by resisted ulnar deviation and forced radial deviation. Normally, firm fusiform swelling of the sixth compartment is present (35,38,39). Subluxation of the ECU may be elicited with supination and ulnar deviation of the wrist. This deviation can result in a painful snap over the dorsal ulnar wrist (40). Splinting the wrist in extension, pronation, and radial deviation, plus antiinflammatory medication, relieves the symptoms in most cases without severe subluxation tendency. An ECU subluxation may not be immediately apparent because of swelling, and the injury may be misdiagnosed as a wrist sprain. If tendon subluxation continues with unrelieved symptoms, surgical reconstruction of the ulnar wall of the compartment should be performed by creating a sling of the extensor retinaculum or with a free retinacular graft (41).

Flexor Compartment Tendinopathies

Flexor Carpi Radialis Tendinitis

Flexor carpi radialis (FCR) tendinitis is an uncommon cause of radial-volar wrist pain. The comparatively high prevalence of other disorders in this region, combined with a low index of suspicion of FCR tendinitis, may result in a failure to diagnose the condition and to provide appropriate treatment (42). It may be a primary condition as a part of an overuse syndrome or a secondary condition associated with soft tissue or osseous abnormalities adjacent to the tendon. The FCR passes through a synovial tunnel bordered by the scaphoid tuberosity, trapezial ridge, and transverse carpal ligament deviating 30° dorsally over the volar pole of the scaphoid. It has been suggested that this angulation may create mechanical irritation and predispose to tenosynovitis in repetitive wrist motions (43).

Several authors have described FCR tendinitis as a nonspecific tenosynovitis, occasionally associated with arthritis of the scaphotrapezial joint (44,45). If a nodule develops, it can block wrist rotation and produce a trigger wrist (46). Rupture of the tendon may be the end result of invasive synovitis. Tenosynovial ganglia around the FCR can also be painful (Fig. 8.3). Wrist immobilization, antiinflammatory medication, and a corticosteroid injection are often successful treatment modalities. Surgery may be needed in refractory cases. Surgical release should be carried far enough distally to confirm that the tunnel has been completely decompressed. The intraoperative findings include adhesions, attrition or rupture of the tendon, exostosis, stenosis, and anomalous tendon slips (44). In FCR rupture, simple debridement of the stump without reconstruction can provide effective pain relief (1).

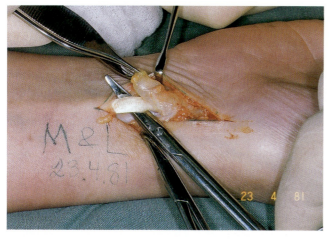

FIGURE 8.3. Tenosynovial ganglion of the flexor carpi radialis tendon.

Linburg's Syndrome

An anomalous tendinous interconnection between the flexor pollicis longus (FPL) and index finger profundus causing pain and tenderness in the distal forearm with repetitive use was described by Linburg and Comstock (47). The pathonomonic sign is simultaneous index finger interphalangeal joint flexion when the thumb is flexed actively across the palm. This anomalous interconnection is rather common; cadaveric studies revealed a 25% incidence of interconnections (47). However, only a few people develop clinical symptoms. Similar symptoms may also exist with synovial hypertrophy and tendon adhesions between the FPL and index finger profundus without any anomaly (48).

In cases of chronic Linburg's syndrome with clinical evidence of the anomaly, surgical excision of the anomalous tendinous interconnection and tenosynovectomy to restore independent motion of the index finger and thumb should be considered.

Flexor Carpi Ulnaris Tendinitis

The most common wrist flexor to become involved with tendinitis is the flexor carpi ulnaris (FCU). Tendinitis of the FCU presents with pain along the volar-ulnar side of the wrist with activities that require repetitive wrist flexion in ulnar deviation. Pain, tenderness, and swelling in this area, especially in the distal part just on the pisiform bone, may also be caused by arthrosis of the pisiform–triquetrial joint or old fractures of the pisiform bone (49,50). Both of those are associated with a positive pisotriquetral grind test. With a positive test, crepitus is noted when sliding the pisiform radially and ulnarly on the triquetrum. With FCU tendinitis, the pain is particularly exacerbated by wrist flexion and ulnar deviation against resistance. Calcific deposits are occasionally present in the FCU tendon (51–53).

In addition to standard treatment, a dorsal splint with 25° of wrist flexion may be helpful. If surgical treatment is required, it is the same for tendinitis and arthritis, involving removal of the pisiform and an optional 5-mm Z-plasty lengthening of the FCU (49,50,54). The ulnar neuromuscular bundle lies on the radial border of the pisiform and must be protected during surgery. After removal of the pisiform, the hand may still exhibit a reduction in strength as well as pain in conjunction with stress (50).

COMPRESSION NEUROPATHIES

Compression neuropathies, or nerve entrapment syndromes, result from chronic compression of the nerve inducing ischemia of the nerve (55). Endoneurial pressure increases after compression, leading to venous congestion, relative ischemia, increased vascular permeability, and a change in local ionic composition that alters conduction. Nerve entrapment may result from a single violent force or from repetitive stress causing swelling of the nerve and surrounding tissues or from more chronic, even rather slight, compression.

The degree of nerve injury in a compression neuropathy may vary. It may be only slight conduction block, a very temporary loss of axial excitability in acute nerve compression that can recover in a few seconds or minutes after compression. A typical example is transient peroneal nerve symptoms when sitting cross-legged. In real neurapraxia, a loss of axon excitability is caused by segmental demyelination. Prognosis is good, resulting in complete recovery over a few days or weeks, depending on the duration of injury and the need for remyelination. Axonotmesis implies axonal injury where the connective tissue supporting the structure of the nerve remains intact. It is a more chronic form of nerve injury, but prognosis is still good, providing there is adequate early release of the nerve. Recovery time depends on the distance from the lesion site to the end organ, axonal growth being approximately 1 mm per day. Sunderland's fourth-degree injury, in which the nerve is physically in continuity but not functioning because the nerve continuity is maintained only with scar tissue, may be the end result of severe longstanding nerve compression. Neurotmesis is a complete disruption of the structure of the nerve and requires surgical intervention with nerve repair. Because of the tendency of a nerve compression injury to worsen over time, it is important in many cases to consider early surgical treatment. On the other hand, diagnosis of nerve entrapment should be reliably confirmed, and suitable methods of conservative treatment should have been offered before surgery is performed.

The patient's symptoms are related to the motor and sensory functions of the nerve. In mild nerve compression, the symptoms are not persistent; there is no muscle wasting or abnormal moving or two-point discrimination. Tinel's sign is negative, and the patient will generally complain of abnormal sensibility and weakness. In moderate entrapment, the symptoms still are not persistent but are more troublesome through the day. In the severe category, the patient has persistent sensory changes, muscle wasting, and abnormal two-point discrimination. The signs and symptoms may vary according to use of the extremity and the degree of ischemia, demyelination, and degeneration occurring in the involved nerve (56).

The diagnosis of nerve entrapment is based on history, symptoms, clinical findings, and electrodiagnostic studies.

Carpal Tunnel Syndrome

Carpal tunnel syndrome (CTS) is the most common compressive neuropathy. Compression of the median nerve in the osteofibrous carpal tunnel is caused by the transverse carpal ligament and carpal bones. The contents of the carpal tunnel include the nine flexor tendons and the median nerve. The volume of the tunnel is only slightly greater than the volume of its soft tissue contents. Any process decreasing the volume of the tunnel, such as deformity after a fracture, or increasing the volume of its contents, as with synovial proliferation or even simple fluid retention or fat deposition, may cause nerve compression. The position of the wrist may be decisive. The pressure inside the carpal tunnel can significantly increase with the wrist in extreme extension or flexion (57).

The median nerve at the wrist is 94% sensory and only 6% motor (58). Therefore, dysfunction usually is manifested by sensory changes such as dysesthesia or pain, paresthesia, numbness, or a pins-and-needles sensation with tingling in the $3^{1}/_{2}$ radial digits. The most commonly involved finger is usually the middle finger. Nocturnal paresthesias and pain are almost universal for CTS. The condition may awaken the patient at night, is worse with activities, and is helped when the hand is elevated or rested. Shaking the hand usually helps, too. The patients frequently complain of clumsiness and weakness when performing grip-related activities. The symptoms may come and go. The patient may feel a tight band around the wrist. Sometimes, intensive shoulder pain may be caused by CTS. A more severe degree of the CTS results in abnormal two-point discrimination with weakness and atrophy of the thenar muscles.

The most common cause of CTS is flexor tenosynovitis usually associated with repeated forced hand movements or continuous flexion or extension of the wrist, as noted in electronics assembly workers, typists, cutters, musicians, packers, and carpenters, and associated with many kinds of sports, such as lacrosse, gymnastics, cycling, and racquet sports. There is an increased incidence of CTS in patients with diabetes, thyroid disease, rheumatoid arthritis and in pregnancy. Obesity is also a remarkable predisposing factor for CTS, and, in fact, according to my personal experience, 10% loss of body weight may eliminate the symptoms even in a moderate degree of CTS. In rare cases, the cause of symptoms may be a tumor mass compressing the nerve (Fig. 8.4).

Although the diagnosis of CTS may be very clear in severe and even in moderate cases, electrodiagnostic studies are important because such studies actually represent the only completely objective test for this condition. Before performing surgery, it is important to have positive electromyelogram (EMG) findings for CTS, especially in mild cases. If EMG and nerve conduction studies are normal, it is not wise to operate. The cause of symptoms may originate from other structures or more proximally. On the other hand, the lack of an abnormal nerve conduction test does not exclude a diagnosis of CTS, especially early in the course of the process.

Initial treatment of CTS consists of activity modification, rest, antiinflammatory medication, and splinting at night. Corticosteroid injections may provide relief in most

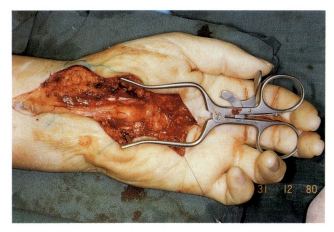

FIGURE 8.4. Lipoma in the carpal tunnel beneath the median nerve causing symptoms.

patients, but this relief is often temporary (59). Surgery is indicated if symptoms progress, there is no improvement within 3 months, or thenar muscle weakness or atrophy is present. There are various methods to divide the transverse carpal ligament, including endoscopy and limited incision techniques.

Carpal tunnel release (CTR) is among the most frequently performed surgical procedures. The transverse carpal ligament forms a 5-cm tunnel extending from the transverse wrist crease to the midpalm. The potential existence of anatomic variations of the median nerve, including variations in the course of the thenar branch and high divisions of the median nerve, is one argument for performing open CTR. I prefer an axillary block. A pneumatic tourniquet is placed on the arm and inflated 80 to 90 mm Hg above the systolic blood pressure. My approach is a straight incision of 3 to 4 cm in the midline just distal to the distal transverse wrist crease. The transverse carpal ligament is divided sharply longitudinally along its ulnar border until its distal edge. If the ligament is very thick, it may be beneficial to resect 2 to 3 mm of its radial part to avoid recurrences. Other adjunctive procedures such as synovectomy, epineurotomy, or internal neurolysis are seldom indicated (60). The results of open CTR are usually favorable, with 96% success (61). In fact, if adequate CTR does not alleviate the patient's symptoms, it is reasonable to consider another etiology of the symptoms.

Endoscopic carpal tunnel release (ECTR) has become a popular alternative for open CTR. It was introduced by three independent surgeons: Agee, Chow, and Okutsu (62–64). Indications for the use of ECTR are the same for treatment of this condition by other surgical means. Absolute contraindications include known anatomic abnormalities and a stiff wrist. Relative contraindications include revision surgery, synovial hyperplasia, and previous tendon surgery.

There are two different techniques for ECTR, the one-portal Agee (62) or Okutsu (64) techniques and the two-portal Chow technique (63). The objective of ECTR is to release the median nerve in the same way as in open surgery, by complete release of the carpal canal under complete endoscopic visualization with minimal surgical invasiveness (see Chapter 9). The technique of ECTR depends on adequate visualization of the transverse fibers of the carpal ligament and a thorough knowledge of the topographical landmarks. Many complications have been reported in association with ECTR, including transection of the median nerve or its branches, the ulnar nerve, and the superficial palmar arch (65–67). On the other hand, after ECTR, patients show greater grip and pinch strength with less scar and pillar tenderness at earlier postoperative periods than do patients after open CTR (62). In experienced hands, complications of ECTR are few (68).

"Intermediary" techniques have also been described, such as the short-incision open technique and the short-incision "device" technique. In Nathan's technique, CTR surgery consists of a short incision of 2 to 2.5 cm, never extending closer that 1.5 cm distal to the distal wrist crease (69). The incision is covered with a soft dressing; splints are not used. In Strickland's technique (70), the transverse carpal ligament is divided by a special device, the "Indiana tome," through a 2- to 2.5-cm palmar incision. The short term results were 92% success.

Guyon's Syndrome

Ulnar nerve entrapment at the wrist most commonly occurs in Guyon's canal or tunnel. It is usually caused by a ganglion arising from the triquetrohamate joint. Guyon's canal is approximately 4 cm in length, extending from the proximal edge of the palmar carpal ligament to the fibrous arch of the hypothenar muscles (71). The motor fascicles are the ulnarmost fascicles in the ulnar nerve as it approaches the wrist. Distal to the pisiform bone, the motor fascicles lie deep to the sensory fascicles to enter the deep tunnel crossing the pisohamate ligament and go beneath the fibrous arch of the hypothenar muscles as the deep motor branch (56). Gross and Gelbermann (71) divided Guyon's tunnel into three zones to correlate clinical symptoms with the anatomic features of this region. The zones are based on a relationship between the internal topography of the nerve and the structures surrounding it. Zone I consists of the portion of the ulnar tunnel proximal to the bifurcation of the nerve; zone II includes the area surrounding the deep motor branch; and zone III includes the space through which the superficial branch of the nerve extends. Mackinnon and Dellon (56), however, believe that description of the patient's symptom complex in terms of motor and sensory distribution of the complaints and findings, and the relationship of these findings to the anatomic site along the ulnar nerve, can best be described in relation to the known anatomic landmarks, such as the pisiform and the hamate. Anatomic variations of the ulnar nerve and

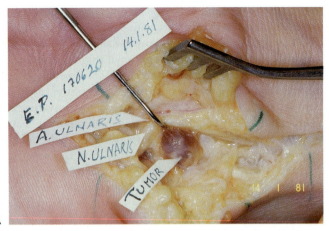 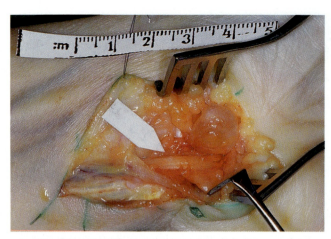

FIGURE 8.5. Ganglion compressing the ulnar nerve in Guyon's canal **(A)** and proximal to it **(B)**.

adjacent tissues at the wrist level are not infrequent and may contribute to entrapment of the nerve, complicating the diagnosis. The deep motor branch may anastomose with the median nerve (72). A part of the deep motor branch may pass through the carpal tunnel (73). Variations in the sensory distribution of the ulnar nerve have been described by many authors. The sensory distribution of the ulnar nerve may extend to the radial aspect of the middle finger (74). Anomalous muscle bellies of the normally existing muscles with abnormal variations in size, shape, or location or anomalous accessory muscles may cause entrapment of the ulnar nerve at the wrist level (75–77). An anomalous extension of the palmaris longus or an accessory palmaris muscle is one such example (78).

Ganglia have been reported to be responsible for more than 85% of nontraumatic cases of Guyon's syndrome (79). Most ganglia arise from the volar aspect of the carpus (Fig. 8.5). A cystic mass may not be palpable but can easily be detected by ultrasound, computed tomography, or magnetic resonance imaging. Of course, any tumor may occur along the course of the ulnar nerve at the wrist level, such as lipomas and rheumatoid synovial cysts.

Fractures of the hook of the hamate and distal radius or ulna are the most common traumatic causes of ulnar nerve compression at the wrist level (80,81). Fractures of the hook of the hamate may be especially difficult to diagnose without computed tomography. Removal of the nonunited fragment may be needed. A malunited fracture, or even a united fracture without malunion, may cause impingement as a result of subsequent scarring during healing.

Repetitive strain injury, occupational or work-related trauma with repetitive blows, or vibratory trauma can also cause Guyon's syndrome. In hypothenar hammer syndrome, repetitive blows to the hypothenar region result in thrombosis of the ulnar artery (Fig. 8.6) with typical symptoms and signs: chronic pain in the hypothenar region, loss of strength, cold sensitivity, and inability to use the hand normally. In performing an Allen's test, circulation through the ulnar artery is not found. Treatment is resection and reconstruction of the ulnar artery, but resection of only the thrombosed 2- to 3-cm part of artery may alleviate symptoms sufficiently.

Typical compression neuropathy or ulnar neuropathy may occur in bicycle riders from the hypothenar eminence pressing against the bicycle during long rides (82). This palsy normally resolves by avoiding bicycling.

Various other conditions, such as burns (83) and electrical injuries, may cause ulnar nerve entrapment at the wrist. In CTS, coexisting distal ulnar nerve symptoms and signs are very common (84). Thus, some authors have advocated simultaneous decompression of both nerves when operating on CTS. However, I consider this unnecessary, even harmful.

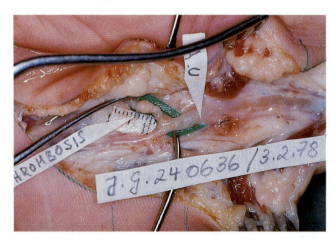

FIGURE 8.6. Thrombosis of the ulnar artery in hypothenar hammer syndrome.

Wartenberg's Syndrome

Entrapment of the radial sensory nerve was first introduced by Robert Wartenberg in 1932 (85). The site of entrapment is the point where the nerve emerges between the tendons of the ECRL and brachioradialis in the distal third of the forearm. The radial sensory nerve begins to branch after it has become subcutaneous. Its branches go to the dorsoradial aspect of the thumb, to the web space between the thumb and index finger, and to the proximal interphalangeal level of the dorsal aspect of the index, middle, ring, and little fingers. There is extensive overlap from dorsal sensory branches of the ulnar nerve and from branches of the lateral antebrachial cutaneous nerve (86). Dellon et al. believe the radial sensory nerve is tethered, causing a "scissoring" effect as it becomes superficial between the named tendons (56). The patient complains of pain, numbness, or tingling over the dorsoradial aspect of the hand. Symptoms of Wartenberg's syndrome or cheiralgia paresthetica are paresthesias or dysesthesias over the dorsoradial aspect of the forearm, wrist, and hand. On physical examination, a Tinel's sign may be positive along the course of the radial sensory nerve. There may also be a positive Finkelstein's test despite the position of the thumb. Repetitive supination and pronation as well as extensive wrist movements predispose to symptoms as in repetitive occupational tasks or sports such as rowing. This compression can occur also from the so-called handcuff neuropathy. Dellon and Mackinnon (56) described a provocative test in which the patient places his arm in front and hyperpronates the forearm with the wrist in ulnar deviation. With a positive test, the patient feels numbness and tingling over the dorsoradial aspect of the hand within 1 minute. There is often a history of trauma of the dorsolateral aspect of the forearm.

The diagnosis can be established by nerve conduction studies. One should take into account the normal overlapping between the radial sensory nerve and lateral antebrachial cutaneous nerve and be sure to measure both nerves. Nonoperative treatment, such as rest in overuse cases and steroid injections, may be very helpful. If surgery is needed, the fascia between the brachioradialis and ECRL tendons is split, and the radial sensory nerve is freed through a short incision on the dorsal radial aspect of the forearm. According to Mackinnon and Dellon (56), entrapment of the radial sensory nerve is surely more common than it has been diagnosed. They believe, as do I, that this entity is most commonly misdiagnosed as de Quervain's disease.

Thoracic Outlet Syndrome

TOS may be a cause of wrist pain. It results from compression of the nerves and/or vessels supplying the upper limb at the level of the thoracic outlet, that is, from the interscalene interval to the level of the coracoid process. Patients' clinical complaints reflect which structures are being compressed within the thoracic outlet. Most patients have symptoms as a result of nerve compression.

The mean age of the TOS patients needing surgical treatment is approximately 35 years (87), but, especially in younger patients, TOS should be considered in cases with chronic vague symptoms involving the wrist. If a 20-year-old woman has been operated on for tendinitis at the wrist without success and still without any specific clinical findings, a proximal cause of the symptoms is likely.

The symptoms of TOS vary from patient to patient. However, the history of the syndrome often reveals the same modalities, including pain and numbness or tingling in the involved area, mostly on the dorsum of the hand and the middle, ring, and little fingers. The patient has difficulties using the hand above the shoulder level, as when combing hair or adjusting curtains. Reading a newspaper or book in supine position may also be difficult, as well as driving a car, because of easy fatigability of the arm. The sensory findings are often subtle and usually occur on both the ulnar and dorsal aspects of the hand and wrist and the medial aspect of the forearm.

The diagnosis of TOS is often based on the patient's history. Provocative positioning tests should be interpreted carefully. The patient should complain of reproduction of symptoms when the arm is placed in the provocative position. Some tests, including Adson's maneuver and the Roos elevation test, may be positive in totally asymptomatic people.

The treatment of TOS is conservative whenever possible. The cornerstone of conservative treatment is an individually designed and intelligently taught postural reeducation and muscle-strengthening program in which the patient must play an active and intensive role. If conservative treatment does not alleviate symptoms over 6 to 12 months, surgical treatment, including scalenotomy or first rib resection, may be necessary (88).

EDITORS' COMMENTS

Most surgeons familiar with de Quervain's disease and radial wrist symptoms frequently prompt unnecessary release of this first dorsal tunnel. Common confusion arises between the positive articular–nonarticular (ANA) junction pain of the scaphoid, de Quervain's tunnel, and the carpometacarpal (CMC) joint (Editors' Fig. 8.1). These lie within a centimeter of one another but are not difficult to differentiate. The radialmost edge of the scaphoid hides behind the styloid in radial deviation and is asymptomatic under direct pressure. With ulnar deviation, the ANA junction is exposed, and if synovitis is present, this area will be acutely tender. The first compartment tunnel is prominent and lies proximal on the radius. The CMC joint lies distal and having positive abduction, adduction and grind maneuvers is more eas-

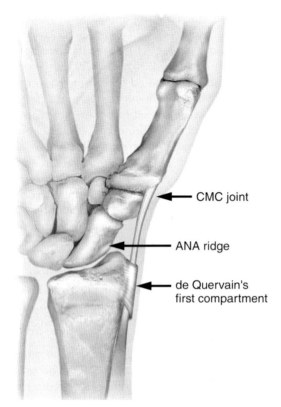

EDITORS' FIGURE 8.1. A common clinical confusion involves identification of three quite proximate areas: the carpometacarpal (CMC) joint, the articular–nonarticular (ANA) junction of the scaphoid, and de Quervain's first compartment. A simple approach is to identify each anatomic area accurately and place a small ink dot over the CMC joint, the ridge, and 5 or 6 mm proximal to the distal edge of the de Quervain's tunnel. With these in place, palpable tenderness is accurately discernible.

ily differentiated. In the normal wrist, there is some tenderness at the ANA junction in everyone. This should not be confusing once the examiner is aware of these three areas capable of producing pain on the radialmost side of the wrist.

Intertendinous connections, particularly in the distal portion of the forearm, are the norm. Most people demonstrate some form of intertendinous connections. The most common are demonstrated by the hitchhiker sign, wherein tendinous connections run from distally on the FPL to proximally on the flexor digitorum profundus of the index. Holding the thumb in maximum hyperextension abduction and making a tight fist will produce pain in the volar aspect of the distal forearm and wrist. There is a similar connection running from distally on the flexor digitorum profundus of the index to proximally on the FPL. Maintaining all four fingers in maximum active hyperextension and then bringing the thumb's tip as far down the fifth metacarpal as possible reproduces the burning sensation. Supernumerary muscle belly syndrome is the pain produced in the forearm by abnormal tendon connections. Burning pain occurs normally from the profundus interconnections if a single digit is held fully extended while the other fingers make a powerful fist. The patient will recognize this pain in the normal arm as being the same as the symptomatic problem in the involved opposite arm in supernumerary muscle belly syndrome.

Small symptomatic ganglia can occur around the wrist and arise within the tendinous structure. These are very rare. Their etiology is not clear. They are easily identified by the fact that they move with the complete excursion of the tendon within which they exist. They demonstrate no connection to a joint.

Extensor brevis manus is an aberrant muscle, typically lying on the dorsum of the wrist, frequently misdiagnosed as a ganglion or synovial mass. Simple excision is sufficient treatment. If an extensor brevis manus is noticed at surgery being carried out for other reasons, it should be excised.

There is a condition with highly localized pain and tenderness at the point where the FCR enters the tunnel in the trapezium. The etiology is not clear. It is effective to remove the trapezium bony roof over the FCR. There is commonly a separate insertion of a portion of the FCR into the trapezium, and this is transected. This condition is not the typical FCR tendinitis, which is more diffuse and involves the tendon.

REFERENCES

1. Kiefhaber TR, Stern P. Upper extremity tendinitis and overuse syndromes in the athlete. *Clin Sports Med* 1992;11:39–55.
2. Bahm J, Szabo Z, Foucher G. The anatomy of de Quervain's disease. A study of operative findings. *Int Orthop* 1995;19:209–211.
3. Leao L. De Quervains's disease. *J Bone Joint Surg Am* 1958;40:1063–1070.
4. Giles KW. Anatomic variations affecting the surgery of de Quervain's disease. *J Bone Joint Surg Br* 1960;42:352–355.
5. Jackson WT, Viegas SF, Coon TM, et al. Anatomic variations in the first extensor compartment of the wrist. *J Bone Joint Surg Am* 1986;68:923–926.
6. De Quervain F. Über eine Form von chronischer Tendovaginitis. *Korrespbl Schweizer Ärzte* 1895;25:389.
7. Weinzweig J, Watson HK, Wiener B, et al. Hemangioma of the extensor pollicis brevis in the first dorsal compartment: An unusual cause of bilateral de Quervain's disease. *J Hand Surg [Am]* 1996;21:256–258.
8. Gillet P, Hestin D, Renoult E, et al. Fluoroquinolone-induced tenosynovitis of the wrist mimicking de Quervain's disease. *Br J Rheum* 1995;34:583–584.
9. Fromm B, Martini A, Schmidt E. Osteoid osteoma of the radial styloid mimicking stenosing tenosynovitis. *J Hand Surg [Br]* 1992;17:236–238.
10. Finkelstein H. Stenosing tendovaginitis at the radial styloid process. *J Bone Joint Surg* 1930;12:509.
11. Louis DS. Incomplete release of the first dorsal compartment—a diagnostic test. *J Hand Surg [Am]* 1987;12:87–88.
12. Harvey FJ, Harvey PM, Horsley MW. De Quervain's disease:

Surgical or nonsurgical treatment. *J Hand Surg [Am]* 1990;15: 83–87.
13. Witt J, Pess G, Gelberman RH. Treatment of de Quervain's tenosynovitis. *J Bone Joint Surg Am* 1991;73:219–222.
14. Weiss A-PC, Akelman E, Tabatabai M. Treatment of de Quervain's disease. *J Hand Surg [Am]* 1994;19:595–598.
15. Murphy ID. An unusual form of de Quervain's syndrome. *J Bone Joint Surg Am* 1949;31:858–859.
16. Loomis LK. Variations of stenosing tenosynovitis at the radial styloid process. *J Bone Joint Surg Am* 1951;33:340–346.
17. Bruner JM. Optimum skin incision for the surgical relief of stenosing tenosynovitis in the hand. *Plast Reconstr Surg* 1966;38:197–201.
18. Alegado RB, Meals RA. An unusual complication following surgical treatment of de Quervain's disease. *J Hand Surg [Am]* 1979; 4:185–186.
19. Dobyns JH, Sim FH, Linscheid RL. Sports stress syndromes of the hand and wrist. *Am J Sports Med* 1978;6:236–253.
20. Howard NJ. Peritendinitis crepitans: A muscle-effort syndrome. *J Bone Joint Surg* 1937;19:447–459.
21. Grundberg AB, Reagan DS. Pathologic anatomy of the forearm: Intersection syndrome. *J Hand Surg [Am]* 1985;10:299–302.
22. Wood MB, Linscheid RL. Abductor pollicis bursitis. *Clin Orthop* 1973;93:293–296.
23. Williams JGP. Surgical management of traumatic non-infective tenosynovitis of the wrist extensors. *J Bone Joint Surg Br* 1977;59: 408–410.
24. Hunter SC, Poole RM. The chronically inflamed tendon. *Clin Sports Med* 1987;6:371–388.
25. Lanzetta M, Howard M, Conolly WB. Post-traumatic triggering of extensor pollicis longus at the dorsal radial tubercle. *J Hand Surg [Br]* 1995;20:398–401.
26. Dums F. Uber Trommlerlahmungen. *Dtsch Mil Zeitschr* 1896; 25;145.
27. Denman EE. Rupture of the extensor pollicis longus—a crush injury. *Hand* 1979;11:295–298.
28. Engkvist O, Lundborg G. Rupture of the extensor pollicis longus tendon after fracture of the lower end of the radius—a clinical and microangiographic study. *Hand* 1979;11:76–86.
29. Ritter MA, Inglis AE. The extensor indicis proprius syndrome. *J Bone Joint Surg Am* 1969;51:1645–1648.
30. Cauldwell EW, Anson BJ, Wright RR. The extensor indicis proprius muscle: A study of 263 consecutive specimens. *Q Bull Northwestern Univ Med School* 1943;17:267–279.
31. Spinner M, Olshansky K. The extensor indicis proprius syndrome. *Plast Reconstr Surg* 1973;51:134–138.
32. Drury BJ. Traumatic tendovaginitis of the fifth dorsal compartment of the wrist. *Arch Surg* 1960;80:554.
33. Ambrose J, Goldstone R. Anomalous extensor digiti minimi proprius causing tunnel syndrome in the dorsal compartment. *J Bone Joint Surg Am* 1975;57:706–707.
34. Hooper G, McMaster MJ. Stenosing tenovaginitis affecting the tendon of the extensor digiti minimi at the wrist. *Hand* 1979; 11:299–301.
35. Crimmins CA, Jones NF. Stenosing tenosynovitis of the extensor capri ulnaris. *Ann Plast Surg* 1995;35:105–107.
36. Spinner M, Kaplan EB. Extensor carpi ulnaris. Its relationship to the stability of the distal radioulnar joint. *Clin Orthop* 1970;68: 124–129.
37. Burkhart SS, Wood MB, Linscheid RL. Posttraumatic recurrent subluxation of the extensor carpi ulnaris tendon. *J Hand Surg [Am]* 1982;7:1–3.
38. Kip PC, Peimer CA. Release of the sixth dorsal compartment. *J Hand Surg [Am]* 1994;19:599–601.
39. Steffens K, Koob E. Die Diagnosis und Therapie der Tendovaginitis des Extensor carpi ulnaris (Stenose VI. Streckerfach). *Z Orthop* 1994;132:437–440.
40. Stern PJ. Tendinitis, overuse syndrome, and tendon injuries. *Hand Clin* 1990;6:467–476.
41. Eckhardt WA, Palmer AK. Recurrent dislocation of extensor carpi ulnaris tendon. *J Hand Surg [Am]* 1981;6:629–631.
42. Bishop AT, Gabel G, Carmichael SW. Flexor carpi radialis tendinitis. *J Bone Joint Surg Am* 1994;76:1009–1014.
43. Weeks PM. A cause of wrist pain: Non-specific tenosynovitis involving the flexor carpi radialis. *Plast Reconstr Surg* 1978;62: 263–266.
44. Gabel G, Bishop AT, Wood MB. Flexor carpi radialis tendinitis. *J Bone Joint Surg Am* 1994;76:1015–1018.
45. Fitton JM, Shea FW, Goldie W. Lesion of the flexor carpi radialis tendon and sheath causing pain in the wrist. *J Bone Joint Surg Br* 1968;50:359–363.
46. Lemon RA, Engber WD. Trigger wrist: A case report. *J Hand Surg [Am]* 1985;10:61–63.
47. Linburg RM, Comstock BE. Anomalous tendon slips from the flexor pollicis longus to the flexor digitorum profundus. *J Hand Surg [Am]* 1989;4:79–83.
48. Lombardi RM, Wood MB, Linscheid RL. Symptomatic restrictive thumb–index finger flexor tenosynovitis: Incidence of musculotendinous anomalies and results of treatment. *J Hand Surg [Am]* 1988;13:337–340.
49. Palmieri TH. Pisiform area pain treatment by pisiform excicion. *J Hand Surg [Am]* 1982;7:477–480.
50. Vastamäki M. Pisiform–triquetral osteoarthritis as cause of wrist pain. *Ann Chir Gynaecol* 1986;75:280–282.
51. Carrol RE, Coyle MP. Dysfunction of the pisotriquetral joint: Treatment by excision of the pisiform. *J Hand Surg [Am]* 1985; 10:703–707.
52. Dilley DF, Tonkin MA. Acute calcific tendinitis in the hand and wrist. *J Hand Surg [Br]* 1991;16:215–216.
53. Archer B, Friedman L, Stilgenbauer S, et al. Symptomatic calcific tendinitis at unusual sites. *Can Assoc Radiol J* 1992;43:203–207.
54. Nüesch B, Sennwald G, Segmüller G. Pisiformeexstirpation: Indikation und Resultate. *Handchir Mikrochir Plast Chir* 1993; 25:42–45.
55. Lundborg G, Meyers R, Powell H. Nerve compression and increased fluid pressure: A "miniature compartment syndrome." *J Neurosurg Psychiatry* 1983;46:119–124.
56. Mackinnon SE, Dellon AL. *Surgery of the peripheral nerve.* New York: Thieme, 1988.
57. Sicuranza MJ, McCue FC: Compressive neuropathies in the upper extremity of athletes. *Hand Clin* 1992;8:263–273.
58. Verdon ME. Overuse syndromes of the hand and wrist. *Orthopedics* 1996;23:305–319.
59. Gelberman RH, Aronson D, Weisman MH. Carpal tunnel syndrome: Results of a prospective trial of steroid injection and splinting. *J Bone Joint Surg Am* 1980;62:1181–1184.
60. Gelberman R, Pfeffer G, Galbraith R, et al. Results of treatment of severe carpal tunnel syndrome without internal neurolysis of the median nerve. *J Bone Joint Surg Am* 1987;69:896–903.
61. Osterman A: The double-crush syndrome: Cervical radiculopathy and carpal tunnel syndrome. *Orthop Clin North Am* 1988;19:147–155.
62. Agee JM, McCarroll HR, Tortosa RD, et al. Endoscopic release of the carpal tunnel: A randomized prospective multicenter study. *J Hand Surg [Am]* 1992;17:987–995.
63. Chow JCY. Endoscopic release of the carpal ligament: A new technique for carpal tunnel syndrome. *Arthroscopy* 1989;5: 19–24.
64. Okutsu I, Ninomiya S, Hamanaka I, et al. Measurement of pressure in the carpal canal before and after endoscopic management of carpal tunnel syndrome. *J Bone Joint Surg Am* 1989;71: 679–683.
65. Brown RA, Gelberman RH, Seiler JG, et al. Carpal tunnel

65. release: A prospective randomized assessment of open and endoscopic methods. *J Bone Joint Surg Am* 1993;75:1265–1274.
66. Connolly WB. Endoscopic carpal tunnel release. *Med J Aust* 1994;160:102–103.
67. Cobb TK, Cooney WP. Significance of incomplete release of the distal portion of the flexor retinaculum. Implications for endoscopic carpal tunnel surgery. *J Hand Surg [Br]* 1994;19:283–285.
68. Chow JCY. Endoscopic carpal tunnel release: Chow 2 portal technique. In: Vastamäki M, ed. *Current trends in hand surgery.* Amsterdam: Elsevier, 1995;305–308.
69. Nathan PA. Advantages of carpal tunnel release with short incision and early postoperative rehabilitation. In: Vastamäki M, ed. *Current trends in hand surgery.* Amsterdam: Elsevier, 1995; 309–312.
70. Lee WPA, Plancher KD, Strickland JW. Carpal tunnel release with a small palmar incision. *Hand Clin* 1996;12:271–284.
71. Gross MS, Gelberman RH. Anatomy of the distal ulnar tunnel. *Clin Orthop* 1985;196:238–247.
72. Riche P. Le nerf cubital et les muscles de l'eminence thenar. *Bull Mem Soc Anat Paris* 1897;5:251–252.
73. Lass R, Shrewsbury MM. Variation in the path of the deep motor branch of the ulnar nerve at the wrist. *J Bone Joint Surg Am* 1975; 57:990–991.
74. Spinner M. *Injuries to the major branches of the peripheral nerves of the forearm.* Philadelphia: WB Saunders, 1978.
75. Gloobe H, Pecket P. An anomalous muscle in the canal of Guyon. *Anat Anz* 1973;133:477–479.
76. Swanson AB, Biddulph SL, Baughman FA, et al. Ulnar nerve compression due to an anomalous muscle in the canal of Guyon. *Clin Orthop* 1972;83:64–69.
77. Salgeback S. Ulnar tunnel syndrome caused by anomalous muscles. A case report. *Scand J Plast Reconstr Surg* 1977;11:255–258.
78. Thomas CG. Clinical manifestations of an accessory palmaris muscle. *J Bone Joint Surg Am* 1958;40:929.
79. Gelberman RH. *Operative nerve repair and reconstruction.* Philadelphia: JB Lippincott, 1991.
80. Nisenfield FG, Neviaser RJ. Fracture of the hook of the hamate: a diagnosis easily missed. *J Trauma* 1974;14:612–616.
81. Vance RM, Gelberman RH. Acute ulnar neuropathy with fractures at the wrist. *J Bone Joint Surg Am* 1978;60:962–965.
82. Hoyt CS. Letter: Ulnar neuropathy in bicycle riders. *Arch Neurol* 1976;33:372.
83. Fissette J, Onkelinx A, Fandi N. Carpal and Guyon tunnel syndrome in burns at the wrist. *J Hand Surg [Am]* 1981;6:13–15.
84. Silver MA, Gelberman RH, Gellman H, et al. Carpal tunnel syndrome: associated abnormalities in ulnar nerve function and the effect of carpal tunnel release on these abnormalities. *J Hand Surg [Am]* 1985;10:710–713.
85. Wartenberg R. Cheiralgia paresthetica (Isolierte Neuritis des Ramus Superficialis Nerve Radialis). *Z Ges Neurol Psychiatr* 1932;141:145–155.
86. Mackinnon SE, Dellon AL. The overlap pattern of the lateral antebrachial cutaneous nerve and the superficial branch of the radial nerve. *J Hand Surg [Am]* 1985;10:522–526.
87. Gockel M, Vastamäki M, Alaranta H. Long-term results of primary scalenotomy in the treatment of thoracic outlet syndrome. *J Hand Surg [Br]* 1994;19:229–233.
88. Leffert RD. Thoracic outlet syndrome. In: Gelberman RH, ed. *Operative nerve repair and reconstruction.* Philadelphia: JB Lippincott, 1991.

9

CARPAL TUNNEL SYNDROME

JAMES C.Y. CHOW

HISTORY

The first carpal tunnel syndrome was described in 1854 by Sir James Paget, as median nerve compression following a fracture of the distal radius (1,2). In 1880, James Putman, a neurologist from Boston, described the symptoms suffered by a group of his patients. Although the term "carpal tunnel syndrome" was not used then, the symptoms he described would be considered classic for carpal tunnel syndrome today (3). In 1913, Marie P. Foix performed an autopsy on a patient and described advanced atrophy of the thenar muscle with no history of trauma or injury to the wrist region. There was enlargement of the median nerve, which was described as neuropathy, proximal to the transverse carpal ligament. It was her opinion that release of the transverse carpal ligament probably would have prevented paralysis of the thenar muscles (4). The first surgical release of the transverse carpal ligament was described by Sir James Learmonth in 1933 (5). In 1946, Cannon and Love reported 38 cases of tardy median nerve palsy (6). In 1947, W. Russell Brain, along with his colleague Marcia Wilkinson and the surgeon Dickson Wright, published the first paper that described the details of the clinical signs, diagnosis, and pathophysiology of spontaneous compression of the median nerve in the carpal canal. Based on their findings, Brain, Wilkinson, and Wright recommended early release of the transverse carpal ligament to prevent muscle or nerve deficits (7).

In the 1950s, George Phalen made decompression of the median nerve of the wrist a well-known procedure to the surgeons of North America through a series of articles (8–15). He also described Tinel's sign and Phalen's sign to aid diagnosis.

ANATOMY OF THE CARPAL LIGAMENT

The transverse carpal ligament is a continuation of the deep fascia of the forearm, and is made of compact, collagen fibers. In cross-section, it has an appearance of an airplane wing, with a thicker, rounded edge distally and a thinner edge proximally. The thicker portion (distal portion) usually measures about 4 to 5 mm while the thinner edge (proximal portion) measures from 1 to 2 mm. On cadaveric dissection it has been noted that some carpal ligaments may be as thick as 8 mm, especially in a large hand, or if there is some disease of the carpal ligament. The transverse carpal ligament extends across the opening on the palmar side of the wrist joint. This forms a roof over the transverse arch of the carpal bones, creating the canal called the carpal tunnel. This tunnel contains nine flexor tendons and the median nerve. The flexor tendons are usually covered by the synovial sheath, which allows movement during flexion of the wrist. Two bursae, ulnar and radial, can also be identified in the canal, with a thin bursal membrane on the top of the tendon sheath. The median nerve has numerous variances, including those of the motor branch, as described in the excellent work of Lanz in 1977 (16–25). In this article, he described how the motor branch exits the carpal canal. For example, in 46% of his patients, it branched past the carpal canal and curved back to the thenar muscle. In 31% of his patients, the motor branch exited under the carpal ligament after passing through the distal edge of the carpal ligament, and then curved back to the thenar muscles. In 23% of his patients, the motor branches were actually transligamental, passing through the carpal ligament, then entering the thenar muscles.

Of course, there are other rare circumstances. For example, a high division of the median nerve, or more than one motor branch exiting from the median nerve to the thenar muscle, is present in less than 1% of patients. During cadaveric dissections of the carpal ligament, it is possible to find two distinct layers: a superficial layer attached to the tubercle of the trapezium, and a deep layer attached to the median lips of the groove of the trapezium (26). Guyon's canal is formed on the ulnar side of the hook of hamate between the two layers of fiber that form a triangular shape in cross section. The ulnar nerve, ulnar artery, and ulnar vein are contained in this canal. The transverse carpal ligament extends 3.5 to 4 cm beyond the distal crease of the wrist. The principal source of the blood supply to the

---

J. C. Y. Chow: Department of Surgery, Southern Illinois University School of Medicine, Springfield, Illinois 62701, and Orthopaedic Center of Southern Illinois, Mount Vernon, Illinois 62864.

transverse carpal ligament can be divided into superficial and deep networks. The superficial network is formed by branches of the ulnar artery; the deep network is formed by branches of the superficial palmar arch (27).

PATHOPHYSIOLOGY

The term "carpal tunnel syndrome" is now applied to all conditions that produce irritations or compression of the median nerve within the carpal canal. Basically, the condition occurs when either the space is too small for the contents or the contents are too large for the space, and pressure is applied to the median nerve itself. Lundborg et al. described their belief that the small capillary flow of the median nerve is shut down when pressure is applied, causing an ischemic factor (28). The majority of the patients that we have seen exhibited idiopathic, or spontaneous, carpal tunnel syndrome. I believe that some people may have inherited a genetically narrow space at birth and developed this problem at a later date. Any other conditions which reduce the capacity of the carpal canal will produce symptoms, such as a deformed Colles' fracture, edema or swelling of the tendon sheath, soft tissue tumors in the canal, or increased thickness of the carpal ligament itself from repetitive trauma. In recent years, repetitive motion in the workplace has also become thought of as an etiologic factor of this problem. Many other systemic conditions may be related to the symptoms, including obesity, diabetes, thyroid dysfunction, Raynaud's dysfunction and disease, scleroderma, rheumatoid disease, systemic lupus erythematosus (SLE), or any other collagen disease. The last trimester of pregnancy is also known to produce carpal tunnel symptoms. Of course, there are many rare and unusual conditions cited in the literature that could also be related to, or produce, carpal tunnel syndrome.

DIAGNOSIS

Because carpal tunnel syndrome is a subjective condition, the patient's history is most important in the diagnosis. Patients usually complain of paresthesia, tingling and numbness involving the long fingers, and are characteristically nocturnal. Patients may have pain referred to the forearm, upper arm, and even the shoulder and neck regions. They usually complain of decreasing grip strength, dropping things, and an inability to feel fine objects. Most predominant are the nocturnal symptoms. Patients indicate that they have problems sleeping at night because they wake up with numbness in the hand and have to rub their fingers to get relief. Sometimes, a patient may wake up several times in a single night, resulting in very little sleep (8–15).

Carpal tunnel syndrome can be divided into three stages: early, progressive, and late. In the early stage, the symptoms appear only when provoked, and are related to specific daytime activities. The majority of the symptoms are sensory related without motor involvement. In the progressive stage, the symptoms are noticeable regardless of the daytime activities. The sensory findings are more pronounced and the motor weakness begins to affect the hand. This is the stage when patients usually seek medical assistance, because symptoms suddenly worsen and begin to disturb sleep and daily activities. In the late stage, usually after symptoms have been present for years, muscle atrophy and weakness become noticeable. Patients sometimes believe that their symptoms are getting better, because the pain and tingling sensations appear to have decreased; however, in reality, the condition has not really improved, and permanent nerve injury has resulted. Patients usually demonstrate classical thenar muscle atrophy and loss of pinch and grip strength, an inability to oppose the thumb, and persistent numbness in the long fingers. In this stage, a nerve conduction velocity (NCV) study may have a marked delay in the distal latency and, at times, may even be nonresponsive in either or both the motor and sensory distal latency of the median nerve, which may suggest permanent nerve damage (27).

Physical examination will assist in evaluation. In classic carpal tunnel syndrome, the small finger is the only finger not involved. In an acute case, there is tenderness along the carpal canal area. Light percussion over the median nerve, at the level of the wrist, produces the Tinel's sign: a tingling sensation that will radiate to the long fingers and will follow the median nerve distribution. Phalen's sign, or the wrist flexion test, is observed by having the patient hold the forearm vertically and drop both hands into complete flexion of the wrist. In this position, the median nerve is squeezed between the proximal edge of the carpal ligament, the adjacent flexor tendons, and the radius. If this produces tingling in the fingers within 60 seconds, the findings are considered positive. Other examinations should include the monofilament test, two point discriminations, reverse Phalen's test, and tourniquet test. Some suggest a direct measurement of the pressure in the carpal canal. In the late stages of the disease, with thenar muscle atrophy, one can observe muscle wasting in the thenar area (8–15,28). Electromyography (EMG) and NCV studies will also help to detect this condition. Surgery should not be indicated based solely on the results of nerve conduction studies, especially when the results are normal but the patient complains of persistent symptoms with classic carpal tunnel syndrome present clinically (29–34). A delay of the distal latency of the median nerve of 7.0 msec or over represents significant compression of the median nerve. If this is present, surgery should be considered without further delay. A careful examination should be performed by the physician to exclude the possibility of cervical disk pathology, thoracic outlet syndrome, pronator compression syndrome in the forearm, or other central nervous system diseases (35–38). Wrist radiography should be done routinely, including anteroposterior (AP), lateral, and carpal tunnel views, to rule out any possibility of any bone or joint deformity, abnormality, or pathology. If a more extensive study is indicated, magnetic resonance imaging (MRI), computed tomography (CT), ultrasound, bone scan, and an arthrogram of the wrist may be necessary (27,39–45).

CONSERVATIVE TREATMENT

Patients in the early stages of carpal tunnel syndrome normally respond quite well to conservative treatment. Conservative treatment includes the use of night splints, nonsteroidal antiinflammatory oral medication, rest of the affected hand, alteration of daily activities, antivibration or protective work gloves, avoidance of repetitive movement or persistent pressure to the palm region, physical therapy, or even steroid injections in the carpal canal (46–50). Patients in the advanced or progressive stage of the condition usually do not respond well to conservative treatment. Most of these patients have suffered for some time, and surgery is often indicated. Patients in the late stage have had tingling and numbness sensations of the hands for years with a marked delay, or no response, of the distal latency on the NCV and thenar muscle atrophy. Some patients in this stage have lost the ability to button a shirt and cannot distinguish between one and two points during the 2-point discrimination. When the patient has reached this stage, surgical decompression of the carpal ligament would be indicated without further delay. For the late stage patient with signs of permanent nerve injury, the prognosis following surgery is guarded.

OPEN CARPAL TUNNEL RELEASE

There are numerous approaches to the standard open surgical procedure (51–63). In general, open carpal tunnel release is performed using a longitudinal curved incision over the palm region, ulnar and parallel to the thenar crest. Some surgeons prefer to extend the incision proximal to the flexor crease of the wrist joint, forming the shape of a lazy "S." The reason for having the incision form a curve, or angle, to the flexor crease is that an incision straight across the crest would form a painful scar postoperatively. Some surgeons prefer to use magnification loupes to preserve all small branches of the cutaneous nerve fibers as much as possible. The deep structures are exposed, and the median nerve is traced to the carpal ligament, which is then released under direct visualization (64). Following the surgery, a compression dressing, volar splint, or both are applied to avoid bowstringing of the tendons or nerve. Another surgical technique involves a transverse incision over the distal wrist crease. The incision is approximately 5 cm in length, cutting straight across the wrist area. Scissors or a knife are then used to cut the carpal ligament proximally to distally. This surgical technique involves a blind cut toward the distal carpal ligament. The danger with this technique is either cutting too far distally, increasing the chance of injury to the digital nerve or superficial palmar arch, or undercutting the ligament resulting in an incomplete release of the carpal ligament. Many surgeons have recommended abandoning this method (64).

In the past few years, endoscopic techniques have been developed in an attempt to decrease postoperative pain, pillar pain, and the painful scar of the open procedure. It has been proven that there is much less postoperative discomfort and a faster recovery with the endoscopic technique than with the open procedure. However, it is a dangerous arthroscopic procedure in the wrong hands (65–68); there have been devastating complications reported by surgeons who have used the endoscopic carpal tunnel technique (69–72). This has raised controversy regarding the value of endoscopic release of the carpal ligament. Many hand surgeons feel that the dangers of the procedure outweigh the benefits to the patient. Obviously, all surgical procedures are dangerous when done by inexperienced hands. It has also been shown that endoscopic carpal ligament release can be performed safely in experienced hands, giving both patients and surgeons a great deal of satisfaction. Personally, my results are much better, and the complications are a lot lower for the endoscopic release compared to my own open procedure for carpal tunnel syndrome (70–77).

ENDOSCOPIC RELEASE OF THE CARPAL LIGAMENT

History

When I began working on my technique in 1985, I did not know that Dr. Ichiro Okutsu, of Japan, or Dr. John Agee, in California, were working with similar goals at approximately the same time. Through trial and error of different approaches, the breakthrough of the idea of the slotted cannula came around late 1986. The procedure was completed in May, 1987, after 4 to 5 months of persistent practice on cadavers, and was applied to the first patient in September, 1987. Since that time, continued efforts have been made toward the improvement of this procedure.

The three original techniques could be summarized as follows: The Chow procedure uses a slotted cannula through dual portals, which introduced the scope at one end and the instrumentation at the other end, allowing for release of the carpal ligament with direct visualization (69–77). Dr. Okutsu used a clear plastic tube to introduce the scope so the carpal ligament could be visualized. A hook knife was then brought alongside the plastic tube to release the ligament (78). Dr. Agee used a transverse incision to introduce a specially designed device. Under arthroscopic visualization, he would pull a trigger which elevated the blade to cut the ligament (78,79). The common denominator of these three procedures is that we all utilized the current advancement of arthroscopic technology, enabling visualization of the surgery by a television monitor with the use of a camera. Although our methods varied, the ideas were similar in that we were attempting to treat carpal tunnel syndrome and preserve the normal hand structures.

Chow Technique

Thanks to the effort of the Seven University Study Group (80,81), the original technique has been modified in an attempt to decrease the complications and the learning curve. The following is a description of the current dual portal technique.

Setup

The patient is placed in a supine position and a hand table is used. Two video monitors are preferred, but some surgeons perform the procedure with only one. One monitor should face the surgeon and the other should face the assistant. The surgeon sits on the ulnar side of the patient and the assistant faces the surgeon. Standard preparations and draping are performed.

Anesthesia

Local anesthesia and intravenous medication are recommended for this procedure. The use of local anesthesia allows the patient and surgeon to communicate. An alert patient can inform the surgeon of any variance of nerve structure during the procedure (17–21). Usually, when the patient first comes into the room, 1-2 mg of Versed [midazolam hydrochloride (Roche, Nutley, NJ)] is given intravenously to help the patient relax and be more comfortable during the preparation and draping. Two hundred µg of Alfenta [alfentanil hydrochloride (Janssen Pharmaceutica, Inc., Piscataway, NJ)] is given intravenously when the surgeon begins to mark the hand. This is a short-acting analgesic with a peak action of 5 to 10 minutes. Usually, the surgical time of the procedure is less than 10 minutes. An injection of 1% Xylocaine (Astra, Westboro, MA) without epinephrine is used at the entry and exit portals, but only in the skin, to avoid affecting the nerve by penetrating too deeply.

Entry Portal

The proximal end of the pisiform is palpated and marked with a small circle. A 1.5 to 2 cm line is drawn radially from the proximal pole of the pisiform, depending on the size of the hand. A second line is drawn approximately 0.5 cm proximally to the end of the first line, keeping to a 1:3 ratio with the first line. A small dotted line, approximately 1 cm

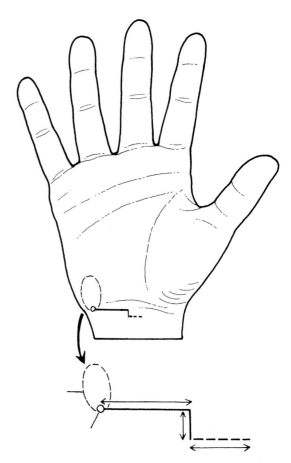

FIGURE 9.1. The entry portal is made by drawing a 1.5 to 2 cm line radially from the proximal pole of the pisiform, then drawing a second line approximately 0.5 cm proximally to the end of the first line, keeping to a 1:3 ratio with the first line. A small, dotted line, approximately 1 cm (7 to 10 mm) in length, is drawn from the end of the second line to complete the location of the entry portal.

(7 to 10 mm) in length is drawn from the end of the second line to create the entry portal. If the palmaris longus is present, the center of the entry portal should be located at the ulnar border of the palmaris longus (Fig. 9.1).

Exit Portal

With the thumb in full abduction, a line is drawn from the distal border, perpendicular to the long axis of the forearm. A second line is drawn from the third web space, parallel to the long axis of the forearm. These two lines should be at a right angle to each other. A bisecting line is drawn from the junction of these two lines proximally 1 cm to locate the distal portal. The surgeon should be able to palpate the hook of hamate. The exit portal should fall into the soft spot in the center of the palm and line up with the ring finger, just slightly radial to the hook of the hamate (Fig. 9.2).

Chapter 9: Carpal Tunnel Syndrome

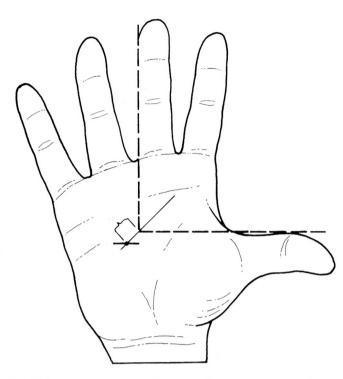

FIGURE 9.2. The exit portal is located by placing the patient's thumb in full abduction and drawing a line across the palm from the distal border of the thumb to approximately the center of the palm. A second line is drawn from the web between the second and third fingers down to the 1st line, forming a right angle. The third line is drawn bisecting this angle and extending proximally from the vertex, 1.0 cm. The exit portal should be 1 cm in length and line up with the ring finger, just slightly radial to the hook of hamate.

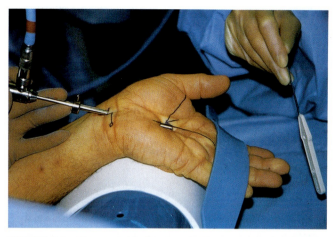

FIGURE 9.3. The assembled unit exits through the distal portal and the trocar is then removed so that the slotted cannula remains in position under the carpal ligament. The hand is then stabilized in the hand holder.

Procedure

One percent Xylocaine is injected at both the entry and exit portals, approximately 1 cc at each portal. A small, transverse 1 cm (7 to 10 mm) incision is made at the entry portal mark. A hemostat is used for blunt dissection. Small digital nerves and vessels are pushed away (25,59,82–85). A tourniquet is usually not required if this dissection is handled properly. The fascia, with its distinct fibers, should be visible. A knife is used to make a small, longitudinal opening. This cut is extended with small Stephen's curved tenotomy scissors. If the palmaris longus is present, the longitudinal cut should be along the ulnar border of the palmaris longus. Care should be taken as sometimes there are two layers of fascia. Both layers must be cut and the ulnar bursa should be seen from underneath. With small retractors, the distal border of the skin is lifted to create a vacuum that will separate the carpal ligament and the ulnar bursa. A curved dissector is used to gently push through a thin membrane and enter the carpal canal. When the dissector is maneuvered back and forth, the rough undersurface of the carpal ligament, described as a "washboard" or "railroad track" effect, can be felt. A curved dissector/slotted cannula assembly unit is then slipped under the carpal ligament. With the tip of this unit touching the hook of hamate, the surgeon picks up the patient's fingers and hand and, maintaining this position, gently hyperextends the fingers and wrist. The assistant brings the hand the rest of the way down so that the patient's hand rests comfortably on the frame. The slotted cannula assembly is gently advanced distally, pointing toward the exit portal. A small transverse or oblique incision is made cutting only the skin. Arch suppressors are used to press down the structures, and the assembled unit exits through the distal portal. The trocar is then removed so that the slotted cannula remains in position under the carpal ligament. The hand is then stabilized in the hand holder (Fig. 9.3).

Endoscopic Examination

The specially designed endoscope is inserted from the proximal opening of the slotted cannula. This is a short, 30-degree scope with a light post that points up in the same direction of the 30-degree angle to be sure that the light post does not hit the forearm. The camera and scope should rest comfortably in the first web space of the surgeon's hand. Usually, the surgeon braces the middle and ring fingers on the forearm, or any firm object, to avoid shaking or moving the endoscope and allow full control of the camera. A cotton swab can be inserted into the tube to clean the lens, then the focus is adjusted to maximize visualization (Fig. 9.4). A blunt hook probe is inserted to palpate the undersurface of the carpal ligament proximally to distally. If any soft tissue appears in the opening of the slotted cannula, the blunt probe is used to carefully palpate it. If the median nerve is present (Fig. 9.5), the patient will feel sharp or shooting pain to the fingers when it is probed, and he or

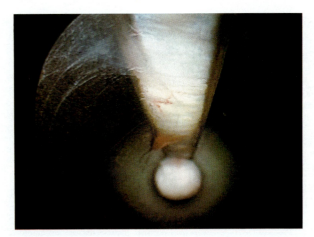

FIGURE 9.4. A cotton swab can be inserted into the tube to clean the lens, then the focus is adjusted to the best visualization.

she will be able to inform the surgeon. Otherwise, it could either be synovial tissue or a portion of the ulnar bursa. If there is a lot of soft tissue noted in the opening of the slotted cannula, surgery should not be carried out. The slotted cannula may need to be reinserted for better visualization; however, to avoid irreversible damage, surgery should never be carried out if there are tendons or other important structures caught between the slotted cannula and the undersurface of the carpal ligament.

If there is only a minimal amount of synovium obstructing the view, the trocar can be reinserted into the slotted cannula. The slotted cannula unit can then be rotated radially about 355 to 360 degrees to push the synovial tissue out of the way. I always emphasize to physicians who attend my workshops and ECTRA course that a surgeon should not hesitate to convert an endoscopic procedure to an open, standard procedure if they are not able to achieve adequate visualization.

Ligament Cutting Technique

With the scope in the proximal opening of the slotted cannula and the instrumentation in the distal opening, the distal border of the carpal ligament is identified with the probe. The probe can also be used to palpate any nonligamentous structure to ensure that it is not the median nerve. The probe knife is used to make the first cut, cutting distally to proximally. Anything beyond the distal border of the carpal ligament should not be excised. The scope is withdrawn proximally about 1 cm (10 mm) and the triangle knife is used to make a small opening in the midsection of the carpal ligament. The retrograde knife is brought in and placed in the second cut. Once the retrograde knife is well-seated, it is pulled distally to join the first two cuts. Now the distal portion of the carpal ligament is completely released (Fig. 9.6).

The scope is removed from the proximal opening of the slotted cannula and inserted in the distal opening. The camera view on the screen now forms a mirror affect. The surgeon should realize that the previous ulnar side is now the radial side. By moving the scope proximally and distally, the previous distal cut is identified. The probe knife is inserted and any soft tissue present is retracted to identify the proximal border of the carpal ligament. A small cut is then made with the probe knife proximally to distally. The probe knife is withdrawn and the retrograde knife is inserted and seated in the proximal edge of the distal cut. It is then pulled proximally to join the proximal cut to completely excise the proximal carpal ligament (Fig. 9.7). The surgeon can use the triangle knife, or any other knife that feels appropriate, to release any fibers that may remain in

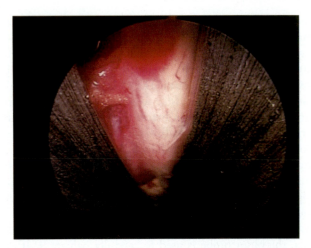

FIGURE 9.5. Transligmental branch of the median nerve as seen through the slotted cannula.

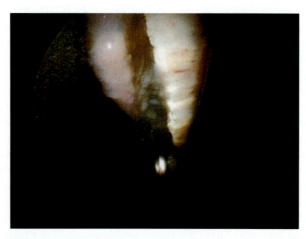

FIGURE 9.6. The retrograde knife is placed in the second cut and pulled distally to join the two previous cuts.

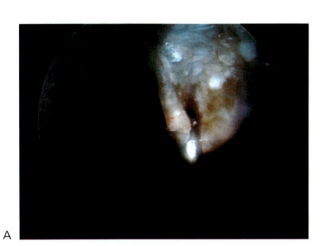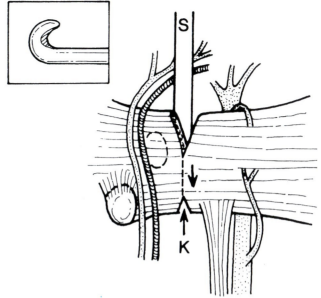

FIGURE 9.7. A,B: The retrograde knife is inserted and seated in the proximal edge of the distal cut. Pulling proximally will join the distal cut and proximal edge cut, completing the excision of the carpal ligament.

place until he or she is satisfied that a complete release has been performed.

Due to the position of the hand, the cut edges of the carpal ligament should spring apart and disappear from the opening of the slotted cannula. If the edges can still be seen through the opening, the release is incomplete. While the assistant fully abducts the patient's thumb, the uncut portion of the ligament can be identified and the surgeon can complete the resection. By rotating the slotted cannula, the completely cut ligament can be seen endoscopically. There is a continuation fan volar to the carpal ligament that should be preserved, as well as the opponens digiti minimi and the palmaris brevis muscle, if present. This thin, fibrous continuation fan from the thenar to the lesser thenar muscles will prevent bowstringing of the flexor tendons and preserve muscle strength. There is seldom any bleeding and only one suture is required for closing each portal. Immediately following the procedure, the surgeon can examine the patient while still in a sterilized environment. If any intraoperative complications have occurred requiring exposure of the hand, it can be performed at the same time.

Cooney et al. performed a study with the dissection of nine cadaver hands (86). They discovered instances involving the distal Guyon's canal in which the ulnar nerve bundle passed radial to the hook of hamate, superficial to the opponate digiti minimus muscle. Preservation of these muscle fibers during endoscopic surgery will avoid damage to these important structures.

Postoperatively, active exercise begins immediately. The patient is advised to avoid heavy lifting or pushing down on the palm region until the discomfort disappears, usually within 2 to 3 weeks. Active movement of the fingers decreases the formation of scar tissue in the wrist region and, therefore, avoids adhesions on the tendons or nerves at the surgical site. Sutures are usually removed in one week. If the patient engages in heavy lifting too soon following surgery, there may be some swelling and prolonged pain in the palm region. If these occur, fluidotherapy treatment for 20 minutes per day helps to decrease the condition within two weeks.

The carpal ligament does not have a rich blood supply or nerve fiber distribution; therefore, cutting only the carpal ligament definitely decreases postoperative pain, bleeding and scarring. The palmaris longus tendon extension and muscle fibers are preserved by the endoscopic technique, which prevents bowstringing of the flexor tendons and the median nerve, thereby preserving pinch and grip strength (82–86).

Alternative Chow Technique

Many hand surgeons are very uncomfortable with the blind insertion of the trocar exiting distally without seeing the distal superficial palmar arch and distal digital nerves; therefore, they may want to make the distal portal larger in order to identify these structures prior to introducing the slotted cannula. This alternative technique is designed for those surgeons who are willing to take the time to explore the distal portal, especially for hand surgeons who use loupe magnification. To allow visualization of these important distal structures, the slotted cannula would be placed in the same way but inserted distally to proximally.

Procedure

The setup and marking of the portal setups are the same as described above. A regional block or local anesthesia is used according to the surgeon's preference; however, we strongly recommend the use of local anesthesia. The entry portal is made with a small oblique incision (1 to 1.5 cm) over the distal palm region at the mark for the exit portal in the above method. Loupe magnification is used while carefully dissecting down to identify the superficial palmar arch curving ulnarly to radially. Further careful dissection allows identification of the median or digital nerves in the area.

The distal carpal ligament is identified and the slotted cannula, with the curved side pointing upwards, is inserted under the carpal ligament. The assembly should be touching the hook of hamate, gliding proximally. The "washboard" texture of the carpal ligament should be palpable with the curved dissector as the cannula is aimed towards the center of the wrist and the exit portal. The exit portal should be on the ulnar border of the palmaris longus, if it exists; otherwise, it should be aimed towards the center of the wrist, marked as previously described, approximately 0.5 to 1.0 cm proximal to the wrist flexion crease. The fingers and the rest of the hand are then hyperextended and the hand is placed in the hand holder. The surgeon should be able to palpate the curved dissector tip. A small transverse incision is then made and the slotted cannula assembly is brought outside proximally. The rest of the procedure and cutting techniques can be carried out as previously described.

Japanese Technique

Dr. Okutsu and colleagues developed a blunt, clear plastic tube, with an outer diameter of 6 mm, an inner diameter of 4 mm, and a barrel length of 175 mm (78). This tube is inserted into the carpal canal through a transverse incision made in the forearm, ulnar to the palmaris longus. The arthroscope is brought in through this clear, plastic tube and the carpal ligament is identified. A hook knife is passed along the ulnar side of the plastic tube to the distal border of the carpal ligament. The knife is "hooked" onto the carpal ligament and withdrawn to release the carpal ligament.

Agee Technique

Dr. John Agee, in cooperation with the 3M Corporation (Minneapolis, MN), developed a surgical device shaped like a hand pistol (80,87). This device is used to release the carpal ligament under direct visualization. This technique requires an incision that closely resembles the standard transverse incision on the wrist for carpal tunnel syndrome. However, instead of cutting blindly, the pistol-shaped instrument allows the surgeon to visualize the undersurface of the carpal ligament while it is being cut. The instrument has a camera hookup located at the back of the handle and a disposable tip which allows for viewing through an open window. Squeezing the trigger of the pistol-shaped instrument elevates a blade through the window and withdrawing the entire instrument distally to proximally releases the carpal ligament.

CLINICAL RESULTS

From September 1987 to September 1997, in Mt. Vernon, Illinois, 2,020 wrists of 1,530 patients with carpal tunnel syndrome underwent endoscopic release of the carpal ligament using the dual portal Chow technique. Of these patients, 1,231 were female and 724 were male. Their ages ranged from 14 to 96 years, with a mean of 51 years. There were 594 right-hand surgeries, 259 left-hand surgeries, and 551 bilateral cases. All of the patients in this series were carefully examined for other associated problems, including cervical disk or thoracic outlet syndrome, and a number of cases had double crush syndrome. All of the patients exhibited classic carpal tunnel syndrome symptoms including diminished sensation in the median nerve distribution, nocturnal pain, decreased pinch and grip strength, weakness of the hand, and persistent waking during the night. The duration of symptoms ranged from one month to 60 years, with the majority (96%) having a positive NCV test. All of the patients had failed to respond to conservative treatment prior to surgery.

Two hundred sixty-seven cases (190 patients) were lost to follow-up due to change of address or death; therefore, the results of this report are based on the remaining 1,753 cases (wrists) and 1,340 patients. We contacted the 1,340 patients by telephone, mail, or repeat clinical examination in order to answer a questionnaire. The clinical data and questionnaire responses were analyzed to reveal that 1,327 patients (1,736 of 1,753 cases) had no complaints or problems following the surgery, for a success rate of 99%. There were 13 patients (17 of 1,753 cases) who complained of symptoms, for a failure rate of 0.97%. Eight patients experienced a recurrence of carpal tunnel syndrome, one bilaterally (9 of 1,753 cases), for a recurrance rate of 0.51%.

Of the 1,753 cases, 591 (34%) had returned to normal activities in 1 week; 1,065 (61%) in 2 weeks; 1,313 (75%) in 3 weeks; and 1,490 (85%) in 4 weeks. Overall, 1,736 (99%) returned to normal activities and work. Eleven of the 1,753 cases (1%) never returned to their presurgical normal activity or work.

Four hundred thirty-one of the 1,753 cases were claimed as workers' compensation (21%). Of these cases, 420 (97%) were engaged in heavy work; 51 (12%) returned to work or normal activities within 1 week, 140 (32%) within 2 weeks, 209 (48%) within 3 weeks, 285 (65%) within 4 weeks, and 425 (99%) after 4 weeks.

Of the 1,322 remaining non–workers' compensation cases, 321(28%) patients were engaged in heavy work, 347 (24%) were engaged in light work, and 654 (49%) were retired, no longer working, or homemakers who did not have to return to a specific workplace. Of these 1,322 cases, 540 (41%) returned to work or normal activities within 1 week, 925 (70%) within 2 weeks, 1,104 (83%) within 3 weeks, 1,205 (91%) within 4 weeks, and 1,311 (99%) after 4 weeks.

Pinch and Grip Study

A pinch and grip study was performed pre- and postoperatively. To avoid confusion, the number of patients, not the number of cases (wrists), was used in this study. Because of geographic distance, only 327 of the 2,020 cases (16%) returned to complete the study. Preoperative strength was used in unilateral cases and the better hand of the two hands was used as a control in bilateral cases. The pinch and grip tests began one week after surgery and repeated each week until the patient regained normal or better than normal strength.

Of the 327 patients who returned for testing, 76 (23%) regained their pinch and grip strength within one week postoperatively; 191 (58%) within two weeks; 233 (71%) within three weeks; and 260 (81%) in four or more weeks.

Complications

The following discussion of complications involves the Chow technique and should not be confused with complications of the other endoscopic techniques. There was no permanent nerve or vessel damage, hematoma, or tendon laceration found in my series. One patient did have an incomplete release of the carpal ligament, 1 patient had a superficial infection of the sutures, and 2 patients experienced transient ulnar neuropraxia early in the series which recovered spontaneously, for an overall complication rate of 0.22% (4/1,753). Since the direction of the retractor was changed, there have not been any cases of neuropraxia.

Although I have not experienced any serious complications, there have been several reports of severe complications reported throughout the US using this technique (70–72, 88–92). A survey of ECTRA course participants resulted in the review of 10,640 cases (72). There were some serious complications reported which included median and ulnar nerve injuries, transections of the ulnar neurovascular bundle, digital nerve injuries, tendon lacerations, and lacerations of the superficial palmar arch and the ulnar artery. This study found a total complication rate of 2.6%. It was interesting to note that the surgeons who performed less than 25 cases had a complication rate of 5.6% and those who performed more than 100 cases had a complication rate of less than 1%. The most common problems are lack of experience and placement of the entry portal too ulnarly. These can be corrected by learning the procedure properly and checking the location of the entry and exit portals prior to performing the surgery. If any problems occur with visualization, the procedure should be abandoned.

DISCUSSION

It took years for arthroscopists to convince knee surgeons that an arthrotomy is not required to treat a meniscus tear, either by partial menisectomy or suturing of the meniscus. I believe it will take years to convince hand surgeons that wide exposure of the hand and wrist is not necessary to treat simple, idiopathic carpal tunnel syndrome. While some surgeons believe that endoscopic decompression of the carpal ligament is dangerous because of complications that have occurred, the learning curve is a major factor in any procedure. Once the surgeon is familiar with the technique and aware of the potential dangers, he or she can avoid them.

What is the fundamental difference between the standard open procedure and the endoscopic procedure for release of the transverse carpal ligament? The open procedure is operating from the outside in, and the endoscopic technique is from the inside out. Endoscopic techniques allow the surgeon to visualize the undersurface of the carpal ligament before any cuts are made. For example, if there is an extremely ulnar exit of a transligamental motor branch of the median nerve (2.5 mm to 3 mm radial to the hook of hamate), the endoscopic technique allows visualization of this anatomical variance before injury occurs. I have performed over 2,500 cases of endoscopic release of the carpal ligament in over 13 years. During that time, I have encountered an extremely ulnar transligamental motor branch of the median nerve 10 times for an incidence of <0.4% (±1:250).

Any surgeon who has performed a large number of carpal tunnel syndrome surgeries knows that reflex sympathetic dystrophy (RSD) is one of the most unfortunate and devastating complications of decompression of the transverse carpal ligament. As of this time I have not had a single case of RSD with endoscopic carpal tunnel release. Preservation of the normal anatomical structures above the transverse carpal ligament may be credited for this result. As surgeons pass the learning curve for endoscopic release of the carpal ligament, I believe that complications will decrease, and the procedure will be fully recognized as a very valuable procedure for treating carpal tunnel syndrome.

EDITORS' COMMENTS

Carpal tunnel syndrome occurs primarily as thickening of the transverse carpal ligament (TCL), but can occur from space-occupying tissue within the carpal tunnel. So-called "idiopathic" or "classic" carpal tunnel syndrome follows certain patterns and is endemic in people with certain occupations, such as hairdressers, dental hygienists, and keyboard operators. From variable etiologies, synovitis develops in both the lining of the tunnel and the covering of the tissues that traverse the tunnel. Inflammation of this synovium over a period of time causes thickening of the roof of the tunnel (flexor retinaculum), combined with conversion to a denser, firmer, more grizzle-like collagen. In rheumatoid arthritis, carpal tunnel syndrome presents in a somewhat different manner, the symptoms are more prolonged and varied with the state of the patient's arthritis, medication, etc. The symptoms are more due to the space-occupying synovium in the tunnel than they are to the thickening of the roof of the tunnel. An acute example of the space-occupying synovium etiology is the 18-year-old college student who takes on two summer jobs after doing no manual activity during the year, and over a two-week period of time develops major carpal tunnel syndrome, typically bilaterally, with significant thenar weakness, which is always totally amenable to conservative treatment. The nerve symptoms are entirely secondary to the synovial pressure. These cases rarely progress to chronic carpal tunnel syndrome.

Carpal tunnel syndrome can be classified as follows:

Type IA (idiopathic): Gradual onset, thick flexor retinaculum.

Type IB: Age over 70, severe night component, sensory deficit, significant thenar weakness, poor return of median nerve.

Type II: Space-occupying tissue or impingement within the tunnel.

    A. Synovial overgrowth (e.g., tumor, rheumatoid arthritis).

    B. Synovitis only (e.g., the young patient with activity overload).

    C. Bone deformity - extrinsic impingement of the tunnel (e.g., Colles' fracture).

Type III: Normal tunnel, but increased sensitivity of the median nerve (e.g., neuropathy).

Type IV: Endocrinologic conditions (e.g., pregnancy, diabetes).

The etiology of classic (Type IA) carpal tunnel syndrome is initiated by synovitis in the tunnel. There are certain activities which appear to produce this synovitis. It is generally accepted, for instance, that the millions of typists in the days prior to computers had a much lower incidence of carpal tunnel syndrome. The difference may be that the power of the finger setters (the sublimi) was necessary to activate a mechanical typewriter keystroke. These muscles are not required for modern ultralight computer keyboards. The profundus tendons lie dorsal to the sublimus tendons in the carpal tunnel; stroking an electric key may require only profundus activity. The profundus tendons then migrate volarly through the relaxed sublimi. At 80 words per minute times five letters per word, this will occur some 24,000 individual times in an hour of keyboarding. This migration displacement phenomenon would be exacerbated by slight wrist flexion. Though less total energy is required, the mechanics may be such that more synovial inflammation occurs within the carpal tunnel with keyboarding than with the use of a mechanical typewriter.

The senior editor currently has performed 7,178 carpal tunnel syndrome operations in his practice. The female to male ratio is 72%:28%. In idiopathic carpal tunnel (Type IA), there is often a long history of simple numbness and tingling in the tips of the index, middle, or thumb digits, which can be relieved with a simple shake of the hand. Gradually, more wrist-fixed activities produce symptoms that are less easily relieved. In women, there is often a history of numbness and tingling with pregnancy, followed by no symptoms for 10 to 15 years. A familial component can exist where entire families develop carpal tunnel syndrome in their middle-aged years. This finding does not mean that the patient's occupation was not the etiology of the carpal tunnel syndrome, but simply that there is an unstudied patient predisposition based on congenital tunnel size. Carpal tunnel syndrome occurs more commonly in patients who are overweight.

Diagnosis

There are three clinical components to the diagnosis of carpal tunnel syndrome, which set it aside from almost any other clinical condition of the upper extremity. The first component occurs at night: The patient will experience numbness and tingling in the milder cases and pain radiating to the medial aspect of the elbow in more severe cases. These symptoms are secondary to a gradual, progressive, localized ischemia of the median nerve. Without tendon motion, the TCL displaces all vascularity from the area of the nerve beneath it. This problem is made more severe by wrist flexion which occurs with the common fetal sleep position. It takes several hours for the severity of symptoms to awaken the patient, usually around 2:00 a.m., not infrequently followed by several more awakenings as the night progresses and the sleep level is less deep. The localized ischemia of the median nerve can be mitigated in part by wrist splints, which maintain the wrist in a neutral or slightly dorsiflexed position and prevent the wrist flexion that places the nerve against the TCL, subjecting it to compression by the normal tone of the flexor tendons dorsal to it.

The second diagnostic component occurs in the morning. This is comprised first of localized ischemia to the median nerve, similar to the nighttime component, and the patient will frequently awaken with numbness and tingling. The second part of the morning component is the inability to open and close the fingers immediately. The patient may need two or three openings to provide complete closure or may require up to several hours of active finger manipulation to achieve full flexion. This is an important phenomenon in that it is not nervous, but tendinous in nature. Because of carpal tunnel irritation, the peritendinous synovium takes on fluid proximal and distal to the flexor retinaculum. This fluid in the peritendinous synovium prevents the excursion of the tendons through the tunnel. The fluid is gradually milked proximally and distally away from the tunnel with attempted flexion/extension until full finger excursion can be achieved. This is a fluid mechanical phenomenon independent of nerve symptoms, which localizes the problem to the carpal tunnel.

The third diagnostic component is wrist-fixed activities. Wrist-fixed activities include driving, reading, and writing. These activities produce ischemia of the sensitive median nerve from pressure or arm elevation. The nerve is compressed against the retinaculum by the flexor tendons which lie dorsal to it when the wrist is maintained in one position for any length of time, particularly if that position includes wrist flexion. Elevation of the extremity above the level of the heart produces a decrease in the arterial hydrostatic pressure and contributes to the ischemia. Among the most common manifestations are inability to place the hands on the top of the steering wheel while driving, and inability to hold a blow dryer or accomplish grooming activities of the hair or face. Writing, small object manipulation, holding a telephone, and holding a book while reading all produce symptoms. Occupational activity above the shoulders is particularly difficult. Opening jars becomes increasingly difficult as the median-innervated thenar muscles weaken.

These three clinical components, night, morning, and wrist-fixed symptoms, comprise the diagnosis of carpal tunnel syndrome. It is important to listen to what the patient is telling you, not what they "say." Patients on occasion will say that the entire arm is numb, or may report that the forearm is numb at the elbow, or pain and numbness occur in the wrist, but if the numbness complaint fits the above description (it occurs at night, has a morning component of carpal tunnel syndrome and wrist-fixed activities reproduce the symptoms), then the diagnosis is carpal tunnel syndrome, despite the nonanatomic description of numbness or pain. Sometimes there is little or no complaint of numbness, only pain. The patient will complain of pain and ache in the wrist or forearm, but it will follow the pattern of nighttime and morning symptoms, and wrist-fixed daytime activities. Of 2,504 patients with carpal tunnel syndrome reviewed, 0.92% had only pain symptoms with no numbness or sensory complaints.

Physical Examination

The appearance and feel of the palm is important. If the skin is tight and cannot be pinched by the examiner, then diabetes is probable. If there is an associated stenosing tenosynovitis or trigger finger, there is a 90% chance that there is diabetes in the family, even though the patient may not have diabetes.

Phalen's test is accomplished by passive flexion of the wrist. If this is painful, it often indicates that the Phalen's test will be positive. A positive Phalen's test produces numbness, tingling, or pins-and-needles sensation in the fingertips within 30 seconds. The more inflamed the nerve, the faster the onset of numbness. A forearm compression test is accomplished with the examiner's thumb compressing the median nerve at the pronator level. This will produce numbness and tingling in the fingers, typically somewhat faster than with Phalen's test, and simply indicates that the nerve is inflamed and under pressure within the carpal tunnel. It is inflamed along its entire course and will "read" as such (see following section on double crush syndrome). Moving two-point discrimination is used to evaluate sensation. This is faster and more reliable than the static two-point and should read under four millimeters.

The most valuable clinical examination in carpal tunnel syndrome is evaluation of the median-innervated thenar muscles. The test is done with the wrist straight while the hand is maintained on the tabletop, palm up. The thumb is brought into full opposition and the examiner's fingers press the radial side of the interphalangeal joint of the thumb, following its arc back to the plane of the fingers. It is important not to be on the dorsum of the thumb, where one is testing the extrinsic extensors, and not to be on the flexor surface of the thumb, where one is testing the extrinsic flexor. The abductor pollicis brevis is the main muscle in the evaluation. If the thumb in a normal adult can be depressed back into the plane of the fingers with the examiner's little finger, it represents about 50% loss of thenar power.

A five-point scale is useful, where number 1 is total paralysis in which the thumb lies in the plane of the fingers and cannot be actively raised; at point 2, the thumb can just reach the full opposition position, but cannot maintain it against any resistance; at point 3, the thumb can be put down to the plane of the fingers with difficulty but by the examiner's little finger; at point 4, the thumb has good power, but less than the first dorsal interosseous muscle. The first dorsal interosseous represents one-third to one-half of the power of the median-innervated thenar muscles. The powerful radially-deviated index finger can be compared to, and should be exceeded by, the full opposition power of the thumb. At point 5, the thumb has full opposition power and can not be collapsed without the use of the examiner's arm musculature. Thenar weakness is the first objective sign of carpal tunnel syndrome. It is the most valuable guide for evaluation of response to conservative therapy and if thenar weakness is significant and persists, it indicates the need for surgery. Evaluation of thenar power supercedes and, for the most part, eliminates the need for nerve conduction studies.

Compensable Carpal Tunnel Syndrome

Carpal tunnel syndrome is commonly and properly deemed a compensable problem. There is no such thing as repetitive stress syndrome in the upper extremity. The body is designed to deal with repetitive insult by improving tissue strength and load tolerance and meeting the needs of a repetitive activity. Our hands have developed a design capable of dealing with repetitive activity. The first factor is power; the patient must have sufficient power to accomplish the task. An 85-year-old woman can no longer successfully operate the assembly line she worked as a 30-year-old. The second factor is adaptive time; tissues require adequate time to adapt to load requirements. These two factors are far more important than whether the activity is done repetitiously. Too much load over too long a period of time can damage tissue, so adequate job rotation or break periods are valuable. The public is currently being led to believe that there is a medical diagnosis called "repetitive stress syndrome" when no such diagnosis exists.

The problem for the clinician is often a clarification of insurance carrier responsibility for compensable carpal tunnel syndrome. The following are guidelines for compensation cases.

1. Etiologic responsibility dates back six months from the time carpal tunnel symptoms are obvious to the patient.
2. If there has been a change in the patient's job description between 1 week and 6 months prior to symptom onset, then the etiology date may be considered to be the date of job change.
3. The compensable etiology lies with the employer of record when symptoms occur, even though the patient may have been doing a similar job for different companies for years, or within the six months of the symptom onset. It is assumed for this dictum that there are some unknown factors, which are extant on the new employment or changed job, that are responsible for the rapid onset of carpal tunnel syndrome.
4. Once symptoms have been medically recorded, whether by the employer's health facility or physician, no subsequent employment is responsible, even though the patient may work at similar jobs with different companies through many subsequent years. The total compensable responsibility remains with the carrier of record when the symptoms were recorded. Once the tunnel roof has begun to "grizzelize," carpal tunnel syndrome will progress on its own, producing peritendinous synovitis in the tunnel with less and less stimulus and a gradual increasing grizzelizing of the roof, even if the patient retires.
5. Sudden trauma may produce tunnel synovitis sufficient to act as the etiology for carpal tunnel syndrome. This is probably combined with wrist joint synovitis from synovial tear or ligament injury. If carpal tunnel symptoms do not occur within three months of a motor vehicle accident/trauma, then the carpal tunnel syndrome is probably not related to that accident or incident.

Wrist Problems Producing Carpal Tunnel Syndrome

Carpal tunnel symptoms are commonly associated with wrist pathology. Chronic synovitis in the wrist secondary to predynamic rotary subluxation, for instance, will produce synovitis in the carpal tunnel. Usually resolution of the wrist problem is the proper approach without carpal tunnel surgery. Occasionally, the process has a long history, and the TCL has grizzelized; in these cases the carpal tunnel should be released at the time of wrist surgery. The single determinant for this decision is thenar weakness. More than fifty percent loss (thenar scale 3 or less) of the median-innervated thenar muscles indicates a need for carpal tunnel release at the time of definitive wrist surgery.

Old Age

The onset of carpal tunnel syndrome in patients aged 70 or older should be recognized as an independent entity. The onset is often rapid. Night symptoms are the predominant feature, often with a severe night component of rapid and distressing onset. Thenar power loss is rapid. Contrary to the younger patient, sensory loss is a problem and recovers poorly. A moving two-point of greater than 7 mm often indicates that there will be some permanent sensory deficit. No conservative treatment is indicated in this age group and any sensory widening of the two-point or decreased thenar power is an indication for surgery.

Nerve Conduction Studies

Nerve conduction studies are generally not indicated in carpal tunnel syndrome. The thenar weakness is a far more accurate evaluation and a more important surgical determinant. There are many false negatives and fewer false positives with the electrodiagnostic studies. It is important that all of the prescribed components for testing be accurately present; it is well accepted that they seldom are. Many factors influence the outcome of electrodiagnostic studies, including the time of day. False negative studies would fall off sharply if the test were performed when the patient first awakens, when there is some ischemia in the nerve. Skin temperature and room temperature are important. The patient's state of relaxation, and the skill and experience of the examiner all play a role in the inaccuracy of nerve conduction studies. The ability to differentiate carpal tunnel syndrome from cubital tunnel syndrome, cervical lesions, peripheral neuropathy, and nerve trauma is often valuable. Surgery is indicated regardless of the study result if thenar weakness persists despite adequate conservative treatment.

Ulnar Nerve Association

Ulnar nerves are commonly inflamed at the medial epicondylar groove in association with carpal tunnel syndrome. This is true before and after carpal tunnel release. The ulnar nerve typically produces symptoms, but has normal power for all motor units and normal sensory components. Such cubital tunnel nerve symptoms are best treated conservatively with nonsteroidal antiinflammatory medication and avoidance of contact or compression on the medial epicondylar area, as occurs when reading in bed. The typical inflammatory picture produces aching in the forearms toward the end of the day. It is a nerve-type ache which is diffuse, deep, difficult for the patient to explain, and nonlocalizing. It is accompanied by numbness and tingling in the ring and little fingers. Most will improve or disappear by nine months post-carpal tunnel surgery. On rare occasions, a simple neurolysis of the ulnar nerve at the elbow is indicated (93).

Double Crush Syndrome

The median nerve under pressure at the carpal tunnel level will produce symptoms along its entire course. It is common to have neck symptoms from carpal tunnel syndrome. The clinical exam will mimic inflammation of the median nerve at the cervical area. It is this inflammation that occurs along the entire course of a nerve secondary to compression at any level that is responsible for the so-called "double crush phenomenon." Pathologic phenomena do not occur simultaneously in different areas of the same nerve. The nerve becomes inflamed from compression at one site and then responds as if compressed at any site.

Peripheral Neuropathy

Diabetes and other metabolic conditions can produce peripheral neuropathy which will present clinically as carpal tunnel syndrome. Since the carpal tunnel is anatomically the most restrictive area for the median nerve, inflammation of the nerve secondary to systemic disease will produce carpal tunnel symptoms and a carpal tunnel syndrome picture. Fortunately, surgery at the carpal tunnel level will relieve these symptoms. The clinical picture will clear for the most part by removing the normally restrictive anatomic area of the carpal tunnel and providing relief for the inflamed median nerve, even though that inflammation is intrinsic to the nerve.

Conservative Treatment

The primary and most effective conservative treatment consists of night splints that prevent the wrist from flexing. A splint should be light, comfortable, and easily applied and removed. The flexor tendons lie dorsal to the median nerve and flexion of the wrist over anything longer than a short period of time produces local ischemia in the nerve as the tendons compress it against the TCL. As noted at surgery, the compression area is extremely short, typically measuring 5 to 6 mm of the median nerve. It is rare to see a nerve compressed over a longer area. Nonsteroidal antiinflammatory drugs are a standard part of conservative therapy, and help to reduce the edema and inflammation of the synovium in the tunnel. A permanent cure is rare by conservative means when the following factors exist: age over forty, significant symptoms for more than six months, obesity, and significant weakness of the median-innervated thenar muscles.

Thirty-three years of experience treating carpal tunnel syndrome, with more than 7,000 patients undergoing surgery, has convinced us that cortisone has no place in the treatment of idiopathic (type IA) carpal tunnel syndrome. The results of cortisone in the flexor compartment rarely last more than two and a half months. If used in a young patient with a short duration of symptoms, there may be no recurrence of symptoms. However, this result is better achieved with night splints and nonsteroidal antiinflammatory drugs. Repeated cortisone is damaging to the tissues. Our current position is that cortisone in any joint, tendon synovium, or localized area should seldom exceed three injections over the life of the patient.

It has been well-documented that changing activities, such as providing exercise, interruption of activities, modifying the ergonomics of the activity, whether assembly line work or keyboarding, are all extremely effective in preventing carpal tunnel syndrome. In a local ski factory, we reduced the incidence of carpal tunnel syndrome from 2 to 3 per year to none by extensive modification of the hand tools used in the ski manufacturing process.

Currently, we will use a minimum of six weeks of night splinting and nonsteroidal antiinflammatory drugs unless the patient is elderly with sensory and motor deficits. The nighttime symptoms are almost always improved with a night splint. If there is improvement in the clinical picture, we will continue the conservative therapy program. Persistent thenar weakness is a concern. With thenar weakness greater than 50% documented for 9 months, we suggest surgery in spite of subjective symptom improvement.

Surgery

Because the surgery is brief in duration, we use a Propofol light general anesthesia. A palmar incision is made in line with the radial aspect of the ring finger. The incision is usually 3 cm long and is almost never more than 4 cm, even in a large hand. The skin incision begins proximally at the most proximal aspect of the palmar rugae and extends straight distally. The knife incision is carried down to the palmar fascia. The superficial arterial arch lies in a line with the distal edge of the fully abducted thumb. This line intersects the incision directly over the superficial arch. The fascia overlying the superficial arch is incised, releasing the roof of the canal of Guyon. There is usually an area of yellow fat that lies between the artery and the distal edge of the retinaculum. Spreading technique in this fat will demonstrate the ulnar side of the tunnel. It is important that all structures in the tunnel be retracted radially so that one is visualizing the ulnarmost aspect of the tunnel. The TCL is then incised distal to proximal on its ulnar aspect until the normal thin retinaculum is reached at the wrist crease. The TCL is then reflected. Blunt dissection separates the median nerve from the tunnel roof and identifies the motor branch distally. The proximal TCL may be pierced by aberrant nerves. A 1- to 3-mm wide band is resected from the radial aspect of the TCL. The nerve is inspected for a sleeve. If there is a fascial sleeve around the nerve, it is opened with spreading technique. In some cases, the sleeve is extremely thick and one cannot see the fascicular bundles. If fascicular bundles are easily visible, then there is minimal sleeve around the nerve and it may be ignored. If there is significant synovial reaction in the tunnel, a partial synovectomy around the flexor tendons is carried out. This is a rare component to the surgery. The skin is closed with 5-0 Ethilon. A bulky dressing is applied, using fluffs covered by bias cut stockinette or hand wrap. The dressing is removed in 48 hours and full active use is allowed. The patients are routinely told that they "may run a chain saw" as a way of making clear to them that there are no activities that are limited beyond the 48-hour period. Therapists usually instruct them in massaging the wound with a vitamin E cream and give them some putty for manipulation.

No one doubts the efficacy of properly done endoscopic carpal tunnel surgery (ECTS) in releasing the pressure on the median nerve. There is a slight difference in postoperative morbidity. The problems lie in two areas: recurrence of carpal tunnel syndrome and aberrant motor nerve branches. The collagen fibers of the TCL run transversely in the palm. All releases of this structure cut the fibers perpendicular to their long axis. Linear collagen bundles, be they tendon or ligament, leave what Dr. Boyes called "unsatisfied tendon/collagen end." A significant repair response is elicited under these conditions and a simple transverse cut can allow the TCL to heal and reproduce pressure on the median nerve. The recurrence rate for ECTS is unknown, but our personal experience leads us to believe it is significant.

When endocarpal tunnel release recurs, it follows a pattern. The patient's nighttime symptoms usually clear immediately following surgery. At about three months postoperatively, the patient will again notice the onset of nighttime symptoms. This is followed by a full compliment of carpal tunnel complaints and findings, all of which are typically less severe than the preendoscopic carpal tunnel release picture. Objective thenar weakness is present. Carpal tunnel syndrome recurrence can occur after open carpal tunnel syndrome, if resection of a section of the TCL is not carried out. The senior author's (H.K.W.) experience with over 7,000 open carpal tunnel releases, all with resection of a 2 to 4 mm band of TCL, demonstrates a nonexistent recurrence rate in the 2,504 cases reviewed to date. The inability to remove a section of TCL is our main contraindication to ECTS.

The second and more severe problem is the transection of aberrant motor nerve branches, because its effects are permanent. In the senior editor's practice twenty to 30 open carpal tunnel releases are condensed into one morning in two or three operating rooms. We are usually able to demonstrate one patient with an aberrant median nerve piercing the TCL well proximal to its midpoint. Most are adjunctive and smaller than the main motor branch distally, but rarely they will comprise most of the motor fibers. It is our contention that these motor branches are commonly transected with an endocarpal technique, but being purely motor, their deficiency is not picked up postoperatively. In addition, there are learning curve complications with ECTS. Our current position is that there is little indication for endoscopic carpal tunnel release. The potential for even one nerve laceration introduces too great a risk when compared with open carpal tunnel release, the reliability and safety of which are close to 100%.

REFERENCES

1. Pfeffer GB, Gelberman RH, Boyes JH, et al. The history of carpal tunnel syndrome. *J Hand Surg [Br]* 1988;13:28–34.
2. Paget J. *Lectures on surgical pathology delivered at the Royal College of Surgeons of England, 2nd American ed.* Philadelphia: Lindsay & Blakiston, 1860.
3. Putman JJ. A series of paraesthesia, mainly of the hand, of periodical recurrence, and possibly of vaso-motor origin. *Arch Med* 1880;4:147–162.
4. Marie P, Foix C. Atrophie Isolee de L'eminence Thenar d'Origin Nervitique. Role du Ligament Annulaire Anterieur du Carpe dans la Pathogenie de la Lesion. *Rev Neurol* 1913;26:647–649.
5. Learmonth JR. The priniciple of decompression in the treatment of certain disorders of peripheral nerves. *Surg Clin North Am* 1933;13:905–913.
6. Cannon BW, Love JG. Tardy median palsy: median thenar neuritis amenable to surgery. *Surgery* 1946;20:210–216.
7. Brain WR, Wright AD, Wilkinson M. Spontaneous compression of both median nerves in the carpal tunnel: six cases treated surgically. *Lancet* 1947:277–282.
8. Phalen GS, Gardner W, Lalonde A. Neuropathy of the median nerve due to compression beneath the transverse carpal ligament. *J Bone Joint Surg Am* 1950;32:109–112.
9. Phalen GS. Spontaneous compression of the median nerve at the wrist. *JAMA* 1951;145:1128–1133.
10. Phalen GS, Kendrick J. Compression neuropathy of the medial nerve in the carpal tunnel. *JAMA* 1957;164:524–530.
11. Phalen GS. The carpal tunnel syndrome: seventeen years experience in diagnosis and treatment of six hundred fifty-four hands. *J Bone Joint Surg Am* 1966;48:211–228.
12. Phalen GS. Reflection on 21 years' experience with carpal tunnel syndrome. *JAMA* 1970;212:1365–1367.
13. Phalen GS, Kendick J, Rodriguez J. Lipomas of the upper extremity. *Am J Surg* 1971;121:298–306.
14. Phalen GS. The carpal tunnel syndrome: clinical evaluation of 598 hands. *Clin Orthop* 1972;83:29–40.
15. Phalen GS. The birth of a syndrome, or carpal tunnel revisited. *J Hand Surg [Am]* 1981;6:109–110.
16. Mannerfelt L, Hybbinette CH. Important anomaly of the thenar motor branch of the median nerve. *Bull Hosp Joint Dis* 1972;33:15–21.
17. Caffee HH. Anomalous thenar muscle and median nerve: a case report. *J Hand Surg [Am]* 1979;4:446–447.
18. Ogden J. An unusual branch of the median nerve. *J Bone Joint Surg Am* 1972;54:1779–1781.
19. Papathanassiou BT. A variant of the motor branch of the median nerve in the hand. *J Bone Joint Surg Br* 1968;50:156–157.
20. Lanz U. Anatomical variations of the median nerve in the carpal tunnel. *J Hand Surg [Am]* 1977;2:44–53.
21. Eiken O, Carsta N, Eddeland A. Anomalous distal branching of the median nerve. *Scand J Plast Reconstr Surg* 1971;5:149–152.
22. Johnson RK, Shrewsbury MM. Anatomical course of the thenar branch of the median nerve—usually in a separate tunnel through the transverse carpal ligament. *J Bone Joint Surg Am* 1970;52:269–273.
23. Seradge H, Seradge E. Median innervated hypothenar muscle: anomalous branch of median nerve in the carpal tunnel. *J Hand Surg [Am]* 1990;15:356–359.
24. Tountas CP, Birhle DM, MacDonald CJ, et al. Variations of the median nerve in the carpal canal. *J Hand Surg [Am]* 1987;12(pt 1):708–712.
25. Carroll RE, Green DP. The significance of the palmar cutaneous nerve at the wrist. *Clin Orthop* 1972;83:24.
26. Cobb TK, Dalley BK, Posteraro RH, et al. Anatomy of the retinaculum. *J Hand Surg [Am]* 1977;2:44–53.
27. Chow JCY. Endoscopic carpal tunnel release. In: Whipple T, ed. *Arthroscopy of the wrist.* Philadelphia: JB Lippincott, 1993: 157–169.
28. Lundborg G, Dahlin LB. The pathophysiology of nerve compression. *Hand Clin* 1992;8:215–227.
29. Braun RM, Davidson K, Doehr S. Provocative testing in the diagnosis of dynamic carpal tunnel syndrome. *J Hand Surg [Am]* 1989:14:195–197.
30. Berman AT, Straub RR. Importance of preoperative and postoperative electrodiagnostic studies in the treatment of carpal tunnel syndrome. *Orthop Rev* 1974;3:57.
31. Grundberg AB. Carpal tunnel decompression in spite of normal electromyography. *J Hand Surg [Am]* 1983;8:348–349.
32. Shivde AG, Dreizin I, Fisher MA. The carpal tunnel syndrome: a clinical electrodiagnostic analysis. *Electromyogr Clin Neurophysiol* 1981;21:143.
33. Jackson DA, Clifford JC. Electrodiagnosis of mild carpal tunnel syndrome. *Arch Phys Med Rehabil* 1989;71:199–204.
34. Cioni R, Passero S, Paradiso C, et al. Diagnostic specificity of sensory and motor nerve conduction variables in early detection of carpal tunnel syndrome. *J Neurol* 1989:236:208–213.
35. Carroll RE, Hurst LC. The relationship of the thoracic outlet syndrome and carpal tunnel syndrome. *Clin Orthop* 1982;164:149–153.
36. Osterman AL. Double crush and multiple compression neuropathy. In: Gelberman RH, ed. *Operative nerve repair and reconstruction.* Philadelphia: JB Lippincott, 1991;1211–1229.
37. Wood VE, Biondi J, Linda L. Double-crush nerve compression in thoracic-outlet syndrome. *J Bone Joint Surgery Am* 1990;72:85–87.
38. Jones NF, Ming NL. Persistent median artery as a cause of pronator syndrome. *J Hand Surg [Am]* 1988;13:728–732.
39. Dellon AL, Fine IT. A noninvasive technique for diagnosis of chronic compartment syndrome in the first dorsal interosseous muscle. *J Hand Surg [Am]* 1990;15:1008–1009.
40. Durkan JA. A new diagnostic test for carpal tunnel syndrome. *J Bone Joint Surg Am* 1991;73:535–538.
41. Molitor PJ. A diagnostic test for carpal tunnel syndrome using ultrasound. *J Hand Surg [Br]* 1988;13:40–41.
42. Murphy RX, Chernofsky MA, Osborne MA, et al. Magnetic resonance imaging in the evaluation of persistent carpal tunnel syndrome. *J Hand Surg [Am]* 1993;18:113–120.
43. Mesgarzadeh M, Schneck CD, Bonakdarpour A, et al. Carpal tunnel: MR imaging. Part II: Carpal tunnel syndrome. *Radiology* 1989;171:749–754.
44. Szabo RM, Gelberman RH, Dimick MP. Sensibility testing in patients with carpal tunnel syndrome. *J Bone Joint Surg Am* 1984;66:60–64.
45. Richman JA, Gelberman RH, Rydevik B, et al. Carpal tunnel volume determination by magnetic imaging 3-D reconstruction. *J Hand Surg [Am]* 1987;12:712–717.
46. Gelberman RH, Aronson D, Weisman MH. Carpal tunnel syndrome: results of a prospective trial of steroid injection and splinting. *J Hand Surg [Am]* 1992;17:1003–1008.
47. Gelberman RH, Rydevik BL, Pess GM, et al. Carpal tunnel syndrome: a scientific basis for clinical care. *Orthop Clin North Am* 1988;19:115–124.
48. Wood MR. Hydrocortisone injections for carpal tunnel syndrome. *Hand* 1980;12:62–64.
49. Stransky M, Rubin A, Lavaa NS, et al. Treatment of carpal tunnel syndrome with vitamin B6: a double-blind study. *South Med J* 1989;82:841–842.
50. Weiss AC, Sachar K, Gendreau M. Conservative managment of carpal tunnel syndrome: a re-examination of steroid injection and splinting. *J Hand Surg [Am]* 19:410–415.
51. Heckler FR, Jabaley ME. Evolving concepts of median nerve decompression in the carpal tunnel. *Hand Clin* 1986;2:723–735.
52. Jakab E, Ganos D, Cook FW. Transverse carpal ligament recon-

struction in surgery for carpal tunnel syndrome: a new technique. *J Hand Surg [Am]* 1991;16:202–206.
53. Lowry WE, Follender AB. Interfascicular neurolysis in severe carpal tunnel syndrome: a prospective, randomized, double-blind, controlled study. *Clin Orthop* 1988;227:251–254.
54. Mackinnon SE, McCabe S, Murray JF, et al. Internal neurolysis fails to improve the results of primary carpal tunnel decompression. *J Hand Surg [Am]* 1991;16:211–218.
55. Nissenbaum M, Kleinert HE. Treatment considerations in carpal tunnel syndrome with coexistent Dupuytren's disease. *J Hand Surg [Am]* 1980;5:544–547.
56. O'Malley MJ, Evanoff M, Terrono AK, et al. Factors that determine re-exploration treatment if carpal tunnel syndrome. *J Hand Surg [Am]* 1992;17:638–641.
57. Rowland SA. A palmar incision for release of the carpal tunnel. *Clin Orthop* 1974;103:89–90.
58. Freshwater MF, Arons MS. The effect of various adjuncts on the surgical treatment of carpal tunnel syndrome secondary to chronic synovitis. *Plast Reconstr Surg* 1978;61:93–96.
59. Taleisnik J. The palmar cutaneous branch of the median nerve and the approach to the carpal tunnel. *J Bone Joint Surg [Am]* 1973;55:1212–1217.
60. Gelberman RH, Pfeffer GB, Galbraith RT, et al. Results of treatment of severe carpal tunnel syndrome without internal neurolysis of the median nerve. *J Bone Joint Surg Am* 1987;69:896–903.
61. Garland H, Sumner D, Clark JMP. Carpal tunnel syndrome: with particular reference to surgical treatment. *Br Med J* 1963;1:581.
62. Clayton M, Linscheid R. Carpal tunnel surgery: should the incision be above or below the wrist? *Orthopedics* 1988;2:819–821.
63. Curtis RM, Eversmann WW Jr. Internal neurolysis as an adjunct to the treatment of the carpal tunnel syndrome. *J Bone Joint Surg Am* 1973;55:733–740.
64. Wright PE II, Milford LW. Carpal tunnel and ulnar tunnel syndromes and stenosing tenosynovitis. In: Crenshaw AH, ed. *Campbell's operative orthopaedics*. St Louis: Mosby, 1976;3435–3438.
65. Levy HJ, Spofer TB, Kleinbart FA, et al. Endoscopic carpal tunnel release: an anatomic study. *Arthroscopy* 1993;9:1–4.
66. Rotman MB, Manske PR. *Anatomical relationships of an endoscopic carpal tunnel device to surrounding structures.* Joseph A. Boyes Award paper presented at the 47th Annual Meeting of the American Society for Surgery of the Hand, Orlando, FL, October, 1991.
67. Seiler J III, Barnes K, Gelberman RH, et al. Endoscopic carpal tunnel release: an anatomic study of the two-incision method in human cadavers. *J Hand Surg [Am]* 1992;17:996–1002.
68. Schwartz TJ, Waters PM, Simmons BP. Endoscopic carpal tunnel release: a cadaveric study. *Arthroscopy* 1993;9:209–213.
69. Luallian SR, Toby EB. Incidental Guyon's canal release during attempted endoscopic carpal tunnel release: an anatomical study and report of two cases. *Arthroscopy* 1993;9:382–386.
70. Malek MM, Chow JCY. *National study of the complications of over 10,000 cases of endoscopic carpal tunnel release.* Presented at the 61st Annual Meeting of the American Academy of Orthopaedic Surgeons, New Orleans, LA, February 24–28, 1994.
71. Chow JCY, Malek MM. *Complications of endoscpic release of the carpal ligament using the Chow technique.* Presented at the 60th Annual Meeting of the American Academy of Orthopaedic Surgeons, San Francisco, CA, February 18–23, 1993.
72. Chow JCY, Malek M, Nagle D. *Complications of endoscopic release of the carpal ligament using the Chow technique.* Presented at the 4th Annual Meeting of the American Society for Surgery of the Hand, Phoenix, AZ, November 12, 1992.
73. Chow JCY. Endoscopic release of the carpal ligament: a new technique for carpal tunnel syndrome. *Arthroscopy* 1989;5:19–24.
74. Chow JCY. *Endoscopic carpal tunnel release—clinical results of 149 cases.* Presented at the the 9th Annual AANA Meeting, Orlando, FL, April 26–29, 1990.
75. Chow JCY. Endoscopic release of the carpal ligament: 22-month clinical results. *Arthroscopy* 1990;6:388–396.
76. Chow JCY. *Endoscopic release of the carpal ligament: analysis of 300 cases.* Presented at the 58th Annual Meeting of the American Academy of Orthopaedic Surgeons, Anaheim, CA, March 9, 1991.
77. Chow JCY. The Chow technique of endoscopic release of the carpal ligament for carpal tunnel syndrome: four years of clinical results. *Arthroscopy* 1993;9:301–314.
78. Okutsu I, Nonomiya S, Takatori Y, et al. Endoscopic management of carpal tunnel syndrome. *Arthroscopy* 1989;5:11–18.
79. Agee JM, McCarroll HR Jr, Tortosa RD, et al. Endoscopic release of the carpal tunnel: a randomized prospective multicenter study. *J Hand Surg [Am]* 1992;17:987–995.
80. Nagle DJ, Fischer T, Hastings H, et al. *A multicenter prospective study of 641 endoscopic carpal tunnel releases using the Chow extrabursal technique.* Presented at the 47th Annual Meeting of the American Society for Surgery of the Hand, Phoenix, AZ, November, 1992.
81. Nagle D, Fischer T, Harris GD, et al. A multi-center prospective review of 640 endoscopic carpal tunnel releases using the Chow technique. *Arthroscopy* 1996;12:139–143.
82. Kessler I. Unusual distribution of the median nerve at the wrist. *Clin Orthop* 1969;67:124–126.
83. Kleinert J. The nerve of Henle. *J Hand Surg [Am]* 1990;15:784–788.
84. Shimizu K, Iwasaki R, Hosihkawa H, et al. Entrapment neuropathy of the palmar cutaneous branch of the median nerve by the fascia of flexor digitoum superficialis. *J Hand Surg [Am]* 1988;13:581–583.
85. Engber WD, Gmeiner JG. Palmar cutaneous branch of the ulnar nerve. *J Hand Surg [Am]* 1980;5:26–29.
86. Cobb, TK, Carmichael SW, Cooney, WP. The ulnar neurovascular bundle at the wrist. A technical note on endoscopic carpal tunnel release. *J Hand Surg [Br]* 1994;19:24–26.
87. Agee JM, Tortsua RD, Palmer CA, et al. *Endoscopic release of the carpal tunnel: a prospective randomized multicenter study.* Presented at the 45th Annual Meeting of the American Society of the Hand, Toronto, Canada, September 24–27, 1990.
88. Ritter MA. The anatomy and function of the palmar fascia. *Hand* 1973;5:263–267.
89. Shrewsbury MM, Johnson RK, Ousterhout DK. The palmaris brevis—a reconsideration of its anatomy and possible function. *J Bone Joint Surg [Am]* 1972;54:344–348.
90. Viegas S, Pollard A, Kaminksi K. Carpal arch alteration and related clinical status after endoscopic carpal tunnel release. *J Hand Surg [Am]* 1992;17:1012–1016.
91. Garcia-Elias M, Sanches-Freijo J, Salo J, et al. Dynamic changes of the transverse carpal arch during flexion-extension of the wrist: effects of sectioning the transverse carpal ligament. *J Hand Surg [Am]* 1992;17:1017–1019.
92. Richman JA, Gelberman RH, Rydevik BL, et al. Carpal tunnel syndrome: morphologic changes after release of transverse carpal ligament. *J Hand Surg [Am]* 1989;14:852–857.
93. Caputo AE, Watson HK. Subcutaneous anterior transposition of the ulnar nerve for failed decompression of cubital tunnel syndrome. *J Hand Surg [Am]* 2000;25:544–551.

10

CONGENITAL ANOMALIES OF THE WRIST

DIETER BUCK-GRAMCKO

The wrist is involved in many congenital malformations of the hand and in most anomalies of the forearm. In a few congenital deformities, the wrist alone is involved, as in carpal coalitions. They are usually found not as isolated anomalies but in combination with other malformations of the upper extremity.

Unlike most malformations of the hand, congenital anomalies of the wrist are not detectable at birth or even in the first years of life. This is not only because they will not produce gross deformities, with the exception of a few malformations such as radial club hand, but because their radiologic appearance is not detected in the early years. Carpal bones and the distal ends of the radius and ulna are cartilaginous at birth and in the first years of life. Ossification occurs over a span of many years; it starts in some bones in the first year but is completed after the age of 12 to 14 years. In some disorders, skeletal maturation is retarded. Form and shape of the bones are used for assessment of the skeletal age and as an indicator of normal or abnormal development of the child.

Because of the tendency to surgically correct many congenital malformations of the hand and forearm in the first 2 or 3 years of life, it may be difficult to see the natural course of the pathologic development of the carpal bones. They are altered by many of the procedures. Therefore, I have tried to find x-ray films of my patients treated 30 years before—an era in which children with congenital malformations were often not referred before the age of 8 to 10 years. I have looked for patients who were examined radiologically several times during their growth period, so that it is possible to demonstrate bony development over a period of many years. The following sections describe the different anomalies.

CARPAL SYNOSTOSIS

The most frequent congenital anomaly of the wrist is synostosis of the carpal bones. It is also called carpal coalition or fusion, although this deformity probably arises not by fusion but rather by nonseparation of the two bones. In most cases, only two bones of the same carpal row are involved; synostoses of three or more bones crossing the midcarpal joint are very rare. Carpal synostoses occur as isolated deformities or in association with other malformations or syndromes. The real incidence is unknown because many of the asymptomatic synostoses will never be detected; the majority of diagnoses are made by radiologic examinations for other reasons or during population studies. Symptoms such as pain or restriction of motion result only following injuries with pseudarthrosis or arthrotic changes; in cases of massive synostoses, the range of motion is restricted in all directions. Classifications into incomplete and complete synostoses or forms with only a notch have no practical value or consequences.

Lunotriquetral synostosis (Fig. 10.1) is the most common type of synostosis, involving only two carpal bones, followed by synostosis of the capitate and hamate (Fig. 10.2A–D) and then between trapezium and trapezoid. These types of carpal synostoses are more common in black than in white people.

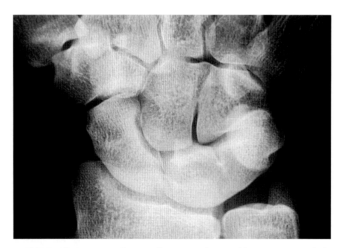

FIGURE 10.1. Lunotriquetral synostosis. In this case a notch is seen at the site of the usual joint space between these bones.

D. Buck-Gramcko: Department of Surgery, University of Hamburg; and Department of Hand Surgery, Wilhelmstift Children's Hospital, D-22149 Hamburg, Germany.

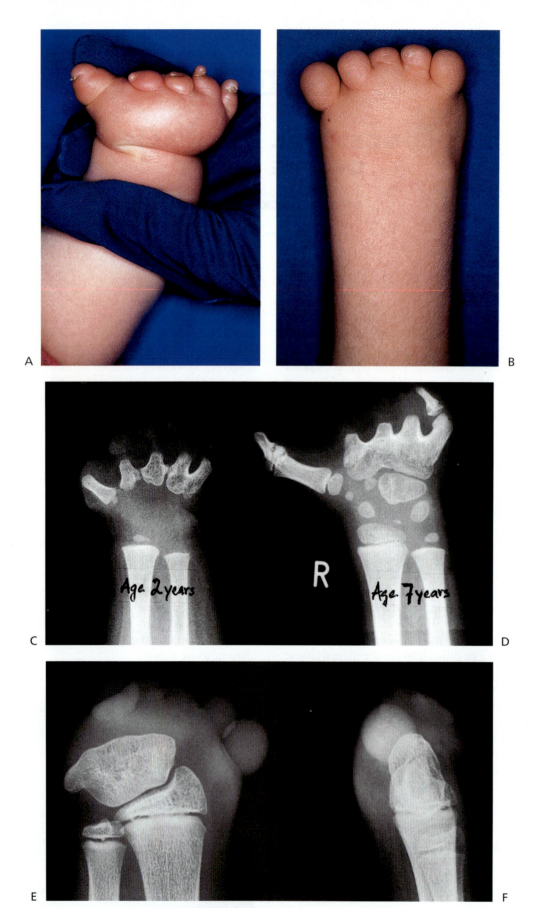

FIGURE 10.2. Clinical and radiologic appearance of two cases of symbrachydactyly. **A,B:** Clinical photos. **C,D:** The radiographs of the hand shown in **A** at the ages of 2 and 7 years show the development of the metacarpal synostoses and the retarded ossification of the carpal bones with a capitohamate synostosis. **E,F:** In this peromelic type (hand in **B**) in a 12-year-old girl, all carpals form a bone block with a relatively good radiocarpal joint.

Synostoses among multiple carpal bones, with the metacarpal bones or even the radius and ulna, are rare and are seen mostly in association with other anomalies or syndromes. In many cases of radial and ulnar deficiencies, these types can occur in symbrachydactyly. In the more advanced grades of this deformity, one can find synostoses not only of the bases of multiple metacarpals (Fig. 10.2A–D) but also of all of the carpals, which form a single bone block (Fig. 10.2E,F).

Of special interest is the association of symphalangism of the interphalangeal joints with multiple carpal and tarsal synostoses. These can also include the first metacarpal (Fig. 10.3). With multiple synostoses syndrome (*La maladie des synostoses multiples* of Maroteaux), a combination of carpal and tarsal coalitions, short first metacarpals and metatarsals, proximal symphalangism, elbow ankylosis or dysplasia, and conductive deafness is described. It is inherited as an autosomal dominant trait.

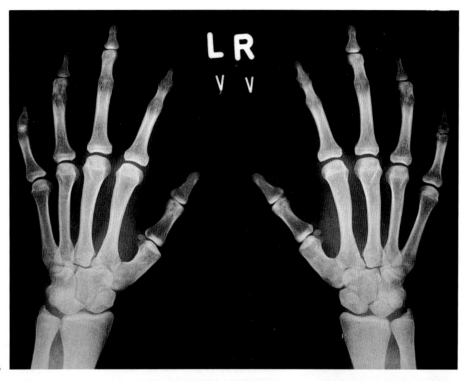

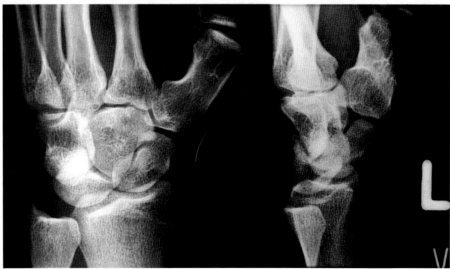

FIGURE 10.3. A,B: Association of symphalangism and carpal coalitions. In addition to the multiple carpal synostoses, the bilateral synostosis between trapezium and first metacarpal is particularly unusual.

ASEPTIC NECROSIS

Aseptic necrosis of a hypoplastic scaphoid bone is an extremely rare disease. In a fully developed scaphoid, aseptic necrosis (Preiser's disease) is very rare, but in a hypoplastic bone it has, to the best of my knowledge, never been described.

Case Report

A girl was born in January 1960 with hypoplasia of both thumbs (right grade I, left grade IIIB). In the anamnesis there were no particular data or mention of thalidomide ingestion by the mother. She was referred in 1965 and treated in December of that year by excision of the hypoplastic thumb and pollicization of the index finger on the left side. The postoperative course was uneventful with the exception of a small area of necrosis of the wound margin. At that time, the scaphoid was not yet ossified (Fig. 10.4A). The patient developed excellent function with her new thumb. In 1977 she complained of some pain with motion at the radial side of the wrist where there was some swelling and tenderness. She had no injury. Radiologic examination demonstrated some sclerosis in the small

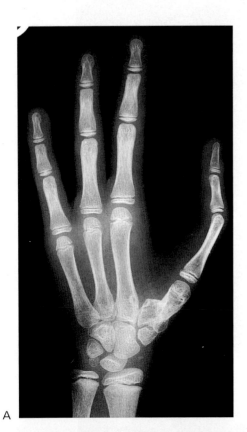

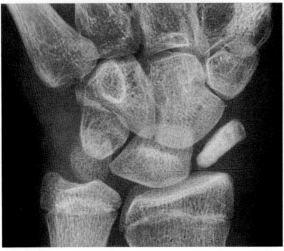

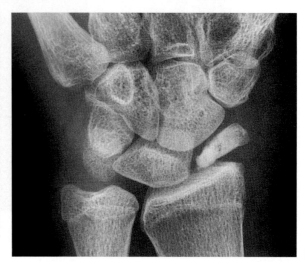

FIGURE 10.4. Aseptic necrosis of a hypoplastic scaphoid in a case of thumb hypoplasia, grade IIIB. **A:** Left hand 6 years after pollicization of the index finger; the scaphoid is beginning to ossify, which was retarded for about 6 years in this 12-year-old girl. **B:** Some sclerosis of the scaphoid at the time of onset of symptoms (April 1977). **C,D:** Disintegration, especially in the proximal half of the scaphoid (October and November 1977).

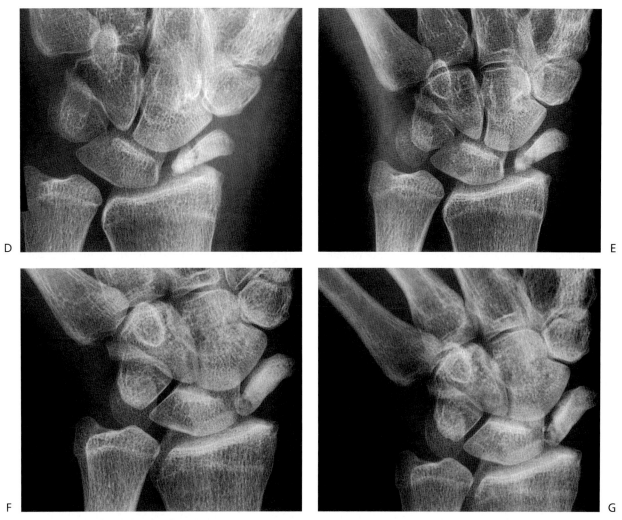

FIGURE 10.4. (continued) E: Unchanged radiologic findings despite clinical improvement following immobilization (April 1978). **F:** Some bone consolidation 1 year later (May 1979). **G:** Radiograph at the follow-up examination 20 years after onset of the symptoms still demonstrates incomplete bone healing.

hypoplastic scaphoid (Fig. 10.4B). During the following months, the left wrist became more painful, even at rest; it was, therefore, immobilized with a plaster splint. X-ray films during the last four months of 1977 showed increasing irregularities with interruption of the bone structure, especially of the proximal half of the scaphoid (Fig. 10.4C,D). After 3 months of immobilization, the complaints decreased, although the radiologic signs of bone necrosis had not yet changed (Fig. 10.4E). About 1 year after the onset of symptoms, the patient was free of complaints (Fig. 10.4F). Radiologic examination 20 years later (1997) showed a sclerotic scaphoid with irregularities in its proximal pole (Fig. 10.4G); clinically, the patient was free of symptoms and able to use her new thumb without problems.

The cause of the aseptic necrosis of the hypoplastic scaphoid remains uncertain. There was no injury in the years before the onset of symptoms. The small size of the scaphoid and the altered biomechanics of the wrist in radial deficiencies with index finger pollicization may be a possible cause but are not probable because I have not seen such changes in any of the other approximately 600 hands and wrists with radial deficiencies I have treated.

RADIAL DEFICIENCY

Congenital anomalies on the radial side of the hand and forearm are not uncommon and are seen in my patients twice as frequently as ulnar deficiencies. In previous years, most of these cases were related to thalidomide ingestion by the mother during the first weeks of pregnancy. There are many variations, ranging from slight hypoplasia of the thumb to a radial club hand with aplasia of the radius. In all cases, the wrist is involved, so that one can find many interesting variations. In earlier years the referral of children was very late, and it was possible to study the anomalies in a stage of advanced ossification of the carpal bones.

In addition to the bone deformities, all soft tissue structures on the radial half of the hand and forearm are involved. Muscles and tendons are missing, hypoplastic, or have abnormal insertions. Blood vessels and nerves run along an abnormal course or are absent. The muscle anomalies play an especially important role in the deformity and influence its surgical correction. Involvement of the soft-tissue structures is seen only in the ulnar deficiency malformations discussed in this chapter; the others have this, if ever, only to a minor extent. Because of partial or complete aplasia of the radius, there is no radiocarpal joint in a radial club hand. The proximal carpal bones form an unphysiologic articulation with the distal ulna (Fig. 10.5), which may show an indentation at the site of this new articulation (Fig. 10.5B). Number, shape, or presence of synostoses of the carpal bones does not depend on the severity of the deformity of the radius. In cases with complete or partial aplasia of the radius, there is always an absence of the scaphoid and trapezium, but the other carpals may be either synostotic (Fig. 10.5A) or normal in shape and separated (Fig. 10.5B). Similar variations are found in cases with hypoplasia of the radius, in which the radius is only slightly shorter than the ulna (Fig. 10.6). In these deformities, the distal end of the radius looks like an ulna; it is not broadened and shows no inclination. Even if the radius is about the same length as the ulna, its distal end is not as broad as in normal wrists. The styloid process is missing in almost all cases of radial deficiency (Figs. 10.4 and 10.6–10.8).

The scaphoid bone is often completely absent (Fig. 10.8) or severely deformed and exists only as an ossicle (Fig. 10.7). Only in relatively few cases it is present, and when it is present, it is hypoplastic to different degrees (Figs. 10.4 and 10.9B). In these wrists, ossification is retarded for several years. The place of the scaphoid can be radiologically "empty" or filled by the distal end of the radius (Fig. 10.8).

The presence of a trapezium depends to a certain degree on the grade of thumb hypoplasia. In hands with aplasia of the thumb, the trapezium is also absent (Fig. 10.9), although with hypoplasia of the thumb a small trapezium often may be present (Figs. 10.8 and 10.10). There are also

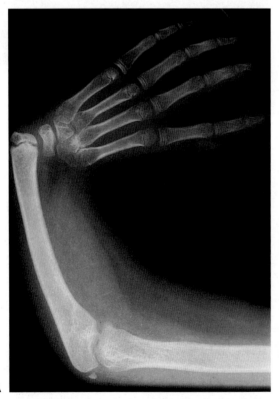
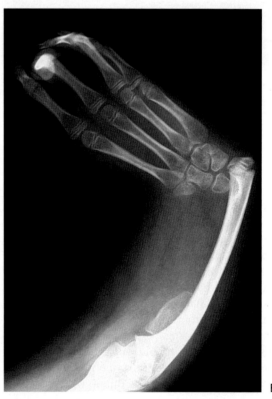

FIGURE 10.5. In untreated radial club hands of adolescents, the carpus articulates with the radial side of the distal ulna. The carpal bones in these hands of two 11-year-old girls may show either synostoses **(A)** or almost normal development **(B)**.

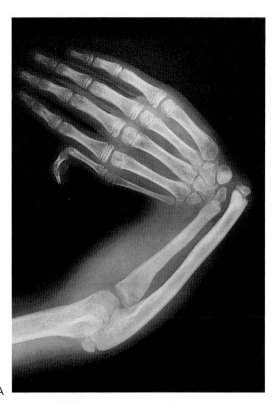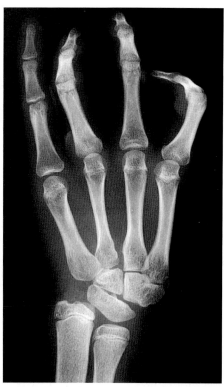

FIGURE 10.6. In hypoplasia of the radius, not only is the degree of radial deviation different, but also the state of the carpal bones. They may be normal with the exception of the scaphoid and trapezium **(A)** or may show multiple synostoses **(B)**.

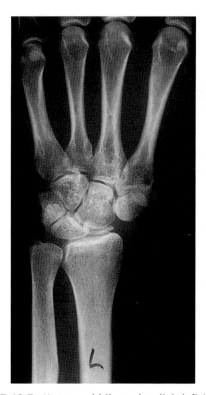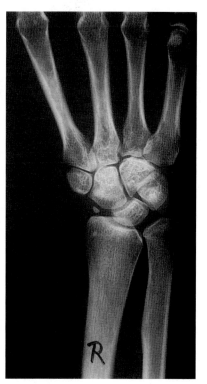

FIGURE 10.7. Untreated bilateral radial deficiency in a female patient aged 25 with absence of the thumb ray including trapezium and styloid process. The scaphoid exists only as a small ossicle.

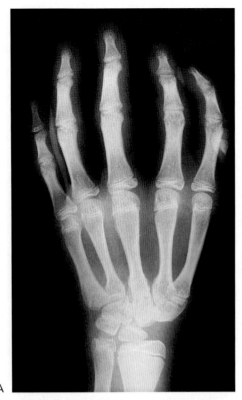 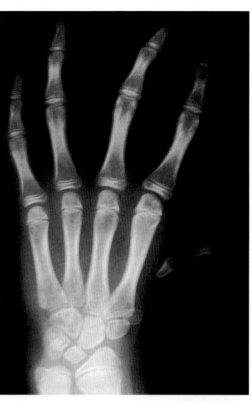

FIGURE 10.8. Aplasia of the scaphoid and presence of the trapezium in cases of a five-finger hand **(A)** and a thumb hypoplasia grade IIIB **(B)**. The articulation between the carpus and the radius is quite different in the two hands.

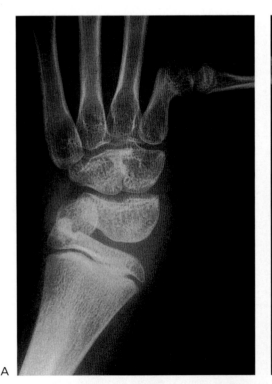 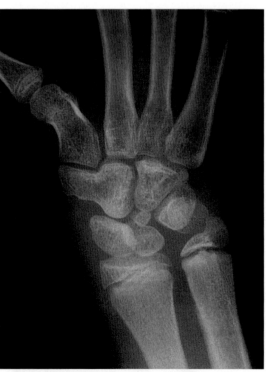

FIGURE 10.9. A,B: In aplasia of the thumb (in both hands of a 15-year-old boy after index finger pollicization), the trapezium is also absent. In the clinically better right hand **(B)**, only the capitate and trapezoid are synostotic. Several carpal bones of the proximal and distal row of the opposite hand form a bone block **(A)**. In the left arm there are distal and proximal radioulnar synostoses; in the right wrist an "os centrale" is seen.

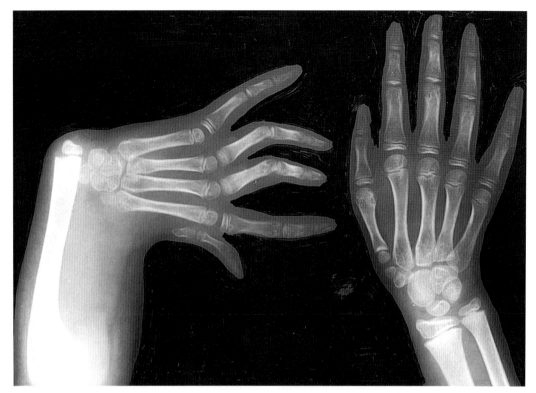

FIGURE 10.10. A small trapezium is present in both hands of this 10-year-old girl with thumb hypoplasia, grade II right and grade IIIB left, despite the severe club hand with aplasia of the radius.

cases of an absent trapezium, although a hypoplastic thumb exists (Fig. 10.11). In a five-finger hand, a trapezium is usually present, even if the scaphoid is missing (Figs. 10.8 and 10.12). It is interesting that minor differences between triphalangeal thumbs are also reflected in the development of the carpal bones (Fig. 10.12).

The configuration of the central and ulnar carpal bones in cases of radial deficiencies with a hypoplastic radius is quite different, even if the same number of bones and no synostoses exist. In some wrists, the size and position appear normal (Figs. 10.5A, 10.10, and 10.13A); in others, the bones of the distal row (capitate and hamate) show some radial "shift," while the lunate is pushed ulnarwards and the triquetrum occupies a more distal position (Figs. 10.7, left hand in 10.12, and 10.13B). The amount of this translation is variable; sometimes the capitate articulates directly with the radius (Fig. 10.13B). The influence of these changes on the range of motion is not significant because in all these wrists, motion is limited in all directions.

Synostoses associated with radial deficiencies usually involve only the carpal bones (Figs. 10.5B, 10.9B, 10.11, and 10.14), sometimes in both rows. Massive synostoses, in which distal and proximal carpals form a block on both sides of the midcarpal joint, are very rare and always associated with other anomalies (in Fig. 10.9A, with distal and proximal radioulnar synostosis).

The development of such synostosis is demonstrated in serial x-ray films of a girl born in August 1961 with bilateral hypoplastic triphalangeal thumbs (with syndactyly of the right hand) following thalidomide ingestion by the mother early in the pregnancy. Our first radiograph of November 1967 (see right hand in Fig. 10.11) shows no ossification center of the scaphoid, and the synostosis between trapezoid and capitate is already completed. This had not changed by June 1968, about half a year after removal of the hypoplastic triphalangeal thumb and pollicization of the index finger (Fig. 10.14A). In October 1970, a quite different configuration was seen: a synostosis of the lunate and a nonossified scaphoid of remarkable size (Fig. 10.14B). Eight years later, these two "fused" bones have increased in size (Fig. 10.14C) and show an excellent congruent articulation to the distal radius (without a styloid process).

Surgical procedures for correction will not concern the wrist if only the thumb is involved (e.g., in pollicization) but will change the carpal bones and the distal end of the ulna considerably in cases of radial club hand.

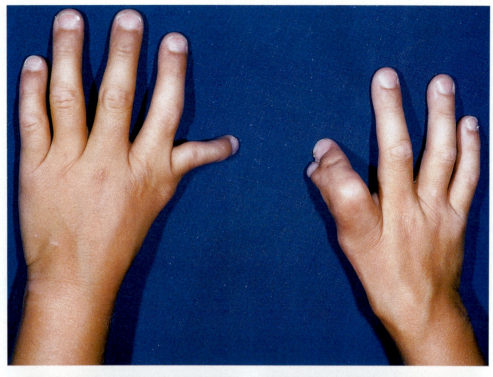
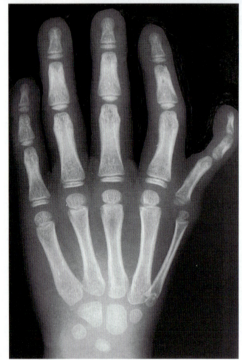
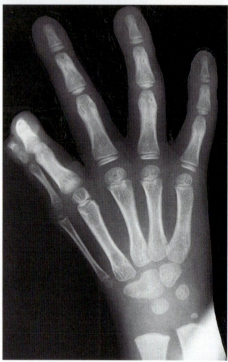

FIGURE 10.11. A,B: A trapezium can be missing even in cases of hypoplastic triphalangeal thumb. In the right hand in this 6-year-old girl, a synostosis between capitate and trapezoid is seen, and in the left hand the existing carpals appear normal.

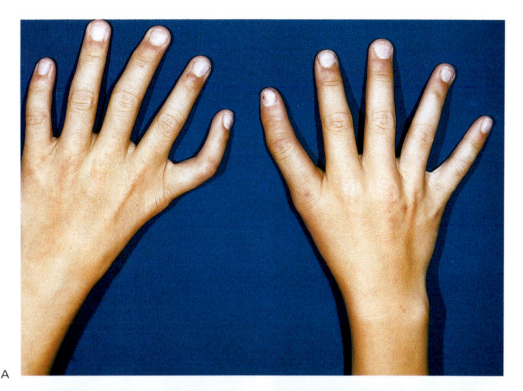
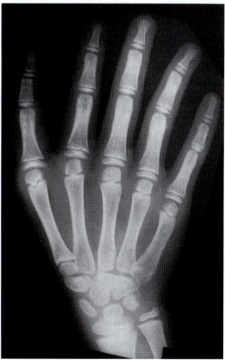

FIGURE 10.12. A,B: Triphalangeal thumbs in both hands of a 12-year-old boy. In the left hand, the radial digit is more hypoplastic than in the right hand; this difference is also seen in the development of the radial carpal bones.

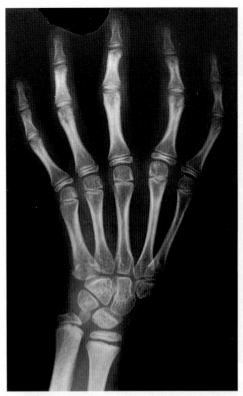
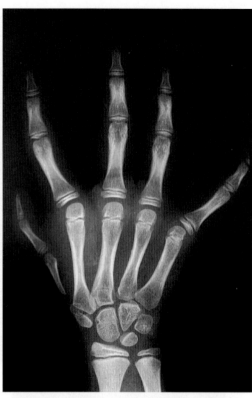

FIGURE 10.13. The configuration of the carpal bones and their correlation to the distal ends of the hypoplastic radius and the ulna can be quite different in radial deficiencies. There are cases with an almost normal carpus except for the absence of the scaphoid **(A)**, but in other cases there is some "distortion" with a radial shift of the distal bones, so that the capitate articulates with the radius **(B)**.

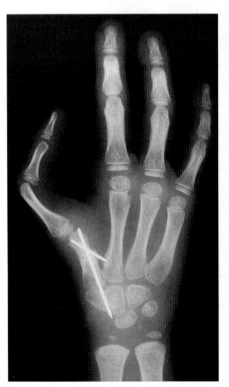
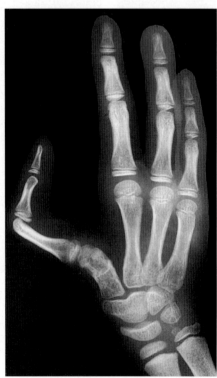
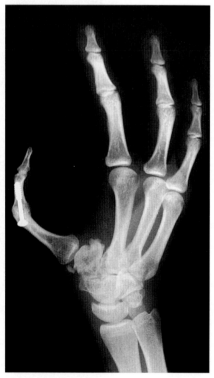

FIGURE 10.14. Development of carpal synostosis in radial deficiencies. At the age of 7, the scaphoid is not yet ossified, and the synostosis between capitate and trapezoid is already established **(A)**. Two years later, the scaphoid is of remarkable size and "fused" with the lunate **(B)**. Eight years later, some further growth of this synostosis has occurred; the pollicized index finger was corrected with shortening of the metacarpal remnant and arthrodesis of the deformed former proximal interphalangeal joint **(C)**.

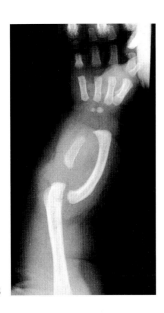
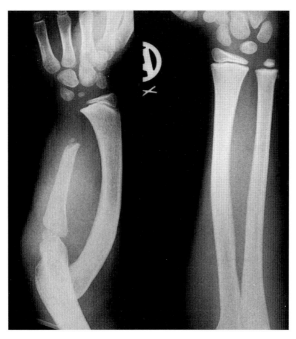

FIGURE 10.15. Ulnar deficiency with partial aplasia of the ulna, dislocation of the radial head, and bowing of the radius with obliquity of its distal articular surface. The length of the forearm is considerably reduced. In a comparison between the radiographs at birth **(A)** and 9 years later **(B)**, retarded ossification of the ulna is seen.

A,B

ULNAR DEFICIENCY

In regard to the wrist, ulnar deficiencies demonstrate some similarities to radial deficiencies. Synostoses and lack of the full complement of carpal bones, often only one forearm bone at the wrist level, and soft-tissue involvement are seen. Additional changes affecting the wrist occur with severe deformities and in cases of reduced numbers of digital rays. The length of the forearm is, in most cases, reduced, as in a radial club hand, which is caused not only by shortening of the bones but also by congenital dislocation of the head of the radius, which is further shortened by its bowing (Fig. 10.15). Ulnar deviation of the wrist is caused by this bowing, by a slant of the articular surface of the radius, often seen in many cases of partial or complete aplasia of the ulna, and probably by the slowly growing fibrocartilaginous anlage of the distal ulna.

The missing carpal bones are related to the absent ulnar digital rays, but often in a quite different way. The wrists of the two hands shown in Fig. 10.16 consist of different

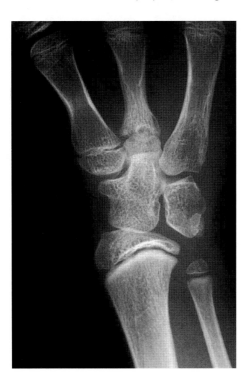
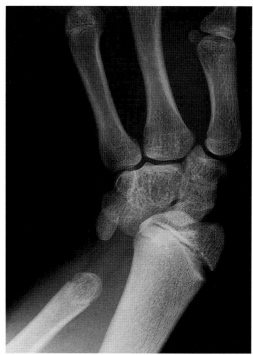

FIGURE 10.16. Shapes and number of carpal bones in ulnar deficiencies differ, unrelated to the number of digital rays. Although the ulnar digits are missing, the pisiform bone is always present, whereas other carpals are difficult to designate.

numbers of carpals, although in both hands there are three digital rays. Shape and synostoses of the carpal bones are often irregular; sometimes it is difficult to designate them correctly (Fig. 10.16). It may be of particular interest that the pisiform bone is always present, as is the flexor carpi ulnaris muscle and its tendon.

DISTAL RADIOULNAR SYNOSTOSIS

A synostosis between the distal ends of the radius and ulna is—as far as I know—almost always combined with a proximal synostosis (Fig. 10.17) or is a part of a rare complete fusion of these bones. Although an isolated proximal synostosis between the two forearm bones has no influence on the radiologic configuration of the wrist, a distal synostosis changes at least the radio- and ulnocarpal artic-ular surface. Both bones form either a common joint surface (Figs. 10.9A and 10.18) or the distal ends of the radius and ulna show some divergence (Fig. 10.19). The carpal bones are irregular in shape and number and often synostotic.

In all cases of combined distal and proximal radioulnar synostosis, there are other associated congenital anomalies, such as radial deficiencies (Figs. 10.9A and 10.17), symbrachydactyly (Fig. 10.17), or severe deformities such as a Cenani syndactyly (Fig. 10.19).

The radiologic development of a distal radioulnar synostosis can be demonstrated in Fig. 10.17. At birth, the radiograph showed only a relatively small bone bridge, which had grown in the next 4 years to a broad fusion. Ossification of the carpal bones occurred normally, at least until the last follow-up examination at the age of 7 years.

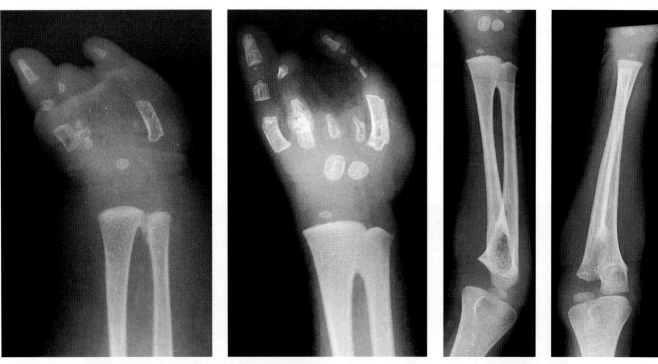

FIGURE 10.17. Development of a broad distal radioulnar synostosis in the course of 4 years **(A,B)** in a patient with symbrachydactyly (cleft hand type) and combined distal and proximal radioulnar synostoses **(C)**.

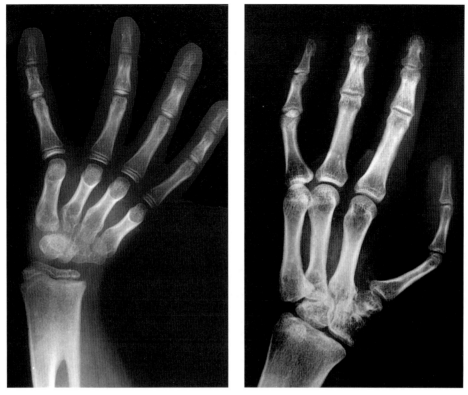

FIGURE 10.18. Distal radioulnar synostosis (proximal synostosis not shown) at the age of 12 with thumb aplasia and deformity of the wrist **(A)**. Result 20 years after pollicization of the index finger and partial resection of carpal bones for axial correction **(B)**.

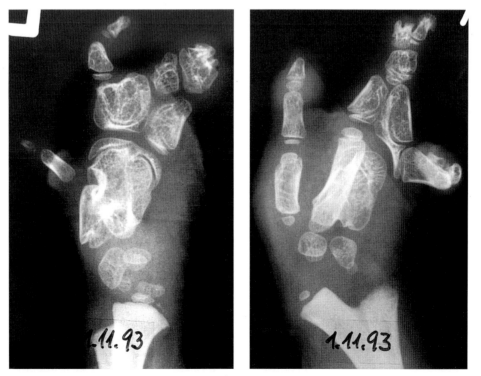

FIGURE 10.19. Bilateral complete radioulnar synostosis with split and divergent distal ends of the forearm bones and severe deformities of the metacarpals and phalanges, including multiple bones with longitudinal epiphyseal brackets ("delta-bones") in a boy with Cenani syndactyly.

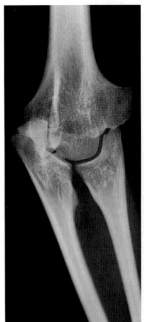
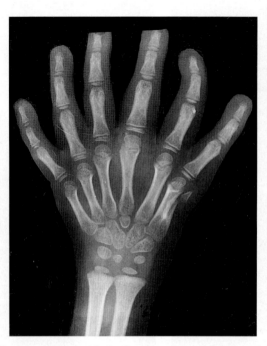
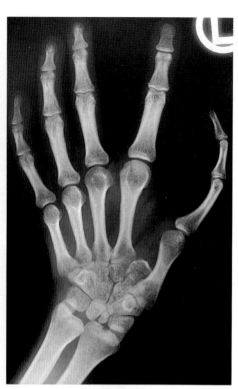

FIGURE 10.20. Mirror hand with duplication of the ulna **(A)** and the ulnar part of the hand. The duplication of the ulnar carpal bones is demonstrated radiographically at the age of six (preoperatively) **(B)** and at 49 years (43 years postoperatively) **(C)**.

MIRROR HAND

This extremely rare anomaly consists of a duplication of the ulna and the ulnar half of the hand and absence of the radius and the thumb. Restriction of motion in the elbow and wrist is caused not only by the bony deformities but also by muscle anomalies. These deformities result in considerable disorders in all parts of the wrist. The proximal articulation surface is composed of two ulnae and shows, at least radiologically, no real congruence to the carpals (Fig. 10.20). These are arranged symmetrically; in their center, there are ossicles, which may be designated as lunate and trapezoid.

Treatment consists of pollicization of the largest of the radial digits, removal of the supernumerary digital rays, and transposition of the flexor tendons of the ablated digits for use as wrist extensors. Figure 10.20 shows the late result of my very first pollicization (out of about 550) in 1959, in which the metacarpal was not as shortened as in the standard technique developed later.

POLYDACTYLY WITH RADIUS DUPLICATION

Triplication of the thumb is the most infrequent form of radial polydactyly. Among my six patients, there was one patient with an accompanying incomplete duplication of the radius (Fig. 10.21A). Although the ulna was of approximately normal size and shape, the radius was approximately twice as broad as usual; its distal end was split. The carpal bones—not completely ossified at the time of the last follow-up examination at the age of 5 years—show an increase in number at the radial side, but it is not possible to determine their correct anatomic names (Fig. 10.21B).

MADELUNG DEFORMITY

This wrist deformity, which bears the name of Otto Wilhelm Madelung, occurs most often bilaterally and is four times as frequent in girls as in boys. It is under discussion whether or not it is a forme fruste of dyschondrosteosis (Léry-Weill). Even if in most cases the diagnosis is not made before the age of 6 to 13 years, Madelung deformity has to be included in the group of congenital anomalies. The main argument is the pattern of heredity in about one-third of cases; the transmission follows an autosomal dominant pattern. In these families the disease can be detected by periodic radiographic examinations in early years; in the majority of patients the first symptom is pain in the wrist without any history of injury or infection. Radiographs reveal the typical signs: an increased ulnar and palmer slant of the distal articular surface of the radius; a bowing of the distal radius to the palmar and ulnar side and, therefore, a dorsal prominence of the ulnar head; and a widening of the distance between radius and ulna

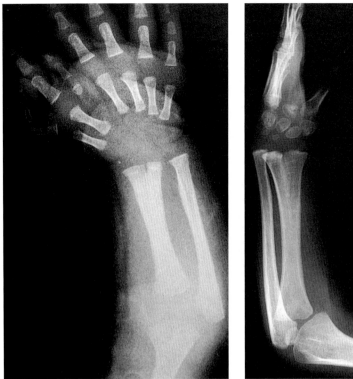
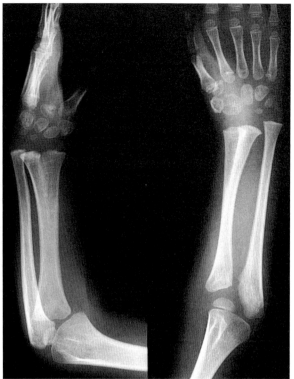

FIGURE 10.21. Thumb triplication with partial duplication of the radius at the time of birth **(A)** and 5 years later **(B),** 4 years after removal of the radial and ulnar thumbs and pollicization of the central thumb.

with a wedge-shaped deformity of the proximal carpal row (Figs. 10.22–10.25). These bone deformities vary considerably according to the stage of development of the disease. At first, only a slightly increased tilt of the ulnar half of the articular surface of the radius is observed (Fig. 10.23). Sometimes an exostosis at the ulnar part of the radius metaphysis is seen (Figs. 10.23 and 10.24A). It is said that it is the origin of a pathologic ligament that is causative of the deformity and pulls the lunate proximally so that the carpal bones grow in a funnel shape (Fig. 10.24B). In late cases, a severe deformity has developed in which the radius is bent palmarly and the ulnar head protrudes dorsally (Fig. 10.25).

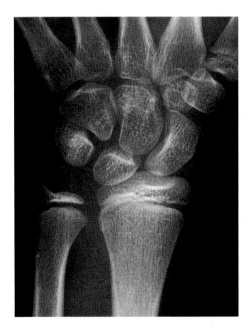
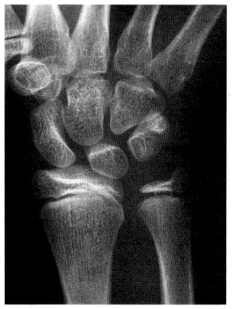

FIGURE 10.22. Madelung deformity of both wrists at an early stage in a 9-year-old girl.

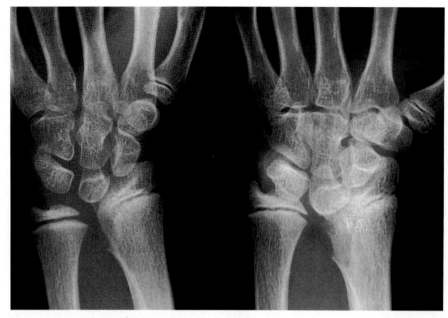

FIGURE 10.23. Development of a Madelung deformity, demonstrated in radiographs with an interval of about 3 years in a girl aged 9 **(left)** and 12 **(right)** years.

The carpal bones are originally normal, but during the progressive development of the deformity of the distal ends of the two forearm bones, they grow abnormally. The proximal row enters the widened gap between radius and ulna like a wedge. The lunate changes its normal relation to the adjacent bones and grows in a more wedge-like shape (Figs. 10.23 and 10.24). The scaphoid rotates palmarly as in a dorsal intercalated segment instability (DISI).

The surgical treatment is difficult and can never normalize an already established deformity. In the first stage of the disease, resection of the ulnar zone of the radius physis and its replacement with autologous fat ("physiolysis") together with resection of the abnormal ligament can give good results and will prevent further progression of the deformity. In late stages, some improvement is possible by osteotomies of the radius and shortening of the ulna (Figs. 10.25 and 10.26),

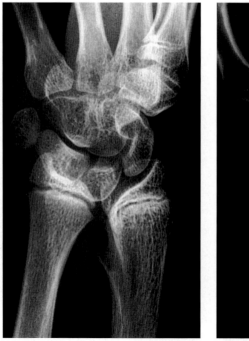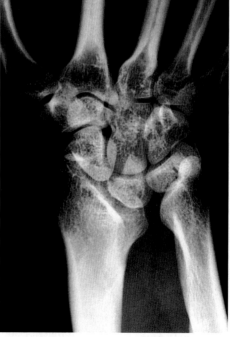

FIGURE 10.24. Madelung deformity. In some cases, an exostosis at the radial metaphysis is seen as a radiographic sign of the origin of a pathologic ligament **(A)**, which pulls the lunate during growth between the radius and ulna **(B)**.

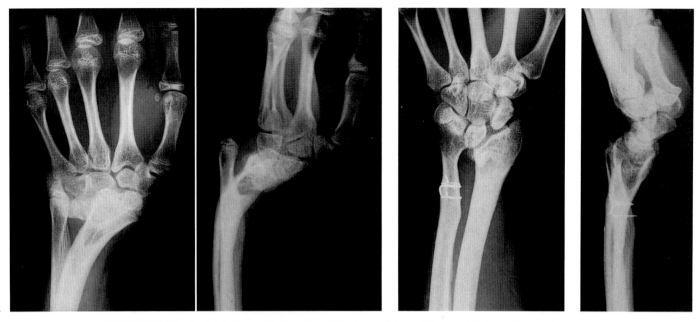

FIGURE 10.25. A right: Severe deformity of the left wrist in a 13-year-old girl with an untreated Madelung deformity. B: Result 7 years following corrective osteotomy of the radius and shortening of the ulna.

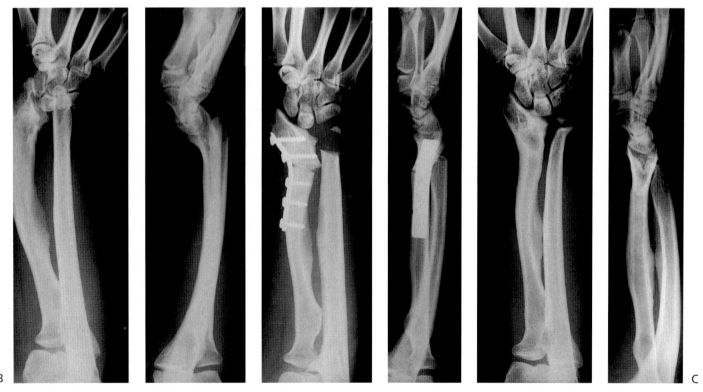

FIGURE 10.26. Madelung deformity with severe deformation of the right wrist in a 20-year-old female patient **(A)**. Treatment with radius osteotomy, plate fixation, and resection of the ulna head **(B)**. Result 15 years later with fairly good correction of the deformity **(C)**.

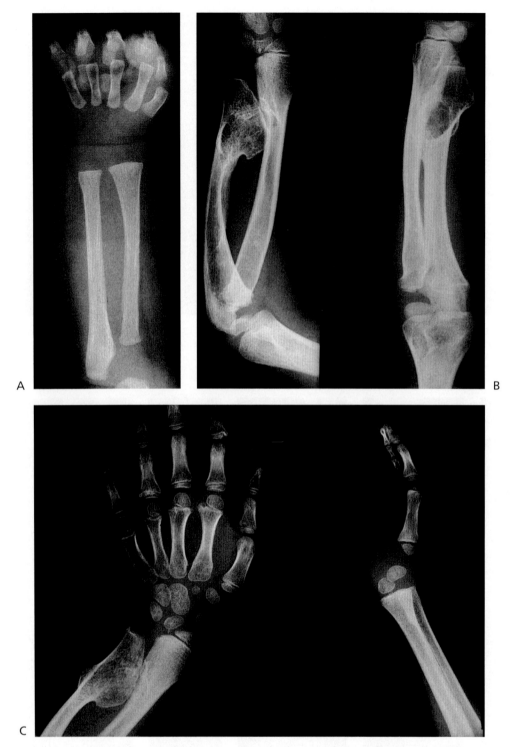

FIGURE 10.27. Hereditary multiple exostoses. At birth, no pathologic findings exist **(A)**, but at the age of 6 years massive exostoses of the ulna have developed **(B)**, which cause shortening of the ulna and deviation of the hand **(C)**. The opposite hand shows only one digital ray.

but this will not correct the funnel-shaped carpus. In some cases, a Kapandji operation gives good results.

HEREDITARY MULTIPLE EXOSTOSES

Similar to the Madelung deformity, the development of bone lesions in multiple cartilaginous exostoses also occurs during the first years of life. At birth, radiographs usually appear normal (Fig. 10.27A). The pattern of transmission is autosomal dominant with a very high penetrance, particularly in boys. The exostoses grow out in the metaphysis and disturb the joint function. In the forearm, the distal ulna is involved early with disturbance of the epiphyseal growth. This results in ulna shortening. Because the radius is tethered by the capsular structures of the distal radioulnar joint to the distal ulna, its further growth is more and more convex (Fig. 10.27). Its distal articular surface becomes oblique, and the hand deviates ulnarward (Fig. 10.27B,C). The next step in the progression is dislocation of the radial head at the elbow—a severe complication that should be prevented by early surgical treatment. Another serious complication is sarcomatous degeneration, which occurs in about 5% of patients.

Surgical treatment of the forearm lesions is difficult because it is not possible to reconstruct the distal radioulnar joint. Excision of the chondromata, lengthening of the ulna, either in a one-stage procedure with an iliac bone graft or by callus distraction, and correction of the bowing of the radius by a closing wedge osteotomy with plate fixation will improve the gross deformity. A preexisting dislocation of the radial head is rarely permanently reduced.

BONE DYSPLASIAS

The wrist is involved in numerous bone diseases, which are usually hereditary and, fortunately, very rare. It is impossible to mention all or even many of them; they are well described in the literature. There are osteolytic as well as tumor-like lesions, many as part of, or associated with, systemic diseases.

The carpal bones are not commonly involved; most of the lesions involve the forearm and/or metacarpal bones with consequences involving the wrist. This is the case, for example, in metaphyseal chondrodysplasia (Jansen type). The radiograph shows intact carpals and epiphyses of both forearm bones; the main lesions are located in the metaphyses of the radius and ulna and in the metacarpals and phalanges (Fig. 10.28). Consequently, the wrist is unstable, and its mobility is restricted. Treatment is performed for symptomatic relief.

Of the different mucopolysaccharidoses, type I-H (Hurler disease) is the most severe in regard to skeletal deformities. In the hand and wrist, radiographs again show

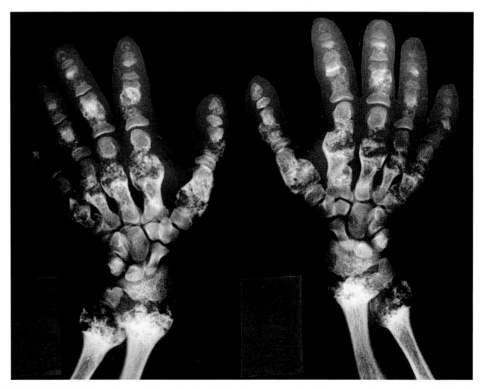

FIGURE 10.28. Metaphyseal chondrodysplasia (Jansen type) with severe destruction of all tubular bones, but with intact carpal bones.

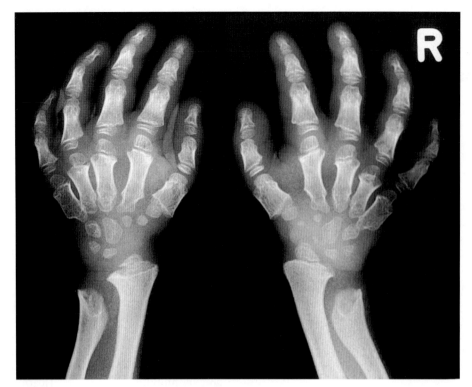

FIGURE 10.29. Mucopolysaccharidosis I-H (Hurler disease) with deformation of the distal ends of the radius and ulna.

the carpal bones to be more or less normal, but the distal ends of the forearm bones are deformed—in the presented case, the ulna more than the radius (Fig. 10.29). The growth centers are involved, and the metacarpals and phalanges are deformed. Surgical treatment is rarely indicated, particularly because of the poor prognosis.

EDITORS' COMMENTS

Congenital hypoplasia of the thumb may be noted clinically by nothing more than absence of some thenar musculature and a more distal positioning of the radial aspect of the palmar wrist crease. Even with this mildest form of congenital hypoplasia of the thumb, there will be some changes in the radial carpals, and an x-ray will almost always show that the epiphyses of the radius and ulna are approximately at the same level. This finding indicates some hypoplasia of the radius. These hands may never be a clinical problem.

The preaxial hypoplasia is a spectrum condition from minimal hypoplasia of the thumb as noted above to the vagaries of radial club hand to humeral involvement, shoulder involvement, rib and vertebral involvement, and, in its most severe form, hemithoracic and hemicardiac structures incompatible with life. Throughout this spectrum, the preaxial hypoplasia progresses cleanly as if one were gradually melting away structures from the radial aspect of the hand and wrist and forearm. We are concerned here only with the segment of the spectrum that involves significant hypoplasia of the thumb, hypoplasia of the radial carpals, and radial club hand.

A 32-year-old woman with congenital hypoplasia of the radial aspect of the wrist was able to function nearly normally as a nurse into her third decade, at which time load capacity deteriorated and pain developed (Editors' Fig. 10.1). Scapholunate advanced collapse (SLAC) reconstruction was performed, producing a symptom-free wrist and return to load activities (Editors' Fig. 10.2). Any treatment of adult radial wrist carpal hypoplasia should be based solely on clinical dysfunction.

Radial club hand is a condition that requires early treatment and surgical intervention in order to maximize the adaptive capability of a young child. The initial treatment following birth is manipulation of the hand by the mother into an ulnar deviation position on a daily basis. The more one can stretch out the radial soft tissue structures, the more effective will be the surgical approach. At 6 months of age, it will be clear that centralization is required, and molded plaster casting much like club foot casting is carried out. The prime restriction to adequate centralization is the combined radial median nerve, which lies on the radialmost aspect of the wrist. Because it is made of components of radial and median nerve, it

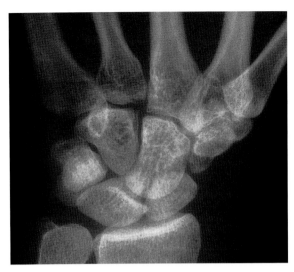

EDITORS' FIGURE 10.1. This patient demonstrates a positive ulnar variance typical of the preaxial hypoplasia. The radius is short. The carpals are hypoplastic on the radial side, in particular the scaphotrapeziotrapezoid. The thumb is hypoplastic with hypoplasia of the thenar musculature.

can not be displaced volarly or dorsally, nor can it be divided or split. Any gain in its length from manipulation and/or casting before surgery pays great dividends in the surgical approach. The second component of concern is the skin. There will be abundant skin on the ulnar aspect of the wrist and a paucity on the radial aspect of the wrist.

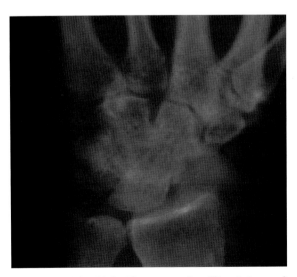

EDITORS' FIGURE 10.2. There was insufficent bone for a triscaphe limited wrist arthrodesis. A capitate–scaphoid arthrodesis was performed. The scaphoid rapidly destroyed itself against the radius, and scapholunate advanced collapse (SLAC) reconstruction was carried out. This was a very early SLAC reconstruction, and silicone scaphoid replacement was carried out simultaneously. There was never an indication for use of a silicone scaphoid, and several years following this x-ray, the silicone scaphoid was removed. The patient has remained functional and asymptomatic.

The key to adequate release of the wrist for proper alignment over the distal ulna is to removal of all the fibrous remnant of the dysplastic radius in the distal forearm. This fibrous analog was consistently the main structure limiting free ulnar movement of the hand. When the radius is absent, it is better to completely centralize early than to accept a radially deviated wrist that is not centered on the ulna and will present a long-term problem of stability and strength with proximal wrist migration under load. The earlier the operation is performed, the better the remodeling potential.

Under pneumatic tourniquet control, two skin incisions are made. The radial incision is a standard 60° Z-plasty with a longitudinal central limb to obtain length along the longitudinal axis of the forearm. The ulnar incision is a similar Z-plasty but with a transverse central limb to take up skin redundancy; the excess tissue is transferred to the deficient radial side of the wrist. Once the skin incisions are completed, dissection is begun on the radial side, and the median/radial nerve is identified. It should be noted that the radial nerve frequently ends at the elbow, and the median nerve has an abnormal location, usually being the most superficial structure on the radial side of the forearm and supplying sensation to usual areas of radial nerve distribution. Identification and preservation of the "median–radial" nerve are vital to the resulting functional capacity of the hand. Dissection is continued ulnarward, resecting the fibrotic distal radial anlage, which acts as a restricting band maintaining the hand in radial deviation. Attenuation is now directed to the ulnar incision. The ulnar nerve and accompanying artery are identified and preserved. Complete capsular release of the ulnocarpal joint is performed, preserving the epiphyseal plate and entire distal ulna. At this point, the hand should be fully movable, attached to the forearm only by the skin, the dorsal and palmar tendons, and the neurovascular structures.

It is important to remove all the fibrotic material in the "center" of the wrist and forearm area. The ulna and ulnar incision should be clearly visible from the radial incision, and vice versa. We have not found it necessary to remove any carpal bones or to remodel the distal ulna to centralize the hand. A 0.045 Kirschner wire is passed through the lunate, capitate, and third metacarpal, exiting through the metacarpophalangeal joint. The hand is centralized in the desired position, and the Kirschner wire is placed retrogradely into the ulna. A bulky hand dressing with a dorsal plaster splint extending above the elbow is used for the first 2 weeks. At this time, the dressing is changed, the sutures are removed, and a long arm cast is placed to complete 6 weeks of immobilization. The Kirschner wire is removed after 6 weeks, and short arm casting is continued for another 3 weeks. At the end of this period, night splinting may be used, if necessary, and may be continued throughout the growing years to epiphyseal closure of the ulna.

If there is a tendency to recurrence, tendon structures can be shifted to the ulnar side of the ulnar carpal axis. The ulnar carpal articulation will gradually resemble a radius carpal articulation with increasing bone shape stability. Centralization is probably best accomplished at about 6 months of age.

Postaxial hypoplasia or absence of the ulnar structures is not a clean anatomic phenomenon. The thumb may be absent even though the postaxial deficiencies are ulnar-sided. The main feature to be handled early is the cartilaginous analog running distally from the distal end of the ulna. This structure may connect the distal end of the ulna with the ulnar aspect of the wrist. First, it may have its major effect on the carpals through the soft tissue structures and produce severe ulnar deviation of the hand. Second, the analog may attach to the radius, producing an increasing ulnar slope of the distal radial articular surface. Third, it may produce bowing of the radius, occasionally into a complete "C" shape. Fourth, it may produce dislocation of the radial capitellar joint, in which case the degree of bowing in the radius is usually less. And, last, the pressure may be so great as to have already fused the radius to the humerus at the radial capitellar joint *in utero*. Under any and all of the above circumstances, the earliest possible resection of the distal ulna analog is indicated. The analog is made up of a spectrum of tissues beginning with bone proximally, progressing to cartilage, then fibrocartilage and finally collagenous fibrous tissue at its most distal aspect. The insertions and effects may be singular, as noted above, or multiple and combined.

During fetal development, the cartilage mass is gradually divided into the separate carpal bones. The most likely joint to undergo incomplete development is the triquetral–lunate joint. The joint develops in the distal-to-proximal direction, and incomplete development results in two separate bones but inadequate cartilage in the most proximal aspect of the triquetral–lunate joint. The more severely involved joint has bony bridging proximally between the triquetrum and lunate and then finally total congenital arthrodeses between the two. Total arthrodesis is typically asymptomatic.

Statistically, the most common congenital abnormalities producing symptoms in the adult wrist are this incomplete development of the triquetral–lunate joint and carpal boss. The symptomatic triquetral–lunate joint is more common. Typically, wrist pain develops in the third or fourth decade with ulnar wrist pain and synovitis localizing to the triquetral–lunate joint. X-rays demonstrate a classic, incomplete development of the triquetral–lunate joint with an open, fully developed joint distally between the two bones and bone protruding into the space where cartilage should be in the proximal portion of the joint. This produces the pathognomonic "fluted champagne glass" appearance of incomplete joint development. There is almost always some change in this joint in the opposite wrist. The incompletely developed joint has had a thin area of cartilage over the proximal opposing bone surfaces. After 20 or 30 years, this cartilage is unable to replace itself, and localized degenerative arthritis develops. Arthrodesis of the triquetral–lunate joint is the only appropriate treatment.

Carpal boss is a wrist problem in which a congenitally abnormal bone, typically an os styloideum, rests on the dorsal portion of the capitate–trapezoid–index metacarpal–middle metacarpal joint combination. It is often fused to one of the four bones, most commonly to the middle metacarpal. It may, however, simply overlie portions of this joint area. This small, abnormal bone produces a localized degenerative arthritis on the dorsum of the joint by the third or fourth decade. There is activity pain and postactivity ache not often well localized historically. Localized tenderness, an associated ganglion, and pain on malaligning the index and middle metacarpals make the diagnosis. Flexing the index metacarpal while extending the middle metacarpal or vice versa will cause sharp reproduction of the symptoms. Similar symptoms can be produced by flexing the metaphalangeal joint of the index and little fingers and then adducting and abducting the proximal phalanges in relation to one another. This produces a rotary moment on the metacarpals. Alone, the prominence of bone in this area is not diagnostic, as the bases of the three odd-numbered metacarpals are prominent. X-rays demonstrate two opposing prominent osteophytes seen best on a slightly supinated lateral image. The degenerative arthritis is highly localized dorsally and may be resected with dental rongeurs down to good cartilage between all four bones. There is no problem with stability following this approach. Significant bone resection is often necessary. Full activity is encouraged 48 hours after surgery.

Madelung's deformity is primarily a growth deformity and seldom evident at birth. Madelung-like deformities may be present at birth. Their etiologies are multiple and include congenital preaxial hypoplasia as just described, multiple osteochondromatosis with involvement of the distal radial epiphysis on its ulnar side, and any systemic diseases or congenital phenomena that involve the epiphysis. The main thrust in all of these conditions is to obtain maximum growth length from the forearm and only secondarily to consider the angular deformity of the distal radius. Epiphyseal lysis procedures may be indicated.

BIBLIOGRAPHY

I have put together a selection of recommendable literature for better understanding and facilitation of further and more detailed studies. This includes, of course, important articles and books in languages other than English.

General References

Bergsma D, ed. *Birth defects. Atlas and compendium.* Baltimore: The National Foundation—March of Dimes, Williams & Wilkins, 1973.
Buck-Gramcko D, ed. *Congenital malformations of the hand and forearm.* Edinburgh, New York: Churchill Livingstone, 1998.
Flatt AE. *The care of congenital hand anomalies,* 2nd ed. St Louis: Quality Medical Publishing, 1994.
Greulich WW, Pyle SI. *Radiographic atlas of skeletal development of the hand and wrist,* 2nd ed. Stanford, CA: Stanford University Press, 1959.
Kelikian H. *Congenital deformities of the hand and forearm.* Philadelphia: WB Saunders, 1974.
Köhler A, Zimmer EA. *Grenzen des Normalen und Anfänge des Pathologischen im Röntgenbild des Skeletts,* 13th ed (Schmidt H, Freyschmidt J, Holthusen W, eds.). Stuttgart: Thieme 1989 (available in English as: *Borderlands of the normal and early pathologic in skeletal roentgenology,* 3rd Eng ed. New York: Grune & Stratton, 1968).
O'Rahilly R. A survey of carpal and tarsal anomalies. *J Bone Joint Surg Am* 1953;35:626–642.
O'Rahilly R. Development deviations in the carpus and the tarsus. *Clin Orthop* 1957;10:9–18.
Poznanski AK. The carpals in congenital malformation syndromes. *Am J Roentgenol* 1971;112:443–459.
Schmid F, Moll H. *Atlas der normalen und pathologischen Handskeletentwicklung.* Berlin: Springer, 1960.
Smith DW. *Recognizable patterns of human malformation. Genetic, embryologic and clinical aspects,* 3rd ed. Philadelphia: WB Saunders, 1982.
Taybi H. *Radiology of syndromes.* Chicago: Year Book, 1975.
Temtamy SA, McKusick VY. The genetics of hand malformations. *Birth Defects Orig Artic Ser* 1978;14:i–xviii, 1–619.
Upton J. Congenital anomalies of the hand and forearm. In: McCarthy JG, ed. *Plastic surgery, vol 8, part 2.* Philadelphia: WB Saunders, 1990:5213–5398.
Werthemann A. Die Entwicklungsstörungen der Extremitäten. In: Lubarsch O, Henke F, Rössle R, eds. *Handbuch der speziellen und pathologischen Anatomie und Histologie, Band 9, Teil 6.* Berlin, Göttingen: Springer, 1952.

Carpal Synostoses

Albrecht A. Beitrag zum Vorkommen der Synostosen am Hand- und Fußwurzelskelett. *Z Orthop* 1968;105:215–235.
Cockshott WP. Carpal fusions. *Am J Roentgenol* 1963;89:1260–1271.
Förstner H. Das Os lunato-triquetrum. *Z Orthop* 1989;127:174–182.
Hughes PCR, Tanner JM. The development of carpal bone fusion as seen in serial radiographs. *Br J Radiol* 1966;39:943–949.
Maroteaux P, Bouvet JP, Briard ML. La maladie des synostoses multiples. *Nouv Presse Méd* 1972;45:3041–3047.
Mestern J. Erbliche Synostosen der Hand- und Fußwurzelknochen. Erbliches Os tibiale externum. *Röntgenpraxis* 1934;6:594–600.
Mortier JP, Kuhlmann JN, Baux S. Synostoses radio-scapho-lunaires dans le cadre des synostoses carpiennes congénitales. *Ann Chir Main* 1986;5:323–327.
Nixon JR. The multiple synostoses syndrome. A plea for simplicity. *Clin Orthop* 1978;135:48–51.
Weinzweig J, Watson HK, Herbert TJ, et al. Congenital synchondrosis of the scaphotrapezio-trapezoidal joint. *J Hand Surg [Am]* 1997;22:74–77.

Radial Deficiencies

Blauth W. Zur Morphologie und Therapie der radialen Klumphand. *Arch Orthop Unfall-Chir* 1969;65:97–123.
Buck-Gramcko D. Angeborene Fehlbildungen. In: Nigst H, Buck-Gramcko D, Millesi H, eds. *Handchirurgie, vol I.* Stuttgart: Thieme, 1981:12.1–12.115 (Eng ed: New York: Thieme, 1988).
Buck-Gramcko D. Radialization as a new treatment for radial club hand. *J Hand Surg [Am]* 1985;10:964–968.
Heikel HVA. Aplasia and hypoplasia of the radius. *Acta Orthop Scand [Suppl]* 1959;39:1–155.
Lamb DW. Radial club hand. A continuing study of sixty-eight patients with one hundred and seventeen club hands. *J Bone Joint Surg Am* 1977;59:1–13.
Manske PR, McCarroll HR, Swanson K. Centralization of the radial club hand: An ulnar surgical approach. *J Hand Surg [Am]* 1981;6:423–433.
O'Rahilly H. Morphological patterns in limb deficiencies and duplications. *Am J Anat* 1951;89:135–187.
Skerik SK, Flatt AE. The anatomy of congenital radial dysplasia. *Clin Orthop* 1969;66:125–143.
Stoffel A, Stempel E. *Anatomische Studien über die Klumphand.* Stuttgart: Enke, 1909.
Watson HK, Beebe RD, Cruz NI. A centralization procedure for radial club hand. *J Hand Surg [Am]* 1984;9:541–547.
Wulle C. Naviculo-radiale Synostose bei Hypoplasie des Daumenstrahles. *Handchirurgie* 1971;3:117–118.

Ulnar Deficiencies

Broudy AS, Smith RJ. Deformities of the hand and wrist with ulnar deficiency. *J Hand Surg [Am]* 1979;4:304–315.
Buck-Gramcko D. Ulnar deficiency. In: Saffar P, Amadio PC, Foucher G, eds. *Current practice in hand surgery.* London: Martin Dunitz, 1997.
Carroll RE, Bowers WH. Congenital deficiency of the ulna. *J Hand Surg [Am]* 1977;2:169–174.
Frantz CH, O'Rahilly R. Ulnar hemimelia. *Artif Limbs* 1971;15:25–35.
Horii E, Miura T, Nakamura R. Ulnar ray deficiency. A report of a family. *J Hand Surg [Br]* 1994;19:244–247.
Lausecker H. Der angeborene Defekt der Ulna. *Virchows Arch Pathol Anat* 1954;325:211–226.
Marcus NA, Omer GE. Carpal deviation in congenital ulnar deficiency. *J Bone Joint Surg Am* 1984;66:1003–1007.
Pardini AG. Congenital absence of the ulna. *J Iowa Med Soc* 1967;57:1106–1112.
Swanson AB, Tada K, Yonenobu K. Ulnar ray deficiency: Its various manifestations. *J Hand Surg [Am]* 1984;9:658–664.

Mirror Hand

Barton NJ, Buck-Gramcko D, Evans DM. Soft-tissue anatomy of mirror hand. *J Hand Surg [Br]* 1986;11:307–319.
Barton NJ, Buck-Gramcko D, Evans DM, et al. Mirror hand treated by true pollicization. *J Hand Surg [Br]* 1986;11:320–336.
Buck-Gramcko D. Operative behandlung einer spiegelbild-defor-

mität der hand ("mirror hand"—doppelte ulna mit polydaktylie). *Ann Chir Plastique* 1964;9:180–183.

Radioulnar Synstosis

Buck-Gramcko D, Ogino T. Congenital malformations of the hand: Nonclassifiable cases. *Hand Surg* 1996;1:45–61.

Cenani A, Lenz W. Totale Syndaktylie und totale radioulnare Synostose bei zwei Brüdern. Ein Beitrag zur Genetik der Syndaktylien. *Z Kinderheilkd* 1967;101:181–190.

Simmons BP, Southmayd WW, Riseborough EJ. Congenital radioulnar synostosis. *J Hand Surg* 1983;6:829–838.

Madelung Deformity

Angelini LC, Leite VM, Faloppa F. Surgical treatment of Madelung disease by the Sauvé-Kapandji technique. *Ann Chir Main* 1996; 15:257–264.

Anton JI, Reitz GB, Spiegel MB. Madelung's deformity. *Ann Surg* 1938;108:411–439.

De Smet L, Fabry G. Treatment of Madelung's deformity by Kapandji's procedure and osteotomy of the radius. Case report. *J Pediatr Orthop (Part B)* 1993;2:96–98.

Ducloyer P, Saffar P. La maladie de Madelung. Revue générale à propos de 17 cas. In: Gilbert A, Buck-Gramcko D, Lister G, eds. *Les malformation congénitales du membre supérieur. Monographies du Groupe d'Etude de la Main.* Paris: Expansion Scientifique Française, 1991:51–61.

Lamb D. Madelung deformity. Editorial. *J Hand Surg [Br]* 1988;13: 3–4.

Murphy MS, Linscheid RL, Dobyns JH, et al. Radial opening wedge osteotomy in Madelung's deformity. *J Hand Surg [Am]* 1996;21: 1035–1044.

Sakuma T, Ogino T. Caractéristiques de la maladie de Madelung et résultats cliniques apres chirurgie. In: Gilbert A, Buck-Gramcko D, Lister G, eds. *Les malformations congénitales du membre supérieur. Monographies du Groupe d'Etude de la Main.* Paris: Expansion Scientifique Française, 1991:43–50.

Vickers D, Nielsen G. Madelung deformity: Surgical prophylaxis (physiolysis) during the late growth period by resection of the dyschondrostenosis lesion. *J Hand Surg [Br]* 1992;17:401–407.

Hereditary Multiple Exostoses

Fogel GR, McElfresh EC, Peterson HA, et al. Management of deformities of the forearm in multiple hereditary osteochondromas. *J Bone Joint Surg Am* 1984;66:670–680.

Jiya TU, Pruijs JEH, Van Der Eijken JW. Surgical treatment of wrist deformity in hereditary multiple exostosis. *Acta Orthop Belg* 1997; 63:256–261.

Masada K, Tsuyuguchi Y, Kawai H, et al. Operations for forearm deformity caused by multiple osteochondromas. *J Bone Joint Surg Br* 1989;71:24–29.

Pritchett JW. Lengthening the ulna in patients with hereditary multiple exostoses. *J Bone Joint Surg Br* 1986;68:561–565.

Saunders C, Szabo RM, Mora S. Chondrosarcoma of the hand arising in a young patient with multiple hereditary exostoses. *J Hand Surg [Br]* 1997;22:237–242.

Wood VE, Sauser D, Mudge D. The treatment of hereditary multiple exostosis of the upper extremity. *J Hand Surg [Am]* 1985;10: 505–513.

Bone Dysplasia

Stranger JW, Langer LO, Wiedemann HR. *Bone dysplasias. An atlas of constitutional disorders of skeletal development.* Stuttgart: Gustav Fischer, 1974.

11

PEDIATRIC PROBLEMS INVOLVING THE WRIST

JAIYOUNG RYU
BRUCE F.C. GOMBERG

Pediatric wrist problems remain understudied and are often poorly understood. Diagnosis of wrist pathology before skeletal maturity continues to be facilitated by newer imaging techniques and better understanding of wrist kinematics. However, children continue to challenge surgical and radiographic advances by earlier and more intense participation in high-energy activities. This chapter focuses on noncongenital wrist pathology seen in the pediatric population until physiologic epiphysiodesis, including Madelung's deformity, the carpal boss, juvenile arthritis (JA), neoplastic processes, and trauma to the skeletally immature carpus and distal forearm.

OSSIFICATION OF THE NORMAL CARPUS AND DISTAL FOREARM

By the tenth gestational week, the carpus develops into eight distinct entities (1,2). Carpal bones generally undergo membranous ossification in a well-known, predictable pattern (1–4). By the fourth or fifth postnatal month, the ossification centers of the capitate and hamate are radiologically evident. The triquetrum appears during the second year of life; the lunate appears around the fourth year and is closely followed by the scaphoid, ossifying distally and progressing proximally. The trapezium closely follows ossification of the scaphoid and, along with the trapezoid, becomes radiographically apparent in the fifth year. The pisiform lags behind, normally undergoing ossification at age 9 years or later (1,2).

The triangular distal radial epiphysis undergoes ossification at about 7 months of age. The distal ulnar epiphysis, however, does not appear until midchildhood, about age 6 or 7, beginning at the base of the ulnar styloid and ossifying radially. Physiologic epiphysiodesis in the distal forearm occurs between 17 and 19 years of age (Fig. 11.1).

THE CARPAL BOSS

First described as *"carpe bossu"* by the French physician Foille, the carpal boss is a protuberance between the base of the second and/or third metacarpals and the articulating trapezoid and/or capitate (5–8). Usually, the patient complains of an asymptomatic palpable mass on the dorsum of the carpus without a history of trauma; however, it may be the source of considerable pain (5,9). The diagnostic workup should include the metacarpal stress test as described by Fusi et al. (10). Pain is elicited by distraction and pronosupination of the index and middle finger metacarpals with the metacarpophalangeal joints flexed, distorting the relationships of the quadrangular (capitate–trapezoid–metacarpal) joint.

Repetitive trauma may be the underlying etiology of the carpal boss, but more likely it is a periostitis near the insertion of the extensor carpi radialis brevis. Cuono and Watson (7) demonstrated that the etiology is related to anomalous osseous development in the region of the quadrangular joint, predisposing it to premature degeneration. A vast majority of cases involve an os styloideum, more often than not fused to the second or third metacarpal (6,10). The carpal boss is often confused with a dorsal wrist ganglion. In fact, 30% of all cases have a small ganglion associated with them, which must be treated as well (5,7).

Posteroanterior (PA) and lateral x-rays of the wrist are appropriate and may help rule out some ominous diagnoses. However, the radiographic series must include a "carpal boss view" to best profile the bony anomaly. It is a lateral x-ray of the wrist with the forearm supinated 30° to 40° and the wrist ulnarly deviated 20° to 30° to account for the radiodorsal angulation of the protuberance and the obliquity of the capitometacarpal joint (Fig. 11.2) (5–7).

J. Ryu and B. F. C. Gomberg: Department of Orthopedics, West Virginia University, Morgantown, West Virginia 26506.

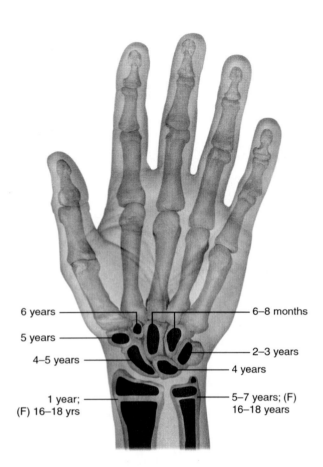

FIGURE 11.1. Age of onset of radiographically apparent ossific nuclei. The pisiform is not shown but ossifies at 6 to 8 years of age. (From Graham TJ, O'Brien ET. Fractures and dislocations of the hand and carpus in children. In: Rockwood CA, Wilkins KE, Beaty JH, eds. *Fractures in children.* Philadelphia: Lippincott–Raven Publishers, 1996;323–447, with permission.)

Treatment

Treatment may be either operative or nonoperative. Nonoperative treatment consists of analgesics, immobilization, and intraarticular injections of corticosteroids and local anesthetic. Operative treatment is aimed at excision of the entire palpable protuberance and the associated ganglion if present (Fig. 11.3) (5,7). A transverse or oblique incision centered on the second and/or third carpometacarpal joints is used to approach the bony prominence. The extensor digitorum communis and extensor indicis proprius tendons are retracted. The associated ganglion, if present, is exposed and excised. Each affected joint is approached by subperiosteal dissection. Complete excision of the osteophyte should extend to normal cartilage and cancellous bone. Soft tissues are then reapproximated with care taken to invert all layers. In refractory cases, complete fusion of the quadrangular joint may provide relief (11). Citteur et al. (9) demonstrated that loss of the dorsal restraints of the carpometacarpal joint during excision of the carpal boss may predispose the joint to abnormal kinematics and loads, subsequent degenerative changes, and pain. Cuono and Watson (7) provide an excellent overview of the surgical technique. Postoperative cast immobilization for 4 to 6 weeks allows for ligamentous healing. Persistence of the mass is

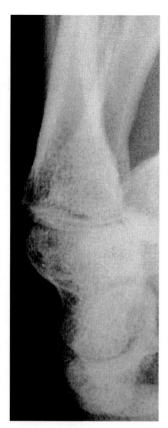

FIGURE 11.2. Carpal boss view highlighting the profile of the protuberance. (From Fusi S, Watson HK, Cuono CB. The carpal boss. *J Hand Surg [Br]* 1995;20:405–408, with permission.)

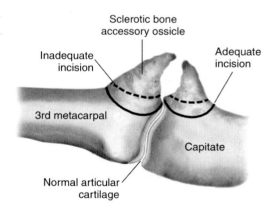

FIGURE 11.3. Technique for excision of the carpal boss. (Modified from Fusi S, Watson HK, Cuono CB. The carpal boss. *J Hand Surg [Br]* 1995;20:405–408, with permission.)

the most frequent complication and often correlates well with pain.

MADELUNG'S DEFORMITY

Madelung's deformity is a congenital anomaly of the wrist that becomes clinically apparent at about age 8 or 9 years, although occasionally not until adolescence. It is seen four times more often in girls than boys and is bilateral in a majority of cases (12,13). The deformity is caused by an arrest of the ulnar and volar portions of the distal radial physis. The etiology of this premature physeal arrest remains unclear, although repetitive trauma, nutritional status, vascular insufficiency, muscular disorders, and tethering of the physis have been postulated (14–17). In addition to the growth arrest, Vickers and Nielsen (17) noted an abnormal, thickened volar ligament tethering the lunate to the radius.

Clearly, there is an association with dyschondrosteosis, a mild mesomelic shortening of the long bones and short stature first described in 1929 by Leri and Weill, now known as Leri-Weill syndrome (16,18–21). The syndrome is transmitted as an autosomal dominant trait with incomplete penetrance (12,22). Some authors consider Madelung's deformity a feature of dyschondrosteosis, consisting of clinical manifestations that range from the full syndrome to the presence of the wrist deformity alone (23,24). Others believe that Madelung's deformity is a completely separate entity that may follow infection or trauma. One report suggests that long-term repetitive trauma to the adolescent radius may lead to a Madelung-like deformity (25). It may be associated with inherited disorders such as dyschondrosteosis, Turner's syndrome, Hurler's mucopolysaccharidosis, multiple hereditary enchondromatosis, or Ollier's dyschondroplasia (12,24,26,27). It is now believed that girls with Madelung's deformity may or may not possess the additional features of the full-blown syndrome, whereas boys always do (21,28). Madelung's deformity should not, however, be confused with Madelung's disease, which is symmetric lipomatosis of the neck and thorax (13,24).

Two forms of the deformity have been reported (22,26). The typical deformity is that of a shortened, bowed distal radius with a prominent dorsal ulnar head (Fig. 11.4). The ulnar head is actually in the normal anatomic position, and the hand and wrist are subluxed volarward. Wrist motion is usually limited but initially may not be painful. Wrist extension and supination are more severely affected than flexion and pronation (12). Pronosupination is hampered by displacement of the carpus between the radius and ulna and resultant diastasis (22). In the atypical or reverse Madelung's deformity, the distal end of the radius tilts dorsally and results in the volar subluxation of the ulnar head (Fig. 11.5) (13,22,26). In this case, extension increases relative to flexion. Fagg (26) reported a case of reverse Madelung's deformity with an associated median neuropathy secondary to deformity of the carpal canal.

According to the radiology literature, 12 criteria must be met to diagnose Madelung's deformity:

1. Absolute and relative radial shortening.
2. A deficient ulnar aspect of the distal radial epiphysis, resulting in its exaggerated wedge shape.
3. Triangular configuration of the proximal carpal row with the lunate at its apex.
4. An ulnar, volar inclination of the distal radius.
5. Distal radioulnar joint (DRUJ) dislocation or subluxation.
6. Carpal arching aligning with the bowed radius.
7. Lateral and dorsal bowing of the radius.
8. Diastasis of the radius and ulna.
9. Epiphysiodesis of the ulnar portion of the distal radius.
10. Decreased bony density of the ulnar border of the radius.
11. An exostosis on the ulnar side of the distal radius.
12. Condensed trabeculations in the ulnar head (15,19,24, 29–31).

Apparently, only the first three are consistently noted in the routine AP wrist x-ray. Cook et al. (32) confirmed by computed tomography (CT) that the distal radius growth arrest was caused by a physeal bar consistently located on the volar ulnar aspect of the radius. In addition, they noted that the bar was completely osseous in those patients with dyschondrosteosis and incompletely ossified and probably fibrous in those without the syndrome. Thomas et al. (24) warned that the dyschondrosteosis lesion of the distal radius may be mistaken for a space-occupying lesion in the distal radius.

Treatment

Treatment should be directed toward relief of pain and restoration of function. Surprisingly, many patients go without surgical correction as long as they are fully functional and have minimal pain. Van Demark and Van Demark (33) attributed long-term success to surgical reconstruction and job retraining to decrease reliance on wrist strength while maximizing reliance of finger dexterity. With a mild deformity, surgical treatment is rarely necessary. Ultimately, the amount of deformity is governed by the onset of epiphysiodesis, and progression is similar to that in tibia vara (Blount's disease). Late complications of untreated asymptomatic deformity include loss of motion and spontaneous extensor tendon rupture (3,11,34,35). However, as the deformity progresses, ulnocarpal abutment usually limits motion and causes enough pain to warrant surgical treatment. Surgical treatment is usually delayed until 11 to 13 years of age, although there is considerable debate about whether or not to operate before or after physeal closure (36).

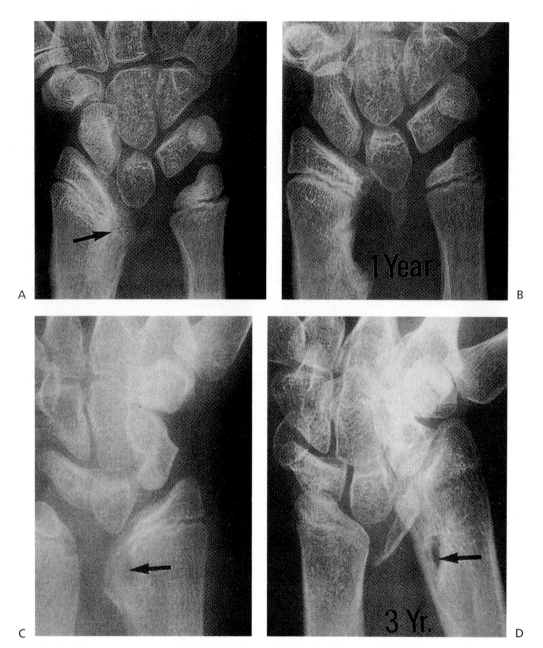

FIGURE 11.4. A: Madelung's deformity of the right wrist. **B:** Same wrist 1 year postoperatively shows excision of the fusion of the ulnar portion of the radial physis. **C,D:** Three-year postoperative image shows marked improvement of the deformity. *Arrows* denote metaphysis in each figure. (From Tachdjian MO. Madelung's deformity. In: Tachdjian MO, ed. *Pediatric orthopedics, 2nd ed.* Philadelphia: WB Saunders, 1990, with permission.)

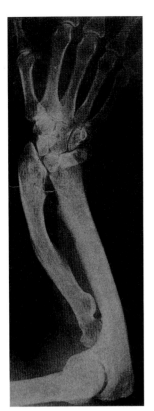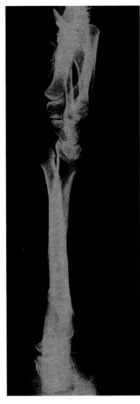

FIGURE 11.5. Reverse Madelung's deformity in which nerve compression was reported. (From Fagg PS. Reverse Madelung's deformity with nerve compression. *J Hand Surg [Br]* 1988;13: 23–27, with permission.)

Most surgical procedures entail ulnar shortening, radial osteotomy, or radiocarpal arthrodesis (Fig. 11.6) (13,14, 37). A Darrach procedure is advocated by some, although late ulnar translation of the carpal bones may be a complication (31,37,38). Others advocate radioulnar fusion. Epiphysiodesis of the distal ulna may be accomplished in the skeletally immature. Milch's cuff resection can be attempted in children (39).

The distal radius may be osteotomized to correct its deformity. Watson et al. (36) advocate a biplanar osteotomy to preserve length in the skeletally mature patient. Various authors use an opening or closing wedge osteotomy; however, these invariably result in lost radial length and require that a matched ulnar resection or a simultaneous ulnar shortening procedure be performed to compensate (22).

The Langenskiöld procedure is one in which the fused physis is excised and replaced by interposition of fat or silastic in the skeletally immature patient (40). Vickers and Nielsen (17) reported success with physiolysis in addition to transection of the abnormal radiolunate tethering ligament, counting on growth left in the distal radius to compensate for the relatively long ulna, thus obviating the need for a formal ulnar shortening procedure (Fig. 11.7). Ideally, the surgical procedure must take into account the relatively long ulna or short radius, attempt to preserve radial length and carpal stability, and maintain functionality while minimizing pain.

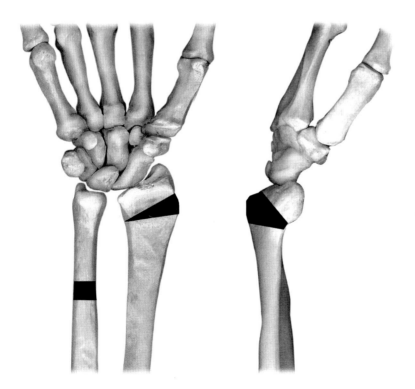

FIGURE 11.6. Usual sites of radial and ulnar osteotomies (*darkened areas*). (Modified from dos Reis FB, Katchburian MV, Faloppa F, et al. Osteotomy of the radius and ulna for the Madelung deformity. *J Bone Joint Surg Br* 1998;80: 817–824, with permission.)

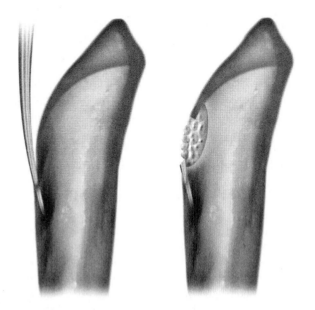

FIGURE 11.7. Vickers' technique of epiphysiodesis of the distal radius and release of the radiolunate tethering ligament. (Modified courtesy of David Vickers, M.B.B.S., F.R.A.C.S., Brisbane, Australia.)

CEREBRAL PALSY AND ARTHROGRYPOSIS

Cerebral palsy and arthrogryposis can result in significant flexion and ulnar deviation contractures of the wrist, flexion contractures of the metacarpophalangeal joints, and adducted thumbs in untreated affected children (41). Early intervention of a multidisciplinary team including occupational and physical therapists, neurologists, urologists, neurosurgeons, physiatrists, orthopedic surgeons, and equipment engineers will help keep all joints supple and realize the full potential of the patient. All team members should primarily be concerned with maximization of the patient's potential, particularly self-feeding, toileting, writing, and mobilization (42–44). Of particular prognostic importance are the psychosocial capabilities of the patient. Arthrogrypotics, who have normal intelligence, and cerebral palsied patients with normal or near-normal intelligence tend to do much better and are more creative in finding ways to perform activities of daily living.

Wrist contractures must be dealt with in conjunction with all other joints of the limb and not in isolation (44,45). Some finger function must be present in order to realize the full potential benefit of wrist reconstruction. In refractory cases, shortening osteotomies of the radius and ulna in combination with a volar wrist capsulotomy and tendon transfers may aid in placing the hand in a more functional position (42,46). Some authors recommend proximal row carpectomy, but outcomes of this procedure are variable (42,47).

GYMNAST'S WRIST

In evolutionary terms, the wrist made the transformation from a weight-bearing structure to one specialized for suspensory locomotion—brachiation—somewhere between 57 and 18 million years ago (48). The physical demands placed on the wrist of a gymnast are such that the wrist once again becomes a weight-bearing joint during high-energy activities, incurring up to 2.4 times the gymnast's body weight under some circumstances (49–51). Nationwide, the population of gymnasts continues to explode, and there are now an estimated 2 to 4 million participants in gymnastics at all skill levels (50,52). Most of this large and rapidly expanding population are preteen. Peak involvement extends into the teenage years, corresponding to the period of maximum growth rate for most young athletes. Retirement from the sport is virtually always before the age of 20 (53). With a general increase in the intensity of training in a population of skeletally immature athletes, it is not surprising that injuries specific to the skeletally immature carpus are now frequent (51–56). Mandelbaum et al. (55) reported an 87.5% incidence of wrist pain in male gymnasts and a 55% incidence in female gymnasts. Aronen (57) reported that wrist pain is so common in gymnastics, it should be considered a normal part of the sport. In gymnasts with wrist pain, symptoms are bilateral approximately one-third of the time (52).

Because the wrist is exposed to abnormally high loads in gymnastics, a spectrum of wrist injuries is seen in gymnasts, ranging from contusions to open fractures, depending on the particular event, duration and intensity of training, participant's level of expertise, and whether the gymnast is practicing or competing (53,58–61). Pettrone and Ricciardelli (59) and Gabel (52) identified the high-risk gymnast as the 12- to 14-year old girl who participates at the elite level, on floor or beam exercises, practicing over 20 hours per week. It is not unusual, however, for elite gymnasts to train for up to 60 hours per week (54). Recent studies report high incidences of wrist injuries in nonelite athletes and overweight recreational gymnasts as well (50).

The gymnast's wrist is prone to both chronic and acute injuries to the soft tissue architecture and carpal bones (52,53). Distal radioulnar and carpal joint instability, triangular fibrocartilage complex (TFCC) tears, and acute and stress fractures of the skeletally immature carpus and distal forearm are covered later in this chapter. Here we focus on the well-studied result of repetitive loading of the skeletally immature distal radial physis, commonly known as "gymnast's wrist."

The physes of the distal radius and ulna are specialized structures composed of an intricate osteochondral and vascular architecture programmed to produce circumferential and longitudinal growth (53,62,63). Repetitive trauma damages this delicate structure, especially the vascularity, consisting of vessels and open channels (53,58,63). The

TABLE 11.1. EFFECTS OF DIFFERENT GYMNASTIC EVENTS ON LOADING OF THE WRIST

Event	Load	Position
Pommel horse	Compression, rotation	Dorsiflexion, pronation, radial–ulnar deviation
Vault	Compression ± rotation	Dorsiflexion
Beam	Compression	Dorsiflexion
Uneven parallel bars	Compression, traction (especially with dowel grip)	Dorsiflexion, neutral
Floor exercise	Compression	Dorsiflexion
Parallel bars	Compression	Dorsiflexion, neutral
Rings	Compression	Neutral

From Dobyns JH, Gabel GT. Gymnast's wrist. *Hand Clin* 1990; 6:493–505, with permission.

and floor exercises, during which the wrist is in extremes positions, incurring abnormally high rotational and compressive loads (62). Most pain results from repetitive trauma to the distal radius in dorsiflexion and compression (55), with the exception of traction incurred by bar activities, rotation while on the pommel horse, and the neutral wrist position during ring exercises. Dobyns and Gabel (53) detailed the specific mechanism of loading of the wrist in each gymnastic event (Table 11.1). One report detailed a clinical and radiographic course similar to chronic physeal compression injury in a gymnast involved in high-bar activities and symptomatic only when hanging from the high bar with the radial physis in tension (65).

It is noteworthy that grip injuries are not unusual and can be quite serious. Thirty-six percent of surveyed gymnastics coaches confirmed such injuries to their team (66). Insertion of a small dowel or crease in the midfinger region of the grips aids in grasping the bar, essentially fastening the gymnast onto it and decreasing the amount of forearm muscular contraction necessary to sustain a grip (Fig. 11.8) (53,61,65). Grips allow the fingers and hand to passively snag the bar, transferring tension forces to the wrist and distal forearm. "Grip lock" occurs when the dowel or crease becomes lodged between the palm and bar. The grip instantly clutches the bar, preventing hand rotation around the bar, while the gymnast continues to rotate. This has

result is dysfunctional ossification as evidenced by persistence of poorly mineralized cartilage at the metaphyseal side of the physis (52,53,64).

Significant injury to the wrist results from peculiar joint positioning and high loads incurred during gymnastic events. This is especially common during pommel horse

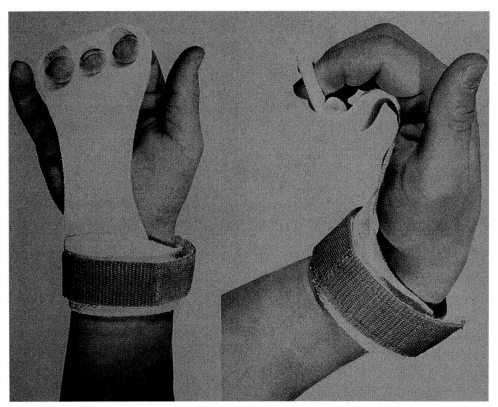

FIGURE 11.8. Dowel grip, utilized during bar events, allows passive suspension of the gymnast from the hand and wrist. (From Dobyns JH, Gabel GT. Gymnast's wrist. *Hand Clin* 1990;6:493–505, with permission.)

been the reported source of quite serious injuries, including open fractures, radiocarpal dislocations, and ligamentous instability. A more frequent complaint, however, is wrist pain in the gymnast who uses dowel grips (65). Yong-Hing et al. (65) recommended that skeletally immature gymnasts refrain from using dowel grips.

Radiology

Consistent radiographic changes are present in the distal radial epiphysis of the symptomatic gymnast. These changes include physeal widening, especially on the radial volar aspect of the physis, cystic changes in the periphyseal metaphysis, a beaked effect of the distal epiphysis, and haziness within the physis (Fig. 11.9) (51–54,67). Positive ulnar variance is another common finding. The etiology of ulnar variance has been the subject of recent debates. Early reports demonstrated premature epiphysiodesis of the distal radius and subsequent positive ulnar variance, which increased with the number of years involved in gymnastics (55). Recently, however, DiFiori et al. (50) noted that positive ulnar variance is prevalent even among nonelite gymnasts. Their report suggested that positive ulnar variance is in part secondary to ulnar overgrowth stimulated by repetitive loading.

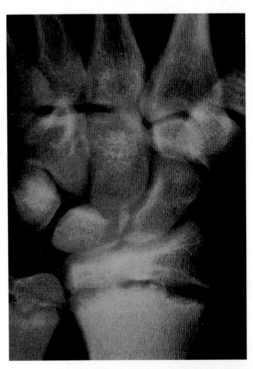

FIGURE 11.9. Sixteen-year-old gymnast showing physeal widening and irregularity of the metaphyseal margins. (From Carter SR, Aldridge MJ, Fitzgerald R, et al. Stress changes of the wrist in adolescent gymnasts. *Br J Radiol* 1988;61:109–112, with permission.)

Staging and Treatment

Stage I

Studies confirm that gymnasts who are symptomatic but have no radiographic changes or physeal injury should avoid axial loading of the extremity until there is a normal pain-free range of motion and no local tenderness (52). This cohort usually returns to competition pain-free and at their preinjury level after about 1 month of rest. Careful monitoring on return to activity is necessary because recurrence of symptoms should prompt immediate reinstitution of the treatment regimen.

Stage II

Gymnasts with symptomatic wrists and radiographic changes consistent with physeal stress injury and no secondary positive ulnar variance take at least 3 months to heal. Multiple authors report that permanent physeal injury will occur if symptoms are not treated appropriately (55). Premature physeal arrest and positive ulnar variance have been reported (50,68). Gymnasts in this group take longer to heal than those in stage I, but full recovery can be expected if the patient complies with the treatment regimen, which frequently necessitates cast immobilization to ensure compliance.

Stage III

A clinically painful wrist, radiographic changes to the physis, and secondary positive ulnar variance define this stage. Ultimately, abutment syndromes have been reported as sequelae of this late presentation (68). Formal ulnar shortening extinguishes pain in gymnasts who were at this advanced stage. Vender and Watson (25) reported the case of one gymnast whose wrist developed a Madelung's-like deformity over time. Although it cannot be concluded that theirs was not a case of idiopathic Madelung's deformity, it is implied that the deformity resulted from chronic subclinical physeal injury. In conclusion, wrist pain in the gymnast should alert the coach, trainers, and involved physicians to a potentially serious problem with long-term sequelae. It is imperative to diagnose this entity and implement appropriate management early.

CARPAL FRACTURE

Fracture of the carpal bones in children is rare. Reports suggest that the skeletally immature carpus is protected by the favorable biomechanics of its developing cartilage (69–72). Isolated reports detail carpal fractures with and without distal radius fractures in children. Clearly, it requires an enormous amount of energy to damage the structures of the pediatric wrist. It has been suggested that these injuries are more common than previously thought (70,73,74). This could be the case, as clinical diagnosis of acute injury to the pediatric wrist is difficult for several reasons (3). First, the child is frequently scared, experiencing pain, and uncooperative. Second, the subcutaneous fat of the child's wrist is often sufficient to minimize any local edema. Third, the examiner's fingers are significantly larger than the structures to be examined.

Carpal fractures are almost never seen in the pediatric population, but current diagnostic modalities lack sensitivity when applied to the pediatric population. Radiographic interpretation of the immature wrist is difficult. There are multiple cartilaginous centers, each undergoing eccentric ossification, which distort radiographic interpretation of intracarpal relationships. Static instability patterns of the pediatric carpus are nearly impossible to demonstrate radiographically (3).

Scaphoid Fractures

Scaphoid fractures are the most common carpal fractures seen in the pediatric population but are still relatively uncommon, accounting for only 2.9% of all hand and wrist fractures seen in the population younger than 15 years of age and 0.34% of all fractures seen in children (74,75). It is extremely uncommon for a child younger than 7 to 10 years of age to incur a scaphoid fracture (69,71,76). The incidence of fracture increases after that, corresponding to ossification of the scaphoid, which appears radiographically at around age 5 or 6 and is not complete until age 13 to 15 years. During the intervening period, the scaphoid is covered with a thick layer of cartilage and ossifies eccentrically (4,70,77). After ossification, the incidence of scaphoid fractures parallels that of the adult population (3). The scaphoid is fractured during the application of an axial load to the wrist with a markedly dorsiflexed wrist in combination with ulnar deviation and wrist pronation (71). Occasionally, a scaphoid fracture is seen in conjunction with another injury, such as fracture of the distal radius or other intracarpal injury, after an extremely large force was imparted onto the carpus (78,79). Rarely, a direct blow is responsible for the injury.

Although fracture at the waist is the most commonly seen scaphoid fracture pattern in adults, this is not so in children. The vast majority of scaphoid fractures in children occur in the distal one-third of the bone. In Mussblicher's (74) series, distal-one-third fractures were seen in 94 of 108 cases, and avulsions of the distal scaphoid constituted 52% of the scaphoid fractures seen. Vahvanen and Westerlund (76) reported that 49% of the fractures in their series were distal-one-third fractures, while 38% were distal avulsions. Greene et al. (70) reported that six of nine scaphoid fractures seen were distal-one-third or avulsions.

Radiographs

Anteroposterior (AP) and true lateral radiographs of the wrist are imperative. In addition, a tangential lateral oblique view with the forearm in maximal pronation will highlight the tubercle fracture in children (70,71,74). Two radiographic soft tissue signs, dorsal wrist swelling and the scaphoid fat stripe sign, are indicative of acute scaphoid fracture in a child (80). The scaphoid fat stripe is a small triangular fat density between the radial collateral ligament and the tendons of the first dorsal wrist extensor compartment. When this is obliterated or radially displaced, it indicates a fracture of the scaphoid, radial styloid, or base of the thumb metacarpal (80). However, it is usually unreliable or absent in children younger than age 12. Contralateral comparison views may be helpful, but only if they are selectively taken. The difficulty of radiographic diagnosis in pediatric carpal fractures was mentioned earlier. Greene et al. (70) reported that half the radiologists reported the sclerosis, cystic changes, and eventual remodeling of a healing fracture to be suggestive of osteochondrosis, such as Prieser's disease (74,81). Cook et al. (80) reported that magnetic resonance imaging (MRI) of the wrist had a 100% negative predictive value and suggested that MRI may be useful in the early diagnostic workup of a scaphoid fracture in children (Fig. 11.10).

Treatment

Aggressive treatment should be instituted even for suspected scaphoid fractures without radiographic evidence to support the diagnosis because delay in treatment can result in significant complications, such as nonunion, avascular necrosis, instability, and arthrosis (82). In the event of no radiologic evidence of fracture and clinical tenderness over the anatomic snuff box and scaphoid tubercle, cast immobilization and repeat radiographs in 10 to 14 days are warranted (71). When pain persists, other diagnostic tools may be employed to confirm the diagnosis of scaphoid fracture, such as computer-assisted tomography, arthrography, MRI, or bone scan.

Closed treatment is usually sufficient for treatment of the scaphoid fracture in the child. Avulsion fractures may be adequately treated in a short arm thumb–spica cast for as little as 3 to 4 weeks (76). Children usually completely heal these fractures within 5 weeks (71). For transverse nondisplaced fractures of the scaphoid, a short arm thumb–spica cast for 4 to 12 weeks is usually sufficient (69,71,76,83,84). In cases of delayed treatment, longer periods of immobilization may be necessary. Operative treatment by open reduction and internal fixation is

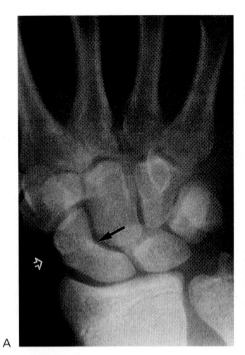 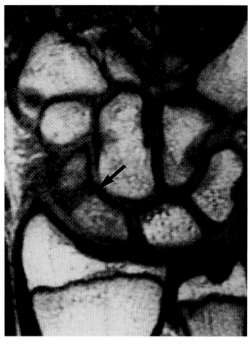

FIGURE 11.10. A: Eleven-year-old boy 4 weeks after fall onto outstretched hand. Initial x-ray was normal. *Closed arrow* denotes cortical disruption; *open arrow* denotes scaphoid fat stripe. **B:** Magnetic resonance image 2 days after injury clearly shows scaphoid fracture *(arrow)*. (From Cook PA, Yu JS, Wiand W, et al. Suspected scaphoid fractures in skeletally immature patients: Application of MRI. *J Comput Assist Tomogr* 1997;21:511–515, with permission.)

reserved for the rare cases of displaced fractures or nonunions (75).

Complications

Nonunion

Nonunion of a scaphoid fracture in adults results in a predictable pattern of late osteoarthrosis, the so-called scaphoid nonunion advanced collapse (SNAC) pattern, and should be treated (85). Nonunion of a scaphoid fracture in the pediatric population is extremely rare, most probably because most fractures in this population are through the distal third of the bone (86). Given the known problems after nonunion in adults, it is probably wise to prevent or repair a nonunion, especially a symptomatic nonunion, in a child. Most scaphoid nonunions in children result from displaced waist or proximal-third fractures (71). This is not surprising because the scaphoid's vasculature is established early and stays constant through skeletal maturity. The blood supply enters the scaphoid at the distal pole and flows proximally, putting the proximal portion of the scaphoid at risk after fracture (84). However, even a distal-third scaphoid fracture may result in delayed union, as reported by Wilson-MacDonald (84). Multiple authors state that scaphoid nonunions result primarily from undiagnosed injury (Fig. 11.11) (71,72,85).

Management of a symptomatic, persistent, or displaced scaphoid nonunion in a child should be treated similarly to that in an adult. Bone grafting is the most common method of treatment employed (72,87), but De Boeck et al. (85) reported a case of a scaphoid nonunion treated successfully with a long arm thumb–spica cast immobilization for 2 months. If the fracture is displaced, internal fixation with bone graft and subsequent plaster immobilization is the treatment of choice. If the fracture is not displaced, a trial of cast immobilization with or without electrical stimulation should be undertaken.

Congenital bipartite scaphoid is nomenclature seen almost exclusively in the literature of the 1970s and continues to be controversial. It was previously thought that failure of fusion of the proximal and distal poles of the scaphoid resulted in bipartite scaphoid. Louis et al. (88) reported several cases of asymptomatic pseudoarthrosis of the scaphoid undoubtedly secondary to fractures that were previously diagnosed as congenital bipartite scaphoids. It remains that congenital bipartite scaphoid probably does not exist and that the only source of bipartition is scaphoid fracture and subsequent pseudarthrosis (89).

Posttraumatic Instability

Posttraumatic carpal instability is rarely diagnosed in a child. Gerard (90) reported one case of posttraumatic

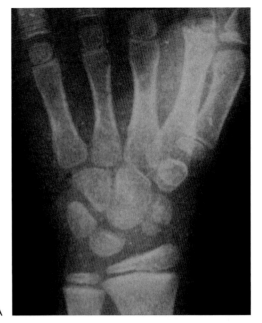 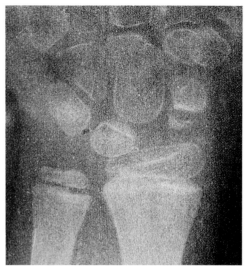

FIGURE 11.11. **A:** Proximal third scaphoid fracture in a child. **B:** Ten weeks postinjury, showing bone resorption and sclerosis at the fracture site. (From Pick RY, Segal D. Carpal scaphoid fracture and non-union in an eight-year-old child. *J Bone Joint Surg Am* 1983;65:1188–1189, with permission.)

scapholunate dissociation in a 7-year-old child who subsequently responded well to surgical reconstruction. Given the difficulties in diagnosing roentgenographic evidence of carpal instability in the skeletally immature carpus, another technique, such as MRI or arthrography, should be used to confirm any clinical suspicion of posttraumatic carpal instability in a child.

FRACTURES OF OTHER CARPAL BONES IN THE IMMATURE WRIST

Carpal fractures other than scaphoid fractures in children are exceptionally uncommon but may be more common than previously thought. Letts and Esser (91) reported that the triquetrum was the second most commonly fractured carpal bone in children included in their study. They identified 15 patients younger than 16 years of age with a diagnosed triquetral fracture, most of whom were between 11 and 13 years of age. Avulsion-type fractures of the triquetrum were present in 12 of the 15 cases, and body fractures were found in the remaining three cases. Compson (92) reported three cases of carpal fractures in children, one of whom was a 13-year-old boy with a scaphoid fracture and an additional late diagnosis of a nondisplaced triquetral body fracture. Larson et al. (89) reported the case of a 5-year-old boy who presented with a nondisplaced triquetrum body fracture and a late diagnosis of a concomitant scaphoid waist fracture, which ultimately went on to nonunion.

Triquetrum fractures result from several mechanisms (91). In extension, the ulnar styloid is thought to act as a chisel on the dorsum of the triquetrum. Also, extreme wrist extension could force the hamate into the dorsoradial portion of the triquetrum, resulting in a shear-type fracture. In flexion, the ulnotriquetral or radiocapitate triquetral ligaments may result in an avulsion. The generalized ligamentous laxity of childhood may predispose children to this fracture pattern. If an acute injury to the triquetrum exists, the patient always complains of localized tenderness at a point just distal to the ulnar styloid on examination. Because the triqetrum in children may be largely cartilaginous, there may be little or no radiographic evidence of a fracture on the standard PA and lateral views, making oblique views imperative. Diagnosis may be made by sufficient clinical suspicion, and regardless of radiographic evidence, treatment should consist of 3 weeks of immobilization in a short arm cast.

Other carpal bones are rarely injured in children, and fracture should be considered when clinical suspicion is high, even if radiographic evidence is absent. Capitate fractures may displace significantly and, without anatomic reduction, will result in nonunion (93). Difficulty interpreting plain radiographs of the injured immature carpus may necessitate contralateral views or MRI of the affected wrist.

TRIANGULAR FIBROCARTILAGE COMPLEX TEARS

The anatomy, biomechanics, and function of the TFCC have been previously documented (94,95). Palmer's (95) classification of TFCC tears is the most universally used. In the adult, the TFCC may be the source of significant ulnar-sided wrist pain and dysfunction if damaged either by direct tear or degenerative pattern. Reports on TFCC injuries in children are exceedingly rare. It is becoming more apparent through recent case reports that TFCC lesions in the pediatric population can occur, despite the notion that this injury does not occur in children. Terry and Waters (96) presented a retrospective review of 29 children (average age, 13.4 years) with surgically confirmed TFCC tears. They found that the average time to surgery (2.4 years) was prolonged by inaccurate or delayed diagnosis. Almost all injuries occurred after a fall onto an outstretched hand, and 52% sustained a distal radius fracture at the time of their initial injury. Ten of the 29 patients had no initial fracture. All had ulnar-sided wrist pain. Seventy-nine percent had an ulnar-sided click on examination, and 41% had clinical evidence of DRUJ instability. Forty-one percent had an ulnar styloid nonunion, and 31% of patients had positive ulnar variance on preoperative radiographs. There was a predominance of type IB (ulnar avulsion) TFCC tears in their cohort. Previous authors (94,97) reported that this lesion was rare in the adult population, with an incidence of 15% in their study.

Kuntz et al. (98) reported the case of an 11-year-old girl with a history of a fall and acute injury to her wrist. Initial radiographs were normal. Eight months later, she had an exacerbation of her initial injury while performing a cartwheel. Again, radiographs were normal. Clicking was present on pronosupination. An arthrogram confirmed the diagnosis of TFCC. Subsequent arthroscopic debridement of a type IC tear (avulsion of the TFCC from its insertion onto the lunate and/or triquetrum) resulted in an excellent outcome. Left untreated, a TFCC tear may result in progressive wrist pathology (96,99).

Initial radiographs are part of a complete examination. Although they will probably appear normal, careful inspection of the radiographs for coexisting wrist pathology must be performed. The role of MRI in the wrist is controversial, and Terry et al. (96) reported a 50% false-negative rate after MRI studies were performed on 10 wrists that ultimately had surgically documented TFCC tears. The benefits of wrist arthrography have been previously documented. However, wrist arthrography is invasive, may not be tolerated well in a child, will have quality that is operator dependent, and will not accurately define the anatomy of a TFCC tear (100). For these reasons, we recommend moving directly to arthroscopy.

Treatment

Treatment of TFCC tears in children should address not only the TFCC pathology but any coexisting pathology as well. Ulnar styloid nonunions should be excised to decrease ulnocarpal abutment and facilitate repair of the TFCC. Ulnar shortening procedures should be considered to remedy ulnar positive variance. Radial osteotomy should be considered in the case of partial epiphysiodesis. DRUJ instability should be corrected. Terry and Waters (96) recommend repair of all IB, (TFCC avulsion from distal ulna with associated fragment of bone), IC (TFCC avulsion from its distal bony insertion on the lunate and/or triquetrum), and ID (avulsion of TFCC from radical origin with or without bony fragment) tears.

FRACTURES OF THE DISTAL RADIUS AND ULNA

The distal forearm is the area most commonly fractured in children (101–106). These fractures virtually always result from a fall onto an outstretched hand. They occur most frequently in boys 13 to 14 years old and girls 9 to 10 years old (107). Reports suggest that a period of relatively reduced mineralization during the adolescent growth spurt puts the distal radius and ulna at risk for fracture (107,108). In contrast to adults, fractures of the distal radius and ulna in children virtually always heal rapidly without functional disability and with minimal intervention (103). However, distal forearm fractures in the child must be thoroughly analyzed because several factors may influence the choice of treatment and outcome.

Distal Radial Physeal and Epiphyseal Fractures

The distal radial physis is the most commonly injured physis in the body (103). Distal radial physeal fractures account for 2% of all children's fractures but 40% of all physeal injuries (109,110). Salter-Harris II injuries are seen most commonly, accounting for over 50% of distal radial physeal injuries (35,102,103,108,109). Careful inspection for intraarticular components of an epiphyseal injury must be performed, as they may result in late arthrosis (111).

Treatment

Most distal radius fractures in children reduce adequately with manual traction. The intact dorsal periosteum provides the hinge with which to reduce the fracture and prevents overcorrection (102). A distal radial fracture without an ulnar fracture is uncommon. Signs of the injury to the nonossified distal ulna are often seen on follow-up x-rays (102,106). Frequently, the result is excellent despite the appearance of an ulnar styloid nonunion.

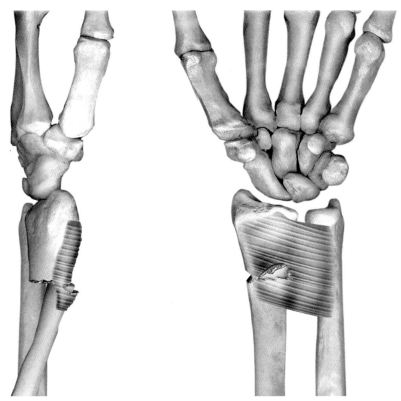

FIGURE 11.12. Entrapment of the pronator quadratus in a distal radius fracture. (Modified from Holmes JR, Louis DS. Entrapment of pronator quadratus in pediatric distal radius fractures: Recognition and treatment. *J Pediatr Orthop* 1994;14:498–500, with permission.)

When closed reduction of a distal radius fracture cannot be accomplished, the distinct possibility of soft tissue entrapment must be considered. The pronator quadratus may block reduction of fractures of the distal radius, although these are usually metaphyseal fractures (Fig. 11.12) (105). Manoli (112) reported a case of a boy with an irreducible Salter-Harris type II injury in which the distal radius and ulna were buttonholed through all volar structures. Karlsson and Appelqvist (35) and Evans et al. (113) reported cases of Salter-Harris type II injuries in which reduction was impossible because of interposition of extensor tendons (Fig. 11.13). Neurologic injury is rare, but radiating pain or paresthesias in the hand indicates irritation of the median nerve by the volar proximal fracture spike (110). Reduction usually results in alleviation of symptoms, which may take months depending on the severity of the neurapraxia (110,112).

In the younger age groups, between 6 and 10 years of age, there is significant remodeling potential of the distal radius and ulna. A useful heuristic is that the distal forearm will regain 1° per month or 10° per year (114). Bayonet apposition in a child younger than 10 years old is acceptable, as it is aligned and more stable than a fracture with less than 50% bone apposition, which has a tendency to deform (102). These young children tend to remodel sufficiently, and healing takes place without functional limitation.

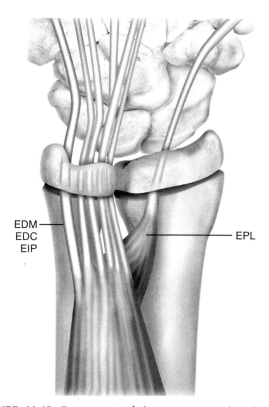

FIGURE 11.13. Entrapment of the extensor tendons between the fractured metaphysis and epiphysis. *EDC,* extensor digitorum communis; *EDM,* extensor digitorum minimi; *EIP,* extensor indicis proprius; *EPL,* extensor pollicis longus. (Modified from Karlsson J, Appelqvist R. Irreducible fracture of the wrist in a child. *Acta Orthop Scand* 1987;58:280–281, with permission.)

Distal Ulnar Physeal and Epiphyseal Fractures

Fracture of the distal ulnar physis accounts for about 5% of all physeal injuries (104,110,115). This structure is probably protected by the cushioning effect of the TFCC and the fact that only 20% of the load through the carpus is borne by the ulna. Distal ulna fractures are seen in conjunction with distal radius fractures about 50% of the time. In the absence of an injury to the radius, ulna fractures occur in conjunction with extreme ulnar deviation during impact (115). The incidence of ulnar styloid fractures with all types of distal radial fractures is 33% (110). Frequently the distal ulna fracture is overlooked and diagnosed only on premature closure of the physis (104).

Physeal Injuries

Physeal injuries can look benign but may cause significant complications (23,116,117). Although premature growth arrest is uncommon after distal radius and ulna fractures in children, it did occur in 7% of all cases (104,109). Most growth arrests result from Salter II injuries, as they are most common, but also follow Salter V injuries—crush of the physis—which are difficult to detect acutely (102). Arrest of the distal radius is more common than in the distal ulna and may result in a Madelung's-like deformity that requires late reconstruction (23,116). Ulnar growth arrest was reported by Nelson et al. (115) Their report detailed four cases of seemingly benign injuries to the ulna with growth arrest evident on follow-up examinations. In the series presented by Golz et al. (104) and Nelson et al. (115), all patients with ulnar growth arrest ultimately had acceptable functional results despite a displeasing cosmetic result. Consideration of ulnar-sided wrist anatomy is important. Growth arrest of the ulna may result in DRUJ pathology and an ulna minus variance. In a series of DRUJ pathology after forearm fractures in children, it was noted that a shortening of 3 mm could result in symptoms related to DRUJ pathology (Fig. 11.14) (118). In addition, ulnar growth arrest may cause a tethering effect on the distal radius, leading to radial bowing and soft tissue contractures of the ulnar side of the wrist (104,115).

Despite anatomic reduction, growth arrest can occur after any physeal injury. It is imperative that the family is made aware of the potential for growth arrest immediately after the injury. They are apt to be more involved in follow-up care and more accepting of this complication if they were initially informed of its possibility. Follow-up x-rays should be inspected closely for Park-Harris growth arrest lines. These sclerotic lines are usually laid down parallel and any deviation from parallel indicates growth arrest.

Growth arrest is associated with repeated, forceful manipulations after 2 to 3 weeks, severe trauma with loss of tissue, and surgical techniques (102,109). Surgical pins or screws should not cross the physis if possible. Pin size, the presence of threads, the angle of penetration of the physis, and where in the physis pins are placed all influence the chance of iatrogenic growth arrest. When pins must cross the physis, the smallest chance of growth arrest follows insertion of small, smooth pins placed perpendicular to the central physeal region for a short time (109).

Galleazzi Fracture in Children

The classic Galleazzi fracture involves a fracture of the radius and disruption of the DRUJ. In children and the elderly, a Galleazzi-equivalent fracture is seen (119). It consists of a distal radius fracture and Salter I injury to the ulnar physis, resulting in an unstable DRUJ (Fig. 11.15) (119,120). The mechanism of injury is a fall onto an outstretched hand with extreme forearm pronation (119). It is seen uncommonly, occurring in 2% to 5% of all fractures of the distal radius in children (119,120). Once the fracture is reduced, it is stable, as the DRUJ soft tissues were not violated. Closed reduction and cast immobilization in full supination for 4 to 6 weeks is usually sufficient (102). The long-term complications relate to failure of the initial treatment in full supination or malreduction of the ulnar epiphysis (119).

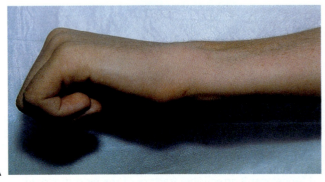
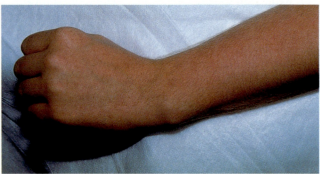

FIGURE 11.14. Voluntary DRUJ dislocation in a 13-year-old boy 3 years after a distal radius fracture.

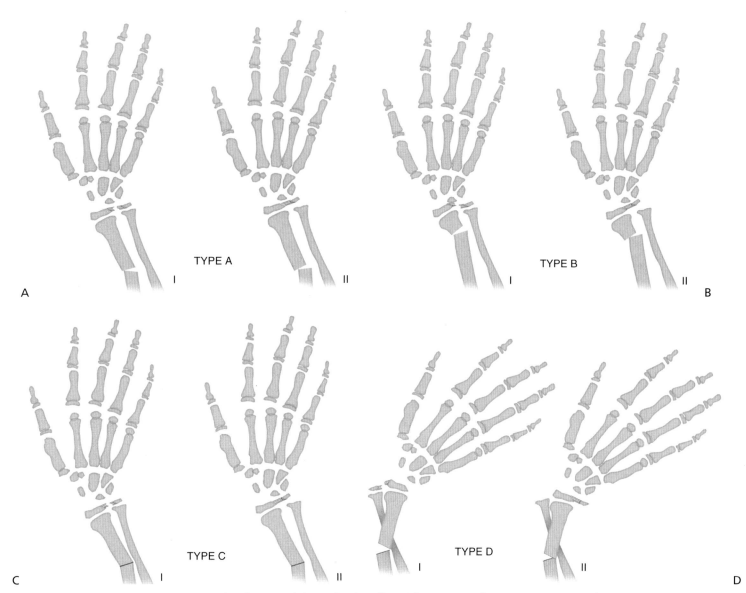

FIGURE 11.15. Classification of the pediatric Galleazzi fracture complex types. **A:** Fracture of the radius at the junction of the distal and middle thirds. **B:** Fracture of the distal third of the radius. **C:** Greenstick fracture of the radius with radial bowing. **D:** Fracture of the distal radius with volar angulation. (Modified from Letts M, Rowhani N. Galeazzi-equivalent injuries of the wrist in children. *J Pediatr Orthop* 1993;13:561–566, with permission.)

DRUJ instability may go undiagnosed if no associated fracture is evident. Care must be taken to assess the DRUJ in a true lateral radiograph as well as a PA radiograph of the wrist. The true lateral may demonstrate dorsal or volar subluxation of the distal ulna. The PA view may show abnormal widening of the DRUJ with dorsal subluxation. Superimposition of the distal radius and distal ulna may represent a distal ulna volar dislocation (121).

GANGLION

Ganglia are benign, mucinous cysts, often attached to the underlying joint capsule, tendon, or tendon sheath. Patients usually seek the attention of a physician because of the presence of a mass and not for pain, as ganglia are frequently painless. In a series of 543 patients with ganglia of the hand and wrist, only 20% of patients were younger than 20 years of age (122).

The exact etiology of the ganglion remains a mystery. Many hypotheses have been proposed, but the most accepted theory of the pathogenesis of ganglia is a mucinous degeneration of fibrous tissue probably secondary to repetitive stress (34).

Dorsal wrist ganglia virtually always arise from the scapholunate joint (5,34,123). Additional dorsal wrist ganglia may be extensions of the scapholunate ganglion attached by a long pedicle. Careful palpation may reveal their interconnectivity. Conversely, volar wrist ganglia, which represent about 20% of wrist ganglia, usually arise from scaphotrapezial or radiocarpal ligaments (5).

Rosson and Walker (124) commented on the natural history of ganglia in children. Of their population of 29 patients, 15 had ganglia at the wrist, 11 on the foot, and three on the hand. At the time of follow-up, 22 of 29 ganglia had resolved spontaneously. Surely, expectant treatment is the treatment of choice in the asymptomatic child. Frequently, parental assurance is all that is required. Other forms of nonoperative treatment, including rupture with a Bible or digital pressure and injection, result in unacceptably high rates of recurrence.

Persistent pain may be an indication for surgical excision of a ganglion. Care must be taken, however, to thoroughly examine the wrist, as a ganglion may be present in association with, or signify, additional wrist pathology that may necessitate treatment. A thorough history should include previous wrist injuries. Preoperative x-rays are appropriate and may result in a change in the surgical plan.

Dorsal wrist ganglia should be approached through a transverse incision centered over the mass, usually at the scapholunate joint. The ganglion must be excised completely with a small rim of capsule. Accessory ganglia on pedicles must also be excised and may be approached through a separate incision and tunneled under the extensor tendons to the site of the primary ganglion. The capsule is left open, and skin reapproximated using a mattress stitch.

Volar ganglia are exposed through an incision that must have extensile options. Otherwise, surgical excision proceeds as in dorsal ganglion excision. Care must be taken to avoid all neurovascular structures. The ganglion is traced to the volar joint capsule, and excision of a portion of a surrounding rim of joint capsule is performed.

Complications after ganglion excision include a 3% to 50% recurrence rate, stiffness, infection, and neuroma formation (34). Scapholunate dissociation is a rare postoperative complication of ganglion surgery secondary to transection of the scapholunate interosseous ligament, especially in a patient with previously weakened volar wrist ligaments (34,123).

NEOPLASTIC DISEASE OF THE PEDIATRIC WRIST

Very few reports in the literature detail neoplastic processes in the child's wrist. Aside from ganglia, the most common neoplastic entities of the wrist in the pediatric age group are osteochondromas and enchondromas, which may affect the ulnar portion of the distal radial metaphysis, resulting in bowing of the radius, premature growth arrest, and subsequent DRUJ problems (125). These are best seen on plain x-ray. Malignant degeneration of enchondromatous lesions of the child's hand and wrist have yet to be reported (126). Maffucci syndrome is the association of multiple enchondromata with hemangiomas, and malignant degeneration in adults is frequently seen. Osteochondromas and enchondromas are virtually always cured by complete excision (125). It is exceedingly rare to find other benign tumors in the child's wrist. Malignant tumors of the child's wrist are also extremely rare, and the reader is referred to an orthopedic oncology textbook for an overview of these diseases.

ANEURYSM

Aneurysms of the upper extremity are very rare, but not unheard of in the pediatric population (127). Usually, patients present complaining of pain in the hand and a pulsatile mass in the palm that is increasing in size. Aneurysms may be true or false. A false aneurysm does not possess all layers of the normal artery and usually results from penetrating trauma that damages only a portion of the arterial wall. The damaged artery thromboses then recanalizes through the hematoma, which is relined with endothelial cells (128–131). However, blunt trauma can cause a false aneurysm, when the ulnar artery is damaged as it passes through the pisohamate ligament and sharply dives deep into the palm (129).

A true aneurysm is one that contains all three arterial layers and results from an injury to the lamina elastica media, the layer that imparts elasticity and stability to the arterial wall (132). These most often result from blunt trauma, either from a single episode or repetetive trauma, to the hypothenar eminence as in adult jackhammer operators with "hypothenar hammer syndrome." True aneurysms usually result in palmar pain and a pulsatile fusiform mass noted on examination.

Digital ischemia may result from embolic showers from both true and false aneurysms. Additionally, an expanding mass may result in compression symptoms of a nearby nerve.

Treatment

An Allen's test at the initial examination will help determine the patency of the involved artery. Contrast angiography is more definitive but controversial, as it possesses the inherent risk of thrombosis. However, it may be indicated under certain circumstances. Microvascular reconstruction is indicated for both true and false aneurysms. Excision of the hematoma and arterial reconstruction is the treatment of choice for a false aneurysm. Some advocate only ligation of a true aneurysm, especially in the absence of digital ischemia. However, restoration of the normal vascular anatomy by vein graft may prevent cold intolerance and digital ischemia (Fig. 11.16).

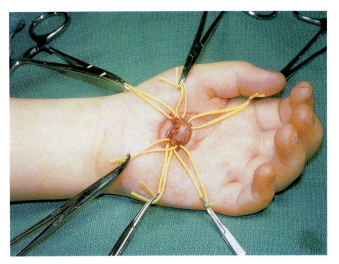

FIGURE 11.16. Excision of a true aneurysm of the superficial palmar arch in a 5-year-old child.

JUVENILE ARTHRITIS

The American Rheumatism Association defines JA as chronic, idiopathic synovitis and objective evidence of arthritis in at least one joint for 6 consecutive weeks in a child younger than 16 years of age. Other diseases must have been excluded (133). It is the most common connective tissue disorder in children (133–136). The prevalence in the United States is estimated to be between 57 and 113 per 100,000 children. The total affected American population is roughly 200,000 to 250,000 children (137). Juvenile rheumatoid arthritis is a major cause of childhood illness and disability. There are three types of disease, designated by their symptoms at onset: pauciarticular JA, polyarticular JA, and systemic JA (Table 11.2). The onset is usually between ages 1 and 3, except in systemic JA, whose onset has no predilection for early ages. Girls are affected at about twice the rate as boys, except in systemic JA, in which boys and girls are equally affected. Active disease persists into adulthood in 50% of cases. More than 30% of JA patients will have significant limitations after 10 or more years of follow-up. Mortality rates range from 0.29 to 1.1 per 100 patients (135).

Etiology

Many hypotheses concerning the etiology of JA have been put forth, including dysfunctional immunoregulation and latent viral infection. The association between arthritis and certain viral infections, especially rubella and parvovirus, has been documented. Additionally, reports of immunodeficiency are compelling. The true etiology of JA, however, remains unknown.

Classification of Onset

Pauciarticular Juvenile Arthritis

Children with pauciarticular JA comprise 40% to 60% of all patients with JA and by definition have arthritis in four or fewer joints, most often the knees and ankles. There are two distinct subgroups: early and late onset (135). Early-onset pauciarticular JA typically affects girls between 1 and 5 years of age. Fifty percent of these patients are antinuclear antibody (ANA) positive. Extraarticular symptoms are uncommon except for ophthalmologic complications (134). Chronic eye inflammation (iridocyclitis) develops in 20% to 50% (133,134). In those with ocular manifestations, 80% are asymptomatic. Delayed ophthalmologic

TABLE 11.2. TYPES OF ONSET OF JUVENILE RHEUMATOID ARTHRITIS

	Polyarthritis	Oligoarthritis	Systemic Disease
Relative frequency (%)	30	60	10
Number of joints involved	≥5	≤4	Variable
Sex ratio (F:M)	3:1	5:1	1:1
Extraarticular involvement	Moderate	Not present	Prominent
Chronic uveitis (%)	5	20	Rare
Seropositivity			
Rheumatoid factors (%)	15[a]	Rare	Rare
Antinuclear antibodies (%)	40	85[b]	10
Clinical course	Systemic disease generally mild; articular involvement often unremitting	Systemic disease absent; major cause of morbidity is uveitis	Systemic disease often self-limited; arthritis chronic and destructive in half
Prognosis	Moderately good	Excellent	Moderate

[a]Rheumatoid factor seropositivity forms a risk group in children with polyarthritis who presented at an older age.
[b]Antinuclear antibody seropositivity forms a risk group for chronic uveitis in children with oligoarthritis who presented at a young age.
From Cassidy JT. Juvenile rheumatoid arthritis. In: Kelly WN, Ruddy S, Harris ED, et al., eds. *Textbook of rheumatology*, 5th ed. Philadelphia: WB Saunders, 1997.

evaluation may lead to irreversible ocular damage and blindness. Therefore, early referral to an ophthalmologist and continued long-term ocular surveillance are imperative. Late-onset pauciarticular JA occurs more commonly in boys, with large joints more often affected. Prognosis is generally excellent in this variant, as more than 70% of cases remit with little or no functional impairment 15 years after onset (133).

Polyarticular Juvenile Arthritis

Thirty to fifty percent of patients present with arthritis in five or more joints (133–135). Polyarticular JA usually presents insidiously and symmetrically in larger joints, such as knees, wrists, elbows, and ankles. The presence or absence of rheumatoid factor (RF) distinguishes the two subgroups of polyarticular JA. RF-positive patients are almost exclusively female with onset after 8 years of age (135). These patients are more likely to have poor long-term functional outcomes. The disease and course often resemble adult-onset rheumatoid arthritis (133,135,138).

Systemic Onset (Still's Disease)

About 10% to 20% of children present with systemic onset of the disease, with or without arthritis (136). Typically, these children present with high, spiking fevers that spike daily (quotidian) or twice daily (double quotidian) (133,134). A rheumatoid rash consisting of erythematous morbilliform macules most commonly on the trunk and proximal extremities when the child is febrile, is diagnostic (133,135). These children often have multiple extraarticular components to their disease, such as growth delay, osteopenia, diffuse lymphadenopathy, hepatosplenomegaly, pericarditis, pleuritis, anemia, leukocytosis, and thrombocytosis (133,135).

Carpal Pathology in Juvenile Arthritis

The child's wrist, in addition to other joints, is susceptible to the effects of stiffness and deformity of JA, most often seen in the polyarticular variant (138). Intermittent bouts of stiffness, synovitis, and tenosynovitis occur. Pain and instability are not usually seen as often as in adult onset rheumatoid arthritis (133).

The pediatric carpus is prone to loss of extension and radial deviation, resulting in a flexion/ulnar deviation deformity. Often, patients with JA undergo spontaneous ankylosis of intracarpal joints. Radiocarpal articulation is frequently spared, but motion is limited nonetheless (138). Volar inclination of the distal radial articular surface in combination with ligamentous laxity produce net forces that contribute to volar subluxation of the carpus. Soft tissue laxity may result from intrinsic ligament destruction by the inflammatory process or from erosion of the articular surface, which results in relative laxity of the supporting ligamentous structures (136). DRUJ involvement may result in pain, decrease in pronosupination, and subluxation. Differential epiphyseal overgrowth of the radius results in DRUJ incongruence and the not unusual finding of negative ulnar variance (136).

Radiographs

Radiographic evaluation of the wrist of a child may be aided by evaluation of carpal size using standardized comparison radiographs (137). Particularly in the younger age groups, this technique helps determine whether or not cartilage has been lost. Common early radiographic evidence of JA include soft tissue swelling, effusions, periosteal new bone formation, lucent metaphyseal bands, and periarticular osteopenia (134,137). Later in the disease, erosions, joint space narrowing, intracarpal fusions, decreased carpal

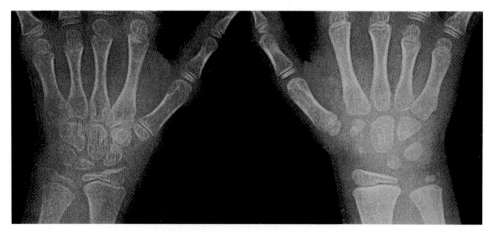

FIGURE 11.17. Accelerated maturation of the left carpus in a nine-year-old with arthritis for 7 years. Carpal bones on the left are more mature and already smaller than those on the right. (From Cassidy JT. Juvenile rheumatoid arthritis. In: Kelley WN, Ruddy S, Harris ED, et al., eds. *Textbook of rheumatology*, 5th ed. Philadelphia: WB Saunders, 1997, with permission.)

height (139), and premature epiphysiodesis and ossification centers are seen (134,137). The latter two phenomena result from chronic hyperemia of the region. Negative ulnar variance results from relative overgrowth of the distal radius (Fig. 11.17).

Treatment

The keys to effective treatment of JA are accurate early diagnosis and family-centered, multidisciplinary team management of the disease (Table 11.3) (134,136). The orthopedic surgeon should closely monitor the patient to detect and correct problems before they become irreversible (136). Children with JA, and particularly those with pauciarticular JA, should be referred immediately for a baseline ophthalmologic examination whether or not they have ocular symptoms. A rheumatology referral is appropriate for medical management of the disease. Early implementation of physical and occupational therapy may prolong joint motion. Stretching and splinting in functionally advantageous positions will minimize joint deformities, mechanical stress, and contractures (133,135). Preservation of wrist function should be addressed before finger deformities to improve overall hand function (136). Management should progress logically from conservative to more aggressive measures only as conservative measures fail.

Pharmacologic Treatment

Nonsteriodal antiinflammatory drugs (NSAIDS) are the mainstay of pharmacologic treatment for JA and should be instituted immediately on diagnosis of the disease. The chronic inflammation of JA can be counteracted only by doses of NSAIDS large enough to obtain an antiinflammatory effect. Frequently, this dose is twice the analgesic dose. Fifty percent of children with JA who will respond to a particular NSAID will do so after 2 weeks of treatment (135). An additional 25% will respond within 8 to 12 weeks of additional therapy (135). The efficacy of each NSAID is about equal, and a particular patient's response is unpredictable. Aspirin dosage is typically 75 to 90 mg/kg per day, depending on the child's age and weight. Other drugs used in the United States are tolmetin (25 mg/kg per day), naproxen (15 mg/kg per day), and ibuprofen (35 mg/kg per day). Complications include gastrointestinal irritation and rarely ulceration, tinnitus, and transient transaminasemia (101). Pseudoporphyria is an unusual sign of naproxen toxicity (134). About one-third of patients are sufficiently treated with NSAIDS alone (135). Advanced pharmacologic treatment is beyond the scope of this chapter.

Surgical Treatment

Operative intervention is warranted when conservative measures fail. Synovectomy of the wrist may decrease active inflammation of the joint but is controversial. It can relieve pain but probably does not increase range of motion or prevent further loss of motion (136). Synovectomy during a period of active synovitis results in adhesions and should not be performed (133). Recurrence after synovectomy is not common. A joint-leveling procedure should be considered to correct an incongruous DRUJ in conjunction with synovectomy of the wrist. Tenosynovectomy of the wrist should probably be considered if surgery is to be performed for tenosynovitis of the finger flexors. Contracture releases may also be necessary to relieve soft tissue deforming forces. Late in the course of the disease, corrective osteotomies should be considered if ankylosis occurs in a disadvantageous or painful position. Closing wedge osteotomy of the distal radius avoids the need for bone grafting. Arthrodesis of the DRUJ (Sauvé-Kapandji procedure) may provide relief of pain and limitations of motion about this joint.

ACKNOWLEDGMENTS

We wish to thank Eric T. Jones, M.D., Ph.D. for his critical review and helpful comments and Suzanne Smith for her administrative assistance during the preparation of this chapter.

TABLE 11.3. MANAGEMENT OF JUVENILE ARTHRITIS

Basic program
   Nonsteroidal antiinflammatory drug
   Physical and occupational therapy
   Education and counseling of family and patient
   Involvement of school and community agencies
   Nutrition
Advanced drug therapy
   Hydroxychloroquine, sulfasalazine, methotrexate
   Gold compounds, d-penicillamine
   Intraarticular steroids
Glucocorticoids
Immunosuppressive therapy
Experimental therapy
Orthopedic surgery
   Preventive surgery
   Reconstructive surgery

From Cassidy JT. Juvenile rheumatoid arthritis. In: Kelley WN, Ruddy S, Harris ED, et al., eds. *Textbook of rheumatology*, 5th ed. Philadelphia: WB Saunders, 1997, with permission.

EDITORS' COMMENTS

Scaphoid fracture in the pediatric population is probably more common than previously thought. Treatment may be conducted along the lines of a more mature wrist with one exception. The pediatric scaphoid can be significantly nonosseous, creating the illusion that the bone has undergone significant necrosis. This is not the case. Because the loss of scaphoid support is such a major functional deficit in the adult, scaphoid nonunions should be opened and grafted under all circumstances in the pediatric population.

A 9-year-old boy with a scaphoid nonunion was felt to have had complete scaphoid necrosis (Editors' Fig. 11.1). At the time of operation, the cartilage scaphoids were extant and structurally sound with good cartilage. The scaphoid was bone grafted at age 9, and x-ray demonstrates the wrist in this patient with a healed functional scaphoid 6 years later (Editors' Fig. 11.2).

The pediatric wrist, as with most other aspects of pediatric trauma, has excellent capacity to heal and recover, and the approach should be one of accepting nothing less than near-normal joint alignment with open surgery as necessary.

Juvenile rheumatoid arthritis can produce a most debilitating loss of function of the wrist. The wrist will frequently dislocate completely off the end of the radius and ulna, sliding proximal in the forearm. We have been pleased with the use of the rheumatoid nonunion procedure in children where essentially a cancellous concavity is formed in the distal radius combined with a matched ulnar arthroplasty. A cancellous surface is formed on the proximal scaphoid and lunate with or without some resection of the triquetrum, and the wrist is cross-pinned for 2 weeks and then mobilized. On occasion, if the wrist is very stable, one may place the extensor ligaments of the wrist in the concavity of the radius before the scaphoid and lunate are seated, assuring a greater nonunion effect and increased mobility. This procedure is described more completely in Chapter 61.

Treatment of symptomatic Madelung's requires careful analysis and is a difficult analytic problem for the wrist surgeon. The pain is diffuse and activity related, along with a postactivity ache component. The examiner must determine what part of this imbalanced wrist is causing the pain.

A common cause of pain in the Madelung's wrist is carpal impaction against the ulna (Editors' Fig. 11.3). This can produce a highly localized area of cartilage loss. There will be localized tenderness and compression of the ulna against the carpals from different positions, and supination and pronation can identify this highly localized degenerative area. X-rays can show the localized area of sclerosis, and if this is the case, treatment is a matter of bone resection relieving the impaction area. It is especially important to identify this phenomenon, as treatment is simple and effective, whereas if one assumes that it is the slope of the radius, treatment may be extensive and unnecessary. The Madelung's wrist does tolerate a distal radial articular surface that is nearly in line with the long axis of the forearm. The upslope ligaments

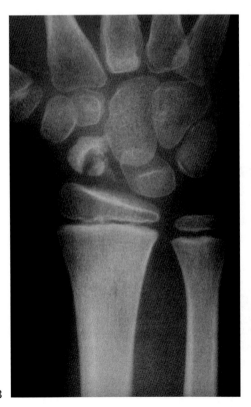
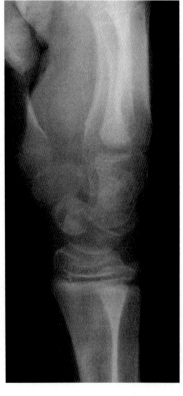

EDITORS' FIGURE 11.1. A: X-ray of a 9-year-old boy demonstrates what appears to be dissolution of the scaphoid following nonunion from a fracture 4 months previously. **B:** The lateral x-ray demonstrates a D-type lunate and fracture loss of scaphoid support for the lunate, allowing it to assume its neutral anatomy position of dorsiflexion.

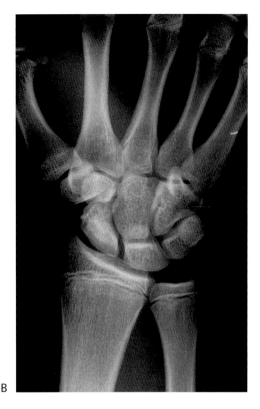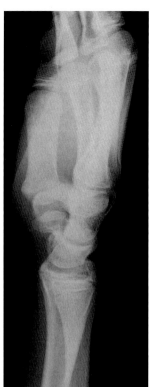

EDITORS' FIGURE 11.2. A: Six years following bone grafting and healing, the scaphoid has reestablished itself as a load component on the radial side of the wrist. The scapholunate interosseous system appears to be intact clinically and by x-ray. B: The lateral x-ray demonstrates a much-improved capitate–lunate alignment. This dorsal intercalated segment instability (DISI) has been basically corrected, and the lunate is now collinear with the capitate. The scapholunate angle remains at 64°.

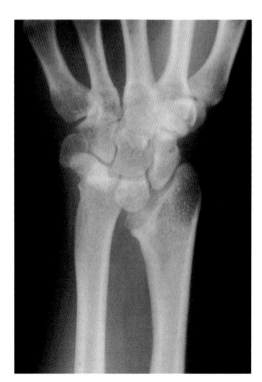

EDITORS' FIGURE 11.3. Madelung's deformity producing significant symptomotology is to some extent the result of carpal impaction against the ulna.

maintain the carpals and tolerate significant symptom-free activity. If it is determined that the symptoms are radial-carpal in nature and that stability will solve the problem, and there are no areas of cartilage loss between radius and carpals, then the nonlengthening, nonshortening osteotomy of the distal radius can be accomplished.

A word of caution is in order in evaluating wrist pain in children. Girls between the ages of 10 and 15 seem to develop an inordinate number of wrist complaints. This overplay is usually not for secondary gain, not always female, and often based on some real low-grade symptom complex such as dorsal wrist syndrome from scapholunate activity overload or rapid bone growth producing transient soft tissue symptoms. It is our experience that significant pathology is rare and that follow-up evaluation is probably the best course. Major diagnostic studies are probably not indicated, as they tend to fix the symptom complaints in the patient's mind. Triangular fibrocartilage problems should be diagnosed with caution and almost never treated. Muscle complaints from forearm growth are common. Occasionally ulnar impaction syndrome after epiphyseal closure will be significant enough to require stepcut shortening osteotomy, but then only if the problem clearly interferes with function.

REFERENCES

1. Esposito PW, Crawford AH. Wrist disorders in children. In: Lichtman DM, ed. *The wrist and its disorders*. Philadelphia: WB Saunders, 1988;385–403.
2. Graham TJ, O'Brien ET. Fractures and dislocations of the hand and carpus in children. In: Rockwood CA, Wilkins KE, Beaty KE, eds. *Fractures in children*. Philadelphia: Lippincott–Raven Publishers, 1996;323–447.
3. Grad JB. Children's skeletal injuries. *Orthop Clin North Am* 1986;17:437–449.
4. Stuart HC, Pyle SI, Cornoni J, et al. Onsets, completions and spans of ossification in the 29 bone-growth centers of the hand and wrist. *Pediatrics* 1962;29:237–249.
5. Angelides AC. Ganglions of the hand and wrist. In: Green DP, ed. *Operative hand surgery*. New York: Churchill-Livingstone, 1993.
6. Conway WF, Destouet JM, Gilula LA, et al. The carpal boss: An overview and radiologic evaluation. *Radiology* 1985;156:29–31.
7. Cuono CB, Watson HK. The carpal boss: Surgical treatment and etiological considerations. *Plast Reconstr Surg* 1979;63:886–888.
8. Frangiadakis EG. Carpal bossing. In: Tubiana R, ed. *The hand*. Philadelphia: WB Saunders, 1988.
9. Citteur JME, Ritt MJPF, Bos KE. Carpal boss: Destabilization of the third carpometacarpal joint after wedge excision. *J Hand Surg [Br]* 1998;23:76–78.
10. Fusi S, Watson HK, Cuono CB. The carpal boss. *J Hand Surg [Br]* 1995;20:405–408.
11. Herbert TJ, Conolly WB, Clarke AM. Treatment of the carpal boss by carpometacarpal arthrodesis. In: Saffar P, Amadio PC, Foucher G, eds. *Current practice in hand surgery*. London: Martin-Dunitz, 1997;105–107.
12. Bayne LG, Costas BL, Lourie GM. The upper limb. In: Morrissy RT, Weinstein SL, eds. *Lovell and Winter's pediatric orthopaedics, 4th ed.* Philadelphia: Lippincott–Raven Publishers, 1996:781–847.
13. Dobyns JH, Wood VE, Bayne LG. Congenital hand deformities. In: Green DP, ed. *Operative hand surgery, 3rd ed.* New York: Churchill-Livingstone, 1993:251–548.
14. dos Reis FB, Katchburian MV, Faloppa F, et al. Osteotomy of the radius and ulna for the Madelung deformity. *J Bone Joint Surg Br* 1998;80:817–824.
15. Lamb D. Madelung deformity. *J Hand Surg [Br]* 1988;13:3–4.
16. Matev I, Karagancheva S. The Madelung's deformity. *Hand* 1975;7:152–158.
17. Vickers D, Nielsen G. Madelung deformity: Surgical prophylaxis (physiolysis) during the late growth period by resection of the dyschondrosteosis lesion. *J Hand Surg [Br]* 1992;17:401–407.
18. Beals RK, Lovrien EW. Dyschondrosteosis and Madelung's deformity. *Clin Orthop* 1976;116:24–28.
19. Fagg PS. Wrist pain in the Madelung's deformity of dyschondrosteosis. *J Hand Surg [Br]* 1988;13:11–15.
20. Golding JSR, Blackburne JS. Madelung's disease of the wrist and dyschondrosteosis. *J Bone Joint Surg Br* 1976;58:350–352.
21. Nielsen JB. Madelung's deformity. *Acta Orthop Scand* 1977;48:379–384.
22. Tachdjian MO. Madelung's deformity. In: Tachdjian MO, ed. *Pediatric orthopedics, 2nd ed.* Philadelphia: WB Saunders, 1990;210–222.
23. Dobyns JH, Cooney WP. The child's wrist: diagnostic and treatment problems. In: Cooney WP, Linscheid RL, Dobyns JH, eds. *The wrist*. St Louis: CV Mosby, 1998:1002–1030.
24. Thomas RD, Fairhurst JJ, Clarke NMP. Madelung's deformity masquerading as a bone tumour. *Skel Radiol* 1993;22:329–331.
25. Vender MI, Watson HK. Acquired Madelung-like deformity in a gymnast. *J Hand Surg [Am]* 1988;13:19–21.
26. Fagg PS. Reverse Madelung's deformity with nerve compression. *J Hand Surg [Br]* 1988;13:23–27.
27. Tlacuilo-Parra JA, Salazar-Paramo M, Davalos IP, et al. Madelung's deformity from a rheumatologist's point of view. Letter to the editor. *Br J Rheum* 1997;36:924–925.
28. Gelberman RH, Bauman T. Madelung's deformity and dyschondrosteosis. *J Hand Surg [Am]* 1980;5:338–340.
29. Ducloyer P, Leclercq C, Lisfranc R, et al. Spontaneous ruptures of the extensor tendons of the fingers in Madelung's deformity. *J Hand Surg [Br]* 1991;16:329–333.
30. Goodwin DRA, Michels CH, Weissman SL. Spontaneous rupture of extensor tendons in Madelung's deformity. *Hand* 1979;11:72–75.
31. Murphy MS, Linscheid RL, Dobyns JH, et al. Radial opening wedge osteotomy in Madelung's deformity. *J Hand Surg [Am]* 1996;21:1035–1044.
32. Cook PA, Yu JS, Wiand W, et al. Madelung deformity in skeletally immature patients: Morphologic assessment using radiography, CT, and MRI. *J Comput Assist Tomogr* 1996;20:505–511.
33. Van Demark RE, Van Demark RE. Long-term results after the surgical treatment of Madelung's deformity: A case report. *J Hand Surg [Am]* 1993;18:1008–1011.
34. Duncan KH, Lewis RC. Scapholunate instability following ganglion cyst excision. *Clin Orthop* 1988;228:250–253.
35. Karlsson J, Appelqvist R. Irreducible fracture of the wrist in a child. *Acta Orthop Scand* 1987;58:280–281.
36. Watson HK, Pitts EC, Herber S. Madelung's deformity. *J Hand Surg [Br]* 1993;18:601–605.
37. White GM, Weiland AJ. Madelung's deformity: treatment by osteotomy of the radius and Lauenstein procedure. *J Hand Surg [Am]* 1987;12:202–204.
38. Ranawat CS, DeFiore J, Straub LR. Madelung's deformity. An end-result study of surgical treatment. *J Bone Joint Surg Am* 1975;57:772–775.
39. Milch H. Cuff resection of the ulna for malunited Colles' fracture. *J Bone Joint Surg Am* 1941;23:311–313.
40. Langenskiöld A. Surgical treatment of partial closure of the growth plate. *J Pediatr Orthop* 1981;1:3–11.
41. Sarwark JF, MacEwen GD, Scott CI. Amyoplasia (a common form of arthrogryposis). *J Bone Joint Surg Am* 1990;72:465–469.
42. Bayne LG. Hand assessment and management of arthrogryposis multiplex congenita. *Clin Orthop* 1985;194:68–73.
43. Thompson GH, Bilenker RM. Comprehensive management of arthrogryposis multiplex congenita. *Clin Orthop* 1985;194:6–14.
44. Williams PF. Management of upper limb problems in arthrogryposis. *Clin Orthop* 1985;194:60–67.
45. Goldberg MJ. Syndromes of orthopaedic importance. In: Morrissey RT, Weinstein SL, eds. *Lovell & Winter's pediatric orthopaedics, 4th ed.* Philadelphia: Lippincott–Raven Publishers, 1996:255–304.
46. Brown LM, Robson MJ, Sharrard WJW. The pathophysiology of arthrogryposis multiplex congenita neurologica. *J Bone Joint Surg Br* 1980;62:291–296.
47. Wenner SM, Saperia BS. Proximal row carpectomy in arthrogrypotic wrist deformity. *J Hand Surg [Am]* 1987;12:523–525.
48. Russell GV, Stern PJ. The phylogeny of the wrist. *Am J Orthop* 1998;27:494–498.
49. De Smet L, Claessens A, Lefevre J, et al. Gymnast wrist: an epidemiologic survey of ulnar variance and stress changes of the radial physis in elite female gymnasts. *Am J Sports Med* 1994;22:846–850.

50. DiFiori JP, Puffer JC, Mandelbaum BR, et al. Distal radial growth plate injury and positive ulnar variance in nonelite gymnasts. *Am J Sports Med* 1997;25:763–768.
51. Roy S, Caine D, Singer KM. Stress changes of the distal radial epiphysis in young gymnasts. *Am J Sports Med* 1988;13:301–308.
52. Gabel GT. Gymnastic wrist injuries. *Clin Sports Med* 1998;3:611–621.
53. Dobyns JH, Gabel GT. Gymnast's wrist. *Hand Clin* 1990;6:493–505.
54. Caine D, Roy S, Singer KM, et al. Stress changes of the distal radial growth plate. *Am J Sports Med* 1992;20:290–298.
55. Mandelbaum BR, Bartolozzi AR, Davis CA, et al. Wrist pain syndrome in the gymnast. *Am J Sports Med* 1989;17:305–317.
56. McAuley E, Hudash G, Shields K, et al. Injuries in women's gymnastics. *Am J Sports Med* 1987;15S:S124–S131.
57. Aronen JG. Problems of the upper extremity in gymnasts. *Clin Sports Med* 1985;4:61–71.
58. Mendez AA, Bartal E, Grillot MB, et al. Compression (Salter-Harris type V) physeal fracture: an experimental model in the rat. *J Pediatr Orthop* 1992;12:29–37.
59. Pettrone FA, Ricciardelli E. Gymnastic injuries: The Virginia experience 1982–1983. *Am J Sports Med* 1987;15:59–62.
60. Weiker GG. Club gymnastics. *Clin Sports Med* 1985;4:39–43.
61. Weiker GG. Hand and wrist problems in the gymnast. *Clin Sports Med* 1992;11:189–202.
62. Markiewitz AD, Andrish JT. Hand and wrist injuries in the preadolescent athlete. *Clin Sports Med* 1992;11:203–225.
63. Oni OOA. The microvascular anatomy of the physis as revealed by osteomedullography and correlated histology. *Orthopedics* 1999;22:239–241.
64. Albanese SA, Palmer AK, Kerr DR, et al. Wrist pain and distal growth plate closure of the radius in gymnasts. *J Pediatr Orthop* 1989;9:23–28.
65. Yong-Hing K, Wedge JH, Bowen CVA. Chronic injury to the distal ulnar and radial growth plates in an adolescent gymnast. *J Bone Joint Surg Am* 1988;70:1087–1089.
66. Samuelson M, Reider B, Weiss D. Grip lock injuries to the forearm in male gymnasts. *Am J Sports Med* 1996;24:15–18.
67. Carter SR, Aldridge MJ, Fitzgerald R, et al. Stress changes of the wrist in adolescent gymnasts. *Br J Radiol* 1988;61:109–112.
68. Tolat AR, Sanderson PL, De Smet L, et al. The gymnast's wrist: Acquired positive ulnar variance following chronic epiphyseal injury. *J Hand Surg [Br]* 1992;17:678–681.
69. Beatty E, Light TR, Belsole RJ, et al. Wrist and hand skeletal injuries in children. *Hand Clin* 1990;6:723–738.
70. Greene MH, Hadied A, LaMont RL. Scaphoid fractures in children. *J Hand Surg [Am]* 1984;9:536–541.
71. Light TR. Injury to the immature carpus. *Hand Clin* 1988;4:415–424.
72. Southcott R, Rosman MA. Non-union of carpal scaphoid fractures in children. *J Bone Joint Surg Br* 1977;59:20–23.
73. DeCoster TA, Faherty S, Morris AL. Pediatric carpal fracture dislocation. *J Orthop Trauma* 1994;8:76–78.
74. Mussblicher H. Injuries of the carpal scaphoid in children. *Acta Radiol* 1961;56:361–368.
75. Mintzer C, Waters PM. Acute open reduction of a displaced scaphoid fracture in a child. *J Hand Surg [Am]* 1994;19:760–761.
76. Vahvanen V, Westerlund M. Fracture of the carpal scaphoid in children. *Acta Orthop Scand* 1980;51:909–913.
77. Gamble JG, Simmons SC. Bilateral scaphoid fractures in a child. *Clin Orthop* 1982;162:125–128.
78. Anderson WJ. Simultaneous fracture of the scaphoid and capitate in a child. *J Hand Surg [Am]* 1287;12:271–273.
79. Stother IG. A report of 3 cases of simultaneous Colles' and scaphoid fractures. *Injury* 1976;7:185–188.
80. Cook PA, Yu JS, Wiand W, et al. Suspected scaphoid fractures in skeletally immature patients: Application of MRI. *J Comput Assist Tomogr* 1997;21:511–515.
81. McCauley RGK, Schwartz AM, Leonidas JC, et al. Comparison views in extremity injury in children: An efficacy study. *Radiology* 1979;131:95–97.
82. Fisk GR. An overview of injuries of the wrist. *Clin Orthop* 1980;149:137–144.
83. Campbell RM. Operative treatment of fractures and dislocations of the hand and wrist reqgion in children. *Orthop Clin North Am* 1990;21:217–243.
84. Wilson-MacDonald J. Delayed union of the distal scaphoid in a child. *J Hand Surg [Am]* 1987;12:520–522.
85. De Boeck H, Van Wellen P, Haentjens P. Nonunion of a carpal scaphoid fracture in a child. *J Orthop Trauma* 1991;5:370–372.
86. Pick RY, Segal D. Carpal scaphoid fracture and non-union in an eight-year-old child. *J Bone Joint Surg Am* 1983;65:1188–1189.
87. Littlefield WG, Friedman RL, Urbaniak JR. Bilateral non-union of the carpal scaphoid in a child. *J Bone Joint Surg Am* 1995;77:124–126.
88. Louis DS, Calhoun TP, Garn SM, et al. Congenital bipartite scaphoid—fact or fiction? *J Bone Joint Surg Am* 1976;58:1108–1111.
89. Larson B, Light TR, Ogden JA. Fracture and ischemic necrosis of the immature scaphoid. *J Hand Surg [Am]* 1987;12:122–127.
90. Gerard FM. Post-traumatic carpal instability in a young child. *J Bone Joint Surg Am* 1980;62:131–133.
91. Letts M, Esser D. Fractures of the triquetrum in children. *J Pediatr Orthop* 1993;13:228–231.
92. Compson JP. Trans-carpal injuries associated with distal radial fractures in children: A series of three cases. *J Hand Surg [Br]* 1992;17:311–314.
93. Minami M, Yamazaki J, Chisaka N, et al. Nonunion of the capitate. *J Hand Surg [Am]* 1987;12:1089–1091.
94. Cooney WP, Linschied RL, Dobyns JH. Triangular fibrocartilage tears. *J Hand Surg [Am]* 1994;19:143–154.
95. Palmer AK. Triangular fibrocartilage complex lesion: A clssification. *J Hand Surg [Am]* 1989;14:594–606.
96. Terry CL, Waters PM. Triangular fibrocartilage injuries in pediatric and adolescent patients. *J Hand Surg [Am]* 1998;23:626–634.
97. Linschied RL, Dobyns JH. Athletic injuries of the wrist. *Clin Orthop* 1985;198:141–151.
98. Kuntz DG, Shah MA, Sotereanos DG. Traumatic triangular fibrocartilage tear in an 11-year old patient. *Orthopedics* 1999;22:253–254.
99. Tehranzadeh J, Labosky DA, Gabriele OF. Ganglion cysts and a tear of triangular fibrocartilages of both wrists in a cheerleader. *Am J Sports Med* 1983;11:357–359.
100. Schers TJ. Evaluation of chronic wrist pain. Arthroscopy superior to arthrography: Comparison of 39 patients. *Acta Orthop Scand* 1995;66:540–542.
101. Cheng JCY, Shen WY. Limb fracture pattern in different pediatric age groups: a study of 3,350 children. *J Orthop Trauma* 1993;7:15–22.
102. Crawford AH. Pitfalls and complications of fractures of the distal radius and ulna in childhood. *Hand Clin* 1988;4:403–413.
103. Dicke TE, Nunley JA. Distal forearm fractures in children. *Orthop Clin North Am* 1993;24:333–340.
104. Golz RJ, Grogan DP, Greene TL, et al. Distal ulnar physeal injury. *J Pediatr Orthop* 1991;11:318–326.
105. Holmes JR, Louis DS. Entrapment of pronator quadratus in pediatric distal radius fractures: Recognition and treatment. *J Pediatr Orthop* 1994;14:498–500.
106. Roy DR. Completely displaced distal radius fractures with intact ulnas in children. *Orthopedics* 1989;12:1089–1092.

107. Bailey DA, Wedge JH, McCulloch RG, et al. Epidemiology of fractures of the distal end of the radius in children as associated with growth. *J Bone Joint Surg Am* 1989;71:1225–1231.
108. Guero S. Fractures and epiphyseal fracture-separation of the distal bones of the forearm in children. In: Saffar P, Cooney WP, eds. *Fractures of the distal radius.* London: Martin-Dunitz, 1995.
109. Boyden EM, Peterson HA. Partial premature closure of the distal radial physis associated with Kirschner wire fixation. *Orthopedics* 1991;14:585–588.
110. Wilkins KE, O'Brien E. Fractures of the distal radius and ulna. In: Rockwood CA, Wilkins KE, Beaty JH, eds. *Fractures in children, 4th ed.* Philadelphia: Lippincott–Raven Publishers, 1996: 451–514.
111. Simmons BP, Stirrat CR. Treatment of traumatic arthritis in children. *Hand Clin* 1987;3:611–625.
112. Manoli A. Irreducible fracture-separation of the distal radial epiphysis. *J Bone Joint Surg Am* 1982;64:1095–1096.
113. Evans DL, Stauber M, Frykman GK. Irreducible epiphyseal plate fracture of the distal ulna due to interposition of the extensor carpi ulnaris tendon. *Clin Orthop* 1990;251:162–165.
114. Rang M. *Children's fractures, 2nd ed.* Philadelphia: JB Lippincott, 1983.
115. Nelson OA, Buchanan JR, Harrison CS. Distal ulnar growth arrest. *J Hand Surg [Am]* 1984;9:164–171.
116. Burgess RC. Use of the Ilizarov technique to treat radial nonunion with physeal arrest. *J Hand Surg [Am]* 1991;16: 928–931.
117. Giddins GEB, Shaw DG. Lunate subluxation associated with a Salter-Harris type 2 fracture of the distal radius. *J Hand Surg [Br]* 1994;19:193–194.
118. Creasman C, Zaleske DJ, Ehrlich MG. Analyzing forearm fractures in children. *Clin Orthop* 1984;188:40–53.
119. Letts M, Rowhani N. Galeazzi-equivalent injuries of the wrist in children. *J Pediatr Orthop* 1993;13:561–566.
120. Walsh HPJ, McLaren CAN, Owen R. Galeazzi fractures in children. *J Bone Joint Surg Br* 1987;69:730–733.
121. Garcia-Elias M, Dobyns JH. Dorsal and palmar dislocations of the distal radioulnar joint. In: Cooney WP, Linscheid RL, Dobyns JH, eds. *The wrist.* St Louis: CV Mosby, 1998.
122. Nelson CL, Sawmiller S, Phalen GS. Ganglions of the wrist and hand. *J Bone Joint Surg Am* 1972;54:1459–1464.
123. Crawford GP, Taleisnik J. Rotary subluxation of the scaphoid after excision of dorsal carpal ganglion and wrist manipulation—a case report. *J Hand Surg [Am]* 1983;8:921–924.
124. Rosson JW, Walker G. The natural history of ganglia in children. *J Bone Joint Surg Br* 1989;71:707–708.
125. Peterson HA. Multiple hereditary osteochondromata. *Clin Orthop* 1989;239:222–230.
126. Azouz EM, Babyn PS, Tuuha SE, et al. MRI of the abnormal pediatric hand and wrist with plain film correlation. *J Comput Assist Tomogr* 1998;22:252–261.
127. Ho PK, Weiland AJ, McClinton MA, et al. Aneurysms of the upper extremity. *J Hand Surg [Am]* 1987;12:39–46.
128. Newmeyer WL. Vascular disorders. In: Green DP, ed. *Operative hand surgery, 3rd ed.* New York: Churchill-Livingstone, 1993: 2251–2308.
129. Palmiere TJ. Vascular tumors of the hand and forearm. *Hand Clin* 1987;3:225–240.
130. Simeonov LG. A false aneurysm in the hand of a child. *J Hand Surg [Br]* 1998;4:555–556.
131. Yetman RJ, Black CT. Traumatic false aneurysms of peripheral arteries in children. *South Med J* 1992;85:665–666.
132. Rieck B, Mailander P, Kuske M, et al. True aneurysms of the palmar arch of the hand: a report of two cases. *Microsurgery* 1996;17:102–105.
133. Sherry DD, Mosca VS. Juvenile rheumatoid arthritis and seronegative spondyloarthropathies. In: Morrissy RT, Weinstein SL, eds. *Lovell & Winter's pediatric orthopaedics, 4th ed.* Philadelphia: Lippincott–Raven Publishers, 1996:393–422.
134. Cassidy JT. Juvenile rheumatoid arthritis. In: Kelley WN, Ruddy S, Harris ED, et al, eds. *Textbook of rheumatology, 5th ed.* Philadelphia: WB Saunders, 1997:1207–1224.
135. Lovell DJ. Juvenile rheumatoid arthritis and juvenile spondyloarthropathies. In: Klippel JH, ed. *Primer on the rheumatic diseases, 11th ed.* Atlanta: Arthritis Foundation, 1997:393–398.
136. Simmons BP, Nutting JT. Juvenile rheumatoid arthritis. *Hand Clin* 1989;5:157–168.
137. Feinstein KA, Poznanski AK. Evaluation of joint disease in the pediatric hand. *Hand Clin* 1991;7:167–182.
138. Ruby LK. Other arthritides. In: *Hand surgery update.* 1994: 197–205.
139. Poznanski AK, Hernandez RJ, Guire KE, et al. Carpal length in children—a useful measurement in the diagnosis of rheumatoid arthritis and some congenital malformation syndromes. *Radiology* 1978;129:661–668.

12

CARPAL BONE FRACTURES (EXCLUDING SCAPHOID FRACTURES)

MARC GARCIA-ELIAS

Despite prognostic uncertainty often similar to that of scaphoid fractures, fractures of the other carpal bones tend to be underestimated both in the literature and in clinical practice (1–7). Indeed, the exponential increase of information generated regarding scaphoid injuries in recent years has not been accompanied by a proportional increase in awareness of the potential adverse effects that other carpal fractures may have, especially if inadequately treated. Certainly, some carpal fractures may be as challenging as scaphoid fractures with regard to their diagnosis, treatment, and rates of complications.

Despite their obvious differences, most carpal bone fractures share a number of features.

1. They commonly affect young individuals who place high functional demands on their wrists (8–10).
2. Because of lack of awareness and suboptimal clinical and/or radiographic examination, these injuries are frequently missed at presentation (11–14) and, thus, are often incorrectly treated. As a consequence, a substantial functional impairment may result.
3. Carpal fractures involve small, short, and irregularly vascularized bones, which complicates their surgical reduction while potentially damaging their blood supply (15, 16).
4. Displaced carpal fractures often affect, and sometimes severely disrupt, the congruency of the articular surfaces. The risk of posttraumatic degenerative disease is significantly increased if these fractures are not anatomically reduced (17,18).
5. When unstable, most carpal fractures appear associated with variable adjacent ligamentous injury, often the source of a secondary intracarpal instability that must be recognized and properly treated (19).
6. Carpal bones share a close relationship with important tendinous and neurovascular structures. Consequently, the incidence of secondary entrapment neuropathies

(20–23) or tendon ruptures caused by friction over unreduced bone fragments (24,25) should not be underestimated.

MECHANISMS OF INJURY

Most carpal fractures are the consequence of a fall on the outstretched hand. If the distal radial metaphysis resists the tensile stress from hyperextension, the energy may be focused on the distal carpal row, which is suddenly forced into abnormal extension and variable degrees of radial or ulnar deviation. This creates strong extension moments on the proximal row bones via the palmar midcarpal crossing ligaments. Such ligaments may either disrupt or, more frequently, result in substantial shear stress within the area around the lunate, known as the "greater arc," and result in a fracture (26). In most cases such fractures are initiated palmarly under tensile stress; dorsal cortical comminution occurs from subsequent shear stress.

In addition to hyperextension, several other mechanisms may be responsible for producing carpal bone fractures (27). These may be direct or indirect mechanisms (Fig. 12.1). An example of the former is a direct impact of an unyielding object on the carpal area, causing an open fracture, usually associated with variable soft tissue injury (28). Fractures that occur as a result of an indirect force seldom are open injuries, although they may appear associated with substantial soft tissue derangement (19–25). Tensile forces are involved in most linear fractures, whereas comminution is usually the result of compressive and shear forces. Ligament avulsions occur frequently, especially from the dorsal (29–32) and palmar (19) aspects of the triquetrum, where important ligament connections exist.

INCIDENCE

According to a recent statistical review of 1,000 consecutive hand fractures recorded over a 10-month period in the city

---

M. Garcia-Elias: Hand and Upper Extremity Surgery, Institut Kaplan, 08022 Barcelona, Spain.

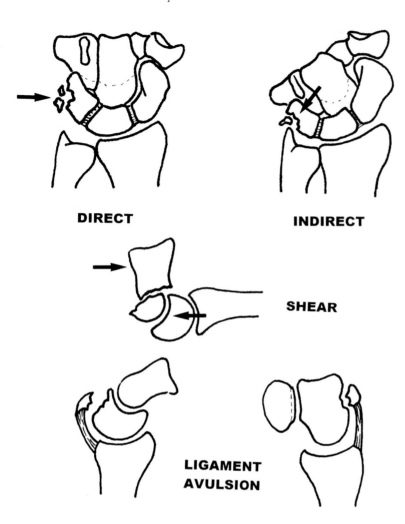

FIGURE 12.1. Mechanisms of production of carpal fractures.

of Bergen, Norway (population 215,000), 183 (18%) involved the carpal bones, the scaphoid being most commonly fractured (58%) (33). A similar incidence of carpal bone fractures has been recorded by Larsen et al. (34). Based on this, the relative incidence of carpal bone fractures, excluding the scaphoid, is approximately 1.1% of all fractures; their estimated annual incidence is 36 per 100,000 inhabitants per year.

The relative incidence of each carpal bone fracture still remains controversial. Some authors contend that lunate fractures are the second most frequent fracture (1,14), but others state that most of them are not true traumatic injuries but the result of a preexisting necrotic process (2–7). Obviously, the first authors tend to include cases of Kienböck's disease in their series.

The frequency of triquetrum fractures has also been controversial. The series of carpal fractures published by Snodgrass (1) and by Auffray (35) demonstrated this point (Table 12.1). Both reported 144 scaphoid fractures. Snodgrass, however, recognized only seven triquetrum fractures, while Auffray reported 72 fractures. In a personal series of 10,400 consecutive wrist injuries seen in the emergency room over a 10-year period (36), we found that, excluding the scaphoid, triquetrum fractures are by far the most common fracture, followed in incidence by the trapezium. Trapezoid fractures are the least common. A similar incidence has been published by Amadio and Taleisnik (37).

TABLE 12.1. RELATIVE INCIDENCE OF CARPAL BONE FRACTURES ACCORDING TO DIFFERENT AUTHORS

Source	S[a]	L	Tq	P	Tr	Td	C	H	Total
Snodgrass (1)	144	11	7	1	3	1	2	1	170
Franz (60)	81	13	6	4	8	1	6	3	122
Borgeskov (2)	102	2	29	1	5	1	2	1	143
Auffray (35)	144	10	72	1	10	—	4	4	245
Dunn (3)	59	1	5	1	2	—	—	4	72
Garcia-Elias (36)	153	2	64	5	15	1	5	4	249

[a]S, scaphoid; L, lunate; Tq, triquetrum; P, pisiform; Tr, trapezium; Td, trapezoid; C, capitate; H, hamate.

FRACTURES OF THE TRAPEZIUM

Trapezium fractures were first described by Kindl in 1910 (38), and the largest series of patients was reported by Pointu et al. (27), who reviewed 34 cases. Trapezial fractures are the third most common type of carpal bone fracture, with an estimated incidence of 6% with respect to the total number of carpal bone fractures (36). Isolated trapezial fractures occur infrequently (39,40). They commonly are associated with fractures of other bones, typically the first metacarpal or the radius (41,42). According to Walker et al. (43), five different patterns of fracture exist: (a) vertical transarticular, (b) horizontal, (c) fracture of the dorsoradial tuberosity, (d) fracture of the anteromedial ridge, and (e) comminuted fracture. The most common pattern is the vertical transarticular fracture (39,40,42,44) (Fig. 12.2), followed by fracture of the dorsolateral tuberosity.

According to Manon's hypothesis (45), dorsoradial trapezium fractures could be the result of vertical shear, with the trapezium being caught by the metacarpal and the tip of the radial styloid. In 1963, Monsche [cited by Pointu et al. (27)] theorized that these fractures could be produced by a commissural shearing force applied to the first web space by an object held within the hand (e.g., the handlebar of a motorcycle when colliding head-on with an oncoming car). Depending on the angle of shear, a fracture of the trapezium, a Bennett's fracture of the thumb metacarpal base, or both may occur. This explanation may be substantiated by the relative frequency with which both a Bennett's fracture and a trapezium fracture appear associated (41,42) and also by the fact that most body fractures have a vertical orientation, certainly the type of fracture one would expect from a vertical shear force (44).

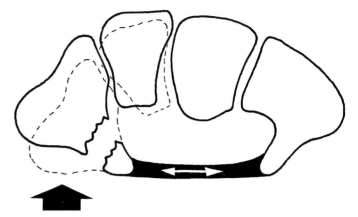

FIGURE 12.3. Trapezial ridge fractures may be the result of a dorsally directed force into the trapezium *(black arrow)*, producing excessive traction of the transverse carpal ligament *(white arrows)* with a subsequent avulsion fracture.

The trapezial ridge is a longitudinal palmar projection of the bone located on the palmar and medial corner of the trapezium and serves as origin of the superficial fibers of the transverse carpal ligament. Although often unrecognized, fractures of the trapezial ridge are probably more common than previously thought (46,47). They may be secondary to direct injury during a fall on the outstretched hand or the result of an avulsion by the transverse carpal ligament produced by a dorsopalmar crush mechanism (48,49) (Fig. 12.3). In the latter case, there is flattening of the carpal concavity, thus inducing either a trapezial ridge avulsion, a hook of the hamate fracture, or a combination of both.

According to Palmer (46), two types of trapezial ridge fractures exist: type I, fractures through the base of the ridge; and type II, avulsion fractures of the tip of the ridge. Type I fractures tend to heal if properly immobilized. Type II fractures, by contrast, often result in painful nonunions that may eventually require excision of the fragments.

FRACTURES OF THE TRAPEZOID

In the transverse plane, the trapezoid has a wedge-shaped configuration, widest dorsally, perfectly adapted to its role as the cornerstone of the carpal arch. Strong ligaments tightly bind the trapezoid to the adjacent bones. As a result of its highly guarded position, very seldom does an isolated fracture of the trapezoid occur, unless produced by a direct impact (50,51). In fact, most cases reported were caused by an indirect mechanism consisting of an axial or bending force transmitted by the second metacarpal and resulting in

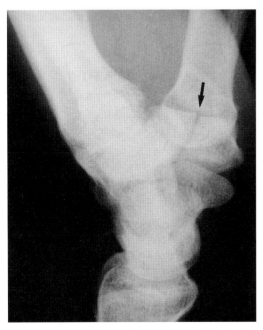

FIGURE 12.2. Vertical transarticular fracture of the body of the trapezium *(arrow)*. Both the trapeziometacarpal and the scaphotrapezial joints are involved. An axially directed force from the thumb metacarpal into the trapezium often produces this injury. (From Garcia-Elias M, Henriquez A, Rossignani P, et al. Bennett's fracture combined with fracture of the trapezium. *J Hand Surg [Br]* 1993;18:523–526, with permission.)

a transtrapezoid fracture-dislocation (52). Probably fewer than 20 isolated cases have been reported in the literature.

FRACTURES OF THE CAPITATE

Fractures of the capitate occur infrequently, accounting for fewer than 2% of all carpal bone fractures (36,37,53,54). The first case was published by Harrigan in 1908 (55). In an extensive review of the literature in 1962, Adler and Shaftan (53) found 72 previously published cases and added 12 of their own. Since then, probably no more than 100 cases have been reported, most being transverse fractures of the neck of the capitate associated with a scaphoid fracture, the so-called "scaphocapitate fracture syndrome" popularized by Fenton in 1956 (56–59).

Four major patterns of fracture have been observed: (a) transverse fracture of the proximal pole, (b) transverse fracture of the body of the capitate, (c) verticofrontal fracture, and (d) parasagittal fracture (36). The second fracture type has been the most frequently reported (56–59). In most cases, transverse fractures of the body present with complete separation of the proximal fragment, sometimes with rotation of up to 180° with the rough surface of the fracture facing proximally (58). The pathomechanics of this peculiar type of fracture-dislocation was investigated in cadaver specimens by Stein and Siegel in 1969 (57). According to these authors, this fracture is the consequence of wrist hyperextension, with the capitate being caught against the dorsal rim of the radius. Proximal migration of the distal portion of capitate may induce a rotation of the proximal fragment as the hand is realigned relative to the forearm, as earlier postulated by Fenton in 1956 (56) (Fig. 12.4). This proximal fragment may be of different sizes and may appear displaced in different directions, representing either an incomplete form or a self-reduced form of the perilunate pattern of the injury (58,59). If poorly reduced and stabilized, transverse fractures of the capitate easily evolve into a nonunion, the proximal pole becoming sclerotic, presumably from osteonecrosis; although it seldom undergoes fragmentation, there is always shortening of the bone (Fig. 12.5). In these cases, if proximal migration of the distal row occurs, progressive overloading and dysfunction at both the scaphotrapezialtrapezoidal and triquetrohamate joints are likely (54). In such circumstances, a bone graft to restore both capitate length and proper midcarpal function is necessary (7).

Magnetic resonance imaging (MRI) is rarely needed for diagnosis of carpal bone fractures. Proximal pole fractures of the capitate would be an exception, as MRI may provide evidence of the vascular and healing status of the capitate head.

Aside from fractures of the neck of the capitate, wrist hyperextension may also induce a coronal fracture of the dorsum of the body of the capitate (52). In such fractures, a combination of a lever-type force applied on the palm and an axial load transmitted along the shaft of the third metacarpal may result in increasing joint compressive force

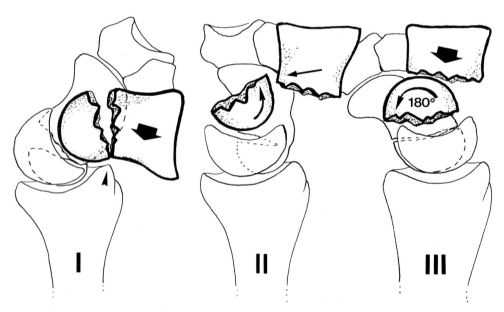

FIGURE 12.4. Mechanism of production of fractures of the neck of the capitate and their subsequent rotational displacement. *I,* The neck of the capitate, once the scaphoid has fractured, may impact on the dorsal ridge of the radius and fracture as a result of tensile forces on its palmar aspect. *II,* When the wrist recovers its neutral position, shortening of the carpus prevents reduction of the fracture. *III,* As the capitate regains its normal alignment with respect to the radius, it exerts a flexion moment to the proximal pole that may result in complete rotation, with the fracture site facing the distal aspect of the lunate.

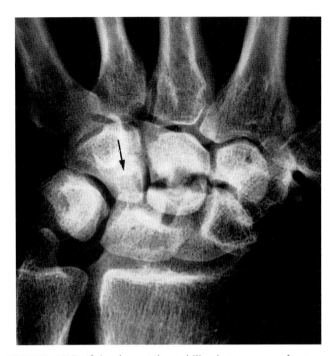

FIGURE 12.5. If inadequately stabilized, transverse fractures may remain ununited, with corresponding proximal migration of the entire distal carpal row. Note the degenerative changes within the proximal pole of the hamate *(arrow)*, the result of lunohamate abutment. Also note the rotatory subluxation of the scaphoid as a result of the overload generated at the scapho-trapeziotrapezoidal joint.

on the dorsal aspect of the articular surface. Cyclists appear to be particularly prone to this type of injury. In such cases, a posteroanterior (PA) radiograph does not show the fracture but just an abnormal location of the bases of the central metacarpals, and a lateral view only demonstrates increased depth of the carpus. Lateral (parasagittal) tomograms or computed tomography (CT) scans are both ideal methods to evaluate the morphology, articular congruency, and amount of displacement of these injuries (52) (Fig. 12.6).

FRACTURES OF THE HAMATE

According to Franz (60), fractures of the hamate were first discussed by Rutherford in 1891 on the occasion of an incidental finding during a necropsy. Since then, no more than 100 cases have been reported (36,60–63). Different patterns of fracture exist and can be divided into two major groups: those affecting the hook of the hamate and those affecting the body of the hamate (Fig. 12.7).

Fractures of the Hook of the Hamate (Hamulus Hamati)

Fractures of the hook are common injuries in stick-handling sports, usually the result of a direct blow produced by the end of a golf club (when missing a shot), a baseball bat, or a tennis racquet (stress fractures caused by repetitive contusions to

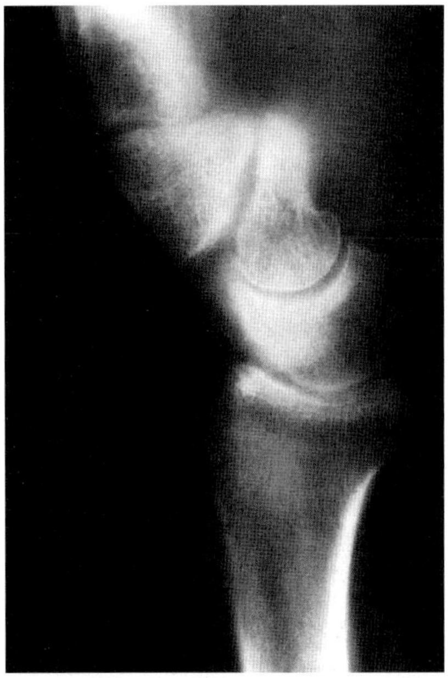

FIGURE 12.6. Parasagittal tomogram of a transcapitate carpometacarpal dislocation. (From Garcia-Elias M, Bishop AT, Dobyns JH, et al. Transcarpal carpometacarpal dislocations, excluding the thumb. *J Hand Surg [Am]* 1990;15:531–540, with permission.)

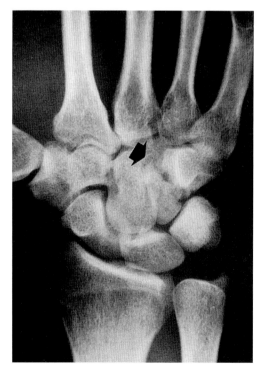

FIGURE 12.7. Sagittal oblique fracture of the body of the hamate *(arrow)*, the result of a dorsopalmar crush injury.

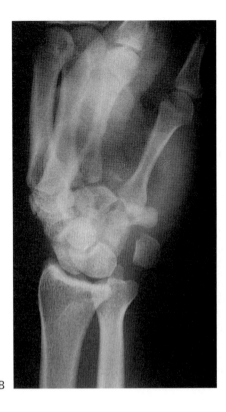
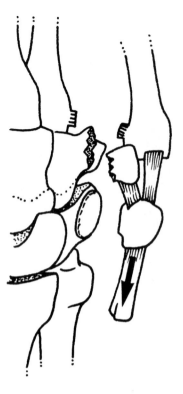

FIGURE 12.8. Avulsion fracture of the hook of the hamate associated with a palmar dislocation of the fifth metacarpal and proximal dislocation of the pisiform **(A)**, the result of violent contraction of the flexor carpi ulnaris muscle **(B)**. (From Garcia-Elias M, Rossignani P, Cots M. Combined fracture of the hook of the hamate and palmar dislocation of the fifth carpometacarpal joint. *J Hand Surg [Br]* 1996;21:446–450, with permission.)

the hook) or any other similar object (64–67). Indirect avulsions are also possible. They may be the consequence of a violent contraction of the flexor carpi ulnaris muscle, with concomitant proximal dislocation of the pisiform and avulsion of the pisohamate ligament (68) (Fig. 12.8), or the result of severe traction of the tranverse carpal arch in crush injuries with flattening of the transverse carpal arch (47,49).

Patients with fractures of the hook of the hamate may present with weakness and pain over the base of the hypothenar eminence that is increased during forceful grasping of an object (65–67). The injury may easily be missed at presentation unless clinically suspected and investigated with special views, such as the carpal tunnel view or the oblique semisupinated projection (11–13). A fracture of the hook of the hamate should be suspected when tenderness is elicited by deep palpation over the tip of the hook in the palm (just distal and radial to the pisiform), and especially if there is increased pain at the base of the hypothenar area when flexing the little finger against resistance despite normal x-rays. In such cases a transverse CT scan is recommended (67) (Fig. 12.9). Indeed, tomograms are the best way to evaluate the extent and nature of these injuries.

According to Milch (61), there are three different types of fractures of the hook of the hamate: avulsion fractures of the tip of the hook, fractures through the base, and fractures through the so-called waist of the hook.

The hamate bone has three arterial systems ensuring its blood supply: two groups of vascular pedicles (palmar and dorsal) enter the bone along the midcarpal capsular attachments and form an intraosseous arterial network that supplies the body of the hamate, and one group of small nutrient arteries, branching from the ulnar artery at the level of Guyon's canal, supplies the hook of the hamate (69,70). Few anastomoses exist between the two systems. As a consequence, there is a poorly vascularized area adjacent to the base of the hook (the so-called "waist of the hook"), with a relatively greater risk of developing a nonunion if a fracture at this level is not properly immobilized (65–71) (Fig. 12.10).

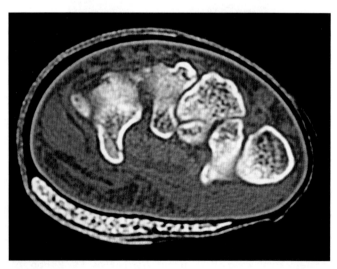

FIGURE 12.9. Transverse computed tomography scan of the carpal tunnel, demonstrating an undisplaced fracture of the hook of the hamate.

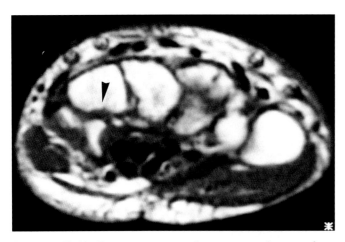

FIGURE 12.10. Transverse magnetic resonance image of an ununited fracture of the hook of the hamate *(arrowhead)*, obtained 8 months after a direct blow to the hypothenar area. The fracture was missed at presentation and left untreated. Despite the nonunion, good vascularity of the hook was present; it was grafted, stabilized with K-wires, and healed uneventfully.

Although it was initially thought that hook excision in fresh or ununited fractures provided quick recovery of painless function (64,65,71), a case against such a procedure has recently been made by Watson and Rogers (72). Indeed, the hook of the hamate constitutes the medial wall of the carpal concavity, acting as an important pulley that enhances the action of the flexor tendons of the little finger by increasing its moment arm. Therefore, excision of the hook should not be regarded as a harmless procedure.

As demonstrated by different authors, despite poor vascularization, if properly immobilized, fresh undisplaced fractures of the waist of the hook may consolidate (7,73,74). Nonunions are frequent when not correctly diagnosed at presentation (11,12). Published complications of unstable nonunions include ulnar neuropathy (20,21,23), median nerve entrapment (22) and flexor tendon ruptures (24,25). To prevent such complications, preservation of the hook through bone grafting and internal fixation is recommended (72). Usually a palmar approach to the canal tunnel, with exploration of the Guyon's canal, is necessary to fix these types of fractures (68,72). A medial approach can also be used (75).

Fractures of the Body of the Hamate

Although less common than the fractures of the hook, fractures of the body of the hamate are not uncommon injuries. They can be classified into four major groups: (a) proximal pole fractures, (b) fractures of the medial tuberosity, (c) sagittal oblique fractures, and (d) dorsal coronal fractures (36).

Small osteochondral fractures of the proximal pole of the hamate are not uncommon in severe fracture-dislocations of the wrist and are likely the result of shear forces during the dislocation process (6,26). These small fragments of bone may remain unnoticed and act as loose intraarticular bodies that may be revealed through the arthroscope.

Fractures of the medial tuberosity of the hamate, at the base of the fifth metacarpal, are usually the result of a direct blow on the ulnar border of the wrist (62).

Most sagittal oblique fractures are produced by a dorsopalmar crush mechanism (63,76) (Fig. 12.7). High-energy trauma with severe flattening of the transverse carpal arch may result in a fracture of the hamate bone, which typically has an oblique direction from distal-radial to proximal-ulnar, just proximal to the base of the hook. Injury to the ulnar nerve as a complication of this type of fracture has been reported by Howard (20).

Coronal fractures of the dorsal aspect of the hamate are more difficult to diagnose (52,77–80). They represent a somewhat similar injury as discussed above for the capitate and usually are associated with a variable degree of dorsal subluxation of the base of the fourth and/or fifth metacarpals. This type of fracture is often the result of an axial force transmitted through the metacarpal bone, not infrequently the result of a fist fight. In these cases, a PA view of the wrist often shows only an overlapping of the articular surfaces indicating a fifth carpometacarpal (CMC) dislocation (79). A sagittal tomogram, however, demonstrates dorsal displacement of the metacarpal together with a fragment of the hamate. These injuries are also called transcarpal carpometacarpal dislocations, and those affecting the hamate are the most frequently reported (52).

FRACTURES OF THE LUNATE

Fractures of the lunate are controversial. Some authors defend their relative frequency (1,14,60,81), but others state that most fractures of the lunate are probably pathologic fractures, the result of repetitive trauma on a weakened, osteonecrotic bone in early stages of Kienböck's disease (82, 83) (Fig. 12.11). Fresh traumatic fractures, however, do exist and in most series account for about 1% of all carpal fractures (2,3,36,81,84).

Teisen and Hjarbaek (83) proposed a classification of fresh lunate fractures into five groups: (a) frontal fractures of the palmar pole with involvement of the palmar nutrient arteries, (b) osteochondral fractures of the proximal articular surface without substantial damage to the nutrient vessels, (c) frontal fractures of the dorsal pole, (d) transverse (horizontal) fractures of the body, and (e) transarticular frontal fractures of the body of the lunate. The latter is probably the most frequently reported.

Although often misdiagnosed as lunate fractures, most dorsal chip fractures of the carpus correspond to avulsions or shear fractures of the dorsal ridge of the triquetrum (30–32). Small avulsions of the dorsal ridge of the lunate, however, may occur, usually as a result of shear force by the capitate in perilunate dislocations. Also

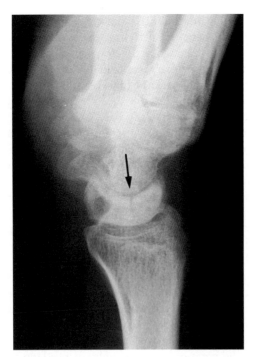

FIGURE 12.11. Vertical transarticular fracture of the lunate without a previous traumatic event *(arrow)*. These types of injuries are almost always the result of the weakening effects of Kienböck's disease.

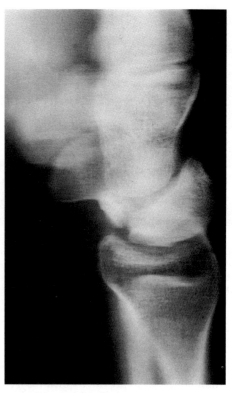

FIGURE 12.12. Parasagittal tomogram of a fracture of the palmar pole of the lunate, with rotatory subluxation of the body of the lunate into flexion. Because of its intrinsic instability, these fractures always need to be surgically reduced and stabilized with a compression screw.

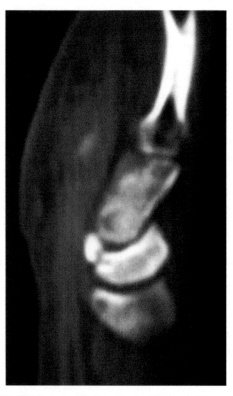

FIGURE 12.13. Parasagittal computed tomography scan of an ununited fracture of the palmar pole of the lunate.

relatively frequent are small avulsion fractures of the scapholunate ligament off the lunate in acute rotatory subluxation of the scaphoid. Although distal pole fractures are relatively benign injuries, avulsions of the dorsal scapholunate ligament need to be addressed surgically in order to reattach the ligament and prevent further destabilization (83).

Frontal, transarticular fractures are probably the result of an extension injury to the wrist, with the palmar pole being avulsed by the short radiolunate ligament as the hyperextended capitate is axially loading the dorsal portion of the bone towards extension. Once unconstrained by the palmar ligaments, the dorsal fragment tends to shift dorsally and ulnarly, while the capitate, as a wedge, promotes separation of the two fragments, thus increasing the chances for an unstable nonunion to develop (7,85,86) (Fig. 12.12). If undisplaced, these fractures are easily missed at presentation, as they are difficult to see in standard lateral projections. When they are suspected, tomograms are recommended (Fig. 12.13). Failure to heal these injuries can lead to chronic palmar subluxation of the capitate, with resultant arthrosis.

Although frequently occurring as isolated injuries, frontal fractures of the lunate may also be seen with high-energy global carpal dislocation, usually a palmar perilunate dislocation (85). Certainly, open internal fixation is recommended in such instances, both to decrease the risk of wrist instability and to minimize the chances of developing osteonecrosis (85,86).

Horizontal fractures involving separation of the proximal articular surface from the body of the lunate are usually the result of subchondral necrosis in Kienböck's disease. They typically appear in the form of a detached osteocartilaginous fragment, radiologically demonstrated by a "crescent line," parallel to the proximal outline of the bone (14). In rare occasions, a horizontal shear stress may induce a radiocarpal fracture-dislocation, including a displaced transverse fracture of the lunate (87,88).

FRACTURES OF THE TRIQUETRUM

If we exclude scaphoid fractures, fractures of the triquetrum are by far the most common carpal injuries, accounting for almost one-fourth of all carpal fractures (36,37). As pointed out by Bartone and Grieco (89), the reason for some old series showing a much lower incidence (1,2) can probably be explained by the fact that dorsal chip fractures were long believed not to be avulsions of the dorsal ridge of the triquetrum, but dorsal pole fractures of the lunate (Fig. 12.14).

According to Auffray (35), the first reported triquetrum fracture was published in 1904 by Wittek. Since then, numerous papers have been published, not only case reports of isolated injuries (90,91,92–94) but also a few series including all types of fractures (36,89,95) as well as specific analyses of the pathomechanics of the dorsal chip fractures (19,29–32).

Fractures of the triquetrum can be divided into two major groups: chip fractures of the dorsal rim and fractures through the body of the triquetrum. The latter group may be subdivided into five categories: (a) fractures of the medial tuberosity, (b) sagittal fractures, (c) transverse fractures of the proximal pole, (d) transverse fractures of the body, and (e) comminuted fractures.

Isolated fractures of the body of the triquetrum are rare injuries, the most common being the ones produced by a direct blow to the ulnar border of the wrist causing a medial tuberosity fracture, not infrequently involving the palmar articular surface of the triquetrum. Sagittal fractures are commonly associated with axial dislocations, the result of a severe dorsopalmar crush mechanism involving flattening of the transverse carpal arch (76,94) (Fig. 12.15). Small fractures of the proximal pole are frequently associated with perilunate dislocations (83). Indeed, such small avulsion fractures are to be regarded as a sign of detachment of the triquetral insertion of the palmar lunotriquetral ligaments, thus carrying a much worse prognosis than just an isolated chip fracture, as emphasized by Smith and Murray. (19). Transverse fractures affecting the body of the triquetrum also appear to be connected to other carpal injuries, commonly scaphoid fractures, certainly the result of a transverse shear stress from a medial to lateral force, the proximal pole of the scaphoid being protected by the radial styloid process (36).

Chip fractures of the dorsal ridge of the triquetrum are quite frequent injuries. When totally displaced, these fractures represent a partial or total detachment of the dorsal radiotriquetral ligament, and this, unless properly treated, may result

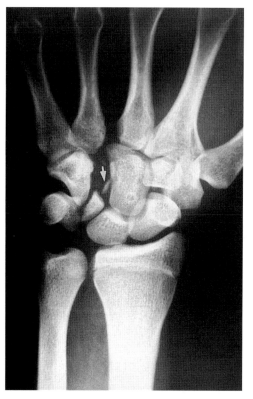

FIGURE 12.15. Sagittal fractures of both the triquetrum and the proximal pole of the hamate (arrow) in the context of an axial–ulnar dislocation of the carpus. These injuries involve a transverse dissociation of the carpus with flattening of the transverse carpal arch. The entire ulnar column becomes unstable and displaces in a proximal and ulnar direction.

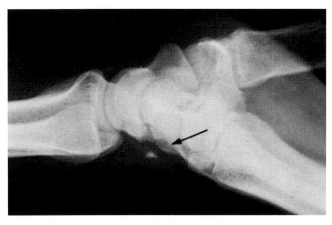

FIGURE 12.14. Chip fracture of the dorsum of the triquetrum (arrow).

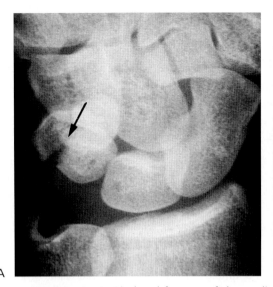
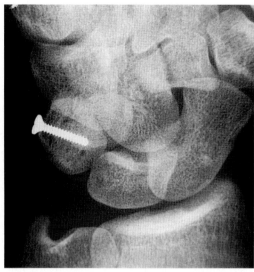

FIGURE 12.16. Displaced fracture of the medial tuberosity of the triquetrum *(arrow)*. **A:** This portion of bone contains important ligamentous attachments. **B:** In this case, open reduction and lag screw fixation were used to avoid destabilizing these ligaments.

in chronic pain as well as persistent instability, as demonstrated by Auffray and others (19,29–32). Chip fractures of the triquetrum have long been assumed to be avulsion fractures. However, the only mechanism by which such an avulsion could occur would be a fall on a hyperflexed and radially deviated wrist. Yet, most of them appear after a hyperextension and ulnar deviation injury. Levy et al. (30) and Garcia-Elias (31) have suggested these fractures to be the result of the chisel action of the tip of the ulnar styloid process impacting on the dorsum of the triquetrum, thus producing a compression fracture of the dorsal ridge of this bone. Höcher and Menschik (32), by contrast, believe that these fractures result from impaction of the hamate against the dorsal rim of the triquetrum during forceful hyperextension. Whatever the mechanism, the fact is that such apparently benign injuries may result in prolonged ulnar-sided tenderness unless adequately recognized and treated with cast immobilization. Only in selected cases might surgery be indicated (Fig. 12.16).

Unlike body fractures, which rarely develop a nonunion (96), dorsal chip fractures may remain ununited and cause permanent tenderness because of instability of the medial insertion of both the dorsal radiotriquetral and dorsal intercarpal ligaments.

FRACTURES OF THE PISIFORM

Although frequently regarded as a true proximal carpal row bone, the pisiform functions as a sesamoid bone within the sheath of the flexor carpi ulnaris (FCU). Distally it is attached to different structures including the flexor and extensor retinaculum, the abductor digiti minimi muscle,

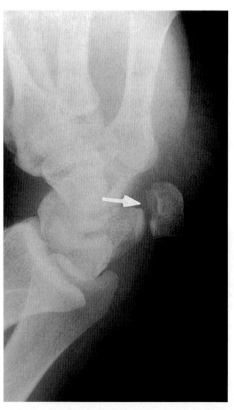

FIGURE 12.17. Pisotriquetral joint impaction fracture *(arrow)*. This type of injury does not violate the continuity of the distal insertions of the flexor carpi ulnaris tendon but creates substantial joint incongruency, resulting in progressive degeneration that eventually will require a pisiformectomy.

and the pisihamatum and pisimetacarpicum ligaments (97, 98). Fracture of the pisiform, therefore, may affect, and sometimes severely disrupt, the distal continuity of the FCU distal tendinous attachments.

Pisiform fractures are not as infrequent as previously thought (99–101) and account for 2% of all fractures of the carpal bones. Alsberg (102) described the first case in 1908. Since then, about 200 cases have been published, most of them presented as a case report, as if they were rare injuries, when they are not (98–104).

Four different types of pisiform fracture exist: (a) transverse, (b) parasagittal, (c) comminuted, and (d) pisotriquetral impaction fractures (Fig. 12.17). Transverse fractures are the most common, probably the result of a combined sudden contraction of the FCU while the pisiform is blocked by the triquetrum against the floor during a fall on the palm. When these fractures are severely displaced, the continuity of the flexor carpi ulnaris tendon may be disrupted, thus making for substantially altered tendon function (101,103). By contrast, longitudinal fractures, usually affecting the ulnar rim of the pisiform, do not involve the continuity of the FCU and thus carry a much more benign prognosis (Fig. 12.18). Comminuted fractures, usually the result of a direct blow at the base of the hypothenar area, may be associated with substantial soft tissue injury, including ulnar neurovascular injuries. In all types, a residual pisotriquetral incongruity may result, yielding an increased risk of developing degenerative arthritis at this level. In such instances, enucleation of the pisiform, with reconstruction of the continuity of the FCU tendon, is the method of choice (104–106).

TREATMENT OF CARPAL BONE FRACTURES

As already stated, most carpal bone fractures share several common features such that a unified concept for treatment can be recommended.

For succesful treatment and optimal results, diagnosis must be accomplished as early as possible following injury. Knowledge of carpal bone topography will help in discovering localized areas of tenderness through pinpoint palpation of all protruding portions of bones. With this, a high level of suspicion will be achieved, and adequate radiologic tests requested. Indeed, the best treatment of complications is prevention, and this is possible only through an early and thorough understanding of the nature and extent of the injury.

The treatment of choice for undisplaced, relatively stable fractures is cast immobilization for 4 to 6 weeks, except for vascular compromised areas (head of the capitate, waist of the hook of the hamate), in which open reduction and solid internal fixation may be recommended. If there is no substantial damage to the articular surfaces, no late degenerative arthrosis is anticipated.

If the fracture is unstable and/or severely affects joint congruity, open anatomic restoration of the articular surfaces, ligament repair when feasible, and stable fixation may be indicated. Lag screw fixation is advocated when the insertion point does not involve any articular surface, as it provides excellent compression of the fracture fragments (7, 36,42,107,108) (Fig. 12.16B). In all other circumstances, a fixation allowing the head of the screw to be buried within the bone is recommended (Herbert, Herbert-Whipple, Acutrak, etc.) (93,109). Sometimes the fracture can be reduced by closed means, in which case percutaneous K-wire fixation, or even cannulated screws, may be very helpful (68,83). K-wires usually do not allow immediate mobilization, but the advantage of their easy removal makes them very convenient in most cases.

Unstable, comminuted trapezial fractures may not be good candidates for open reduction and internal fixation. In those cases, the use of continuous oblique traction has yielded acceptable results (110,111). Alternatively, complete removal of the bone and a suspensionplasty of the thumb metacarpal with a portion of FCR may also be considered. This latter option should not be used in unstable comminuted fractures of the other distal carpal row bones. In such special instances, bone reconstruction using bone grafts and external fixation is recommended.

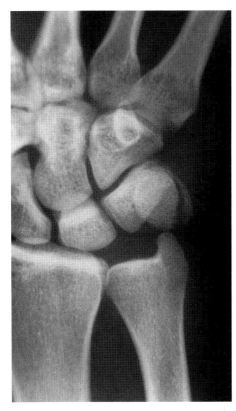

FIGURE 12.18. Longitudinal fracture of the medial edge of the pisiform, probably the result of a sudden contraction of the abductor digiti minimi while the wrist was forcefully extended and radially deviated. Conservative treatment produced healing of the fracture and an excellent functional result.

In badly comminuted fractures of the lunate and proximal pole of the scaphoid, resection of the proximal carpal row may be utilized as a salvage procedure. Aside from this, the only carpal bone that can be resected without a major functional penalty is the pisiform (106). Eventually, symptomatic ununited fractures of the tip of hook of the hamate can be excised to eliminate the residual pain (65–67). Similarly, fractures of the palmar ridge of the trapezium (type II) (46,47) and ununited avulsion fractures of the dorsal rim of the triquetrum may also be excised in order to eliminate the continous discomfort that usually accompanies such unstable fragments (5).

EDITORS' COMMENTS

The hook of the hamate serves as the turning pulley particularly for the ulnar finger flexors. Magnetic resonance imaging in full ulnar deviation power grip position will demonstrate an 80° turn of the tendons around the hook of the hamate. Loss of this pulley by excision significantly decreases grip power in certain positions. In a professional athlete, particularly a golfer, the importance of the hook of the hamate requires that bone grafing rather than excision be done.

The following is our operative technique for bone grafting a nonunion of the hook of the hamate (Editors' Fig. 12.1). A longitudinal palmar incision is made in line with the radial aspect of the ring finger, never extending more proximal than the rugae pattern of the palm. A 2- to 3-cm incision is sufficient. The hook of the hamate is easily palpated; the section is carried deep on the distal edge of the hook of the hamate as the motor branch of the ulnar nerve is in a constant relationship to the distal base of the hook of the hamate. The nerve is identified and traced proximally, releasing the muscle fibers that overlay it until the motor branch can be retracted ulnarward with the ulnar nerve. Subperiosteal dissection is carried down both sides of the hook of the hamate which is long in its proximal-to-distal measurement and short in its transverse dimension. The nonunion site is identified, and subperiosteal dissection is carried out for a few millimeters onto the body of the hamate or dorsal to the nonunion site. A tiny pointed pin or small drill is used to make an initial 1-mm or so sized hole from proximal to dorsal in the body of the hamate. This drill hole is gradually enlarged with increasing sized drills. The volar segment of the hamate maintains its stability primarily because of its soft tissue attachments proximally. This hole is enlarged to the maximum allowable by the width of the hook, usually 3 mm and occasionally 4 mm. Bone graft is then obtained from the distal radius in standard fashion, but the cortical window is utilized as a peg. This cortical cancellous peg is shaped with dental rongeurs or bone cutters until it can be driven down the hook of the hamate and into the body of the hamate. An 0.035-in or 0.045-in pin is placed proximal or distal to the bone graft peg after it has been driven in to stabilize the hook to the body of the hamate. This pin is driven just through the dorsal cortex of the hamate and is cut off just below skin level but left prominent on the volar surface of the hook for removal at 6 weeks. Cancellous bone graft that has been taken from the distal radius is then packed around the nonunion site medially and laterally.

A major component of surgery is maintaining the radial deviation position of the hand from the time of surgery until healing has occurred. The radial deviation position prevents the ulnar finger flexors from pressing ulnarward on the hook of the hamate. Normal tone and contractions of the flexors will tend to rock the hook of the hamate at the nonnion site if the hand is in ulnar deviation. This radial deviation position must be maintained for 6 weeks, at which point there is usually sufficient healing. The pin may be removed, and the patient may be started on gradually increasing activities. Postoperative dressing is a standard bulk dressing with plaster included from the fingertips to the upper forearm. The patient is allowed supination and pronation. At 48 hours the gauntlet cast is applied. The fingers may be left free of the plaster as long as the wrist is maintainted in the radially deviated position.

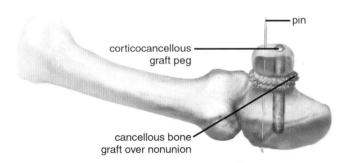

EDITORS' FIGURE 12.1. A corticocancellous peg is used to stabilize the hook of the hamate to the main body of the hamate along with a temporary pin. Cancellous bone graft is packed around the nonunion site after the periosteum has been peeled back. The pin is removed after initial healing occurs.

REFERENCES

1. Snodgrass LE. Fractures of the carpal bones. *Am J Surg* 1937;38: 539–548.
2. Borgeskov S, Christiansen B, Kjaer A, et al. Fractures of the carpal bones. *Acta Orthop Scand* 1966;37:276–287.
3. Dunn AW. Fractures and dislocations of the carpus. *Surg Clin North Am* 1972;52:1513–1538.
4. Bryan RS, Dobyns JH. Fractures of the carpal bones other than lunate and navicular. *Clin Orthop* 1980;149:107–111.
5. Botte MJ, Gelberman RH. Fractures of the carpus, excluding the scaphoid. *Hand Clin* 1987;3:149–161.

6. Buterbaugh GA, Palmer AK. Other carpal fractures. In: Barton NJ, ed. *Fractures of the hand and wrist.* Edinburgh: Churchill Livingstone, 1988;243–250.
7. Cohen MS. Fractures of the carpal bones. *Hand Clin* 1997;13: 587–599.
8. Compson JP. Trans-carpal injuries associated with distal radial fractures in children: A series of three cases. *J Hand Surg [Br]* 1992;17:311–314.
9. Letts M, Esser D. Fractures of the triquetrum in children. *J Pediatr Orthop* 1993;13:228–231.
10. Stark HH, Jobe FW, Boyes JH, et al. Fracture of the hook of the hamate in athletes. *J Bone Joint Surg Am* 1977;59:575–582.
11. Neviaser RJ. Fracture of the hook of the hamate: A diagnosis easily missed. *J Trauma* 1974;14:612–616.
12. Polivy KD, Millender LH, Newberg A, et al. Fractures of the hook of the hamate—a failure of clinical diagnosis. *J Hand Surg [Am]* 1985;10:101–104.
13. Abbitt PL, Riddervold HO. The carpal tunnel view: helpful adjuvant for unrecognized fractures of the carpus. *Skel Radiol* 1987;16:45–47.
14. Beckenbaugh RD, Shives TC, Dobyns JH, et al. Kienböck's disease: the natural history of Kienböck's disease and consideration of lunate fractures. *Clin Orthop* 1980;149:98–106.
15. Gelberman RH, Panagis JS, Taleisnik J, et al. The arterial anatomy of the human carpus. Part I: The extraosseous vascularity. *J Hand Surg [Am]* 1983;8:367–375.
16. Panagis JS, Gelberman RH, Taleisnik J, et al. The arterial anatomy of the human carpus. Part II: The intraosseous vascularity. *J Hand Surg [Am]* 1983;8:375–382.
17. Jenkins SA. Osteoarthritis of the pisiform–triquetral joint. *J Bone Joint Surg Br* 1951;33:532–534.
18. Green DP. Pisotriquetral arthritis: A case report. *J Hand Surg [Am]* 1979;4:465–467.
19. Smith DK, Murray PM. Avulsion fractures of the volar aspect of triquetral bone of the wrist: A subtle sign of carpal ligament injury. *Am J Roentgenol* 1996;166:609–614.
20. Howard FM. Ulnar-nerve palsy in wrist fractures. *J Bone Joint Surg Am* 1961;43:1197–1201.
21. Baird DB, Friedenberg ZB. Delayed ulnar-nerve palsy following a fracture of the hamate. *J Bone Joint Surg Am* 1968;50: 570–572.
22. Manske PR. Fracture of the hook of the hamate presenting as carpal tunnel syndrome. *Hand* 1978;10:181–183.
23. Rouhart F, Fourquet I, Tea SH, et al. Lesion of the deep branch of the ulnar nerve caused by fracture of the hook of the hamate. *Neurophysiol Clin* 1990;20:253–258.
24. Okuhara T, Matsui T, Sugimoto Y. Spontaneous rupture of flexor tendons of a little finger due to projection of the hook of the hamate. A case report. *Hand* 1982;14:71–74.
25. Milek MA, Boulas HJ. Flexor tendon ruptures secondary to hamate hook fractures. *J Hand Surg [Am]* 1990;15:740–744.
26. Johnson RK. The acutely injured wrist and its residuals. *Clin Orthop* 1980;149:33–44.
27. Pointu J, Schwenck JP, Destree G, et al. Les fractures du trapeze. Mecanisme, anatomo-pathologie et indications thérapeutiques. *Rev Chir Orthop* 1988;74:454–465.
28. Blair WF, Kilpatrick WC, Omer GE. Open fracture of the hook the hamate. *Clin Orthop* 1980;163:180–184.
29. Fairbank TJ. Chip fractures of the os triquetrum (carpal cuneiform). *BMJ* 1942;2:310–311.
30. Levy M, Fischel RE, Stern GM, et al. Chip fractures of the os triquetrum. The mechanism of injury. *J Bone Joint Surg Br* 1979; 61:355–357.
31. Garcia-Elias M. Dorsal fractures of the triquetrum. Avulsion or compression fractures? *J Hand Surg [Am]* 1987;12:266–268.
32. Höcker K, Menschik A. Chip fractures of the triquetrum. Mechanism, classification and results. *J Hand Surg [Br]* 1994; 19:584–588.
33. Hove LM. Fractures of the hand. Distribution and relative incidence. *Scand J Plast Reconstr Hand Surg* 1993;27:317–319.
34. Larsen CF, Brøndum V, Skov O. Epidemiology of scaphoid fractures in Odense, Denmark. *Acta Orthop Scand* 1992;63: 216–218.
35. Auffray Y. Les fractures du pyramidal. *Acta Orthop Belg* 1970; 36:313–345.
36. Garcia-Elias M. Las fracturas de los huesos del carpo a excepción del escafoides. *Proc XIII Symp MAPFRE* 1987;27:459–476.
37. Amadio PC, Taleisnik J. Fractures of the carpal bones. In: Green DP, Hotchkiss RN, Pederson WC, eds. *Green's operative hand surgery, 4th ed.* New York: Churchill Livingstone, 1999;809–864.
38. Kindl J. Isolierte handwurzelknochen verletzungen. *Beitr Klin Chir* 1910;67:549–569.
39. Cordrey LJ, Ferrer-Torells M. Management of fractures of the greater multangular. *J Bone Joint Surg Am* 1960;42:1111–1118.
40. Jones WA, Ghorbal MS. Fractures of the trapezium. *J Hand Surg [Br]* 1985;10:227–230.
41. Radford PJ, Wilcox DT. Simultaneous trapezium and Bennett's fractures. *J Hand Surg [Am]* 1992;17:621–623.
42. Garcia-Elias M, Henriquez A, Rossignani P, et al. Bennett's fracture combined with fracture of the trapezium. *J Hand Surg [Br]* 1993;18:523–526.
43. Walker JL, Greene TL, Lunseth PA. Fractures of the body of the trapezium. *J Orthop Trauma* 1988;2:22–28.
44. Binhammer P, Born T. Coronal fracture of the body of the trapezium: A case report. *J Hand Surg [Am]* 1998;23:156–157.
45. Manon M. Les fractures du trapèze dans les traumatismes du poignet. *Rev Orthop* 1924;11:127–140.
46. Palmer AK. Trapezial ridge fractures. *J Hand Surg [Am]* 1981;6:561–564.
47. Botte MJ, von Schroeder HP, Gellman H, et al. Fracture of the trapezial ridge. *Clin Orthop* 1992;276:202–205.
48. Ohshio I, Ogino T, Miyake A. Dislocation of the hamate associated with fracture of the trapezial ridge. *J Hand Surg [Am]* 1986;11:658–660.
49. Jensen BV. An unusual combination of simultaneous fracture of the tuberosity of the trapezium and the hook of the hamate. *J Hand Surg [Am]* 1990;15:185–287.
50. Kuhlmann JN, Fournol S, Mimoun M, et al. Fracture du trapezoide. A propos d'une observation. *Ann Chir Main* 1986;5: 133–134.
51. Yasuwaki Y, Nagata Y, Yamamoto T, et al. Fracture of the trapezoid bone. A case report. *J Hand Surg [Am]* 1994;19:457–459.
52. Garcia-Elias M, Bishop AT, Dobyns JH, et al. Transcarpal carpometacarpal dislocations, excluding the thumb. *J Hand Surg [Am]* 1990;15:531–540.
53. Adler JB, Shaftan GW. Fractures of the capitate. *J Bone Joint Surg Am* 1962;44:1537–1547.
54. Rand JA, Linscheid RL, Dobyns JH. Capitate fractures. A long-term follow-up. *Clin Orthop* 1982;165:209–216.
55. Harrigan AH. Fracture of the os magnum. *Ann Surg* 1908;48: 917–922.
56. Fenton RL. The naviculo-capitate fracture syndrome. *J Bone Joint Surg [Am]* 1956;38:681–684.
57. Stein E, Siegel MW. Naviculocapitate fracture syndrome. A case report: New thoughts on the mechanism of injury. *J Bone Joint Surg [Am]* 1969;51:291–295.
58. Vance RM, Gelberman RH, Evans EF. Scaphocapitate fractures. Patterns of dislocation. Mechanism of injury and preliminary results of treatment. *J Bone Joint Surg Am* 1980;62:271–276.
59. Kaulesar Sukul DMKS, Joñahnnes EJ. Transscapho-transcapitate fracture dislocation of the carpus. *J Hand Surg [Am]* 1992; 17:348–353.

60. Franz A. Contributo allo studio della frattura isolata dell'uncinato. *Chir Org Mov* 1952;37:487–495.
61. Milch H. Fracture of the hamate bone. *J Bone Joint Surg Am* 1934;16:459–462.
62. Bowen TL. Injuries of the hamate bone. *Hand* 1973;5:235–238.
63. Ogunro O. Fracture of the body of the hamate bone. *J Hand Surg [Am]* 1983;8:353–355.
64. Cameron HU, Hastings DE, Fournasier VL. Fracture of the hook of the hamate. *J Bone Joint Surg Am* 1975;57:276–277.
65. Carter PR, Eaton RG, Littler JW. Ununited fracture of the hook of the hamate. *J Bone Joint Surg Am* 1977;59:583–588.
66. Foucher G, Schuind F, Merle M, et al. Fractures of the hook of the hamate. *J Hand Surg [Br]* 1985;10:205–210.
67. Bishop AT, Beckenbaugh RD. Fracture of the hamate hook. *J Hand Surg [Am]* 1988;13:135–139.
68. Garcia-Elias M, Rossignani P, Cots M. Combined fracture of the hook of the hamate and palmar dislocation of the fifth carpometacarpal joint. *J Hand Surg [Br]* 1996;21:446–450.
69. Van Demark RE, Parke WW. Avascular necrosis of the hamate: a case report with reference to the hamate blood supply. *J Hand Surg [Am]* 1992;17:1086–1090.
70. Failla JM. Hook of the hamate vascularity: Vulnerability to osteonecrosis and nonunion. *J Hand Surg [Am]* 1993;18:1075–1079.
71. Smith P, Wright TW, Wallace PF, et al. Excision of the hook of the hamate: A retrospective survey and review of the literature. *J Hand Surg [Am]* 1988;13:612–615.
72. Watson HK, Rogers WD. Nonunion of the hook of the hamate: an argument for bone grafting the nonunion. *J Hand Surg [Am]* 1989;14:486–490.
73. Stark HH, Chao EK, Zemel NP, et al. Fracture of the hook of the hamate. *J Bone Joint Surg Am* 1989;71:1202–1207.
74. Whalen JL, Bishop AT, Linscheid RL. Nonoperative treatment of acute hamate hook fractures. *J Hand Surg [Am]* 1992;17:507–511.
75. Mizuseki T, Ikuta Y, Murakami T. Lateral approach to the hook of hamate for its fracture. *J Hand Surg [Br]* 1986;11:109–111.
76. Garcia-Elias M, Dobyns JH, Cooney WP, et al. Traumatic axial dislocations of the carpus. *J Hand Surg [Am]* 1989;14:446–457.
77. Marck KW, Klasen HJ. Fracture-dislocation of the hamatometacarpal joint: a case report. *J Hand Surg [Am]* 1986;11:128–130.
78. Cain JE, Shepler TR, Wilson MR. Hamatometacarpal fracture-dislocation: classification and treatment. *J Hand Surg [Am]* 1987;12:762–767.
79. Gillespy T, Stork JJ, Dell PC. Dorsal fracture of the hamate: distinctive radiographic appearance. *Am J Roentgenol* 1988;151:351–353.
80. Loth TS, McMillan MD. Coronal dorsal hamate fractures. *J Hand Surg [Am]* 1988;13:616–618.
81. Failla JM, Amadio PC. Recognition and treatment of uncommon carpal fractures. *Hand Clin* 1988;4:469–476.
82. Cetti R, Chistensen SE, Reuther K. Fracture of the lunate bone. *Hand* 1982;14:80–84.
83. Green DP, O'Brien ET. Open reduction of carpal dislocations: indications and operative techniques. *J Hand Surg [Am]* 1978;3:250–265.
84. Teisen H, Hjarbaek J. Classification of fresh fractures of the lunate. *J Hand Surg [Br]* 1989;13:458–462.
85. Conway WF, Gilula LA, Manske PR, et al. Translunate, palmar perilunate fracture-subluxation of the wrist. *J Hand Surg [Am]* 1989;14:635–639.
86. Garcia-Elias M, Proubasta I, Cornudella E. Carpal instability secondary to lunate nonunions. *Rev Esp Cir Mano* 1998;25:7–14.
87. Noble J, Lamb DW. Translunate scapho-radial fracture. *Hand* 1979;11:47–49.
88. Ruijters R, Kortmann J. A case of translunate luxation of the carpus. *Acta Orthop Scand* 1988;59:461–463.
89. Bartone NF, Grieco RV. Fractures of the triquetrum. *J Bone Joint Surg Am* 1956;38:353–356.
90. Mark LK. Fractures of the triquetrum. *Am J Roentgenol* 1960;83:676–679.
91. Greening WP. Isolated fracture of the carpal cuneiform. *BMJ* 1942;1:221–222.
92. Wanadurongwan W. Triquetral fracture associated with hamate dislocation: A case report. *Bull Hosp Joint Dis* 1990;50:54–58.
93. Porter ML, Seehra K. Fracture-dislocation of the triquetrum treated with a Herbert screw. *J Bone Joint Surg Br* 1991;73:347–348.
94. Skelly WJ, Nahigian SH, Hidvegi EB. Palmar lunate transtriquetral fracture dislocation. *J Hand Surg [Am]* 1991;16:536–539.
95. DeBeer JV, Hudson DA. Fractures of the triquetrum. *J Hand Surg [Br]* 1987;12:52–53.
96. Durbin FC. Non-union of the triquetrum. *J Bone Joint Surg Br* 1950;32:388–389.
97. Pevny T, Rayan GM, Egle D. Ligamentous and tendinous support of the pisiform, anatomic and biomechanical study. *J Hand Surg [Am]* 1995;20:299–304.
98. Helal B. Racquet player's pisiform. *Hand* 1978;10:87–90.
99. Deane RB. Simple fracture of the pisiform bone. *Ann Surg* 1911;54:228–229.
100. McCarty V, Farber H. Isolated fracture of the pisiform bone. *J Bone Joint Surg Am* 1946;28:90–391.
101. Jacobs LG. Isolated fracture of the pisiform bone. *Radiology* 1948;50:529–531.
102. Alsberg A. Isolierte fraktur des erbsenbeines. *Z Orthop Chir* 1908;20:299–301.
103. Vasilas A, Grieco V, Bartone N. Roentgen aspects of injuries to the pisiform bone. *J Bone Joint Surg Am* 1960;42:1317–1328.
104. Carroll RE, Coyle MP. Dysfunction of the pisotriquetral joint: Treatment by excision of the pisiform. *J Hand Surg [Am]* 1985;10:703–707.
105. Johnston GH, Tonkin MA. Excision of pisiform in pisotriquetral arthritis. *Clin Orthop* 1986;210:137–142.
106. Amer M, Hagberg L. Wrist flexion strength after excision of the pisiform bone. *Scand J Plast Reconstr Surg* 1984;18:241–245.
107. Richards RR, Paitich CB, Bell RS. Internal fixation of a capitate fracture with Herbert screws. *J Hand Surg [Am]* 1990;15:885–887.
108. Freeland AE, Finley JS. Displaced dorsal oblique fracture of the hamate treated with a cortical mini lag screw. *J Hand Surg [Am]* 1986;11:656–658.
109. Freeland AE, Finley JS. Displaced vertical fracture of the trapezium treated with a small cancellous lag screw. *J Hand Surg [Am]* 1984;9:843–845.
110. Gelberman RH, Vance RM, Zakaib GS. Fractures at the base of the thumb: treatment with oblique traction. *J Bone Joint Surg Am* 1979;61:260–262.
111. Foster RJ, Hastings H. Treatment of Bennett, Rolando, and vertical intraarticular trapezial fractures. *Clin Orthop* 1987;214:121–129.

13

DIAGNOSIS AND MANAGEMENT OF SCAPHOID FRACTURES

DAVID M. KALAINOV
A. LEE OSTERMAN

The scaphoid is the most commonly fractured carpal bone (1,2). The injury is seen most frequently in young men, with a peak incidence between the ages of 15 and 35 years (3,4). Approximately 35,000 scaphoid fractures occur annually in the United States, with occult fractures representing 12% to 16% of the total (5–7).

Since the first recognition of this injury over 100 years ago (8), methods and goals of treatment have changed. No longer is union of the scaphoid adequate; union must occur with proper length and alignment of the scaphoid, and associated ligamentous injuries repaired (5,9). Scaphoid fractures with more than 1 mm of displacement are associated with a 55% incidence of nonunion and a 50% rate of avascular necrosis (10–12). If the scaphoid heals in a collapsed configuration, a suboptimal result can be expected, with loss of wrist motion, particularly extension (9,13).

ANATOMY AND FUNCTION

The scaphoid is a peanut-shaped bone with a palmarly directed concave surface. With the wrist in a neutral position, the scaphoid lies at 47° of flexion and 20° of radial deviation to the long axis of the wrist (5). Articular cartilage covers 80% of the surface area, with abundant soft tissue support provided by the dorsal and palmar carpal ligaments (14). The scaphoid serves as a mechanical link between the proximal and distal carpal rows (5,15–18). When the wrist is brought into either extension or ulnar deviation, the scaphoid extends, and with the wrist in flexion or radial deviation, the scaphoid flexes; this motion resembles a gymnast rotating around a bar, the radioscaphocapitate ligament. The bony integrity of the scaphoid is important for maintaining normal wrist motion, carpal alignment, and proper functioning of the wrist flexor and extensor tendons (13,18,19).

The proximal 70% to 80% of the scaphoid is supplied by small branches of the radial artery entering through foramina along the dorsal ridge (20–22) (Fig. 13.1). The distal 20% to 30% of bone is supplied by palmar branches of the radial artery penetrating the distal tubercle. The extraosseous blood supply is augmented by communicating branches from the anterior interosseous artery, with venous drainage occurring through vessels exiting the dorsal ridge foramina (23). Interruption of the dorsal ridge blood supply during injury or surgery may lead to ischemic changes involving a large segment of bone (24).

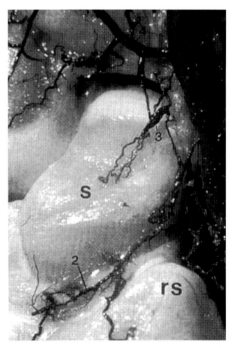

FIGURE 13.1. Vascular injection study demonstrating dorsal branches of the radial artery. *rs*, radial styloid; *s*, scaphoid; *2*, dorsal radiocarpal arch; *3*, branch to the dorsal ridge of the scaphoid; *4*, dorsal intercarpal arch. (From Herndon JH, ed. *Scaphoid fractures and complications.* Rosemont, IL: American Academy of Orthopaedic Surgeons Monograph Series, 1994, with permission.)

D. M. Kalainov: Department of Orthopaedic Surgery, Northwestern University Medical School and Northwestern Memorial Hospital, Chicago, Illinois 60611.

A. L. Osterman: Department of Orthopaedic Surgery, Thomas Jefferson University Hospital, Philadelphia, Pennsylvania; and Philadelphia Hand Center, King of Prussia, Pennsylvania 19406.

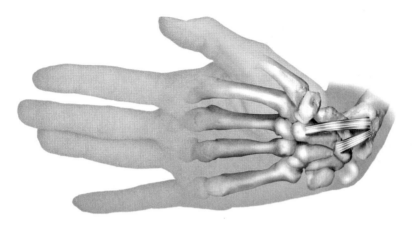

FIGURE 13.2. Mechanism of injury according to Weber and Chao (25). The proximal half of the scaphoid is stabilized amid the radius, capitate, and volar carpal ligaments. A force applied to the radial half of the palm with the wrist in hyperextension may fracture the scaphoid between the proximally supported and distally unsupported regions.

MECHANISM OF INJURY

The usual mechanism of injury involves a sudden impact on the palm with the wrist hyperextended (Fig. 13.2). Weber and Chao, in a cadaveric study, demonstrated consistent reproduction of scaphoid waist fractures with the wrist in 95° to 100° of extension and a force directed against the radial portion of the palm (25). Angulation and displacement were shown to be related to the degree of soft-tissue disruption (12).

Less common mechanisms of injury may involve forced palmar flexion of the wrist (2,26,27) and axial loading of the wrist with the hand in a fisted position (28). Horii et al. reported 18 scaphoid fractures induced by punching with the wrist in neutral to slight palmar flexion (28). The pattern of injury was similar to scaphoid fractures caused by impaction with the wrist in hyperextension.

Intrinsic forces often lead to displacement of a scaphoid fracture into a flexed, "humpback" position; the proximal pole extends with the lunate while the distal pole flexes (17,29–32) (Fig. 13.3). Concurrent deformities include apex radial angulation at the fracture site and pronation of the distal fragment (5,29,30).

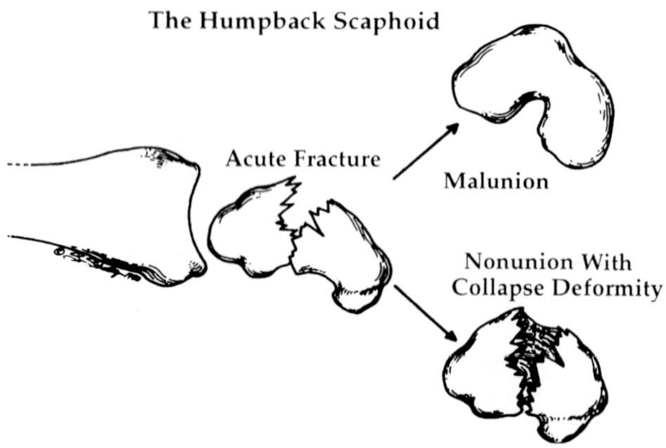

With a significant ulnarly directed force, the injury pattern may be more extensive with involvement of the greater arc as defined by Mayfield and associates (33). Examples include the dorsal transscaphoid perilunate fracture-dislocation and the scaphocapitate syndrome (34–36). These injuries are unstable and may necessitate open reduction and internal fixation with repair of concomitant ligamentous damage. High-energy forces can also result in simultaneous fractures of the distal radius and scaphoid (37,38). Operative fixation of the fractured scaphoid has been recommended with either open or closed treatment of the distal radius injury (37).

DIAGNOSIS

A scaphoid fracture is suspected on recognition of the mechanism of injury and evaluation of the clinical signs and symptoms on presentation. The diagnosis is confirmed by a standard x-ray series with additional imaging studies obtained in equivocal cases.

Clinical Examination

Classically, the patient will present with loss of wrist motion, snuff box tenderness, and pain with resisted forearm pronation and supination. Tenderness in the anatomic snuff box and over the scaphoid tuberosity are sensitive but not specific tests for fracture (6,39). Wrist swelling may be present, but this and other signs of local trauma are not always apparent (40,41).

Additional clinical tests for evaluation of a suspected scaphoid fracture include "intrasound vibration" (42), pain with pronation and ulnar deviation of the wrist (43),

FIGURE 13.3. Humpback deformity with the potential to progress to nonunion or malunion. (From Herndon JH, ed. *Scaphoid fractures and complications.* Rosemont: American Academy of Orthopaedic Surgeons Monograph Series, 1994, with permission.)

the scaphoid shift maueuver (44), and the scaphoid compression test (40,45,46). Although a fracture may be assumed following clinical examination, imaging modalities remain essential for a correct diagnosis. In a study of 12 clinical features for scaphoid injury, Waizenegger and associates found none to be reliable in the diagnosis of a scaphoid fracture (47).

Imaging

Four radiographic views of the wrist should be obtained when evaluating a presumed scaphoid injury; posteroanterior and scaphoid views (posteroanterior view with 30° of ulnar deviation), a true lateral, and an oblique projection (5,48). Most scaphoid fractures can be detected on good quality radiographs at first presentation (49). A radiolucent line through the waist, distal pole, or proximal pole is diagnostic of an acute scaphoid fracture (Fig. 13.4). Resorption at the fracture site and subchondral sclerosis are radiographic findings suggestive of a delayed union or nonunion.

Indirect evidence of a scaphoid fracture in the lateral projection includes an increased scapholunate angle (normal 30° to 60°) or an increased capitolunate angle (normal 0° to 15°), both of which may be associated with fracture displacement and dorsal intercalated segmental instability (DISI) (16,50) (Fig. 13.5). An anteroposterior view with the patient gripping tightly may demonstrate a widened scapholunate interval, indicative of a scapholunate ligament injury (51,52). Lateral displacement or obliteration of the navicular fat stripe on the posteroanterior view can also serve as a clue to the presence of an underlying radial-sided wrist injury (53). Soft tissue signs on x-ray are generally nonspecific (54), however, and care must be taken not to mistake a normal ossification center in a child for a scaphoid fracture.

Several supplementary radiographs are available in cases of a suspected scaphoid injury when initial plain radiographs appear normal. Stress views may demonstrate carpal instability or motion at the fracture site, and x-rays of the contralateral wrist will usually provide a normal template for comparison (55,56). A long-axis projection of the scaphoid can be accomplished with a clenched-fist posteroanterior image (57), an ulnar-deviated oblique view with the beam angled 20° in the cranial direction (58), or an ulnar-deviated posteroanterior image with 10° to 15° of cranial angulation of the x-ray tube (5). "Carpal box" images produce elongated and magnified views of the wrist that can also be helpful in the diagnosis of an occult scaphoid fracture (59,60).

Specialized imaging studies include magnetic resonance imaging, scintigraphy, tomography, and computerized tomography. Both magnetic resonance imaging and scintigraphy have been reported to be highly sensitive and specific in the detection of occult scaphoid fractures (61–66). A three-phase technetium-99m bone scan, however, may not turn positive until 48 to 72 hours after the injury. Magnetic resonance imaging, in contrast, will depict a fracture in the acute setting as a defined region of decreased signal intensity on a T1-weighted image. Magnetic resonance imaging is also valuable in detecting concomitant wrist pathology including osteonecrosis, cartilaginous defects, and ligamentous tears (67) (Fig. 13.6). Tomography is readily available in most medical centers, but true coronal and sagittal images are often difficult to obtain (9,68,69). Computerized tomography affords the distinct advantages of fracture detection in the acute phase with an accurate evaluation of both fracture angulation and displacement (70–72). Liquid crystal thermography and ultrasound have also been reported as diagnostic methods for scaphoid injury, but neither has gained wide clinical acceptance (73–76).

Our current algorithm is to obtain four radiographic views on initial presentation (posteroanterior, lateral, oblique, and scaphoid). If the x-rays are inconclusive and there is a strong suspicion of fracture, the wrist is immobilized with new x-rays taken out of plaster after 2 to 3 weeks (5,7,39,77). If the radiographs remain indeterminate, consideration is given toward additional imaging studies including tomography, comput-

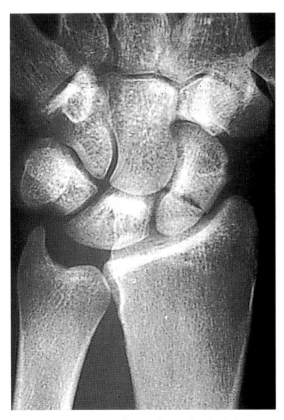

FIGURE 13.4. Posteroanterior radiograph depicting an acute scaphoid fracture at the juncture of the waist and proximal poles.

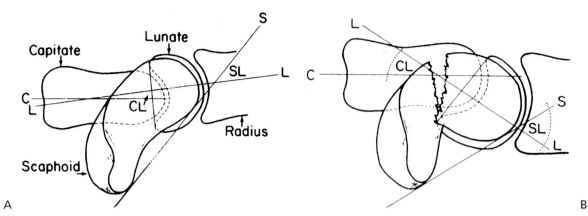

FIGURE 13.5. A: Illustration of normal carpal alignment. *SL,* scapholunate angle (45°); *CL,* capitolunate angle (8°); *L,* longitudinal axis of lunate; *C,* longitudinal axis of capitate; *S,* line paralleling the volar cortices of the proximal and distal convexities of the scaphoid. **B:** Illustration of dorsal intercalated segmental instability alignment with a displaced and angulated scaphoid fracture. *SL,* scapholunate angle (68°); *CL,* capitolunate angle (35°); *L,* longitudinal axis of lunate; *C,* longitudinal axis of capitate; *S,* line paralleling the volar cortices of the proximal and distal convexities of the scaphoid. (From Smith DK, Gilula LA, Amadio PC. Dorsal lunar tilt (DISI configuration): sign of scaphoid fracture displacement. *Radiology* 1990;176:497–499, with permission.)

erized tomography, scintigraphy, or magnetic resonance imaging. Although specialized imaging studies will incur further expense, early detection with a bone scan or MRI may be more cost effective than prolonged empirical immobilization (61,78).

CLASSIFICATION

Classification systems have been developed based on fracture pattern, an assessment of fracture stability, the status of

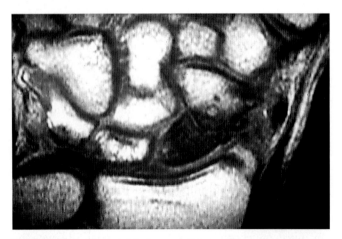

FIGURE 13.6. T1-weighted magnetic resonance image demonstrating a scaphoid waist fracture. Loss of signal intensity within the scaphoid signifies ischemic changes. **Editors' Notes:** *Radiographic evidence of avascular necrosis is not necessarily a contraindication to bone grafting surgery as long as the segment is not significantly crushed or deformed. It is often salvageable.*

bone healing, and the time interval since injury. Acute fractures are considered to be less than 3 weeks old, delayed unions 4 to 6 months old, and nonunions more than 6 months old (48).

Russe divided the scaphoid into three parts to describe fracture location: proximal third, middle third, and distal third (79). Fractures of the middle third were subtyped according to the orientation of the fracture line in relation to the long axis of the bone: transverse, horizontal oblique, and vertical oblique. Cooney and associates separated scaphoid injuries into two types based on stability and anatomic alignment (80). One group included stable and undisplaced fractures, and the second group unstable and displaced fractures. Herbert and Fisher classified scaphoid fractures into four categories: acute stable, acute unstable, delayed union, and nonunion (81). Subclassifications were established to describe the location of the fracture within the bone, the presence of an associated perilunate injury, and the type of nonunion (fibrous or pseudarthrosis).

Various classification systems are often combined in clinical practice to describe the salient features of a scaphoid injury (Fig. 13.7). Fracture location is determined by dividing the scaphoid into thirds: proximal pole, waist, and distal pole. Waist fractures are further denoted as transverse, vertical oblique, or horizontal oblique, and distal pole injuries are subtyped into body, tuberosity, and intraarticular fragments. Stability, displacement, angulation, and comminution of the fracture are noted along with a description of concurrent bone and soft tissue injuries: 63% to 68% of all scaphoid fractures are located in the waist, whereas 16% to 28% occur in the proximal pole, and 6% to 10% occur in the distal pole (82).

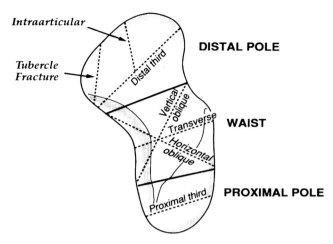

FIGURE 13.7. Scaphoid fracture patterns. (From Herndon JH, ed. *Scaphoid fractures and complications.* Rosemont, IL: American Academy of Orthopaedic Surgeons Monograph Series, 1994, with permission.)

NONOPERATIVE TREATMENT

Closed treatment is indicated for acute, nondisplaced scaphoid fractures and for displaced fractures that are easily reduced and stabilized with external support (Table 13.1). More than 90% of stable scaphoid injuries will heal if diagnosed promptly and immobilized for an adequate duration (1,2,79,83–86). The true incidence of fracture union with conservative treatment, however, is difficult to estimate.

TABLE 13.1. SCAPHOID FRACTURE STABILITY

Acute stable
  Displacement less than 1 mm
  Normal intercarpal alignment
    C-L angle 0–15°[a]
    S-L angle 30–60°[a]
± Distal pole fractures
Acute unstable
  Displacement greater than 1 mm
  Lateral intrascaphoid angulation greater than 35°[b]
  Significant bone loss or comminution
  Arc injuries
  DISI alignment
    C-L angle greater than 15°[a]
    S-L angle greater than 60°[a]
± Proximal pole fractures

[a]Comparison views of the contralateral wrist are important. Typical C-L angulation is 0–15°; 30° is the uppermost limit of normal. Normal S-L angulation is 30–60°; an angle of 61–80° is questionably abnormal, and an angle greater than 80° definitely abnormal (50).
[b]Lateral intrascaphoid angulation is most accurately determined with lateral tomography or computed tomography. Normal lateral intrascaphoid angulation is 24 ± 5°; greater than 45° is associated with an increased risk of functional impairment (9).
C, capitate; L, lunate; S, scaphoid; DISI, dorsal intercalated segmental instability.

Many series do not clearly define the criteria for union or specify the length of follow-up (81). In general, nondisplaced fractures of the distal third and transverse waist fractures heal in 6 to 8 weeks, oblique waist fractures in 8 to 12 weeks, and proximal pole fractures in 12 to 24 weeks (5). Prompt immobilization within 4 weeks of injury is important, as a delay in immobilization may lead to a higher nonunion rate (80,83,87).

Various techniques have been proposed for the closed reduction of displaced scaphoid fractures (88–90). In 1928, Soto-Hall recommended a reduction maneuver involving traction on the thumb with simultaneous "molding" of the anatomic snuff box (88). The scaphoid fragments were impacted and stabilized by applying pressure at the base of the thumb with the wrist positioned in full radial deviation and 20° to 30° of dorsiflexion. More recently, Cooney and associates reported a method of reduction applicable to a dorsally angulated scaphoid fracture (90). Downward pressure is applied to the dorsum of the capitate and lunate, with upward pressure directed over the scaphoid tuberosity (5,90). The reduction is stabilized using K-wires or cast immobilization with pressure maintained at three distinct points (Fig. 13.8).

Opinions are varied regarding the optimum position for immobilization and the number of joints to be incorporated in a cast (2,15,27,41,79,80,86,88,89,91–102).

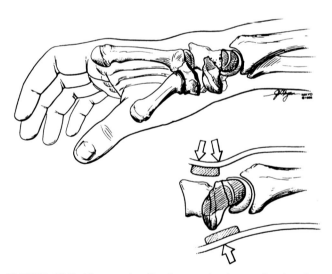

FIGURE 13.8. Three-point fixation method to maintain alignment following closed reduction of a humpback deformity. The cast is molded to provide pressure dorsally over the distal radius and capitate and palmarly along the scaphoid tuberosity. (From Cooney WP, Linscheid RL, Dobyns JH. Fractures and dislocations of the wrist. In: Rockwood CA, Green DP, Bucholz R, eds. *Rockwood and Green's fractures in adults,* 4th ed. Philadelphia: Lippincott–Raven Publishers, 1996, with permission of Mayo Foundation.) **Editors' Notes:** *We feel it is anatomically impossible to control the position of the scaphoid with external molding of plaster. Any significant deformity of an acute scaphoid fracture is probably an indication for surgery.*

This diversity of opinion can be attributed to the successful outcomes reported in several series using different cast configurations (2,27,79,80,85,86,89,92,93,98,99). From experiments on cadaveric wrists, Weber and Chao concluded that nondisplaced scaphoid waist fractures were best immobilized with the wrist in neutral to slight palmarflexion and mild radial deviation (25). Ulnar deviation of the wrist, particularly when combined with dorsiflexion, was found to lead to fracture displacement. Yanni and associates reported similar results, recommending immobilization of scaphoid waist fractures with the wrist in neutral to slight palmarflexion and neutral radial–ulnar deviation (91).

Gellman and associates prospectively studied 51 patients with acute, nondisplaced scaphoid fractures (99). Patients were randomly assigned to treatment with either a long-arm or a short-arm thumb–spica cast. After 6 weeks, the hands that were initially treated with a long-arm cast were placed in a short-arm cast. For nondisplaced fractures of the proximal pole and waist, there was a shorter time to union and a decreased incidence of nonunion with long-arm cast treatment. No loss of elbow motion was observed when the cast extended above the elbow for the recommended 6-week period of immobilization.

Failla and associates studied the effects of forearm rotation on scaphoid fragment displacement in a cadaveric model (103). Scaphoid waist osteotomies were created in four upper extremity specimens, preserving the dorsal and volar carpal ligaments. Radiographic markers were placed in the distal radius and proximal and distal scaphoid fragments for each specimen, and a short-arm thumb–spica cast was applied with the wrist in neutral position. The specimens were mounted on a specially designed x-ray frame, and images were obtained at different degrees of forearm rotation. Fracture displacement of up to 4.19 mm in the coronal plane was noted when the forearms were rotated from 60° pronation to 60° supination.

For nondisplaced fractures of the waist and large proximal pole fragments, we treat our patients with a well-fitted, long-arm thumb–spica cast. The elbow is flexed to 90° with the forearm and wrist positioned in neutral (Fig. 13.9). The cast extends to the interphalangeal joint of the thumb, allowing for some motion at this joint, and the cast is checked regularly for adequacy of fit. If there is marked swelling, a temporary above-elbow splint is applied for the first 7 to 10 days. After 3 weeks, the long-arm cast is converted to a short-arm thumb–spica cast for the additional period of time necessary to achieve union. In some patients with early radiographic signs of healing, we have switched from a short-arm thumb–spica cast to a scaphoid mobilization splint (104) (Fig. 13.10).

Nondisplaced fractures of the scaphoid tuberosity are treated differently. A short-arm thumb–spica cast is applied at the time of diagnosis and discontinued 3 to 6 weeks later, provided the patient is comfortable and there are no radiographic signs of fracture displacement. Gellman and associates found no difference in healing rates of distal-third scaphoid fractures with use of either a long-arm or short-arm thumb–spica cast (99). Prosser and associates, however, reported one nonunion and frequent malunions in a series of 37 distal articular scaphoid fractures treated conservatively (105).

The recommended period of immobilization should continue despite the appearance of sclerotic changes in the proximal pole. Plain radiographs are not very accurate in the detection of avascular necrosis (106), and an increased density in the proximal pole may proceed to uncomplicated fracture union (79,107,108). When avascular necrosis of the scaphoid is suspected, MRI provides the best means for confirming the diagnosis (106,109), outside of visualization of punctate bleeding at surgery (107).

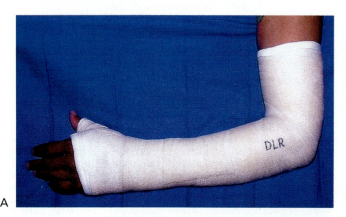
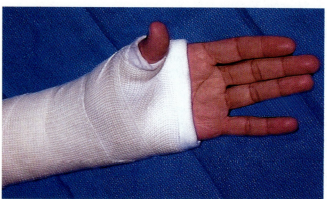

FIGURE 13.9. Fiberglass long-arm thumb–spica cast for the treatment of stable waist and proximal pole fractures. **Editors' Notes:** *Immobilization of the carpal bones whether following limited wrist arthrodesis or fracture requires a long-arm cast with the thumb included to the tip and the index and middle proximal phalanges included in the plaster and flexed at the metacarpophalangeal joints.*

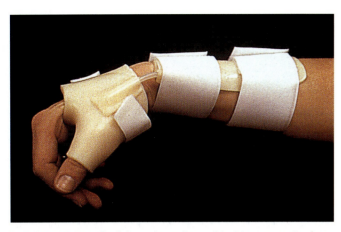

FIGURE 13.10. Flexible wrist splint with hinges made from polypropylene rods. The splint permits approximately 30° of wrist flexion and extension while limiting radial and ulnar deviation.

Electrical Stimulation and Ultrasound

Pulsed electrical stimulation has been shown experimentally to enhance both neovascularization and osteogenesis (110). Noninvasive electrical stimulation can be helpful in the treatment of select scaphoid delayed unions and nonunions (111–113). Electromagnetic field stimulation as an adjunct in the treatment of acute scaphoid fractures, however, has no proven benefits to date.

Pulsed low-intensity ultrasound has been shown to accelerate healing of acute distal radial and tibial diaphyseal fractures (114–116). Ultrasound pressure waves impart a mechanical strain on injured bone tissue that appears to influence both bone formation and resorption (114). Low-intensity ultrasound in the management of scaphoid fractures requires further investigation to determine its value and effectiveness.

OPERATIVE TREATMENT

Surgical intervention is indicated for acute scaphoid fractures that are unstable and not amenable to closed reduction and cast treatment (Table 13.1). Scaphoid fracture instability is defined as displacement greater than 1 mm in any direction (80,83,117), significant bone loss or comminution, increased angulation at the fracture site with a lateral intrascaphoid angle exceeding 35° (9), fractures associated with DISI (17), and arc injuries, including transscaphoid perilunate fracture-dislocations and the scaphocapitate syndrome (34–36,118–121) (Fig. 13.11).

Relative indications for surgical treatment in the acute setting include polytrauma and prolonged immobilization that is unacceptable to the patient for social or economic reasons. Internal fixation may permit earlier return to sport for a professional athlete who requires maximum manual dexterity (122–124). Delayed union of more than 4 months for a waist fracture and 6 months for a proximal pole fracture may also benefit from operative intervention (5).

The treatment of acute proximal pole fractures is debated. In our opinion, fractures involving less than 25% of bone are best treated by open reduction and internal fixation. The healing time with closed treatment of proximal pole injuries is prolonged, and the potential for developing avascular necrosis and/or nonunion is increased. Operative stabilization with early wrist mobilization may decrease joint stiffness and lessen the degree of osteoporosis and muscle wasting commonly associated with extended cast treatment.

Methods

Kirschner wires provide a relatively simple and inexpensive method for scaphoid fracture fixation. Wires are useful in

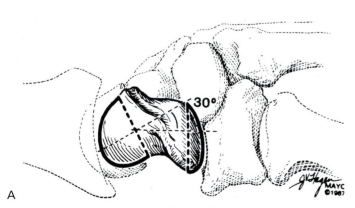
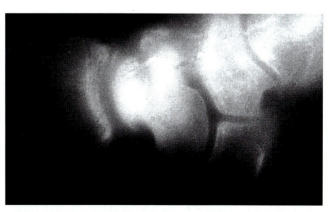

FIGURE 13.11. A: Technique for measuring lateral intrascaphoid angulation. (From Amadio PC, Berquist TH, Smith DK, et al. Scaphoid malunion. *J Hand Surg [Am]* 1989;14:679–687, with permission of Mayo Foundation.) **B:** Lateral tomogram of a proximal pole fracture demonstrating an increased intrascaphoid angle of 60°.

the treatment of comminuted scaphoid fractures, acute carpal instability, and for fracture stabilization when bone grafting is necessary to fill a structural defect. Wires are also helpful as an adjunct with other methods of internal fixation to provide rotational stability. The major disadvantage of pin fixation, however, is the need for concomitant external support, with the attendant problems of prolonged immobilization.

Given the intraarticular nature of scaphoid fractures, many surgeons have advocated fixation devices that allow for early wrist motion and an earlier return to activities. Preliminary results using a trapeziolunate external fixator were reported by Gunal and associates (125). The fixator bridges the scaphoid fracture and permits motion at the radiocarpal and carpometacarpal joints. However, normal motion of the scaphoid is restricted, disrupting intercarpal kinematics.

Staples (126,127) and the Ender compression blade plate (128,129) have been reported in limited series for the treatment of delayed unions and nonunions. These devices are applied on the external surface of the scaphoid and, consequently, may impinge on adjacent wrist structures, necessitating a second operation for hardware removal. Cannulated and noncannulated headed screws permit intramedullary placement with compression across the fracture site achieved by lag insertion (97,130–135). Correct screw placement can be technically demanding, however, and protrusive screw heads may also interfere with surrounding wrist structures.

In 1984, Herbert and Fisher introduced a headless screw and an alignment guide that allowed for both fracture compression and controlled implant insertion (81). The screw is buried beneath articular cartilage, curtailing the problems of impingement from a prominent screw head. The Herbert screw and headless screws of similar design have become the standard for intramedullary fixation of scaphoid fractures. Mobilization is encouraged within the first few weeks postoperatively, and union rates are similar to those reported for closed cast treatment (81,136–138).

Technique: Volar and Dorsal Exposures

The volar approach is recommended for internal fixation of waist and distal pole fractures; this approach affords excellent exposure of the undersurface of the scaphoid without violating the dorsal ridge vessels (79,81). A straight 4-cm skin incision is made in the interval between the flexor carpi radialis tendon and radial artery, centered over the tubercle of the scaphoid and directed toward the base of the thumb (Fig. 13.12). The flexor carpi radialis tendon sheath is divided, and the tendon is retracted ulnarly to expose the underlying wrist capsule. The wrist capsule is opened sharply, cutting across the radioscaphocapitate and long radiolunate ligaments. Hematoma and debris are cleaned from the fracture site, and an anatomic reduction is performed, incorporating provisional K-wire fixation when

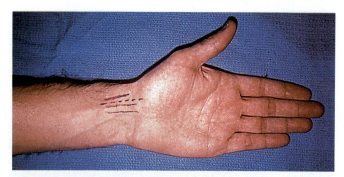

FIGURE 13.12. Volar incision for open reduction and internal fixation of waist and distal pole fractures.

needed. If a standard Herbert screw is used, the Huene alignment guide is placed around the proximal and distal poles of the scaphoid, perpendicular to the fracture line (Fig. 13.13). Herbert recommends releasing the scaphotrapezial ligament and elevating the distal pole of the scaphoid for accurate seating of the compression jig (81). This has raised concerns about the potential for developing early arthritic changes in the scaphotrapezial joint (139). The amount of scaphoid mobilization can be decreased by removing the volar tubercle of the trapezium with an osteotome or rongeur.

Fracture reduction and proper positioning of the alignment guide are confirmed with image intensification (140). The tract for the Herbert screw is then created, and the appropriately sized screw is inserted. The alignment guide is disengaged, and the accuracy of fracture reduction and screw placement is assessed (Fig. 13.14). The volar capsule and carpal ligaments are repaired and the wound edges reapproximated. Several modifications of this technique

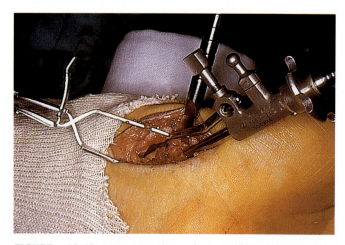

FIGURE 13.13. Intraoperative photograph of the volar approach. A self-retaining retractor is positioned in the wound, and a Huene alignment guide is placed around the proximal and distal poles of the scaphoid. A blunt elevator is used to carefully elevate the distal pole.

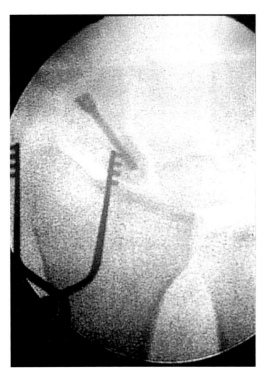

FIGURE 13.14. Intraoperative image of anterograde Herbert screw fixation.

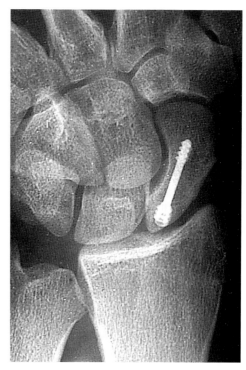

FIGURE 13.15. Posteroanterior radiograph demonstrating retrograde Herbert screw placement.

have been described to assist with accurate jig and screw placement (141–143).

In the case of a proximal pole fracture involving less than 25% of the scaphoid, a dorsal approach with retrograde Herbert screw or K-wire placement is preferred (138,144,145). A mini Herbert screw is particularly useful in this situation (138). A 4-cm longitudinal incision is made over the dorsoradial aspect of the wrist, ending proximally at Lister's tubercle. The extensor retinaculum is divided between the second and third extensor compartments, and the extensor pollicis longus and extensor carpi radialis brevis tendons retracted radially. The fourth extensor compartment is then elevated subperiostially and retracted in an ulnar direction to expose the dorsal wrist capsule. The capsule is opened sharply for a short distance to gain access to the proximal pole of the scaphoid; vessels entering the scaphoid along the dorsal ridge may be at risk if the capsule is divided too far distally. The wrist is flexed, and the proximal pole fracture is reduced and stabilized with a K-wire and/or Herbert screw. Proper implant placement is confirmed radiographically (Fig. 13.15). The capsule and extensor retinaculum are then closed, repositioning the extensor pollicis longus tendon ulnar to Lister's tubercle. If the proximal pole fragment is small and ischemic, vascularized bone grafting, simple debridement, or debridement with soft tissue interposition may be indicated (48,133,139,146).

The wrist is supported in a volar plaster splint immediately following surgery, and sutures are removed 7 to 10 days later. After the first postoperative week, we provide the majority of our patients with a scaphoid mobilization splint, which permits early protected wrist motion (104) (see Fig. 13.10). The splint may also be used as a step-down measure in treating scaphoid fractures nonoperatively. By the eighth week after surgery, patients are allowed to resume most activities without protection if wrist range of motion is near normal and grip strength is 80% of the contralateral side (5).

Arthroscopically Assisted Fixation

Wrist arthroscopy is a minimally invasive technique that may enhance our ability to diagnose and treat acute scaphoid fractures. Arthroscopy permits visualization of the fracture site, confirmation of fracture reduction, and a direct assessment of concomitant cartilage and ligamentous injuries. Whipple reported 20 consecutive scaphoid fractures reduced with arthroscopic assistance and stabilized using a new alignment guide and a cannulated version of the Herbert screw (147). Jig placement required a radial-sided arthroscopic portal and a small volar incision, allowing for preservation of the radioscaphocapitate and long radiolunate ligaments. Nineteen fractures had healed without complication at 12-month follow-up.

The arthroscopic technique involves standard wrist arthroscopy equipment and portal placement. The scaphoid fracture is most clearly visualized from the midcarpal perspective, whereas ligamentous damage is best evaluated through the radiocarpal portals. Our series of 15 patients treated with arthroscopic assistance over a 5-year period has been rewarding; these cases represented fewer than 1% of all scaphoid fractures seen during that same time interval. The union rate has been 100%, and an early return to function, especially sports, has been realized. The procedure, however, is difficult and time consuming, with operative times ranging from 1 to 3 hours. Advanced arthroscopy skills are mandatory, and, in our opinion, this technique should still be considered investigational.

Percutaneous Fixation

There are relatively few reports describing the technique and results of percutaneous scaphoid fracture fixation (133,148,149). Wozasek and Moser published a series of 198 scaphoid injuries treated with cannulated screws through a limited volar incision (133). After a mean postoperative period of 83 months, union was noted in 89% of acute fractures, 81.8% of fractures with delayed or nonunion, and 42.8% of those with sclerotic nonunion. Bone grafting following the primary procedure was required in an unspecified number of delayed and nonunion cases, and overall radiographic results were much worse than in a previously published report.

We believe percutaneous screw fixation can be useful for the stabilization of nondisplaced or easily reducible scaphoid fractures in the acute setting, particularly in patients who are unable to tolerate prolonged cast treatment. The procedure requires a good understanding of the three-dimensional anatomy of the scaphoid, however, and should be reserved for fractures without bone loss or comminution. The technique may be best used in conjunction with arthroscopic scaphoid evaluation.

Transscaphoid Perilunate Fracture-Dislocations

Operative stabilization with at least 6 weeks of immobilization is the preferred treatment for this complex injury pattern (5). A combined volar–dorsal approach has been recommended to provide full exposure of the injury (34,35). Sotereanos and associates reported six transscaphoid perilunate fracture-dislocations treated by screw and wire fixation through volar and dorsal incisions (35). At an average follow-up of 22 months after surgery, all scaphoid fractures united, and five patients demonstrated a satisfactory outcome.

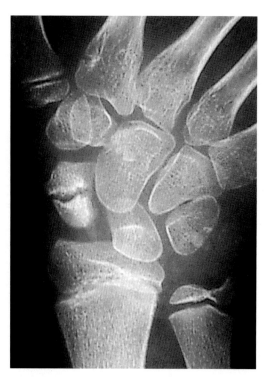

FIGURE 13.16. Scaphoid waist fracture in an adolescent boy. The fracture was not recognized until several months after the injury.

PEDIATRIC FRACTURES

Ossification of the scaphoid is generally not complete until age 13 in girls and age 15 in boys (150). Fractures of the scaphoid account for only 0.45% of upper extremity fractures in children (150,151). Approximately two-thirds of these fractures occur in the distal pole region, whereas one-third occur in the waist (150) (Fig. 13.16). Fracture displacement is rare, and most fractures will heal with 3 to 6 weeks of immobilization. If union is not achieved by 6 months after injury, a bone-grafting procedure may be considered (150,152).

COMPLICATIONS

Complications following surgical management of scaphoid fractures include capsular contractures and joint stiffness, scar hypertrophy, improper implant placement, hardware failure, and infection (Fig. 13.17). Additional complications following both operative and nonoperative treatment include neurovascular injury, tendon rupture, carpal instability, posttraumatic arthritis, delayed union, nonunion, malunion, and avascular necrosis (9,17,31,32,109, 153–163). Estimates for the incidence of avascular necrosis following fractures of the scaphoid range between 13% and

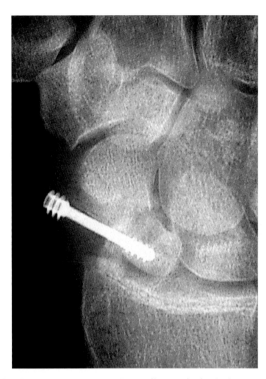

FIGURE 13.17. Posteroanterior radiograph depicting nonunion of a scaphoid fracture with cutout of the Herbert screw.

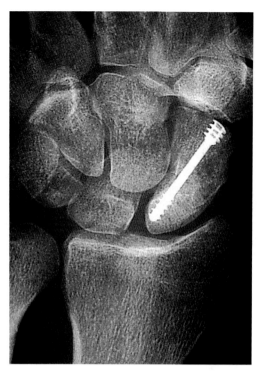

FIGURE 13.18. Posteroanterior radiograph showing sclerotic changes in the proximal pole of the scaphoid. Tomography confirmed union.

40% (5,11). Proximal pole fractures are at the highest risk of developing ischemic changes.

DETERMINING UNION

Assessment of scaphoid fracture healing can be problematic, and the time to union quite variable (139,164,165). Of the 116 acute waist fractures in the Dickison and Shannon series, only 74% were healed at 4 months (165). The remaining 26% of cases required up to 9 months to unite.

Fracture union is based on both clinical and radiographic criteria. However, tenderness over the fracture site and pain with active wrist motion may dissipate with time in both delayed unions and nonunions. Fracture healing is best assessed with the same radiographic series used to diagnose the initial injury (posteroanterior, lateral, oblique, and scaphoid views). The radiographs are generally obtained at 4-week intervals until healing is assured, with union based on the finding of osseous trabeculae crossing the fracture line in at least one projection (Fig. 13.18). Fluoroscopy is helpful in deciding whether there is motion at the injury site, and long-axis CT or tomograms may be useful in equivocal cases. Failure of union following internal fixation is assumed when there is evidence of screw loosening, such as a lucency around the screw threads (81). Follow-up for a minimum of 1 year after injury is recommended in all cases.

EDITORS' COMMENTS

Surgeons of the wrist have gradually accepted more indications for an open approach to acute scaphoid fractures. The scaphoid is responsible for almost all degenerative arthritis of the wrist and is involved in instability in the great majority of cases. A scaphoid not properly aligned and/or restrained produces symptoms and function loss. The scaphoid must, therefore, be approached with the great respect it deserves. Satisfactory union is no longer an end measurement for successful treatment. Normal scaphoid alignment and ligament restraints are mandatory.

Following the evolutionary process of articular fractures of the distal radius, most scaphoid fractures should be considered for early open reduction. Surgery includes a dorsal transverse incision with its minimal scarring and direct alignment and pinning of scaphoid fractures, with or without bone graft from the ipsilateral distal radius. We think this approach is indicated in all but the totally undisplaced scaphoid fracture.

The acute completely undisplaced scaphoid fracture, though it requires careful observation, can be treated with short arm casting. We have used external splints that can be sterilized and have allowed surgeons to continue operating on undisplaced scaphoid fractures.

Any discussion of scaphoid fracture is first a discussion of healing. The scaphoid is the poorest healing bone in the body. Immobilization of this fracture goes back to the earliest medicine. It is important to have a feel for what immobilization means. Tiny capillaries are attempting to bridge the fracture site. The slightest motion between the fractured components will rupture these capillaries, and the process must begin anew. Fortunately, in most bones, an amalgam of material (callus) is produced that holds the bone sufficiently that vascular continuity can eventually be established, even without adequate external support. Unfortunately for the scaphoid, the periosteum is a major part of this process, and because of the paucity of noncartilage surface in the scaphoid, healing occurs as an internal process. The effect of compression is not so much to change the manner in which the healing process occurs but to provide a more absolute form of immobilization. This allows for the process of vascular bridging and the development of a substructure on which osteoid and eventually bone can be laid. If one recognizes the effect of microscopic motion in disrupting this initial vascular bridging, then the need for early near-absolute immobilization becomes obvious. We feel that in fracture healing, as with limited wrist arthrodesis, there is actual healing by 3 weeks, at which point the immobilization can be relative as long as loads are not applied to the healing area sufficient to produce disruption of the bridging mechanism. Scaphoid nonunion is treated much as limited wrist arthrodesis, with 3 weeks of long arm "Groucho Marx" casting followed by 3 weeks of protective short arm gauntlet casting.

There are two principles guiding the procedures for scaphoid nonunion surgery. They are the correction of angular deformity between the distal and proximal segments and the reestablishment of scaphoid length. The angulation problem is obvious, but the collapse and loss of bone stock at the nonunion site, particularly in waist and distal scaphoid nonunions, has perhaps not been as well addressed. Our preferred approach to scaphoid nonunion is a dorsal transverse incision with cancellous bone grafting from the distal radius, as demonstrated in Chapter 68. The dorsal approach allows use of the capitate as a template and facilitates establishment of normal scaphoid architecture. We have used only a dorsal approach for over 30 years and have yet to produce an avascular necrosis of the proximal pole. Kauer's work on the volar radial scapholunate ligament implies that this ligament is a vascular ligament filled with coiled vessels, capable of extreme elongation. There are also nerve endings that probably serve to call on increased muscle control of the carpals as loads increase and the ligament is stretched. Contrary to Gelberman's work (20), there appears to be adequate blood supply to the proximal pole in most cases, independent of the dorsal ridge vascular attachment.

The principle of the surgery is identical to that for limited wrist arthrodeses, where the gap between the proximal and distal portions of the scaphoid is simply filled with cancellous bone. This technique does not lend itself to any form of compression, as the bone is being maintained out to length with the interposition of cancellous bone. The small proximal pole fracture is really an avulsion fracture and puts the injury into the category of a scapholunate dissociation. The scapholunate interosseous ligament does not rupture but tears off a small proximal pole. This small piece, however, is the ligament support system for the scaphoid, and rotary subluxation will occur to the distal fragment. This is true for all scaphoid nonunions and explains the complete destruction of the rotated distal segment against the radius with no articular cartilage loss between the unrotated proximal pole and the radius. This is true throughout the realm of scaphoid nonunion: the distal pole destroys itself against the radius. The capitate shears the cartilage and destroys the capitate proximal pole joint just as with the capite–lunate joint in other scapholunate advanced collapse (SLAC) wrists. With this in mind, therefore, there is no indication for removing the proximal pole, which has the ligamentous attachments. It is mandatory that the small proximal pole be fused to the scaphoid body or, at the very least, that fibrous union occur to prevent rotation of the distal segment. All scaphoid nonunions follow this pattern.

Because all scaphoid nonunions will destroy themselves, producing the SLAC wrist, it is incumbent on the hand surgeon to advise surgery for scaphoid nonunions even though they are often asymptomatic. This has always been a difficult decision, but we think the total quality of life for the patient is best served by open reduction and bone grafting of the nonunion before changes occur. Some professional athletes require special considerations. On occasion failed bone graftings of nonunions have produced sufficient fibrous stability that a professional athlete can play out his career. For some, these are the only high-income years in their lives, and this takes precedence over future degenerative arthritis in the wrist. A SLAC reconstruction once the professional years are over is satisfactory. In children, a scaphoid nonunion will often result in apparent dissolution of the bone. The radiograph may show no scaphoid bone in one segment or the other. Open surgery and bone grafting should still be considered. Fusion will usually occur, and ossification will demonstrate a good scaphoid years later (see Editors' Comments in Chapter 11).

REFERENCES

1. Dunn AW. Fractures and dislocations of the carpus. *Surg Clin North Am* 1972;52:1513–1538.
2. Leslie IJ, Dickson RA. The fractured carpal scaphoid. Natural history and factors influencing outcome. *J Bone Joint Surg Br* 1981;63:225–230.
3. Gumucio CA, Fernando B, Young VL, et al. Management of scaphoid fractures: a review and update. *South Med J* 1989;82:1377–1388.
4. Larsen CF, Brondum V, Skov O. Epidemiology of scaphoid fractures in Odense, Denmark. *Acta Orthop Scand* 1992;63:216–218.
5. Herndon JH, ed. *Scaphoid fractures and complications.* Rosemont: American Academy of Orthopaedic Surgeons Monograph Series, 1994.
6. Freeland P. Scaphoid tubercle tenderness: a better indicator of scaphoid fractures? *Arch Emerg Med* 1989;6:46–50.
7. Mittal RL, Dargan SK. Occult scaphoid fracture: a diagnostic enigma. *J Orthop Trauma* 1989;3:306–308.
8. Destot EAJ. *Injuries of the wrist: a radiological study.* New York: Paul B. Hoeber, 1926. Atkinson FRB, translator.
9. Amadio PC, Berquist TH, Smith DK, et al. Scaphoid malunion. *J Hand Surg [Am]* 1989;14:679–687.
10. Dabezies EJ, Mathews R, Faust DC. Injuries to the carpus: fractures of the scaphoid. *Orthopedics* 1982;5:1510–1521.
11. Szabo RM, Manske D. Displaced fractures of the scaphoid. *Clin Orthop* 1988;230:30–38.
12. Weber ER. Biomechanical implications of scaphoid waist fractures. *Clin Orthop* 1980;149:83–89.
13. Burgess RC. The effect of a simulated scaphoid malunion on wrist motion. *J Hand Surg [Am]* 1987;12:774–776.
14. Berger RA. The ligaments of the wrist: a current overview of anatomy with considerations of their potential functions. *Hand Clin* 1997;13:63–82.
15. Fisk GR. Carpal instability and the fractured scaphoid. *Ann R Coll Surg Engl* 1970;46:63–76.
16. Fisk GR. An overview of injuries of the wrist. *Clin Orthop* 1980;149:137–144.
17. Smith DK, Cooney WP III, An KN, et al. The effects of simulated unstable scaphoid fractures on carpal motion. *J Hand Surg [Am]* 1989;14:283–291.
18. Linscheid RL, Dobyns JH, Beabout JW, et al. Traumatic instability of the wrist: diagnosis, classification, and pathomechanics. *J Bone Joint Surg Am* 1972;54:1612–1632.
19. Tang JB, Ryu J, Han JS, et al. Biomechanical changes of the wrist flexor and extensor tendons following loss of scaphoid integrity. *J Orthop Res* 1997;15:69–75.
20. Gelberman RH, Menon J. The vascularity of the scaphoid bone. *J Hand Surg [Am]* 1980;5:508–513.
21. Gelberman RH, Panagis JS, Taleisnik J, et al. The arterial anatomy of the human carpus. Part 1: the extraosseous vascularity. *J Hand Surg [Am]* 1983;8:367–375.
22. Taleisnic J, Kelly PJ. The extraosseous and intraosseous blood supply of the scaphoid bone. *J Bone Joint Surg Am* 1966;48:1125–1137.
23. Handley RC, Pooley J. The venous anatomy of the scaphoid. *J Anat* 1991;178:115–118.
24. Botte MJ, Mortensen WW, Gelberman RH, et al. Internal vascularity of the scaphoid in cadavers after insertion of the Herbert screw. *J Hand Surg [Am]* 1988;13:216–222.
25. Weber ER, Chao EY. An experimental approach to the mechanism of scaphoid waist fractures. *J Hand Surg [Am]* 1978;3:142–148.
26. Shestak K, Ruby LK. An unusual fracture of the scaphoid. *J Hand Surg [Am]* 1983;8:925–928.
27. Clay NR, Dias JJ, Costigan PS, et al. Need the thumb be immobilized in scaphoid fractures? A randomized prospective trial. *J Bone Joint Surg Br* 1991;73:828–832.
28. Horii E, Nakamura R, Watanabe K, et al. Scaphoid fracture as a "puncher's fracture." *J Orthop Trauma* 1994;8:107–110.
29. Belsole RJ, Hilbelink DR, Llewellyn JA, et al. Computed analysis of the pathomechanics of scaphoid waist nonunions. *J Hand Surg [Am]* 1991;16:899–906.
30. Nakamura R, Imaeda T, Horii E, et al. Analysis of scaphoid fracture displacement by three-dimensional computed tomography. *J Hand Surg [Am]* 1991;16:485–492.
31. Nakamura R, Hori M, Horii E, et al. Reduction of the scaphoid fracture with DISI alignment. *J Hand Surg [Am]* 1987;12:1000–1005.
32. Mack GR, Bosse MJ, Gelberman RH, et al. The natural history of scaphoid non-union. *J Bone Joint Surg Am* 1984;66:504–509.
33. Mayfield JK, Johnson RP, Kilcoyne RK. Carpal dislocations: pathomechanics and progressive perilunar instability. *J Hand Surg [Am]* 1980;5:226–241.
34. Cooney WP, Bussey R, Dobyns JH, et al. Difficult wrist fractures; perilunate fracture-dislocations of the wrist. *Clin Orthop* 1987;214:136–147.
35. Sotereanos DG, Mitsionis GJ, Giannakopoulos PN, et al. Perilunate dislocation and fracture dislocation: a critical analysis of the volar–dorsal approach. *J Hand Surg [Am]* 1997;22;49–56.
36. Vance RM, Gelberman RH, Evans EF. Scaphocapitate fractures: patterns of dislocation, mechanisms of injury, and preliminary results of treatment. *J Bone Joint Surg Am* 1980;62:271–276.
37. Trumble TE, Benirschke SK, Vedder NB. Ipsilateral fractures of the scaphoid and radius. *J Hand Surg [Am]* 1993;18:8–14.
38. Hove LM. Simultaneous scaphoid and distal radial fractures. *J Hand Surg [Br]* 1994;19:384–388.
39. Zarnett R, Martin C, Barrington TW, et al. The natural history of suspected scaphoid fractures. *Can J Surg* 1991;34:334–337.
40. Grover R. Clinical assessment of scaphoid injuries and the detection of fractures. *J Hand Surg [Br]* 1996;21:341–343.
41. Perkins G. Fracture of the carpal scaphoid. *BMJ* 1950;1:536–537.
42. Finkenberg JG, Hoffer E, Kelly C, et al. Diagnosis of occult scaphoid fractures by intrasound vibration. *J Hand Surg [Am]* 1993;18:4–7.
43. Powell JM, Lloyd GJ, Rintoul RF. New clinical test for fracture of the scaphoid. *Can J Surg* 1988;31:237–238.
44. Watson HK, Ashmead D, Makhlouf M. Examination of the scaphoid. *J Hand Surg [Am]* 1988;13:657–660.
45. Chen SC. The scaphoid compression test. *J Hand Surg [Br]* 1989;14:323–325.
46. Esberger DA. What value the scaphoid compression test? *J Hand Surg [Br]* 1994;19:748–749.
47. Waizenegger M, Barton NJ, Davis TR, et al. Clinical signs in scaphoid fractures. *J Hand Surg [Br]* 1994;19:743–747.
48. Simonian PT, Trumble TE. Scaphoid nonunion. *J Am Acad Orthop Surg* 1994;2:185–191.
49. Jacobsen S, Hassani G, Hansen D, et al. Suspected scaphoid fractures. Can we avoid overkill? *Acta Orthop Belg* 1995;61:74–78.
50. Smith DK, Gilula LA, Amadio PC. Dorsal lunar tilt (DISI configuration): sign of scaphoid fracture displacement. *Radiology* 1990;176:497–499.
51. Dobyns JH, Linscheid RL, Chao EYS, et al. Traumatic instability of the wrist. *Instr Course Lect* 1975;24:182–199.
52. Jones WA. Beware the sprained wrist. The incidence and diagnosis of scapholunate instability. *J Bone Joint Surg Br* 1988;70:293–297.
53. Terry DW Jr, Ramin JE. The navicular fat stripe: a useful roentgen feature for evaluating wrist trauma. *Am J Roentgenol* 1975;124:25–28.

54. Dias JJ, Finlay DB, Brenkel IJ, et al. Radiographic assessment of soft tissue signs in clinically suspected scaphoid fractures: the incidence of false negative and false positive results. *J Orthop Trauma* 1987;1:205–208.
55. Abdel-Salam A, Eyres KS, Cleary J. Detecting fractures of the scaphoid: the value of comparative x-rays of the uninjured wrist. *J Hand Surg [Br]* 1992;17:28–32.
56. Herbert TJ. *The fractured scaphoid.* St. Louis: Quality Medical Publishing, 1990.
57. Stecher WR. Roentgenography of the carpal navicular bone. *Am J Roentgenol* 1937;37:704–705.
58. Ziter FMH. A modified view of the carpal navicular. *Radiology* 1973;3:706–707.
59. Tiel-van Buul MM, Van Beek EJ, Dijkstra PF, et al. Radiography of the carpal scaphoid: experimental evaluation of the "carpal box" and first clinical results. *Invest Radiol* 1992;27:954–959.
60. Roolker W, Tiel-van Buul MM, Bossuyt PM, et al. Carpal box radiography in suspected scaphoid fracture. *J Bone Joint Surg Br* 1996;78:535–539.
61. Gaebler C, Kukla C, Breitenseher M, et al. Magnetic resonance imaging of occult scaphoid fractures. *J Trauma* 1996;41:73–76.
62. Thorpe AP, Murray AD, Smith FW, et al. Clinically suspected scaphoid fracture: a comparison of magnetic resonance imaging and bone scintigraphy. *Br J Radiol* 1996;69:109–113.
63. Hunter JC, Escobedo EM, Wilson AJ, et al. MR imaging of clinically suspected scaphoid fractures. *Am J Roentgenol* 1997;168:1287–1293.
64. Brown JN. The suspected scaphoid fracture and isotope bone imaging. *Injury* 1995;26:479–482.
65. Tiel-van Buul MM, Van Beek EJ, Borm JJ, et al. The value of radiographs and bone scintigraphy in suspected scaphoid fracture. A statistical analysis. *J Hand Surg [Br]* 1993;18:403–406.
66. Tiel-van Buul MM, Van Beek EJ, Broekhuizen AH, et al. Radiography and scintigraphy of suspected scaphoid fracture. A long-term study in 160 patients. *J Bone Joint Surg Br* 1993;75:61–65.
67. Lepisto J, Mattila K, Nieminen S, et al. Low field MRI and scaphoid fracture. *J Hand Surg [Br]* 1995;20:539–542.
68. Tehranzadeh J, Davenport J, Pais MJ. Scaphoid fracture: evaluation with flexion–extension tomography. *Radiology* 1990;176:167–170.
69. Linscheid RL, Dobyns JH, Younge DK. Trispiral tomography in the evaluation of wrist injury. *Bull Hosp Joint Dis Orthop Inst* 1984;44:297–308.
70. Sanders WE. Evaluation of the humpback scaphoid by computed tomography in the longitudinal axial plane of the scaphoid. *J Hand Surg [Am]* 1988;13:182–187.
71. Jonsson K, Jonsson A, Sloth M, et al. CT of the wrist in suspected scaphoid fracture. *Acta Radiol* 1992;33:500–501.
72. Bain GI, Bennett JD, Richards RS, et al. Longitudinal computed tomography of the scaphoid: a new technique. *Skel Radiol* 1995;24:271–273.
73. Hosie KB, Wardrope J, Crosby AC, et al. Liquid crystal thermography in the diagnosis of scaphoid fractures. *Arch Emerg Med* 1987;4:117–120.
74. DaCruz DJ, Taylor RH, Savage B, et al. Ultrasound assessment of the suspected scaphoid fracture. *Arch Emerg Med* 1988;5:97–100.
75. Christiansen TG, Rude C, Lauridsen KK, et al. Diagnostic value of ultrasound in scaphoid fractures. *Injury* 1991;22:397–399.
76. Hodgkinson DW, Nicholson DA, Stewart G, et al. Scaphoid fracture: a new method of assessment. *Clin Radiol* 1993;398–401.
77. Amadio PC. Scaphoid fractures. *Orthop Clin North Am* 1992;23:7–17.
78. Tiel-van Buul MM, Broekhuizen TH, Van Beek EJ, et al. Choosing a strategy for the diagnostic management of suspected scaphoid fracture: a cost-effectiveness analysis. *J Nucl Med* 1995;36:45–48.
79. Russe O. Fracture of the carpal navicular: diagnosis, nonoperative treatment and operative treatment. *J Bone Joint Surg Am* 1960;42:759–768.
80. Cooney WP, Dobyns JH, Linscheid RL. Fractures of the scaphoid: a rational approach to management. *Clin Orthop* 1980;149:90–97.
81. Herbert TJ, Fisher WE. Management of the fractured scaphoid using a new bone screw. *J Bone Joint Surg Br* 1984;66:114–123.
82. Jupiter JB. Scaphoid fractures. In: *American society for surgery of the hand: hand surgery update.* Rosemont, IL: American Academy of Orthopaedic Surgeons, 1996;77–84.
83. Eddeland A, Eiken O, Hellgren E, et al. Fractures of the scaphoid. *Scand J Plast Reconstr Surg* 1975;9:234–239.
84. London PS. The broken scaphoid bone. The case against pessimism. *J Bone Joint Surg Br* 1961;43:237–244.
85. Soto-Hall R, Haldeman KO. The conservative and operative treatment of fractures of the carpal scaphoid (navicular). *J Bone Joint Surg* 1941;23:841–850.
86. Stewart MJ. Fractures of the carpal navicular (scaphoid): a report of 436 cases. *J Bone Joint Surg Am* 1954;36:998–1006.
87. Langhoff O. Anderssen JL. Consequences of late immobilization of scaphoid fractures. *J Hand Surg [Br]* 1988;13:77–79.
88. Soto-Hall R. Recent fractures of the carpal scaphoid. *JAMA* 1945;129:335–338.
89. King RJ, Mackenney RP, Elnur S. Suggested method for closed treatment of fractures of the carpal scaphoid: hypothesis supported by dissection and clinical practice. *J R Soc Med* 1982;75:860–867.
90. Cooney WP, Linscheid RL, Dobyns JH. Fractures and dislocations of the wrist. In: Rockwood CA, Green DP, Bucholz RW, et al, eds. *Rockwood and Green's fractures in adults, 4th ed.* Philadelphia: Lippincott–Raven, 1996.
91. Yanni D, Lieppins P, Laurence M. Fractures of the carpal scaphoid: a critical study of the standard splint. *J Bone Joint Surg Br* 1991;73:600–602.
92. Goldman S, Lipscomb PR, Taylor WF. Immobilization for acute carpal scaphoid fractures. *Surg Gynecol Obstet* 1969;129:281–284.
93. Thomaidis VT. Elbow–wrist–thumb immobilization in the treatment of fractures of the carpal scaphoid. *Acta Orthop Scand* 1973;44:679–689.
94. Berlin D. Position in the treatment of fracture of the carpal scaphoid. *N Engl J Med* 1929;201:574–579.
95. Friedenberg ZB. Anatomic considerations in the treatment of carpal navicular fractures. *Am J Surg* 1949;78:379–381.
96. Hosford JP. Prognosis in fractures of the carpal scaphoid. *Proc R Soc Med* 1931;24:92–94.
97. Alho A, Kankaanpaa U. Management of fractured scaphoid bone: a prospective study of 100 fractures. *Acta Orthop Scand* 1975;46:737–743.
98. Broome A, Cedell CA, Colleen SA. High plaster immobilization for fracture of the carpal scaphoid bone. *Acta Chir Scand* 1964;128:42–44.
99. Gellman H, Caputo RJ, Carter V, et al. Comparison of short and long thumb–spica casts for non-displaced fractures of the carpal scaphoid. *J Bone Joint Surg Am* 1989;71:354–357.
100. Dehne E, Deffer PA, Feighney RE. Pathomechanics of the fracture of the carpal navicular. *J Trauma* 1964;4:96–114.
101. Verdan C. Fractures of the scaphoid. *Surg Clin North Am* 1960;40:461–464.

102. Kuhlmann JN, Boabighi A, Kirsch JM, et al. An experimental study of plaster immobilization for fractures of the carpal scaphoid: a clinical investigation. *Fr J Orthop Surg* 1987;1: 43–50.
103. Failla JM, Tashman S, Kaneshiro SA. *Quantification of scaphoid fracture displacement with forearm rotation in short-arm thumb spica cast.* Paper presented at the American Society for Surgery of the Hand Annual Meeting, Denver, CO, September 13, 1997.
104. Bora FW Jr, Culp RW, Osterman AL, et al. A flexible wrist splint. *J Hand Surg [Am]* 1989;14:574–575.
105. Prosser AJ, Brenkel IJ, Irvine GB. Articular fractures of the distal scaphoid. *J Hand Surg [Br]* 1988;13:87–91.
106. Perlik PC, Guilford WB. Magnetic resonance imaging to assess vascularity of scaphoid non-unions. *J Hand Surg [Am]* 1991;16: 479–484.
107. Green DP. The effect of avascular necrosis on Russe bone grafting for scaphoid nonunion. *J Hand Surg [Am]* 1985;10: 597–605.
108. Mulder JD. The results of 100 cases of pseudarthrosis in the scaphoid bone treated by the Matti-Russe operation. *J Bone Joint Surg Br* 1968;50:110–115.
109. Trumble TE. Avascular necrosis after scaphoid fracture. A correlation of magnetic resonance imaging and histology. *J Hand Surg [Am]* 1990;15:557–564.
110. Aaron RK, Ciombar DM, Jolly G. Stimulation of experimental endochondral ossification by low-energy pulsing electromagnetic fields. *J Bone Miner Res* 1989;4:227–233.
111. Beckenbaugh RD. Noninvasive pulsed electromagnetic stimulation in the treatment of scaphoid nonunion. *Orthop Trans* 1985; 9:444.
112. Adams BD, Frykman GK, Taleisnik J. Treatment of scaphoid nonunion with casting and pulsed electromagnetic fields: a study continuation. *J Hand Surg [Am]* 1992;17:910–913.
113. Frykman GK, Taleisnik J, Peters G, et al. Treatment of nonunited scaphoid fractures by pulsed electromagnetic field and cast. *J Hand Surg [Am]* 1986;11:344–349.
114. Kristainsen TK, Ryaby JP, McCabe J, et al. Accelerated healing of distal radial fractures with the use of specific, low-intensity ultrasound. *J Bone Joint Surg Am* 1997;79:961–973.
115. Cook SD, Ryaby JP, McCabe J, et al. Acceleration of tibia and distal radius fracture healing in patients who smoke. *Clin Orthop* 1997;337:198–207.
116. Heckman JD, Ryaby JP, McCabe J, et al. Acceleration of tibial fracture-healing by non-invasive, low-intensity pulsed ultrasound. *J Bone Joint Surg Am* 1994;76:26–34.
117. Cooney WP III, Dobyns JH, Linscheid RL. Nonunion of the scaphoid: analysis of the results from bone grafting. *J Hand Surg [Am]* 1980;5:343–354.
118. Viegas SF, Bean JW, Schram RA. Transscaphoid fracture/dislocations treated with open reduction and Herbert screw internal fixation. *J Hand Surg [Am]* 1987;12:992–999.
119. Moneim MS. Management of greater arc carpal fractures. *Hand Clin* 1988;4:457–467.
120. Inoue G, Tanaka Y, Nakamura R. Treatment of trans-scaphoid perilunate dislocations by internal fixation with the Herbert screw. *J Hand Surg [Br]* 1990;15:449–454.
121. Kaulesar-Sukal DMKS, Johannes EJ. Transscapho-transcapitate fracture dislocations of the carpus. *J Hand Surg [Am]* 1992;17: 348–353.
122. Huene DR. Primary internal fixation of carpal navicular fractures in the athlete. *Am J Sports Med* 1979;7:175–177.
123. Rettig AC, Kollias SC. Internal fixation of acute stable scaphoid fractures in the athlete. *Am J Sports Med* 1996;24:182–186.
124. Rettig AC, Weidenbener EJ, Gloyeske R. Alternative management of midthird scaphoid fractures in the athlete. *Am J Sports Med* 1994;22:711–714.
125. Gunal I, Oztuna V, Seber S. Trapezio-lunate external fixation for scaphoid fractures. *J Hand Surg [Br]* 1994;19:759–762.
126. Korkala OL, Antti-Poika IU. Late treatment of scaphoid fractures by bone grafting and compression staple osteosynthesis. *J Hand Surg [Am]* 1989;14:491–495.
127. Korkala OL, Kuokkanen HOM, Eerola MS. Compression-staple fixation for fractures, non-unions, and delayed unions of the carpal scaphoid. *J Bone Joint Surg Am* 1992;74:423–426.
128. Ender HG. Treatment of problem fractures and nonunion of the scaphoid. *Tech Orthop* 1986;1:74–78.
129. Huene DR, Huene DS. Treatment of nonunions of the scaphoid with the Ender compression blade plate system. *J Hand Surg [Am]* 1991;16:913–922.
130. McLaughlin HL. Fracture of the carpal navicular (scaphoid) bone: some observations based on treatment by open reduction and internal fixation. *J Bone Joint Surg Am* 1954;36:765–774.
131. Gasser H. Delayed union and pseudarthrosis of the carpal navicular treated by compression-screw osteosynthesis. *J Bone Joint Surg [Am]* 1965;47:249–266.
132. Maudsley RH, Chen SC. Screw fixation in the management of the fractured carpal scaphoid. *J Bone Joint Surg Br* 1972;54:432–441.
133. Wozasek G, Moser KD. Percutaneous screw fixation of fractures of the scaphoid. *J Bone Joint Surg Br* 1991;73:138–142.
134. Leyshon A, Ireland J, Trickey EL. The treatment of delayed union and non-union of the carpal scaphoid by screw fixation. *J Bone Joint Surg Br* 1984;66:124–127.
135. Heim U, Pfeiffer KM. *Internal fixation of small fractures: technique recommended by the AO–ASIF Group, 3rd ed.* Berlin: Springer-Verlag, 1988.
136. Bunker TD, McNamee PB, Scott TD. The Herbert screw for scaphoid fractures. A multicenter study. *J Bone Joint Surg Br* 1987;69:631–634.
137. Herbert TJ, Fisher WE, Leicester AW. The Herbert bone screw: a ten year perspective. *J Hand Surg [Br]* 1992;17:415–419.
138. Filan SL, Herbert TJ. Herbert screw fixation of scaphoid fractures. *J Bone Joint Surg Br* 1996;78:519–529.
139. Barton NJ. Twenty questions about scaphoid fractures. *J Hand Surg [Br]* 1992;17:289–310.
140. Compson JP, Heatley FW. Imaging the position of a screw within the scaphoid: a clinical, anatomical and radiological study. *J Bone Joint Surg Br* 1993;18:716–724.
141. Botte MJ, Gelberman RH. Modified technique for Herbert screw insertion in fractures of the scaphoid. *J Hand Surg [Am]* 1987;12:149–150.
142. Chun S, Wicks BP, Meyerdierks E, et al. Two modifications for insertion of the Herbert screw in the fractured scaphoid. *J Hand Surg [Am]* 1990;15:669–671.
143. Heaps RJ, Degnan G. A modification for the insertion of the Herbert screw in the fractured or nonunited scaphoid. *J Hand Surg [Am]* 1996;21:922–924.
144. Alnot JY, Bellan N, Oberlin C, et al. Fractures and nonunions of the proximal pole of the carpal scaphoid bone: internal fixation by a proximal to distal screw. *Ann Chir Main* 1988;7:101–108.
145. DeMaagd RL, Engber WD. Retrograde Herbert screw fixation for treatment of proximal pole scaphoid nonunions. *J Hand Surg [Am]* 1989:14:996–1002.
146. Amadio PC, Taleisnik J. Fractures of the carpal bones. In: Green DP, Hotchkiss RN, eds. *Operative hand surgery.* New York: Churchill Livingstone, 1993;799–860.
147. Whipple TL. The role of arthroscopy in the treatment of intra-articular wrist fractures. *Hand Clin* 1995;11:13–18.
148. Wozasek GE, Moser KD. Indications for percutaneous screw fixation of scaphoid fractures. *Unfallchirurg* 1991;94:342–345.

149. Streli R. Perkutane Verschraubung des Hand Kahnbeines mit Bohrdrahtkompressionsschraube. *Zentralbl Chir* 1970;95:1060–1078.
150. Christodoulou AG, Colton CL. Scaphoid fractures in children. *J Pediatr Orthop* 1986;6:37–39.
151. Armstrong PF, Joughin VE, Clarke HM. Pediatric fractures of the forearm, wrist, and hand. In: Green NE, Swiontkowski MF, eds. *Skeletal trauma in children.* Philadelphia: WB Saunders, 1994;127–211.
152. Southcott R, Rosman MA. Non-union of carpal scaphoid fractures in children. *J Bone Joint Surg Br* 1977;59:20–23.
153. Culp RW, Lemel M, Taras JS. Complications of common carpal injuries. *Hand Clin* 1994;10:139–155.
154. Harvey FJ, Harvey PM. Three rare causes of extensor tendon rupture. *J Hand Surg [Am]* 1989;14:957–962.
155. Cross AB. Rupture of the flexor pollicis longus tendon resulting from the non-union of a scaphoid fracture. *J Hand Surg [Br]* 1988;13:80–82.
156. Smith DK, An KN, Cooney WP III, et al. Effects of a scaphoid waist osteotomy on carpal kinematics. *J Orthop Res* 1989;7:590–598.
157. Lindstrom G, Nystrom A. Incidence of post-traumatic arthrosis after primary healing of scaphoid fractures: a clinical and radiologic study. *J Hand Surg [Br]* 1990;15:11–13.
158. Ruby LK, Stinson J, Belsky MR. The natural history of scaphoid non-union: a review of fifty-five cases. *J Bone Joint Surg Am* 1985;67:428–432.
159. Dias JJ, Brenkel IJ, Finlay DBL. Patterns of union in fractures of the waist of the scaphoid. *J Bone Joint Surg Br* 1989;71:307–310.
160. Vender MI, Watson HK, Wiener BD, et al. Degenerative changes in symptomatic scaphoid nonunion. *J Hand Surg [Am]* 1987;12:514–519.
161. Birchard D, Pichora D. Experimental corrective scaphoid osteotomy for scaphoid malunion with abnormal wrist mechanics. *J Hand Surg [Am]* 1990;15:863–868.
162. Nakamura P, Imaeda T, Miura T. Scaphoid malunion. *J Bone Joint Surg Br* 1991;73:134–137.
163. Lynch NM, Linscheid RL. Corrective osteotomy for scaphoid malunion: technique and long-term follow-up evaluation. *J Hand Surg [Am]* 1997;22:35–43.
164. Dias JJ, Taylor M, Thompson J, et al. Radiographic signs of union of scaphoid fractures: an analysis of inter-observer agreement and reproducibility. *J Bone Joint Surg Br* 1988;70:299–301.
165. Dickison JC, Shannon JG. Fractures of the carpal scaphoid in the Canadian army: a review and commentary. *Surg Gynecol Obstet* 1944;79:225–239.
166. Taleisnik J. *The wrist.* New York: Churchill Livingstone, 1985.

14

CARPAL DISLOCATIONS AND INSTABILITY

RICHARD S. IDLER

Carpal dislocation may be defined as the loss of contact at one or more articulations involving one or more carpal bones. Carpal dislocation occurs most frequently as a result of trauma but may also develop secondary to inflammatory arthropathy, congenital ligamentous laxity, or connective tissue disease. Traumatic carpal dislocations are only part of a spectrum of injuries that can occur about the wrist. Mayfield pointed out that injuries about the wrist will be influenced by the direction of loading, the magnitude and direction of force, and the properties of the involved bones and ligaments (1). The magnitude of force required for acute carpal ligament disruption is considerable (2). To create a carpal dislocation, these forces must be applied to a population of patients in whom the ligamentous structures of the wrist are at least as vulnerable, if not more vulnerable, to failure as the adjacent osseous structures. These factors tend to select a predominantly young to middle-aged adult male population involved in vehicular accidents, falls, or crush injuries as the prime candidates for carpal dislocation.

Based on common pathomechanics and anatomic patterns of injuries, carpal dislocations may be classified into perilunar, radiocarpal, midcarpal, axial, and isolated carpal dislocations (Fig. 14.1). By far the most frequent traumatic carpal dislocations are perilunar dislocations and fracture dislocations. Less common are radiocarpal and axial pattern carpal dislocations. Although isolated dislocation of every carpal bone has been reported, these remain unusual injuries in their pure form. Midcarpal dislocation must be an extremely rare, traumatic occurrence, as a pure dislocation has yet to be reported (3).

Following reduction of a carpal dislocation, the resultant ligamentous disruption may leave the carpus unstable. It is now understood that certain patterns of carpal dislocation represent a terminal event in an injury sequence that can be staged into intermediate levels of injuries. Common patterns of carpal instability, therefore, can occur as a result of an intermediate level of injury or incomplete recovery from carpal dislocation (Table 14.1).

Compared with the incidence of other types of injuries about the wrist, carpal dislocations are relatively infrequent and are not fully understood by all health care providers called on to treat such injuries. When these injuries are overlooked or misdiagnosed, there is a predictably poor prognosis. Although greater understanding of these injuries has led to a more aggressive approach to treatment, the ability to repair ligament disruption and cartilage damage, and to prevent joint arthrofibrosis secondary to trauma and immobilization remains limited. Carpal dislocations are significant wrist injuries, and even when they are correctly diagnosed and treated, there may be residual impairment and the potential for secondary complications.

PERILUNAR DISLOCATION

Perilunar dislocations are the most common type of carpal dislocation (4–6). They are part of a staged pattern of injury centered around the lunate. Perilunar dislocations can be further subdivided into pure ligamentous injuries, also referred to as lesser arc injuries, which include both lunate and perilunate dislocations, and greater arc injuries, which comprise a transosseous pattern involving one or more carpal bones in the injury path about the lunate (7) (Fig. 14.2). Perilunar dislocations are produced by high-energy injuries, most frequently resulting from motor vehicle accidents, sports injuries, and falls from substantial heights. The population primarily at risk is male young adults.

Within the group of lesser arc injuries are perilunate and lunate dislocations. Both have been shown to be produced by the same mechanism of injury, with the lunate dislocation representing a more extensive form of injury (1,8). The difference between the two patterns of dislocation is best defined by the relationship of the lunate with the radius. In

---

R. S. Idler: Indiana Hand Center, Indiana University Medical School, Indianapolis, Indiana 46280

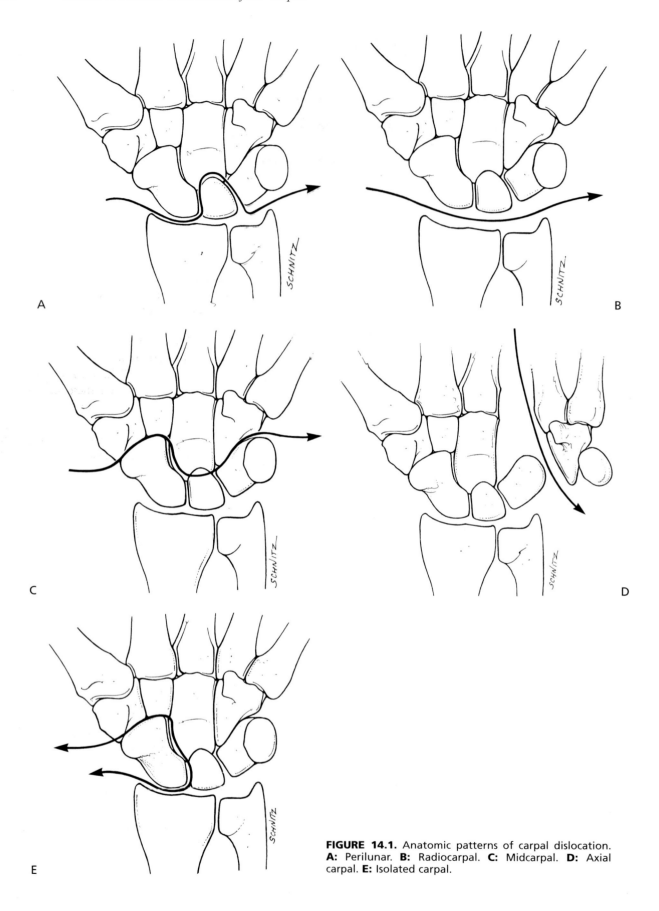

FIGURE 14.1. Anatomic patterns of carpal dislocation. **A:** Perilunar. **B:** Radiocarpal. **C:** Midcarpal. **D:** Axial carpal. **E:** Isolated carpal.

TABLE 14.1. CARPAL INSTABILITY PATTERNS ASSOCIATED WITH TYPES OF CARPAL DISLOCATION

Carpal Dislocation	Carpal Instability
Perilunar	Scapholunate dissociation
	Lunatotriquetral dissociation
	Dorsal intercalated segmental instability
	Volar intercalated segmental instability
Radiocarpal	Palmar carpal subluxation
	Ulnar translation

lunate dislocation, the proximal articular surface of the lunate is dislocated from that of the distal radius. In perilunate dislocation, the proximal articular surface of the lunate retains contact with the distal radius, and it is the remainder of the carpus that is dislocated. Both palmar and dorsal patterns of perilunate and lunate dislocation have been reported (Fig. 14.3). The dorsal–perilunate/volar–lunate dislocation is considerably more common than the volar–perilunate/dorsal–lunate dislocation (9,10).

Greater arc injuries are defined as a perilunar pattern of dislocation that includes a transosseous path involving at least one carpal bone (7,11,12). The simplest and perhaps most common form of greater arc injury or perilunate fracture dislocation is the transscaphoid pattern (6,9,13–17). In its most extensive form, the osseous pattern begins at the radial styloid and transverses through the scaphoid, capi-

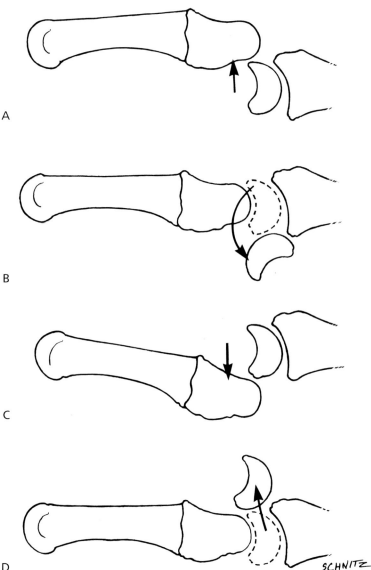

FIGURE 14.3. Patterns of lesser arc injuries. **A:** Dorsal perilunate dislocation. **B:** Palmar lunate dislocation. **C:** Palmar perilunate dislocation. **D:** Dorsal lunate dislocation.

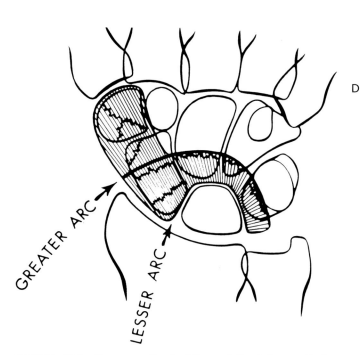

FIGURE 14.2. Diagrammatic depiction of the injury path for greater and lesser arc perilunar dislocations. (From Johnson RP. The acutely injured wrist and its residual. *Clin Orthop* 1980;149: 33–36, with permission.)

tate, hamate, and triquetrum and terminates through the ulnar styloid. Between these two extremes are numerous other fracture dislocation patterns. As with lesser arc injuries, in greater arc injuries there is the potential for the lunate to remain aligned with the distal radius or to be part of the component that is dislocated. In specific injury patterns, there may be both palmar and dorsal variants of the dislocation.

In the original investigation and description of lesser arc injuries by Mayfield et al. (8), the potential for associated radial styloid fractures was documented. This has generated some confusion as to how to interpret an injury pattern that includes both a radial styloid fracture and a perilunate pattern of dislocation (11). Small styloid tip and palmar radial avulsion fractures in association with a perilunate or lunate dislocation are consistent with a lesser arc injury. Larger styloid fractures, as suggested by Mayfield, may also result from the same injury mechanism that creates a perilunate dislocation but may also be explained by other mechanisms as well (18) (Fig. 14.4). There is increasing documentation of intrinsic and extrinsic carpal ligament injuries with both intra- and extraarticular fractures of the distal radius (19,20). When the primary focus of the instability of the injury becomes the distal radius, it is best to consider this a variation of a distal radius fracture-dislocation as opposed to a carpal fracture-dislocation.

Of all types of carpal dislocation, the most extensively studied is the perilunar pattern (1,2,7,8). In the now classic work of Mayfield, Johnson, and Kilcoyne, the pathomechanics and progressive stages leading toward perilunate instability were defined (8). Both greater and lesser arc injuries could be produced with an axial load to the wrist producing hyperextension, ulnar deviation, and intercarpal supination. A greater arc injury is most likely to result when the initial load places the wrist in hyperextension, causing the scaphoid to fracture through an extension bending force. When this is followed by ulnar deviation and intercarpal supination, a transscaphoid perilunate dislocation is created. When the most significant load occurs in ulnar deviation and intercarpal supination, a pure ligamentous lesser arc injury is more likely. These investigators were able to show that lunate dislocation was the end stage in a spectrum of injuries produced by the same pathomechanic mechanism. They classified perilunate instability into four stages: stage I, scaphoid dislocation; stage II, capitate dislocation; stage III, triquetral dislocation (perilunate dislocation); and stage IV, lunate dislocation. These stages of perilunate injury are associated with specific ligament injuries and patterns of carpal instability. Stage I injury will produce a scapholunate dissociation. Stage II injury will result in scapholunate dissociation with dorsal intercalated segmental collapse. Stage III injury creates a dorsal perilunate pattern of dislocation. Palmar lunate dislocation will be seen following stage IV injury.

Other loading sequences may produce a perilunar dislocation (Fig. 14.4).

Wrist hyperflexion has been proposed as a mechanism for volar–perilunate/dorsal–lunate dislocations (21–23). It has been suggested that a perilunar injury may be initiated from the ulnar side of the wrist (24–26). Intermediate stages of such an injury pattern would explain lunatotriquetral dissociation and volar intercalated segmental collapse. To date, the experimental reproduction of such an injury pattern in the laboratory similar to the work performed by Mayfield, Johnson, and Kilcoyne has yet to be reported. The necessary wrist position and sequence of loading for such an injury have yet to be defined.

As noted by Mayfield, an important key component in the occurrence of perilunar dislocation is the properties of the involved bone and ligaments (1). These injuries are rare in children and elderly adults. Perilunate dislocations and fracture-dislocations are sufficiently infrequent in the pediatric population to warrant case reports (27–31). Both populations represent situations in which the distal radius with injury is at greatest risk of failure because of the presence of a growth plate or osteoporotic bone.

Evaluation

Because the majority of perilunar dislocations will result from high-energy accidents such as vehicular crashes and falls from significant heights, these patients must undergo a comprehensive examination for the presence of injuries other than just to the wrist. The occurrence of associated life-threatening trauma may divert attention away from the wrist injury and lead to a delay in diagnosis and treatment.

Evaluation of the injured wrist should begin with inspection for open wounds or penetrating trauma. This not only influences the timing of treatment but may also be a prognostic indicator of a potentially worse result (9). Significant swelling and deformity will be found in both greater and lesser arc injury patterns. In a perilunate dislocation or fracture-dislocation, the hand will not be collinear with the forearm. In a volar or dorsal lunate dis-

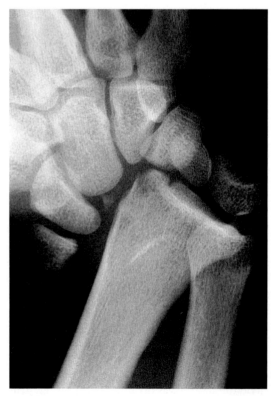

FIGURE 14.4. An example of a perilunate dislocation with a significant radial styloid fracture. It is likely this injury occurred secondary to loading of the wrist in radial deviation with a compression shear fracture of the radial styloid.

location, the hand–forearm alignment may appear normal, but a prominence or swelling may be noted either palmarly or dorsally, depending on the direction of lunate dislocation. Symptoms of median nerve injury are common with perilunar dislocations; therefore, a thorough neurologic examination is important. It is extremely difficult to distinguish clinically among median nerve dysfunction caused by elevated carpal tunnel pressures, median nerve compression from carpal displacement, and direct median nerve injury secondary to contusion or stretch. Postreduction carpal tunnel pressure measurements are of benefit in this situation.

Radiographic evaluation should consist of posteroanterior (PA) and lateral neutral-rotation views of the wrist. The injured wrist is easily positioned for these views. The lateral projection is most helpful and will demonstrate the abnormal relationship among the lunate, distal radius, and capitate. As recommended by Hill, *always watch the lunate* (32). In the case of perilunate dislocation on the lateral view, the lunate maintains its articulation with the radius, but the capitate will be displaced either palmarly or dorsally from the lunate. On a PA view with a perilunate dislocation, the carpus will be foreshortened, there will be overlap of the lunate and capitate, and the normal carpal arcs of Gilula will be disrupted (33) (Fig. 14.5). Klein described the "crowded" carpal sign in association with palmar perilunate dislocations (34). This involves an overlap of the proximal and distal carpal rows on PA radiographs (Fig. 14.6). With a lunate dislocation on the lateral view, the lunate will be dislocated palmarly or dorsally to the distal radius and capitate. The capitate will remain collinear with the radius. The lunate pivots on a hinge of proximal capsule, rotating its articular surfaces 90° to the longitudinal axis of the wrist, creating what is known as the "spilled teacup sign" (35). On the PA view with a lunate dislocation, there is disruption of Gilula's lines with a lunate that is triangular in shape and overlaps the capitate (Fig. 14.7).

Greater arc injuries will appear radiographically similar to perilunate dislocations with the inclusion of one or more carpal fractures and/or radial–ulnar styloid fractures. The most common pattern of greater arc injury is the transscaphoid perilunate fracture dislocation (Fig. 14.8). Another pattern that requires careful evaluation is the transscaphoid, transcapitate, perilunate fracture-dislocation. This pattern is sometimes also referred to as the scaphocapitate fracture syndrome (11,15,36–38) (Fig. 14.9). With this specific fracture dislocation, it is possible for the proximal fragment of the capitate to rotate up to 180°. The radiographic interpretation of unreduced greater arc injuries is even more challenging than lesser arc injuries. Determination of the extent of osseous pathology may be difficult on prereduction injury films. Obtaining radiographs of the acutely injured wrist in traction (the so-called exploded view of the wrist) can be quite beneficial in documenting the path of injury (34). More detailed information provided by computed tomography (CT) scans and

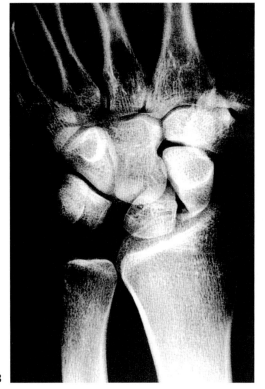
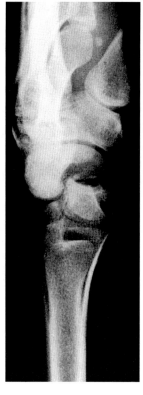

FIGURE 14.5. Posteroanterior (PA) **(A)** and lateral **(B)** radiographs of a dorsal perilunate dislocation. On the lateral view, note the loss of the normal collinear relationship of the capitate and radius. The PA view shows a disruption of Gilula's lines with overlap of the lunate by the head of the capitate.

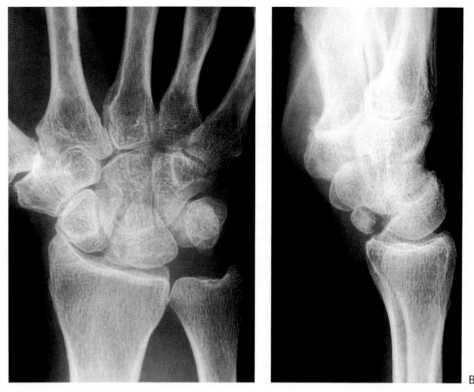

FIGURE 14.6. Posteroanterior **(A)** and lateral **(B)** radiographs of a palmar perilunate dislocation. The degree of overlap between the proximal and distal rows is greater with the palmar perilunate dislocation than the dorsal perilunate dislocation, creating the "crowded" carpal sign described by Klein (34).

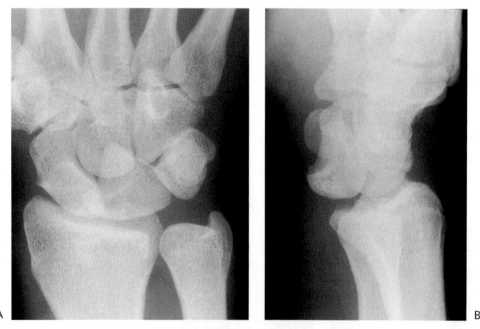

FIGURE 14.7. Posteroanterior (PA) **(A)** and lateral **(B)** radiographs of a palmar lunate dislocation. The PA view demonstrates disruption of Gilula's lines with a triangular lunate that overlaps the capitate. The lateral view demonstrates the palmarly dislocated lunate. **Editors' Notes:** *This is the extreme example of a volar intercalated segment instability (VISI) position but makes the point nicely that if the lunate is triangular, it is volarflexed whether dislocated as seen here or still located in the wrist. A severe dorsal intercalated segment instability (DISI) position of the lunate will demonstrate a quadrangular-shaped lunate on the PA view.*

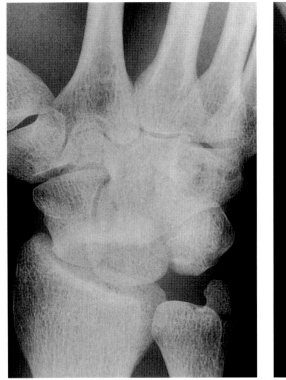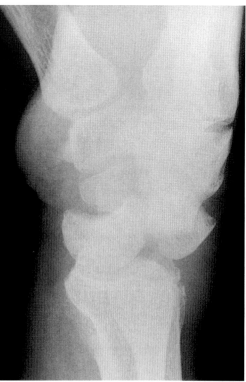

FIGURE 14.8. Posteroanterior (PA) **(A)** and lateral **(B)** radiographs of a dorsal transscaphoid perilunate dislocation. The scaphoid fracture is more apparent on the postreduction PA view.

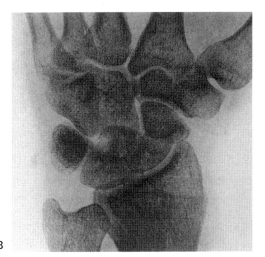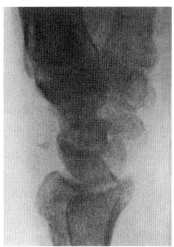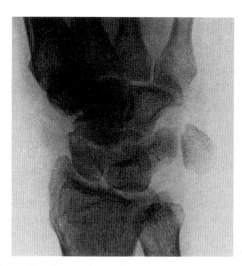

FIGURE 14.9. Posteroanterior **(A)**, lateral **(B)**, and oblique **(C)** radiographs of a scaphocapitate fracture syndrome. The position of the proximal capitate head is highlighted. Note the 180° rotation in its position. (From Fenton RL. The naviculocapitate fracture syndrome. *J Bone Joint Surg Am* 1956;38:681–684, with permission.)

tomography can be helpful in the analysis of both acute and chronic carpal fracture dislocations.

Treatment

Factors that have been shown to influence results in the treatment of perilunar dislocations include open injury, delayed treatment, and nonanatomic reduction (9,16). In general, an open injury is a reflection of a higher-energy trauma. The negative influence of this occurrence on the outcome of treatment probably relates to greater osseous displacement and associated soft tissue trauma. Delayed treatment of perilunar dislocations is not an uncommon phenomenon given the high frequency with which the diagnosis is initially missed. The frequency with which this occurs in reported case series varies from 25% to 43% (6,9,16,39,40). A multicenter series of perilunar dislocations reported by Garcia-Elias et al. noted a statistically significant impact on results when treatment was delayed longer than 1 week (16). In a similar multicenter study reported by Herzberg et al., this effect on outcome was not noted until a delay in treatment of more than 45 days (9). Although a nonanatomic reduction does not preclude a satisfactory result, numerous authors have noted the association between a poor result and a nonanatomic reduction (5,6,9,14,16,41). Failure to achieve an anatomic reduction in the management of perilunar dislocation may result in the occurrence of scapholunate dissociation, lunatotriquetral dissociation, and intercalated segmental collapse. In perilunar fracture-dislocations, in addition to the potential for carpal instability, the incidence of fracture nonunion and avascular necrosis is greater.

There has been some controversy in the literature as to whether or not there is a difference in outcome between perilunate dislocations and perilunate fracture-dislocations. Case series reported in the earlier literature suggested a worse prognosis for perilunate fracture dislocation (6,14, 41–43), whereas more recent case series have shown no statistical difference in results between the two injury patterns (9,16,39). Review of the earlier literature reveals a more conservative approach toward management, with a high percentage of cases being managed closed. More recent techniques for management of a perilunate fracture dislocation have involved open techniques with rigid internal fixation, which has decreased the occurrence of nonanatomic reduction and carpal nonunion.

Commonly recommended treatment options for perilunar dislocation and fracture-dislocation include closed reduction and cast immobilization, percutaneous pinning, or open reduction and internal fixation. Historically, closed reduction and cast immobilization has been the most common form of treatment for perilunar dislocation (4,6,14,15, 32,39,41,44). Good results have been reported with this conservative form of treatment, but concerns have been raised regarding its predictability. Numerous investigators have reported on the failure of closed techniques to maintain an anatomic reduction (12,13,15,44–47). In the management of perilunate dislocation, this loss of reduction leads to residual carpal instability and, in the case of perilunate fracture-dislocations, increases the likelihood of fracture nonunion and avascular necrosis. Although closed reduction and cast immobilization remain an acceptable method for treatment of perilunar dislocation, alternative measures must always be considered if a nonanatomic reduction cannot be achieved and/or maintained.

Percutaneous pinning is an alternative to cast immobilization if an anatomic reduction can be achieved. A small number of cases of percutaneous pinning have been reported among the various case series reviewing treatment for perilunar dislocations (9,16,48). There are no large or prospective studies comparing this technique with other forms of treatment for perilunate dislocation. The series reported by Rabb compared five cases of closed reduction and percutaneous pinning to five cases of open reduction and internal fixation for perilunate dislocation in football players (48). The study indicated that the players treated with percutaneous pinning were able to return to competitive play earlier than the players treated by open technique. Long-term outcome with both forms of treatment, however, was not reported. Percutaneous pinning can be technically difficult, particularly in the management of perilunate fracture dislocation. The exact role for closed reduction and percutaneous pinning in the management of perilunar dislocation remains uncertain, but it is probably best reserved as supplemental stabilization reduction in the management of perilunate dislocations that can be easily reduced and are relatively stable to provocative stress.

Based on the unpredictability of closed reduction with cast immobilization and the technical difficulty associated with percutaneous pinning, open reduction with internal fixation is currently the recommended treatment of choice for both perilunar dislocations and fracture-dislocations (9,12,13,49–51). Open treatment permits direct assessment of the anatomic pathology; facilitates carpal manipulation, allowing for more accurate reduction; and provides the opportunity for ligament repair, augmentation, or reconstruction. Internal fixation enhances stabilization during the healing process required for both bone and ligament. The more recent use of medullary compression screws has improved the success rate for fracture union. The surgical approach for open reduction will vary with the direction and severity of the dislocation. A palmar approach has been recommended for the management of transscaphoid perilunate dislocations (52,53). Moneim has recommended the use of a dorsal approach in the management of most perilunate dislocations and fracture-dislocations, and this approach has been used successfully by others as well (12,13,15,44,49,52). Most recently, investigators have been stressing the importance of ligament repair in the management of both perilunar dislocation and fracture-dislocation. For this reason, a combined palmar and dorsal approach has been recommended. Review of the literature by Sotereanos et al. comparing wrist score reports following open treatment for perilunar dislocations and fracture dislocations found there was no significant difference in the percentage of patients with satisfactory results when surgery was performed by a volar, dorsal, or combined approach (51).

Among the more frequent injuries associated with perilunar dislocation are median neuropathy and avascular necrosis. The incidence of median neuropathy occurring with perilunar dislocation ranges from 11% to 45% in reported case series. Of interest is the fact that in these series a palmar or combined open approach was used infrequently. The majority of median nerve symptoms resolved spontaneously and only on rare occasion required secondary carpal tunnel decompression (13,16,42,44,49,51). Although it would be assumed that avascular necrosis of the lunate would be a significant risk following lunate dislocation, this is actually an unusual occurrence. When it does occur, it is probably related to the degree of initial lunate displacement and injury to the capsular flap on which the lunate normally hinges (9,15–17,42,54). On the other hand, with a perilunar fracture dislocation, avascular necrosis of the proximal pole of the scaphoid, and occasionally the lunate, is not infrequently seen (15,16,42).

Review of the literature for assessment of outcome following treatment for perilunar dislocation is difficult because most case series include multiple injury types with mixed treatment methods and limited long-term follow-up. It is known that no treatment because of a missed diagnosis leads to poor wrist function and posttraumatic arthrosis (9,39,55,56). Despite the fact that diminished results can be expected with delayed treatment, attempts at open reduction and internal fixation for unreduced perilunar dislocations are recommended up to 4 months postinjury (44,57). When indicated, alternative forms of treatment for the unreduced, chronic perilunar dislocation include proximal row carpectomy and wrist arthrodesis. Patients with closed perilunar dislocations treated in a timely fashion by closed or open methods and able to achieve and maintain an anatomic reduction can expect a satisfactory outcome (9,11,15,16,49,51). Some loss of wrist motion and grip strength can be expected, but most patients will recover a functional range that will permit a return to work (15,51). Of concern is the fact that, despite a favorable early clinical result, radiographic evaluation in these same patients shows a high frequency of residual carpal instability and posttraumatic arthritis (9,5,11). Longer-term follow-up studies are needed to assess the impact these radiographic findings will ultimately have on the clinical result.

Closed Reduction

The ideal setting for an attempted closed reduction is in the operating room with an axillary block anesthetic, tourniquet control, and image intensification. The muscle relaxation achieved with an axillary block makes closed reduction much easier. Tourniquet control minimizes swelling during manipulation. Image intensification will allow for detailed examination of associated fractures and stress loading of the reduction to assess its instability. In a situation where operating time is unavailable and there is concern about neurovascular compromise, an attempt at closed reduction may be made under wrist-level regional anesthetic or bier block. Without muscle relaxation, reduction may be difficult to achieve, and persistent attempts should not be made if initial attempts are unsuccessful.

Once adequate anesthesia has been achieved, the arm is suspended in finger trap traction with 10 to 15 lb of weight. After 10 to 15 minutes to allow for muscle relaxation, closed reduction may be attempted. For a dorsal perilunate dislocation, the lunate is stabilized by placing the thumb volarly. With the axial traction, the wrist is hyperextended to unlock any soft tissue entrapment, and then, with flexion, the capitate is reduced to its articulation with the lunate. For a lunate dislocation, after application of longitudinal traction, it may be possible to achieve reduction by direct pressure to the lunate. If this is not successful, a simultaneous translation force should be applied to the distal carpal row and lunate converting it to a perilunate dislocation. The lunate is now stabilized to the radius (by manual pressure or percutaneous pinning) and the distal carpal row reduced as described with a perilunate dislocation. If a closed reduction cannot be achieved, open reduction is required.

Operative Treatment

The surgical management for perilunate dislocation involves both a palmar and dorsal approach. The availability of sterile horizontal traction is beneficial for this surgical procedure. The wrist is first approached through a dorsal midline incision. The third compartment is incised, and the extensor pollicis longus tendon transposed. The second and fourth dorsal compartments are mobilized by subperiosteal dissection, preserving the proximal origins of the wrist capsule. The wrist capsule is carefully inspected for evidence of dorsal ligament disruption. Incorporating the original capsular injury with a ligament-sparing dorsal capsulotomy as proposed by Berger and Bishop allows maximum preservation of wrist capsular structures for dorsal capsulodesis (58). With the carpus exposed, the sites and degree of interosseous ligament disruption within the proximal row can be assessed. If the carpus has not yet been reduced, this can be accomplished with axial traction and direct manipulation of the involved carpal bones.

An extended carpal tunnel incision is used to approach the palmar aspect of the wrist. In the case of a palmar lunate dislocation, great care must be taken when dividing the transverse carpal ligament not to injure the median nerve, which will be intimately against the deep surface of the ligament and may be displaced from its normal position. Division of the transverse carpal ligament can be facilitated by first identifying the median nerve proximal to the carpal canal and then placing an elevator or hemostat between the nerve and transverse carpal ligament before dividing the transverse carpal ligament. The median nerve should be carefully inspected after release of the transverse carpal ligament for findings that suggest direct trauma to the nerve, as this may have a different prognosis than simple nerve compression or transient ischemia. With the extended carpal tunnel approach, the contents of the carpal canal can be easily manipulated for exposure of the palmar wrist capsule.

If the patient has a greater arc injury with carpal fractures requiring internal fixation, or should there be substantial radial and/or ulnar styloid fractures, these injuries are best addressed at this time. Carpal fractures may be addressed from a dorsal approach, although some scaphoid fractures are more easily managed from a palmar exposure. Most fractures can be stabilized with K-wires; however, when possible, intramedullary screws are preferred to obtain rigid internal fixation and to eliminate the need for secondary hardware removal. The availability of a cannulated screw system facilitates hardware placement. Radial styloid fractures can be openly reduced and stabilized by two 0.45 K-wires or a combination of a pericutaneous compression screw and a supplemental K-wire to prevent rotation. To avoid injury to the dorsoradial sensory nerve and radial artery, this fixation is best placed through a small incision over the safe zone of the anatomic snuff box (59). Ulnar styloid fractures are approached through a separate longitudinal incision placed just palmar to the sixth dorsal compartment. A tension band technique is usually sufficient for stabilization of the ulnar styloid.

Attention is next directed to the palmar wrist capsule. An effort is made to identify the radioscaphocapitate ligament, the long radiolunate ligament, and the volar lunatotriquetral ligament for repair. Because the radiocapitate and long radiolunate ligaments are intraarticular structures, their initial identification is facilitated through the dorsal incision. Repair is then accomplished with a 3-0 or 2-0 nonabsorbable suture.

In the treatment of a perilunate dislocation, the scapholunate ligament is of primary concern. Berger identified the dorsal component as the primary stabilizer (60). The specific site of injury is identified, and ligament repair is performed using a 3-0 nonabsorbable suture. Our intraoperative experience has been that the ligament usually detaches from the scaphoid, although it may tear intrasubstance or detach from the lunate. With an intrasubstance tear, direct ligament repair is attempted using figure-of-eight or mattress sutures. If the ligament detaches from bone, ligament repair through drill holes placed in the bone is preferred over suture anchors. The technique of ligament repair to the scaphoid as described by Taleisnik is ideal, but technically difficult (61). We have concentrated our efforts on repair of the dorsal portion of the scapholunate ligament and can typically place only two or three mattress sutures to accomplish this. Suture passage through the drill holes in bone can be facilitated with the use of a meniscal repair needle and wire suture passer (Fig. 14.10). In the presence of dorsal intercalated segmental collapse, the lunate tends to assume a dorsiflexed position. Placement of a stout K-wire into the dorsum of the lunate as a joystick is helpful in controlling its position. Once manipulated into a neutral position, the lunate can be temporarily transfixed to the capitate by K-wire fixation, and the joystick eliminated. Next, 0.54-in. K-wires are placed pericutaneously from the safe zone of the anatomic snuff box into the scaphoid directed toward the lunate and more distally toward the capitate. The position of these pins is carefully checked to make certain they do not interfere with the preplaced ligament sutures. Under fluoroscopic control, the scaphoid is reduced relative to the capitate and the lunate by palmar pressure applied to the distal pole of the scaphoid with dorsal manipulation of the proximal pole of the scaphoid using a dental pick or similar instrument. Once the scaphoid is in a reduced position, the preplaced K-wires are driven across the scapholunate and scaphocapitate joints. The position of the reduction is confirmed with care taken to make certain that the scapholunate reduction is 2 mm or less. Once an acceptable reduction has been confirmed, the ligament sutures are tied. If it is found that there is deficient tissue for scapholunate ligament repair, a triquetral-based segment of the dorsal scaphotriquetral or radiotriquetral ligament can be mobilized for incorporation into the scapholunate ligament repair. An alternative is to perform a ligament reconstruction using a tendon transfer or transverse carpal ligament graft (62).

To further stabilize the scaphoid, a dorsal scaphoid capsulodesis is performed. Depending on the surgical approach to the dorsum of the wrist and available tissue, this may be

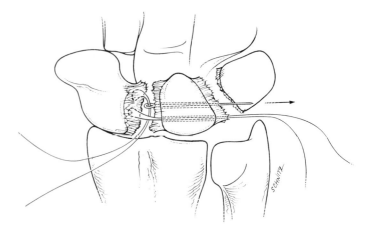

FIGURE 14.10. Technique of suture passage for scapholunate ligament repair using a wire loop or suture passer.

accomplished with a proximally based capsulodesis as suggested by Blatt (63) or using a portion of the scaphotriquetral ligament as described by the Mayo Clinic group (64). Alternatively, a distally based tenodesis can be performed as suggested by Braun using a strip of the extensor carpi radialis brevis tendon (64) (Fig. 14.11) or flexor carpi radialis tendon as described by Brunelli (65). If the capsulodesis is to be anchored to the distal pole of the scaphoid, a small trough is made transversely across the dorsum of the scaphoid just proximal to the articular surface of the distal pole. Drill holes are then placed from the trough emerging out the palmar aspect of the distal pole of the scaphoid. The necessary length of the tissue for the capsulodesis is determined, and it is trimmed to length. A 3-0 or 2-0 nonabsorbable suture is placed at the end of the capsular flap using a horizontal mattress stitch and passed through the drill holes on Keith needles. A small palmar incision over the distal pole of the scaphoid allows this suture to be tied directly over bone.

For stabilization of the lunatotriquetral ligament disruption, two 0.45 K-wires are placed pericutaneously from an ulnar approach across the joint. Based on the work of Viegas et al. indicating that the volar lunatotriquetral ligament is the most important for stabilization of the lunatotriquetral joint, this ligament is repaired through the palmar exposure (26). If there is a volar intercalated segmental collapse, efforts are made to repair the dorsal radiotriquetral ligament and any injury to the palmar ulnar midcarpal ligaments.

After ligament repairs and internal stabilization have been completed, any fixation K-wires are cut subcutaneously, and the palmar and dorsal incisions are closed over suction drains. The extremity is immobilized in a long arm thumb–spica dressing or cast for 6 weeks. This is followed by 4 weeks in a short arm thumb–spica. Tomograms are obtained at this time when required to confirm healing of associated carpal fractures. Subcutaneous pins are removed after 10 to 12 weeks. Wrist mobilization and strengthening are then progressed as tolerated (Fig. 14.12).

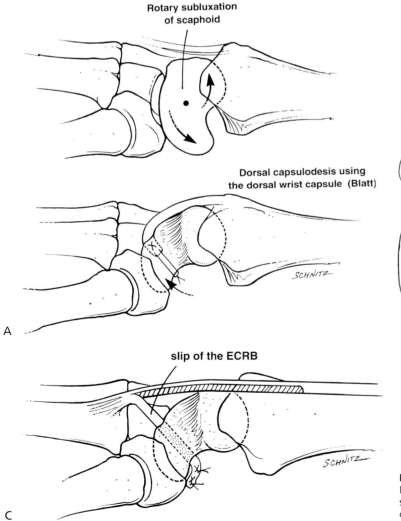
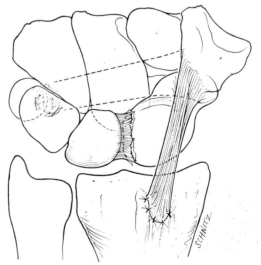

FIGURE 14.11. Technique for scaphoid capsulodesis. **A:** Proximally based dorsal wrist capsule (63). **B:** Distally based scaphotriquetral ligament (64). **C:** Distally based extensor carpi radialis brevis tenodesis (64).

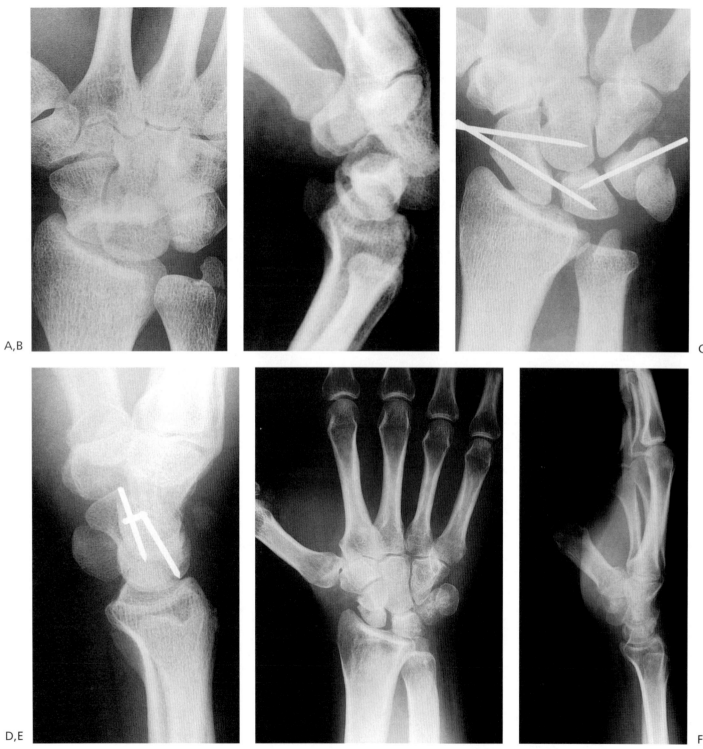

FIGURE 14.12. A 35-year-old construction worker who sustained a crush injury of his left wrist with open dorsal perilunar dislocation of his left wrist **(A,B)**. He was treated with wound debridement, open reduction, scapholunate ligament repair using a transferred portion of the dorsal scaphotriquetral ligament, and a Blatt capsulodesis. Internal fixation was achieved with three 0.45 K-wires. **C,D:** Through an extended carpal tunnel incision, the palmar lunatotriquetral ligament was repaired. **E,F:** Final follow-up at 7 months postinjury.

RADIOCARPAL DISLOCATION

For purposes of this discussion, a dislocation of the radiocarpal joint will be defined as loss of articular contact between the proximal carpal row and distal radius not in association with a biomechanically significant fracture of the distal radius. The important distinction being made between a dislocation and a fracture-dislocation is the primary site of injury: loss of stability is ligamentous in the dislocation and osseous in the fracture-dislocation. Moneim et al. have classified radiocarpal dislocations into two groups. Type I radiocarpal dislocation occurs with the proximal row intact. Type II radiocarpal dislocation occurs with a concurrent proximal row dissociative injury (66) (Fig. 14.13).

By this strict definition, these injuries are quite rare, and their occurrence still justifies a case report. Both palmar and dorsal radiocarpal dislocations have been reported, and all cases of dorsal radiocarpal dislocation have been associated with avulsion fractures of the dorsal rim of the radius (66–68).

The exact mechanism of injury involved in a radiocarpal dislocation is not known. Forces similar to those required to produce a perilunate dislocation have been implicated, as have distraction and shear forces (67–70). Rosado, in a case report of a palmar radiocarpal dislocation, stated that dorsiflexion with a shear force was responsible (69). He speculated that radiocarpal dislocation was an intermediate stage in the pathomechanics of a lunate dislocation. Weiss et al., using a cadaver model, produced a dorsal radiocarpal dislocation with disruption of the distal radioulnar joint, similar to his case report, by a compression and torsion force applied to a hyperextended, pronated wrist (68). Regardless of the mechanism involved, dislocation of the proximal row of the carpus from the distal radius and ulna requires disruption of the radiocapitate, long and short radiolunate, ulnocarpal, and dorsal radiotriquetral ligaments (70,71).

Evaluation

When unreduced, radiocarpal dislocations produce noticeable deformity of the hand–forearm unit with the carpus and hand translated palmar or dorsal to the forearm axis unit, depending on the direction of dislocation. Given the energy required to create this dislocation and the amount of translation involved, neurovascular injury may be associated. PA and lateral neutral rotation views of the wrist are adequate for initial evaluation. On the PA views, the carpus will be found overlapping the distal radius. On the lateral view, the proximal carpal row will be found perched palmar or dorsal to the distal radial articular surface. Diagnosis of a radiocarpal dislocation that has spontaneously reduced is more difficult and requires an index of suspicion. Findings of palmar carpal subluxation and/or ulnar translation are an indication of the magnitude of such an injury. Periarticular rim fractures of the distal radius and/or radial and ulnar styloid avulsion fractures may also be present. Stress loading of the radiocarpal joint under an appropriate anesthetic and fluoroscopic control is valuable in ascertaining the presence of this injury. In cases of spontaneous reduction of radiocarpal dislocation, it is quite possible this diagnosis will initially be missed.

Treatment

Treatment of radiocarpal dislocations has included closed reduction with cast immobilization or percutaneous

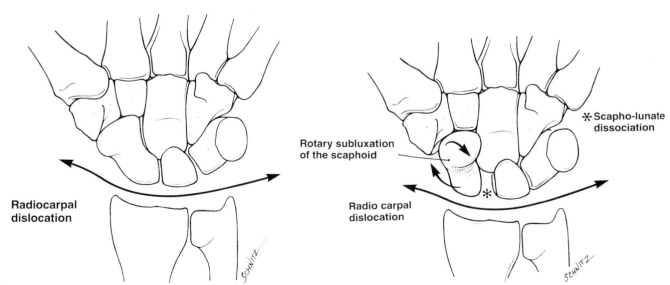

FIGURE 14.13. Moneim classification of radiocarpal dislocations. **A:** Type I, radiocarpal dislocation with intact proximal carpal row. **B:** Type II, radiocarpal dislocation with dissociative lesion of the proximal carpal row.

pinning (66,67,69,70,72–74); open reduction with cast immobilization (75); open reduction, internal fixation with ligament repairs (66,68,71,76); and radiocarpal fusion (10). Moneim et al., based on their experience in treating radiocarpal dislocations, recommended attempted closed reduction and cast immobilization for type I injuries and open reduction, internal fixation and ligament repair in type II injuries (66). A review of cases reported in the literature indicates that the most common method of treatment for radiocarpal dislocation has been closed reduction with cast immobilization. Although the length of follow-up has been short, outcomes have been considered reasonable.

The Mayo Clinic group, based on their difficulties managing late instability seen after radiocarpal dislocations, have recommended palmar and dorsal approaches for ligament repair of the radiocapitate, long radiolunate, ulnocarpal, and dorsal radiotriquetral ligaments (Fig. 14.14). When direct ligament repair cannot be accomplished, particularly in the case of the radiocapitate ligament, tendon augmentation is recommended. The ligament repair is protected by transfixation pinning of the radiocarpal joint and immobilization in a long arm cast for 6 to 8 weeks. Following pin removal, progressive mobilization occurs over 6 weeks (64,71). To date, there are no results to document the outcome of such treatment.

Complications seen following the treatment of radiocarpal dislocation include posttraumatic arthritis, intercarpal instability, palmar radiocarpal subluxation, and ulnar translation. Taleisnik described two types of ulnar translation (10). Type I involves ulnar translation of the entire carpal row relative to the distal radius. Radiographically, a V-shaped widening can be appreciated between the radial styloid area and the scaphoid. In type II ulnar translation, the radioscaphoid articulation remains intact with the translation occurring through the scapholunate interval (Fig. 14.15). Taleisnik's classification of ulnar translation is consistent with the type of ulnar translation expected from the injuries described by the Moneim classification of radiocarpal dislocation. Rayhack et al. reported on the results of ligament repair or reconstruction for the treatment of posttraumatic radiocarpal subluxation (71). The technique used was as recommended for acute management of radiocarpal dislocation. They considered their results disappointing, with recurrent ulnar translation occurring in nearly all cases. Despite this, three of their eight cases were judged good results. Taleisnik, based on his personal experience

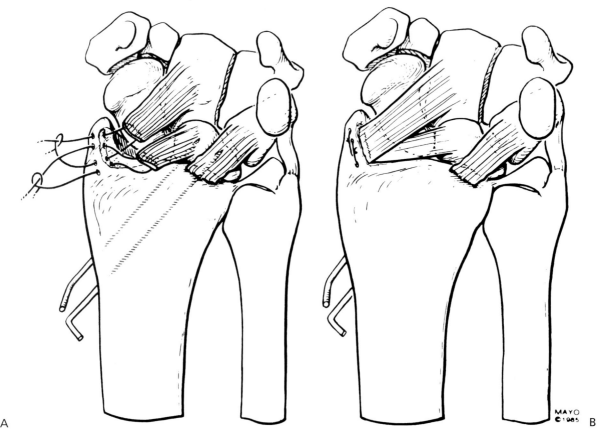

FIGURE 14.14. A,B: Technique for ligament repair following radiocarpal dislocation. (From Rayhack JM, Linscheid RL, Dobyns JH, et al. Posttraumatic ulnar translation of the carpus. *J Hand Surg [Am]* 1987;12:180–189, with permission.)

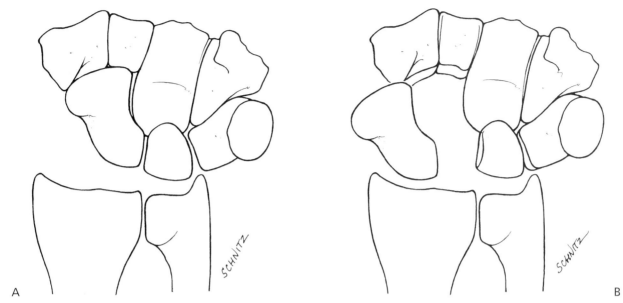

FIGURE 14.15. Taleisnik classification of ulnar translation. **A:** Type I. Ulnar translation of the entire proximal carpal row as an intact unit. Note the V-shaped space between the ulnar styloid and scaphoid. **B:** Type II. The radius and scaphoid maintain a normal relationship while the remainder of the carpus translates ulnarly.

with late management of radiocarpal subluxation, has recommended radiocarpal fusion for treatment of this complication (10).

Given the limited experience with this dislocation, there does not appear to be an ideal means of treatment. Moneim's recommendations for management seem reasonable at this time. Initial treatment should commence with an attempt at closed reduction under axillary block and fluoroscopic control. Following reduction, the wrist should be evaluated for occult fracture and the presence of dissociative lesions within the proximal carpal row. Stress loading under fluoroscopy or, even better, arthroscopy, may be used to identify intercarpal ligament injuries. If it is determined that the proximal carpal row has remained intact, the stability of the reduction should be assessed with traction released. If this is felt to be stable, closed treatment with long arm cast immobilization may be considered. A more secure form of immobilization would be percutaneous pinning of the radiocarpal joint and cast immobilization or external fixation of the radiocarpal joint. If, when traction is released, the wrist joint falls into a pattern of palmar radiocarpal subluxation and/or ulnar translation; or there are findings of dissociative lesions involving the proximal carpal row, open reduction with internal fixation and ligament repair is indicated. A palmar and dorsal approach similar to that previously described for management of perilunate instability is used. The radiocarpal joint is initially stabilized by pin fixation. Repair of the dorsal radiotriquetral and palmar radiocapitate, radiolunate, and ulnocarpal ligaments is performed. When indicated, tendon augmentation is used to supplement the ligament repairs. Immobilization can be accomplished with a long arm thumb–spica cast or external fixation crossing the radiocarpal joint. We would recommend a postoperative treatment program similar to that for a perilunar dislocation.

AXIAL DISLOCATIONS OF THE CARPUS

Axial dislocation represents longitudinal disruption of the carpus and respective metacarpals. In most cases, it is the distal carpal row that is disrupted, although on occasion the disruption will extend into the proximal row, most commonly involving the hamate and/or pisiform (76,77). Axial dislocations have been subclassified by Garcia-Elias et al. into axial radial, axial ulnar, and axial radial–ulnar disruption (78) (Fig. 14.16). With axial radial dislocation, it is the radiocarpal bones and their respective metacarpals that are disrupted and displaced from the remainder of the hand. With axial ulnar, it is the ulnar carpometacarpal (CMC) column that is displaced. In axial radial–ulnar dislocation, both axial radial and axial ulnar disruptions are present.

As with other types of carpal dislocation, a high-energy injury is required to produce axial dislocation. The most commonly reported mechanisms are blast or crush injuries that flatten the carpal arch. It is this flattening of the carpal arch that produces the axial displacement. Given the mechanism of injury, it is not surprising that axial dis-

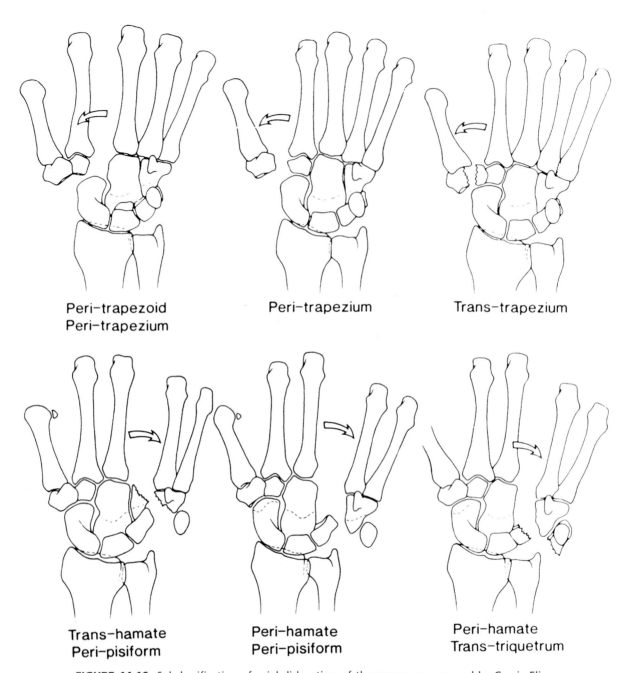

FIGURE 14.16. Subclassification of axial dislocation of the carpus as proposed by Garcia-Elias. (From Garcia-Elias M, Dobyns JH, Cooney WP, et al. Traumatic axial dislocations of the carpus. *J Hand Surg [Am]* 1989;14;446–457, with permission.)

locations of the carpus have a high incidence of associated osseous and soft tissue trauma (79). Fractures of the trapezial ridge and hook of hamate are commonly seen. CMC dislocations, metacarpal fractures, and phalangeal fractures may be present as well. Burst injuries of the intrinsic muscles occur almost universally. In addition, flexor and extensor tendon injuries as well as neurovascular trauma may occur. Nerve injuries are more frequent with axial ulnar dislocation.

Evaluation

On examination of the hand with an axial dislocation of the carpus, there is always significant swelling. These are usually open injuries. As a result of osseous disruption as well as associated soft tissue trauma, there is marked limitation in wrist and digital motion. With ulnar axial dislocation, rotational malalignment of the ulnar digits may be present.

Standard PA and lateral neutral rotation views of the hand and wrist should be adequate to establish the pattern of dislocation. More subtle components of the osseous pathology such as hook of the hamate or trapezial ridge fractures can be detected by CT scan or tomography. They may also be detected intraoperatively using fluoroscopy or special x-ray views, which are better tolerated when the patient is anesthetized.

Treatment

The treatment for axial dislocation will depend on whether the wound is open or closed and the extent of associated osseous and soft tissue trauma. The goal in all forms of treatment is to restore mobility of the hand and wrist as quickly as possible to minimize the effect of the crush or blast injury. Closed treatment may be considered for closed dislocations without other injuries. Reduction can usually be accomplished by longitudinal traction and manipulative reduction. Percutaneous pinning will enhance the stability of the reduction and may permit early active motion. If an anatomic reduction cannot be achieved, open management is indicated. Treatment concerns for open injuries are multifactorial. The blast or crush injury typically produces extensive devitalization of both skin and muscle. This requires radical debridement to minimize the risk of infection. Extensive skin loss may create the need for wound coverage using local or distant flaps. Careful intraoperative assessment is necessary to define the full extent of osseous pathology. The technique selected for management of fractures and stabilization of the dislocation will be dependent on the state of the surrounding soft tissues, the ability to achieve primary wound coverage, and the potential for initiation of early wrist and finger motion. All vascular injuries must be addressed primarily. Whenever possible, nerve injury and associated tendon injury should be addressed primarily as well. As might be expected from the mechanism of injury, axial dislocations of the carpus are devastating injuries to the hand. In the series reported by Garcia-Elias, residual functional impairment existed in all patients with few good results. The factor that was determined to be the most significant in determining outcome was the presence or absence of associated nerve injury (78–81).

ISOLATED CARPAL DISLOCATION

Trapezoid Dislocation

The trapezoid sits as a keystone between the trapezium and capitate in the distal carpal row. It is bound to its adjacent carpal bones by stout intercarpal ligaments, particularly on its palmar aspect. It is also bound proximally to the scaphoid by the scaphotrapezoidal ligament and distally to the second metacarpal. The trapezoid has nutrient vessels that enter its palmar and dorsal surfaces. The dorsal circulation is dominant, supplying the dorsal 70% of this carpal bone. There are no intraosseous anastomoses between the palmar and dorsal systems (82).

Isolated dislocation of the trapezoid is one of the more commonly reported carpal bone dislocations (83–98). Both palmar (92,93,95–98) and dorsal (83–91,94) isolated dislocations of the trapezoid have been reported. Dislocation of the trapezoid with an intact articulation with the second metacarpal can also occur, producing a peritrapezoidal pattern of axial carpal dissociation (94). Because of the dorsally flaring wedge shape of the trapezoid, dorsal dislocations are more common. Dorsal dislocations may be produced by direct trauma or indirectly from a blow to the second metacarpal with the wrist flexed. With wrist flexion, the scaphoid rotates palmarly, leaving the proximal articular surface of the trapezoid relatively uncovered. Palmar dislocation of the trapezoid has been reported primarily after direct trauma. It has been speculated that a dorsal blow to the distal row flattens the carpal arch, widening the palmar space and allowing palmar extrusion of the trapezoid (93). An alternate explanation offered by Rhoades is forced wrist and second metacarpal extension (96).

A dorsal dislocation of the trapezoid will create a fullness at the base of the index finger metacarpal. A palmar dislocation will not have such an obvious presentation, but, given the mechanism of injury, diffuse swelling and pain with manipulation of the second CMC can be anticipated. With either direction of dislocation, direct trauma over the base of the second metacarpal or hypermobility of the second CMC joint should raise suspicion regarding the possibility of this injury. Standard PA and lateral views of the wrist are usually adequate to make an initial diagnosis. An empty space will be seen at the base of the second metacarpal. The trapezium may be superimposed over the scaphoid or second metacarpal base. When necessary, tomograms or a CT scan can be obtained.

Treatment for dorsal dislocation of the trapezoid has included closed reduction (83,86,87), open reduction (84,85,88,91,94–96,98), excision (80,90,97), and fusion (92). In the acute situation, closed reduction under adequate anesthesia should be attempted. This can usually be accomplished by longitudinal traction and manipulation of the trapezoid by dorsally applied pressure. Palmar flexion of the wrist may also prove beneficial until reduction is achieved, at which point the wrist is extended to rotate the scaphoid into a position to help stabilize the trapezoid. The stability of the reduction should then be assessed. If it is stable, a short arm cast is applied for 4 to 6 weeks. If, however, there is any question regarding the stability of the reduction, the trapezoid should be percutaneously pinned in place and supplemented by cast immobilization. In the event the trapezoid cannot be reduced by closed methods, an open dorsal approach for reduction and pinning is necessary. Intraoperatively, the articular surfaces of the trapezoid can be inspected for injury. The soft tissue attachments to the trapezoid should be preserved to protect its blood supply. Postoperative immobilization is maintained for 4 to 6 weeks.

In the management of palmar dislocations, open reduction is necessary. The palmarly displaced trapezoid may initially be approached palmarly or dorsally, but a combined approach may be necessary. The reduction should then be stabilized with K-wires and cast immobilization. Once stabilized, treatment is the same as for a dorsal dislocation.

Although excision is a reported technique for management of trapezoidal dislocation, it is best reserved for the management of a delayed diagnosis in which there has been proximal migration of the second metacarpal to obliterate the space formerly occupied by the trapezoid. Excision might also be considered if there is extensive articular damage to the trapezoid. An alternative to excision is arthrodesis.

With a stable reduction, good results can be achieved. Complications of this injury include recurrent instability, posttraumatic arthritis and avascular necrosis. Avascular necrosis may occur as the result of the original injury or may be precipitated by surgical intervention. The occurrence of avascular necrosis does not necessarily indicate a bad outcome. Of all isolated carpal bone dislocations, avascular necrosis has been most frequently reported in the trapezoid (88,91,94,96).

Scaphoid Dislocations

The scaphoid is a highly mobile carpal bone with secure ligamentous attachments at its proximal and distal poles. Proximally, the scaphoid is bound to the lunate through its interosseous ligament. Distally, the scaphoid is stabilized by the scaphotrapezial and scaphocapitate ligaments (99). The radioscaphocapitate ligament has been described as a fulcrum for rotation of the scaphoid; however, with displacement of the scaphoid in a palmar radial direction, rupture of this ligament must occur (100).

The scaphoid normally receives its blood supply from branches of the radial artery. These branches enter the palmar surface at the distal pole of the scaphoid and along its dorsal nonarticular surface. Typically a single intraosseous blood supply progresses from distal to proximal. This situation creates the potential for avascular necrosis (101).

Palmar radial (102–110) and dorsal (111) dislocations of the scaphoid have been reported. Direct trauma, blast injuries, and high-speed motor vehicle accidents are among the most common precipitating events associated with isolated scaphoid dislocation. Inoue (111) and Szabo (100) have proposed that some cases of isolated scaphoid dislocation occur as the result of the same forces implicated in producing a perilunar dislocation. Thus, a scaphoid dislocation may represent a potential outcome of a stage I lesser arc injury as described by Mayfield.

Clinical presentation will vary with the direction of dislocation. In most instances, the proximal pole dislocates into a subcutaneous position, hinging on residual soft tissue attachments at the scaphotrapeziotrapezoid joint. With palmar dislocation, median nerve injury has been reported (109). Wrist range of motion will be limited and painful. PA and lateral neutral-rotation x-rays supplemented by a scaphoid view are adequate for evaluation. With palmar radial dislocation, the scaphoid fossa is vacant with the proximal pole of the scaphoid perched on the rim of the distal radius (Fig. 14.17). With dorsal dislocation on the PA view, the proximal pole of the scaphoid appears to remain in its fossa. The lateral view, however, demonstrates a perpendicular orientation of the scaphoid to the longitudinal axis of the forearm with the proximal pole displaced dorsal to the rim of the radius (Fig. 14.18).

Treatment options for isolated scaphoid dislocation have included closed reduction (105,108), closed reduction with percutaneous pinning (100), and open reduction with and without internal fixation (101,102, 104–107). Although excellent results have been reported with simple closed reduction (105,108), scapholunate dissociation and rotational instability of the scaphoid may persist (106). Szabo has proposed a spectrum of ligamentous injuries that may occur, with scaphoid dislocation commencing with rupture of the radioscaphocapitate ligament and progressing to complete ligament disruption at both the proximal and distal ends of the scaphoid (100). At the initial end of the spectrum, conservative management with simple closed reduction and 6 weeks of immobilization in a thumb–spica cast may be sufficient. As the severity of ligament injury increases, greater stabilization of the scaphoid is required. Szabo has recommended arthroscopic assessment of the ligament injuries if closed reduction can be accomplished. If global ligament disruption is present or closed reduction cannot be accomplished, open reduction, internal fixation, and scapholunate ligament repair are indicated. Following open treatment, fixation pins are removed at 6 to 8 weeks, and immobilization is continued in a thumb–spica cast until 10 to 12 weeks postsurgery.

Potential complications following an isolated scaphoid dislocation are residual carpal instability (106,112) and posttraumatic arthrosis (104). Although avascular necrosis is an anticipated risk, its occurrence has been rare (100,107,113).

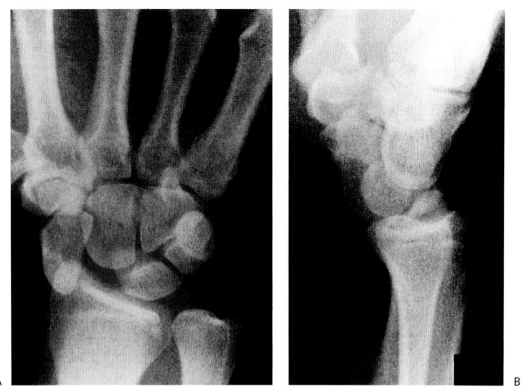

FIGURE 14.17. Posteroanterior **(A)** and lateral **(B)** radiographs of a palmar radial dislocation of the scaphoid. (From Szabo RM, Newland CC, Johnson PG, et al. Spectrum of injury and treatment options for isolated dislocation of the scaphoid. *J Bone Joint Surg Am* 1995;77:608–615, with permission.)

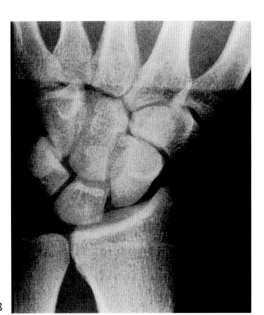
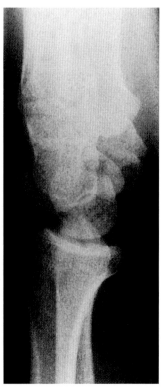

FIGURE 14.18. Posteroanterior **(A)** and lateral **(B)** radiographs of a dorsal dislocation of the scaphoid. (From Inoue G, Maeda N. Isolated dorsal dislocation of the scaphoid. *J Hand Surg [Br]* 1990;15:368–369, with permission.)

Simultaneous Scaphoid and Lunate Dislocation

All reported cases of simultaneous scaphoid and lunate dislocations have dislocated in a palmar direction (114–118). The injury has most frequently occurred as a result of a substantial fall or motor vehicle accident. The pathomechanics of the dislocation is thought to be a variation of a major arc injury. The dislocation requires disruption of the dorsal radiotriquetral and scaphotriquetral ligaments as well as the palmar radiocapitate, long and short radiolunate ligaments, and the lunatotriquetral interosseous ligament. The scapholunate ligament may be found intact (115) or ruptured (114,116).

Clinical examination typically demonstrates a significant swelling of the wrist. A palpable mass and palmar radial wrist tenderness may be present. Dysfunction in the median nerve may be noted (115). Lateral radiographs show a palmar displacement of the scaphoid and lunate. The scaphoid may retain partial contact with the trapezium and trapezoid. On the PA view, proximal migration of the carpus is noted, with the scaphoid and lunate overlapping the distal radius. A substantial gap is noted between the lunate and triquetrum (Fig. 14.19).

Treatment for this dislocation has included closed reduction with long arm cast immobilization (117,118), open reduction and cast immobilization (114), and open reduction and internal fixation (115,116). The initial treatment for this condition should be an attempted closed reduction under adequate anesthesia. An assessment should be made of the stability of the reduction with stress testing under fluoroscopy. Examination should also determine if there are other sites of ligament injury not initially detected. This evaluation can be enhanced by the use of arthroscopy. To assure the stability of the reduction, K-wire fixation is recommended with 6 to 8 weeks of thumb–spica immobilization. If a closed reduction cannot be achieved, or there is evidence of gross instability, open reduction with K-wire internal fixation and ligament repair through palmar and dorsal approaches is necessary. Postoperatively, the wrist is immobilized in a thumb–spica for 3 months with pin removal at 8 weeks. Complications associated with this injury have included scapholunate dissociation (114,116), palmar (117,118) or dorsal (116) intercalated segmented instability, ulnar translation (116), and avascular necrosis of the lunate (115,116).

Trapezium Dislocation

The trapezium may dislocate in isolation or together with the thumb metacarpal (119–122). Palmar and dorsal radial dislocations of both have been described (123–126). Dislocation of the trapezium and thumb metacarpal as a unit has

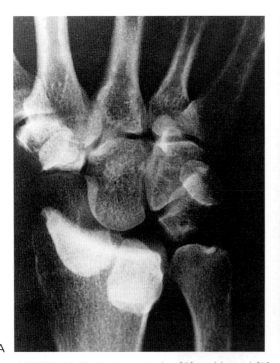
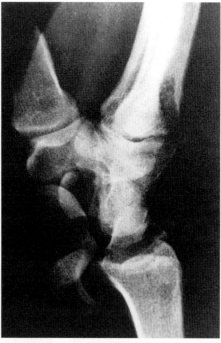

FIGURE 14.19. Posteroanterior **(A)** and lateral **(B)** radiographs of a simultaneous palmar dislocation of the scaphoid and lunate. (From Kupfer K. Palmar dislocation of scaphoid and lunate as a unit: Case report with special reference to carpal instability and treatment. *J Hand Surg [Am]* 1986;11:130–134, with permission.)

been classified by Garcia-Elias as a pattern of axial radial carpal dislocation (78). Isolated dislocation of the trapezium requires disruption of the radial and palmar scaphotrapezial ligament, trapezial–trapezoid interosseous ligament, as well as the capsular ligaments between the trapezium and first metacarpal, and its attachments to the transverse carpal ligament. The trapezium receives its blood supply from nutrient arteries that enter from its palmar, dorsal, and lateral surfaces. The trapezium has consistent intraosseous anastomoses of its blood supply, which make it resistant to avascular necrosis (100).

Crush injuries and motor vehicle accidents are the most commonly reported causes of these injuries. Direct trauma is a mechanism for producing either a palmar or dorsal radial dislocation of the trapezium. A force applied indirectly through the thumb metacarpal producing supination and either flexion or extension may result in a dislocation of the trapezium with or without the first CMC joint remaining intact (121,123,124,126). With isolated dorsal radial dislocation, a palpable mass may be present at the base of the thumb. Pain and instability of the first CMC joint may be noted. Limited range of motion of the first CMC joint may be present if the thumb metacarpal dislocates with the trapezium. Palmar dislocation of the trapezium has been associated with avulsion of the thenar branch of the median nerve (122,123). A hyperpronated view and lateral of the first CMC joint should be adequate to assess the injury. A gap will be found between the distal pole of the scaphoid and base of the thumb metacarpal on the hyperpronated view. The lateral view will show whether the dislocation is palmar or dorsal (Fig. 14.20).

Treatment options for this injury have included closed reduction with percutaneous pinning (4), open reduction and internal fixation (119–126), fusion (119), and excision of the trapezium (120,127). For initial management of closed dislocations, an attempted closed reduction under anesthesia is indicated. Reduction can usually be accomplished by longitudinal traction and gentle manipulation. To assure the stability of the reduction, percutaneous K-wire fixation is appropriate. For the management of open injuries or irreducible closed injuries, open reduction and internal fixation is necessary. In instances where median nerve dysfunction is present, particularly with loss of thenar muscle function, decompression of the carpal canal and exploration of the median nerve is required. Whenever possible, repair of the periarticular ligamentous structures should be accomplished. When not dictated by associated open wounds, a Wagner palmar radial approach offers extensile exposure for either a palmar or dorsal dislocation. Immobilization in a thumb–spica cast for 4 to 6 weeks is followed by a program of progressive mobilization.

Following trapezial dislocation, potential complications include basilar joint instability, arthrofibrosis (121,122), and posttraumatic arthritis. Avascular necrosis of the trapezium has not reported as a consequence of this injury. Two cases of median nerve thenar motor branch rupture have been reported with isolated trapezial dislocation (122,123).

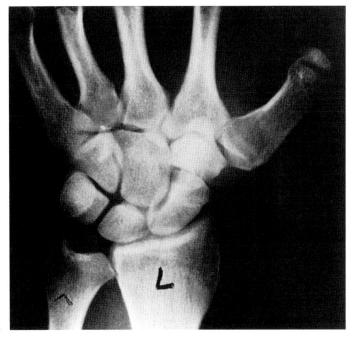
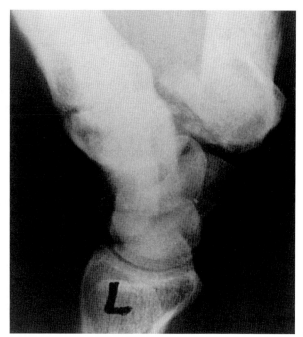

FIGURE 14.20. Anteroposterior **(A)** and lateral **(B)** views of a palmar dislocation of the trapezium. (From Goldberg I, Amit S, Bahar A, et al. Complete dislocation of the trapezium (multangulum majus). *J Hand Surg [Am]* 1981;6:193–195, with permission.)

Triquetrum Dislocation

Both palmar (128,129) and dorsal (130–133) dislocations of the triquetrum have been documented. The typical precipitating event has been a major fall, motor vehicle accident, or crush injury. The pathomechanics of a dorsal or palmar dislocation can be explained on the basis of direct trauma (128,131). Dorsal dislocation may also be produced by wrist hyperflexion and pronation (133) secondary to a perilunar dislocation or a variant of an ulnar axial loading injury (132). It is proposed that with forced wrist hyperextension, the proximal pole of the hamate rides dorsally on the triquetrum, exerting a palmar force leading to a palmar dislocation of the triquetrum (129). Dislocation of the triquetrum requires disruption dorsally of the radiotriquetral and scaphotriquetral ligaments and palmarly of the ulnocarpal ligament, lunatotriquetral ligament, lunatotriquetral intraosseous ligament, triquetral hamate ligament, and triquetral capitate ligament (130). The triquetrum receives nutrient arteries through both its palmar and dorsal surfaces. Although the dorsal system is usually dominant, consistent intraosseous anastomoses limit its risk for avascular necrosis (100).

On examination, swelling will be noted about the ulnar aspect of the wrist. There may be evidence of direct trauma to the area. If the dislocation is dorsal, it may be possible to palpate the displaced triquetrum. With palmar dislocation, neurovascular compromise can occur (128,129). PA and lateral neutral-rotation views of the wrist are adequate for radiographic evaluation (Fig. 14.21). On the PA projection, the triquetrum will be absent from its normal postion adjacent to the lunate. The lateral view provides information on the direction of dislocation.

Treatment for triquetral dislocation has included excision (128,129), closed reduction (131), and open reduction and internal fixation (130,132,134). Good results have been reported with all treatment options. (130–133). Initial management of a triquetral dislocation begins with an attempted closed reduction under general or regional anesthesia and fluoroscopic control. If a closed reduction can be achieved, the intercarpal alignment should be assessed for other sites of ligament injury and the general stability of the reduction. To prevent redislocation and the late development of carpal instability, percutaneous pinning of the triquetrum to the lunate and to the hamate or capitate is recommended. If the injury is open or closed reduction cannot be achieved, open reduction and internal fixation is required. The initial approach should be from the direction of dislocation, although combined palmar and dorsal approaches may be necessary. Pin fixation of the reduced triquetrum with ligament repair is performed. To minimize torsional and translation forces through the ulnocarpal joint, long arm or Muenster cast immobilization for 4 to 6 weeks is appropriate. This is followed by pin removal and

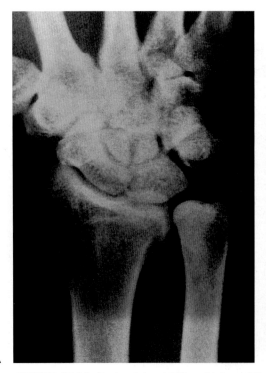
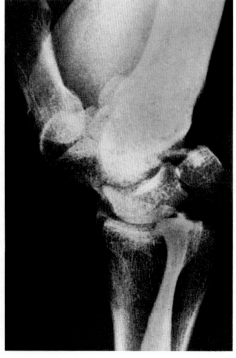

FIGURE 14.21. Posterolateral **(A)** and lateral **(B)** radiographs of a dorsal dislocation of the triquetrum. (From Inoue G. Dorsal dislocation of the triquetrum: A case report. *Ann Hand Surg* 1992;11:233–236, with permission.)

gradual mobilization over 4 to 6 weeks. Excision of the triquetrum as a form of treatment should be reserved for extensive articular trauma or delayed diagnosis.

Triquetral dislocation has been seen in conjunction with other injuries such as scapholunate dissociation (131) and dislocation of the distal radioulnar joint (133). Palmar intercalated segmental collapse has been reported following triquetral dislocations (133). There have been no reported cases of avascular necrosis following treatment of a triquetral dislocation.

Hamate Dislocation

Isolated dislocation of the hamate is a rare carpal dislocation (134–137). Both palmar (136) and dorsal (135,137) dislocations of the hamate have been reported. Hamate dislocation with the pisiform has been reported as a form of axial instability (78,138). The usual mechanism of injury is direct trauma (135). Hyperextension has also been implicated (136). Dislocation of the hamate requires disruption of the triquetrohamate ligament, pisohamate ligament, and capitohamate interosseous ligament as well as the fourth and fifth CMC joint capsules. The hamate lacks an intraosseous anastomosis of its nutrient vessels and, therefore, can be at risk for avascular necrosis (100).

Clinical examination reveals swelling about the ulnar aspect of the hand. There may be evidence of direct trauma to the area. Depending on the direction of dislocation, palmar or dorsal fullness may be noted. Manipulation of the fourth and fifth CMC joints may reveal pain, crepitance, or instability. Given the nearby presence of the ulnar neurovascular bundle, injury to this structure might be anticipated; however, this has not been noted as a problem in prior case reports (136). PA and lateral neutral rotation views of the wrist are adequate for diagnosis. Most noticeable will be a gap between the proximal pole of the hamate and its articulation with the triquetrum and lunate.

Treatment options include closed reduction (136), open reduction with or without internal fixation (135–137), and excision (136). Good results have been reported with all forms of treatment. Treatment of a hamate dislocation should commence with attempted closed reduction under appropriate anesthesia and fluoroscopic control. If a reduction can be achieved, its stability should be assessed fluoroscopically. To prevent recurrent dislocation, percutaneous pinning is reasonable. The extremity should be immobilized in a short arm cast for 4 to 6 weeks. Following pin removal, mobilization can be commenced. If the injury is open, or closed reduction cannot be achieved, an open approach from the direction of dislocation is necessary. Once reduction has been accomplished, pin fixation and ligament repair are performed. Postoperative immobilization and rehabilitation are the same as for closed reduction. Hamate excision and intercarpal arthrodesis are best reserved for cases of severe articular injury or delayed diagnosis.

Pisiform Dislocation

The pisiform lies as a sesamoid within the flexor carpi ulnaris tendon. The pisiform serves as a source of attachment for the pisohamate ligament, abductor digiti minimi, transverse carpal ligament, as well as the joint capsule to the triquetrum. Dislocation of the pisiform occurs relative to its articulation with the triquetrum. The precipitating event may be direct trauma or indirect, when a flexed wrist is forced into extension (139–141).

Clinical examination may demonstrate swelling in the area or a depression over the palmar aspect of the triquetrum. Hypermobility and crepitance may be detected at the pisotriquetral joint. PA and lateral neutral rotation views of the wrist as well as a pisotriquetral view are appropriate for evaluation of this injury. Typically, the displaced pisiform will be seen adjacent to the hamate, distal to its normal position over the triquetrum.

Treatment options for dislocation of the pisiform include closed reduction (139,142), open reduction (143), and excision (140,144). For treatment of a pisiform dislocation, closed reduction should be pursued as the initial form of treatment. This requires regional anesthesia and is assisted by fluoroscopy. Closed reduction usually requires maximum wrist flexion with manual manipulation of the pisiform back into position. This reduction can be aided by placing the forearm in pronation (142). Postreduction immobilization for a minimum of 3 weeks in a radially deviated short arm cast (139) or a long arm cast holding the wrist flexed and forearm pronated (142) has been recommended. The choice should be made by assessing the stability of the pisiform in each position. Pisiform excision is reserved for the management of open injuries with severe articular injury or when diagnosis is delayed or dislocation is a recurrent problem.

Capitate Dislocation

True isolated dislocation of the capitate is an extremely rare event (145–147). The injury requires disruption of the interosseous ligaments to the adjacent trapezoid and hamate. In addition, it requires disruption of the ligaments stabilizing its CMC joint distally and proximally disrupting the radiocapitate and capitotriquetral ligaments. Although the capitate receives palmar and dorsal nutrient vessels, most frequently the dorsal system dominates. A single dominant intraosseous blood supply may be present, potentially placing the capitate at risk for avascular necrosis.

The proposed mechanism of injury is wrist extension and axial compression. Direct trauma may also play a role, as it does with other isolated carpal dislocations. Of the three cases reported in the literature, all have been palmar dislocations. One case was a massive open injury associated with multiple other carpal and metacarpal fracture-dislocations. This case was treated with open reduction and internal fixation (145). The other two cases were closed, and both had other adjacent associated injuries. One case was treated closed (147), and the other with open reduction and K-wire fixation (146). Both cases resulted in findings of residual palmar midcarpal instability. On follow-up, the open capitate dislocation had findings of posttraumatic arthrosis.

Miscellaneous Patterns of Dislocation

Carpal dislocation may occur in units of adjacent bones. The most common pattern is combined scaphoid and lunate (114–118). The trapezium and trapezoid may dislocate from the scaphoid, most commonly as a variant of radial axial carpal dislocation (78,148,149). Other reported patterns are lunate and triquetrum (150), hamate and pisiform (138), and lunate, triquetrum, and hamate (151).

These unusual patterns of dislocation are most likely the result of direct trauma and appropriately grouped with isolated carpal dislocations. The exception is the scaphoid and lunate combined dislocation, which may occur as a variation of a major arc perilunar dislocation.

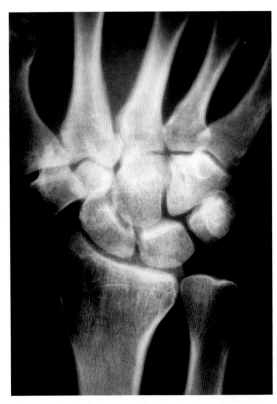

EDITORS' FIGURE 14.1. Dislocation has occurred between the index and middle metacarpals, between the trapezoid and the capitate, and out through the triscaphe joint. This two-digit, two-carpal dislocation is a common result of crush injuries to the hand that occur in a radioulnar direction.

EDITORS' COMMENTS

Carpal dislocations are manifestations of significant trauma. In general, percutaneous pinning is not an accepted mode of treatment. The interosseous ligament systems are short and require anatomic reduction of the carpals under direct visualization. The major forces required to produce these injuries often produce unrecognized components of ligament tear involving other parts of the wrist. Open reduction, direct visualization, anatomic reduction with pinning, or other secure fixation is mandatory. Prolonged immobilization, usually a minimum of 8 weeks, is necessary.

A carpal dislocation pattern involving the triscaphe joint can be seen with crush force injuries in which force is applied in a radioulnar direction and associated with a dorsiflexion mechanism of injury (Editors' Fig. 14.1).

REFERENCES

1. Mayfield JK. Mechanism of carpal injuries. *Clin Orthop* 1980; 149:45–54.
2. Mayfield JK, Williams WJ, Erdman AC, et al. Biomechanical properties of human carpal ligaments. *Orthop Trans* 1979;3: 143–144.
3. Nunn D. Trans-triquetral mid-carpal dislocation. *J Hand Surg [Br]* 1986;11:432–433.
4. Dunn AW. Fractures and dislocation of the carpus. *Surg Clin North Am* 1972;52:1513–1538.
5. Pai CH, Wei DC, Hu ST. Carpal bone dislocations: an analysis of twenty cases with relative emphasis on the role of crushing mechanisms. *J Trauma* 1993;35:28–35.
6. Russell TB. Inter-carpal dislocations and fracture dislocations: a review of 59 cases. *J Bone Joint Surg Br* 1949;31:524–531.
7. Johnson RP. The acutely injured wrist and its residuals. *Clin Orthop* 1980;149:33–44.
8. Mayfield JK, Johnson RP, Kilcoyne RK. Carpal dislocations: Pathomechanics and progressive perilunar instability. *J Hand Surg [Am]* 1980;5:226–241.
9. Herzberg G, Comtet JJ, Linscheid RL, et al. Perilunar dislocations and fracture dislocations: a multicenter study. *J Hand Surg [Am]* 1993;18:768–779.
10. Taleisnik J. Dislocations and fracture—dislocations of the carpus. In: Taleisnik J. *The wrist*. New York: Churchill Livingstone, 1985;195–228.
11. Kohut G, Smith A, Giudici M, et al. Greater arc injuries of the wrist treated by internal and external fixation—six cases with mid-term follow-up. *Hand Surg* 1996;1:159–166.
12. Moneim MS. Management of greater arc carpal fractures. *Hand Clin* 1988;4:457–467.
13. Adkison JW, Chapman MW. Treatment of acute lunate and perilunate dislocations. *Clin Orthop* 1982;164:199–207.
14. Altissimi M, Mancini GB, Azzara A. Perilunate dislocations of the carpus: a long-term review. *Ital J Orthop Traumatol* 1987;13: 491–500.
15. Cooney WP, Bussey R, Dobyns JH, et al. Difficult wrist fractures. *Clin Orthop* 1987;214:136–147.
16. Garcia-Elias M, Irisarri C, Henriquez A, et al. Perilunar dislocation of the carpus: a diagnosis still often missed. *Ann Chir Main* 1986;5:281–287.

17. Morawa LG, Ross PM, Schock CC. Fractures and dislocations involving the navicular–lunate axis. *Clin Orthop* 1976;118:48–53.
18. Mugdal C, Hastings H II. Scapholunate diastasis in fractures of the distal radius: pathomechanics and treatment options. *J Hand Surg [Br]* 1993;18:725–729.
19. Richards RS, Bennett JD, Ross JH, et al. Arthroscopic diagnosis of intra-articular soft tissue injuries associated with distal radius fractures. *J Hand Surg [Am]* 1997;22:772–776.
20. Geissler WB, Freeland AE, Savoie FH, et al. Intracarpal soft tissue lesions associated with an intra-articular fracture of the distal end of the radius. *J Bone Joint Surg Am* 1996;78:357–365.
21. Roman A, Sendino M, Salomon G, et al. A rare case of carpal dislocation. *Ann Chir Main Memb Super* 1994;13:207–213.
22. Aitken AP, Nalebuff EA. Volar transnavicular perilunar dislocation of the carpus. *J Bone Joint Surg Am* 1960;42:1051–1057.
23. Pournaras J, Kappas A. Volar perilunate dislocation: A case report. *J Bone Joint Surg Am* 1979;61:625–626.
24. Reagan DS, Linscheid RL, Dobyns JH. Lunotriquetral sprains. *J Hand Surg [Am]* 1984;9:502–514.
25. Trumble TE, Bour CJ, Smith RJ, et al. Kinematics of the ulnar carpus related to the volar intercalated segment instability pattern. *J Hand Surg [Am]* 1990;15:384–392.
26. Viegas SF, Patterson RM, Peterson PD, et al. Ulnar-sided perilunate instability: an anatomic and biomechanic study. *J Hand Surg [Am]* 1990;15:268–278.
27. DeCoster TA, Faherty S, Morris AL. Pediatric carpal fracture dislocation. *J Orthop Trauma* 1994;8:76–78.
28. Hokan R, Bryce GM, Cobb NJ. Dislocation of scaphoid and fractured capitate in a child. *Injury* 1993;24:496–497.
29. Peiro A, Martos F, Mut T, et al. Transcaphoid perilunate dislocation in a child. *Acta Orthop Scand* 1981;52:31–34.
30. Zimmerman NB, Weiland AJ. Scapholunate dissociation in the skeletally immature carpus. *J Hand Surg [Am]* 1990;15:701–705.
31. Anderson WA. Simultaneous fracture of the scaphoid and capitate in a child. *J Hand Surg [Am]* 1987;12:271–273.
32. Hill NA. Fractures and dislocations of the carpus. *Orthop Clin North Am* 1970;1:275–284.
33. Gilula LA, Weeks PM. Post-traumatic ligamentous instabilities of the wrist. *Radiology* 1978;129:641–651.
34. Klein A, Webb LX. The crowded carpal sign in volar perilunar dislocation. *J Trauma* 1987;27:82–84.
35. Green DP, O'Brien ET. Classification and management of carpal dislocations. *Clin Orthop* 1980;149:55–72.
36. Kaulesar Sukul DM, Johannes EJ. Transscapho-transcapitate fracture dislocation of the carpus. *J Hand Surg [Am]* 1992;17:348–353.
37. Fenton RL. The naviculocapitate fracture syndrome. *J Bone Joint Surg Am* 1956;38:681–684.
38. Stein F, Siegel MW. Naviculocapitate fracture syndrome: A case report. New thoughts on the mechanism of injury. *J Bone Joint Surg Am* 1969;51:391–395.
39. Campbell RD, Lance EM, Chin BY. Lunate and perilunar dislocations. *J Bone Joint Surg Br* 1964;46:55–72.
40. Rawlings ID. The management of dislocations of the carpal lunate. *Injury* 1981;12:319–330.
41. Wagner CJ. Fracture dislocations of the wrist. *Clin Orthop* 1959;15:181–196.
42. Panting AL, Lamb DW, Noble J, et al. Dislocations of the lunate with and without fracture of the scaphoid. *J Bone Joint Surg Br* 1984;66:391–395.
43. MacAusland WR. Perilunar dislocation of the carpal bones and dislocation of the lunate bone. *Surg Gynecol Obstet* 1944;79:256–266.
44. Green DP, O'Brien ET. Open reduction of carpal dislocations: Indications and operative techniques. *J Hand Surg [Am]* 1978;3:250–265.
45. Engel A, Keeman JN. Transcaphoid perilunate fracture dislocation and pseudarthrosis of the scaphoid. *Neth J Surg* 1990;42:128–130.
46. Hawkins L, Torkelson R. Transnavicular perilunar fracture of the wrist. *J Bone Joint Surg Am* 1979;56:1087.
47. Woodward AH, Neviaser RJ, Nisenfeld F. Radial and volar perilunate trans-scaphoid fracture dislocation. *South Med J* 1975;68:926–928.
48. Raab DJ, Fischer DA, Quick DC. Lunate and perilunate dislocations in professional football players: a five year retrospective analysis. *Am J Sports Med* 1994;22:841–845.
49. Moneim MS, Hofammann KE, Omer GE. Transscaphoid perilunate fracture dislocation: result of open reduction and pin fixation. *Clin Orthop* 1984:190:227–235.
50. Minami A, Kaneda K. Repair and/or reconstruction of scapholunate interosseous ligament in lunate and perilunate dislocations. *J Hand Surg [Am]* 1993;18:1099–1106.
51. Sotereanos DG, Mitsionis GJ, Giannakopoulos PN, et al. Perilunate dislocation and fracture dislocation: a critical analysis of the volar–dorsal approach. *J Hand Surg [Am]* 1997;22:49–56.
52. Inoue G, Inagaki Y. Isolated palmar dislocation of the trapezoid associated with attritional rupture of the flexor tendon: a case report. *J Bone Joint Surg Am* 1990;72:446–448.
53. Viegas SF, Bean JW, Schram RA. Trans-scaphoid fracture dislocations treated with open reduction and Herbert screw internal fixation. *J Hand Surg [Am]* 1987;12:992–999.
54. Mamon JF, Tan A, Pyati P, et al. Unusual volar dislocation of the lunate into the distal forearm: case report. *J Trauma* 1991;31:1316–1318.
55. Howard FM, Dell PG. The unreduced carpal dislocation. *Clin Orthop* 1986;202:112–116.
56. Stern P. Multiple flexor tendon ruptures following an old anterior dislocation of the lunate: a case report. *J Bone Joint Surg Am* 1981;63:489–490.
57. Siegert JJ, Frassica FJ, Amadio PC. Treatment of chronic perilunate dislocations. *J Hand Surg [Am]* 1988;13:206–212.
58. Berger RA, Bishop AT. A fiber-splitting capsulotomy technique for dorsal exposure of the wrist. *Tech Hand Upper Extremity Surg* 1997;1:2–10.
59. Steinberg BD, Plancher KD, Idler RS. Percutaneous Kirschner wire fixation through the snuff box: an anatomic study. *J Hand Surg [Am]* 1995;20:57–62.
60. Berger RA. The gross and histologic anatomy of the scapholunate interosseous ligament. *J Hand Surg [Am]* 1996;21:170–178.
61. Lavernia CJ, Cohen MS, Taleisnik J. Treatment of scapholunate dissociation by ligamentous repair and capsulodesis. *J Hand Surg [Am]* 1992;17:354–359.
62. Palmer AK, Dobyns JH, Linscheid RL. Management of post-traumatic instability of the wrist secondary to ligament rupture. *J Hand Surg [Am]* 1978;3:507–532.
63. Blatt G. Capsulodesis in reconstructive hand surgery. *Hand Clin* 1987;3:81–102.
64. Cooney WP, Linscheid RL, Dobyns JH. Fractures and dislocations of the wrist. In: Rockwood CA, Green DP, Bucholz RW, et al, eds. *Rockwood and Green's fractures in adults.* Philadelphia: Lippincott–Raven Publishers, 1996;745–854.
65. Brunelli GA, Brunelli GR. Une nouvelle intervention pour la dissociation scapho-lunaire proposition d'une nouvelle technique chirurgicale pour l'instabilité carpienne avec dissociation scapho-lunaire (11 cas). *Ann Chir Main Memb Super* 1995;14:207–213.

66. Moneim MS, Bolger JT, Omer GE. Radiocarpal dislocation—classification and rationale for management. *Clin Orthop* 1985;192:199–209.
67. Reynolds IS. Dorsal radiocarpal dislocation. *Injury* 1980;12:48–49.
68. Weiss C, Laskin RS, Spinner M. Irreducible radiocarpal dislocation. *J Bone Joint Surg Am* 1970;52:562–564.
69. Rosado AP. A possible relationship of radiocarpal dislocation and dislocation of the lunate bone. *J Bone Joint Surg Br* 1966;48:504–506.
70. Bellinghausen HW, Gilula LA, Young LV, et al. Post-traumatic palmar carpal subluxation. *J Bone Joint Surg Am* 1983;65:998–1006.
71. Rayhack JM, Linscheid RL, Dobyns JH, et al. Posttraumatic ulnar translation of the carpus. *J Hand Surg [Am]* 1987;12:180–189.
72. Fehring TK, Milek MA. Isolated volar dislocation of the radiocarpal joint. *J Bone Joint Surg Am* 1984;66:464–466.
73. Gomez W, Grantham SA. Radial carpal–volar lunate dislocation. *Orthopedics* 1988;11:937–940.
74. Richards RS, Bennett JD, Roth JH. Scaphoid dislocation with radial axial carpal disruption. *AJR* 1993;160:1075–1076.
75. Lourie JA. An unusual dislocation of the lunate and the wrist. *J Trauma* 1982;22:966–967.
76. Apergis E, Dimitrakopoulos K, Chorianopoulos K, et al. Late management of post-traumatic palmar carpal subluxation: a case report. *J Bone Joint Surg Br* 1996;78:419–421.
77. Sides D, Laorr A, Greenspan A. Carpal scaphoid: radiographic pattern of dislocation. *Radiology* 1995;195:215–216.
78. Garcia-Elias M, Dobyns JH, Cooney WP, et al. Traumatic axial dislocations of the carpus. *J Hand Surg [Am]* 1989;14:446–457.
79. Garcia-Elias M, Abanco J, Salvador E, et al. Crush injury of the carpus. *J Bone Joint Surg Br* 1985;67:286–289.
80. Norbeck DE, Larson B, Blair SJ, et al. Traumatic longitudinal disruption of the carpus. *J Hand Surg [Am]* 1987;12:509–514.
81. Gunther SF, Bruno PD. Divergent dislocation of the carpometacarpal joints: a case report. *J Hand Surg [Am]* 1985;10:197–201.
82. Panagis JS, Gelberman RH, Taleisnik J, et al. The arterial anatomy of the human carpus. Part II: the intraosseous vascularity. *J Hand Surg [Am]* 1983;8:375–382.
83. Bendre DV, Baxi VK. Dislocation of trapezoid. *J Trauma* 1981;21:899–900.
84. Ostrowski DM, Miller ME, Gould JS. Dorsal dislocation of the trapezoid. *J Hand Surg [Am]* 1990;15:874–878.
85. Cuenod P, Della Santa DR. Open dislocation of the trapezoid. *J Hand Surg [Br]* 1995;20:185–188.
86. Frix JM, Levine MI. Isolated dorsal dislocation of the trapezoid. *Orthop Rev* 1993;22:1329–1331.
87. Meyn MA, Roth AM. Isolated dislocation of the trapezoid bone. *J Hand Surg [Am]* 1980;5:602–604.
88. Milch H. Isolated luxation of the lesser multangular. *Bull Hosp Joint Dis* 1943;4:36–40.
89. Sampson DA. Isolated dislocation of the lesser multangular bone. *Am J Roentgenol Radium Ther* 1948;59:712–716.
90. Peterson TH. Dislocation of the lesser multangular: Report of a case. *J Bone Joint Surg* 1940;22:200–202.
91. Stein AH. Dorsal dislocation of the lesser multangular bone. *J Bone Joint Surg Am* 1971;53:377–379.
92. Goodman ML, Shankman GB. Update: palmar dislocation of the trapezoid—a case report. *J Hand Surg [Am]* 1984;9:127–131.
93. De Tullio V, Celenza M. Isolated palmar dislocation of the trapezoid. *Int Orthop* 1992;16:53–54.
94. Dunkerton M, Singer M. Dislocation of the index metacarpal and trapezoid bones. *J Hand Surg [Br]* 1985;10:377–378.
95. Kopp JR. Isolated palmar dislocation of the trapezoid. *J Hand Surg [Am]* 1985;10:91–93.
96. Rhoades CE, Reckling FW. Palmar dislocation of the trapezoid—case report. *J Hand Surg [Am]* 1983;8:85–88.
97. Lewis HH. Dislocation of the lesser multangular. *J Bone Joint Surg Am* 1962;44:1412–1414.
98. Yao L, Lee JK. Palmar dislocation of the trapezoid: case report. *J Trauma* 1989;29:405–406.
99. Drewniany JJ, Palmer AK, Flatt AE. The scaphotrapezial ligament complex: an anatomic and biomechanical study. *J Hand Surg [Am]* 1985;10:492–498.
100. Szabo RM, Newland CC, Johnson PG, et al. Spectrum of injury and treatment options for isolated dislocation of the scaphoid. *J Bone Joint Surg Am* 1995;77:608–615.
101. Gelberman RH, Menon J. The vascularity of the scaphoid bone. *J Hand Surg [Am]* 1980;5:508–513.
102. Antuna SA, Antuna-Zapico JM. Open dislocation of the carpal scaphoid: a case report. *J Hand Surg [Am]* 1997;22:86–88.
103. Amamilo SC, Uppal R, Samuel AW. Isolated dislocation of carpal scaphoid. *J Hand Surg [Br]* 1985;10:385–388.
104. Engkvist O, Ekenstam F. Closed dislocation of the scaphoid. *Scand J Plast Reconstr Surg* 1986;20:239–242.
105. Maki NJ, Chuinard RG, D'Ambrosia R. Isolated, complete radial dislocation of the scaphoid. *J Bone Joint Surg Am* 1982;64:615–616.
106. Murakami Y. Dislocation of the carpal scaphoid. *Hand* 1977;9:79–81.
107. Stambough JL, Mandel RJ, Duda JR. Volar dislocation of the carpal scaphoid: case report and review of the literature. *Orthopedics* 1986;9:565–570.
108. Thomas HO. Isolated dislocation of the carpal scaphoid. *Acta Orthop Scand* 1977;48:369–372.
109. Takami H, Takahashi S, Ando M. Dislocation of the carpal scaphoid associated with median nerve compression: case report. *J Trauma* 1992;33:921–923.
110. Thompson TC. Campbell RD, Arnold WD. Primary and secondary dislocation of the scaphoid bone. *J Bone Joint Surg Br* 1964;46:73–82.
111. Inoue G, Maeda N. Isolated dorsal dislocation of the scaphoid. *J Hand Surg [Br]* 1990;15:368–369.
112. McNamara MG, Corley FG. Dislocation of the carpal scaphoid: an 8 year follow-up. *J Hand Surg [Am]* 1992;17:496–498.
113. Milankov M, Somer T, Jovanovic A, et al. Isolated dislocation of the carpal scaphoid: two case reports. *J Trauma* 1994;36:752–754.
114. Cleak DK. Dislocation of the scaphoid and lunate bones without fracture: A case report. *Injury* 1982;14:278–281.
115. Coll GA. Palmar dislocation of the scaphoid and lunate. *J Hand Surg [Am]* 1987;12:476–480.
116. Kupfer K. Palmar dislocation of scaphoid and lunate as a unit: Case report with special reference to carpal instability and treatment. *J Hand Surg [Am]* 1986;11:130–134.
117. Sarrafian SK, Breihan JH. Palmar dislocation of scaphoid and lunate as a unit. *J Hand Surg [Am]* 1990;15:134–139.
118. Taleisnik J, Malerich M, Prietto M. Palmar carpal instability secondary to dislocation of scaphoid and lunate: Report of case and review of the literature. *J Hand Surg [Am]* 1982;7:606–612.
119. Brewood AFM. Complete dislocation of the trapezium: a case report. *Injury* 1985;16:303–304.
120. Goldberg I, Amit S, Bahar A, et al. Complete dislocation of the trapezium (multangulum majus). *J Hand Surg [Am]* 1981;6:193–195.
121. Seimon LP. Compound dislocation of a trapezium. *J Bone Joint Surg Am* 1972;54:1297–1300.

122. Siegel MW, Hertzberg H. Complete dislocation of the greater multangular (trapezium). *J Bone Joint Surg Am* 1969;51: 769–772.
123. Ehara S, El-Khoury GY, Blair WF. Scaphotrapezial dislocation: a case report. *J Trauma* 1988;28:1587–1589.
124. Holdsworth BJ, Shackleford I. Fracture dislocation of the trapezio-scaphoid joint—the missing link? *J Hand Surg [Br]* 1987;12:40–42.
125. Sherlock DA, Phil D. Traumatic dorsoradial dislocation of the trapezium. *J Hand Surg [Am]* 1987;12:262–265.
126. Boe S. Dislocation of the trapezium (multangulum majus). *Acta Orthop Scand* 1979;50:85–86.
127. Peterson CL. Dislocation of the multangulum majus or trapezium (and its treatment in two cases with extirpation). *Arch Chir Neerl* 1950;2:369–376.
128. Frykman E. Dislocation of the triquetrum. *Scand J Plast Reconstr Surg* 1980;14:205–207.
129. Soucacos PN, Hartofilakidis-Garofalidis GC. Dislocation of the triangular bone: Report of a case. *J Bone Joint Surg Am* 1981;63: 1012–1014.
130. Bieber EJ, Weiland AJ. Traumatic dislocation of the triquetrum: A case report. *J Hand Surg [Am]* 1984;9:840–842.
131. Goldberg B, Heller AP. Dorsal dislocation of the triquetrum with rotary subluxation of the scaphoid. *J Hand Surg [Am]* 1987;12:119–122.
132. Ikpeme JO, Hankey S. Dorsal dislocation of the triquetrum: a rare complication of perilunate dislocation. *Injury* 1995;26: 497–499.
133. Inoue G. Dorsal dislocation of the triquetrum: A case report. *Ann Chir Main Memb Super* 1992;11:233–236.
134. Bowen TL. Injuries of the hamate bone. *Hand* 1973;5:235–238.
135. Geist DC. Dislocation of the hamate bone. *J Bone Joint Surg* 1939;21:215–217.
136. Gunn RS. Dislocation of the hamate bone. *J Hand Surg [Br]* 1985;10:107–108.
137. Mathison GW, MacDonald RI. Irreducible transcapitate fracture and dislocation of the hamate. *J Bone Joint Surg Am* 1975; 57:1166–1167.
138. Gainor BJ. Simultaneous dislocation of the hamate and pisiform: A case report. *J Hand Surg [Am]* 1985;10:88–90.
139. Immerman EW. Dislocation of the pisiform. *J Bone Joint Surg Am* 1948;30:489–492.
140. Demartin F, Quinto O. Isolated dislocation of the pisiform. A case report. *Chir Organi Mov* 1993;78:121–123.
141. Mather JH. Dislocation of the pisiform bone. *Br J Radiol* 1993; 18:195–196.
142. Sharara KH, Farrar M. Isolated dislocation of the pisiform bone. *J Hand Surg [Br]* 1993;18:195–196.
143. Minami M, Yamazaki J, Ishii S. Isolated dislocation of the pisiform: A case report and review of the literature. *J Hand Surg [Am]* 1984;9:125–127.
144. Ishizuki M, Nakagawa T, Itoh S, et al. Positional dislocation of the pisiform. *J Hand Surg [Am]* 1991;16:533–535.
145. Lowrey DG, Moss SH, Wolff TW. Volar dislocation of the capitate. Report of a case. *J Bone Joint Surg Am* 1984;66: 611–613.
146. Hirata H, Sasaki H, Ogawa A, et al. Rotatory dislocation of the capitate: a case report. *J Hand Surg [Am]* 1997;22:89–90.
147. Ruijters R, Kortmann J. A case of translunate luxation of the carpus. *Acta Orthop Scand* 1988;59:461–463.
148. Maxwell HA, Morris MA. Scaphotrapeziotrapezoidal dislocation: A case report. *Acta Orthop Scand* 1993;64:385–386.
149. Rockwell WB, Wray RC. Simultaneous dorsal trapezium–scaphoid and trapezoid–carpal subluxations. *J Hand Surg [Am]* 1992;17:376–378.
150. Fowler JL. Dislocation of the triquetrum and lunate: brief report. *J Bone Joint Surg Br* 1988;70:665.
151. Lundkvist L, Larsen CF, Juul SM. Dislocation of the lunate, triquetral and hamate bones. *Scand J Plast Reconstr Surg* 1991;25: 83–85.

15

OPEN REDUCTION AND LIGAMENTOUS REPAIR OF CARPAL FRACTURE-DISLOCATIONS

ROBERT R. SLATER, JR.
ROBERT M. SZABO

Lunate and perilunate dislocations and fracture-dislocations constitute about 10% of all carpal injuries (1). Other forms of carpal dislocations are far less common. Axial dislocations, for instance, were reported in only 1.4% of 1,140 patients treated for any form of carpal fracture, dislocation, or subluxation at one institution (2). Carpal fracture-dislocations are usually high-energy injuries and can result in significant long-term wrist pain and dysfunction, particularly if inappropriately treated or misdiagnosed.

In this chapter the anatomic features and the pathomechanics of carpal dislocations and fracture-dislocations are detailed. Specific injury patterns and treatment recommendations are reviewed; pitfalls to avoid and likely outcomes are considered.

ANATOMY

The anatomy and biomechanics of the wrist are described in Chapters 2 and 4 of this text, but certain concepts that may help explain the pathogenesis of carpal dislocations and fracture-dislocations warrant review. Several theories of carpal bone arrangements into different functional units have been proposed. The traditional theory is that the carpals are arranged in two rows, proximal and distal, and that motion occurs both between and within the rows (3), with the scaphoid acting as a bridge to stabilize the "link joint" between the carpal rows (4). Navarro considered the carpus in three columns: the lateral (mobile) column, composed of the scaphoid, trapezium, and trapezoid; the central (flexion–extension) column, composed of the lunate, capitate, and hamate; and the medial (rotation) column, composed of the triquetrum and pisiform (5). Taleisnik (6) modified that theory and proposed that the pisiform could be eliminated from consideration in any column because it does not participate meaningfully in carpal motion, and that the trapezium and trapezoid could be considered as an integral part of the central flexion–extension unit. Therefore, according to Taleisnik, there is a central flexion–extension unit made up of the trapezium, trapezoid, capitate, hamate, and lunate. The scaphoid is still considered the link stabilizing the midcarpal joint, and the triquetrum is the point around which the rest of the wrist and hand pivot. Weber (7) advanced a different concept of columns, considering them as a central force-bearing column and an ulnar-sided control column and highlighting the helicoid configuration of the triquetrohamate joint as the important controlling unit. Lichtman (8) describes the carpus as a ring with two mobile links permitting reciprocal motion between the proximal and distal rows during radial and ulnar deviation. According to Lichtman, a break in the ring anywhere, whether ligamentous or bony, will result in abnormal motion and carpal instability. Uniform to all conceptual views of wrist mechanics is the importance of a delicate balance inherent in the wrist and how easily injuries can disrupt the balance.

Knowledge of the ligamentous anatomy is critical in understanding and treating carpal dislocations. The wrist ligaments are intracapsular, which makes them difficult to visualize at surgery because they are covered by joint capsule. They are best seen arthroscopically (Fig. 15.1). By current nomenclature (9) there are five important palmar ligaments and two dorsal ligaments. The palmar ligaments are thicker and more substantial structures and are thought to be more important functionally. Palmarly three principal structures secure the carpus to the radius: the radioscaphocapitate (RSC), long radiolunate (LRL), and short radiolunate (SRL) ligaments. The RSC originates from the radial styloid and attaches to the palmar capitate via a groove in the palmar scaphoid waist. It can be thought of as having two subunits, based more on fiber insertion than discrete anatomic divisions. The radioscaphoid subunit runs between the proximal pole of the scaphoid and the distal

---

R. R. Slater, Jr. and R. M. Szabo: Department of Orthopaedic Surgery, University of California, Davis, Sacramento, California 95817.

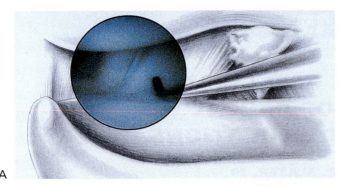
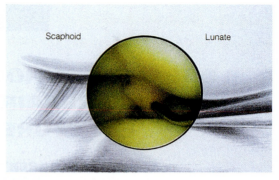

FIGURE 15.1. Arthroscopic view of the palmar radiocarpal ligaments. **A:** The probe is on the long radiolunate ligament, and the radioscaphocapitate ligament is seen to its left. **B:** The probe is on the synovial tuft (once called the ligament of Testut) found opposite the palmar edge of the scapholunate interosseous ligament. (From Whipple T. *Arthroscopic surgery: the wrist.* Philadelphia: JB Lippincott, 1992;73–90, with permission.)

radius and serves as a prime stabilizer of the proximal pole of the scaphoid. Rotary subluxation and dislocation of the scaphoid cannot occur unless this ligament and the scapholunate interosseous ligament (SLIL) are torn (10,11). The other subunit is the scaphocapitate ligament, which contributes to the link between proximal and distal carpal rows. The LRL ligament courses from the palmar rim of the distal radius to the radial margin of the palmar horn of the lunate. The SRL ligament attaches from the palmar rim of the radius at the level of the lunate facet to the palmar surface of the lunate, where it blends in with fibers from the triangular fibrocartilage complex (TFCC).

A structure historically called the ligament of Testut or radioscapholunate ligament was thought to contribute important additional stability to the radial side of the wrist. Further study (9,10), however, showed it is actually a neurovascular pedicle with small branches off the radial and anterior interosseous arteries and anterior interosseous nerve passing to the scapholunate ligament. It lies between the long and SRL ligaments and is best seen arthroscopically (Fig. 15.1B). The remaining two important palmar ligaments originate from the ulna as part of the TFCC and attach to the lunate and triquetrum, the ulnolunate and ulnotriquetral ligaments, respectively. Just distal to the insertion of the ligaments on the lunate and between the LRL and RSC ligament is an area of relatively thin areolar tissue palmar to the capitolunate articulation, first described by Poirier and Charpy in 1926 (12). It is through this potential weak spot, the "space of Poirier" that the lunate usually dislocates.

The dorsal ligaments have been described (5,13) as two thickenings of the dorsal wrist capsule. The dorsal radiocarpal ligament originates from the radius, runs obliquely over the lunate and inserts primarily on the triquetrum. The dorsal intercarpal ligament runs more transversely across the wrist and attaches primarily to the triquetrum and the trapezium.

The intrinsic ligaments in the proximal carpal row, the scapholunate and lunotriquetral interosseous ligaments, allow some rotation and translation between bones. The lunotriquetral interosseous ligament is a thin fibrocartilaginous structure with poor intrinsic vascularity (14). The SLIL has been characterized by Berger (15) as having three distinct regions: the dorsal portion is thickest, with short, transversely oriented collagen fibers; the proximal region is primarily fibrocartilage; and the palmar region is thin and composed of obliquely oriented collagen fibers. These morphologic features have implications for tissue repair and healing potential after injury. For example, a dorsal approach to a perilunate dislocation may allow suture repair of the stoutest portion of the SLIL.

The carpal bones of the distal row are aligned in an arch with the convexity dorsal. The arch is regarded as a relatively rigid structure, with only slight rotational motions occurring between carpal bones as the wrist moves (16). The interosseous ligaments in the distal row keep it functioning and moving as a single unit (2,11,17). The capitohamate joint provides the major stability to the arch. It is stabilized by three ligaments: the dorsal, palmar, and deep interosseous ligaments. The longitudinal interosseous ligament attaches from the capitohamate interosseous recess to the bases of the long and ring finger metacarpals (16,18). Recently, Ritt et al. (16) described the anterior interconnecting bands that originate from the palmar interosseous ligament and insert at the recess between the capitate and hamate. All of these structures are thought to provide additional stability to the capitohamate joint and the articulations between the distal carpal row and the adjacent metacarpal bases.

BIOMECHANICS

Forces acting on the wrist and how these forces are distributed as they are transmitted are referred to as "kinetics."

The complexity of wrist motions comprises "kinematics." Appreciation of both wrist kinetics and kinematics is fundamental to understanding and treating carpal dislocations and fracture-dislocations.

Based on analytic models of human hand forces, An et al. (19) and Schuind et al. (20) have calculated that the total force transmitted by all the metacarpals to the distal carpal row when grasping an object can reach 10 times the force applied at the tips of the fingers. The average maximum grip strength is 137 lb (62 kg) for men and 81 lb (37 kg) for women (21); therefore, it is evident that the wrist may bear compressive forces as high as 1,370 lb in men and 810 lb in women with everyday activities. Forces to produce significant wrist trauma may therefore be even higher.

Once forces have been transferred across the carpometacarpal (CMC) joint, they are distributed through the wrist following specific patterns depending on their magnitude, direction, and point of application as well as the orientation and shape of the carpal bones and the joint surfaces through which they act (19). Pooling data from a variety of studies, Garcia-Elias (17) summarized the force distribution as follows: in neutral wrist position, 50% to 60% of the load borne by the distal row is transmitted through the capitate to the scaphoid and lunate. In the radiocarpal joint, peak pressures are higher in the scaphoid fossa than in the lunate fossa (1.5:1) when the wrist is neutral, but the radiolunate fossa becomes overloaded with ulnar deviation (22–24). These studies help explain the injury patterns seen clinically, which can be altered based on the position of the wrist at impact.

The kinematics of the wrist are dictated by the interactions of carpal bone anatomy, joint articulations, and ligamentous attachments (Figs. 15.2 and 15.3). With axial load, the distal carpal row migrates proximally as a unit, stabilized by the strong intercarpal ligaments. Partly because of its oblique orientation across the carpal rows, the scaphoid is forced to rotate into palmar flexion as the distal row slides proximally (Fig. 15.2A). If the SLIL is intact, this flexion moment on the scaphoid is transmitted to the lunate. Simultaneously, tension in the scaphocapitate ligament while the scaphoid is flexing causes palmar translation of the proximal capitate, which amplifies the force causing lunate flexion (Fig. 15.2B). Meanwhile, the loaded triquetrum is subjected to two opposite moments. If the lunotriquetral ligament is intact, a flexion moment is imparted by the rest

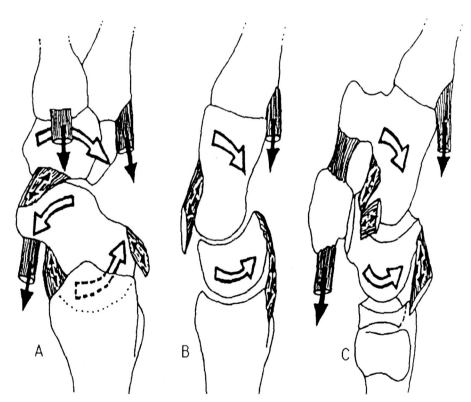

FIGURE 15.2. Schematic illustration of rotations in the sagittal plane occurring in the loaded wrist. **A:** The scaphoid tends to flex while the distal carpal row (trapezium and trapezoid) extends. The constraining ligaments *(double-headed arrows)* are the palmar scaphotrapezial ligaments and the scapholunate interosseous ligament. **B:** The lunate is pulled into flexion by the moment generated by the scaphoid, with only the dorsal capsule constraining this displacement. **C:** The triquetrum follows the predominant flexion moment transmitted by the scaphoid and lunate. The palmar triquetrohamate and triquetrocapitate and the dorsal radiocarpal ligaments constrain this moment. (From Garcia-Elias M. Carpal kinetics. In: Buchler U, ed. *Wrist instability.* London: Martin Dunitz, St Louis: CV Mosby, 1996, with permission.)

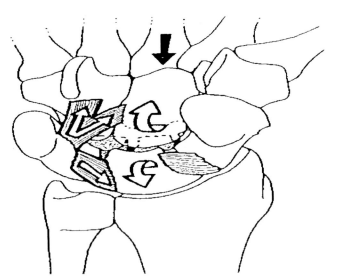

FIGURE 15.3. Schematic illustration from a palmar perspective showing how the loaded midcarpal joint is subjected to two opposite moments: extension generated by the wrist extensors and flexion generated by the obliquely oriented scaphoid, assuming the interosseous ligaments are intact. (From Garcia-Elias M. Carpal kinetics. In: Buchler U, ed. *Wrist instability*. London: Martin Dunitz, St. Louis: CV Mosby, 1996, with permission.)

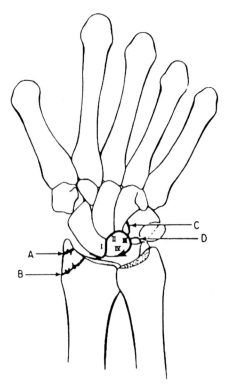

FIGURE 15.4. Mayfield's scheme of progressive lunate instability occurs in four stages: stage I begins with injury to the scapholunate interosseous ligament; stage II includes failure of the midcarpal portion of the radioscaphocapitate ligament (or alternatively fracture of the scaphoid); stage III includes injury of the lunotriquetral and ulnotriquetral ligaments; stage IV includes rupture of the dorsal radiocarpal ligament, allowing palmar dislocation of the lunate. Associated fractures may include A, radial styloid tip; B, radial styloid body; C, lunotriquetral ligament avulsion; or D, ulnotriquetral ligament avulsion. (From Mayfield JK, Johnson RP, Kilcoyne RK. Carpal dislocations: pathomechanics and progressive perilunar instability. *J Hand Surg [Am]* 1980;5:226–241, with permission.)

of the proximal row, but the helicoid articulation between hamate and triquetrum applies extension force as the distal row and hamate are pushed proximally and into extension. Of the opposite moments, the one transmitted by the lunate predominates (17) (Fig. 15.2C). In the normal condition, therefore, under axial load, the three proximal carpal bones have a tendency to rotate into flexion, radial deviation, and slight supination. Note that this is nearly the reverse direction of the force thought to produce lunate and perilunate dislocations: extension, ulnar deviation, and extreme supination (25–27), as explained further below.

Injury Patterns

Analysis of cadaver loading experiments led Mayfield et al. (25–27) to propose a theory of "progressive perilunar instability." No one has been able to refute this theory, and it still proves to be useful in considering the spectrum of injuries seen clinically. The injury mechanism includes extension, ulnar deviation, and intercarpal supination, forces likely produced by falling on the thenar eminence. The pattern of ligamentous disruptions starts on the radial aspect of the wrist and progresses distally and then circumferentially around the lunate (Fig. 15.4). Mayfield's four stages of instability are (I) scapholunate dissociation, caused by disruption of the SLIL and RSC ligaments; (II) capitate dislocation, with disruption of the capitolunate joint through the space of Poirier; (III) triquetral dislocation, with disruption of the lunotriquetral ligament; and (IV) lunate dislocation, with tearing of the dorsal capsule and radiocarpal ligament. In stage IV, the lunate may be flipped into the carpal tunnel (28) or, even more proximally, displaced in the forearm (29).

The result of a traumatic force applied to the extended wrist will depend on the direction and point of impact of that force, hand position at the time of impact, and the relative strength of the carpal bones and ligaments. In light of Mayfield's staging scheme, the following scenario, as iterated by Moneim (30), likely explains the frequent injury patterns recognized clinically. If the point of impact is the base of the thumb, then the scaphoid extends while it is tethered proximally by the scapholunate ligament and distally by the scaphotrapezial and scaphocapitate portion of the RSC ligaments. Progression of the force will produce one of two results: either the scaphoid will fracture as it impinges against the dorsal rim of the radius, or the scapholunate ligament will tear. As the force is applied, the lunate also extends but is locked in by the distal radius. During ulnar deviation, the distal edge of the RSC ligament

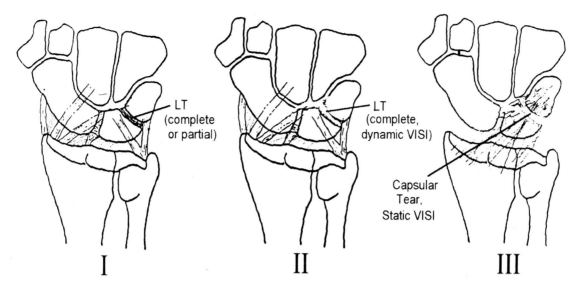

FIGURE 15.5. Classification of ulnar-sided perilunate instability. Stage I is disruption of the lunotriquetral interosseous (LT) ligament, partial or complete, in which dynamic volar intercalated instability (VISI) deformity may or may not be evident. Stage II is disruption of the palmar ulnotriquetral in addition to complete disruption of the LT ligament with dynamic VISI deformity. Stage III is capsular tear and disruption of the dorsal radiocarpal ligament with static VISI deformity. (Modified from Viegas SF, Patterson RM, Patterson PD, et al. Ulnar sided perilunate instability: An anatomic and biomechanic study. *J Hand Surg [Am]* 1990;15:268–277, with permission.)
Editors' Notes: *What is not demonstrated in this figure is the significant spreading moment that occurs between the volar scaphoid and lunate, resulting in the most common of wrist injuries, the tear of the volar scapholunate interosseous ligament.*

is taut, firmly supporting the waist of the scaphoid and tethering the scaphoid and capitate together, while the proximal (radioscaphoid) portion is lax, allowing the capitate to ride dorsally on the lunate.

If the extension and ulnar deviation forces continue and intercarpal supination is added, then a tear develops in the capsular fibers in the space of Poirier between the lunate and capitate, and the capitate is dislocated from the lunate. The force continues toward the triquetrum and either the lunotriquetral ligament ruptures or the bone fractures and a perilunate dislocation occurs. If the force continues, then the lunate will displace palmarly in the carpal canal, causing the distal carpal row to realign with the distal radius. If a fracture occurs through the scaphoid, the proximal pole of the scaphoid may travel with the lunate while the distal pole remains with the capitate. In very rare cases, the scaphoid may fracture, and the scapholunate ligament may also tear, in which case the proximal pole of the scaphoid and the lunate may both be displaced palmarly out of the wrist and found separately (31).

This concept of progressive perilunar instability is consistent with the most common injury patterns seen, where the primary dislocation occurs at the midcarpal joint and the capitate is initially displaced dorsal to the lunate. Instability limited to the ulnar side of the wrist is seen clinically but is not explained by Mayfield's original theory. Viegas (14) described a staging system for ulnar-sided perilunate instability (Fig. 15.5): (I) partial or complete disruption of the lunotriquetral ligament, although radiographic evidence of dynamic or static instability may or may not present; (II) complete lunotriquetral ligament tear with clinical and radiographic evidence of dynamic volar intercalated segment instability (VISI); and (III) static VISI deformity.

Finally, isolated scaphoid dislocations may be considered as resulting from yet another distribution of forces (Fig. 15.6). Based on intraoperative observations made while

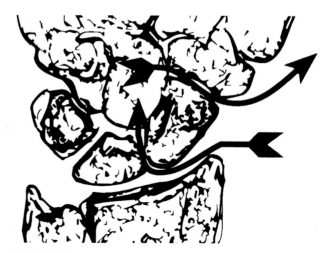

FIGURE 15.6. Diagram of the postulated sequence of ligamentous failure in scaphoid dislocation. (From Szabo RM, Newland CC, Johnson PG, et al. Spectrum of injury and treatment options for isolated dislocation of the scaphoid. *J Bone Joint Surg Am* 1995;17:608–615, with permission.)

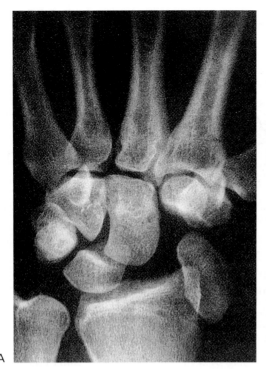 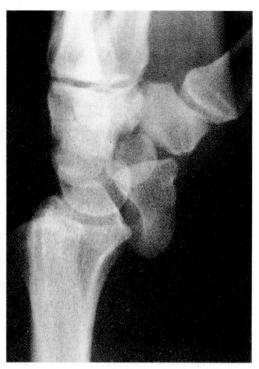

FIGURE 15.7. Isolated scaphoid dislocation. Anteroposterior **(A)** and lateral **(B)** radiographs showing a complete radiopalmar dislocation of the scaphoid. (From Szabo RM, Newland CC, Johnson PG, et al. Spectrum of injury and treatment options for isolated dislocation of the scaphoid. *J Bone Joint Surg Am* 1995;77:608–615, with permission.)

treating three cases (Fig. 15.7), one of us (R.M.S.) (32) described how isolated scaphoid dislocations may result from a sequence of ligamentous failure that starts at the radiopalmar aspect of the proximal pole of the scaphoid with failure of the RSC and SLIL, progresses to the LRL ligament, and ends with the scaphotrapezial ligament.

DIAGNOSIS

Making the diagnosis of a carpal dislocation clinically begins with the history of the injury mechanism. The key element of the history is a significant force applied to the outstretched hand, usually from a fall or motor vehicle accident. Physical examination after most carpal dislocations and fracture-dislocations reveals diffuse wrist swelling and tenderness. It is often difficult to localize maximum areas of tenderness, but specific areas should be palpated including the radial styloid, scaphoid, lunate, scapholunate joint, triquetrum, and carpal tunnel. The initial clinical evaluation must include a careful assessment of the neurovascular status of the hand because median nerve injury is present in approximately 40% of these injuries (30,33–35).

Diagnostic Imaging

The diagnosis of carpal dislocations and fracture-dislocations is confirmed primarily on the basis of radiographs. Routine posteroanterior (PA), lateral, and oblique views usually suffice. Gilula has stressed the importance of examining the PA view for three smooth arches: along the proximal and distal edges of the proximal carpal row and the proximal edge of the distal carpal row (36) (Fig. 15.8A). Any break in continuity of any arch suggests an abnormality at the site of the broken arch. Either flexion or extension of the lunate can make it appear more triangular in shape on the PA view and cause a break in Gilula's lines, suggesting an abnormality (36–38). These lines must be interpreted with caution, however, because a more recent study by Peh and Gilula (39) showed the arcs to be commonly disrupted even in normal wrists if the wrist is not strictly in neutral position (Fig. 15.8B,C).

Carpal bone alignment is measured on the lateral radiograph. Guidelines for measuring and interpreting the scapholunate, capitolunate, and radiolunate angles have been defined and are considered a routine part of establishing carpal malalignment (38,40,41). The angles can be measured from the lateral radiograph using one of two methods (Fig. 15.9). The axial method uses the midpoints of the proximal and distal articular surfaces of the carpals to

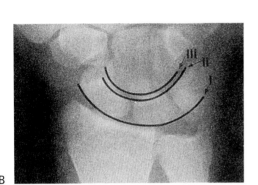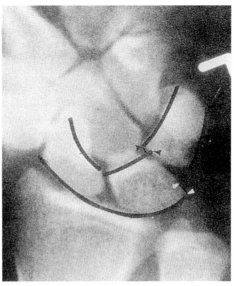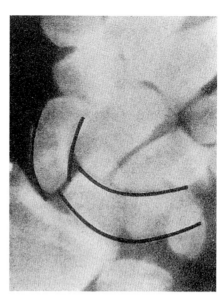

FIGURE 15.8. The carpal arcs according to Gilula. **A:** Normally, three concentric arcs can be drawn along the cortical outlines of the scaphoid, lunate, and triquetrum *(arcs I and II)* and the proximal edges of the distal carpal row *(arc III)*. One must be careful that the wrist is in neutral position when the x-ray is obtained because the arcs may be disrupted even in normal wrists in radial **(B)** and ulnar **(C)** deviation. (From Peh WCG, Gilula LA. Normal disruption of carpal arcs. *J Hand Surg [Am]* 1996;21:561–566, with permission.)

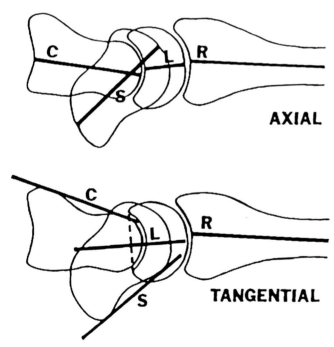

FIGURE 15.9. Two methods of determining carpal angles on a lateral x-ray, using the radius *(R)*, lunate *(L)*, scaphoid *(S)*, and capitate *(C)* as landmarks. The axial method uses the midpoints of the proximal and distal articular surfaces of the carpals to obtain the longitudinal axis. The tangential method determines the axis using lines tangential to the palmar outline of the scaphoid, the distal end of the lunate, and the dorsal outline of the capitate. (From Garcia-Elias M, An K, Amadio PC, et al. Reliability of carpal angle determinations. *J Hand Surg [Am]* 1989;14:1017–1021, with permission.)

obtain the bones' longitudinal axes. The tangential method determines carpal axis using lines drawn tangential to the palmar outline of the scaphoid, the dorsal outline of the capitate, and the distal outline of the lunate. Neither method is superior in terms of statistical significance. Interobserver variation averages ±5.2° for both methods, and measurements are an average of 7.4° different from true measurements of carpal angle (40). Nonetheless, the following guidelines have been established: normal capitolunate angle is 0°, and anything greater than 15° is abnormal; normal scapholunate angle is less than 60°, and anything greater than 80° is abnormal; normal radiolunate angle is 0°, and an angle greater than 15° is abnormal. The values between abnormal and the upper limits of normal are considered "gray zones."

Special views are helpful in some cases. Distraction radiographs can be obtained with the fingers in finger traps and a 10- to 15-lb counterweight applied to the patient's arm. These x-rays can show the extent of bony damage much more clearly than the initial films, which can be hard to interpret because of the overlap and displacement of the carpal bones. Usually these views are obtained as part of treatment, for example, when preparing to reduce an acute injury, rather than for the sake of diagnosis alone.

In evaluating more subtle, suspected injuries or chronic injuries, other diagnostic methods can be useful. Tomography is most commonly used, either trispiral or computerized (CT scan). Arthrography can confirm suspected ligamentous tears (42–44) but is more applicable to chronic injury states. Magnetic resonance imaging (MRI) is becoming a more important diagnostic tool in wrist injury evaluation. It is an expensive test, but in some cases its use is appealing because it is noninvasive and because it can be used to evaluate the status of carpal fractures and vascularity as well as ligamentous integrity.

CLASSIFICATION

To help plan treatment, we find it useful to classify carpal dislocations according to injury pattern (Table 15.1).

TABLE 15.1. CLASSIFICATION OF CARPAL DISLOCATIONS

I. Dorsal perilunate–palmar lunate dislocation
II. Dorsal transscaphoid–perilunate dislocation
III. Palmar perilunate–dorsal lunate dislocation
IV. Combination injuries
 A. Transradial styloid–perilunate dislocation
 B. Scaphocapitate syndrome
 C. Transtriquetral fracture-dislocation
V. Scaphoid rotary subluxation-dislocation
VI. Axial disruptions

Modified from Green DP, O'Brien ET. Classification and management of carpal dislocations. *Clin Orthop* 1980;149:55–72, with permission.

Dorsal Perilunate Dislocation or Palmar Lunate Dislocation

These entities were once considered separately but probably are best considered to be progressive stages of the same injury, as recommended by Green and O'Brien (33). The lateral radiograph is the most revealing (Fig. 15.10A,B). In a dorsal perilunate dislocation, it shows the capitate dorsal to the longitudinal axis of the radius as well as dorsal rotation of the proximal pole of the scaphoid. This will be further evidenced by the "signet ring" sign on the PA x-ray, which is the radiographic shadow of the distal pole of the scaphoid seen in cross section, indicating its flexed posture. The PA x-ray also will show carpal overlap, disruption of Gilula's lines, and a triangular-shaped lunate (Figs. 15.10C and 15.11).

In a lunate dislocation, the forces causing the injury may have resulted in spontaneous reduction of the capitate and the distal carpal row and complete palmar displacement of the lunate. In this case, the lateral x-ray will show the capitate nearly collinear with the longitudinal axis of the radius, and the lunate's distal articular surface will face palmarly to produce the so-called "spilled teacup" sign (33) (Fig. 15.12). The lateral view will also show dorsal displacement of the triquetrum secondary to the tear in the lunotriquetral ligament. Because of the dissociation between lunate and triquetrum and the loss of extension influence of the triquetrum on the lunate, a static VISI collapse pattern is evident (45).

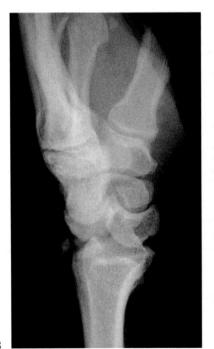
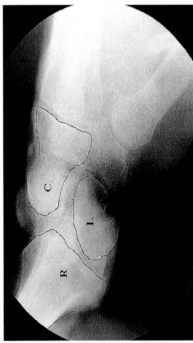
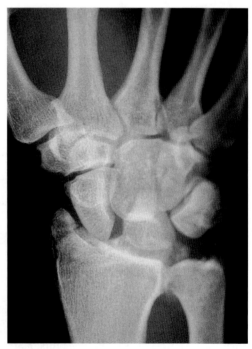

FIGURE 15.10. A: Lateral view radiograph of a dorsal perilunate dislocation variant. **B:** Lateral view (fluoroscopy) of this injury in a cadaver model, labeled for clarity. The capitate *(C)* is dorsal to the longitudinal axis of the radius *(R)*, while the lunate *(L)* remains collinear with the radius. **C:** The posteroanterior view confirms that this is a transradial styloid dorsal perilunate dislocation. There is carpal overlap, complete disruption of Gilula's lines, and a triangular-shaped lunate.

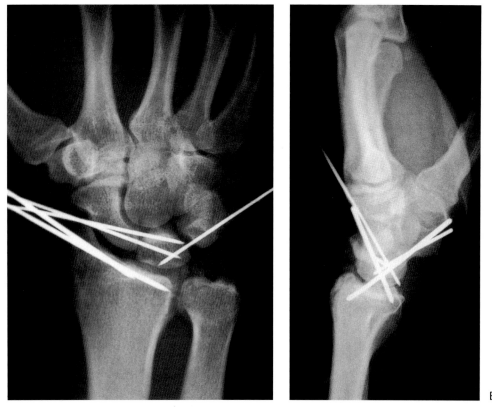

FIGURE 15.11. Posteroanterior **(A)** and lateral **(B)** radiographs after treatment of the injury shown in Fig. 15.10 by open reduction, percutaneous pinning, and ligament repair. Normal carpal alignment has been restored.

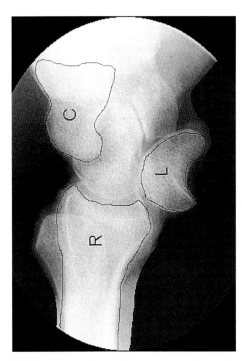

FIGURE 15.12. Lateral view (fluoroscopy) of a palmar lunate dislocation produced in a cadaver. In this case, the capitate remains nearly aligned with the radius, but the lunate is displaced palmarly and tilted in flexion ("spilled teacup" sign). *C,* capitate; *R,* radius; *L,* lunate.

The PA x-ray will still show carpal overlap and disruption of Gilula's lines. The shape and position of the lunate will vary depending on the amount of its displacement. In either a dorsal perilunate or lunate dislocation, there is disruption of the SLIL, which will be reflected in a wide gap between the scaphoid and lunate. This was once called the "Terry Thomas sign" (46) after the British comedian with a wide front tooth diastasis but would perhaps be better updated and renamed the "David Letterman sign."

Dorsal Transcaphoid Perilunate Dislocation

The hallmark of this injury is the displaced scaphoid fracture (Fig. 15.13). In this injury the distal pole of the scaphoid displaces dorsally with the capitate and the lunate remaining attached to the proximal pole of the scaphoid. In a multicenter study of these injuries reported by Herzberg et al. (47), it was determined that the scaphoid fractures through the waist in 95% of cases with comminution in 22%. In 5% of cases there was a proximal pole fracture. The lunotriquetral ligament may be torn in some cases (Mayfield's stage IV equivalent).

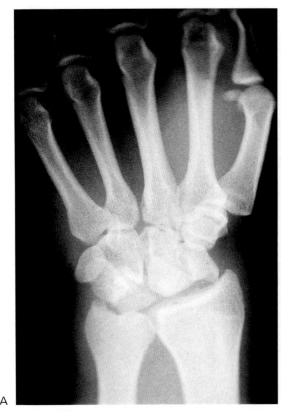 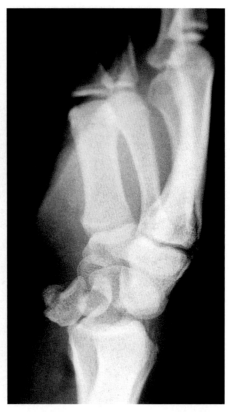

FIGURE 15.13. Anteroposterior **(A)** and lateral **(B)** radiographs of a transscaphoid perilunate dislocation. **Editors' Notes:** *Note on the PA view the discontinuous curvature of the proximal scaphoid and lunate, illustrating the fact that these are extremely difficult to align even under direct visualization. Percutaneous pinning is not indicated in these cases. The key to the anatomic reduction is the reestablishment of normal relationships among the scaphoid, the lunate, and the capitate. Occasionally, in major injuries, the relationship to the radius may require reduction.*

Palmar Perilunate Dislocation or Dorsal Lunate Dislocation

This injury pattern is rare. The mechanism of injury is uncertain and has been debated. Some authors postulate forceful wrist hyperflexion sustained by falling on the back of the hand (48–50). Others suggest that severe wrist hyperextension can produce this injury as well as the more common dorsal perilunate dislocation (5,48–51). In a recent study, Niazi (51) was able to reliably reproduce palmar perilunate dislocations in a series of cadavers by sectioning the scaphotrapezial and palmar radiocarpal ligaments and applying a dorsal shearing force.

Combination Injuries

The most common of these is the *transradial styloid perilunate dislocation* (Figs. 15.12 and 15.13). In this injury, the force is dissipated by fracturing through the radial styloid and SLIL rather than the scaphoid. Isolated radial styloid fractures occur and are sometimes referred to as "chauffeur's" fractures, but if the history suggests a high-velocity fall or axial load, then associated carpal bone fracture and ligamentous instability, specifically of the SLIL, must be ruled out. One should have a high index of suspicion for these associated injuries.

Scaphocapitate syndrome is a rare pattern of wrist injury first described by Nicholson in 1940 (52). Several variants have been described, all usually resulting from severe trauma. The hallmark is transverse fractures of both the scaphoid and the capitate with rotation of the proximal pole of the capitate so that its articular surface faces distally (53). It has been postulated (54) that it occurs most often in extreme wrist extension; the dorsal rim of the radius impinges on the capitate, fracturing it, while the scaphoid fractures as the result of stress between the proximal and distal carpal rows generated by the extreme extension. Midcarpal dislocation then occurs, and the proximal pole of the capitate rotates 90° to 180°. Spontaneous relocation may occur, leaving only the fractured scaphoid and inverted capitate fragment as evidence of this injury. This proposed mechanism does not explain all injury patterns reported, and other mechanisms have been postulated, including axial loading in extreme flexion (53).

Despite the displacement of the capitate fragment, this fracture can be overlooked on routine radiographs and mismanaged as a simple scaphoid fracture. The relationship of the radius to the lunate and fractured capitate should be assessed critically on the lateral x-ray. Distraction view films are sometimes helpful in this situation and will show the squared-off end of the proximal capitate.

Transtriquetral fracture-dislocations occur when the applied force exits through the triquetrum. In such cases, the proximal radial fragment remains with the lunate via its attachment with the lunotriquetral ligament while the distal ulnar fragment displaces with the capitate. This can occur in association with perilunate dislocations (33,55) or in association with scaphocapitate syndrome (56).

Scaphoid Subluxation versus Dislocation

A distinction should be made between the injury historically called "rotary subluxation of the navicular (scaphoid)" and true dislocation of the scaphoid. Several authors (57–62) have shown that primary rotary subluxation of the scaphoid can occur. Taleisnik (6) and Mayfield et al. (13) have suggested that the structure now called the RSC ligament must be torn at least partially in addition to a disruption of the SLIL to allow the rotary subluxation to occur. However, there is no injury to the scaphotrapezial ligaments that support the distal pole of the scaphoid. This may be the first stage of a perilunate dislocation or, in cases where the diagnosis is made late, may represent a partially healed perilunate dislocation. On the lateral x-ray there is an increased scapholunate angle, the lunate tilts dorsally, and the scaphoid is flexed with its proximal pole subluxated dorsally, the so-called dorsal intercalated segment instability (DISI) pattern.

In contrast, dislocation of the scaphoid results from a different pattern of ligamentous injury. In this case, it is postulated (32) that a sequence of ligamentous failure begins with disruption of the RSC and SLIL and then progresses to include the LRL and scaphotrapezial ligaments, resulting in complete instability of the scaphoid (see Fig. 15.6). Displacement of the proximal pole out of the scaphoid fossa is diagnostic of a scaphoid dislocation rather than a perilunate dislocation.

Longitudinal Disruptions

A constellation of uncommon carpal dislocations and instabilities between the radial and ulnar sides of the carpus can be considered together as longitudinal disruptions. *Axial dislocations of the carpus* fall into this category. They are rare and result from blast or crush injuries in which the carpus is separated longitudinally and usually displaced with the respective metacarpals. The hand is flattened with destruction of the normal convex relationship between the metacarpal heads (2). Because of the mechanism of injury, significant soft tissue injuries and thenar lacerations are frequently noted. Garcia-Elias et al. (2,63) have classified these injuries into three variants (Fig. 15.14): axial-radial (most common), axial-ulnar, and combined axial-radial-ulnar (least common). In the axial-radial type, the radial column is displaced radially and proximally while the ulnar column remains stable with respect to the radius. In axial-ulnar disruption, the ulnar column is shifted proximally and ulnarly while the radial column remains relatively stable, and in the combined injuries both columns displace proximally.

TREATMENT

Treatment strategy can be based largely on injury pattern (Fig. 15.15). Treatment must be individualized for each patient, but some general guidelines are useful. Following the initial physical exam and documentation of associated injuries and any neurovascular deficits, if the lunate is displaced in the carpal tunnel or the capitate is not articulating with the lunate, then urgent closed reduction should be done to obtain gross carpal alignment and relieve pressure on the median nerve. Beyond these initial steps, treatment will depend on the classification of injury as described in the following sections.

Perilunate Dislocations

Traction with finger traps is applied using 10 to 15 lb of counterforce at the arm for 10 minutes. At this point distraction x-rays may be obtained to further delineate the pathology. Then the finger traps are removed while longitudinal manual traction is maintained. With one hand, the surgeon extends the patient's wrist while the thumb of the surgeon's other hand stabilizes the patient's lunate palmarly. The patient's wrist is then gradually flexed, which delivers the head of the capitate back into the lunate concavity, usually with a palpable and audible "clunk." The wrist is then splinted in neutral position. PA and lateral postreduction x-rays should then be obtained.

On the postreduction films, the scapholunate angle should be less than 60° on the lateral view and the scapholunate gap less than 2 mm on the PA view. If anatomic reduction is obtained, some have advocated percutaneous pinning utilizing fluoroscopy (5). We prefer open reduction with internal and fixation (ORIF) because truly anatomic reduction is difficult to obtain and rarely maintained (28,34,58,64).

One area of controversy in the literature is the preferred surgical approach: dorsal, palmar, or both. Many authors have recommended a dorsal approach because it offers good exposure of the proximal carpal row and midcarpal joint (25,30,65). Others recommend a palmar approach (28,66), and many recommend routinely utilizing a combined dorsal and palmar approach in all cases (5,55,67–70), arguing

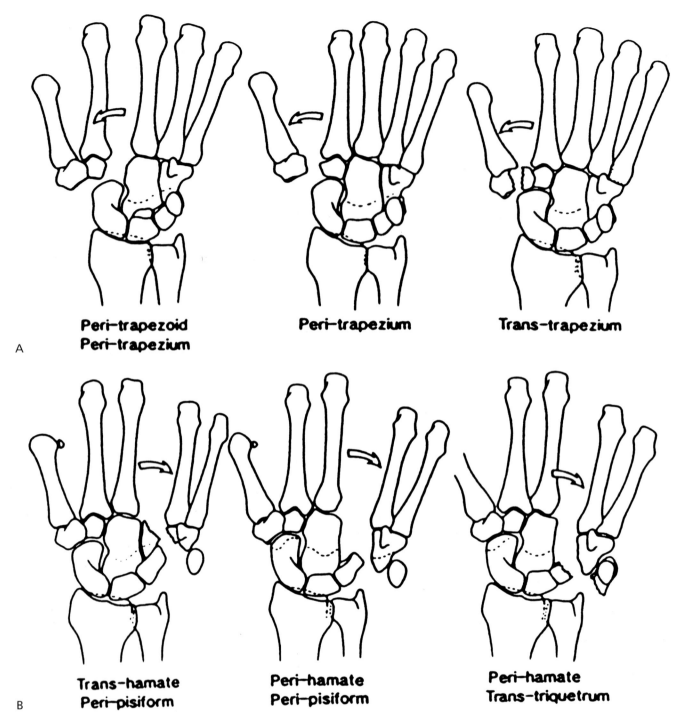

FIGURE 15.14. Longitudinal disruptions of the carpus. The most common types are shown: **(A)** axial–radial disruptions, three types; **(B)** axial–ulnar disruptions, three types. Combined injuries may also rarely occur. (From Garcia-Elias M, Dobyns JH, Cooney WP, et al. Traumatic axial dislocations of the carpus. *J Hand Surg [Am]* 1989;14:446–457, with permission.)

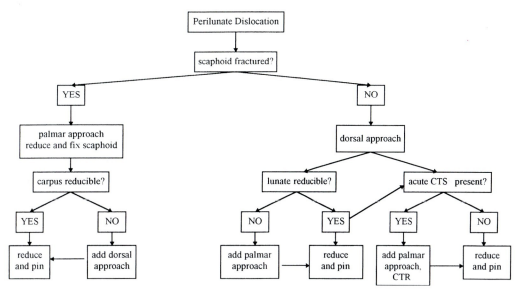

FIGURE 15.15. Treatment algorithm for perilunate dislocations and fracture-dislocations. *CTS,* carpal tunnel syndrome; *CTR,* carpal tunnel release.

that the palmar approach provides an opportunity to visualize and repair the palmar ligaments.

We believe the palmar approach is not necessary for treating most perilunate dislocations. Although the palmar radiocarpal structures are distinct structures when viewed from within the joint, they cannot be distinguished from the palmar side because of the overlying capsule. The traumatic disruption of the normal tissues compounds the problem, making it unlikely that they can be repaired in their correct orientation and under proper tension. Rather, in our experience, attempts to repair them cause shortening and further scarring of the ligaments and ultimately loss of motion of the wrist. Recurrent palmar dislocation after a lunate or perilunate dislocation properly treated via an isolated dorsal approach is unlikely and not something we have ever encountered. In contrast, stiffness is a more common problem. In general, we use a dorsal approach to the wrist when treating perilunate dislocations, with some exceptions, as discussed below.

Technique: Dorsal Approach

Make a dorsal longitudinal skin incision in line with Lister's tubercle. Develop the interval between the third and fourth compartments by dividing the distal portion of the extensor retinaculum and the septum between the compartments. Retract the tendons of the fourth compartment ulnarly and the extensor pollicus longus radially (Fig. 15.16). Incise the dorsal capsule longitudinally in line with Lister's tubercle; if there is already a traumatic rent in the capsule, extend it longitudinally. Elevate the capsular flaps by subperiosteal dissection to expose the scaphoid, lunate, triquetrum, and capitate, but be careful to avoid the blood supply to the scaphoid entering the dorsal ridge.

We create "joysticks" to help manipulate the scaphoid and lunate by placing 0.062-in. Kirschner wires (K-wires) in a dorsal-palmar direction, one wire in the lunate and another in the scaphoid (Fig. 15.17). Drill them deep

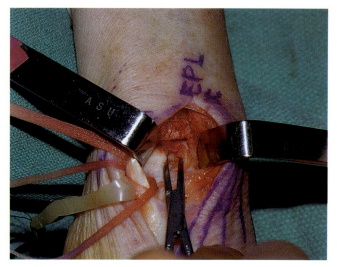

FIGURE 15.16. Dorsal approach to repair a dorsal perilunate dislocation. The interval between the third and fourth extensor compartments is utilized. Umbilical tapes tag the tendons, and a rubber dam protects the superficial branch of the radial nerve. The lamina spreader is in the gap between the scaphoid and lunate that follows from scapholunate interosseous ligament disruption. **Editors' Notes:** *The dorsal approach is preferred even with scaphoid fracture. The scaphoid is more easily visualized from a dorsal approach, and the capitate and lunate act as templates to reestablish anatomic relationships.*

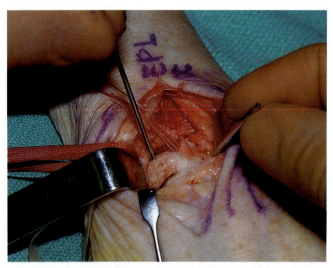

FIGURE 15.17. Joysticks (0.062-in K-wires) are drilled into the lunate and scaphoid and manipulated to achieve anatomic reduction. **Editors' Notes:** *A transverse skin incision allows wide and adequate exposure of the entire carpus while maintaining the extensor retinaculum, which primarily overlies the distal radius.*

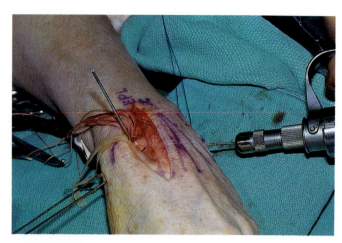

FIGURE 15.18. After placing K-wires from the radial side of the wrist to maintain the scapholunate reduction, an additional K-wire is drilled percutaneously from the ulnar side of the wrist to maintain the lunotriquetral joint.

enough to reach the palmar cortex to provide adequate leverage and control. Manipulate the scaphoid to reduce its palmar flexion and the lunate to reduce its extension; use the joysticks to reduce the interosseous gap. While an assistant maintains the reduction, drill two 0.045-in. K-wires from the radial side of the carpus percutaneously through the proximal pole of the scaphoid into the lunate. Place a third wire of the same size percutaneously, through the scaphoid into the capitate. Make sure there are no chondral fragments or other fracture fragments in the capitolunate joint before placing the third pin.

The dorsal portion of the scapholunate ligament should be repaired if possible, using 4-0 nonabsorbable suture. If the tear is off bone, the ligament can be tacked down with horizontal mattress sutures passed through drill holes in bone as described by Lavernia et al. (71) (see below) or via a suture minianchor.

Examine the lunotriquetral joint and confirm that it is reduced or manipulate the bones as necessary to obtain reduction. Maintain this reduction while driving another 0.045-in. K-wire from the ulnar side of the triquetrum into the lunate (Fig. 15.18). Additional pins are usually not necessary. We do not place any pins across the radiocarpal joint (Fig. 15.19). In those cases where treatment has been delayed by more than 7 to 10 days but typically less than 3 weeks, we reinforce the SLIL repair with a dorsal capsulodesis as discussed below for treatment of chronic injuries.

A few tips on placing the K-wires warrant mention. It is possible to injure sensory branches of the superficial radial nerve and dorsal ulnar nerve and branches of the radial artery when placing percutaneous pins near the wrist. To minimize this risk, make a 3-mm skin incision and spread bluntly down to the capsule with a hemostat. Use a blunted 14-gauge angiocath held in a hemostat as a guide and pass the K-wires through the guide when drilling them into position. Cut the wires beneath the skin to minimize the chance of their becoming infected. It is also helpful to use intraoperative fluoroscopy to place the K-wires to ensure their proper placement with a minimum number of passes through bone and cartilage.

Obtain standard radiographs in the PA and lateral projections once final reduction and pin placement are achieved. Close the capsulotomy incision as well as any other tears in the dorsal capsule with 4-0 nonabsorbable suture, and close the skin in a routine fashion. A drain is usually unnecessary.

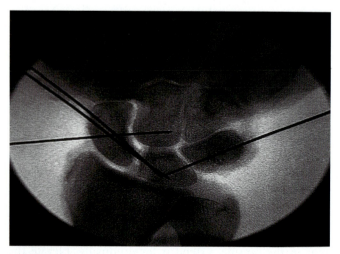

FIGURE 15.19. Anteroposterior radiograph (fluoroscopy) showing the recommended final pin placement for treating a perilunate dislocation.

Postoperatively, immobilize the extremity in a bulky plaster reinforced thumb–spica dressing that extends above the elbow, maintaining the forearm in neutral and the wrist in 15° flexion and 10° radial deviation. Convert this to an above-elbow thumb–spica cast after 10 days when the sutures are removed. At 6 weeks apply a below-elbow thumb–spica cast. Remove the pins after 8 weeks. After a total of 12 weeks of immobilization, a removable splint is used for comfort, and range-of-motion exercises are begun.

Technique: Palmar Approach

We reserve the addition of a palmar approach to the dorsal approach for two situations: first, for those cases where the lunate is dislocated (Mayfield stage IV) and cannot be reduced closed or with the dorsal exposure; second, for acute carpal tunnel syndrome. We use a standard carpal tunnel release extending the incision obliquely and ulnarly across the wrist crease for 1 cm. After complete decompression of the median nerve, reduce the lunate provisionally through the floor of the radiocarpal joint. Then return to the dorsal incision and complete the accurate reduction and fixation in the manner outlined above.

Transcaphoid Perilunate Fracture-Dislocations

Part of this injury always includes a displaced fracture of the scaphoid for which early ORIF is preferred (34,72,73). In contrast to a perilunate or lunate dislocation where a palmar approach is not used routinely, in cases where the scaphoid is fractured, a palmar approach is used routinely to reduce and fix the scaphoid. Bone graft from the distal radius or iliac crest may be added in cases where there is extensive comminution. The addition of a dorsal approach is usually not necessary.

Technique: Palmar Approach

Our standard palmar approach is that described by Russe if the carpal tunnel does not need release. If it does, then a modified carpal tunnel release incision is used, carrying the proximal portion of the incision further radially. The palmar cutaneous branch of the median nerve must be identified, tagged, and protected when the incision extends across the wrist crease. Next, identify and tag the radial artery and the flexor carpi radialis (FCR) tendon and retract both radially. Open the floor of the FCR sheath and the radiocarpal joint capsule longitudinally to expose the scaphoid. Insert 0.045-in. K-wires perpendicular to each fracture fragment to act as joysticks. Manipulate the fracture to achieve reduction and then place a Freer elevator in the radioscaphoid joint to maintain reduction and apply counterforce. Drill two smooth 0.045-inch K-wires percutaneously across the fracture and confirm their position radiographically.

Once the scaphoid is anatomically reduced and fixed, the wrist is examined fluoroscopically. The perilunate dislocation is usually found to be reduced. In stage IV (Mayfield) injuries, the lunotriquetral joint can be reduced and pinned percutaneously by applying palmarly directed pressure to the triquetrum, which is usually displaced dorsally. Sometimes osteochondral fractures, particularly of the capitate, block complete reduction (33). Jasmine et al. (65) reported two cases in which the dorsal capsule was impaled by the fractured scaphoid and blocked reduction from a palmar approach of a transcaphoid perilunate dislocation. In such cases, a dorsal approach is added to remove the offending fragments, debride the involved joint(s) and facilitate reduction. Once the reduction and fixation are satisfactory, close the capsule with 4-0 nonabsorbable suture, and close the skin in a routine fashion.

There is controversy about the benefits of compression screws such as the Herbert screw versus K-wires for fracture fixation (74,75). We prefer K-wires because they are easier to insert and do not require stripping away the important scaphotrapezial and scaphocapitate ligaments to afford exposure for screw placement. Two K-wires also provide better rotational control of the fracture than a single screw, which can be a problem in the face of the comminution frequently seen. If K-wires are used, they should be cut off under the skin and not removed until the fracture is radiographically united as demonstrated by tomography (11). In the small number of cases (5%) where the scaphoid is fractured through the proximal pole, it may be possible to reduce and fix the fracture via an isolated dorsal approach, and in this case screw fixation probably provides more stability. We prefer a small cannulated screw for this purpose.

Other Combination Injuries

For *transradial styloid perilunate dislocations,* fixation of the radial styloid is often possible. Because the important radiocarpal ligaments attach here, it is important to preserve as much bony stability at this corner of the wrist as possible. Single large styloid fragments can be fixed with K-wires or 3.5-mm lag screws or a combination of each.

The scaphocapitate syndrome is usually best addressed surgically because closed reduction and treatment have been largely unsuccessful (53,54,76). A dorsal approach is used. Capitate fractures should be fixed anatomically if possible, and bone graft added where necessary. Similarly, the transtriquetral fracture-dislocations are best treated surgically using a dorsal approach. The triquetral fractures should be stabilized with additional K-wires as necessary. The postoperative management for all of these injuries is the same as for the transcaphoid perilunate fracture-dislocation.

Scaphoid Instability

Treatment of scaphoid dislocation injuries focuses on restoration of the scapholunate relationship. The SLIL should be repaired whenever possible. Sometimes that is possible using the technique of passing sutures through drill holes in bone as described by Lavernia et al. (71) or using suture minianchors in lieu of bone tunnels. The role of arthroscopy in managing these injuries is evolving. In a series of three scaphoid dislocations reported by one of us (R.M.S.) (32), arthroscopy provided useful information about the status of the SLIL and radiocarpal ligaments and allowed thorough joint debridement and removal of loose chondral fragments as part of the definitive management.

Longitudinal Dissociations

In longitudinal injuries, the focus of treatment is directed to the associated soft tissue and neurovascular damage, making it more difficult to establish generalized treatment guidelines. Certain principles apply to all cases, however. Treatment consists of debridement of nonviable tissues, open reduction and fixation of fractures (usually with K-wires), repair of damaged tendons and neurovascular structures where possible, and application of immediate or delayed skin coverage. Cast immobilization for 6 to 8 weeks is usually utilized, after which active hand therapy is started. Secondary procedures such as tenolysis and neurolysis are commonly necessary (2,11).

Late Recognition and Treatment

Unfortunately, many carpal dislocations continue to be misdiagnosed acutely, especially the perilunate dislocations and scaphoid subluxations (5,28,55,67,70,77). In the large series reported by Herzberg et al. (47), the diagnosis was missed initially in 25% of cases. Late treatment of neglected perilunate or lunate dislocation is difficult and controversial (35,70,78,79). There is general agreement that results after long delays in treatment or no treatment for perilunate dislocations or fracture-dislocations are poor (34,47,70,80).

The upper time limit considered consistent with the ability to restore anatomy has been reported to be 6 weeks (55,81–84). Alternative procedures such as ligament reconstructions, proximal row carpectomy, or selective intercarpal or radiocarpal arthrodeses have been recommended for patients who present with dislocations or fracture-dislocations more than 6 weeks old (58,81,84). This remains controversial. For example, Gellman et al. (55) reported successfully treating a dorsal transcaphoid, transtriquetral perilunate wrist dislocation 3 months after injury. Sousa et al. (85) described using an external fixator and slow distraction over 1 week to stretch the soft tissues enough to allow open reduction after missed diagnoses in three patients. We have no experience with this technique.

In general, open reduction may be attempted late, but with the recognition that for those cases where reduction is impossible, proximal row carpectomy may be a good option. Limited or total wrist arthrodesis should be done if symptomatic arthritic changes are already present.

A common scenario is a delay in treating scapholunate ligament disruptions where the scaphoid rotation is not fixed but can be corrected surgically. A variety of ligament reconstruction and augmentation procedures can be useful in this situation. We prefer the technique described by Lavernia, Cohen, and Taleisnik (71), which we have modified slightly as described below.

Technique: Scapholunate Ligament Repair and Capsulodesis

Make a longitudinal skin incision centered over Lister's tubercle. Expose and then incise the extensor retinaculum between the third and fourth compartments. Unroof and retract the extensor pollicis longus (EPL) radially and dissect the fourth compartment subperiosteally to reflect it ulnarly; this should expose the scaphoid and lunate. The remnant of the SLIL is usually avulsed from the scaphoid and remains attached to the lunate. Place horizontal mattress sutures in this tissue with 4-0 nonabsorbable suture (Fig. 15.20). Create a trough in the proximal pole of the

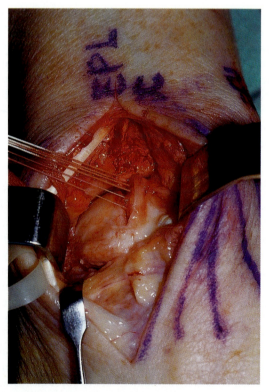

FIGURE 15.20. Scapholunate interosseous ligament (SLIL) repair and capsulodesis: 4-0 nonabsorbable sutures are placed in the remnant of SLIL that remains attached to the lunate.

scaphoid along its lunate facet to accept the ligament. Make drill holes in the proximal scaphoid from this trough to the scaphoid waist just distal to the radial styloid. A 0.045-in. K-wire works well for this (Fig. 15.21). Place two parallel 0.045-in. K-wires percutaneously into the scaphoid in preparation for pinning the reduction. Reduce the scaphoid and lunate, paying careful attention to bringing the scaphoid up out of its flexed posture, and then drill the K-wires across into the lunate. Pass the sutures in the SLIL through the drill holes in the scaphoid and tie them securely (Fig. 15.22). To correct any residual DISI deformity, a third 0.045-in. K-wire may be drilled percutaneously across the scaphoid and into the capitate while palmarly directed force is applied to the capitate manually.

The *capsulodesis* is performed next. Different techniques have been described for this step. Lavernia et al. (71) utilize local capsular tissue in a vest-over-pants fashion as follows (Fig. 15.23). Make a transverse incision in the radial side of the dorsal capsular flap just distal to the waist of the scaphoid. Apply firm tension to the proximal edge of the flap and roughen an area of the scaphoid at the level where the flap will reach it. Suture the flap to this area with 4-0 nonabsorbable suture inserted through drill holes made in the bone and tie over a palmarly placed button. An alternative to using sutures passed through drill holes is to use suture minianchors. Suture the redundant distal portion of the capsular flap over the proximal flap in a vest-over-pants fashion. Repair the longitudinal capsular incision side to side.

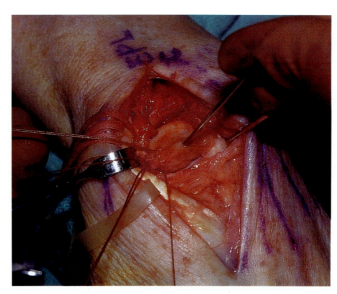

FIGURE 15.22. While the scaphoid and lunate are held reduced, the sutures in the scapholunate interosseous ligament are passed through the drill holes via Keith needles and tied down securely on the radial side of the scaphoid.

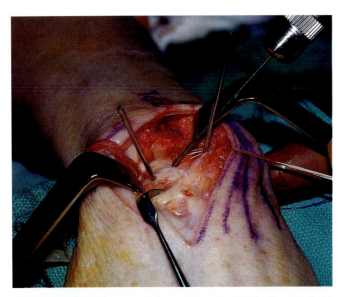

FIGURE 15.21. After preparing a bony trough in the scaphoid to accept the scapholunate interosseous ligament, place drill holes (0.045-in K-wire) from this trough through the bone to exit distal to the scaphoid waist. The joysticks in the scaphoid and lunate are evident.

Another option for augmenting the SLIL reconstruction is to use the capsulodesis recommended by Blatt (86). A 1-cm–wide strip of dorsal capsule is pivoted on its proximal attachment to the radius proximally and reattached to the distal pole of the scaphoid, distal to its axis of rotation (Fig. 15.24). Blatt recently presented evidence that this transferred capsular tissue may hypertrophy over time (87). The problem with the procedure is that it tethers the distal pole of the scaphoid to the distal radius, thus necessarily reducing wrist flexion, particularly if the tissue becomes hypertrophied rather than attenuated. In Blatt's experience (86,88), patients lose up to 20° wrist flexion. In a recent series of patients treated for dynamic scapholunate instability using the capsulodesis, the mean loss of wrist flexion was 12° (89). In addition, the capsulodesis does not treat the scapholunate gap. Blatt suggests that this can be ignored (86,88).

Currently we are investigating an alternative capsulodesis based on the dorsal intercarpal ligament. This ligament, a thickening of the dorsal wrist capsule, normally originates on the dorsum of the triquetrum and inserts on the trapezium and trapezoid. The technique we are investigating is done as follows. Detach the ligament from its insertion onto the trapezium and trapezoid and reflect it ulnarly (Fig. 15.25). Prepare a bony trough in the distal pole of the scaphoid, distal to the axis of rotation. Place a suture anchor in the base of the trough. Hold the scaphoid reduced in a relatively extended posture by applying manual pressure on the palmar side of the wrist or using a K-wire as a joystick and then secure the prepared ligament to the suture anchor (Fig. 15.26).

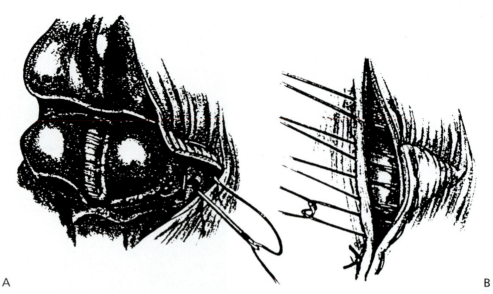

FIGURE 15.23. Capsulodesis recommended by Lavernia et al. A dorsal capsular flap is advanced into place **(A)**, and the redundant capsule imbricated in vest-over-pants fashion **(B)**. (From Lavernia CJ, Cohen MS, Taleisnik J. Treatment of scapholunate dissociation by ligamentous repair and capsulodesis. *J Hand Surg [Am]* 1992;17:354–359, with permission.)

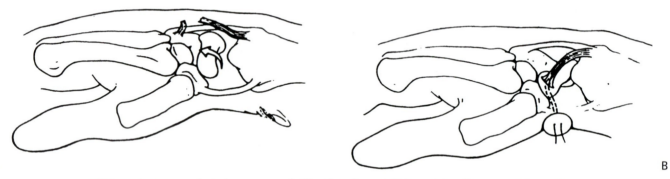

FIGURE 15.24. Capsulodesis recommended by Blatt. (From Wintman BI, Gelberman RH, Katz JN. Dynamic scapholunate instability: Results of operative treatment with dorsal capsulodesis. *J Hand Surg [Am]* 1995;20:971–979, with permission.)

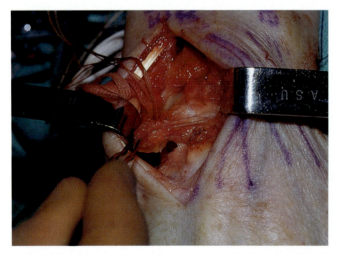

FIGURE 15.25. Authors' modified capsulodesis. A strip of dorsal intercarpal ligament *(in forceps)* is detached from its insertion onto the trapezium and trapezoid and reflected ulnarly to expose the distal pole of the scaphoid.

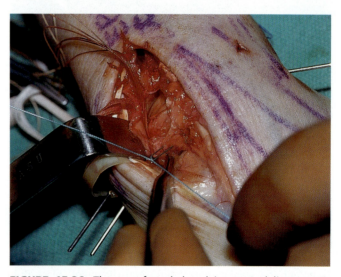

FIGURE 15.26. The transferred dorsal intercarpal ligament is placed in a bony trough created in the distal pole of the scaphoid and secured with a suture anchor (*green* suture shown).

We hypothesize that this capsulodesis will be advantageous because it will prevent gapping (lateral displacement) of the scapholunate articulation better than other capsulodeses by tethering the triquetrum to the scaphoid, keeping the proximal row functioning as a unit. It may also allow more wrist flexion because there is no tether to the distal radius. The transferred ligament lies over the proximal pole of the capitate like a pulley and may prevent the scaphoid from dropping into excessive flexion (DISI pattern).

Postoperatively, immobilize the extremity in a plaster-reinforced above-elbow thumb–spica dressing for 10 days, followed by 3 weeks in an above-elbow thumb–spica cast and then a below-elbow thumb–spica cast for an additional 4 weeks. Remove the K-wires after 8 weeks. Begin gentle range-of-motion (ROM) exercises under supervision at that time while a removable protective splint is worn between exercise sessions. Discontinue immobilization 3 months after surgery. Forceful axial loading of the wrist, particularly in extension such as with bench pressing, should be avoided for 6 months.

Expected Outcomes

Minami et al. (90) were among the first to report a correlation between clinical results and radiographic carpal instabilities. In a small series, patients with more than 3 mm residual scapholunate gap or lunotriquetral incongruity had poor clinical results. In the large multicenter study reported subsequently by Herzberg et al. (47), the prognosis of perilunate dislocations and perilunate fracture-dislocations was more influenced by whether the injury was open or closed and by the delay in treatment than by the anatomic type. Based on a clinical score assessing pain, ROM, grip strength, and activities, the best results were obtained in patients who had closed injuries treated within 1 week, averaging 80 out of 100 possible points. Panting et al. (91) noted that patients with simple dislocations (group A) fared better than those with fracture-dislocations (group B). In group A, 24 of 29 (83%) patients had a good or satisfactory result, whereas 13 of 19 (68%) patients in group B had a good or satisfactory result.

In the study by Sotereanos et al. (68), a critical assessment was made of patients' subjective and objective results after perilunate dislocation and fracture-dislocation. It should be noted that a combined dorsal and palmar approach was used in all patients. After an average of 30 months, patient satisfaction was high in 82% of cases, but only 5 of 11 patients had returned to their previous occupations without limitation. The ROM averaged 71% of that in the opposite wrist. Grip strength averaged 77% of that of the opposite hand. Radiographs showed all fractures healed, and 2 of 11 developed posttraumatic arthritis.

SLIL repair combined with dorsal capsulodesis has advantages over other operative treatments for scapholunate dissociation, including dynamic instability. Specifically, triscaphe arthrodesis has been recommended as an alternative treatment (92,93), even for predynamic instability (94). However, the loss of wrist motion can be significant after this limited arthrodesis. In a series of long-term results of triscaphe arthrodesis reported by Kleinman (92), 45% of normal wrist flexion and 25% of normal wrist extension were lost following STT fusion. Watson et al. (95) also noted that their patients lost an average of 25% extension, 16% flexion, 45% radial, and 27% ulnar deviation postoperatively. In our opinion, it is better to try to stabilize the scapholunate dissociation with soft tissue procedures such as the dorsal capsulodesis rather than resorting to arthrodeses, which destroy the STT joints when they are potentially normal, especially in the setting of dynamic or predynamic instability.

There are less data available for outcomes after other types of carpal dislocations. In the axial distraction group of injuries, however, Garcia-Elias et al. noted that the factor most useful for prognosis was the neurovascular injury sustained at the time of accident (2). In a series of 15 patients for whom there was adequate follow-up, none achieved an excellent result, four had a good result, and the results were considered fair in six and poor in five. There were three good and six fair results among patients with no nerve involvement; only one good and five poor results were obtained in patients with major nerve injury. The authors also noted that the 10 patients who had immediate reduction, fixation, and primary repair of all damaged structures had a better final outcome (mean functional score 71 of 100 possible points) than those five patients treated in delayed fashion (mean score 66).

COMPLICATIONS

Fracture nonunion or malunion may develop, particularly in those cases where the scaphoid is fractured. Comminution of fractures is a risk factor for malunion and development of a "humpback" deformity of the scaphoid. Bone grafting defects at the time of fracture fixation may avoid this potential problem. In all cases, union should be confirmed radiographically, preferably by trispiral or CT, before hardware removal. Bridging trabeculae confirm healing, but plain films are unreliable when making this judgment (96).

Posttraumatic avascular necrosis (AVN) of the carpal bones has been reported by several authors. In the lunate this is usually a transient phenomenon. With progressive healing, revascularization and resolution of the AVN may occur without carpal fragmentation or collapse. This was noted by White et al. (97) in all three of the 24 wrists they treated that developed AVN. As a striking example of this, Ekerot (29) reported a case in which the lunate was stripped of all soft tissue attachments but showed no collapse after

70 months, and an MRI did not demonstrate osteonecrosis.

Other potential complications relate to the soft tissue injuries often associated with carpal dislocations and fracture-dislocations. Median nerve deficits usually resolve after reduction or carpal tunnel release where indicated. Those that do not suggest additional nerve contusion occurred at the time of injury. They should be observed expectantly, although complete recovery cannot be guaranteed. Persistent ligamentous instability is uncommon if K-wires are left in place for 8 weeks and the wrist is immobilized for a total of 12 weeks. Displacement following wire removal after 6 weeks is uncommon but has been reported (73). Stiffness is a far more common problem. Because the mechanical properties of scar are different from original ligament, some loss of motion is unavoidable.

Direct cartilage injury is another concern in carpal dislocations, and arthritis may be considered an unavoidable end result rather than a complication. Iatrogenic injury can be minimized by avoiding multiple passage of K-wires through joint surfaces and forced vigorous reduction maneuvers. Additional cartilage wear from abnormal joint biomechanics and incongruous reductions may explain the faster onset and progression of posttraumatic arthritis in some cases (98).

Kirschner wires used to stabilize fractures and dislocations are frequently problematic. If the wires are left protruding through the skin, they are easy to remove after healing is complete, but soft tissue irritation, problems with pin caps, drainage, and pin tract infections are common. On a related note, authors who use thin wire external fixators for other reasons report pin tract problems and drainage as "events" almost to be expected during treatment rather than as complications (99). On the other hand, if the wires are left buried beneath the skin, they are more difficult to remove and may even require another procedure in the operating room to retrieve them safely, and they can still cause soft tissue irritation and ulcerations. We generally prefer to leave the wires buried. The perfect solution to this problem awaits discovery.

SUMMARY

Success in managing carpal dislocations and fracture-dislocations comes from accurate diagnosis based on careful examination of the patients' wrists and radiographs, and early treatment. The goal should always be to restore the anatomy of the injured wrist. For the more common perilunate and lunate dislocations and fracture-dislocations, that means restoring the relationships among three key elements: the scaphoid, the lunate, and the capitate. Some loss of motion and grip strength as well as some degree of pain should be expected after these injuries, even with optimum treatment, and patients should be counseled early accordingly.

EDITORS' COMMENTS

The norm for major trauma to the wrist has become open reduction and direct visualization, reduction, and repair. This is a terribly important transformation that has gradually occurred, dictated by the poor results of minimalist treatment. If major trauma is not dissipated in fracturing the distal radius, it dissipates through fracture and/or ligamentous destruction in the carpus. Diagnosis of major acute injuries to the wrist is usually not difficult. That there has been major insult is immediately evident based on the clinical appearance of the wrist. No wrist demonstrating major soft tissue reaction should be treated as a "sprain" and sent out with a simple splint in the face of normal x-rays. Hemarthrosis, swelling, and pain are evidence of major trauma, and it is the responsibility of the surgeon to determine the locale and pattern of that trauma. On the other side of this same coin, the patient whose x-ray in the Emergency Room demonstrates rotary subluxation of the scaphoid but no ecchymosis, minimal swelling and minimal clinical evidence of trauma after a dorsiflexion injury probably represents a preexisting tear and does not warrant open reduction and attempted acute ligament reconstruction. In reviewing the etiology for compensable injuries, the description of the degree of soft tissue response as was seen in the Emergency Room helps to determine whether, indeed, the problem preexisted the trauma.

Plain x-rays in acute circumstances are important. When viewing an x-ray of suspected carpal trauma, it is important to find a parallel surface to match each joint surface. If the partner surface either is not there or demonstrates a lack of parallelism, then there has been disruption of the relationship of the two bones involved. A lack of parallelism between those two surfaces we have designated as a positive "V sign," as it usually produces a converging or diverging of the articular surfaces that should otherwise be parallel to one another.

Sclerosis can often be spotted better, especially at the handfellow level, by backing away four feet from the x-ray and squinting until the details are slightly blurred.

Another useful maneuver is to take the lateral x-ray and rotate it until the lunate sits as a "bowl of cereal on a table" along the lower edge of the view box. The lunate "line" is then vertical. A quick mental line from the volar aspect of the proximal articular surface of the scaphoid to the volar edge of the distal pole can then be compared to the horizontal. This allows a rapid and quite accurate reading of the scapholunate angle without protractor and line drawing. Seventy degrees may be considered the upper limits of normal for the scapholunate angle in a neutral lateral. If some VISI is noted (lunate angled volarly and displaced dorsally), this may or may not represent the neutral anatomy for the lunate. If major ligament injury has occurred at the STT joint and the scaphoid collapses into flexion, the lunate will be forced into VISI because of intact SLILs. If this injury occurs with concomitant or extant complete scapholunate interosseous ligament disruption, the lunate is then free to assume its neutral anatomy position. If the lunate is thinner dorsally (67% of normal lunates) DISI positioning will occur. If the lunate is thinner volarly (23% of normal lunates), VISI positioning will occur. RSS can, therefore, be the same basic ligament injury as a midcarpal instability associated with a V-type lunate (see Chapter 31).

Loads across the carpals are significantly increased by positions of flexion, extension, or deviation. Much more is demanded of the ligament system in angular positions. Wrist angulation is the multiplier that contributes to ligament rupture under load in almost all cases.

REFERENCES

1. Dobyns HH, Linscheid RL. Carpal injuries. In: Rockwood CA, Green DP, eds. *Fractures in adults*. Philadelphia: JB Lippincott, 1984;451–509.
2. Garcia-Elias M, Dobyns JH, Cooney WP, et al. Traumatic axial dislocations of the carpus. *J Hand Surg [Am]* 1989;14:446–457.
3. Ruby LK, Cooney WP, An KH, et al. Relative motion of selected carpal bones: a kinematic analysis of the normal wrist. *J Hand Surg [Am]* 1988;13:1–10.
4. Gilford WW, Bolton RH, Lambrinudi C. The mechanism of the wrist joint with special reference to fractures of the scaphoid. *Guy's Hosp Rep* 1943;92:52–59.
5. Green DP. Carpal dislocations and instabilities. In: Green DP, ed. *Operative hand surgery*. New York: Churchill Livingstone, 1993;861–928.
6. Taleisnik J. Wrist: anatomy, function and injury. In: *AAOS Instructional Course Lectures*. St Louis: CV Mosby, 1978;61–87.
7. Weber ER. Wrist mechanics and its association with ligamentous instability. In: Lichtman D, ed. *The wrist and its disorders*. Philadelphia: WB Saunders, 1988;41–52.
8. Lichtman D, Schneider JE, Swafford AR, et al. Ulnar midcarpal instability—clinical and laboratory analysis. *J Hand Surg [Am]* 1981;6:515–523.
9. Berger RA, Landsmeer JMF. The palmar radiocarpal ligaments: A study of adult and fetal human wrist joints. *J Hand Surg [Am]* 1990;15:847–854.
10. Berger RA, Blair WF, Crowninshield RD, et al. The scapholunate ligament. *J Hand Surg [Am]* 1982;7:87–91.
11. Szabo RM, Sutherland TB. Acute carpal fractures and dislocations. In: Peimer CA, ed. *Surgery of the hand and upper extremity*. New York: McGraw-Hill, 1996;711–726.
12. Poirier P, Charpy A. *Traite d'anatomie humaine*. Paris: Masson, 1926.
13. Mayfield JK, Johnson RP, Kikoyne RF. The ligaments of the human wrist and their functional significance. *Anat Rec* 1976; 186:417.
14. Viegas SF, Patterson RM, Patterson PD, et al. Ulnar sided perilunate instability: An anatomic and biomechanic study. *J Hand Surg [Am]* 1990;15:268–277.
15. Berger RA. The gross and histologic anatomy of the scapholunate interosseous ligament. *J Hand Surg [Am]* 1996;21:170–178.
16. Ritt MJPF, Berger RA, Kauer JMG. The gross and histologic anatomy of the ligaments of the capitohamate joint. *J Hand Surg [Am]* 1996;21:1022–1028.
17. Garcia-Elias M. Carpal kinetics. In: Buchler U, ed. *Wrist instability*. St Louis: CV Mosby, 1996:9–13.
18. Zancolli EA, Cozzi EP. *Atlas of surgical anatomy of the hand*. New York: Churchill Livingstone, 1992.
19. An KN, Chao EYS, Cooney WP, et al. Forces in the normal and abnormal hand. *J Orthop Res* 1985;3:202–211.
20. Schuind R, Garcia-Elias M, Cooney WP, et al. Flexor tendon forces: *in vivo* measurements. *J Hand Surg [Am]* 1992;17:291–298.
21. Crosby CA, Wehbe MA, Mawr B. Hand strength: normative values. *J Hand Surg [Am]* 1994;19:665–670.
22. Hara T, Horii E, An KN. Force distribution across wrist joint: application of pressure-sensitive conductive rubber. *J Hand Surg [Am]* 1992;17:339–347.
23. Viegas SF, Tencer AF, Cantrell J. Load transfer characteristics of the wrist. *J Hand Surg [Am]* 1987;12:971–978.
24. Werner FW, An KN, Palmer AK, et al. Force analysis. In: An KN, Berger RA, Cooney WP, eds. *Biomechanics of the wrist joint*. New York: Springer-Verlag, 1991;77–98.
25. Mayfield JK. Mechanism of carpal injuries. *Clin Orthop* 1980; 149:45–54.
26. Mayfield JK, Johnson RP, Kilcoyne RK. Carpal dislocations: pathomechanics and progressive perilunar instability. *J Hand Surg [Am]* 1980;5:226–241.
27. Mayfield JK. Patterns of injury to carpal ligaments. A spectrum. *Clin Orthop* 1984;187:36–42.
28. Hill NA. Fractures and dislocations of the carpus. *Orthop Clin North Am* 1970;1:275–284.
29. Ekerot L. Palmar dislocation of the trans-scaphoid-lunate unit. *J Hand Surg [Br]* 1995;20:557–560.
30. Moneim MS. Management of greater arc carpal fractures. *Hand Clin* 1988;4:457–467.
31. Eglseder A. Transscaphoid palmar lunate dislocation with scapholunate dissociation. *Mil Med* 1992;157:382–385.
32. Szabo RM, Newland CC, Johnson PG, et al. Spectrum of injury and treatment options for isolated dislocation of the scaphoid. *J Bone Joint Surg Am* 1995;17:608–615.
33. Green DP, O'Brien ET. Classification and management of carpal dislocations. *Clin Orthop* 1980;149:55–72.
34. Campbell RD, Lance EM, Yeoh CB. Lunate and perilunar dislocations. *J Bone Joint Surg Br* 1964;46:55–72.
35. Moneim MS, Hofammann KEI, Omer GE. Transscaphoid perilunate fracture-dislocation. Result of open reduction and pin fixation. *Clin Orthop* 1984;190:227–235.
36. Gilula LA. Carpal injuries: Analytic approach and case exercises. *Am J Roentgenol* 1979;133:503–517.
37. Gilula LA, Destouet JM, Weeks PM, et al. Roentgenographic diagnosis of the painful wrist. *Clin Orthop* 1984;187:52–64.
38. Gilula LA, Weeks PM. Post-traumatic ligamentous instability of the wrist. *Radiology* 1978;129:641–651.
39. Peh WCG, Gilula LA. Normal disruption of carpal arcs. *J Hand Surg [Am]* 1996;21:561–566.
40. Garcia-Elias M, An K, Amadio PC, et al. Reliability of carpal angle determinations. *J Hand Surg [Am]* 1989;14:1017–1021.
41. Linscheid RL, Dobyns JH, Beabout JW, et al. Traumatic instability of the wrist. Diagnosis classification and pathomechanics. *J Bone Joint Surg Am* 1972;54:1612–1632.
42. Palmer AK, Levinsohn EM, Kuzma GR. Arthrography of the wrist. *J Hand Surg [Am]* 1983;8:15–23.
43. Moneim MS, Omer GE. Wrist arthrography in acute carpal injuries. *Orthopedics* 1983;6:299–306.

44. Mikic ZDJ. Arthrography of the wrist joint: An experimental study. *J Bone Joint Surg Am* 1984;66:371–378.
45. Taleisnik J. Triquetrohamate and triquetrolunate instabilities (medial carpal instability). *Ann Chir Main* 1984;3:331–343.
46. Frankel VH. The Terry-Thomas sign (Letter). *Clin Orthop* 1977;129:321–322.
47. Herzberg G, Comtet JJ, Linscheid FL, et al. Perilunate dislocations and fracture-dislocations: A multicenter study. *J Hand Surg [Am]* 1993;18:768–779.
48. Pournaras J, Kappas A. Volar perilunar dislocation—a case report. *J Bone Joint Surg Am* 1979;61:625–626.
49. Saunier J, Chamay A. Volar perilunar dislocation of the wrist. *Clin Orthop* 1981;157:139.
50. Aitken AP, Nalebuff EA. Volar transnavicular perilunar dislocation of the carpus. *J Bone Joint Surg Am* 1960;42:1051–1057.
51. Niazi TBM. Volar perilunate dislocation of the carpus: a case report and elucidation of its mechanism of occurrence. *Injury* 1996;27:209–211.
52. Nicholson CB. Fracture-dislocation of the os magnum. *J R Nav Med Serv* 1940;26:289–291.
53. Vance RM, Gelberman RH, Evans EF. Scaphocapitate fractures: Patterns of dislocation, mechanism of injury, and preliminary results of treatment. *J Bone Joint Surg Am* 1980;62:271–276.
54. Stein F, Seigel MW. Noviculocapitate fracture syndrome: A case report. *J Bone Joint Surg Am* 1969;51:391–395.
55. Gellman H, Schwartz SD, Botte MJ, et al. Late treatment of a dorsal transscaphoid, transtriquetral perilunate wrist dislocation with avascular changes of the lunate. *Clin Orthop* 1988;237:196–203.
56. Weseley MS, Barenfeld PA. Trans-scaphoid transcapitate, transtriquetral, perilunar fracture-dislocation of the wrist. A case report. *J Bone Joint Surg Am* 1972;54:1073–1078.
57. Connell MC, Dyson RP. Dislocation of the carpal scaphoid. *J Bone Joint Surg Br* 1955;37:252–253.
58. Campbell RD, Thompson TC, Lance EM, et al. Indications for open reduction of lunate and perilunate dislocations of the carpal bones. *J Bone Joint Surg Am* 1965;47:915–937.
59. Crittenden JJ, Jones DM, Santarelli AG. Bilateral rotational dislocation of the carpal navicular. *Radiology* 1970;94:629–630.
60. Armstrong GWD. Rotational subluxation of the scaphoid. *Can J Surg* 1968;11:306–314.
61. Parkes JC, Stovell PB. Dislocation of the carpal scaphoid: A report of two cases. *J Trauma* 1973;13:384–388.
62. Tullos HS, Erwin WD, Fain RH. Isolated subluxation of the carpal scaphoid associated with secondary displacement of the capitate. *South Med J* 1973;66:568–574.
63. Garcia-Elias M, Abanco J, Salvador E, et al. Crush injury of the carpus. *J Bone Joint Surg Br* 1985;67:286–289.
64. Adkison JW, Chapman MW. Treatment of acute lunate and perilunate dislocations. *Clin Orthop* 1982;164:199–207.
65. Jasmine MS, Packer JW, Edwards GS. Irreducible transscaphoid perilunate dislocation. *J Hand Surg [Am]* 1988;13:212–215.
66. Miller ST, Smith PA. Volar dislocation of the lunate in a weight lifter. *Orthopedics* 1996;19:61–63.
67. Minami A, Kaneda K. Repair and/or reconstruction of scapholunate interosseous ligament in lunate and perilunate dislocations. *J Hand Surg [Am]* 1993;18:1099–1106.
68. Sotereanos DG, Mitsionis GJ, Giannakopoulos PN, et al. Perilunate dislocation and fracture dislocation: A critical analysis of the volar-dorsal approach. *J Hand Surg [Am]* 1997;22:49–56.
69. Cooney WP, Bussey R, Dobyns JH, et al. Difficult wrist fractures. *Clin Orthop* 1987;214:136–147.
70. Howard FM, Dell PC. The unreduced carpal dislocation. A method of treatment. *Clin Orthop* 1986;202:112–116.
71. Lavernia CJ, Cohen MS, Taleisnik J. Treatment of scapholunate dissociation by ligamentous repair and capsulodesis. *J Hand Surg [Am]* 1992;17:354–359.
72. White SJ, Louis DS, Braunstein EN. Capitate–lunate instability: Recognition by manipulation under fluoroscopy. *Am J Roentgenol* 1984;143:361–364.
73. Green DP, O'Brien ET. Open reduction of carpal dislocations: Indications and operative techniques. *J Hand Surg [Am]* 1978;3:250–265.
74. Herbert TJ, Fisher WE. Management of the fractured scaphoid using a new bone screw. *J Bone Joint Surg [Br]* 1984;66:114–123.
75. Viegas SF, Bean JW, Schram RA. Transscaphoid fracture-dislocation treated with open reduction and Herbert screw fixation. *J Hand Surg [Am]* 1987;12:992–999.
76. Bryan RS, Dobyns JH. Fractures of the carpal bone other than the lunate or navicular. *Clin Orthop* 1980;149:107–111.
77. Weir IGC. The late reduction of carpal dislocations. *J Hand Surg [Br]* 1992;17:137–139.
78. Glickel SZ, Millender LH. Ligamentous reconstruction for chronic intercapal instability. *J Hand Surg [Am]* 1984;94:514–527.
79. Crabbe WA. Excision of the proximal row of the carpus. *J Bone Joint Surg Br* 1964;46:708–711.
80. Stern PJ. Mulitple flexor tendon ruptures following an old anterior dislocation of the lunate: A case report. *J Bone Joint Surg Am* 1981;63:489–490.
81. Russel TB. Inter-carpal dislocations and fracture dislocations: A review of fifty-nine cases. *J Bone Joint Surg Br* 1949;31:524–531.
82. Rawlings ID. The management of dislocations of the carpal lunate. *Injury* 1981;12:319–330.
83. O'Brien ET. Acute fractures and dislocations of the carpus. *Orthop Clin North Am* 1984;15:237–258.
84. Morawa LG, Ross PM, Schock CC. Fractures and dislocations involving the navicular lunate axis. *Clin Orthop* 1976;118:48–53.
85. Sousa HP, Fernandes H, Botelheiro JC. Pre-operative progressive distraction in old transcapho-peri-lunate dislocations. *J Hand Surg [Br]* 1995;20:603–605.
86. Blatt G. Capsulodesis in reconstructive hand surgery. Dorsal capsulodesis for the unstable scaphoid and volar capsulodesis following excision of the distal ulna. *Hand Clin* 1987;3:81–102.
87. Blatt G. *The case for my capsulodesis method.* In: Specialty Day, American Society for Surgery of the Hand, San Francisco, 1997.
88. Blatt G. Scapholunate instability. In: Lichtman DM, ed. *The wrist and its disorders.* Philadelphia: WB Saunders, 1988;251–273.
89. Wintman BI, Gelberman RH, Katz JN. Dynamic scapholunate instability: Results of operative treatment with dorsal capsulodesis. *J Hand Surg [Am]* 1995;20:971–979.
90. Minami A, Ogino T, Ohshio I, et al. Correlation between clinical results and carpal instabilities in patients after reduction of lunate and perilunar dislocations. *J Hand Surg [Br]* 1986;11:213–220.
91. Panting AL, Lamb DW, Noble J, et al. Dislocations of the lunate with and without fracture of the scaphoid. *J Bone Joint Surg [Br]* 1984;66:391–395.
92. Kleinman WB. Long-term study of chronic scapholunate instability treated by scaphotrapeziotrapezoid arthrodesis. *J Hand Surg* 1989;14:429–445.
93. Watson HK. Instabilities of the wrist. *Hand Clin* 1987;3:103–111.
94. Watson HK, Weinzweig J, Zeppieri J. The natural progression of scaphoid instability. In: Nelson DL, ed. *Hand clinics.* Philadelphia: WB Saunders, 1997;39–49.

95. Watson HK, Ryu J, Akelman E. Limited triscaphoid intercarpal arthrodesis for rotatory subluxation of the scaphoid. *J Bone Joint Surg Am* 1986;68:345–349.
96. Dias JJ, Taylor M, Thompson J, et al. Radiographic signs of union of scaphoid fractures: An analysis of inter-observer agreement and reproducibility. *J Bone Joint Surg Br* 1988;70:299–301.
97. White RE, Omer GE. Transient vascular compromise of the lunate after fracture-dislocation or dislocation of the carpus. *J Hand Surg [Am]* 1984;9:181–184.
98. Szabo RM, Newland CC. Open reduction and ligamentous repair for acute lunate and perilunate dislocations. In: Gelberman RH, ed. *The wrist.* New York: Raven Press, 1994;167–182.
99. Fischgrund J, Paley D, Suter C. Variables affecting time to bone healing during limb lengthening. *Clin Orthop* 1994;301:31–37.
100. Whipple T. *Arthroscopic surgery: the wrist.* Philadelphia: JB Lippincott, 1992;73–90.
101. Berger RA. The ligaments of the wrist. In: Nelson DL, ed. *Hand clinics.* Philadelphia: WB Saunders, 1997;63–82.

16

CARPOMETACARPAL FRACTURES AND FRACTURE-DISLOCATIONS

MARC GARCIA-ELIAS

According to a recent epidemiologic study, the incidence of wrist trauma requiring x-ray examination is 58 per 10,000 inhabitants per year (1). Of these, 7.9% are diagnosed with a scaphoid fracture (2). Based on this, and assuming that the percentage of carpometacarpal (CMC) injuries is as found by Hove (3), the estimated annual incidence of fractures affecting the CMC joints would be 40 per 100,000 inhabitants, half of which involve the trapeziometacarpal (TMC) joint. The incidence of pure CMC dislocations is lower, representing 0.18% of all fracture-dislocations of the hand and wrist, according to Dobyns et al. (4). Therefore, the injuries covered in this chapter are not as uncommon as one may think. Nevertheless, despite the emphasis made by numerous recent publications (5–9), the rate of CMC injuries that are missed at presentation is still high, the consequence of which is often a wrist with permanent discomfort and diminished grip and pinch strength because of posttraumatic degenerative arthritis of the CMC joint.

From a pathomechanical and clinical point of view, two well-differentiated areas exist: the thumb and the finger CMC joints (Fig. 16.1). Costagliola et al. (10) used the term "columnar" to refer to the injuries affecting the thumb, as opposed to "spatular" injuries, referring to those involving the four ulnar CMC joints, terminology that is still quite popular in Europe. In this chapter, we use the more anatomic and less confusing terms "trapeziometacarpal" to refer to the basal joint of the thumb and "finger carpometacarpal" to refer to the four ulnar CMC joints.

TRAPEZIOMETACARPAL INJURIES

For the thumb to have both the ability to manipulate fine objects and the strength to resist the important loads that are being transmitted, a perfect interaction among muscle forces, ligament constraints, and articular surface geometry is necessary (11,12). Of the three thumb articulations, the TMC is probably the most important in terms of function, for it provides large multidirectional mobility while resisting substantial stresses during most manual activities of daily living. In terms of incidence of injury, it is certainly one of the most frequently affected by trauma. Indeed, 4.9% of all hand fractures occur at the base of the first metacarpal, most of them implying a substantial degree of thumb instability with the consequent disability unless properly recognized and treated (3). In this section, after a brief anatomic and functional review, the diagnosis and management of the four most frequent intraarticular destabilizing injuries are reviewed: (a) Bennett's fracture-dislocations, (b) Rolando's fractures, (c) pure TMC dislocations, and (d) unstable trapezial fractures.

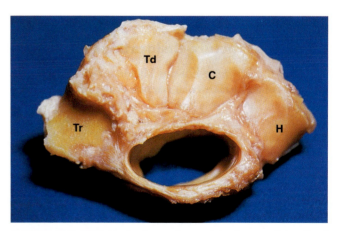

FIGURE 16.1. Distal articular surfaces of the bones of the distal carpal row. The saddle-shaped trapezium *(Tr)* allows substantial motion of the first metacarpal. By contrast, the wedge-shaped trapezoid *(Td)* and capitate *(C)* interlock the second and third metacarpal bases, preventing their mobility. The distal surface of the hamate *(H)* has two facets, allowing some motion to the fourth and fifth metacarpals.

M. Garcia-Elias: Hand and Upper Extremity Surgery, Institut Kaplan, 08022 Barcelona, Spain.

Anatomy and Function of the Trapeziometacarpal Joint

The TMC joint is a true saddle joint composed of two articulating bones with reciprocal saddle-shaped configurations. In the plane of flexion–extension, the convexity of the trapezium fits the concavity of the first metacarpal, and, vice versa, the trapezium concavity in the plane of abduction–adduction matches the convexity of the first metacarpal. On the palmar and medial aspect of the base of the first metacarpal, there is a rounded prominence, called the volar beak or tubercle, which serves as an attachment for two important stabilizers of the TMC joint: the anterior oblique ligament (AOL) and the intermetacarpal ligament (IML) (12). Aside from these two palmarly located ligaments, the TMC joint is constrained by means of a relatively loose capsule and two other capsular reinforcing ligaments: the posterior oblique ligament (POL) and the dorsoradial ligament (DRL) (12,13). The joint cavity is lined by synovial tissue and usually does not communicate with the finger CMC joint cavity.

The TMC joint is comparable to a universal joint with separate axes for flexion–extension and abduction–adduction. The first axis lies within the trapezium, proximal to the joint articular surface, whereas the second is located within the base of the first metacarpal. Because of the offset between the two axes, the resultant circumduction motion of the first metacarpal follows an ellipsoidal cone of motion (12), providing substantial mobility of the TMC joint contact, certainly an inherent factor of joint instability.

With the joint in neutral position, the primary constraints in resisting pronation of the metacarpal are the AOL and the IML. However, when the joint is flexed and adducted (the position in which most fracture-dislocations occur), the POL and DRL are also important in ensuring joint stability (12).

Bennett's Fracture-Dislocations

In 1882, the Irishman Edward Halloran Bennett reported five cases of an intraarticular fracture of the first metacarpal in cadaveric specimens that had healed with an obvious stepoff, resulting in a "partial luxation of the metacarpal bone of the thumb backwards" (14). Four years later, the same author presented two further clinical observations emphasizing the importance of an adequate reduction with cast immobilization in order to succeed with such inherently unstable injuries. Since then, multiple studies have been published, the most outstanding being the comprehensive analysis of 107 such injuries published by Gedda in 1954 (15).

Despite early interpretations of this injury as the result of a shear force produced by an object violently hitting the first web space (16), most authors now agree that Bennett's fracture-dislocations are the result of a combination of leverage applied to the dorsum of the first metacarpal and an axial load transmitted along the shaft (15). The resultant vector from these forces results in an increased joint compressive stress on the palmar aspect of the articular surface, leading to a fracture of the anteromedial prominence, and in a distracting force on the DRL, which causes its avulsion from the trapezium. Subsequent contraction of the abductor pollicis longus and adductor and flexor pollicis brevis would enhance the proximal displacement of the first metacarpal in a dorsoradial direction (Fig. 16.2).

A true lateral projection of the TMC joint is essential for making an accurate diagnosis and assessing its reduction (17) (Fig. 16.3). This is obtained by placing the lateral border of the first metacarpal flat on the x-ray plate while the palm is pronated 30° relative to the plate and the x-ray beam is angled 15° in a distal-to-proximal direction (18). According to Roberts (19), a correct anteroposterior view can be obtained by maximally internally rotating the extended arm and flexing the wrist so that the dorsum of the thumb metacarpal lies flat on the x-ray plate.

The treatment of a Bennett's fracture-dislocation is controversial (20). The advocates of closed reduction and cast immobilization base their preference on an apparently good tolerance of any residual joint displacement in such a mobile joint. Blum (21), in 1941, recommended active early motion in order to facilitate creation of a new joint,

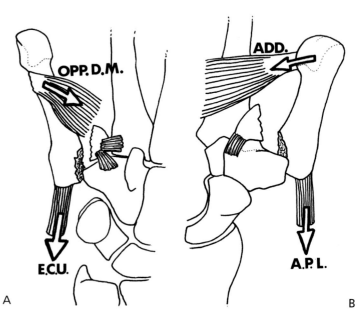

FIGURE 16.2. Most fractures of the base of the fifth metacarpal **(A)** are similar to Bennett's fracture-dislocations **(B)**. They both have a fragment that remains normally attached to the carpal bone by palmar ligaments. The two injuries are inherently unstable because of the pull of a dorsally located tendon [extensor carpi ulnaris (E.C.U.) or abductor pollicis longus (A.P.L.)]. In both cases instability is further enhanced by the action of a distally attached, obliquely oriented muscle [adductor pollicis (ADD.) or opponens digiti minimi (OPP.D.M.)].

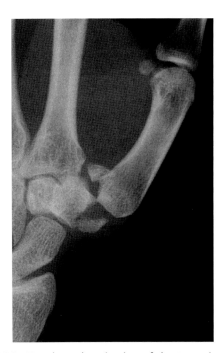

FIGURE 16.3. True lateral projection of the trapeziometacarpal joint demonstrating the association of a Bennett's fracture-dislocation and a displaced fracture of the dorsoradial aspect of the trapezium. This is a relatively frequent injury, particularly unstable, often requiring an open treatment to avoid late degenerative arthritis. (From Garcia-Elias M, Henriquez-Lluch A, Rossignani P, et al. Bennett's fracture combined with fracture of the trapezium. A report of three cases. *J Hand Surg [Br]* 1993;18:523–526, with permission.)

slightly reduced in mobility, but painless and functional. Favoring closed reduction and cast immobilization alone are, among others, Cannon et al. (22), who found no difference in the late subjective outcome between fractures that had been anatomically reduced and those with a residual displacement. In agreement with this view is the recently published laboratory study by Cullen et al. (23), who did not find a biomechanical basis for the development of posttraumatic osteoarthritis after a Bennett's fracture as long as the palmar-medial fragment is small, the residual stepoff is less than 2 mm, and the relationship between the metacarpal shaft and the trapezium has been reestablished. However, the extensive clinical work by Gedda (15) and the most recent long-term analyses of patients by Kjœr-Petersen et al. (24) and Livesley (25) seem to indicate that despite careful cast application, recurrence of the deformity is frequent. This latter work (25), with an average 26-year follow-up of 17 patients treated conservatively, found persistent subluxation and marked degenerative changes in 12 patients, seven of whom had persistent pain, and thus concluded that an accurate reduction and proper stabilization of these injuries was of utmost importance.

Reduction of an acute Bennett's fracture-dislocation is frequently easy to achieve by applying axial traction to the abducted and pronated thumb while exerting direct pressure at the dorsoradially displaced base of the metacarpal. This, however, is seldom stable. The more commonly recommended method of stabilization involves percutaneous pinning of the reduced first metacarpal to the trapezium (Wagner's method) (26) and/or to the second metacarpal (Johnson's technique) (27). In Europe, Iselin's technique (28), consisting of double pinning of the first metacarpal to the second, is still very popular. Because of the size (frequently small) and instability of the medial fragment, percutaneous K-wire fixation of the fracture is not recommended, as it may result in an increased fracture separation. Recent studies have emphasized the importance of an accurate anatomic restoration of the articular surface (20,23–25), which can be achieved by an open reduction and internal fixation with K-wires or, size-permitting, minifragment screws (29), allowing for a more optimistic postoperative outcome. An anterolateral L-shaped surgical approach with partial detachment of the abductor pollicis brevis, as suggested by Gedda (15), which provides excellent visualization for fixation of the fracture, is recommended.

Rolando's Fractures

Displaced three-part, T- or Y-shaped fractures of the base of the first metacarpal were first recognized by Silvio Rolando in 1910 (30). Of the two unstable fragments in which the base is divided, generally the anteromedial fragment remains attached to the AOL, while the dorsolateral fragment appears displaced by the action of the abductor pollicis longus tendon. The principles for a correct diagnosis and treatment of these injuries are similar to those of a Bennett's fracture-dislocation, except that in this case two fragments are to be stabilized, preferably by means of an open reduction. If the two fragments are of a consistent size, a minifragment plate may be used (31). Alternatively, interfragmentary K-wires, supplemented with either the Iselin's intermetacarpal double-pinning technique (28) or an external fixation device (29), may be of help. These, however, are technically demanding operations that, even in experienced hands, seldom achieve complete restoration of joint anatomy. According to Langhoff and associates (32), 6 of the 16 patients followed for an average of 5.8 years had symptoms from secondary osteoarthritis.

Rolando's fractures should not be confused with the severely comminuted intraarticular fractures of the base of the first metacarpal, often with a central impaction of small fragments into the metaphyseal region, resulting from high energy axial compression. In these cases, an open reduction and fixation of such comminuted injuries is rarely successful, and the results are frequently disappointing. Under these circumstances, either oblique traction (Thorén's method) (33) or the use of an external fixator device (29) may be indicated.

Dislocations of the Trapeziometacarpal Joint

Pure TMC dislocations of a traumatic origin are uncommon, with very few cases reported (34–37). Pathomechanically similar to Bennett's injuries, they are usually the result of an indirect mechanism involving an axial force applied on the adducted and flexed first metacarpal, followed by a sudden contraction of the abductor pollicis longus tendon (34). Based on such similarity, Gedda (15) described these injuries as Bennett's injuries without a fracture. The most frequent variety of dislocation is the one displaced in a dorsoradial direction. Occasionally, the metacarpal bone may displace in a strict dorsal or palmar direction making their diagnosis difficult (Fig. 16.4). In most cases, reduction is easily achieved by traction and local manipulation. However, the long-term results of treating these injuries solely by closed reduction and percutaneous K-wire fixation remains controversial. Toupin et al. (36), using this method, achieved good functional recovery with minimal recurrence of instability. By contrast, Simonian and Trumble (37) recommended treating these cases by open reduction and anterooblique ligament reconstruction (Eaton-Littler's method) (38), based on the better outcome achieved when this ligament was reconstructed early, as compared to those treated by closed reduction and pin fixation. When closed treatment is utilized, it is essential to immobilize the first metacarpal in a slight abduction and opposition in order to ensure maximal contact between the two ends of the IML ligament and the AOL. If postreduction x-rays are not satisfactory, soft tissue interposition may be suspected, and then open reduction and ligament reconstruction is advised.

Unstable Fractures of the Trapezium

Unstable displaced intraarticular fractures of the trapezium are not uncommon and may represent a serious problem affecting both the congruity and the stability of the TMC joint (34) (Fig. 16.3). Usually, these injuries involve the distal dorsolateral edge of the bone, although parasagittal fractures affecting both the proximal and distal articular surfaces have also been described. Because of their similarity to Bennett's fracture-dislocations in terms of how they occur, the two injuries are frequently associated (39) (Fig. 16.5A–D). In this case, the trapezial fracture would be the consequence of the distracting force in the DRL, which, instead of suffering a midsubstance rupture, induces an avulsion fracture of the trapezium.

In cases diagnosed early, closed manipulation may be successful by flexing and adducting the thumb while exerting direct pressure to the dorsolateral aspect of the bone. Such reduction, however, is seldom stable and, despite correct immobilization, tends to result in articular incongruency and late joint degeneration (40). Closed reduction and K-wire fixation is considered by most to be the method of choice, although no long-term analysis of results have been published. Interestingly, most of the cases in the literature underwent open treatment for trapezial fracture, and all reported excellent results with patients returning to their previous occupations without any significant limitation in thumb motion, pinch strength, or grasp (39,41) (Fig. 16.5E,F).

FINGER CARPOMETACARPAL INJURIES

The oldest reference to a finger CMC traumatic injury appeared in 1844, when Blandin reported a case that involved a dorsal displacement of the second and third metacarpal bases [cited by Waugh and Yancey (42)]. In 1873, Rivington published a case involving the five metacarpal bases (42), and McWhorter (43) was the first to operate on an isolated little finger CMC dislocation. In 1986, Mueller et al. (44) reviewed 143 previously published cases and found that the most frequently reported combination of CMC injuries consists of dorsal dislocations of the medial four CMC joints (42 cases), followed by isolated dislocations of the fifth metacarpal (37 cases).

Fractures of the distal row of the carpus producing instability of the metacarpals are probably not as rare as the literature would suggest (7–10,45,46–49). In a recent study using sagittal tomograms, in 13 (26%) of 50 finger CMC dislocations, concomitant fractures of one or several bones

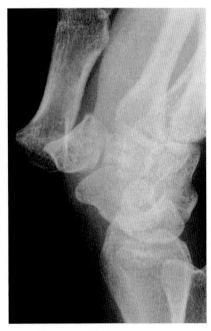

FIGURE 16.4. Oblique semipronated projection of the wrist of a 32-year-old woman who sustained a violent hyperextension and adduction trauma to her right thumb that resulted in an anterolateral trapeziometacarpal dislocation.

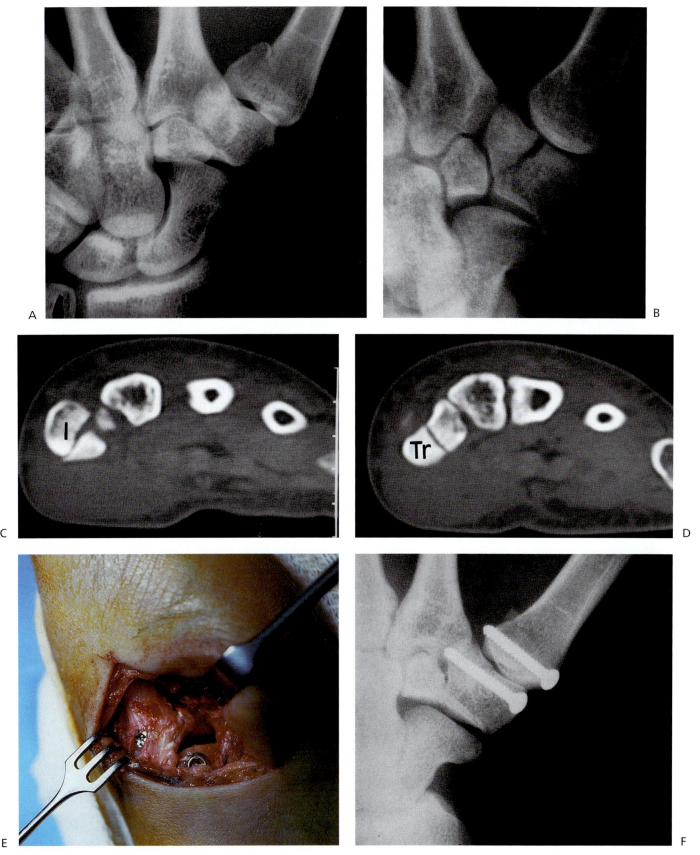

FIGURE 16.5. A,B: Posteroanterior and oblique views showing a Bennett's injury associated with a sagittal fracture of the trapezium. **C,D:** Tranverse computed tomography scans demonstrating the perpendicular direction of the fractures of the metacarpal base *(I)* and the trapezium *(Tr).* **E:** Surgical anterolateral approach, according to the method of Gedda (15). **F:** Seven weeks after stabilization with two lag screws, the fractures appear consolidated. (From Garcia-Elias M, Henriquez-Lluch A, Rossignani P, et al. Bennett's fracture combined with fracture of the trapezium. A report of three cases. *J Hand Surg [Br]* 1993;18:523–526, with permission.)

of the distal carpal row were also found (50). The most frequent carpal fracture involved the dorsal and distal edge of the hamate, an injury that was first described by Rossi in 1937 (51), and whose treatment was emphasized by Cain et al. (52) and others (53–56). Although they are not as frequently reported as the hamatometacarpal fracture-dislocation, similar injuries affecting the central bones of the distal carpal row (capitate and trapezoid) have also been described. Sheldon (57), in 1901, published a case of a dorsal dislocation of the trapezoid together with the second metacarpal as a consequence of a fist fight. Similar cases of fracture-dislocation of the trapezoid and/or capitate producing metacarpal instability have been reported by Russell (58), Rand et al. (59), and others (6,50).

Although certainly not as common as TMC fracture-dislocations, intraarticular displaced fractures of the base of the metacarpals are relatively frequent but unfortunately often underestimated (5–8). According to Hove (3), they represent 1.0% of all hand fractures. Several reports have commented on the instability of these injuries and the necessity of restoration of a congruent joint surface to avoid late degenerative arthritis (6,45,60). In this section, the pertinent anatomy, pathomechanics, classification and treatment of the different types of finger CMC fracture-dislocations is reviewed.

Anatomy and Function of the Finger Carpometacarpal Joints

The proximal epiphyses of the second to fifth (finger) metacarpal bones are broad and somewhat cuboidal. They articulate with each other by means of flat lateromedial facets, with palmar and dorsal IML ligaments connecting their corresponding palmar and dorsal nonarticular surfaces.

The second metacarpal base has a sagittal notch for the trapezoid, with an ulnar and dorsal prominence, called the metacarpal styloid process, matching with the shape of the distal articular facet of the capitate. The proximal articular surfaces of the third, fourth, and fifth metacarpals are flat or just slightly convexoconcave.

The distal articular surface of the trapezoid is wedge-shaped with two facets separated by a sagittal ridge fitting into a deep notch at the base of the second metacarpal (Fig. 16.1). In about one-third of the cases, there is also a small oblique facet for the third metacarpal. The radial and ulnar articular facets of the trapezoid are flat, tightly bound to their corresponding facets of the trapezium and capitate, respectively. The distal articular surface of the capitate has two constant facets: one broad central, sometimes slightly concave facet that articulates with the third metacarpal base and one small lateral facet for the styloid process of the second metacarpal base. A third small facet for the fourth metacarpal base is found in approximately 85% of the population. The hamate articulates distally with the fourth and fifth metacarpal bases through two articular surfaces, separated by a minimally prominent sagittal ridge. The articular surface to the fourth metacarpal base is slightly concave, and the ulnar facet to the fifth metacarpal has a dual configuration (palmarly concave, dorsally convex).

A tight ligamentous complex, both palmar and dorsal, supplemented by the distal insertions of the flexor and extensor carpi radialis tendons, interlock the second and third metacarpal bases to the trapezium, trapezoid, and capitate, constituting a rigid structural unit. By contrast, the ligaments binding the ulnar CMC joints (dorsal, palmar, and intraarticular) are more elastic, allowing 25° to 40° from full extension to a flexed-supinated position in the fifth ray and 10° to 15° of flexion in the fourth. This motion, which is mainly controlled by the hypothenar muscles palmarly and the extensor carpi ulnaris dorsally, is important, as it permits modification of the distal transverse arch and a better grip of different sized objects (20,45).

Mechanism of Injury

When the clenched fist strikes a rigid, unyielding object, a fracture of the metacarpal neck (boxer's fracture) is likely to occur (20). In some instances, however, the resultant axial force is transmitted along the metacarpal shaft, inducing a dislocation of the base of the metacarpal (Fig. 16.6). This

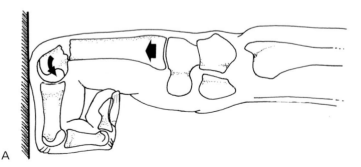
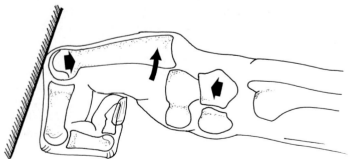

FIGURE 16.6. When the metacarpal head is violently subjected to an axial load, either a fracture of the metacarpal neck (boxer's fracture) **(A)** or a proximal dislocation of the carpometacarpal (CMC) joint **(B)** is likely to result. The latter is more likely when the direction of the impact is somewhat oblique, thus inducing not only an axial load but also a flexion moment to the CMC joint.

mechanism is said to be relatively common in producing the dorsal variety of dislocation of the fourth and fifth metacarpal base (5,6,52,56). In the laboratory, however, this mechanism could be reproduced only if the dorsal and palmar CMC ligaments had been previously sectioned (61).

Aside from the frequent "fist-fight" axial loading, other ways of producing an unstable CMC fracture-dislocation have been postulated. One involves a sharp object penetrating the palm, resulting in a dorsal translation of one or several metacarpal bases, usually in association with injury to the carpal bones and extensive soft tissue lacerations. A blast or crush mechanism, though uncommon, may produce a similar injury (50,62).

Another possible mechanism may involve a force applied to the dorsum of the hand while the wrist is palmarflexed, which can produce a dorsal dislocation of the metacarpals with or without avulsion from the adjacent carpal bones (55,63,64).

Not infrequently, finger CMC injuries are the consequence of a high-energy deceleration (e.g., motorcycle accident) in which the handlebar produces a combination of a lever-type of force applied on the palm and an axial load transmitted along the shaft (42,46,47,54). This results in increasing the joint compressive force on the dorsal aspect of the articular surface, responsible for the fracture, and a distracting force to the palmar CMC ligaments, responsible for the progressive joint disruption (50). A similar mechanism with the wrist in palmarflexion could possibly result in palmar compression and dorsal distraction with dislocation.

A completely different mechanism has recently been hypothesized for the palmarly dislocated fifth metacarpal (65). According to its proponents, such an injury could be the result of a violent contraction of the flexor carpi ulnaris muscle, which would cause a proximal dislocation of the pisiform and, through the pisometacarpal ligament, a palmar displacement of the fifth metacarpal (Fig. 16.7). Through this mechanism, the frequent association of this injury with an avulsion-fracture of the hook of the hamate (66) can also be explained.

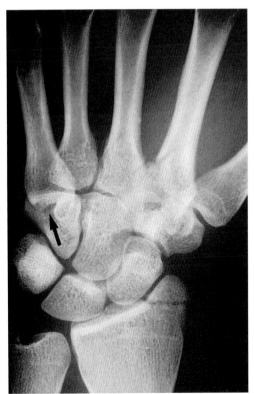 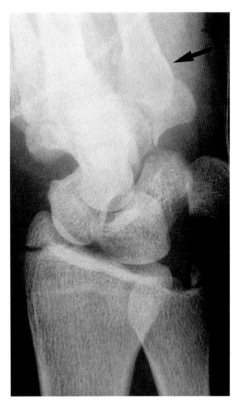 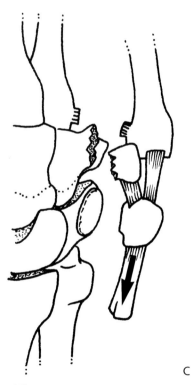

FIGURE 16.7. A: Posteroanterior view of the wrist of a 22-year-old man who was riding a motorbike when he collided with a car that had suddenly stopped in front of him. A proximal displacement of the fifth metacarpal relative to the hamate *(arrow)* and an undisplaced fracture of the radial styloid are evident. **B:** In an oblique semisupinated projection, a proximally displaced fracture of the hook of the hamate *(arrow)* and a proximally subluxed pisiform are clearly seen. **C:** The three problems could be explained as the result of a violent contraction of the flexor carpi ulnaris muscle *(arrow)* while the wrist was blocked into extension by the handle bar. (From Garcia-Elias M, Rossignani P, Cots M. Combined fracture of the hook of the hamate and palmar dislocation of the fifth carpometacarpal joint. *J Hand Surg [Br]* 1996;21:446–450, with permission.)

Classification of Finger Carpometacarpal Injuries

From a descriptive point of view, injuries to the finger CMC joints can be classified according to several parameters: number of rays involved (isolated, multiple compound, multiple divergent), direction of dislocation (palmar, dorsal, ulnar), and severity of the displacement (sprain, subluxation, dislocation).

From a therapeutic viewpoint, however, it is important to recognize how stable the injury will be after reduction. Indeed, if the injury becomes autostable after reduction, the prognosis will be better than for the more unstable injuries. This concept was first suggested by Cain et al. (52), who defined three types of hamate-metacarpal fracture-dislocation. Later, the same concept was modified by Garcia-Elias et al. (50) and extended to include all the rays of the hand (Fig. 16.8). According to this classification, there are three types of metacarpal instability:

Type I (transmetacarpal instability): Metacarpal instability caused by a fracture of the base of the metacarpal, which may be extraarticular (type Ia) or intraarticular (type Ib).

Type II (carpometacarpal instability): Metacarpal instability secondary to a CMC dislocation without adjacent fractures (type IIa) or just small chip avulsion-fractures (type IIb).

Type III (transcarpal instability): Metacarpal instability secondary to a major fracture-dislocation of one or several distal carpal row bones. This can involve only the dorsal and distal corner of the bone (type IIIa) or may be a frontal fracture affecting both the proximal (midcarpal) and distal (carpometacarpal) articulations (type IIIb). Rarely, the instability may be due to a dorsal subluxation of the distal carpal bone with (type IIIc) or without (type IIId) a fracture of its palmar surface.

Difficult to classify are the cases produced by a violent, direct force to the CMC area of a penetrating object, resulting in loss of bone substance at both sides of the joint (Fig. 16.9).

The most typical example of a type Ib CMC injury is the so-called reverse Bennett's fracture-dislocation of the fifth metacarpal base (20,60). It consists of a bipartite articular fracture, the anteroradial fragment of which usually remains attached to the hamate by the palmar CMC, intermetacarpal, and pisometacarpal ligaments, while the metacarpal shaft dislocates dorsally and ulnarly because of the pull of the extensor carpi ulnaris tendon in combination with the adductor moment produced by the opponens digiti minimi (Fig. 16.2). In high-energy accidents, tripartite (reversed Rolando) or multifragmentary, highly unstable, fractures of the fifth metacarpal base may also occur (67,68) (Fig. 16.10).

One of the most frequently reported type II injuries is the isolated fifth CMC dislocation, which may be palmar (65,66) (Fig. 16.7) but more commonly is dorsal

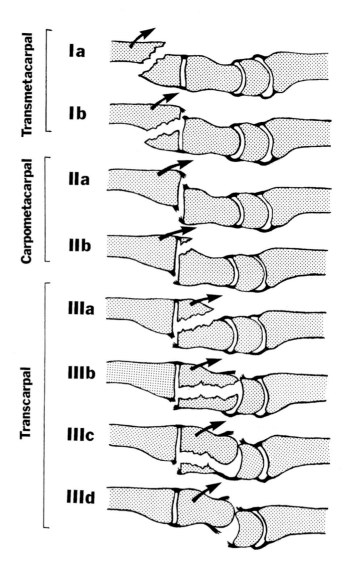

FIGURE 16.8. Mayo Clinic classification of injuries producing metacarpal instability, as reported by Garcia-Elias et al. (50). Although in this figure only the central column (radius-lunate-capitate-III metacarpal) is represented, the classification system can be applied to all the carpometacarpal rays.

(48,60,67). Multiple compound or divergent dislocations of the CMC joints have also been frequently reported (Fig. 16.11) (42,49,69), the most common involving all four CMC joints and the less severe dislocation of the fourth and fifth metacarpals (48,70) (Fig. 16.12). More rarely, all five CMC joints have dislocated (46,71), in which case the thumb tends to displace in a divergent direction relative to the rest of the metacarpals. Adjacent to the base of the dislocated metacarpal, small bone fragments can frequently be observed (type IIb). These fragments represent an avulsion fracture of the corresponding CMC ligaments rather than a midsubstance ligament rupture; therefore, in theory, the chances of achieving a stable joint if it is correctly reduced are better than if the ligament failed.

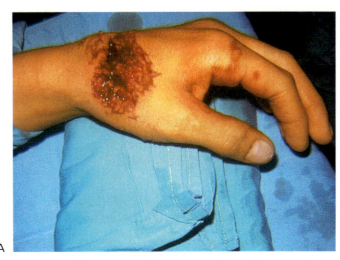
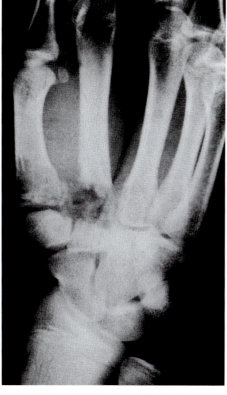

FIGURE 16.9. A: Clinical appearance of the wrist of a 23-year-old-worker who had his right hand caught by a press machine. **B:** Oblique view demonstrating extensive bone loss, including the distal aspect of the trapezoid and the base of the index metacarpal. The case was treated by a carpometacarpal arthrodesis.

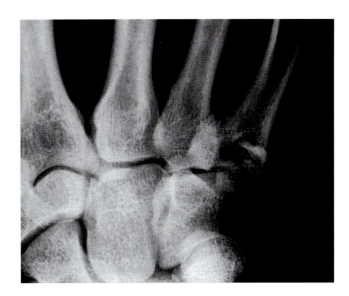

FIGURE 16.10. Y-shaped displaced fracture of the fifth metacarpal base (reverse Rolando's fracture). Note the rotatory displacement of the ulnar fragment, probably a consequence of the action of the extensor carpi ulnaris tendon.

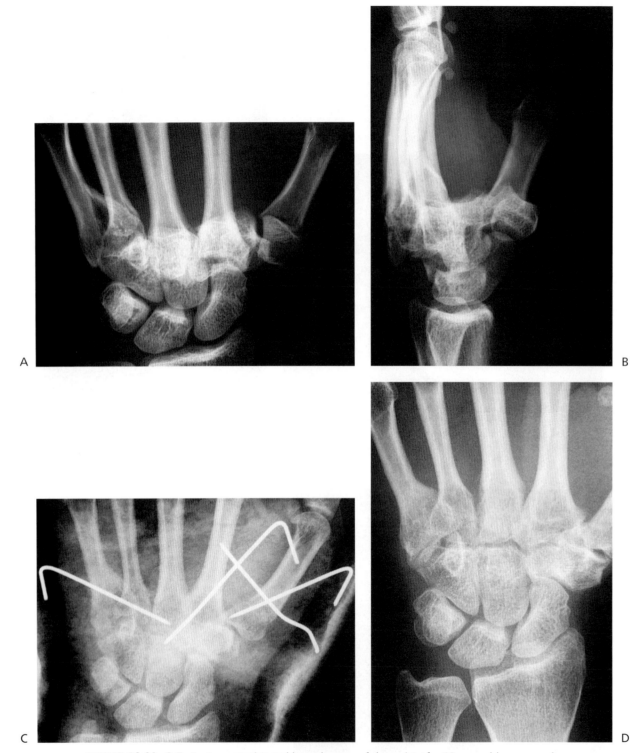

FIGURE 16.11. A,B: Posteroanterior and lateral x-rays of the wrist of a 46-year-old woman who was seen after a car accident. Complete dorsal dislocation of the four ulnar carpometacarpal joints (types IIa for the second, third, and fourth rays; type Ib for the fifth ray) associated with an extraarticular displaced fracture of the first metacarpal base. **C:** X-ray obtained after closed reduction and percutaneous K-wire fixation. All joints had acceptable reduction except for the fifth ray, which remained slightly subluxed. **D:** Three years after the injury, the patient had full range of motion with only a slightly decreased grip strength and mild discomfort at the carpometacarpal of both the first and fifth rays because of posttraumatic degenerative changes.

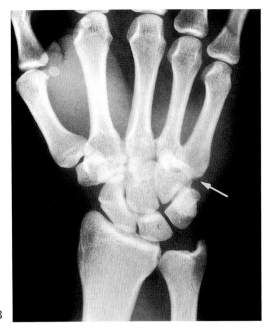 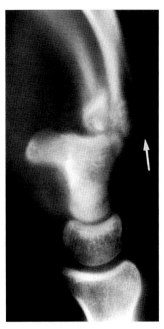 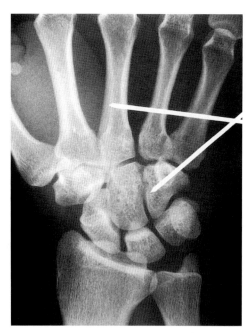

FIGURE 16.12. Dorsal dislocation of the fourth and fifth metacarpals. **A:** Posteroanterior view of the wrist demonstrates mild proximal migration of the fourth and fifth metacarpals. The overlapping outlines of the base of the fifth metacarpal and the hamate bone *(arrow)* denote loss of congruency of that carpometacarpal joint. **B:** Lateral tomogram through the base of the fifth metacarpal view shows the presence of a reverse Bennett's fracture-dislocation (type Ib) with a relatively undisplaced palmar fragment and a dorsal dislocation of the metacarpal shaft *(arrow)*. **C:** Posteroanterior view obtained after open reduction and percutaneous fixation with Kirchner wires. The final functional result was excellent. (From Garcia-Elias M, Bishop AT, Dobyns JH, et al. Trans-carpal carpometacarpal dislocations, excluding the thumb. *J Hand Surg [Am]* 1990;15 531–540, with permission.)

The more common type IIIa injury is that involving a fracture of the dorsomedial aspect of the hamate, which displaces dorsally together with the fifth metacarpal base (50–53) (Fig. 16.13). All other transcarpal types of CMC injury involving the capitate and/or trapezoid (Fig. 16.14) are less common, usually the result of high-energy trauma, and typically are associated with multiple soft-tissue lesions. Because in most instances multiple rays are involved, diagnosis must specify what type is present on each CMC joint as well as the direction and severity of displacement for each unstable segment.

Diagnosis

Injuries to the CMC joints from high-energy trauma (crush or blast mechanism) may present with a dramatic appearance, including tremendous swelling, pain, finger dysfunction, and signs of neurovascular deficiencies. In less severe injuries, especially if a period has elapsed from the time of the accident to examination, swelling may still be substantial enough to obscure any palpable deformity.

Not infrequently, if only standard posteroanterior (PA) and lateral views of an injured wrist are taken, diagnosis of a dislocated CMC joint may be missed on initial examination. The absence of obvious radiologic signs, the rarity of

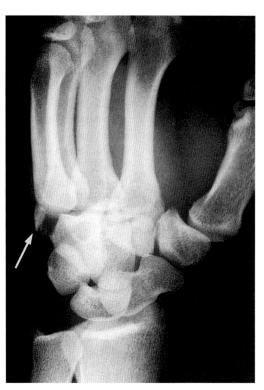

FIGURE 16.13. Semipronated oblique view of the wrist demonstrating a displaced dorsomedial fracture of the hamate *(arrow)* affecting the stability of the fifth carpometacarpal joint (type IIIa).

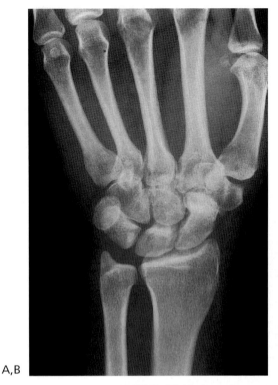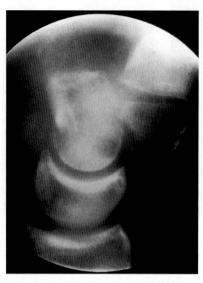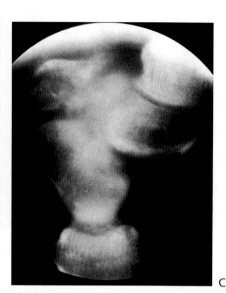

FIGURE 16.14. Dorsal transcapitate, peritrapezoid, second and third carpometacarpal dislocation. **A:** Posteroanterior view shows abnormal location of the bases of the central metacarpals with respect to the capitate and overlapping of the trapezoid and the scaphoid. **B,C:** Lateral trispiral tomograms revealed a dorsally displaced capitate fracture (type IIIa) and a dorsally subluxed trapezoid with a palmar fracture (type IIIc). (From Garcia-Elias M, Bishop AT, Dobyns JH, et al. Trans-carpal carpometacarpal dislocations, excluding the thumb. *J Hand Surg [Am]* 1990;15: 531–540, with permission.)

the condition, and the lack of awareness by the examiner are all factors that may help explain the high incidence of neglected diagnoses reported in most series (8,9,69). Yet, there are subtle x-ray signs on those standard projections that are very suggestive of the presence of these injuries, and they should never be overlooked. Overlapping of opposing articular surfaces of the CMC joint on the PA view, foreshortening of a distal row bone, and increased anteroposterior diameter of the carpus on the lateral view are indirect signs suggesting CMC joint injury (50,70) (Figs. 16.12 and 16.14). When a CMC injury is suspected, the direction and amount of displacement are better seen on oblique views: a 30° pronated view for injuries of the fourth and fifth metacarpals or a 15° supinated view for second and third CMC injuries. Special views in different degrees of wrist flexion with or without traction may also be useful. In unusual cases, where a hook of the hamate or trapezial ridge fracture is suspected, a carpal tunnel view may be indicated (71). If available, however, parasagittal and transverse trispiral tomography or computed tomography scan is by far the most reliable method for evaluation of these injuries, especially when they affect multiple joints (50) (Fig. 16.14).

Treatment

By using the classification system described above, a unified concept for treatment can be developed. The treatment of choice for the relatively stable type II injuries (pure dislocations without adjacent fractures) is early closed reduction, distal-to-proximal pin fixation, and specific cast support. Closed manipulative reduction by traction and pressure on the dorsal aspect of the wrist (or palmar, depending on the direction of displacement) is very seldom a problem. In most series, however, when the reduced wrist was stabilized only with plaster, the incidence of recurrence of the subluxation, leading to residual deformity, local tenderness, decreased grip strength, and late joint degeneration, is quite high (46,47). For this reason, most authors now advocate using percutaneous K-wire fixation routinely to prevent postreduction micromotion (5,7,20,72) (Fig. 16.12C). Indeed, when properly reduced, stabilized, and immobilized for 4 to 6 weeks, the CMC ligaments may heal, and if no substantial damage to the articular surfaces exists, an excellent outcome can be expected. Still, complications may appear, including recurrence of the subluxation, irreducibility from soft-tissue incarceration (73), or neuropraxis of the deep branch of the ulnar nerve (74,75). In all these complicated cases an early operative treatment is advised.

Types I and III, by contrast, because of the presence of a displaced fracture involving the joint, are inherently unstable and may severely affect the long-term function of the CMC and/or midcarpal joint. Accordingly, open treatment to achieve anatomic restoration of the articular surfaces, avoidance of soft tissue interposition, and proper stabilization, when feasible, is the method of choice (6–8). K-wires are the most frequent means of fracture fixation, although AO or Herbert screws have also been used succesfully (50, 55). In severely comminuted fractures, anatomic restoration of the joint surface may not be possible. Even in this case, however, an open attempt to reassemble the joint fragments, using bone graft when necessary, is likely to achieve better long-term results than accepting an incongruous articulation (76). Obviously, when these injuries are associated with other soft-tissue damage, early neurovascular or tendinous repair is advocated, an intervention that should also include reduction and stable fixation of the dislocated bone fragments. As noted by Bora and Didizian (60), painful posttraumatic osteoarthritis secondary to suboptimal reduction is not uncommon and frequently requires either a CMC fusion (45,77) or a resection-interposition arthroplasty (78). When a type I or III fracture-dislocation has been unsuspected and not properly immobilized, nonunion of the carpal fracture from both vascular and mechanical factors may appear (50). Treatment in such circumstances should include stabilization of the ununited bone and inclusion of an intercalary graft (59).

REFERENCES

1. Larsen CF, Lauritsen J. Epidemiology of acute wrist trauma. *Int J Epidemiol* 1993;22:911–916.
2. Larsen CF, Brøndum V, Skov O. Epidemiology of scaphoid fractures in Odense, Denmark. *Acta Orthop Scand* 1992;63:216–218.
3. Hove LM. Fractures of the hand. *Scand J Plast Reconstr Hand Surg* 1993;27:317–319.
4. Dobyns JH, Linscheid RL, Cooney WP. Fractures and dislocations of the wrist and hand, then and now. *J Hand Surg [Am]* 1983;8:687–690.
5. Gunther SF. The carpometacarpal joints. *Orthop Clin North Am* 1984;15:259–277.
6. Dobyns JH. Fractures and dislocations at the base of the metacarpals. In: Barton JN, ed. *Fractures of the hand and wrist.* Edinburgh: Churchill Livingstone, 1988;125–133.
7. Lawlis JF, Gunther SF. Carpometacarpal dislocations. Long-term follow-up. *J Bone Joint Surg Am* 1991;73:52–59.
8. Henderson JJ, Arafa MAM. Carpometacarpal dislocation. An easily missed dislocation. *J Bone Joint Surg Br* 1987;69:212–214.
9. Pullen C, Richardson M, McCullough K, et al. Injuries to the ulnar carpometacarpal region: are they being underdiagnosed? *Aust NZ J Surg* 1995;65:257–261.
10. Costagliola M, Micheau PH, Mansat CH, et al. Les luxations carpo-métacarpiennes. *Ann Chir* 1966;20:1466–1481.
11. Cooney WP, Chao EYS. Biomechanical analysis of static forces in the thumb during hand function. *J Bone Joint Surg Am* 1977;59:27–36.
12. Imaeda T, An KN, Cooney WP. Functional anatomy and biomechanics of the thumb. *Hand Clin* 1992;8:9–15.
13. Kauer JMG. Functional anatomy of the carpometacarpal joint of the thumb. *Clin Orthop* 1987;220:7–13.
14. Bennett EH. On fracture of the metacarpal bone of the thumb. *BMJ* 1886;2:12–13.
15. Gedda KO. Studies on Bennett's fracture: Anatomy, roentgenology, and therapy. *Acta Chir Scand [Suppl]* 1954;193:1–114.
16. Pointu J, Schwenck JP, Destree G, et al. Fractures of the trapezium. Mechanism, pathology and indications for treatment. *Fr J Orthop Surg* 1988;2:380–391.
17. Pellegrini VD Jr. Fractures at the base of the thumb. *Hand Clin* 1988;4:87–102.
18. Billing L, Gedda KO. Roentgen examination of Bennett's fracture. *Acta Radiol* 1952;38:471–476.
19. Roberts N. Fractures of the phalanges of the hand and metacarpals. *Proc R Soc Med* 1938;31:793–794.
20. Wolfe SW, Elliott AJ. Metacarpal and carpometacarpal trauma. In: Peimer CA, ed. *Surgery of the hand and upper extremity.* New York: McGraw-Hill, 1996;883–920.
21. Blum L. The treatment of Bennett's fracture-dislocation of the first metacarpal bone. *J Bone Joint Surg Am* 1941;23:578–580.
22. Cannon SR, Owd GSE, Williams DH, et al. A long-term study following Bennett's fracture. *J Hand Surg [Br]* 1986;11:426–431.
23. Cullen JP, Parentis MA, Chinchilli VM, et al. Simulated Bennett fracture treated with closed reduction and percutaneous pinning. *J Bone Joint Surg Am* 1997;79:413–420.
24. Kjœr-Petersen K, Langhoff O, Andersen K. Bennett's fracture. *J Hand Surg [Br]* 1990;15:58–61.
25. Livesley PJ. The conservative management of Bennett's fracture-dislocation: A 26-year follow-up. *J Hand Surg [Br]* 1990;15:291–294.
26. Wagner CJ. Methods of treatment of Bennett's fracture-dislocation. *Am J Surg* 1950;80:230–231.
27. Johnson EC. Fractures of the base of the thumb: A new method of fixation. *JAMA* 1944;126:27–28.
28. Iselin M. Fractures. In: Iselin M, ed. *Atlas of hand surgery.* New York: McGraw-Hill, 1964;38–42.
29. Howard FM. Fractures of the basal joint of the thumb. *Clin Orthop* 1987;220:46–51.
30. Rolando S. Fracture de la base du premier métacarpien, et principalement sur une variété non encore décrite. *Presse Med* 1910;33:303–304.
31. Foster RJ, Hastings H II. Treatment of Bennett, Rolando and vertical intra-articular trapezial fractures. *Clin Orthop* 1987;214:121–129.
32. Langhoff O, Andersen K, Kjær-Petersen K. Rolando's fracture. *J Hand Surg [Br]* 1991;16:454–459.
33. Gelberman RH, Vance RM, Zakaib GS. Fracture of the base of the thumb: Treatment with oblique traction. *J Bone Joint Surg Am* 1979;61:260–262.
34. Foucher G. Les traumatismes de l'articulation trapézo-métacarpienne. *Ann Chir Main* 1982;1:168–179.
35. Péquignot JP, Giordano PH, Boatier C, et al. Luxation traumatique de la trapézo-métacarpienne. *Ann Chir Main* 1988;7:14–24.
36. Toupin JM, Milliez PY, Thomine JM. Luxation trapézo-métacarpienne post-traumatique récente. A propos de 8 cas. *Rev Chir Orthop* 1995;81:27–34.
37. Simonian PT, Trumble TE. Traumatic dislocation of the thumb carpometacarpal joint: early ligamentous reconstruction versus closed reduction and pinning. *J Hand Surg [Am]* 1996;21:802–806.
38. Eaton RG, Littler JW. Ligament reconstruction for the painful

38. thumb carpometacarpal joint. *J Bone Joint Surg Am* 1973;55:1655–1666.
39. Garcia-Elias M, Henriquez-Lluch A, Rossignani P, et al. Bennett's fracture combined with fracture of the trapezium. A report of three cases. *J Hand Surg [Br]* 1993;18:523–526.
40. Jones WA, Ghorbal MS. Fractures of the trapezium. A report on three cases. *J Hand Surg [Br]* 1985;10:227–230.
41. Cordrey LJ, Ferrer-Torells M. Management of fractures of the greater multangular. *J Bone Joint Surg Am* 1960;42:1111–1118.
42. Waugh RL, Yancey AG. Carpometacarpal dislocations, with particular reference to simultaneous dislocation of the bases of the fourth and fifth metacarpals. *J Bone Joint Surg Am* 1948;30:397–404.
43. McWhorter GL. Isolated and complete dislocation of the fifth carpometacarpal joint: Open operation. *Surg Clin Chicago* 1918;2:793–796.
44. Mueller JJ. Carpometacarpal dislocations: Report of five cases and review of the literature. *J Hand Surg [Am]* 1986;11:184–188.
45. Clendenin MB, Smith RJ. Fifth metacarpal/hamate arthrodesis for posttraumatic osteoarthritis. *J Hand Surg [Am]* 1984;9:374–378.
46. Shephard E, Solomon DJ. Carpometacarpal dislocation. *J Bone Joint Surg Br* 1960;42:772–777.
47. Hazlett JW. Carpometacarpal dislocations other than the thumb: A report of 11 cases. *Can J Surg* 1968;11:315–323.
48. Hsu JD, Curtis RM. Carpometacarpal dislocations on the ulnar side of the hand. *J Bone Joint Surg Am* 1970;52:927–930.
49. Hartwig RH, Louis DS. Multiple carpometacarpal dislocations. *J Bone Joint Surg Am* 1979;61:906–908.
50. Garcia-Elias M, Bishop AT, Dobyns JH, et al. Trans-carpal carpometacarpal dislocations, excluding the thumb. *J Hand Surg [Am]* 1990;15:531–540.
51. Rossi F. Lussazioni e frattura dell' uncinato. *Atti Mem Soc Lomb Chir* 1937;5:1019–1022.
52. Cain JE, Shepler TR, Wilson MR. Hamatometacarpal fracture-dislocation: Classification and treatment. *J Hand Surg [Am]* 1987;12(part 1):762–767.
53. Loth TS, McMillan MD. Coronal dorsal hamate fractures. *J Hand Surg [Am]* 1988;13:616–618.
54. Kinnett JG, Lyden JP. Posterior fracture-dislocation of the IV metacarpal hamate articulation: case report. *J Trauma* 1979;19:290–291.
55. Roth JH, de Lorenzi C. Displaced intra-articular coronal fracture of the hamate treated with a Herbert screw. *J Hand Surg [Am]* 1988;13:619–621.
56. Kimura H, Kamura S, Akai M. An unusual coronal fracture of the body of the hamate bone. *J Hand Surg [Am]* 1988;13:743–745.
57. Sheldon JG. Dorsal dislocation of the trapezoid. *Am J Med Sci* 1901;121:85–89.
58. Russell TB. Carpal dislocations and fracture-dislocations. A review of fifty-nine cases. *J Bone Joint Surg [Br]* 1949;31:524–531.
59. Rand JA, Linscheid RL, Dobyns JH. Capitate fractures. A long-term follow-up. *Clin Orthop* 1982;165:209–216.
60. Bora FW, Didizian NH. The treatment of injuries to the carpometacarpal joint of the little finger. *J Bone Joint Surg Am* 1974;56:1459–1463.
61. Shorbe HB. Carpometacarpal dislocations. Report of a case. *J Bone Joint Surg Am* 1938;20:454–457.
62. Garcia-Elias M, Dobyns JH, Cooney WP, et al. Traumatic axial dislocations of the carpus. *J Hand Surg [Am]* 1985;14:446–457.
63. Milch H. Isolated luxation of the lesser multangular. *Bull Hosp Joint Dis* 1943;4:36–40.
64. Bendre DV, Baxi VK. Dislocation of trapezoid. *J Trauma* 1981;21:899–900.
65. Garcia-Elias M, Rossignani P, Cots M. Combined fracture of the hook of the hamate and palmar dislocation of the fifth carpometacarpal joint. *J Hand Surg [Br]* 1996;21:446–450.
66. North ER, Eaton RG. Volar dislocation of the fifth metacarpal. *J Bone Joint Surg Am* 1980;62:657–659.
67. Domisse IG, Lloyd GJ. Injuries to the fifth carpometacarpal region. *Can J Surg* 1979;22:240–242.
68. Chmell S, Light TR, Blair SJ. Fracture and fracture dislocation of ulnar carpometacarpal joint. *Orthop Rev* 1982;11:73–80.
69. Guimaraes RM, Benaïssa S, Moughabghab M, et al. Les luxations carpo-métacarpiennes des doigts longs. A propos de 26 cas dont 20 cas revus. *Rev Chir Orthop* 1996;82:598–607.
70. Fischer MR, Rogers LF, Hendrix RW. Systematic approach to identifying fourth and fifth carpometacarpal joint dislocations. *Am J Roentgenol* 1983;140:319–324.
71. Hsu KY, Wu CC, Wang KC, et al. Simultaneous dislocation of the five metacarpal joints with concomitant fractures of the tuberosity of the trapezium and the hook of the hamate. *J Trauma* 1993;35:479–483.
72. Foster RJ. Stabilization of ulnar carpometacarpal dislocations or fracture dislocations. *Clin Orthop* 1996;327:94–97.
73. Mehara AK, Bhan S. Rotary dislocation of the second carpometacarpal joint: Case report. *J Trauma* 1993;34:464–466.
74. Gore DR. Carpometacarpal dislocation producing compression of the deep branch of the ulnar nerve. *J Bone Joint Surg Am* 1971;53:1387–1390.
75. Murphy TP, Parkhill WS. Fracture-dislocation of the base of the fifth metacarpal with an ulnar motor nerve lesion: Case report. *J Trauma* 1990;30:1585–1587.
76. Kjœr-Petersen K, Jurik AG. Intra-articular fractures at the base of the fifth metacarpal. A clinical and radiographical study of 64 cases. *J Hand Surg [Br]* 1992;17:144–147.
77. Joseph RB, Linscheid RL, Dobyns JH, et al. Chronic sprains of the carpometacarpal joints. *J Hand Surg [Am]* 1981;6:172–180.
78. Proubasta I, Lluch AL. [Treatment of posttraumatic degenerative arthritis of the carpometacarpal joint of the small finger by silicone implant arthroplasty.] *Rev Ortop Trauma* 1994;38:66–68.

17

TRANSCARPAL AND RADIOCARPAL WRIST AMPUTATION AND REPLANTATION

DAVID L. CANNON
JAMES R. URBANIAK

The incidence of traumatic wrist amputation is not well known. The majority of reports that have been published regarding amputation and replantation address mainly digits and thumb, with hand replantations also being included. One of the largest reports on upper extremity replantations is that of Tamai, in which there were 273 upper limb replantations, 15 involving the hand, and six of which involved a completely amputated hand (1). Over the past 15 years, our institution has replanted over 1,500 traumatically amputated parts. The vast majority of these have been digits and thumbs, but 57 of these were major limb replantation, of which six were replanted at the level of the wrist.

The disability associated with the loss of the hand is quite high. The disability rating for loss of one upper extremity is 50%, and that for loss of just one hand is 45%. Therefore, every attempt should be made for replantation at the level of the wrist because even a hand with partial function is superior to a prosthetic replacement.

HISTORY OF REPLANTATION

Experimental replantation of amputated limbs of animals was successfully performed at the turn of the century (2,3). However, clinical accomplishment of limb replantation was not realized until the 1960s with the introduction of the operating microscope by Jacobson and Suarez in 1960 (4). In Boston in 1962, Malt and McKhann successfully replanted a completely amputated arm of a 12-year-old boy (5). In 1963, the first successful hand replantation was reported by Chen at the Sixth People's Hospital in China (6). In 1968, Komatsu and Tamai of Japan reported the first successful replantation of the completely amputated thumb (7).

For more than 35 years, refinements in the field of microsurgery (operating microscope, ultrafine nonreactive suture material, and precision microcaliber needles) have made successful replantation of digits and hands possible (8–13).

Although many developments have helped to improve the success rate of hand replantations, patient selection and the refinement of the technique for microvascular anastomosis are the main contributors. In a microvascular anastomosis, the key points are minimal stripping of the adventitia, frequent intraluminal irrigation with diluted heparinized solution, interrupted sutures, proper needle placement technique, and nonabsorbable suture material of the correct size (14).

PATIENT SELECTION: INDICATIONS AND CONTRAINDICATIONS

Our criteria for proper patient selection for replantation are based on our team's experience of over 1,500 parts. Even with this knowledge, the decision to replant an amputated part is not always easy. Again, a hand with partial recovery of function is superior to a prosthetic replacement, and, therefore, every attempt is made to salvage an amputated hand at the level of the wrist. Certainly patients with guillotine-type amputations are ideal candidates; however, this type of amputation is uncommon. Most limbs are amputated by crushing or avulsion injury, which makes the surgical repair more difficult and lowers the percentage of viability. Absolute indications for hand replantation are clean-cut guillotine-like amputations with minimal crushing or avulsion, relatively short ischemic time (less than 6 hours of warm ischemic time or 9 to 10 hours of cold ischemic time), and amputations on children.

D. L. Cannon: Department of Surgery, Uniformed Services University of Health Sciences, Bethesda, Maryland 20814; and Department of Orthopaedic Surgery, Navy Medical Center, Portsmouth, Virginia 23708.

J. R. Urbaniak: Division of Orthopaedic Surgery, Department of Surgery, Duke University School of Medicine, Duke University Medical Center, Durham, North Carolina 27710.

Successful replantations at the level of the palm, wrist, and distal forearm result in good hand function (15–18). Proper handling of the amputated hand is essential for successful replantation. The instructions given to the referring physician should be to place the hand in a saline-filled plastic bag that is tightly secure. The bag with the hand should then be placed in a large container filled with crushed ice. The ice should not touch the hand at any time. These instructions are relatively easy to understand over the phone. Another technique that has been described is to place the hand in a gauze wrap soaked in saline then into a sealed bag, and to place the bag in ice (6,15,16). There has not been a difference seen between these two methods as long as the body part was not frozen (19).

Contraindications for hand replantation include severely crushed or mangled part, amputations at multiple levels, amputations in patients with other serious injuries or diseases, amputations with prolonged warm ischemic time (more than 9 to 10 hours) or with freezing of the tissues, and amputations in which the vessels are arteriosclerotic. Amputations in the mentally unstable patient are not uncommon and should be dealt with on a case specific basis with a consultation from psychiatry.

Usually the patient and his or her family desire a replantation and expect a miraculous result. The surgeon must explain to the patient the chances of viability, anticipated function, length of operation and hospitalization, and the amount of time lost from work. The patient and family must know that the final decision for replantation cannot be made until the status of the vessels of the amputated hand is carefully studied under the operating microscope.

TECHNIQUE AND SEQUENCE OF SURGERY

When the patient with an amputated hand arrives in the Emergency Room, the replantation team divides into two subteams in an effort to save time. One team immediately transports the amputated hand to the operating room, where it is cleansed with Hibiclens (Stuart Pharmaceuticals, Wilmington, DE) and sterile Ringer's lactate solution. The amputated hand is placed on a bed of ice covered with a sterile plastic drape.

Under operating loupes or an operating microscope, the hand is carefully debrided. A second set of instruments is used for this procedure. The radial and ulnar arteries as well as a minimum of four dorsal veins along with the ulnar median and superficial radial nerves are identified and trimmed to normal tissue level and tagged with small silver vascular clips (hemoclips). Tagging of the vessels and nerves will prove to be very helpful and time saving when working in a bloody field later. Heparinized saline is used to irrigate the radial and ulnar arteries before they are tagged. Releases of both the carpal tunnel and Guyon's canal are performed. The retraction of the distal dorsal skin allows for easy identification of the dorsal veins located within the subcutaneous tissues. Evaluation of the condition of the cartilage on the carpus is then undertaken. After preparation of the hand has been completed, it is returned to the bed of ice or placed in the refrigerator.

While preparation of the amputated hand is occurring, the other subteam assesses the patient with a routine physical examination, radiographs of the injured extremity and chest, electrocardiogram, blood chemistries, complete blood count, urinalysis, blood type and cross match, and activated partial thromboplastin time. Intravenous fluids are begun, and the patient is given IV antibiotics and tetanus prophylaxis. An indwelling Foley catheter is inserted to monitor urine output.

A combination of general and regional anesthesia is ideal. General anesthesia allows for patient relaxation and proper positioning of the extremity on the table.

Peripheral blood flow to the injured limb is enhanced by the sympathetic block provided by regional anesthesia.

After anesthesia has been administered and the hand has been prepared, the tourniquet is inflated to 250 mm Hg, and the preparation of the stump is undertaken. Under loupe or microscope magnification, the stump is debrided, and the nerves and vessels are identified and tagged in a manner similar to that used on the amputated hand. Once debridement is complete, the articular cartilage of the distal radius is evaluated.

The operative sequence of replantation varies slightly with the level of amputation (digit vs. hand vs. proximal limb), and the type of injury (clean cut, crush, or avulsion). The general operative sequence for a replantation is as follows:

1. Locate and tag the vessels and nerves.
2. Debride.
3. Shorten and fix the bone.
4. Repair the extensor tendons.
5. Repair the flexor tendons.
6. Anastomose the arteries.
7. Repair the nerves.
8. Anastomose the veins.
9. Obtain skin coverage.

The operative sequence is slightly modified for transcarpal replantation of the hand. The first three steps of locating and tagging the vessels and nerves, debriding the amputated hand and the stump appropriately, and shortening and fixing the bones are still done in that order. However, the most important factor in determining the viability as well as the return of the function of the hand is to reestablish blood flow as soon as possible. This is why the next step that is undertaken is to anastomose the ulnar or radial artery first. The tourniquet is then deflated, and flow to the hand is evaluated. It may be necessary to reanastomose both arteries in order to obtain good blood flow to the hand. While working in the vicinity of the ulnar nerve, it is usual to repair it at that time. Once the arterial flow has been reestablished in both radial and ulnar arteries, attention is usually turned toward the dorsum of the hand. A large dorsal vein is then located, and reanastomosis is carried out at this point. After at least one dorsal vein has been reanastomosed, the extensor tendons are then repaired. An attempt is then made to find as many dorsal veins as possible for venous anastomoses. Attention is then returned to the volar aspect of the hand, where the flexor tendons are identified and repaired. The median nerve and superficial radial nerve are then identified and repaired. Skin coverage is then attempted.

It is extremely important to carefully isolate and tag the vessels, nerves, and tendons before carrying out any debridement. Magnification is essential to obtain optimal debridement. A pulsating jet lavage is useful in severely contaminated wounds. Any potentially necrotic tissue must be excised. All severed structures that can possibly be repaired are reconnected during the replantation procedure. Total repair of all structures provides effective stabilization and allows for early motion of the reconstructed hand.

BONE STABILIZATION

Bone shortening and fixation are critical aspects of any replantation (20,21). Sufficient bone must be resected to ensure approximation of normal intima in the vascular anastomosis. The connection of arteries, veins, and nerves must never be performed under tension. Ideally there can be shortening of the bone with maintenance of some wrist motion. If the articular surface from the distal radius is intact, then a proximal row carpectomy can be entertained. However, if the distal radius articular surface has been damaged by the amputation process, then a limited fusion such as a radius-scapholunate arthrodesis can be undertaken. For these two procedures, cross K-wires, usually two on the radial and two on the ulnar aspect, are placed to stabilize the bones (Figs. 17.1–17.3).

If there has been extensive articular surface damage to the carpal bones, then a wrist fusion will need to be undertaken. Because rapid stabilization of the bones is critical, limited plating of the dorsal aspect of the radius to the metacarpals is undertaken with the thought of returning at a later date to add bone graft if necessary.

ARTERIAL REPAIR

The arteries are anastomosed following bone fixation. When possible, we repair both the ulnar and radial arteries. A volar curved incision may be needed for adequate exposure. This is likely to be the same incision as used to expose the flexor tendons. The ulnar and radial arteries are identified, and the hemoclips are removed. Vascular clamps are then placed on the ulnar and radial arteries. The tourniquet is then released.

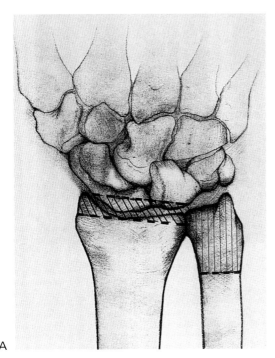
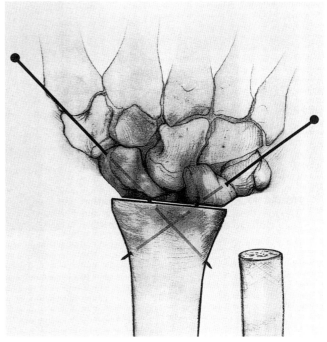

FIGURE 17.1. A,B: The bone fixation for replantation of an amputation through the carpus is most rapidly obtained by cross-pin fixation. Matching cuts are made on the carpus and distal radius for accurate approximation. The ulna has been resected.

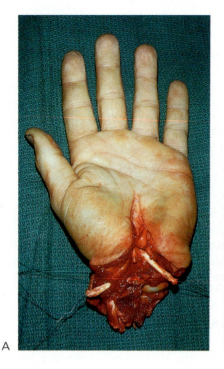
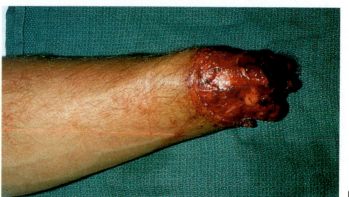
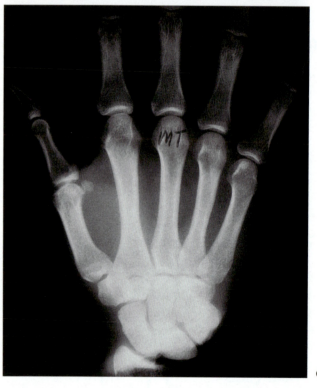

FIGURE 17.2. A–C: A complete amputation through the carpal bones of a 21-year-old man, with radiograph of amputated wrist.

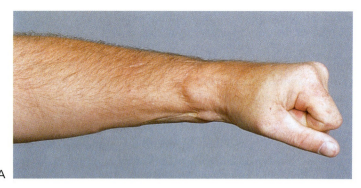
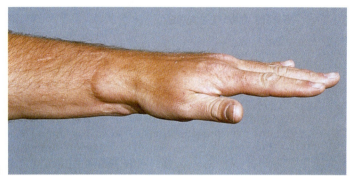
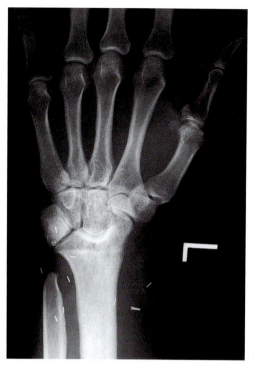

FIGURE 17.3. Fifteen-year follow-up of the replanted hand. **A,B:** The patient has 30° of wrist flexion and extension, full function of all intrinsics and extrinsics, and protective sensation. **C:** The radiograph demonstrates solid fusion between the radius and proximal carpal row and motion between the proximal and distal carpal rows.

The arterial repair should not be attempted until spurting blood flow occurs from the proximal vessel. If a pulsating proximal arterial flow is not evident, steps to induce flow include:

1. Relief of vascular tension or compression.
2. Proximal resection to healthy vessel walls.
3. Warming of the operating room and patient.
4. Adequate hydration of the patient.
5. Elevation of the patient's blood pressure.
6. Irrigation of the proximal vessel with warm Ringer's lactate solution.
7. External application or gentle interluminal flushing with papaverine solution (1 to 20 dilution).
8. Checking with the anesthesiologist about a metabolic problem that could incite vasospasm, e.g., acidosis (22).
9. Being certain that the tourniquet is not inflated.
10. Wait!

The severed arteries must be resected until normal intima is visualized under high-power magnification: only normal intima is reconnected. If this cannot be achieved, an interpositional vein graft is used. The two most critical factors in achieving successful microvascular anastomosis are the skill and expertise of the microsurgeon and easy coaptation of normal intima to normal intima. Two easy anastomoses are quicker and more likely to be successful than one difficult anastomosis under tension.

A pneumatic tourniquet may safely be used for each vascular anastomosis. If the technique of the microvascular anastomsis is skillfully performed, tourniquet ischemia will not diminish patency rate. The tourniquet should be released at the conclusion of each anastomosis. The tourniquet may be inflated and deflated many times during the procedure to allow considerable decrease in operating time and blood loss. If hemorrhage is not excessive or obscuring the visual field, then a tourniquet is not used.

Interposition vein grafts are used in approximately 20% of all our replantations to obtain reapproximation of the healthy arteries and veins. Vein grafts are usually taken from the same or the opposite volar forearm. The distance that is to be bridged is measured so that the length of the vein graft needed can be determined.

Dextran 40 (Kendall McGraw Labs Inc., Irvine, CA) should be given at the completion of the vascular anastomosis.

VEIN REPAIR

An attempt should be made to anastomose four veins, two for each artery. The veins should be debrided back to healthy tissue before anastomosis. If harvesting a vein does not allow coaptation without undue tension, the surgeon should proceed immediately with a vein graft. The radial and middorsal aspect of the hand usually provide large veins that can be repaired successfully.

Some recognized replantation surgeons repair veins before arteries to decrease the blood loss and maintain a bloodless field for better vision (16,23,24). However, by judicious use of the tourniquet, the arteries may be repaired first, and a dry field maintained. This provides the advantages of earlier revascularization and allows easier location of the most functional vein detected by their spurting back flow. If the veins are repaired first, especially in an avulsion type injury, and subsequent arterial anastomosis fails to show adequate arterial inflow, the surgeon has wasted valuable time on a nonsalvageable hand. Additionally, reanastomosing the arteries and allowing for some venous oozing before anastomosis of the vein reduces the amount of ischemic metabolites returned to the general circulation.

NERVE REPAIR

Because the bone has been shortened in replantation, nerve repair is generally not difficult, for there is no tension at the suture line. The median, ulnar, and superficial radial nerves have been identified in both the stump and in the amputated hand. It is usually the case that minimal trimming of the nerve ends is required. The microscope is used for careful fascicular (or bundle) alignment of the freshly injured nerves. The nerves are repaired with 8-0 monofilament nonabsorbable suture by epineural repair after fascicular alignment has been determined. Primary nerve grafting using the sural nerve is performed when end-to-end repair is not possible.

EXTENSOR TENDON REPAIR

All digital extensor tendons including indicis proprius and digiti quinti are repaired when possible. The wrist extensors are also repaired.

Extensor repair is done using a modified Kessler stitch of 4-0 nonabsorbable suture combined with a running epitendinous stitch of 5-0 nonabsorbable suture. To prevent bowstringing of the extensor tendons, reconstruction of the retinaculum is completed by repairing it primarily or by using local tissue for augmentation. The tendons are trimmed back to a healthy tissue level before repair.

FLEXOR TENDON REPAIR

All of the flexor tendons are repaired, including the wrist flexors. Previous dissection of the amputated hand and the volar aspect of the stump allow for visualization of the tendon ends. The tendons are trimmed back to a healthy tissue level.

We prefer to use the Tajima stitch of 4-0 nonabsorbable suture for primary flexor tendon repair in replantation (25). The sutures are placed in all of the proximal and distal tendon stumps before any knots are tied. After appropriate matching is ensured, the tendon ends are connected by securing the knots. A running epidentinous stitch using 5-0 nonabsorbable suture is then used for each tendon.

SKIN COVERAGE

Meticulous hemostasis is obtained after all structures have been repaired and revascularization of the replanted hand has been assured. The skin is loosely approximated with a few interrupted nylon sutures. All damaged skin that may become necrotic is excised, and no tension should be placed on the skin during closure. The vessels should be covered without constriction from the overlying skin or sutures. Coverage of the vessels is important to prevent desiccation of the vessel walls. Split-thickness skin, full-thickness skin, or a local rotational skin flap may be used for coverage. In some instances skin grafting is not able to be accomplished, so a pigskin graft is used temporarily until definitive coverage can be obtained.

DRESSING

The primarily closed wounds are covered with strips of Xeroform gauze. If split-thickness skin grafting was used, a layer of adaptic is placed over the skin graft, with Bunnell's-soaked cotton balls placed on the adaptic. The cotton balls are held in place by an additional layer of adaptic placed over them, and the second adaptic is held to the skin with either staples or silk stays. The upper extremity is then immobilized in a bulky compression hand dressing that extends above the elbow to prevent slippage. Each step of the dressing is carefully designed to prevent circumferential constriction. A dorsal plaster splint extending proximally from the distal interphalangeal joints is applied.

POSTOPERATIVE CARE

Postoperative management is extremely important in achieving a high success rate in replantation. Despite a technically successful replantation, postoperatively the replanted hand may develop vascular insufficiency that can frequently be corrected if detected early.

The hand in the bulky compression dressing is elevated by a foam rubber cradle boot. The elbow usually rests on the bed. If arterial inflow is diminished, the hand may be lowered. If venous outflow is slow, the hand needs elevation.

We prefer the use of some type of anticoagulation in all of our patients. We use dipyridamole (Persantine, 50 mg twice a day). In addition, Dextran 40 (500 cc a day), aspirin (300 g twice a day), and chlorpromazine (Thorazine, 25 mg four times a day), are all used for 1 week. The chlorpromazine is useful as a peripheral vasodilator and tranquilizer to diminish vasospasm secondary to anxiety.

The patient's room should be maintained comfortably warm (approximately 75°F), and cool drafts should be avoided. The patient is not permitted to smoke. Initially the patient is kept NPO so that he or she may be returned to the operating room if vascular exploration is required.

Color, pulp turgor, capillary refill, and warmth are all useful aids in monitoring the replanted hand, but quantitative skin temperature measurements have proven to be the most reliable indicators (26). The digital temperature is monitored with a YSI Tele-Thermometer (Yellow Springs Instrument Company, Yellow Springs, OH) and small surface probes. If the skin temperature of the replanted hand drops below 30°C or is more than 2°C different from the normal hand, poor perfusion of the replanted hand is suspected, and a cause for the compromised circulation must be found and corrected if possible.

It is essential that the patient have adequate hydration in the initial postoperative period. After the first 24 hours following surgery, the patient is begun on a diet that excludes vasoconstrictive agents such as caffeine. The patient is kept at bed rest for 2 to 3 days, and then activity is permitted in accordance with the patient's course, desires, and personality.

If a careful and intelligent postoperative program is employed, it is rarely necessary to return the patient to the operating room for reexploration. If this decision is made, however, it must be carried out within 4 to 6 hours of loss of adequate perfusion. Reexploration with correction of the problem (redoing the anastomoses, removal of thrombi, or vein grafting a previously unrecognized damaged vessel segment) is most effective when acute cessation of arterial inflow is diagnosed.

REHABILITATION

At 5 to 7 days postoperatively, the first dressing change is done. If the dressing is adherent to the incision, warm saline may be used so that the Xeroform gauze can be gently removed. A new dressing and splint are then applied. Gentle passive range of motion of the digits is begun at this time. The patients then progress, with the assistance of occupational therapists, from passive range-of-motion exercises to active assistive and then to active range-of-motion exercises. The wrist is splinted for a varying percentage of time postoperatively, depending on the shortening procedure. If a proximal row carpectomy was performed, the transfixing pins are removed at 6 weeks postoperatively. If a limited fusion was done, then the transfixion pins are removed at approximately 6 to 8 weeks, and splinting continues until there is evidence of a solid fusion. Once the splint has been removed, active range of motion of the wrist is started. If wrist fusion was required, the patient remains in a short arm cast until fusion is evident.

EXPECTATIONS FOLLOWING REPLANTATION

A survival rate of 100% for hand amputations was reported by Tamai (1) (Figs. 17.2 and 17.3). By applying the principles described in this chapter, the experienced and proficient microsurgeon should be able to achieve at least an 80% viability rate in transcarpal hand replantations. The results, based on reports from major replantation centers, should be as follows (6,17,18,27,28):

1. Nerve recovery comparable to that of repair of an isolated severed peripheral nerve. Patients will not report normal sensation after hand replantation.
2. Active range of motion approximately 50% of that on the normal, uninvolved side.
3. Cold intolerance, a definite problem that usually resolves by 2 years' time.
4. Patient satisfaction, usually greater than 90%. The cosmetic appearance is much preferred to amputation revision or prosthesis.
5. Return to work, usually at 3 to 4 months after replantation; however, job modification may be necessary.

WRIST DISARTICULATION FOR REVISION AMPUTATION

When there has been a severe injury to the hand and replantation cannot be completed, or the attempt at replantation has failed, a wrist disarticulation is indicated. Because there is no benefit to retaining the carpal bones, the wrist disarticulation is made at the level of the radius and ulna. Distal radioulnar joint preservation allows for forearm rotation. It is important to be careful to preserve the triangular fibrocartilage complex during disection because this is an vital stabilizer of the distal radioulnar joint. Tenodesis of the major forearm motors stabilizes the muscle unit, which improves the physiologic response and thus improves myoelectric performance. The shape of the stump remains bulbous, thus permitting prosthetic attachment. Although the stump will pronate and supinate, the socket will not permit this axial rotation. This level of amputation is most useful because of the strong, durable stump.

REFERENCES

1. Tamai S. Twenty years experience of limb replantation—Review of 293 upper extremity replants. *J Hand Surg [Am]* 1982;7: 549–556.
2. Carrel A, Guthrie CC. Results of a replantation of a thigh. *Science* 1906;23:393.
3. Hopfner E. Uber Gefassnaht: Gefasstransplantation und Reimplantation von amputierten Extremitaten. *Arch Klin Chir* 1903; 70:417.
4. Jacobson JH, Suarez CL. Microsurgery and anastomosis of the small vessels. *Surg Forum* 1960;11:243.
5. Malt RA, McKhann C. Replantation of severed arms. *JAMA* 1964;189:716.
6. Bunke HJ, Alpert BS, Johnson-Giebink R. Digital replantation. *Surg Clin North Am* 1981;61:383–394.
7. Komatsu S, Tamai S. Successful replantation of a completely cut-off thumb: Case report. *Plast Reconstr Surg* 1968;42:374–377.
8. Acland RD. *Microsurgery practice manual.* St Louis: CV Mosby, 1980.
9. Bright DS. Microsurgical techniques in vessel and nerve repair. *AAOS Instruct Course Lect* 1979;27:1–15.
10. Daniel R, Terzis J. *Reconstructive microsurgery.* Boston: Little, Brown, 1977.
11. Nunley JA. Microscopes and microinstruments. *Hand Clin* 1985;1:197–204.
12. Urbaniak JR, Roth JH, Nunley JA, et al. The results of replantation after amputation of a single finger. *J Bone Joint Surg Am* 1985;67:611–619.
13. Urbaniak JR, Soucacos PN, Adelaar RS, et al. Experimental evaluation of microsurgical techniques in small artery anastomoses. *Orthop Clin North Am* 1977;8:249–263.
14. Tamai S, Hori Y, Tatsumi Y, et al. Microvascular anastomosis and its application on the replantation of amputated digits and hands. *Clin Orthop* 1978;133:106–121.
15. Kleinert HE, Juhala CA, Tsai T-M, et al. Digital replantation—selection, technique, and results. *Orthop Clin North Am* 1977;8: 309–318.
16. Morriason WA, O'Brien BM, MacLeod AM. Digital replantation and revascularization. A long term review of one hundred cases. *Hand* 1978;10:125–134.
17. Tamai S. Digit replantation: Analysis of 163 cases in an 11 year period. *Clin Plast Surg* 1978;5:195.
18. Urbaniak JR. Digit and hand replantation: Current status. *Neurosurgery* 1979;4:551–559.
19. Van Giesen P, Seaber AV, Urbaniak JR. Storage of amputated parts prior to replantation. An experimental study with rabbit ears. *J Hand Surg [Am]* 1983;8:60–65.
20. Urbaniak JR, Hayes MG, Bright DS. Management of bone in digital replantation: Free vascularized and composit bone grafts. *Clin Orthop* 1978;133:184–194.
21. Whitney TM, Lineaweaver WC, Buncke HJ, et al. Clinical results of boney fixation methods in digital replantatrion. *J Hand Surg [Am]* 1990;15:328–334.
22. Dell PC, Seaber AV, Urbaniak JR. The effect of systemic acidosis on perfusion of replanted extremities. *J Hand Surg [Am]* 1980;5: 433–442.
23. Moniem MS. Replantation of the hand. In: Blair WF, ed. *Techniques in hand surgery.* Baltimore: Williams & Wilkins, 1996; 439–449.
24. O'Brien BMcC. *Microvascular reconstructive surgery.* Edinburgh: Churchill Livingstone, 1977.
25. Tajima T. History, current status, and aspects of hand surgery in Japan. *Clin Orthop* 1984;184:41–49.
26. Gelberman RH, Urbaniak JR, Bright DS, et al. Digital sensibility following replantation. *J Hand Surg [Am]* 1978;3:313–319.
27. Urbaniak JR. Replantation in children. In: *Pediatric plastic surgery.* St Louis: CV Mosby, 1984;1168.
28. Weiland AJ, Villarreal-Rios A, Kleinert HE, et al. Replantation of digits and hands: Analysis of surgical techniques and functional results in 71 patients with 86 replantations. *J Hand Surg [Am]* 1977;2:1–12.

BIBLIOGRAPHY

Dell PC, Seaber AV, Urbaniak JR. Effect of hypovolemia on perfusion after digit replantation. *Surg Forum* 1980;31:503.
Fahmy HWM, Moneim MS. The effect of prolonged blood stasis on a microarterial repair. *J Reconstr Microsurg* 1988;4:139–142.
Goldner RD. Postoperative managment. *Hand Clin* 1985;1: 205–215.
Goldner RD, Fitch RD, Nunley JA, et al. Demographics and replantation. *J Hand Surg [Am]* 1987;12:961–965.
Goldner RD, Howson MP, Nunley JA, et al. One hundred eleven thumb amputations: Replantation versus revision. *Microsurgery* 1990;11:243–350.
Goldner RD, Urbaniak JR. Indications for replantation in the adult upper extremity. In: Kasden ML, ed. *Occupational medicine state of the art reviews.* Philadelphia: Hanley & Belfus, 1989;525–538.
Hayes MG, Urbaniak JR. Management of bone in microvascular surgery. In: *AAOS symposium on microsurgical practical use in orthopaedics.* St Louis: CV Mosby, 1979;96.
Moniem MS, Chacon NE. Salvage of replanted parts of the upper extremity. *J Bone Joint Surg Am* 1985;67:880–883.
Morris HB, Seaber AV, Urbaniak JR. *The effect of acute limited normovolemic hemodilution on pH and temperature recovery of ischemic rat extremities.* Paper presented at the 27th Annual Meeting of the Orthopaedic Research Society, Las Vegas, February 1981.
Morris HB, Sylvia AL, Seaber AV, et al. Effect of acute normovolemic Dextran 70 hemodilution on post-ischemic skeletal muscle respiration and perfusion. *Surg Forum* 1981;32:536–538.
Sixth People's Hospital, Shanghai. *Replantation of severed fingers: Clinical experience in 162 cases involving 270 severed fingers (pamphlet).* Shanghai: Sixth People's Hospital, 1963.
Urbaniak JR. Replantation. In: Green DP, ed. *Operative hand surgery, 3rd ed, vol 2.* New York: Churchill Livingstone, 1993;1085–1102.
Urbaniak JR. Replantation of amputated hands and digits. *AAOS Instruct Course Lect* 1978;27:15–26.
Urbaniak JR. Replantation of amputated parts—technique, results, and indications. In: *AAOS symposium on microsurgery practical use in orthopaedics.* St Louis: CV Mosby, 1979;64.
Wheeless CR. Wrist disarticulations. In: Wheeless CR, ed. *Wheeless' textbook of orthopaedic surgery.* www.medmedia.com, 1996.
Yamauchi S, Nomura S, Yoshimura M, et al. A clinical study of the order and speed of sensory recovery after digital replantation. *J Hand Surg [Am]* 1983;8.545–549.
Yoshizu T, Katsumi M, Tajima T. Replantation of untidy amputated finger, hand and arm: Experience of 99 replantaions in 66 cases. *J Trauma* 1978;18:194–200.

18

CLASSIFICATION AND CONSERVATIVE TREATMENT OF DISTAL RADIUS FRACTURES

DIEGO L. FERNANDEZ
CLAUDE J. MARTIN

Fractures of the distal radius continue to attract the attention of many surgeons and represent a constant therapeutic challenge because of the variety of anatomic patterns, the complexity of intraarticular disruption, as well as associated injuries to the adjacent soft tissues, intrinsic and extrinsic carpal ligaments, carpal bones, and radioulnar ligaments. Fracture of the distal radius is the most common fracture of the upper extremity and has been estimated to account for more than one-sixth of all fractures treated in emergency rooms. Although the majority of such fractures, especially the stable extraarticular fractures, the minimally displaced intraarticular fractures, and fractures in the elderly osteoporotic patient, can be adequately treated with nonoperative measures (closed reduction and plaster immobilization), approximately 30% are more complex and will require surgical treatment in order to guarantee a successful functional outcome. Failure to recognize the potentially unstable fractures, the patterns of intraarticular disruption, as well as the associated distal radioulnar joint (DRUJ) and intercarpal ligamentous disruption will lead to painful sequelae soon after the fracture has healed.

In the past decade, there has been an overwhelming evolution and a high degree of sophistication in the diagnosis, evaluation, and treatment concepts concerning distal radius fractures. These include the application of special imaging techniques, arthroscopic assisted reduction, modern plate design adapted for the distal radius, dynamic external fixation, and, more recently, the use of bone substitutes as an alternative to bone-grafting techniques. Because of this substantial increase of different treatment modalities, and because a successful outcome in fracture treatment begins with the recognition of the fracture type and associated soft tissue injuries, there is an urgent need to provide the attending surgeon with a practical and modern distal radius fracture classification. For a classification to be practical, it must provide (a) a reproducible diagnosis (high degree of intraobserver and interobserver reliability), (b) prognostic considerations, (c) account for associated soft tissue lesions, and (d) recommend treatment options.

Furthermore, it should serve as a discriminator for management modalities and outcome expectations.

CLASSIFICATION OF FRACTURES OF THE DISTAL RADIUS

Historical Review

Between 1783 and 1847, most of the fracture types that occurred at the distal end of the radius were recognized on the basis of clinical and postmortem observation. The extraarticular fractures with dorsal or backward displacement were described by Pouteau (1) in 1783 and Colles (2) in 1814. The first description of an extraarticular fracture with anterior or volar displacement was reported by Goyrand (3) in 1832 and later by Smith (4) in 1847. In 1838, both Barton (5) and Letenneur (6) described dorsal and palmar marginal shearing fractures of the joint surface, and Dupuytren (7), in 1839, stressed the point that most wrist injuries were actually fractures of the distal radius and not wrist dislocations. Voillemier (8), a contemporary of Dupuytren, is credited with providing the first case report of a complete dorsal radiocarpal dislocation in 1839.

The recognition of fractures that involve the joint surface was a product of the turn of the nineteenth century, and a more accurate analysis of the intraarticular involvement came with the advent of radiology. However, it is of interest to observe descriptions of compression or impaction-type fractures dating back as early as 1842, when Voillemier mentioned such a fracture in a postmortem examination of a patient who died 4 hours following a fall from a three-story house (8). Publications by Callender (9)

D. L. Fernandez: Department of Orthopaedic Surgery, Lindenhof Hospital, and University of Berne, CH-3012 Berne, Switzerland.

C. J. Martin: Department of Medical Services, Commission of Health and Occupational Safety, Montreal, Quebec, Canada H3C 4E1.

and Cotton (10) soon followed. The latter identified, in 1900, many of the contemporary intraarticular fracture patterns from specimens at the Massachusetts General Hospital. In 1910, Harold C. Edwards (11) reported the mechanism of injury of the fracture of the radial styloid that held the eponym of Chauffeur's or backfire fracture. The lunate load, die punch, or medial cuneiform fracture of the joint surface was originally reported by Rutherford in 1891 and by Cotton in 1900 (10), and Scheck (12) in 1962 coined the term "die punch" to distinguish the fracture that results from impaction of the lunate against the posteromedial aspect of the radius.

Because of the accuracy and richness of these original descriptions, authors' names continue to identify a particular pattern of fracture of the distal radius. These fracture eponyms are routinely used in daily clinical practice. Although this may render communication easy between treating physicians, it may not be effective in analyzing the individual characteristics of specific fracture patterns, especially when dealing with the more complex type of intraarticular fractures. On the other hand, if an eponym is accurately applied with a direct correlation to the radiographic diagnosis, we believe that it may as well continue to be used. The problem arises when intraarticular disruption is misdiagnosed, such as in a minimally displaced die punch fragment, and the fracture is documented as a "simple Colles' fracture." For this reason, contemporary investigators have purposely avoided eponyms and, instead, have grouped fractures numerically or alphabetically based on a wide spectrum of fracture classification parameters.

We divide the classification systems into historical and contemporary. Although most of the classification systems developed and used in the first half of this century are no longer in daily use, we would like to enumerate some of the efforts of our predecessors because these prior classifications have, with no doubt, influenced contemporary authors.

Historical Classifications

As pointed out by Lindström (13), distal radius fracture classifications were based on (a) the fracture line, (b) the direction of displacement of the distal fragment, (c) the degree of displacement, (d) the extent of articular involvement, and (e) any involvement of the DRUJ.

In 1925, Destot (14) differentiated between fractures displaced anteriorly and posteriorly; the direction of the fracture line was then defined within these two main groups. In 1938, Taylor and Parsons (15) also classified these fractures into two main groups; however, considerable interest was given to associated injuries of the triangular fibrocartilage.

The classification systems of Nissen-Lie in 1939 (16) and Gartland and Werley in 1951 (17) were based on the presence or absence of an extra- or intraarticular component, angular deformity, and metaphyseal comminution. Both classifications lacked a grading system to establish the amount of fracture displacement. In 1959, Lindström (13) expanded this criterion, providing six groups to identify the direction of displacement as well as the nature of the articular involvement. Older et al., in 1965, (18) graded the fractures according to the amount of dorsal angulation, extent of comminution, direction and extent of displacement, as well as the presence of shortening of the distal fragment in relation to the distal ulna. Radial shortening has subsequently been considered an important prognostic feature regarding the final functional outcome. Finally, in 1967, Frykman (19) established a classification that incorporated individual involvement of the radiocarpal and radioulnar joints as well as the presence or absence of a frac-

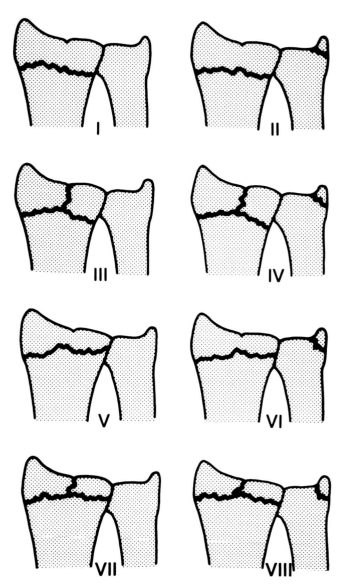

FIGURE 18.1. Frykman classification: type I, extraarticular; type II, a type I with fracture of distal ulna; type III, the radiocarpal joint involved; type IV, a type III with fracture of distal ulna; type V, distal radioulnar joint is involved; type VI, a type V with fracture of distal ulna; type VII, radiocarpal and radioulnar joints are both involved; type VIII, type VII with fracture of distal ulna.

ture of the ulnar styloid process (Fig. 18.1). Although this classification gained universal popularity and was frequently utilized in the literature, it does not reflect initial fracture displacement, the degree of comminution, or shortening of the distal fragment.

It is of interest to state that all the above-mentioned classification systems concentrated on the Colles' type of dorsal displacement fractures and did not include partial articular fractures, radiocarpal fracture-dislocations, or volarly displaced fractures. In 1957, Thomas (20) subclassified the Goyrand-Smith fracture family with palmar displacement into three fracture types: type 1, transverse extraarticular fracture; type 2, an intraarticular, marginal, volarly and proximally displaced fragment; and type 3, oblique, extraarticular palmarly displaced distal radius fracture.

Although all these classifications were published in the Anglo-Saxon literature, a very detailed classification, with an accurate description of both the dorsally displaced and palmarly displaced extra- and intraarticular fractures, was provided by Castaing and Le Club des Dix in 1964 (21). This classification was supported by a French multicenter study of 440 fractures with complete documentation and was the first, to our knowledge, to provide treatment recommendations based on the outcome study of the results (Table 18.1). The authors further included associated osteoarticular and ligamentous injuries and even provided a type 4 "nonclassifiable" fracture type for the rare injuries, usually high velocity, that would not fit into the suggested two main types of compression and extension fractures with posterior displacement, and compression and flexion fractures with anterior displacement.

Contemporary Classifications

Deciding what constitutes a contemporary classification versus a historical one can sometimes be quite difficult, but the search for a more representative and accurate classification system has been the subject of numerous investigations (18,21–31) since the advent of the Frykman classification.

These contemporary classifications are dealt with here in chronological order; this by no means reflects their importance and/or lack of it within the classification hierarchy.

Sarmiento Classification (1975)

This classification system, initially reported in 1962 (28) and later revised and modified in 1975 (32), was based on the radiologic appearance and displacement type of the fracture (Table 18.2). Its most distinguishing feature was that it took into account the involvement or, more importantly, the noninvolvement of the radiocarpal joint. With our expanding knowledge base of kinematics of the radiocarpal joint and our additional recognition of patterns of injury to the radiocarpal ligaments with distal radial fractures, this was one of the first "contemporary" classifications to point this out.

Melone Classification (1984)

This classification system, initially reported in 1984 (33) and later revised (22), was based on articular joint surface involvement of the distal radius. Four major components were described by Melone: (a) the shaft, (b) the radial styloid, (c) the dorsal medial fragment, and (d) the volar medial fragment. Although the initial classification had four types based on the number of articular parts a particu-

TABLE 18.1. CLASSIFICATION OF CASTAING AND LE CLUB DES DIX

Type 1	Compression–extension (posterior displacement)
	Pouteau, Colles
	With posteromedial fragment complex
	a. Sagittal T
	b. With medial component
	c. With lateral component
	d. Posterolateral rim isolated or complex
	e. Frontal T
	f. Cross lines in two planes
	g. Comminuted
	h. Undisplaced
Type 2	Compression–flexion
	Goyrand-Smith
	Anterior rim isolated or anterolateral
	Complex anterior rim
Type 3	Associated osteoarticular injuries
	Ulnar styloid
	Ulnar head
	Ulnar neck
	Radioulnar dislocation
	Radioulnar diastasis
	Carpal injuries
	Other injuries of the upper limb
	Open fracture
	Bilateral
Type 4	Nonclassifiable

From Castaing J. Les fractures récentes de l'extrémité inférieure du radius chez l'adulte. *Rev Chir Orthop* 1964;5:581–696, with permission.

TABLE 18.2. SARMIENTO ET AL. CLASSIFICATION

Group	Characteristics
1	Nondisplaced fractures without radiocarpal joint involvement
2	Displaced fractures without radiocarpal joint involvement
3	Nondisplaced fractures with radiocarpal joint involvement
4	Displaced fractures with radiocarpal joint involvement

Modified from Sarmiento A, Pratt GN, Berry NC, Sinclair WF. Colles' fractures: functional bracing in supination. *J Bone Joint Surg Am* 1975;57:311–317, with permission.

lar fracture had, much like the proximal humerus and the proximal femur, an additional fifth type was introduced in 1993 to incorporate a type of fracture that was extremely comminuted, unstable, and without any large identifiable facet fragments (Fig. 18.2). The extent of separation and displacement of the articular fragments served as the basis for the classification system as well as a prognostic view of the fracture type's reducibility and intrinsic stability. This classification system also brought attention to the medial complex (medial or lunate facet) and its overall importance in functional outcome.

Jenkins Classification (1989)

In an article reviewing prior classifications (26), Jenkins added his own, this one based on the presence, extent, and location of comminution of the fracture (Fig. 18.3). The point emphasized, according to this classification, continued to be the relationship of comminution to the intrinsic stability of a particular fracture following manipulative reduction. In other words, the more comminution the more unstable the fracture was thought to be after reduction.

AO Comprehensive Classification of Fractures (1986, 1990, 1995)

In 1986, the Swiss Association for the Study of Internal Fixation (AO) accepted a new classification system that would make its appearance coincident with the Congress of the International Society of Orthopaedic Surgery (SICOT) in Munich in 1987 (34). The historical aspects of this classification system are well documented and discussed in the preface to the French edition written by Professor Maurice E. Müller. *The Comprehensive Classification of Fractures of Long Bones,* or the AO classification, as it has

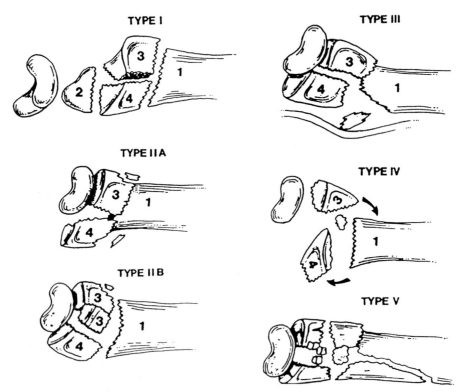

FIGURE 18.2. Melone classification of intraarticular fracture: type I, stable fracture, nondisplaced or variable displacement of the medial complex as a unit, no comminution, stable after closed reduction; type II, unstable "die punch," moderate or severe displacement of the medial complex as a unit with comminution of both anterior and posterior cortices, separation of the medial complex from the styloid fragment, radial shortening more than 5–10 mm, considerable angulation usually exceeding 20° (IIa, reducible; IIb, irreducible); type III, "spike" fracture, unstable, displacement of the medial complex as a unit as well as displacement of an additional spike fragment from the comminuted radial shaft; type IV, split fracture, unstable, medial complex severely comminuted with wide separation and/or rotation of the distal and palmar fragments; type V, explosion injuries. (From Melone CP. Distal radius fracture: patterns of articular fragmentation. *Orthop Clin North Am* 1993;24:239–253, with permission.)

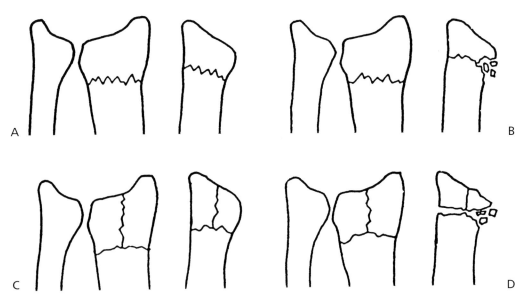

FIGURE 18.3. Jenkins classification based entirely on comminution. **A:** Group 1, no radiographically visible comminution. **B:** Group 2, comminution of the dorsal radial cortex without comminution of the distal fragment. **C:** Group 3, comminution of the fracture fragment without significant involvement of the dorsal cortex. **D:** Group 4, comminution of both the distal fragment and the dorsal cortex. Because the fracture line involves the distal fracture fragments in groups 3 and 4, intraarticular involvement is very common within these groups. Such involvement is not, however, inevitable, nor does it affect the fracture's placement within the classification. (From Jenkins NH. The unstable Colles' fracture. *J Hand Surg [Br]* 1989;14:149–154, with permission.)

come to be recognized and called, was further revised in 1990 (24). This classification system considers the severity of the bone lesion and serves as a basis for treatment and for evaluation of results. In order to classify a fracture in this system, one must determine its morphologic characteristics and its location. The characterization of the morphology of the fracture, that is, the bone lesion, is based on the fact that fractures of all bone segments can be classified into three types, which are subsequently divided into three groups and further subdivided into three subgroups (Fig. 18.4). The three basic types are type A, extraarticular; type B, partial articular; and type C, complete articular. The three groups are organized in order of increasing severity based on the morphologic complexity, the difficulty of treatment, and their prognosis. Therefore, three basic types (A, B, and C), nine main groups (A1, A2, A3, B1, B2, B3, C1, C2, C3), and 27 subgroups (1, 2, and 3) can be identified. If a fracture cannot be assigned to any of the groups, it is placed in a separate group. This corresponds to a D1 type. Documentation of additional ulnar lesions (Fig. 18.5) will produce over 144 possible combinations of distal radial fractures.

This is by far the most detailed classification system to date. However, its reproducibility for both intra- and interobserver reliability have proved to be a problem when the groups and subgroups were evaluated (35–38).

Because of these difficulties in making three choices (type, group, and subgroup), a simplified binary system of questions was developed by M. E. Müller in 1995 (39). This was intended to lead the observer down a logical path of questioning in order to accurately classify the fracture pattern.

The proposed questioning begins by asking whether the fracture is extra- or intraarticular. This would differentiate between type A and B fractures. The next question would be that if the fracture is intraarticular, whether it is partial or complete. This would differentiate between the B type and C type. Further classification for various groups is determined by asking questions about the direction of the fracture line: sagittal (group 1), frontal and dorsal (group 2), or frontal and volar (group 3). It may not be possible to determine all the fracture lines based on standard radiographs; the addition of other projections, standard tomography, or computed tomography may be required. Observations made at the time of surgery may also be required to complete the classification, especially when there is radioulnar joint involvement.

Although this system appears complicated at first, it is structured in such a way that it can be entered directly into a computer for documentation and later analysis, thereby providing a useful tool for multicenter outcome studies.

A1 Extraarticular fracture of the ulna, radius intact

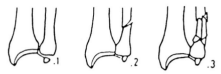

1. styloid process
2. metaphyseal simple
3. metaphyseal multifragmentary

A2 Extraarticular fracture of the radius, simple and impacted

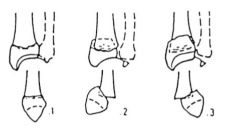

1. without any tilt
2. with dorsal tilt (Pouteau-Colles)
3. with volar tilt (Goyran-Smith)

A3 Extraarticular fracture of the radius, multifragmentary

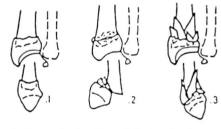

1. impacted with axial shortening
2. with a wedge
3. complex

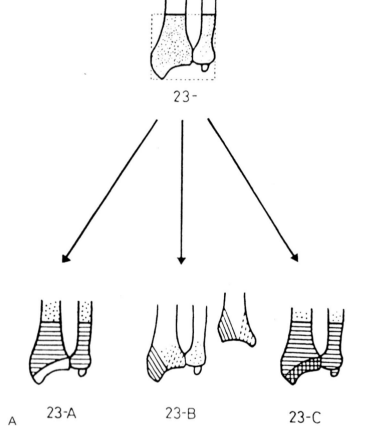

FIGURE 18.4. The comprehensive classification of fractures (AO/ASIF). **A:** Each bone and segment of the individual bone is given a number: the forearm is coded 2, its distal segment 3. The three basic groups are illustrated alone. **B:** Type A, extraarticular fracture.

B1 Partial articular fracture of the radius, sagittal

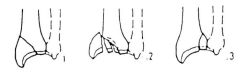

1 lateral simple
2 lateral multifragmentary
3 medial

B2 Partial articular fracture of the radius, dorsal rim (Barton)

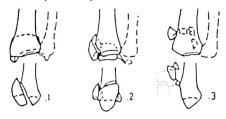

1 simple
2 with lateral sagittal fracture
3 with dorsal dislocation of the carpus

B3 Partial articular fracture of the radius, volar rim (reverse Barton, Goyrand-Smith II)

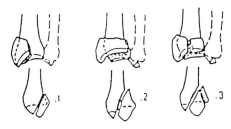

1 simple, with a small fragment
2 simple, with a large fragment
3 multifragmentary

C1 Complete articular fracture of the radius, articular simple, metaphyseal simple

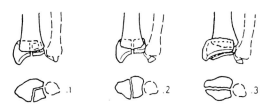

1 postero-medial articular fragment
2 sagittal articular fracture line
3 frontal articular fracture line

C2 Complete articular fracture of the radius, articular simple, metaphyseal multifragmentary

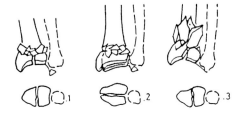

1 sagittal articular fracture line
2 frontal articular fracture line
3 extending into the diaphysis

C3 Complete articular fracture of the radius, multifragmentary

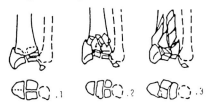

1 metaphyseal simple
2 metaphyseal multifragmentary
3 extending into the diaphysis

FIGURE 18.4. (continued) C: Type B, partial articular fracture. D: Type C, complete articular fracture. In **B–D**, the distal radius is shown in the anatomic position. The reader is looking at the palmar surface in the anteroposterior views and at the radial border of the forearm in the lateral views so that dorsal is to the left and palmar is to the right. Type A, extraarticular fractures affect neither the articular surface nor the radioulnar joints. Type B, simple articular fracture affects a portion of the surface, but the continuity of the metaphysis and epiphysis is intact. Type C, complex articular fracture affects the joint surfaces (radioulnar and/or radiocarpal) and the metaphyseal area. (From Fernandez DL, Jupiter JB. *Fractures of the distal radius. A practical approach to management.* New York: Springer-Verlag, 1995, with permission.)

Mathoulin, Letrosne, and Saffar Classification (1989)

Saffar suggested that distal radius injuries were becoming more prevalent in younger and more active adults, probably in part because of increasing sporting activities and high-velocity trauma. He proposed an additional classification system (Table 18.3) to provide both therapeutic options and prognosis as well as to prevent redisplacement and malunions (40).

Rayhack's Classification (1990): Universal Classification

This additional classification system further emphasized prognostic aspects of the different fracture groupings. Rayhack (41) believed that although the Frykman classification could be considered beneficial because the majority of surgeons were familiar with it, it also had weaknesses in that it did not make a distinction between displaced and nondis-

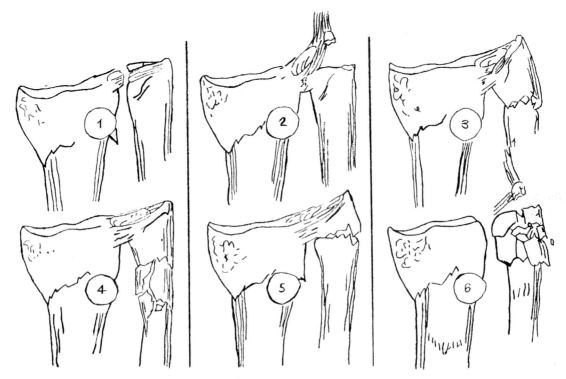

FIGURE 18.5. *1,* Tear of the triangular fibrocartilage and/or distal radioulnar ligaments; *2,* fracture of the ulnar styloid and/or distal radioulnar ligaments; *3,* fracture of the neck of the ulna; *4,* metaphyseal multifragmented fracture of the ulna; *5,* fracture through the ulnar head; *6,* multifragmented articular fracture of the distal ulna. (From Fernandez DL, Jupiter JB. *Fractures of the distal radius. A practical approach to management.* New York: Springer-Verlag, 1995, with permission.)

placed intraarticular fractures, for which treatment modalities vary widely.

Therefore, this classification differentiates extra- and intraarticular fractures, displaced and nondisplaced fractures, and the reducibility and stability of individual fracture patterns (Table 18.4).

TABLE 18.3. MATHOULIN, LETROSNE, AND SAFFAR CLASSIFICATION

Type	Characteristics
1	One articular line in the coronal plane Barton, reverse Barton
2	One articular line in the sagittal plane involving the scaphoid facet the lunate facet the radioulnar joint
3	Two lines associated: one extraarticular horizontal one intraarticular = type 2a,b + other fragments or dorsal comminution (T fractures, die punch)
4	Three lines associated: one extraarticular horizontal two articular, one coronal, one sagittal (posteromedial fragments—T frontal and sagittal)

Modified from Mathoulin CH, Letrosne E, Saffar PH. Classification of intraarticular fractures of the distal radius. In: Saffar PM, Cooney WP, eds. *Fractures of the Distal Radius.* London: Martin Dunitz, 1995;126–130, with permission.

The simplicity of this system is very attractive to guide the surgeon in the course of management. This classification was further modified by Cooney in 1993 (23).

McMurtry and Jupiter Classification (1991)

The relative importance of this classification based on articular joint surface involvement (27) was that it added measured parameters (i.e., amount of displacement in millimeters of an articular part) and recommended various treatment modalities based on a set amount of "acceptable" displacement (Fig. 18.6).

TABLE 18.4. PROPOSED RAYHACK CLASSIFICATION OF DISTAL RADIUS FRACTURES

I.	Nonarticular	Nondisplaced
II.	Nonarticular	Displaced
	A. Reducible[a]	Stable
	B. Reducible[a]	Unstable
	C. Irreducible[a]	
III.	Articular	Nondisplaced
IV.	Articular	Displaced
	A. Reducible[a]	Stable
	B. Reducible[a]	Unstable
	C. Irreducible[a]	

[a]By ligamentotaxis only.
From Rayhack JM. Symposium on distal radius fractures. *Contemp Orthop* 1990;21:71–104, with permission.

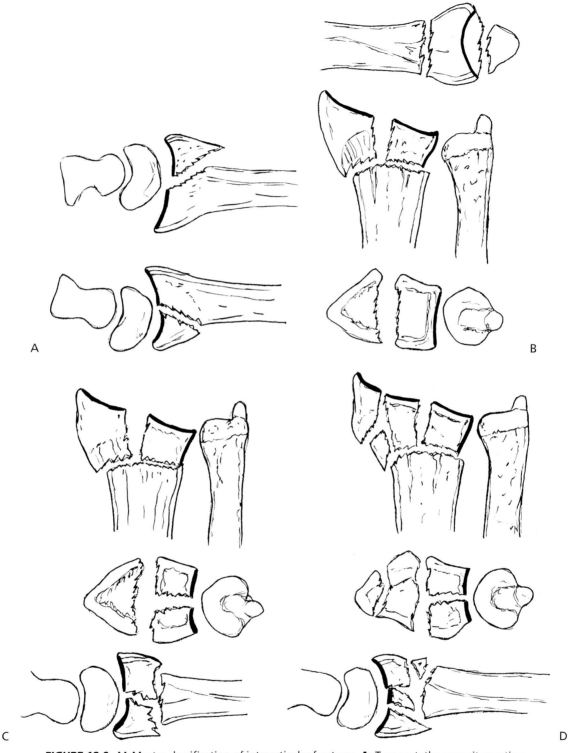

FIGURE 18.6. McMurtry classification of intraarticular fractures. **A:** Two-part: the opposite portion of the radiocarpal joint remains intact. **B:** Three-part: the lunate and scaphoid facets of the distal radius separate from each other and from the proximal portion of the radius. **C:** Four-part: similar to the three-part except that the lunate facet is further divided into volar and dorsal fragments. **D:** Five-part: includes a wide variety of comminuted fragments. (Redrawn from McMurtry RY, Jupiter JB. Fractures of the distal radius. In: Browner B, Jupiter JB, Levine A, et al., eds. *Skeletal trauma*. Philadelphia: WB Saunders, 1991;1063–1094, with permission.)

Mayo Clinic Classification (1992)

The classification system presently used at the Mayo Clinic (42) resembles the one proposed by Rayhack except for a slightly different classification of the location of the articular disruption. This classification system emphasizes the role of specific articular contact areas and was formulated to include specific articular surfaces of the distal radius (Fig. 18.7).

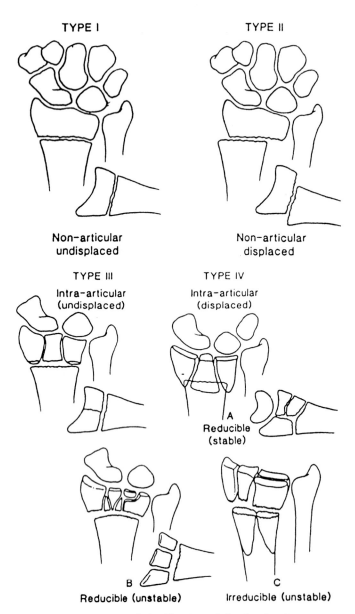

FIGURE 18.7. Universal classification of distal radius fractures as proposed by Cooney et al.: type I, nonarticular, undisplaced; type II, nonarticular, displaced; type III, intraarticular, undisplaced; type IVA, intraarticular, displaced, reducible, stable; type IVB, intraarticular, displaced, reducible, unstable; type IVC, intraarticular, irreducible; type IVD, complex (not illustrated). (From Cooney WP, Agee JM, Hasting H, et al. Symposium: Management of intra-articular fractures of the distal radius. *Contemp Orthop* 1990;21:71–184, with permission.)

The goal was primarily to call attention to the intraarticular components that require treatment beyond the fracture, involving the distal radial metaphysis and radial shaft. Similar to the Rayhack classification, the concepts of stability and/or reducibility are also included.

Fernandez Classification (1993)

One of us (D.L.F.) became interested in classifying fractures of the distal radius according to the mechanism of injury (29,43). It was assumed that a better understanding of the mechanism of injury would provide a better overall assessment of the injury, the associated potential soft tissue damage (tendon, ligament, nerve, vessels), and a better algorithm for treatment modalities and recommendations. This classification system includes the fracture equivalent in children, the degree of stability, and the patterns of articular fragmentation, if present. The fractures are classified in five main types: type I, bending fractures of the metaphysis; type II, shearing fractures of the joint surface; type III, compression fractures of the joint surface; type IV, avulsion fractures or radiocarpal fracture-dislocations; and type V, which are combined fractures associated with high-velocity injuries (Table 18.5).

This fracture classification also provides prognostic information because the complexity of the bone lesion and the probability of associated soft tissue disruption increase consistently from type I through type V fractures.

This classification also provides a separate grouping of the possible associated DRUJ lesions (44) (Table 18.6). Associated DRUJ lesions deserve as much attention as the fracture of the distal radius itself with regard to evaluation, documentation, and initial treatment because one of the most common causes of disability after the fracture has healed is posttraumatic derangement of the radioulnar articulation.

The various DRUJ lesions are placed in three possible categories after the distal radius fracture has been adequately reduced and stabilized. This is based on the residual stability of the DRUJ following anatomic reduction of the sigmoid notch to the ulnar head: type I lesions involve either an avulsion fracture of the tip of the ulnar styloid or a stable fracture at the ulnar neck, representing the likelihood of the DRUJ being congruous and stable following reduction of the radius. Type II lesions represent an unstable injury with subluxation or dislocation of the ulnar head involving either a substance tear of the triangular fibrocartilage complex or palmar and dorsal capsular ligament, or an avulsion fracture of the base of the ulnar styloid. Type III lesions represent potentially unstable injuries involving either extraarticular fracture of the sigmoid notch or an extraarticular fracture of the ulnar head.

Attempts are now being made to provide the user with the possibility of computer documentation and retrieval for analysis. To use a clinical example, a simple reversed Barton type of fracture associated with a fracture of the tip of the ulnar styloid is classified as a type II, unstable, volarly displaced fracture with two fragments. In numeric and alpha-

TABLE 18.5. FERNANDEZ CLASSIFICATION OF FRACTURES OF THE RADIUS

Fracture Types (Adults) Based on the Mechanism of Injury	Fracture Equivalent in Children	Stability/Instability: High Risk of Secondary Displacement after Initial Adequate Reduction	Displacement Pattern	Number of Fragments	Associated Lesions: Carpal Ligament Fractures, Median, Ulnar Nerve, Tendons, Ipsilateral Upper Extremity Fractures, Compartment Syndrome	Recommended Treatment
Type I: bending fracture of the metaphysis	Distal forearm fracture	Stable	Nondisplaced, dorsally Colles, volarly Smith proximal combined	Always two main fragments +	Uncommon	Conservative (stable fractures)
	Salter II	Unstable		Varying degree of metaphyseal comminution (instability)		Percutaneous pinning (extra- or intrafocal) External fixation (exceptionally bone graft)
Type II: shearing fracture of the joint surface	Salter IV	Unstable	Dorsal Barton Radial Chauffeur Volar reverse Barton Combined	Two-part Three-part Comminuted	Less uncommon	Open reduction Screwplate fixation
Type III: compression fracture of the joint surface	Salter III, IV, V	Stable Unstable	Nondisplaced Dorsal Radial Volar Proximal Combined	Two-part Three-part Four-part Comminuted	Common	Conservative Closed, limited, arthroscopic-assisted or extensile open Percutaneous pins, External fixation, Internal fixation plate, bone graft
Type IV: avulsion fractures, radiocarpal fracture-dislocation	Very rare	Unstable	Dorsal Radial Volar Proximal Combined	Two-part (radial styloid, ulnar styloid) Three-part (volar, dorsal margin) Comminuted	Frequent	Closed or open reduction Pin or screw fixation Tension wiring
Type V: Combined fractures (I–II–III–IV), high-velocity injury	Very rare	Unstable	Dorsal Radial Volar Proximal Combined	Comminuted and/or bone loss (frequently intraarticular, open, seldom extraarticular)	Always present	Combined method

TABLE 18.6. FERNANDEZ CLASSIFICATION OF DISTAL RADIOULNAR JOINT LESIONS

	Pathoanatomy of the Lesion	Joint Surface Involvement	Prognosis	Recommended Treatment
Type I: stable (following reduction of the radius, the DRUJ is congruous and stable)	A: Fracture tip ulnar styloid B: Stable fracture ulnar neck	None	Good	A,B: Functional after treatment; encourage early pronation–supination excercises Note: Extraaarticular unstable fractures of the ulna at the metaphyseal level or distal shaft require stable plate fixation
Type II: unstable (subluxation or dislocation of the ulnar head is present)	A: Tear of triangular fibrocartilage complex and/or palmar and dorsal capsular ligaments B: Avulsion fracture base of the ulnar styloid	None	Chronic instability Painful limitation of supination if left unreduced Possible late arthritic changes	A: Closed treatment reduce subluxation, sugar tong splint in 45° supination 4 to 6 weeks A,B: Operative treatment: repair triangular fibro-cartilage complex or fix ulnar styloid with tension band wiring; immobilize wrist and elbow in supination (cast) or transfix ulna/radius with K-wire and forearm cast
Type III: potentially unstable (subluxation possible)	A: Intraarticular fracture of the sigmoid notch B: Intraarticular fracture of the ulnar head	Present	Dorsal subluxation possible together with dorsally displaced die punch or dorso-ulnar fragment Risk of early degenerative changes and severe limitation of forearm rotation if left unreduced	A: Anatomic reduction of palmar and dorsal sigmoid notch fragments; if residual subluxation tendency is present, immobilize as in type II injury B: Functional after treatment to enhance remodeling of ulnar head; if DRUJ remains painful, partial ulnar resection, darrach or Sauvé-Kapandji procedure at a later date

DRUJ, distal radioulnar joint.

betical code terms, this would make it an RIIV2P-UIA, where *R* is radius, *II* means type II (shearing), *V* indicates volar displacement pattern, *2P* means two-part (number of articular fragments), and *U* refers to DRUJ lesions (O; IA, IB; IIA, IIB; IIIA, IIIB) (Table 18.6). Additional soft tissue lesions (skin, tendons, nerves, and vessels) are to be coded separately in written text as well as associated carpal injuries (ligaments, fractures). Ipsilateral injuries and fractures would also be included.

Similar to the AO Comprehensive Classification, we believe that all fractures of the distal radius can be included and classified according to this system, and that it is practical, and treatment-oriented. Unfortunately, to date, being a relatively new classification system, it has not had wide applications in the literature, nor has it been analyzed in studies regarding iets reproducibility, accuracy, and eventual usefulness.

NONOPERATIVE TREATMENT OF FRACTURES OF THE DISTAL RADIUS IN ADULTS

Reduction methods as well as immobilization techniques have many variations that depend on geographic and chronological factors, on individual preferences, and on potential risks and complications associated with one method or another. Faced with the many classification systems available in the literature, the physician dealing with these injuries to the distal radius in the emergency room, the outpatient clinic, or the office should use one that works for him or her from both clinical and scientific points of view. That is, the classification system should help guide the practitioner in decision making, treatment options, and prognosis.

Eponyms may be used as long as the eponym matches the fracture that corresponds to the x-ray and particular injury. Problems begin to arise when multicenter studies are instituted and various clinical results in the literature are compared. For this, a classification system with a high degree of intra- and interobserver reliability is warranted (35). The AO Comprehensive Classification has rated better than the McMurtry and Jupiter, the Mayo Clinic, and the Jakim classification as reported by Altissimi (45). In an additional study by Andersen et al. (37) evaluating the reliability of classification systems, including those of Melone, Frykman, Mayo, and the AO Comprehensive Classification system, only the Comprehensive System approached a statistically significant level. Its reproducibility was also confirmed in an additional study by Kreder et al. (38).

Closed Reduction Techniques

As with any other injuries or fractures of an extremity, the patient as a whole should be evaluated for associated injuries. Thereafter, factors related specifically to the injured distal radius, such as the patient's age, handedness, occupation, daily activity, level, and general medical condition, should be assessed. The fracture should be evaluated as to whether it is open or closed, whether or not vascular compromise is present, the degree of displacement, whether it is extra- or intraarticular, the amount of comminution, and also the neurologic status of the hand and upper extremity.

It also should be kept in mind that even in the hands of skilled physicians dealing with closed reduction techniques and cast immobilization, certain so-called unstable fractures cannot be predictably maintained with the use of splints or circular casts alone. Lafontaine, Hardy, and Delince (46) put forth five factors that could predict instability following fracture reduction: (a) initial dorsal angulation greater than 20°, (b) dorsal metaphyseal comminution, (c) intraarticular disruption, (d) associated ulnar fracture, and (e) patients over 60 years of age and/or those with massive osteoporosis. An additional parameter was put forth by Altissimi and associates (47) and related to the severity of initial radial shortening as the most reliable indication of instability.

Based on a large body of clinical and experimental evidence (48–53), the authors believe that an attempt at an anatomic reduction of a distal radius fracture is warranted. The ability to maintain such a reduction may require additional methods other than closed reduction techniques alone. The principle of reducing a distal radius fracture applies a force opposite to that which produced the injury. Colles' fracture types typically exhibit dorsal tilt, apex volar, shortening, and radial deviation as well as supination of the distal fragment. Smith fracture types exhibit the opposite, with palmar tilt, apex dorsal, pronation of the distal fragment, and varying degrees of radial shortening with respect to the ulna. Therefore, manual reduction techniques as advocated by Sir Robert Jones have been, at least in the author's hands, supplemented by techniques of Böhler (54,55), who advocated longitudinal traction followed by realignment procedures.

Authors' Preferred Method of Closed Reduction

Under sterile conditions, a hematoma block is performed through a dorsal approach. The fracture hematoma is evacuated, and the hematoma is replaced with 5 to 10 cc of 1% lidocaine (Xylocaine) without epinephrine (56). The anesthetic agent is allowed to settle in and diffuse around the fracture site. The patient is warned beforehand that he or she may experience median nerve symptoms such as numbness or paresthesia in that distribution. This method of anesthesia is applicable only to acute fractures. General anesthesia or axillary blocks may be required if the fracture is seen late or if significant soft tissue swelling is seen.

Manual Reduction

Colles' fractures are reduced by applying longitudinal traction, palmar flexion, ulnar deviation, and pronation. Restoration of skeletal length in overlapping fractures is easily obtained by increasing the initial deformity until one cortex engages (Fig. 18.8). This contact point is then used as a fulcrum to realign both fragments with flexion maneuvers. The principle of reduction is based on the application of tension to the soft tissue hinge (periosteum, overlying tendons) located on the concavity of the angulation. Conversely, Smith's fractures require dorsiflexion and supination of the wrist to obtain reduction.

Finger Trap Traction Reduction

With the hand in suspended finger trap traction attached to the thumb, index, and long fingers and countertraction applied to the flexed elbow (Fig. 18.9), thumb pressure is

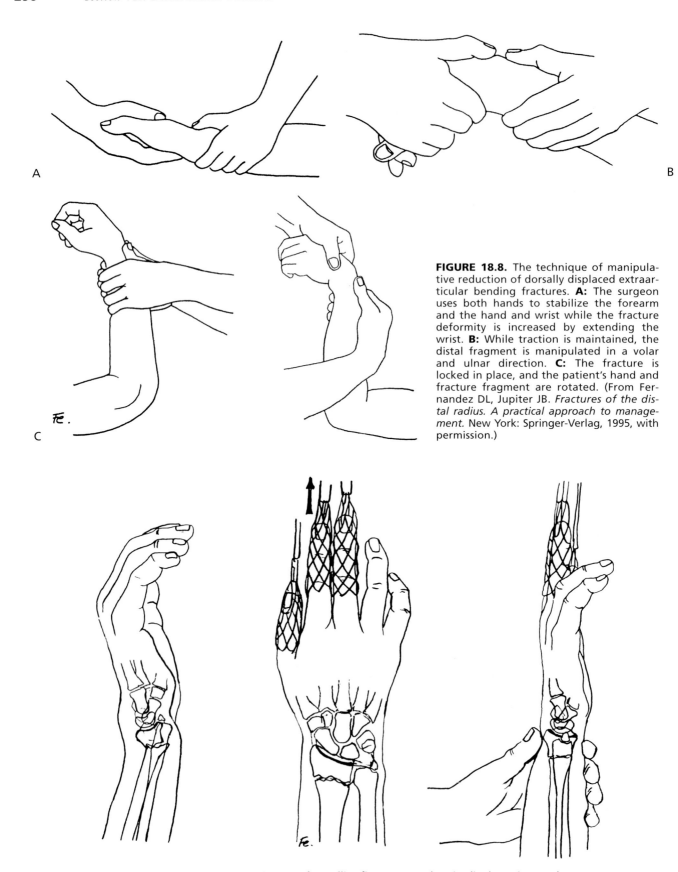

FIGURE 18.8. The technique of manipulative reduction of dorsally displaced extraarticular bending fractures. **A:** The surgeon uses both hands to stabilize the forearm and the hand and wrist while the fracture deformity is increased by extending the wrist. **B:** While traction is maintained, the distal fragment is manipulated in a volar and ulnar direction. **C:** The fracture is locked in place, and the patient's hand and fracture fragment are rotated. (From Fernandez DL, Jupiter JB. *Fractures of the distal radius. A practical approach to management.* New York: Springer-Verlag, 1995, with permission.)

FIGURE 18.9. Since the introduction of metallic "finger traps," longitudinal traction can be provided without the need for assistants. (From Fernandez DL, Jupiter JB. *Fractures of the distal radius. A practical approach to management.* New York: Springer-Verlag, 1995, with permission.)

applied by the treating physician to the distal fragment in a direction that will reduce the displacement.

Therefore, for displaced Colles' fractures, the distal fragment is manipulated with the treating physician's thumb into a flexed, palmarly translocated, and pronated position on the radial shaft. Agee (57) introduced the concept of multiplanar ligamentotaxis in which longitudinal traction is combined with palmar and also radioulnar translocation of the hand on the forearm (Fig. 18.10). Palmar translation creates a sagittal movement of forces that descends the capitate, which in turn rotates the lunate palmarly. This produces a rotatory force that efficiently tilts the distal radial fragment volarly. A similar observation was reported by Gupta in 1991 (58). Agee (57) further advocated radioulnar translation to realign the distal fragment with the radial shaft in the frontal plane. This is controlled by tension on the soft tissue hinge of the first and second dorsal compartment. For adequate reduction in the frontal plane, it is important to restore the anatomic relationship of the sigmoid notch and the ulnar head. The application of a dorsopalmar reduction force to restore volar tilt should be kept in mind because it offers better anatomic restoration with immobilization of the hand in the physiologic and functional position.

These principles of closed fracture reduction, again, apply only to reducible fractures. Impacted, severely displaced, and comminuted fractures that do not respond to ligamentotaxis require additional and supplementary forms of treatment modalities.

Preferred Position for Cast Immobilization

Despite the widespread acceptance of cast immobilization, questions remain regarding the optimal position, the duration of immobilization, and the need to extend the cast above the elbow. The authors favor a position of immobilization for a Colles' fracture that has a slight palmar flexion, ulnar deviation, and neutral forearm rotation (43–61) (Fig. 18.11). The Cotton-Loder position (10), which is the position of acute flexion, extreme pronation, and ulnar deviation, is avoided for fear of problems concerning median nerve compression and finger and wrist stiffness (62). Other distal radial fractures are immobilized accordingly to position the hand and wrist in a deviation opposite to the displacement that occurred in producing the injury. An x-ray is taken to evaluate the reduction obtained.

We prefer to immobilize all acute distal radial fractures in a sugar-tongs splint (61) (Fig. 18.12). This splint is usually applied while the upper extremity is suspended from finger trap traction following the reduction. As the splint sets, the fracture can be further manipulated into the appropriate position. The splint allows swelling to be handled without, one hopes, compromising proper reduction. As the swelling decreases, the splint can be tightened with a 4-in. Kling or Ace bandage (Fig. 18.13).

Neutral forearm rotation is favored except for extraarticular Smith fractures, where a pronation rotational deformity of the distal fragment is always present. Immobilization in extension and supination (45° to 60°) in either a sugar-tongs splint or long arm cast is mandatory for the first 4 weeks (Fig. 18.14).

Sarmiento et al. (32) have favored immobilization of all distal radial fractures with the forearm in supination, postulating that the brachioradialis was not a deforming force in this position, and also because it favors anatomic reduction of the DRUJ. This work has been questioned by Gibson et al. (63), and Sarmiento (32) stated that the method did not entirely prevent collapse of the fracture, especially in comminuted and articular fractures.

For a Colles' type of fracture, the sugar-tongs splint can be changed to a short arm cast or long arm cast at approximately 2 to 3 weeks, depending on the severity of the fracture and the physiology of the patient. The fracture immobilization with the sugar tongs or cast is carried out for approximately 4 to 6 weeks. Thereafter a protective removable

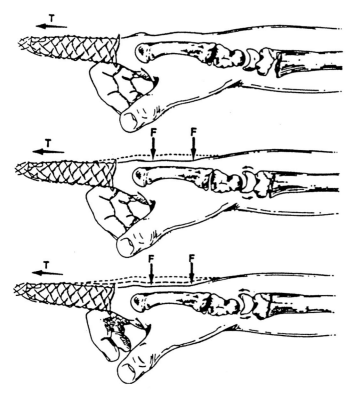

FIGURE 18.10. The longitudinal length can be restored by longitudinal traction. Palmar (volar) tilt of the distal radius articular surface can be obtained and maintained by a palmar translating force. Note that progressive palmar translation transmits this force through the carpus to the distal radius, hinging the distal fragment about the attached dorsal soft tissue hinge. *F,* palmar translation forces; *T,* traction. (From Agee JM. External fixation. Technical advances based upon multiplanar ligamentotaxis. *Orthop Clin North Am* 1993;24:265–274, with permission.)

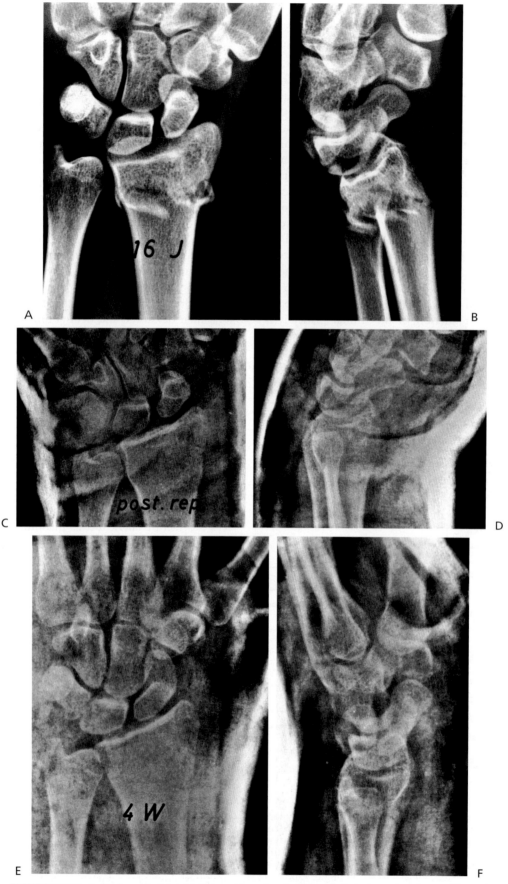

FIGURE 18.11. A displaced but "stable" dorsal bending fracture. **A,B:** Anteroposterior and lateral radiographs of the displaced fracture. Comminution involves only the dorsal cortex. **C,D:** The postreduction radiographs demonstrate an anatomic reduction. Also illustrated is our preferred position of immobilization, that is, slight palmar flexion with ulnar deviation. **E,F:** Control radiographs at 4 weeks postreduction. A well-molded cast has been applied. Note the dorsal molding.

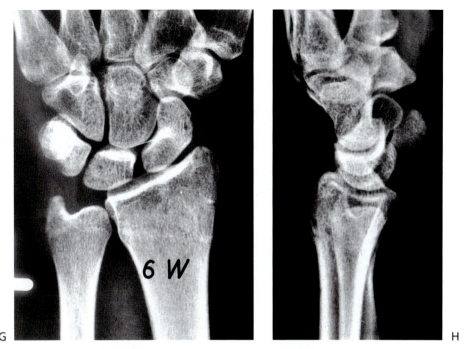

FIGURE 18.11. *(continued)* G,H: Fracture union and anatomic alignment seen at 6 weeks postreduction.

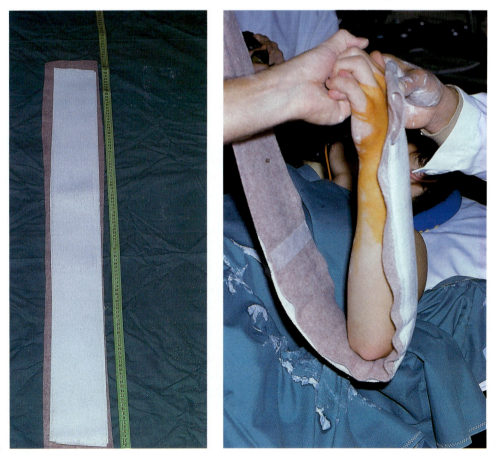

FIGURE 18.12. A: Sugar-tongs splint. **B:** Splint being applied; it is well padded for bony prominences.

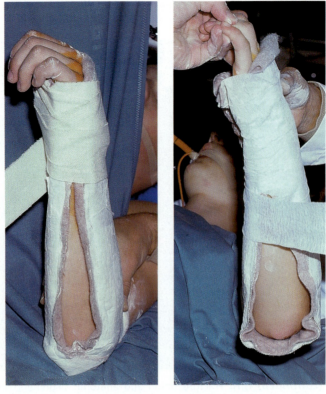

FIGURE 18.13. A,B: Sugar-tongs splint being wrapped with Ace bandage. Notice how posterior aspect of olecranon is free (to allow flexion–extension at the elbow).

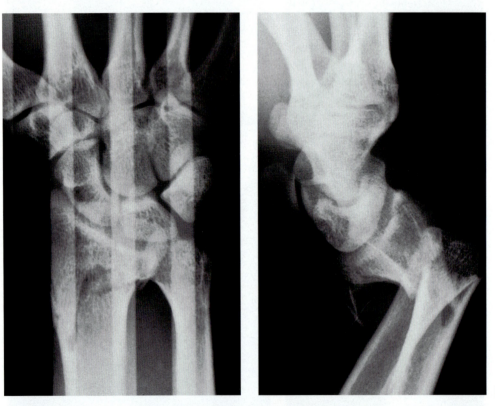

FIGURE 18.14. A displaced intraarticular "palmar bending" or Smith's fracture in a 35-year-old manual laborer. Today, many surgeons would opt for more aggressive modes of intervention, such as open reduction, internal fixation, percutaneous pinning, or external fixation. **A,B:** Anteroposterior and lateral radiographs of the palmarly displaced intraarticular fracture.

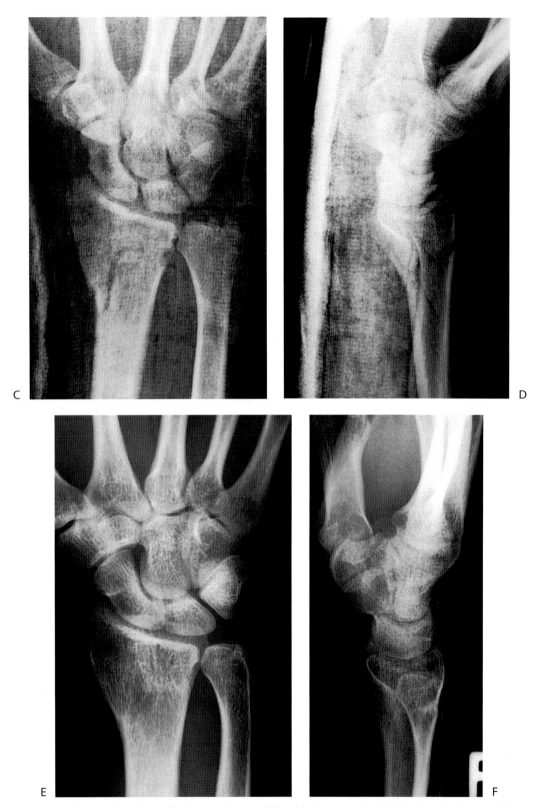

FIGURE 18.14. *(continued)* C,D: Under an axillary block, an anatomic closed reduction could be obtained and confirmed on AP and lateral radiographs. Initially a sugar-tongs splint was applied with the forearm in supination. At 7 days, this was converted to a long arm cast (5 weeks total). **E,F:** Anteroposterior and lateral radiographs at 1 year showing anatomic alignment. Excellent function and range of motion were obtained.

wrist orthosis is worn by the patient for an additional month while active range-of-motion exercises are begun. During that month the patient is progressively weaned from the brace.

During the period of immobilization and also during the period of weaning from the splint, all patients are instructed to keep their fingers mobile by performing the "six pack" exercises, as popularized by Dobyns (61), at least three times a day.

CONCLUSIONS

The desire to obtain and maintain an anatomic reduction of a distal radius fracture constitutes the main goal of treatment. This should not overshadow the fact that maximum mobilization of the surrounding joints should be allowed and that the method of immobilization that will maintain the reduction with a minimum of complications should be employed.

As was presented in this chapter, both historical and contemporary classifications have been proposed over the last 200 years.

A contemporary classification, in order to be useful for reporting and allowing comparative assessment of treatment methods between various groups should include the following characteristics: (a) location, (b) configuration, (c) displacement, (d) ulnar styloid integrity, (e) DRUJ integrity, (f) stability, (g) associated injuries (skin, muscle, tendon, nerve), and (h) management considerations.

By better defining and classifying these fractures, we hope that this will influence both treatment decisions and the evaluation of results. The increased functional expectations of the population at large, coupled with the enthusiasm for "outcome studies" along with the changing regulations of the delivery of health care, make this necessary.

EDITORS' COMMENTS

It would be a significant advantage if one could accurately classify a fracture by some means and then simply look up the exact surgical procedure and apply it to that classification. Unfortunately, no matter how detailed any classification system is, each articular fracture of the radius will have its own persona, and the surgeon's mindset is most important. Accurate anatomic realignment of the articular surface must be achieved. After hours of unsuccessful struggling to realign articular fragments, the surgeon does not have the privilege of saying, "There! That's good enough." Rather better to sit back or even leave the operating room momentarily, reestablish one's mindset that accurate articular alignment is mandatory. Those minutes in the operating room translate into thousands upon thousands of patient activity hours. In a documented experience, a surgeon in the middle of such a case said, "I'm not up to this today," closed the patient, and reoperated several days later—if necessary, an effective approach.

A nursing home patient with limited mental capacity can have his or her distal radius fracture immobilized and allowed to heal in almost any position without compromising functional capacity. A more important issue becomes a cosmetically acceptable forearm to the family. As one moves back from that almost functionless activity level to an elderly patient who lives alone, gardens, plays cards, and cares for her own apartment, one can accept several degrees of dorsiflexion of the distal articular surface. The problems in this type of patient are almost exclusively at the DRUJ. If the DRUJ is symptomatic, a matched ulnar arthroplasty is indicated, typically 3 to 6 months after fracture.

As we move along the spectrum from the elderly to the more active adult population with some sports activity or all the way to those with a full heavy load, athletics, and construction-type occupations, the distal radial articular surface requires some palmar tilt or at least no dorsal tilt. The radial carpal joint has predicted vectors. All loads will result in a volar-ulnar translation of the carpals, no matter the position of the wrist, and the majority of wrist ligaments are what we term "upslope" ligaments. They counter the normal volar-ulnar vector load and support the wrist from this displacement direction. As soon as there is 1° of dorsal tilt of the articular surface, these loads reverse themselves, and one must prevent the wrist from displacing dorsally. With only a degree or two of dorsal displacement, however, there is usually adequate ligament support, even under heavy loads because the articular surface is essentially perpendicular, even though on an absolute basis the wrist is tending to dorsal displacement under loading. Beginning at this position of essentially perpendicular articular surface of the radius, one can derive an equation multiplying the degrees of dorsal articular angulation by the activity level. As one goes up, the other must go down, or their equivalent will result in symptoms. This is a judgment call based on the surgeon's experience, but seldom will a normally loaded wrist including some limited golf or tennis tolerate more than 5° of dorsal articular tilt without symptoms.

There is a variability in elastic fiber content of ligaments between individuals. There are those in whom the metacarpophalangeal (MP) joints can not be hyperextended. Ligament tightness in these patients can compensate for torn ligaments or fracture malalignments.

Immobilization time for closed Colles' fracture is not to be taken lightly in the elderly. It is better to have a nonunion with supple joints without pericapsular fibrosis and permanent restriction than it is to guarantee fracture healing, accompanied by an unacceptable incidence of predystrophy, joint contractures, and functionally deficient wrists. Because of an inordinate number of stiff wrists, not to mention shoulders, elbows, and fingers, the immobilization time in a large New York clinic was cut to 4 weeks in all Colles' fractures. This produced a major reduction in postoperative joint problems, produced no nonunions, and has always been our standard immobilization time in the elderly with Colles' fractures.

REFERENCES

1. Pouteau C. *Oeuvres posthumes de M. Pouteau. Mémoire, contenant quelques réflexions sur quelques fractures de l'avant-bras sur les luxations incomplétes du poignet et sur le diastasis.* Paris: Ph-D Pirres, 1783.
2. Colles A. On the fracture of the carpal extremity of the radius. *Edinb Med Surg J* 1814;10:182–186.
3. Goyrand G. Mémoire sur les fractures de l'extrémité inférieure du radius qui simulant les luxations du poignet. *Gaz Med* 1832;3:664–667.
4. Smith RW. *A treatise on fracture in the vicinity of joints and on certain forms of accidental and congenital dislocations.* Dublin: Hodges and Smith, 1847.
5. Barton JR. Views and treatment of an important injury of the wrist. *Med Examiner* 1938;1:365–368.
6. Letenneur M. *Soc Anat Bull XIV,* 1838:162.
7. Dupuytren G. Des fractures de l'extrémité inférieure du radius simulant les luxations du poignet. In: *Lecons orales du Baron Dupuytren, tome 4.* Paris: Baillié, 1834;161–231.
8. Voillemier M. Histoire d'une luxation complète et récente du poignet en arrière suivit de réflexions sur le mécanisme de cette luxation. *Arch Gen Med* 1839;6:401–417.
9. Callender GW. Fractures injuring joints—fractures interfering with the movements at the wrist and with those of pronation and supination. *Saint Bartholomew's Hosp Rep* 1865;281–298.
10. Cotton FJ. The pathology of fractures of the lower end of the radius. *Ann Surg* 1900;32:194–218.
11. Edwards HC. The mechanism and treatment of backfire fracture. *J Bone Joint Surg Br* 1926;47:724–727.
12. Scheck M. Long term follow-up of treatment of comminuted fractures of the distal end of the radius by transfixation with Kirschner wires and cast. *J Bone Joint Surg Am* 1962;44:337–351.
13. Lindström A. Fractures of the distal radius. A clinical and statistical study of end results. *Acta Orthop Scand [Suppl]* 1959;41:1–95.
14. Destot E, ed. *Injuries of the wrist: a radiological study*. London: Ernest Benn, 1925. Atkinson FRB, translator.
15. Taylor GW, Parsons CL. The role of the discus articularis in Colles' fractures. *J Bone Joint Surg* 1938;20:149–152.
16. Nissen-Lie H. Fracture radic "typica." *Norske Mag* 1939;1:293–303.
17. Gartland JJ, Werley CW. Evaluation of healed Colles' fractures. *J Bone Joint Surg Am* 1951;33:895–907.
18. Older TM, Stabler EV, Cassebaum WH. Colles' fracture: Evaluation and selection of therapy. *J Trauma* 1965;5:469–476.
19. Frykman G. Fracture of the distal radius including sequelae—shoulder–hand–finger syndrome, disturbance in the distal radioulnar joint and impairment of nerve function. *Acta Orthop Scand [Suppl]* 1967;108:1–153.
20. Thomas FB. Reduction of Smith's fracture. *J Bone Joint Surg Br* 1957;39:463–470.
21. Castaing J. Les fractures récentes de l'extrémité inférieure du radius chex l'adulte. *Rev Chir Orthop* 1964;5:581–696.
22. Melone CP Jr. Distal radius fractures: Patterns of articular fragmentation. *Orthop Clin North Am* 1993;24:239–253.
23. Cooney WP. Fractures of the distal radius: A modern treatment-based classification. *Orthop Clin North Am* 1993;24:211–216.
24. Müller ME, Nazarian S, Koch P, et al, eds. *The comprehensive classification of fractures.* New York: Springer-Verlag, 1990;54–63.
25. Jupiter JB. Current concepts review: Fractures of the distal end of the radius. *J Bone Joint Surg Am* 1991;73:461–467.
26. Jenkins NH. The unstable Colles' fracture. *J Hand Surg [Br]* 1989;14:149–154.
27. McMurtry RY, Jupiter JB. Fractures of the distal radius. In: Browner B, Jupiter J, Levine A, et al, eds. *Skeletal trauma.* Philadelphia: WB Saunders, 1991;1063–1094.
28. Sarmiento A, Pratt GW, Berry NC, et al. Colles's fracture: Functional bracing in supination. *J Bone Joint Surg Am* 1962;44:337–351.
29. Fernandez DL. Fractures of the distal radius. Operative treatment. *AAOS Instruct Course Lect* 1993;42:73–88.
30. Bradway JK, Amadio PC, Cooney WP. Open reduction and internal fixation of displaced, comminuted intra-articular fractures of the distal end of the radius. *J Bone Joint Surg Am* 1989;71:839–847.
31. Saffar PH. Current trends in treatment and classification of distal radius fractures. In: Saffar PH, Cooney WP, eds. *Fractures of the distal radius.* London: Martin Dunitz, 1995;12–18.
32. Sarmiento A, Pratt GW, Berry NC, et al. Colles' fractures: Functional bracing in supination. *J Bone Joint Surg Am* 1975;57:311–317.
33. Melone CP Jr. Articular fractures of the distal radius. *Orthop Clin North Am* 1984;15:217–236.
34. Müller ME, Nazarian S, Koch P, eds. *Klassifikation AO der Frakturen.* Berlin: Springer-Verlag, 1987.
35. Burstein AH. Editorial: Fracture classification systems: Do they work and are they useful? *J Bone Joint Surg Am* 1993;75:1743–1744.
36. Andersen GR, Rasmussen JB, Dahl B, Solgaard S. Older's classification of Colles' fractures: Good intraobserver and interobserver reproducibility in 185 cases. *Acta Orthop Scand* 1991;62:463–464.
37. Andersen DJ, Blair WR, Steyers CM, et al. Classification of distal radius fractures. An analysis of interobserver reliability and intraobserver reproducibility. *J Hand Surg [Am]* 1996;21:574–582.
38. Kreder HJ, Hanel DP, McKee M, et al. Consistency of AO fracture classification for the distal radius. *J Bone Joint Surg Br* 1996;78:726–731.
39. Müller ME, ed. *Comprehensive classification of fractures. Pamphlet 1.* Bern: ME Müller Foundation, 1995;1–24.
40. Mathoulin CH, Letrosne E, Saffar PH. Classification of intra-articular fractures of the distal radius. In: Saffar PH, Cooney WP, eds. *Fractures of the distal radius.* London: Martin Dunitz, 1995;126–130.
41. Rayhack JM. Symposium on distal radius fractures. *Contemp Orthop* 1990;21:71–104.
42. Missakian ML, Cooney WP, Amadio PC, et al. Open reduction and internal fixation for distal radius fractures. *J Hand Surg [Am]* 1992;17:745–755.
43. Fernandez DL, Jupiter JB. *Fractures of the distal radius.* New York: Springer-Verlag, 1995.
44. Fernandez DL. Treatment of articular fractures of the distal radius with external fixation and pinning. In: Saffar PH, Cooney WP, eds. *Fractures of the distal radius.* London: Martin Dunitz, 1995;104–117.
45. Altissimi M, Azzara A, Mancini GB, et al. The reliability of clas-

sification of articular fractures of the distal radius. *J Hand Surg [Br]* 1996;21(Suppl 1):31.
46. Lafontaine M, Hardy D, Delince PH. Stability assessment of distal radius fractures. *Injury* 1989;20:208–210.
47. Altissimi M, Mancini GB, Azzara A, et al. Early and late displacement of fractures of the distal radius. The prediction of instability. *Int Orthop* 1994;18:61–65.
48. Martini AK. Die sekundäre Arthrose des Handgelenkes bei der Fehlstellung der verheilten und nicht korrigierten distalen Radiusfraktur. *Akt Traumatol* 1986;16:143–148.
49. Miyake T, Hashizume H, Inoue H, et al. Malunited Colles' fracture. Analysis of stress distribution. *J Hand Surg [Br]* 1994;19: 737–742.
50. Palmer AK, Werner FW. The triangular fibrocartilage complex of the wrist—anatomy and function. *J Hand Surg [Am]* 1981;6: 153–162.
51. Pogue DJ, Viegas SF, Patterson RM, et al. Effects of distal radius fracture malunion on wrist joint mechanics. *J Hand Surg [Am]* 1990;15:721–727.
52. Short WH, Palmer AK, Werner FW, et al. A biomechanical study of distal radial fractures. *J Hand Surg [Am]* 1987;12:529–534.
53. Tanzer TL, Horne JG. Dorsal radiocarpal fracture dislocation. *J Trauma* 1980;20:999–1000.
54. Caldwell JA. Device for making traction on the fingers. *JAMA* 1931;96:1226.
55. King RE. Barton's fracture-dislocation of the wrist. *Curr Pract Orthop Surg* 1975;6:133–144.
56. Carothers RG, Berning DN. Colles' fracture. *Am J Surg* 1950;80: 616–629.
57. Agee JM. Distal radius fractures. Multiplanar ligamentotaxis. *Hand Clin* 1993;9:577–585.
58. Gupta A. The treatment of Colles' fracture: Immobilisation with the wrist dorsiflexed. *J Bone Joint Surg Br* 1991;73:312–315.
59. DePalma AF. Comminuted fractures of the distal end of the radius treated by ulnar pinning. *J Bone Joint Surg Am* 1952;34:651–662.
60. Kihara H, Palmer AK. The effect of dorsally angulated distal radius fractures on distal radioulnar joint-congruency and forearm rotation. *J Hand Surg [Am]* 1996;21:40–47.
61. Palmer AK. Fractures of the distal radius. In: Green DP, ed. *Operative hand surgery, 2nd ed.* New York: Churchill Livingstone, 1988:991–1026.
62. Cooney WP, Dobyns JH, Linscheid RL. Complications of Colles' fractures. *J Bone Joint Surg Am* 1980;62:613–619.
63. Gibson AGF, Bannister GC. Bracing or plaster for Colles' fractures? A randomized prospective controlled trial. *J Bone Joint Surg Br* 1983;65:221.

19

EXTERNAL FIXATION OF DISTAL RADIUS FRACTURES

MICHAEL E. RETTIG
KEITH B. RASKIN
CHARLES P. MELONE, JR.

Fractures of the distal radius constitute one of the most common skeletal injuries treated by orthopedic surgeons. These injuries account for one-sixth of all fractures evaluated in emergency rooms and have often been considered primarily stable extraarticular fractures of the elderly. However, increasing experience has revealed that the vast majority of distal radius fractures are articular injuries resulting in disruption of both the radiocarpal and distal radioulnar joints. Better understanding of the spectrum of distal radial fractures has led to changing concepts of treatment. Prominent among the concepts is that optimal management of distal radial fractures requires differentiation of the relatively low-energy metaphyseal injuries, traditionally called Colles' fractures, from the more violent injuries that disrupt the articular surfaces. The articular injuries are more frequently comminuted and unstable and therefore less suitable for more traditional methods of closed reduction and cast immobilization. Without supplemental skeletal fixation, redisplacement of the fracture—frequently to their prereduction position—is inevitable. Resultant malunion predictably leads to pain, limited range of motion, weakness, and posttraumatic arthritis.

The optimal method of obtaining and maintaining an accurate restoration of distal radial anatomy remains a topic of considerable controversy. A wide array of techniques, including closed, percutaneous, and open methods of reduction and stabilization, have been increasingly advocated as successful treatment. Although these methods have been eloquently described, the fracture, per se, is less frequently defined with precision. It must be recognized that articular fractures comprise a diverse spectrum of injury for which optimal management requires differing methods of treatment. Employment of a single technique for dissimilar injuries is predictably prone to a variable and often disappointing quality of recovery.

Much of the confusion can be eliminated by recognition of specific key fracture characteristics: (a) consistent patterns of articular fracture anatomy, (b) articular fracture stability, and (c) articular fracture reducibility. With prompt detection of these features, an accurate diagnosis can be established, and a rational plan of management based on precise fracture configurations can be formulated for the vast majority of distal radius injuries.

CLASSIFICATION

In our experience with distal radius fractures, radiographic evidence of articular disruption has been present in the majority of cases (1–4). Consistent radiographic observations have led to the formulation of a classification subset of articular injuries that has considerably facilitated their treatment. Stability and reducibility can be determined, and a treatment plan can be formulated based on the analysis of the fracture pattern. Rather than a global classification system, these categories should be considered a subset of more complex articular fractures.

Despite frequent comminution, articular fractures comprise four basic components: (a) the radial shaft, (b) the radial styloid, (c) a dorsal medial fragment, and (d) a palmar medial fragment (Fig. 19.1). To underscore their pivotal position as the cornerstone of both the radiocarpal and radioulnar joints, the two medial fragments along with their strong ligamentous attachments to the carpus and the ulnar styloid have been termed the medial complex. Because even minimal displacement of the key medial fragments is likely to cause a major biarticular disruption with a serious compromise of articular function, anatomic preservation of this complex must be recognized as an absolute requirement for optimal fracture management. Displacement of these strategically positioned medial fragments also forms the

---

M. E. Rettig, K. B. Raskin, and C. P. Melone, Jr.: Department of Orthopedic Surgery, New York University Medical Center, New York, New York 10016

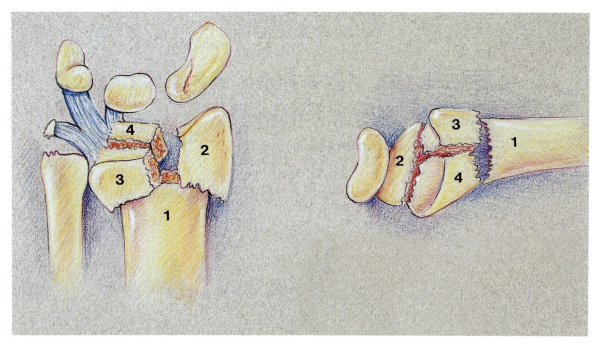

FIGURE 19.1. Articular fractures, despite variable and often extensive comminution, comprise four basic components: *1*, metaphyseal or shaft; *2*, radial styloid; *3*, dorsal medial; and *4*, palmar medial. (From Melone CP Jr. Distal radius fractures: patterns of articular fragmentation. *Orthop Clin North Am* 1993;24:239–253, with permission.)

basis for an increasingly comprehensive system of categorizing articular injuries into precise patterns of fragmentation (Fig. 19.2).

Type I fractures are minimally displaced, stable after closed reduction, and effectively treated by a short period of cast immobilization. Progressive remobilization and strengthening supplement splint immobilization until rehabilitation is complete.

The most common articular fracture is the dorsally displaced type II fracture, the die-punch fracture (Fig. 19.3). In such instances, the lunate selectively impacts the dorsal medial component, resulting in an unstable fracture characterized by greater comminution of the dorsal metaphysis with marked dorsal tilting and considerable shortening of the radius (Fig. 19.4).

Less frequently, greater lunate compression is applied to the palmar medial fragment, resulting in proximal displacement of the medial complex along with the carpus. In the majority of type II fractures, the medial complex is neither widely separated nor rotated and is generally amenable to closed reduction and external skeletal fixation (type IIA).

In contrast, radiographic evidence of these fractures has revealed a recurring variation in the characteristic die-punch pattern that has consistently proved irreducible by closed methods (type IIB). The distinctive pattern of fragmentation is characterized by greater comminution and displacement of the medial fragments, usually in a dorsal direction, with the scaphoid and lunate seen impacting the articular surface (double die-punch) with an offset of the radiocarpal joint exceeding 2 mm (Fig. 19.5).

Radiographic signs of a greater magnitude of injury similarly are observed for the irreducible die-punch fracture with volar displacement. The hallmarks of this fracture pattern are greater comminution and displacement of the palmar medial fragment, resulting in a radiocarpal stepoff exceeding 5 mm as viewed in the sagittal plane.

The type III spike fracture demonstrates articular disruption similar to that in type II injuries as well as displacement of an additional and substantial fracture component, the

text continues on p. 303

FIGURE 19.3. The unstable type II fracture resulting from the die-punch mechanism of injury. In most cases, the lunate selectively impacts the dorsal medial fragment, resulting in dorsal displacement of the articular surfaces. Less frequently, the palmar medial fragment and the carpus demonstrate volar displacement. Regardless of the direction of displacement, these fractures are reducible by closed techniques. *1*, metaphyseal or shaft; *2*, radial styloid; *3*, dorsal medial; *4*, palmar medial. (From Melone CP Jr. Distal radius fractures: patterns of articular fragmentation. *Orthop Clin North Am* 1993;24:239–253, with permission.)

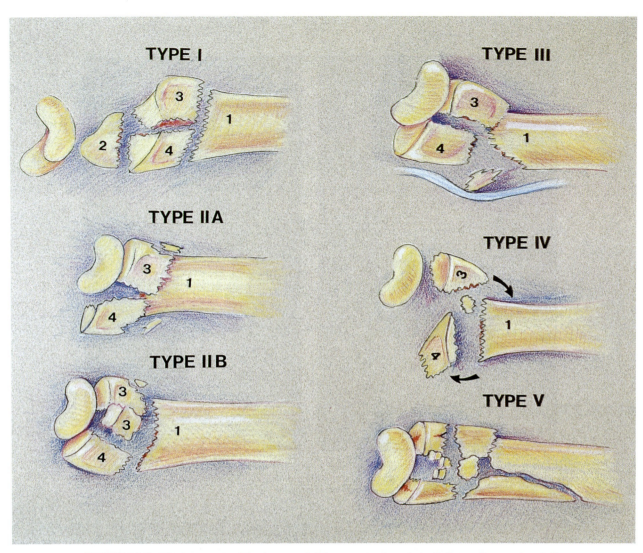

FIGURE 19.2. Displacement of the key medial fragments disrupts both the radiocarpal and distal radioulnar joints and is the basis for an increasingly comprehensive system of categorizing distal radius articular fractures. *1*, metaphyseal or shaft; *2*, radial styloid; *3*, dorsal medial; *4*, palmar medial. (From Melone CP Jr. Distal radius fractures: patterns of articular fragmentation. *Orthop Clin North Am* 1993;24:239–253, with permission.)

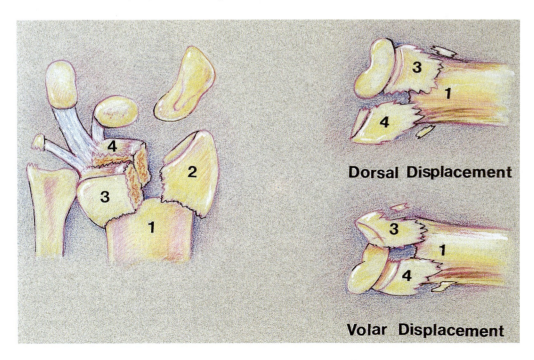

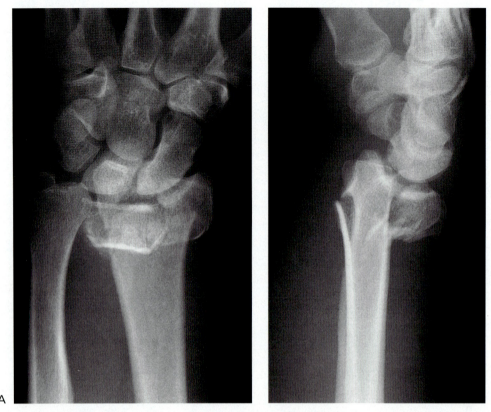

FIGURE 19.4. Typical posteroanterior **(A)** and lateral **(B)** radiographs of an unstable displaced intraarticular die-punch fracture of the distal radius. Significant metaphyseal comminution, as well as dorsal and volar cortical fragmentation, is present.

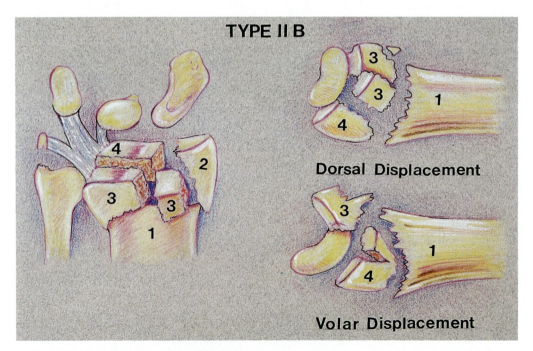

FIGURE 19.5. The unstable type IIB fracture results from a violent compression force, termed the double die-punch mechanism of injury, and demonstrates greater comminution and displacement of the medial fragments, usually in a dorsal direction. This fracture type consistently has proved irreducible by closed methods of reduction. With greater compression and fragmentation of the palmar medial fragment, the less frequently encountered irreducible type IIB fracture with volar displacement occurs. *1,* metaphyseal or shaft; *2,* radial styloid; *3,* dorsal medial; *4,* palmar medial. (From Melone CP Jr. Distal radius fractures: patterns of articular fragmentation. *Orthop Clin North Am* 1993;24:239–253, with permission.)

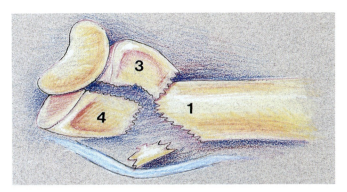

FIGURE 19.6. The type III articular fracture demonstrates displacement of the additional fracture component, the spike fragment from the metaphysis. *1*, metaphyseal or shaft; *3*, dorsal medial; *4*, palmar medial. (From Melone CP Jr. Distal radius fractures: patterns of articular fragmentation. *Orthop Clin North Am* 1993;24:239–253, with permission.)

spike fragment, from the volar metaphysis (Fig. 19.6). Displacement of the fragment may occur at the time of injury or during fracture manipulation and causes not only injury to the adjacent nerves and tendons but also a further compromise in fracture stability.

The type IV fracture pattern is characterized by wide separation or rotation of the dorsal and palmar medial fragments with severe disruptions of the distal radius articulations (Fig. 19.7). Not infrequently, the palmar medial fragment is rotated 180°, causing its articular surface to face proximally toward the radial shaft. This injury also results in extensive concomitant soft tissue and skeletal damage.

An increasingly violent magnitude of injury accounts for the occurrence of an additional pattern of articular disruption called the type V explosion fracture (Fig. 19.8). This severe lesion results from an enormous force comprising both axial compression and direct crush that causes profound comminution, frequently extending from the articular surfaces to the diaphysis. This major skeletal injury usually occurs in association with massive soft tissue trauma that is likely to disrupt skin, nerves, and vascular structures.

Several other classification systems have been advocated for fractures of the distal radius. Frykman devised a classification system based on the differentiation of extraarticular from intraarticular fractures (5). The classification system developed by the AO group was organized to aid in identifying more severe injuries of the distal radius (6). Fernandez has suggested a classification based on the mechanism of injury (7).

Classifications identifying unstable and irreducible fractures and thereby facilitating treatment options based on fracture patterns have recently been formulated (8). These treatment-directed schemes are based on fracture location, displacement, stability, and reducibility.

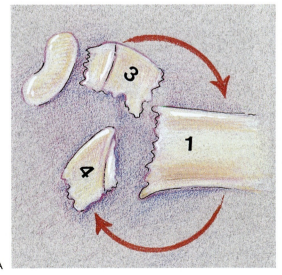
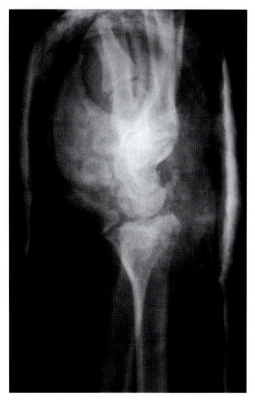

FIGURE 19.7. A: The type IV fracture pattern is characterized by wide separation of the dorsal and palmar medial fragments with severe disruption of the distal radius articulations. (From Melone CP Jr. Distal radius fractures: patterns of articular fragmentation. *Orthop Clin North Am* 1993;24:239–253, with permission.) **B:** This type IV injury demonstrates 180° rotation of the palmar medial fragment, causing a complete reversal of its articular surface toward the radial shaft. *1*, metaphyseal or shaft; *3*, dorsal medial; *4*, palmar medial.

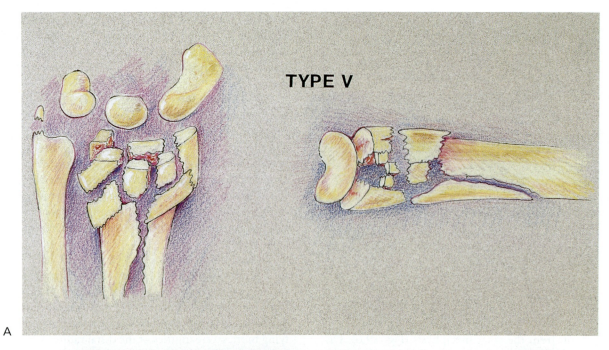
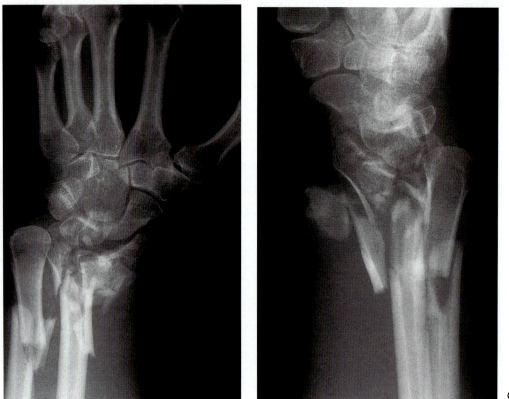

FIGURE 19.8. The type V explosion fracture, demonstrating profound comminution extending from the articular surfaces to the diaphysis. (**A** is from Melone CP Jr. Distal radius fractures: patterns of articular fragmentation. *Orthop Clin North Am* 1993;24:239–253, with permission.)

PRINCIPLES OF MANAGEMENT

The fundamental goal of treatment for distal radius fractures is an accurate and stable reduction. It is generally acknowledged that the reduction may be easily achieved but difficult to maintain (9). Successful treatment requires a method of reduction that restores anatomic relationships between the fractured radius and adjacent ulna and carpus and maintains this alignment until the healing process is complete. More recently, it has also become increasingly acknowledged that a suboptimal outcome is likely to result if seemingly minor alterations of fracture anatomy persist. For example, only 2 mm of articular offset, 10° of dorsal tilt, or 3 to 5 mm of radial shortening is apt to compromise recovery (1,10–17). Although a good functional result can be achieved despite a poor radiographic result, excellent function is more likely to be attained when normal anatomy has been restored. For an articular fracture, precise restitution of the medial complex is essential for the preservation of the distal radius articulations, and this occasionally requires open treatment. Also, because the unstable fractures are frequently complicated by serious concomitant soft tissue and skeletal damage, optimal management requires prompt recognition of these associated injuries.

Understanding the stability of an articular fracture is paramount in selecting the appropriate treatment. Although stable fractures can often be reduced and maintained in a cast, closed techniques are doomed to failure for the unstable fractures. Reduction of the unstable fracture may be possible, but maintenance of the reduction until fracture healing is unlikely. As Gartland and Werley observed in their classic review of articular fractures managed by closed reduction, redisplacement of the unstable fracture, frequently to its prereduction position, is inevitable (18). The quandary is considerably lessened by recognition of those characteristics of articular fragmentation and displacement that render the fracture unstable and, thus, not suitable for treatment solely by manipulation and immobilization. The obvious hallmarks of articular fracture instability are excessive comminution and severity of displacement. Other signs less obvious yet highly suggestive of a fracture prone to redisplacement usually can be identified. First, initial radial shortening in excess of 10 mm is predisposed to further collapse, resulting in both disabling radioulnar instability and ulnocarpal impaction. Lidstrom has indicated that residual shortening of only 6 mm can seriously compromise wrist function (16). Palmer and Short have demonstrated that even a smaller discrepancy in radioulnar length is likely to cause deleterious alterations in load bearing, leading to articular deterioration (19). Because even relatively stable articular fractures tend to collapse several millimeters as a result of impaction of comminuted metaphyseal fragments, a successful reduction should secure the preinjury level of the medial complex and its critical relationships with the radial styloid, the proximal carpus, and the ulnar head. In all fractures, comparison radiographs of the contralateral wrist should be assessed to determine normal length and to avoid misinterpretation related to anatomic variation. Second, angulation or tilting of the distal radial articular surface exceeding 20° in the sagittal plane causes a serious disturbance of radiocarpal collinear alignment as well as incongruity of the distal radioulnar joint. Similar to radial shortening, this typical feature of the unstable articular fracture is exceedingly difficult to correct by casting. Finally, metaphyseal comminution involving both the volar and dorsal radial cortices eliminates an intact bony buttress on which a stable reduction must hinge. Lateral radiographs obtained at the time of injury clearly demonstrate this bicortical comminution, whereas frontal projections taken after attempts at reduction often display an articular surface bereft of a sturdy osseous support as a result of extensive metaphyseal cavitation. Recognition of these radiographic signs of instability is essential for satisfactory management of these injuries.

Because of the unique configuration of the skeletal anatomy and surrounding capsuloligamentous tissue, unstable fractures of the distal radius are amenable to reduction and stabilization by means of ligamentotaxis. This form of management provides both reduction of the fracture fragments by indirect distraction through the extraarticular ligaments of the wrist and neutralization of the detrimental forces of the proximal carpus at the fracture site during the critical acute healing phase.

METHODS OF REDUCTION AND STABILIZATION

A prevalent misconception has been that distal radius articular fractures, regardless of their extent, usually can be managed with equal success by similar techniques. Rational management, however, is contingent on recognition of the variable magnitude of articular disruption and skillful treatment based on specific fracture configurations. Each fracture should be distinguished by its degree of articular displacement, its stability, and its reducibility. After the fracture is thoroughly evaluated, optimal treatment can be instituted.

Minimally displaced distal radius fractures can be reduced by closed manipulation. The reduction is performed after aspiration of the fracture hematoma under sterile conditions and local infiltration of 3 to 5 cc of 2% lidocaine. The reduction is essentially a reversal of the mechanism of injury. Usually a hyperextension–compression force applied to the pronated wrist results in posterior displacement with relative supination of the distal fragments; thus, the reduction is achieved by axial traction of the wrist, followed by palmar flexion, ulnar deviation, pronation of the displaced fracture fragments, and cast immobilization.

A satisfactory reduction requires restoration of normal radial length (usually neutral ulnar variance) and stability provided by accurate apposition of the anterior cortices of the radius. Invariably, the dorsal cortex is comminuted, and stability of the reduction hinges on the buttress of a relatively intact anterior cortex. If both cortices are extensively comminuted, the fracture is unstable, and collapse with loss of reduction is inevitable.

If the fracture is unstable, the frequently encountered dorsally displaced fracture that is unstable and reducible but requires some form of skeletal fixation must be distinguished from the irreducible die-punch fracture. Compared to the reducible type II fracture, the irreducible articular pattern demonstrates greater comminution and displacement of the medial fragments, usually in the dorsal direction, with persistent articular stepoff or gapping greater than 2 mm.

Specific fracture patterns also facilitate a rational choice of operative techniques from the ever-expanding list of methods advocated for the surgical treatment of unstable distal radius fractures. Whereas the unstable type II fracture with relatively mild displacement and comminution can be managed successfully by pins and plaster (20–22) or percutaneous Kirschner wires (23,24), type II injuries with greater articular fragmentation and instability are preferentially stabilized by external fixators (4,25–31). Although the underlying principle of ligamentotaxis for pins and plaster and external fixators is the same, the external fixator affords the distinct advantages of superior mechanical efficiency, a capacity for secondary adjustment in fracture position, and unobstructed access for wound care. For those complex fractures requiring open reduction and internal fixation, the external fixator is an excellent method of providing both supplemental stabilization and secure immobilization during the period of fracture healing.

In most unstable fractures, ligamentotaxis alone successfully restores articular congruity, radial length, and inclination. The stout volar radiocarpal ligaments are credited for this unique capacity of fracture reduction. However, the restoration of normal volar tilt is less successful because of the lack of distractive force from the less developed and obliquely oriented dorsal capsuloligamentous complex (32). External fixators incorporating multiplanar ligamentotaxis (Agee WristJack, Hand Biomechanics Lab, Sacramento, CA) have been developed in an effort to restore volar tilt (33). Fracture reduction is obtained by dorsal–palmar fragment alignment using a dorsal–palmar fixator adjustment mechanism. Palmar translation of the hand restores palmar tilt to the distal fragment. Anatomic volar tilt can be achieved with a uniplanar external fixator by closed manipulation of the distal fragment in conjunction with multiple Kirschner wires. After initial radial length has been restored, correction of volar tilt can be achieved through manipulation of the fracture in conjunction with flexion though the adjustable components of the external fixator. Supplemental Kirschner wires inserted from the volar aspect of the styloid fragment to the dorsal cortex of the intact radial shaft facilitate this maneuver without additional complications. After the fracture reduction is completed and the wires are inserted, the wrist is returned to near neutral alignment, and the adjustable clamp is tightened.

Compared with the reducible, unstable type IIA fracture, the irreducible articular pattern demonstrates greater comminution and displacement of the medial complex, usually in a dorsal direction, persistent articular stepoff or gapping greater than 2 mm, irreversible articular tilting in excess of 20°, and uncorrectable radial shortening exceeding 5 mm. Marked articular incongruity will not be restored adequately with ligamentotaxis alone. Restoration of articular congruity can be accomplished only by open treatment—usually involving a limited dorsal exposure for articular reduction. After primary ligamentotaxis with an external fixator, articular fragments are derotated and reduced to each other and then to the radial metaphysis with Kirschner wires. If larger fragments are present, plates and screws may be used for fixation. Iliac crest bone grafting for restitution of skeletal integrity and support of the articular fragments is essential. Even in the presence of extensive comminution, meticulous fracture reduction can successfully preserve articular contours.

SURGICAL TECHNIQUE

Successful uncomplicated treatment of unstable distal radius fractures is directly related to the precise, reproducible surgical technique used for these injuries. Several key steps of surgical application can significantly reduce the frequently reported pin-related complications. We have learned over the years that percutaneous half-pin placement potentially leads to unnecessary iatrogenic soft tissue, tendon, and nerve injuries. The risk of unicortical pin insertion resulting in metacarpal or radial shaft fracture or subsequent loosening and infection has also been well described (31).

The distal pin site is approached through a short longitudinal incision directly over the dorsoradial border of the index finger metacarpal. The terminal branches of the radial sensory nerve are well visualized and protected as the first dorsal interosseous muscle is reflected. Minimal periosteal stripping is essential and avoids unnecessary devascularization. The presently available common pin sizes range from 3 to 4 mm, and most require predrilling before insertion. A low-speed power drill and minimal irrigation prevent thermal necrosis of the metacarpal during predrilling. The pins are often inserted in a dorsal-to-volar direction of 30° to 45° to avoid encroachment of thumb extension and obscuring of the lateral radiographs when the external fixation frame is applied. Two bicortical pins placed within the index metacarpal alone are satisfactory for reduction ligamentotaxis and maintained fracture alignment.

The proximal pins are similarly inserted through a short longitudinal incision along the dorsoradial border of the radius shaft 3 to 5 cm proximal to the fracture site. In this region, the radial sensory nerve is located beneath the fascial layer between the brachioradialis and the extensor carpi radialis longus and is carefully avoided during pin insertion.

We now commonly insert the pins within the interval between the extensor carpi radialis longus and brevis to provide additional soft tissue protection and to avoid potential iatrogenic radial neuritis. After completion of pin insertion, the external fixation frame is assembled and secured to both sets of fixation pins. Manipulation of the fracture site is then performed while gentle longitudinal traction is applied to the digits with countertraction at the flexed elbow. Finger-trap apparatus and a hanging counterweight are reasonable alternative methods of initial ligamentotaxis fracture distraction. Most contemporary external fixation frames allow for distraction through an adjustable sliding couple-clamp or turn-screw component and fracture reduction at a ball joint or hinge location.

By way of the expanded understanding of the pathoanatomy of the distal radius fracture, enhanced surgical techniques have developed. Percutaneously placed smooth 0.045 Kirschner wires have routinely produced a more stable fracture fixation configuration without additional complications. This allows for reduction of the demands for external fixation alone and the potential carpal overdistraction seen with excessive ligamentotaxis as well as restoration of volar tilt (Fig. 19.9). Excessive wrist flexion and ulnar deviation are inappropriate and should be avoided in the reduction of these unstable fractures.

The correct amount of distraction across the wrist joint to provide the optimally maintained reduction of the distal radius fracture is poorly quantified (Fig. 19.10). Overdistraction can result in permanent functional impairment from capsular tightness and digital stiffness. Underdistraction and loss of reduction lead to radius malunion, carpal instability, and ulnar impaction (10). A useful intraoperative

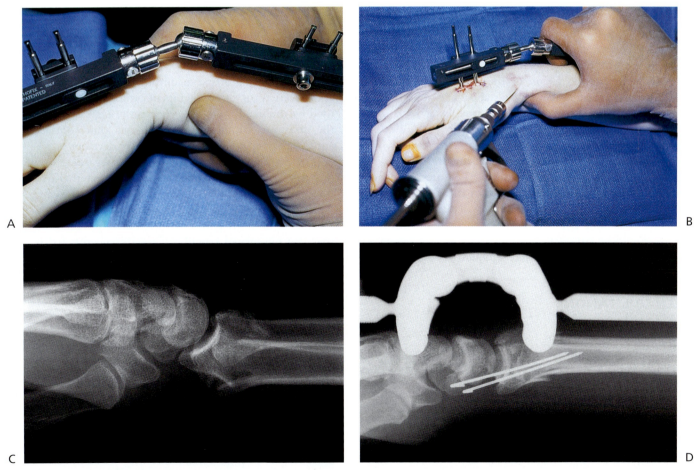

FIGURE 19.9. A: Manual fracture reduction in conjunction with flexion through the adjustable external fixator components restores volar tilt. **B:** Supplemental Kirschner wires maintain the fracture reduction after the wrist is returned to neutral alignment. **C,D:** Radiographic assessment of the reduction of the dorsal angulation deformity and final restoration of volar tilt.

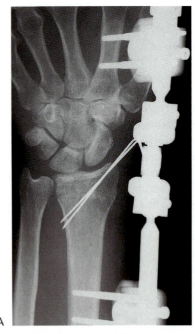
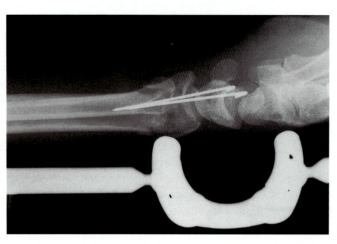

FIGURE 19.10. A,B: Optimal fracture reduction without overdistraction. Radial length, inclination, and volar tilt are restored.

technique of assessment that has achieved good results incorporates clinical and radiographic evaluation. After application of the external fixation frame and fracture reduction, simultaneous passive flexion of the metacarpophalangeal, and interphalangeal joints to the distal palmar crease should be accomplished without difficulty if overdistraction is not present. If it is not possible to complete the passive flexion arc, related extrinsic extensor tendon tightness is present. We have also found that the radiographic finding of a radiocarpal to midcarpal distraction ratio of 2:1 ensures avoidance of overdistraction of the volar radiocarpal capsuloligamentous structures. After ligamentotaxis is reduced, if loss of fracture reduction is observed, than alternative treatment plans should be considered (open reduction, supplemental bone graft, or internal fixation techniques).

REHABILITATION

Attainment of maximum recovery after fracture depends largely on a carefully planned and executed program of therapy. Patients should be cautioned that a perfect reduction does not ensure a satisfactory recovery; they should also be reassured that a motivated patient working with a skilled therapist can often convert a fair anatomic result into an excellent functional result.

Rehabilitation begins immediately after fracture reduction and stabilization; digital, elbow, and shoulder motion is encouraged and must not be impaired by faulty techniques of immobilization (Fig. 19.11). Sling immobilization of the affected limb can contribute to cervical spine discomfort, shoulder capsular adhesions, and elbow flexion contractures and therefore should be avoided. Mobilization of the uninjured finger joints can be enhanced by static and dynamic splinting, massage, antiinflammatory medication, and a variety of other therapeutic modalities commonly used by the hand therapist. With early, aggressive therapy, the disastrous complications of digital joint contractures and reflex sympathetic dystrophy rarely develop.

There are several schools of thought regarding optimal postoperative patient management of the external fixation frame and pin sites. The quality of patient pin care can vary depending on the level of compliance and overall patient acceptance of this routine task. Alternatively, we have found that few pin-related complications are encountered when the external fixator is covered by sterile gauze at the skin contact interface, avoiding the need for daily treatment

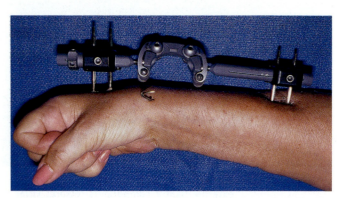

FIGURE 19.11. Active finger motion is encouraged throughout the perioperative period.

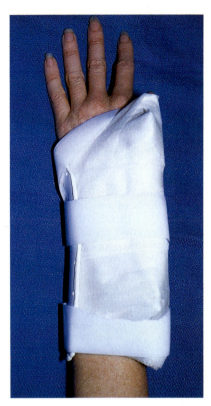

FIGURE 19.12. Protective postoperative sterile dressing and supportive splint.

(Fig. 19.12). The pins are exposed only during dressing changes in the office, approximately four times during the 8-week healing phase. A supplemental volar Orthoplast splint is also supplied to improve patient comfort and limit soft tissue disturbance.

Recently, external fixation frames have been modified to allow for early wrist motion during the acute healing phase in an attempt to prevent potential residual wrist stiffness. Despite this attractive concept, several recent studies have concluded that there is no significant additional benefit to dynamic fixation of these fractures in comparison with the traditional static wrist immobilization until completion of union (34). Further complications have also been incurred as a result of the difficulty in locating the precise center of wrist rotation and subsequent loss of fracture reduction. The accurate anatomic restoration and stable fixation of the distal radius articular surface is the most reliable indicator of successful uncomplicated recovery.

After the fracture is healed, the pins are removed in the physician's office. On removal of the frame and pins, irrigation and curettage of the pin tract sites are performed in a sterile fashion. A protective splint is provided, and mobilization of the wrist is begun. As early motion is restored, incremental resistance is included in the therapy program. During the first several weeks of therapy, we have found it helpful to wear an Orthoplast splint during sleep to maintain neutral position and to prevent flexion contracture.

Because wrist extension is often the most difficult motion to regain, the splint is converted to a dynamic extension or static cock-up splint as indicated during the recovery period. Patients are encouraged to use their hands in activities of daily living with increasing demand as tolerated.

SUMMARY

Distal radius fractures principally result from the die-punch mechanism of injury, which leads to consistent patterns of articular disruption with readily identified radiographic signs of instability and reducibility. Treatment-oriented classifications have replaced the once popular eponym grouping of these diverse injuries. Recognition of fracture instability and irreducibility based on the radiographic evaluation of fragment comminution and displacement as well as articular congruity is the focus of current classifications. Although closed reduction with cast immobilization remains a reliable standard of treatment for stable and minimally displaced articular fractures, similar management for unstable articular disruption is prone to failure.

Ligamentotaxis employing an external fixator, frequently in conjunction with supplemental Kirschner wire internal fixation, has proved to be a reliable means of maintaining an accurate reduction of unstable articular fractures of the distal radius. Critical preoperative evaluation and restoration of articular congruity along with attention to key technical details have resulted in a reproducible successful recovery.

EDITORS' COMMENTS

Unloading the fractured articular surface of the distal radius is a mandatory counterpart to preservation of realignment unless adequate support can be achieved with plate and screws. The tone of the forearm muscles and patient activity can displace the fragments even in the face of good pin fixation and bone graft. This is especially true with impaction of central fragments or lateral explosion of peripheral fragments. There are many external fixators, and the surgeon must be familiar with the device of his choice. The pins should traverse the index metacarpal and on occasion the middle metacarpal, particularly if one is dealing with a large, heavily muscled man.

A transverse incision over the dorsum of the wrist made halfway between the articular surface of the radius and the level of the cortex fracture in the radius allows for visualization into the joint and visualization of the fracture. This approach maintains the external retinaculum in a 1- to 2-cm strip between the two.

Significant traction may be applied at the time of surgery to aid in visualization within the articular compartment and the manipulation of fragments. The traction can then be backed off at least until full passive flexion of all digits is easily accomplished and usually further, as the traction is not holding the reduction, simply keeping pressure off the realigned articular surface. Excessive traction can maintain separation between carpals and prevent torn ligament healing. There is even an advantage under some circumstances in allowing the carpals to make contact with the articular surface, acting as a low-pressure molding template for the fragments of radius without applying excessive pressure. This is particularly true of multiple small fragment explosive-type fractures of the articular surface. Exogenous bone graft has been an effective tool in our hands, filling defects beneath fragments; typically there is adequate support for the articular surface by about $4^1/_2$ weeks for removal of the external fixator.

REFERENCES

1. Melone CP Jr. Articular fractures of the distal radius. *Orthop Clin North Am* 1984;15:217–316.
2. Melone CP Jr. Open treatment for displaced articular fractures of the distal radius. *Clin Orthop* 1986;202:103–111.
3. Melone CP Jr. Distal radius fractures: Patterns of articular fragmentation. *Orthop Clin North Am* 1993;24:239–253.
4. Raskin KB, Melone CP Jr. Unstable articular fractures of the distal radius: Comparative techniques of ligamentotaxis. *Orthop Clin North Am* 1993;24:275–286.
5. Frykman G. Fractures of the distal radius, including sequela of shoulder–hand syndrome: Disturbance of the distal radio-ulnar joint and impairment of nerve function. A clinical and experimental study. *Acta Orthop Scand [Suppl]* 1973;108:1–153.
6. Muller ME, Nazarian S, Koch P. *Classification AO der Fracturen.* Berlin: Springer, 1987.
7. Fernandez DL. *A practical, simplified, comprehensive and treatment oriented classification of fractures of the distal radius.* Paper presented at the 4th International Federation of Societies for Surgery of the Hand, Bone and Joint Injuries Committee, Paris, May 1992.
8. Missakian ML, Cooney WP, Amadio PC. Open reduction and internal fixation for distal radius fractures. *J Hand Surg [Am]* 1992;17:745–755.
9. Abbaszadegan H, Jonsson U, vonSivers K. Prediction of instability of Colles' fractures. *Acta Orthop Scand* 1989;60:646–650.
10. Aro HT, Koivunen T. Minor axial shortening of the radius affects outcome of Colles' fracture treatment. *J Hand Surg [Am]* 1991;16:392–398.
11. Bass RL, Blair WF, Hubbard PP. Results of combined internal and external fixation for the treatment of severe AO-C3 fractures of the distal radius. *J Hand Surg [Am]* 1995;20:373–381.
12. Bassett RL. Displaced intraarticular fractures of the distal radius. *Clin Orthop* 1987;214:148–152.
13. Bradway JK, Amadio PC, Cooney WP. Open reduction and internal fixation of displaced, comminuted intra-articular fractures of the distal radius. *J Bone Joint Surg Am* 1989;71:839–847.
14. Hastings H, Leibovic S. Indications and techniques of open reduction and internal fixation of distal radius fractures. *Orthop Clin North Am* 1993;24:309–326.
15. Knirk JL, Jupiter JB. Intra-articular fractures of the distal end of the radius in young adults. *J Bone Joint Surg Am* 1986;68:647–659.
16. Lidsrom A. Fractures of the distal end of the radius: A clinical and statistical study of end results. *Acta Orthop Scand [Suppl]* 1959;41:1–95.
17. Trumble TE, Schmitt SR, Vedder NB. Factors affecting functional outcome of displaced intra-articular distal radius fractures. *J Hand Surg [Am]* 1994;19:325–340.
18. Gartland JJ Jr, Werley CW. Evaluation of healed Colles' fractures. *J Bone Joint Surg Am* 1951;33:895–907.
19. Short WH, Palmer AK, Werner FW, et al. A biomechanical study of distal radius fractures. *J Hand Surg [Am]* 1987;12:529–534.
20. Carrozzella J, Stern PJ. Treatment of comminuted distal radius fractures with pins and plaster. *Hand Clin* 1988;4:391–397.
21. Chapman DR, Bennet JB, Bryan WJ. Complications of distal radius fractures: Pins and plaster treatment. *J Hand Surg* 1982;7:509–512.
22. Green DP. Pins and plaster treatment of comminuted fractures of the distal end of the radius. *J Bone Joint Surg Am* 1975;57:304–310.
23. Clancy GJ. Percutaneous Kirschner wire fixation of Colles' fractures. *J Bone Joint Surg Am* 1984;66:1008–1014.
24. Greatting MD, Bishop AT. Intrafocal (Kapandji) pinning of unstable fractures of the distal radius. *Orthop Clin North Am* 1993;24:301–307.
25. Cooney WP. External fixation of distal radius fractures. *Clin Orthop* 1983;180:44–49.
26. Cooney WP, Linscheid RL, Dobyns JH. External pin fixation for unstable Colles' fractures. *J Bone Joint Surg Am* 1979;61:840–845.
27. Edwards G. Intraarticular fractures of the distal part of the radius treated with the small AO external fixator. *J Bone Joint Surg Am* 1991;73:1241–1250.
28. Jenkins NH. The unstable Colles' fracture. *J Hand Surg [Br]* 1989;14:149–154.
29. Seitz WH, Froimson AI, Leb R. Augmented external fixation of unstable distal radius fractures. *J Hand Surg [Am]* 1991;16:1010–1016.
30. Szabo RM, Weber SC. Comminuted intraarticular fractures of the distal radius. *Clin Orthop* 1988;230:39–48.
31. Weber SC, Szabo RM. Severely comminuted distal radius fractures as an unsolved problem: Complications associated with external fixation and pins and plaster techniques. *J Hand Surg [Am]* 1986;11:157–165.
32. Bartosh RA, Saldana MJ. Intraarticular fractures of the distal radius: A cadaveric study to determine if ligamentotaxis restores radiopalmar tilt. *J Hand Surg [Am]* 1990;15:18–21.
33. Agee JM. External fixation: Technical advances based upon multiplanar ligamentotaxis. *Orthop Clin North Am* 1993;24:265–274.
34. Sommerkamp TG, Seeman M, Silliman J. Dynamic external fixation of unstable fractures of the distal part of the radius. *J Bone Joint Surg Am* 1994;76:1149–1161.

20

OPEN REDUCTION AND INTERNAL FIXATION OF DISTAL RADIUS FRACTURES

HOWARD A. LIPTON
JESSE B. JUPITER

Fractures of the distal radius are very common (1,2) and continue to challenge the treating surgeon. If certain criteria are not met, patients with these fractures will not do well and may have painfully stiff, dysfunctional wrists (3–15). The titles of this chapter and Chapter 19 should not, however, be construed to imply that there may be a competition between open and closed methods of treatment. The method selected should be one that meets the needs of the specific clinical situation. The surgeon should be familiar with a wide variety of treatment methods and have some understanding of the biomechanical characteristics of a specific fracture pattern that may make one technique or another more or less likely to succeed. A successful outcome represents restoration of a functional hand and wrist, and all the measureable objective criteria such as union rates, anatomic joint restoration, radial height, radial inclination, and volar tilt that may be discussed are simply predictors that good function may still occur, but they are not guarantors.

CRITERIA FOR SUCCESS AND CLINICAL ADVANCES

For most of the more than 180 years since Abraham Colles published his famous paper, and particularly since the advent of radiography about 100 years ago, most of the attention paid to fractures of the distal radius had to do with certain extraarticular characteristics that are relatively easy to measure and appear related to outcome (10,16,17). These criteria include the volar tilt of the distal radius in the sagittal plane, the radial inclination of the articular surface while moving distally in the coronal plane, the radial height or the ulnar variance, and the radial width or shift (which measures the radial displacement of the fragment(s) containing the articular surface relative to the proximal fragment) (11,17–24). Certainly these measurements are useful in assessing treatment and predicting outcome, but even more crucial is the restoration of the articular surface when it is involved (6,11,15,24–36).

As understanding of the importance of an anatomic distal radial articular surface has grown, so has there been an evolution in the techniques commonly employed to treat such a fracture. Traditional cast fixation was supplemented with the pins-and-plaster technique, which itself was later refined into a number of external fixators, some developed solely for the purpose of treating these specific fractures (15,37–52). Both dynamic and static configurations have had their advocates (53–57), and the anatomic basis for ligamentotaxis in maintaining a reduction has been thoroughly examined (37,46,58,59). Kirschner wires (K-wires) were used percutaneously to augment external fixation (26,60–62) (although probably the external fixator was augmenting the K-wires), and limited open reduction techniques for certain articular fragments were developed (50, 63,64).

Following the 1986 publication by Knirk and Jupiter (11) that established the primacy of the articular restoration over extraarticular orientation in predicting outcome for these fractures, with solid evidence that the largest tolerable articular stepoff is 2 mm, the next decade was witness to a proliferation of reported series on open reduction and internal fixation of these articular fractures (27,33,65–71). The results of these series strongly confirm that the better the restoration of the articular surface, the better the outcome. These developments have been very encouraging and suggest that aggressive but judicious operative intervention may result in less pain, stiffness, instability, arthritis, and nerve entrapment and may diminish the necessity for performing

---

H. A. Lipton: Department of Plastic and Reconstructive Surgery, Hadassah-University Hospital, Jerusalem 91120, Israel.
J. B. Jupiter: Department of Orthopaedic Surgery, Harvard Medical School, and Department of Orthopaedics, Massachusetts General Hospital, Boston, Massachusetts 02114.

even more technically difficult osteotomies later (16,17,19, 72–76).

One interpretation of the improved outcomes following joint restoration is that the anatomic joint surface will be subject to less friction and long-term wear and tear. But all fractures of the distal end of the radius have at least two characteristics in common: injury to the soft tissues as well as to the bone. Because joint motion is mediated by soft tissues, the concept of the intertwined injury to bone and soft tissue is absolutely key to successful treatment of intraarticular fractures of the distal radius. The "wrist" represents a complex of multiple joints, each of whose range of motion is dependent on the relative positions of the adjacent component joints. Beyond the inherent limitations on joint motion that are created by the surface topography itself, there is an intricate network of ligamentous connections that serves to stabilize and control wrist motion. The operative repair of an intraarticular fracture of the distal radius includes a restoration of the ligamentous network as accurately as possible, either in the form of direct repair of torn structures or, more commonly, by realignment of the articular anatomy of the end of the radius. We feel that further advances in the successful treatment of these fractures will be dependent on improved treatment of the injured soft tissues.

ASSESSMENT

Perhaps the most important part of the initial evaluation is the condition of the soft tissues. Neurovascular compromise, elevated compartment pressures, and soft tissue disruption or loss must all be diagnosed properly if they are to be treated in a timely fashion (77). Each in its own way may affect the timing and sequence of the steps in treating the underlying fracture. Diminished sensibility, paleness or cyanosis of the distal skin, altered capillary refill, tenseness of the soft tissues, and pain out of proportion to the skeletal injury should all serve to raise our index of suspicion for significant problems involving the soft tissue.

Radiographic evaluation of the fracture is crucial to obtain a good three-dimensional understanding of the fracture pattern. The initial trauma series should include (the patient's condition permitting) true anteroposterior (AP) and lateral views, and an oblique view is usually very helpful because major fracture fragments are often rotated out of their anatomic planes (77). Tomography is a very important tool for assessment of the articular surface fragments because of the curvatures of the articular surfaces and the overlap shadowing that occurs with plain films (78,79). The amount of articular stepoff, the degree of fragment rotation, the presence of additional and possibly occult fracture lines, and the degree of fragment compression may not be appreciated on plain films (80). Routine or trispiral tomography in the AP and lateral planes serves the surgeon's purpose very well with these fractures. Computed axial tomography (CAT), if obtained in the correct planes or with appropriate software for nonfragmented reconstructions, can also provide this information, and three-dimensional representations can be constructed. Knowledge of fragment location, compression, and rotation before the skin incision is made will often permit a more efficient procedure than that originally planned.

Although we emphasize the importance of determining as much as possible about the damage to the articular surface, we do not neglect the more established extraarticular parameters discussed above. The rationale is simply that malorientation of the distal radius will tighten some radiocarpal ligaments and increase the laxity of others, and such changes may produce instability (17), altered joint loading that may lead to osteoarthrosis (16), and decreased ranges of motion. On a posteroanterior (PA) view, the radial inclination is measured as the angle between a line along the distal radial articular surface and a line perpendicular to the long axis of the radius (81), normally 23° to 24° (Fig. 20.1, Table 20.1). On a lateral view the volar (palmar) tilt is measured as the angle between the distal radial articular surface and a line perpendicular to the long axis of the radius, normally 11° to 12° (Fig. 20.2). The radial height is calculated on the PA view by measuring the distance between two lines perpendicular to the axis of the radius, one tangent to the tip of the radial styloid and the second tangent to the flat surface of the ulnar head. The normal distance is 9 to 12 mm (81–83) (Fig. 20.3). Alternatively, this criterion may be measured as the ulnar variance, which is the distance between two parallel lines that are both perpendicular

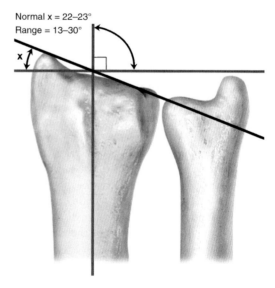

FIGURE 20.1. Radial inclination. This angle is measured in the coronal plane between a line perpendicular to the axis of the radius and a line tangent to the distal radial articular surface. The normal range is 22° to 23°.

TABLE 20.1. RADIOGRAPHIC CRITERIA IN ASSESSMENT OF DISTAL RADIUS FRACTURES

Radial height	9–12 mm
Ulnar variance	0 mm (± 2 mm)
Radial inclination (coronal plane)	23–24°
Volar tilt (sagittal plane)	11–12°
Radial width	Equal to opposite side
Joint surface stepoff	0–2 mm

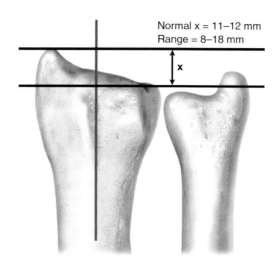

FIGURE 20.3. Radial height. This is the distance in the coronal plane between two lines perpendicular to the axis of the radius, one tangent to the tip of the radial styloid and the second tangent to the ulnar (medial) corner of the distal radial articular surface. The normal range is 9 to 12 mm.

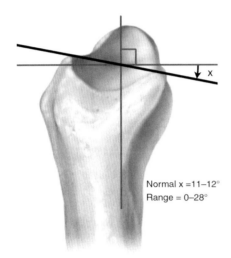

FIGURE 20.2. Volar (palmar) tilt. This angle is measured in the sagittal plane between a line perpendicular to the axis of the radius and a line that connects the dorsal and volar lips of the distal radius as seen in this plane and is essentially parallel to an approximation of the distal radial articular surface. The normal range is 11° to 12°. If the angle reflects actual dorsal tilt, then the measurement is designated as negative, "–."

to the radial axis, one tangent to the medial (ulnar) corner of the distal radius and the other tangent to the lateral (radial) corner of the ulnar head (Fig. 20.4). The normal value for ulnar variance is 0 ± 2 mm. The radial width is the distance between the longitudinal axis in the center of the radius and the most lateral (radial) point of the radial styloid process. Posteroanterior radiographs of both wrists are compared, and the measurements should differ by no more than 1 mm (Fig. 20.5) (20,21,79,82,84).

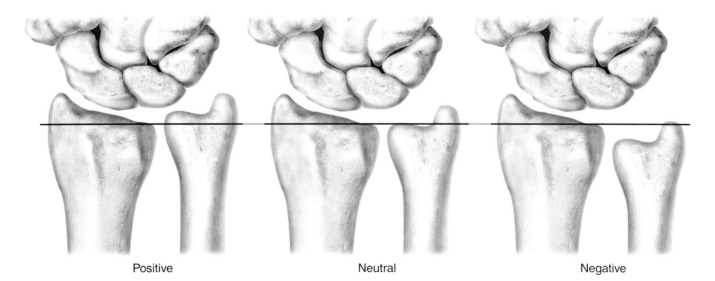

FIGURE 20.4. Ulnar variance. This is the distance in the coronal plane between two lines perpendicular to the axis of the radiuvariance. If the radiuvariance is larger, the distance is positive; if it is the same, neutral; if it is shorter, negative.

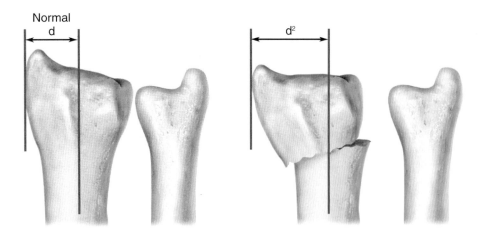

FIGURE 20.5. Radial width (shift). In the coronal plane, the distance is measured between two parallel lines, the midaxis of the radius and a tangent to the radial-most aspect of the displaced radial styloid. This measurement is compared to that of the opposite distal radius, and the normal range is within 1 mm.

CLASSIFICATIONS

A multitude of classification systems has been developed, and their goals are to permit precise communication, aid in selecting a treatment option, and provide a reliable prognosis for outcome. More than 15 classification systems have been proposed in the twentieth century, and there has been a steady evolution in attempts to organize the fracture patterns into related groups.

Frykman's classification (1967) (5) maintained simplicity while emphasizing the crucial significance of distal radioulnar joint (DRUJ) involvement. There were eight types of fracture patterns: (a) extraarticular distal radius fracture; (b) the same, with ulnar styloid fracture; (c) intraarticular radiocarpal joint; (d) the same, with ulnar styloid; (e) intraarticular DRUJ; (f) the same, with ulnar styloid; (g) intraarticular radiocarpal joint and DRUJ; and (h) the same, with ulnar styloid. Although the prognosis worsens as the type number increases, the system suffers because it does not address the key issues of comminution and displacement.

In 1984, Melone described a classification system that reflected both the mechanism and the degree of injury, although it excluded associated distal ulna injuries (32,33). Type 1 fractures were comprised of four components, including the radial styloid, the radial shaft, and the dorsal and volar medial fragments. These fragments were undisplaced, or the medial complex had variable displacement as a unit. As a group, these fractures were minimally comminuted and were stable after closed reduction. In the type 2 fracture, the medial complex was significantly displaced, with comminution of the metaphysis and instability of the fragments. It included die-punch fractures, and if the die-punch fragment was irreducible by closed means, the pattern was called type 2B. Type 3 fractures resembled type 2 regarding displacement and instability, with the addition of a spiked fragment from the radial shaft component that could project into the flexor compartment. Type 4 were characterized by severe disruption of the radial articular surface. The dorsal and volar medial fragments were widely separated or rotated or both, and there could be extensive soft tissue injury, including nerve damage. In 1993, type 5 was added to describe high-energy explosion-type fractures (34).

In 1990, the Universal Classification was based on the presence or absence of articular involvement, reducibility, and stability (85). It prescribes a logical course of treatment based on the defined fracture characteristics. Type 1 includes nondisplaced extraarticular fractures that are treated with cast immobilization. Type 2 fractures are extraarticular but displaced: type 2A are reducible and stable and hence are treated with cast immobilization; type 2B are reducible but unstable and are treated with percutaneous pinning; type 2C are irreducible by closed means, and therefore, they require open reduction with either internal or external fixation. Type 3 fractures are nondisplaced intraarticular fractures treated with percutaneous pinning and cast immobilization. Type 4 fractures are displaced and intraarticular, and their treatment reflects a stepwise progression paralleling type 2. Type 4A are reducible and stable, so they are treated with closed reduction and percutaneous pinning. Type 4B are reducible but unstable, and they are treated with closed reduction, external fixation, and percutaneous pinning. Type 4C fractures are irreducible by closed means, so they are treated with open reduction, internal fixation, external fixation, and percutaneous pinning. The complex fractures fall into category type 4D and require a combination of open reduction, internal (plate) fixation, external fixation, percutaneous pinning, and bone grafting.

The Mayo classification appeared in 1992 (70). Noting that Melone's schema did not account for all fracture patterns, it attempted to subclassify the intraarticular fractures of the distal radius. Mayo type 1 includes nondisplaced articular fractures and is similar to Melone's type 1. Type 2 involves the articular surface of the scaphoid fossa. Type 3 includes the lunate fossa and may also include the sigmoid notch of the DRUJ. Type 4 includes both the scaphoid and lunate fossae and usually involves the sigmoid notch as well.

The two classifications we favor are the Comprehensive Classification of Fractures of Long Bones and the Fernandez Classification. The Comprehensive Classification (86,87) describes 24 patterns of distal radius fractures, three patterns of isolated distal ulna fractures, and six subtypes of distal ulna injury that may accompany each distal radius fracture, and the Fernandez Classification (77,87) groups the fractures of the distal radius into five mechanistic categories, with six subgroups for associated distal ulna injuries.

In the Comprehensive Classification, type A represents extraarticular fractures, type B simple intraarticular fractures, and type C the more complex intraarticular fractures. There are two more sequential levels of subclassification within each type (groups x1, x2, x3, and subgroups xy.1, xy.2, xy.3), and in each case a larger number indicates a greater severity of injury (x can be A, B, or C; y can be 1, 2, or 3). Within type A are the group A1 isolated extraarticular fractures of the distal ulna, the group A2 impacted but noncomminuted extraarticular fractures of the distal radius, and the group A3 comminuted extraarticular fractures of the distal radius, with varying impaction of the metaphysis. Type B includes radial styloid fractures within group B1, dorsal marginal fractures of the distal radius in group B2, and the volar marginal fractures in group B3. For most of the type B fractures there is only one significant articular fragment, although there may be comminution. All type B fractures have at least a portion of the articular surface in continuity with the proximal radius via unfractured bone, in contradistinction to type C, where there is never continuous support between the articular surface and the proximal radius. The type C fractures also always have at least two significant articular components. Group C1 has two articular fragments in addition to the proximal radius and hence is overall a three-part fracture. Group C2 is also a three-part fracture with two articular components, with comminution of the metaphysis or diaphysis. Group C3 has at least four parts, of which three or more are articular.

In the Fernandez Classification of Fractures of the Distal Radius, a type I distal radius fracture is an extraarticular bending fracture in which tensile stresses cause failure of either the dorsal or volar metaphyseal cortex, with the opposite cortex suffering a certain degree of comminution. Type II is a shearing fracture of the articular surface, in conjunction with either a volar or dorsal subluxation of the carpus. The injury force may separate a fracture fragment from the radius in an axial or shearing manner at its radial (B1), dorsal (B2), or volar (B3) margins. When this happens, the fragment may be displaced both proximally and perpendicularly away from the radius. With displacement there is usually concomitant subluxation of the carpus in the direction of the fracture displacement by virtue of the generally intact radiocarpal ligaments at that site.

Type III represents compression fractures where axial loading causes an articular fracture with impaction of the underlying subchondral and metaphyseal bone. Type IV is an avulsion fracture with intact ligamentous attachments from the fragments to the carpus, characteristic of radiocarpal fracture-dislocations. Type V fractures are combined fractures, with components of two or more of the above types, usually resulting from high-energy injuries.

In the Fernandez classification of associated DRUJ injuries, type I represents a stable lesion. The DRUJ is stable to clinical and radiographic examination, with avulsion of the tip of the ulnar styloid (IA) or a stable fracture of the ulnar neck (IB). Type II is an unstable lesion. The DRUJ is dislocated (or subluxated) or easily dislocatable (or subluxatable), with a tear of the substance of the triangular fibrocartilage complex (TFCC) (IIA) or an avulsion fracture at the base of the ulnar styloid (IIB). Type III is a potentially unstable lesion, with a fracture of the radius into the DRUJ (IIIA) or a fracture of the ulna into the DRUJ (IIIB).

By appreciating the type of fracture at the outset, we can immediately rule in or out certain treatment options as appropriate for the case at hand, based on broad experience reported in the literature.

OPERATIVE STRATEGY

The importance of the reconstruction of the articular surface is well documented. In the case of the wrist, failure to do so will result not only in diminished motion but also in pain (11). There are a number of objective measures of the extraarticular mechanical relationships that have been demonstrated to be useful in predicting outcome, including radial height, radial angle, volar tilt, and radial width (see Table 20.1) (11,17–24). Abnormalities in the final values of any of these can lead to a diminished range of motion (ROM), carpal instability, or incongruity in the DRUJ (10,16,17).

Changes in these angles and distances will generally affect the function of the wrist through their effects on the soft tissues, particularly ligaments, that interlink the solid components of the wrist (17). By allowing the ligaments to adapt to resting lengths that are either too long or too short, laxity or tightness, respectively, can be created. These altered relationships can then affect the distribution of force loads across the joint (16). The ligaments attaching the radius to the rest of the carpus are stretched, twisted, and torn by the injury that causes the fracture. Even fibers not directly injured in this fashion will be affected by the regional edema that occurs from the fracture hematoma and the direct contusions of the adjacent tissues. The presence of the edema alone, in conjunction with immobilization, can greatly affect the function of such a ligament later by making it stiff and effectively shorter. In order to reduce such complications, it is incumbent on the surgeon not only to position the fracture fragments appropriately but also to create a construct that will allow soft tissue and joint mobilization as early as possible. Because restoration of the articular surface by correct positioning of the bony fragments, whose soft tissue connections have been preserved, is a most reliable method of anatomic placement of the ligaments, this goal highlights the surgeon's strategy (6,11,15,24–36).

Anesthesia

The anesthesia should be either regional or general. Brachial plexus and axillary blocks provide an anesthetic that is satisfactory for prolonged surgery on the wrist, and they have the additional advantage of creating muscle relaxation for the extremity. Intravenous regional anesthesia may be appropriate for less complex cases that are expected to last less than 1 to 1$\frac{1}{2}$ hours, but it also has the disadvantage of limiting tourniquet release to check for bleeding, as that would terminate the anesthetic.

When regional anesthesia is employed, the anesthesia team must always be prepared to convert to general anesthesia when cancellous bone is harvested from the iliac crest because local anesthetic infiltration is not always adequate to complete this procedure.

Preparation

Tourniquet control is requisite for any open procedure on the upper extremity. We prefer to use a double pneumatic cuff, placed above the elbow, and to alternate cuff inflation at 1-hour intervals, beginning with the distal cuff. The entire upper extremity, and usually the contralateral iliac crest region, are prepared and draped in sterile fashion. Before inflation of the tourniquet we administer an appropriate dosage of a first-generation cephalosporin intravenously, barring allergies.

Closed Reduction

With adequate anesthesia in place, standard reduction maneuvers should be performed. These include both longitudinal traction and, for the dorsally angulated fractures, exaggeration of the deformity followed by traction, flexion, ulnar deviation, and pronation. If a reduction cannot be accomplished or is not stable (for example, it is lost while radiographing the unrestrained wrist), then simple plaster casting will likely not be adequate. Dorsal comminution and an excessive initial dorsal angulation greater than 20° are known indicators of instability (4).

OPERATIVE TECHNIQUE

External Fixation

External fixation is a very useful tool both in achieving reduction and in protecting it, either with or without further internal fixation. It is our preference to apply Kirschner wires to control the reduced articular fragments directly, with external fixation serving primarily to protect the Kirschner wires. Ordinarily the external fixator is applied to the second metacarpal and to the radial shaft. This format obviously prevents radiocarpal wrist motion while it is in place. In some cases of extraarticular fractures, the distal pins may be inserted into the distal fracture fragment and thereby spare immobilization of the wrist.

We prefer to use the Small AO External Fixator, although the principles are the same for any number of other available instrumentations. A fluoroscopic image intensifier is required to accomplish the fixation efficiently. The technique involves direct visualization of the bony surfaces before insertion of the threaded pins, in order to prevent inadvertent damage to sensory nerves, extensor tendons, and vessels. Two 2.5-mm pins threaded distally are placed in the second metacarpal, one in the distal diaphyseal–metaphyseal junction and one in the proximal diaphyseal–metaphyseal junction. At each site, a 5- to 10-mm skin incision is made radial to the metacarpal, and blunt dissection is performed in a plane that will injure neither the first dorsal interosseous muscle nor the extensor tendons. Once the dorsoradial aspect of the metacarpal is revealed, a serrated-tipped soft tissue protector (drill guide) is placed against the cortex and angled at 45° from both the true vertical and the true lateral (radial) planes. Furthermore, it is angled at about 20° to 30° toward the midpoint of the metacarpal, so that the two metacarpal pins will be converging toward each other at an angle of 40° to 60°. It is important to ensure that the tips of the pins will not penetrate the opposite cortex too close to one another, as this would potentiate a stress riser and possibly result in a fracture of the metacarpal. In this fashion four cortices are penetrated in the second metacarpal.

The pins to be inserted into the radius may be either 2.5-mm threaded-tip pins or 4-mm-shaft Schanz pins that step down to 3 mm where threaded. If the larger pins are used, they should be predrilled with a 2-mm drill bit. The radial shaft is approached for placement of the two proximal pins via a 3- to 4-cm incision located proximal to the musculotendinous unit of the abductor pollicis longus. Branches of the superficial radial and lateral antebrachial cutaneous nerves must be protected. The radial cortex is reached along the plane between the brachioradialis and extensor carpi radialis longus. With soft tissue retractors in place, the serrated-tipped drill guide is then oriented as for the metacarpal pins, at 45° from the true vertical and true lateral, and at 20° to 30° toward the site of the other radial pin. Again, care is taken to prevent approximation of the tips of the pins where they penetrate the opposite cortex.

After transfixion of the four radial cortices, all four pin positions are checked with the image intensifier and adjusted as needed regarding depth of penetration. The fixator clamps and connecting bars are then applied, and while the reduction maneuver described earlier is maintained, the clamps are tightened. Of the several configurations available, the most versatile employs short connecting bars between each pair of proximal and distal pins, with the pins being distracted slightly when they are secured to the connecting bar via pin–bar clamps (or bar–bar clamps if 4-mm pins are used), thus creating a prestressed construct that reduces the chance of pin loosening. The two 4-mm connecting bars are then connected to each other via a separate connecting bar and clamps as reduction is maintained. Once a satisfactory reduction is confirmed radiographically, a second connecting bar is placed between the metacarpal and radius groupings to make the entire construct more rigid (Fig. 20.6). The skin incisions should be closed without tension around the pins at the conclusion of the procedure, and any pins that are shortened should be capped to prevent injury.

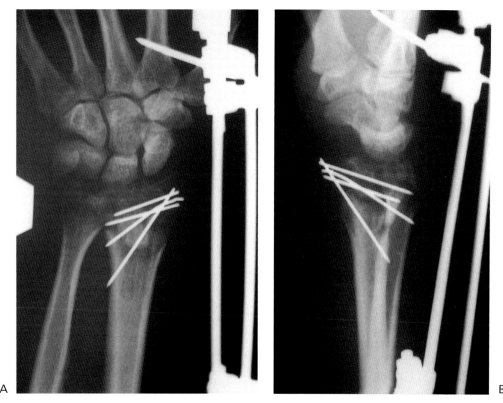

FIGURE 20.6. External fixation. Posteroanterior **(A)** and lateral **(B)** radiographs taken after placement of the fixator. Attention to detail during fixator placement will permit full finger mobilization.

If the reduction is stable and there is no significant dorsal comminution, then external fixation may maintain the reduction (perhaps supplemented with bone graft) until healing is adequate to remove it. Because in most cases we use the external fixator to supplement percutaneous K-wire fixation, one is thereby able to remove the external fixator earlier (at 3 or 4 weeks) because the internal fixation will maintain the reduction. Even in complex cases there may be a role for the external fixator to protect an operative reduction where the degree of comminution or soft tissue injury precludes rigid internal fixation. Often we use the fixator as an intraoperative tool to maintain distraction and a provisional reduction while the formal internal fixation is being applied, and if the internal fixation is sufficiently rigid, the external fixator is removed, and the construct is reexamined for stability intraaoperatively.

Open Percutaneous Pinning

In cases where closed or limited open means can accomplish the reduction, then Kirschner wires (K-wires) of 0.045-in. (1.1 mm) or 0.062-in. (1.5-mm) diameter may be placed to secure the reduction and prevent subsequent settling and loss of reduction. A key point when these pins are placed is to avoid injury to sensory nerves (the superficial radial nerve and the lateral antebrachial cutaneous nerve), to extensor tendons, and to vessels (particularly the radial artery). This is best accomplished by a limited open technique that involves a small incision and blunt dissection down to bone. This is particularly true for pins that must enter the radial styloid because the contents of the first dorsal compartment (abductor pollicis longus and extensor pollicis brevis) may be transfixed at this site.

A 1- to 2-cm incision is made over the radial aspect of the radial styloid. Neural elements are retracted out of the way, and a site for K-wire insertion is selected just dorsal or volar to the first dorsal compartment, depending on the fracture configuration. The selected K-wires are inserted to a depth of 1 cm under direct vision using a power wire driver, and the accuracy of their direction and orientation is confirmed in the coronal, sagittal, and at least one oblique plane using the image intensifier. Once any necessary adjustments are made, the K-wires are then advanced so that they adequately secure the reduced fragment(s). The DRUJ should not be penetrated because this would limit rotation during rehabilitation and perhaps cause additional articular injury.

The initial goal is to secure the distal radius fragment that contains the radial styloid to the radial shaft. This is usually accomplished with two K-wires that angle in a proximal and ulnar direction, about 45° to 60° from the axis of the radius, and penetrate (not excessively) the opposite radial cortex. Following this, two parallel transverse pins can secure a reduced die-punch fragment (Fig. 20.7). These pins should pass just deep to the subchondral bone of the distal radius in

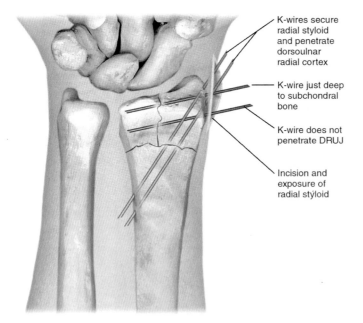

FIGURE 20.7. K-wire placement for a die-punch fragment and a radial styloid fragment. The radial styloid should be exposed through a short incision to avoid neural or tendinous injury.

order to provide adequate buttressing that will prevent collapse. Occasionally, pins may be placed from the dorsoulnar aspect of the radius, aimed radially and proximally, to secure a fragment in that position. Fragments displaced in a palmar direction are *not* amenable to percutaneous fixation because of the risk of injury to volar structures.

The pins may be cut off beneath the skin or left protruding through the skin incison, which would be closed around them. If they are left penetrating the skin, it is important that there not be any tension at the pin–skin interface and that the pin tips be capped to prevent injury to hospital personnel.

Limited Open Reduction

On occasion, closed reduction maneuvers and external fixation can reposition the major fragment(s) of the fracture, but one piece remains out of place. Commonly this fragment is the so-called die-punch fragment, the dorsomedial (dorsoulnar) aspect of the distal radius (89). When this occurs, an incision about 1 cm long can be made between the fourth and fifth compartments, and then blunt dissection through the extensor tendons with an elevator or awl will allow placement of that instrument into the fracture site, as confirmed by fluoroscopy (Fig. 20.8). If the inadequately reduced fragment is the radial styloid, then the

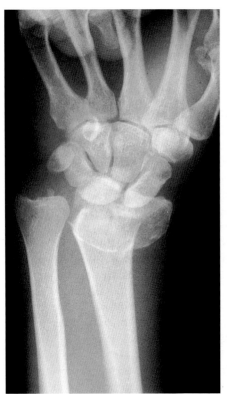
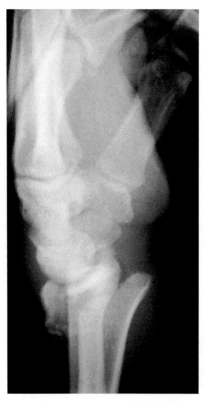
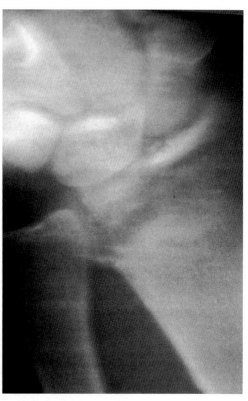

FIGURE 20.8. Limited open reduction in the treatment of a type III (C2.1) fracture suffered by a 32-year-old man who fell 25 feet. Posteroanterior **(A)** and lateral **(B)** radiographs demonstrate dorsal displacement and dorsal tilt, with some metaphyseal comminution seen in the lateral view. **C:** Tomogram showing residual displacement of the medial fragment (lunate fossa) after closed reduction.

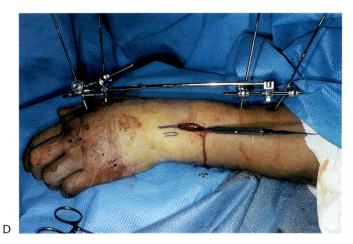

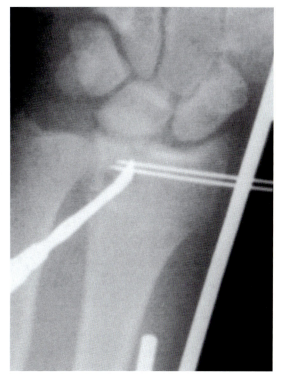

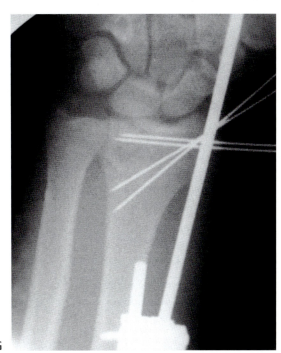

FIGURE 20.8. *(continued)* D: Following application of an external fixator, a short incision was made over the border between the fourth and fifth compartments. An instrument (Freer elevator) was inserted through this incision and placed within the fracture site using fluoroscopic image intensification guidance **(E). F:** Simultaneous fluoroscopic view demonstrates the support by the Freer elevator while the K-wires were inserted. **G:** Addition of two additional oblique K-wires to stabilize the distal radial styloid construct against the diaphysis. The external fixator is kept in place due to the metaphyseal comminution.

approach would be between the first and second extensor compartments. Gentle manipulation and rotation of the instrument under fluoroscopic guidance can often dislodge such an impacted or displaced fragment. It is then manipulated distally until the articular surface is restored. Once the reduction of such an isolated fragment, or occasionally of two fragments, is accomplished, K-wire transfixion is performed as described. In the face of comminution, however, this technique is less effective and may even result in additional fragmentation of the displaced fragment.

SURGICAL APPROACHES

When closed reduction or limited open reduction is inadequate, then the surgeon must consider full open reduction. There are a number of approaches to both the dorsal and volar aspects of the distal radius, and none is necessarily the best for every fracture. The approach must be appropriate to the fracture pattern and allow the surgeon access to all fracture lines and fragments so that reduction and fixation may be accomplished. If the problematic displacement is dorsal, then the approach will be dorsal. If it is volar, then a volar approach may be selected. Not infrequently with high-energy injuries, there is significant displacement both dorsally and volarly, and both approaches must be utilized.

Dorsal Approaches

A dorsal approach is very useful when the facture has a dorsal angulation or when key fragments are located on the dorsal aspect of the distal radius. Nevertheless, the approach may be centered over different sites in order to facilitate expedient exposure with a minimum of soft tissue dissection. The dorsal approaches presented below are summarized in Table 20.2.

Approach between Third and Fourth Compartments (or between Second and Third Compartments)

Traditionally, the most utilitarian of these approaches develop a plane between the third and fourth dorsal compartments. This provides access to the entire dorsal aspect of the distal radius as well as to the carpus and is the most commonly used approach for the comminuted fractures that require open reduction. The skin incision is along a longitudinal line just ulnar to Lister's tubercle and aligned with the radial border of the third metacarpal. The proximal and distal extents are dictated by the fracture configuration and the fixation methods to be employed. With care taken to preserve superficial nerve branches of the radial and lateral antebrachial cutaneous nerves, the extensor retinaculum is revealed. An incision is then made either into the septum between the third and fourth compartments, attempting to avoid entering either compartment (this may reduce postoperative extensor tendon scarring), or, more commonly (because of the thinness of the septum), directly into the third compartment. The tendon of the extensor pollicis longus (EPL), when the third compartment is opened, is gently retracted radially away from the tubercle. With careful attention to the subperiosteal elevation, the third, second, and first compartments may also be raised as a group. The fourth compartment is then elevated subperiosteally from the radius, preserving its integrity.

We have recently modified this approach and now design the incision between the second and third compartments. The third compartment is opened along its radial border, and the EPL tendon is retracted radially. The subperiosteal elevation of the fourth compartment is then begun more radially than in the past, and it is hoped that this will provide additional protection to the extensor tendons in that compartment and thereby reduce further any chances of later tenosynovitis.

Small Hohmann or Bennett retractors may be placed radially and ulnarly to retract the soft tissues away from the radius. Unless the DRUJ is involved in the fracture, it is unnecessary to open its dorsal capsule. Hematoma and entrapped soft tissues are debrided from the fracture site(s), and all fracture beds are irrigated. Gentle manipulation with a curved elevator or a blunt awl can then free the compressed and displaced fragments. Often the radiocarpal joint can be visualized through the fragments as they are manipulated, and any loose fragments may be removed. If necessary, a transverse capsulotomy is made to improve visualization of the articular surface and the reduction. If desired, partial denervation of the wrist joint may be accomplished by performing a neurectomy of the terminal portion of the posterior interosseous nerve (PIN). The PIN is readily accessible along the radial floor of the fourth compartment via a small incision in the compartmental sheath.

Approach between First and Second Compartments

When a fracture of the radial styloid must be exposed, the incision should be longitudinal, overlying the plane

TABLE 20.2. DORSAL SURGICAL APPROACHES TO DISTAL RADIUS FRACTURES

Approach between	To fix
Compartments 1–2	Radial styloid
Compartments 2–3 (formerly 3—4)	Everything
Compartments 4–5	Die-punch
Compartments 5–6	DRUJ, ulnar head
Tendons ECU–FCU	Ulnar styloid, ulnar neck

DRUJ, distal radioulnar joint; ECU, extensor carpi ulnaris; FCU, flexor carpi ulnaris.

between the first and second dorsal compartments, radial to Lister's tubercle. Branches of the superficial and lateral antebrachial cutaneous nerves must be protected. The exposure involves subperiosteal elevation of the extensor compartments, which are then retracted away from the fracture site. If the exposure is carried more distally, then the deep (dorsal) branch of the radial artery must be preserved where it emerges from beneath the first compartment and crosses the floor of the anatomic snuff box. It may be at risk when the proximal carpal row is also exposed for repair of associated carpal fractures (e.g., the scaphoid) or ligamentous disruptions (e.g., the scapholunate interosseous ligament). The radial articular surface can be visualized through a transverse dorsal capsulotomy to confirm an anatomic reduction.

Approach between Fourth and Fifth Compartments

When an isolated dorsoulnar (die-punch) fragment involving the lunate fossa of the distal radius must be reduced through open means, the incision should be directed longitudinally over the septum between the fourth and fifth compartments. In addition to branches of the superficial radial nerve, there may be elements of the dorsal sensory branch of the ulnar nerve in this same territory, and they all must be preserved to prevent painful neuromas postoperatively. If the membrane between the two compartments cannot be split, then the fifth compartment is opened. While the tendon of the extensor digitorum quinti (EDQ) is retracted ulnarly and protected, the fourth compartment is elevated subperiosteally as much as necessary for adequate fracture exposure. A capsulotomy may be necessary to ensure anatomic reduction.

Approach between Fifth and Sixth Compartments

When the DRUJ must be exposed in order to reduce a fracture of either the sigmoid notch of the radius or the distal ulna itself, or if the TFCC is to be repaired, the approach is between the fifth and sixth compartments. This generally entails opening the sixth compartment and retracting the extensor carpi ulnaris (ECU) tendon ulnarward. Branches of the dorsal sensory portion of the ulnar nerve must be protected.

Approach between ECU and FCU Tendons

When the ulnar neck or the ulnar styloid is involved, an approach may be made between the ECU and the flexor carpi ulnaris (FCU), again with care taken to avoid injury to sensory elements of the ulnar nerve. This exposure will allow plating of the ulna as well as tension band repair of ulnar styloid fractures.

Volar Approach over the FCR

The most useful volar approach is initiated with an incision over the tendon of the flexor carpi radialis (FCR) beginning distally at the level of the wrist flexion crease (Fig. 20.9). The sheath of the FCR is exposed and then opened. By staying within the sheath and opening its dorsal surface, it is easy to avoid any injury to the radial artery. Once the dorsal sheath of the FCR is opened, then the muscle of the pronator quadratus is visible. Alternatively, the radial artery is identified radial to the FCR, carefully protected and preserved, and dissection continues in the plane between the two, exposing the pronator quadratus. This muscle is usually filled with considerable hematoma from the underlying fracture and from bleeding within the muscle itself. Blunt dissection reveals the radialmost edge of the pronator quadratus where it inserts into the radius. The insertion is incised sharply, and the pronator is then retracted ulnarly to expose the volar aspect of the radius. If the exposure must be extended more proximally, then the flexor pollicis longus muscle may be elevated from its radial attachment to the radius to avoid injury to the motor fibers of the anterior interosseous nerve that supply it from its ulnar side.

If the carpal tunnel is to be released in conjunction with this approach, there should be a separate incision made in line with the axis of the fourth ray that is not in continuity with the original incision, in order to avoid injury to the palmar cutaneous branch of the median nerve.

Extensile Volar Approach

If the DRUJ is involved and a more extensile volar approach is needed, then a curved incision is made over the distal volar forearm, which may be in continuity with a carpal tunnel incision in the palm. A plane is developed with the median nerve and the tendons of the flexor digitorum superficialis, flexor digitorum profundus, and flexor pollicis longus on the radial side and the ulnar nerve and artery on the ulnar side. As the structures that, more distally, will comprise the contents of the carpal tunnel are retracted radially, the pronator quadratus is revealed. If access only to the volar DRUJ is needed, then the distal portion of the pronator quadratus overlying the DRUJ may be incised. If a broad exposure of the entire volar aspect of the distal radius is needed, then the median nerve and flexor tendons may be retracted radially enough to incise the pronator quadratus at its radial border and elevate it ulnarly. Once the relevant portion of the radial surface is exposed, then debridement of hematoma and entrapped soft tissues, such as fibers of the pronator, may be accomplished. Manipulation of the fracture fragments and reduction are described below.

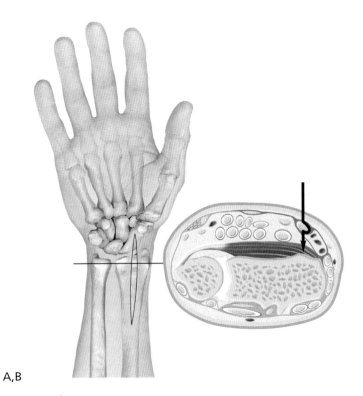
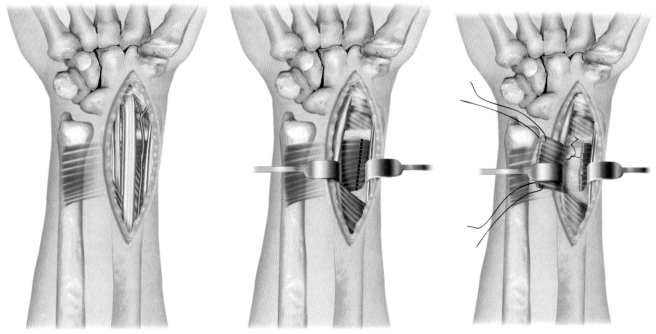

FIGURE 20.9. Standard volar exposure of the distal radius. **A:** The skin incision is located over the tendon of the flexor carpi radialis (FCR). **B:** Cross section of the approach through the FCR sheath to the pronator quadratus muscle. **C:** Exposure of the FCR. **D:** The FCR is retracted ulnarly by a retractor. The flexor pollicis longus tendon and muscle usually are similarly retracted and not visualized. Note the planned incision in the pronator quadratus *(dashed line)*. **E:** The incised pronator quadratus with tagging sutures being retracted ulnarly, exposing the distal radius fracture.

OPERATIVE TECHNIQUE

Bone Graft

There is frequently a defect in the metaphysis after restoration of the articular surface, with or without comminution of the dorsal (or volar) cortex. This occurs as a result of the compression of the cancellous bone of the metaphysis at the time of the injury. When the articular fragments are elevated and moved distally and reduced, there is a gap proximal to the subchondral surfaces and distal to the compacted metaphysis. This situation may lead to late settling of the articular reconstruction, particularly if there is cortical comminution as well. The best way to prevent this complication is by the liberal placement of an autogenous iliac crest cancellous bone graft.

This will not only diminish the tendency to collapse by virtue of the mechanical support but may speed healing and allow earlier removal of an adjunctive external fixator. The graft may be harvested either through a small 3- to 5-cm incision over the anterior iliac crest or with a trephine-type bone biopsy needle with a core of 4 to 5 mm. This procedure may be accomplished under local anesthesia if only a small amount of cancellous bone is necessary. If so, the surgeon should infiltrate both the anterior and posterior periosteum of the crest with an appropriate anesthetic, e.g., bupivacaine with epinephrine, in order to reduce postoperative pain.

Operative Tactics

In this section we discuss the specific approach that is most useful for each particular fracture pattern as defined by the Fernandez and Comprehensive Classifications (denoted within parentheses).

Fernandez Type I Bending Fractures (Compehensive Classification Type A)

Of all the distal radius fractures, the ones most likely to be amenable to nonoperative treatment fall within this category of extraarticular fractures, particularly the type A2 in the Comprehensive Classification. However, when there is significant metaphyseal (or diaphyseal) comminution or dorsal tilting, the reduced fracture is generally not stable, and reduction will often be lost during the first 2 or 3 weeks after treatment if only cast immobilization is used. These fractures can generally be treated without difficulty using either percutaneous pinning, an external fixator, or both. This is because the problem is rarely one of obtaining the initial reduction, which under regional anesthesia is straightforward, but of maintaining it. Loss of reduction can occur, creating a dorsal intercalated segmental instability pattern and subsequently requiring an osteotomy for correction (Fig. 20.10).

Fernandez Type II Shearing Fractures (Comprehensive Classification Type B)

If a radial styloid fracture (group B1) is nondisplaced and stable, it is possible to treat it with only plaster immobilization. However, because these fractures are usually unstable, it may be best to secure the fracture fragments in their anatomic locations with K-wires or (percutaneously placed) lag screws. The displaced radial styloid can sometimes be reduced by closed manipulation that includes distraction and ulnar deviation. When this fails, a limited open reduction may be performed via a small 1-cm incision made between the first and second compartments about 2 cm proximal to the fracture fragment. This location is selected with the help of the image intensifier. A blunt instrument (Freer elevator or awl) is inserted into the incision and manipulated distally toward the fracture site with fluroscopic guidance. It is then used to displace the radial styloid distally until the articular surface is restored radiographically. At this point, the styloid fragment is transfixed to the radial shaft using K-wires (inserted via an open technique). One wire (0.045 in. or 0.62 in.) should be parallel to the distal radial articular surce, and one should be angled proximally and ulnarly to secure the dorsoulnar radial cortex. At least two pins, and perhaps three, are needed. Alternatively, a lag screw may be placed using the same open percutaneous exposure to create an even more rigid fixation, and it may be supplemented by a K-wire to prevent subsequent rotation.

If a limited approach is inadequate to accomplish reduction, then the incision is extended and the fracture site exposed visually. Once hematoma and entrapped soft tissues are removed, the fracture is reduced under direct vision and secured with a pointed bone forceps. (Care must be utilized with any pointed instrument not to entrap or damage adjacent soft tissue structures.) The fixation can then be accomplished with K-wires and/or a lag screw as described above (Fig. 20.11).

The dorsal shearing fractures (group B2) are usually displaced and unstable, with an associated dorsal subluxation of the attached carpus. Because there is only a relatively thin layer of soft tissues (the extensor tendons, subcutaneous tissue, and skin) covering the dorsal radius, it is reasonable to attempt a closed reduction of the fracture by distraction and direct, distally oriented pressure over the fracture edge. If the reduction is accomplished, it must be secured at least with percutaneous pins, which should be applied using the techniques described earlier. Because of the inherent instability of these fractures, the application of an external fixator to protect the reduction of the fracture and the carpus should be considered. Such a fixator can usually be removed after 3 to 4 weeks, when the early stage of fracture healing is progressing.

If the reduction cannot be accomplished closed, then a limited open technique may be appropriate. The incision

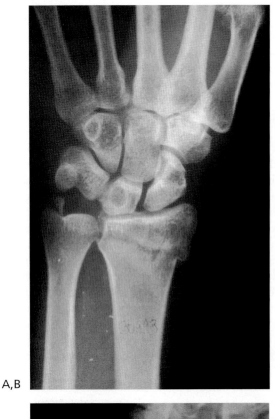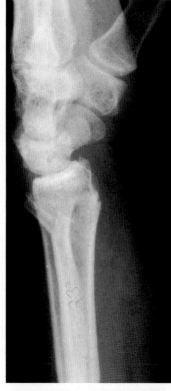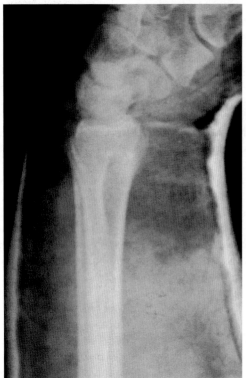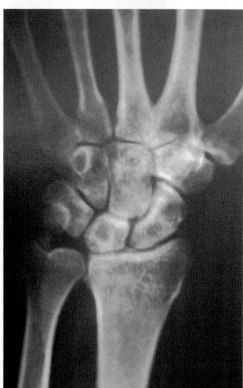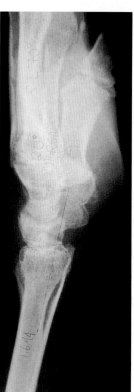

FIGURE 20.10. Example of a type I bending fracture (A3.2) that lost reduction. Posteroanterior **(A)** and lateral **(B)** radiographs of the distal radius of a 52-year-old woman who fell. There is 23° dorsal angulation of the distal fragment. **C:** Lateral view postreduction image shows the restoration of 4° of volar tilt. Posteroanterior **(D)** and lateral **(E)** radiographs 6 months following reduction demonstrate the healed dorsally angulated malunion and a scapholunate angle of 70°. At this point the recommended treatment was a distal radial osteotomy.

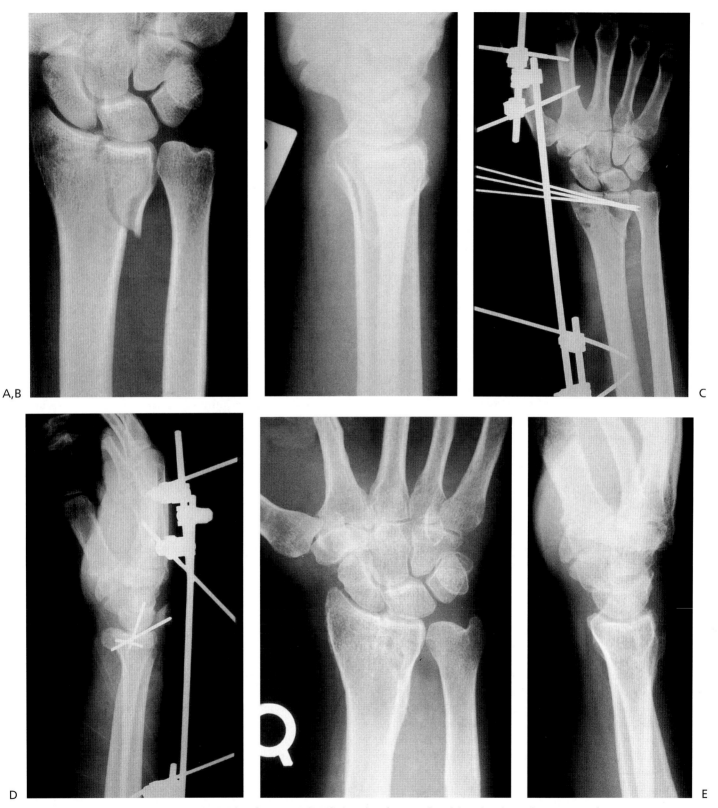

FIGURE 20.11. Example of a type II (B1.3) shearing fracture involving the dorsoulnar aspect of the distal radius. Posteroanterior **(A)** and lateral **(B)** radiographs of a fracture that was very unstable and could not be reduced by limited open reduction. The fracture was exposed via an incision over the septum between the fourth and fifth compartments and directly reduced. Three K-wires were inserted at varying angles through the radial styloid to stabilize the fragment **(C,D)**. The external fixator was maintained for 3 weeks postoperatively because of a lack of complete rigidity. **E:** Posteroanterior and lateral radiographs 6 months later, after healing.

selected should be a limited version of one of the standard approaches so that if a full open exposure is necessary, the same incision may be extended. In many cases a formal dorsal approach is required, either for profound instability or for comminution. In these cases the best fixation might be accomplished with a buttress plate. Depending on the size of the fracture fragments, the selected plate may be a 3.5-mm T- or L-plate, a smaller minifragment T- or L-plate, or another plate of appropriate design such as the π-plate (see later discussion). After reduction of the fragments and provisional fixation with K-wires sited so that they will not interfere with plate placement, any metaphyseal defect should be filled with a cancellous bone graft. In such a case, the distal row of holes of the plate may be secured to the reduced fragment to neutralize it and prevent subsequent settling.

The technique of plate placement involves contouring the selected implant so that the central portion of the plate will rest about 1 mm above the reduced dorsal radius. The distal edge of the plate should not protrude beyond the dorsal rim of the radius. A 21-gauge needle may be used to locate the edge by walking it along the dorsal radius and puncturing the dorsal capsule at its proximal edge. The most proximal screw is then inserted, followed by the second most proximal. As the latter is tightened, it will force the distal plate more volarward, thereby reducing and compressing the distal fragment. The reduction is examined radiographically or through a transverse dorsal capsulotomy. If it is inadequate, the second screw is removed, the fragments are rereduced, and the second screw is reapplied through a new drill hole. Once the reduction is confirmed, additional screws are placed, and if bone graft has been inserted to support the distal fragment, then neutralization screws may be placed in the distal holes of the plate.

The volar shearing fractures (group B3) are more common than the dorsal ones. Because they are almost always displaced and unstable, they are virtually never amenable to closed, or even percutaneous, treatment. The fracture should be approached formally with an incision oriented along the FCR tendon. After elevation of the pronator quadratus muscle, the fracture site is revealed, and debridement and reduction are performed. Placing a rolled towel under the dorsal aspect of the supinated wrist permits the extension and supination of the fracture to facilitate reduction. The joint space can often be visualized during this procedure by further displacement of the volar fragments, and this allows removal of any tiny free fragments that may be present in the joint. It also permits examination of the articular surfaces of the radius, scaphoid, and lunate for chondral defects. However, a transverse capsulotomy should not be made since this will disrupt the radiocarpal ligaments so necessary to normal wrist function. A small 5-mm longitudinal incision may be made between the ligamentous fibers for the insertion of an instrument such as a Freer elevator, and it may be used to palpate the articular surface. For further visualization, we perform a dorsal capsulotomy (through a small dorsal skin incision of 2 to 3 cm if a dorsal surgical approach was not utilized) as described above, and obtain radiographs intraoperatively.

Once the fragment is reduced, it may be secured in place provisionally (if the reduction is unstable) using K-wires that are placed peripherally to the borders of the planned implant, usually a buttressing 3.5-mm T-plate or a newer titanium buttress plate that uses smaller screws. It is important that the distal edge of the plate not extend beyond the volar articular rim of the distal radius because that could adversely affect flexion of the wrist. Direct palpation is an unreliable indicator, so it is useful to walk a 21-gauge needle distally along the volar cortex until it penetrates the volar capsule, thereby identifying the radiocarpal joint space. This will serve as a guide to the distal extent of the plate. If there is comminution of the volar cortex, or if there is a metaphyseal defect present after reduction, then autogenous iliac bone grafting is indicated.

Once an appropriate buttress plate has been selected, whether T-shaped or L-shaped, its contouring must be adjusted by judicious bending so that when it is placed against the provisionally reduced fracture, the plate will rest about 1 mm off the bone in its central portion. This permits more effective buttressing when the plate is secured proximally because as the proximal part of the plate is flattened against the stable proximal fragment, the distal end of the plate is forced dorsally and further reduces the fracture fragments (Fig. 20.12). The first screw to be placed is the proximalmost. Then the next most distal screw is inserted, and this flattens the plate against the volar cortex of the radius and secures the reduction. Once it is in place, the reduction is reexamined to be sure that it is satisfactory. This involves either radiographs or visualization through the dorsal capsulotomy. If the reduction is not adequate, then the second screw is removed. The fragment is remanipulated to establish the reduction, and the second screw is placed in a new drill hole. In most cases, there is no need to place screws in the distal fragment(s), but if there is a sagittal split of the distal fragment that creates instability, then while a bone forceps compresses the radial and ulnar fragments together, additional screws can be inserted into these fragments to neutralize them.

We have recently switched to a lower-profile titanium plate to replace the bulkier stainless steel implants available earlier. Although we advocate replacing the pronator quadratus over the plate and resuturing it in place, the bulk of the standard steel buttress plate and screws usually makes this a difficult goal to achieve. Although the thinner titanium implants alleviate this difficulty considerably, do not be surprised if a complete pronator closure cannot be accomplished. The tourniquet is released before closure, hemostasis is obtained, and closure is accomplished in layers. In most cases, a suction drain is left in place for 24 hours.

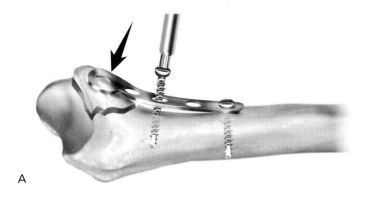
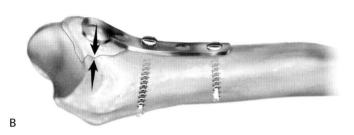
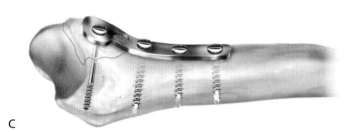

FIGURE 20.12. Technique of volar buttress plating. **A:** After placement of the first screw in the most proximal hole, there is a small preplanned gap between the plate and the radial cortex. As the second screw is tightened, the plate will be apposed to the radial surface. **B:** The plate is flush with the radius, and any gap in the reduction of the volar radial fragment(s) seen in **A** has been compresssed, thus completing the anatomic reduction. **C:** Additional screws have been placed in the longitudinal portion of the plate and in the crossing portion to neutralize a large fragment.

Fernandez Type III Compression Fractures (Comprehensive Classification Type C)

Fernandez type III fractures correspond to the Comprehensive Classification type C fractures. The C1 fractures have three parts, two of which are articular. (The third part is the remaining radius proximally.) The C2 fractures also have two articular fragments, with additional metaphyseal comminution. The C3 fractures have four or more parts, including at least three articular fragments.

The C1 fractures with two articular fragments are common and can usually be treated with a combination of K-wires, limited open reduction, compressing bone forceps, and provisional external fixation (Table 20.3). Among the most frequently seen is the subgroup C1.1, which contains as one of its components the die-punch fragment involving the dorsoulnar (dorsomedial) distal radius. Whereas traction-based ligamentotaxis will often reduce the major distal radius component containing the radial tyloid, the displaced die-punch fragment is difficult to reduce by closed means. A limited open reduction is very useful, although in the face of comminution, this technique is less effective and may even result in additional fragmentation of the displaced fragment.

When the major (or both) fragment(s) is reduced closed, an external fixator may be applied to maintain the reduction during percutaneous pinning and even to protect the fixation during the early postoperative period. To reduce the dorsoulnar fragment by limited open means, an incision about 1 cm long can be made over the fourth compartment, and then blunt dissection through the extensor tendons with an elevator or awl will allow placement of that instrument into the fracture site, as confirmed by fluoroscopy. Gentle manipulation and rotation of the instrument under fluoroscopic guidance can often dislodge such an impacted or displaced fragment. It is then manipulated distally until the articular surface is restored. Once the reduction of such an isolated fragment, or occasionally of two fragments, is accomplished, K-wire transfixion is performed as described earlier. The initial goal is to secure the distal radius fragment that contains the radial styloid to the radial shaft. This is

TABLE 20.3. SUMMARY OF OPERATIVE TACTICS FOR FERNANDEZ TYPE II FRACTURES

Group (Comprehensive Classification)	Techniques	Fixation	Bone Grafting
C1	Limited open, bone forceps	K wires	No
C2	Limited open, bone forceps (articular repair same as C1)	K wires, external fixation (plate)	Yes
C3	Open reduction (multiple articular fragments)	K wires, external fixation (plate)	Usually

usually accomplished with two K-wires that angle in a proximal and ulnar direction, about 45° to 60° from the axis of the radius, and penetrate the opposite radial cortex. Following this, two parallel transverse pins can secure the reduced die-punch fragment. These pins should pass just deep to the subchondral bone of the distal radius in order to provide adequate buttressing that will prevent collapse.

The subgroup C1.2 fractures can be treated in a similar fashion to C1.1, with closed reduction, provisional external fixation, and percutaneous pinning. When the sagittal T-fracture fragments are reduced closed, or by a limited open technique, they may be secured by (open) percutaneous pinning. If it is difficult to reduce the sagittal split, a pointed bone forceps may be used to compress the radial styloid component against the ulnar component of the distal radius. It is best to make a small stab incision and use blunt dissection to clear a path to the radial surfaces to avoid entrapment of neural or tendinous structures. The approach on the radial side is the same as that for the K-wire insertion, and the approach on the dorsoulnar side is over the fifth compartment. After applying the bone forceps, the reduction is examined radiographically. If satisfactory, K-wire fixation is performed.

The subgroup C1.3 fractures can be more difficult to manage, depending on the degree of displacement of the volar fragment. If it cannot be reduced by closed means, or if it does not include an accessible (subcutaneous) portion of the radial styloid, then an open volar approach may be required because application of a bone forceps to the volar fragment will endanger the adjacent soft tissue structures. For an isolated articular fragment that can be reduced and held with pointed bone forceps, satisfactory permanent fixation may occasionally be accomplished with K-wires that are inserted in a proximodorsal direction, through the dorsal cortex, and out through the dorsal skin if desired. They are left protruding about 1 mm from the volar cortex and should not cause irritation on that side. Lag screws are also appropriate for securing and compressing small fragments on the volar surface, and rarely would have to be removed. The most commonly utilized instrumentation on the volar side continues to be a buttress plate, and there are many fewer problems with soft tissue irritation on this side. The dorsal component, as well as the fixation of the articular complex to the proximal radius, can generally be managed as with C1.2 fractures.

The C2 fractures have articular patterns similar to those of C1. There are two articular fragments, with either sagittal or coronal splits in a T configuration. The increased difficulty derives from the metaphyseal and/or diaphyseal comminution. Thus, although the articular injury can be reconstructed using the same techniques as for C1 fractures, either external fixation (6–8 weeks) or plating, both with a supplemental bone graft, must be performed. This is necessary both to restore radial length and orientation, and to prevent postoperative settling of the articular reconstruction.

Because the comminution requires open exposure for placement of the autogenous cancellous bone graft, and because at least a limited open reduction may be necessary to reduce the articular components, it is usually best to treat these fractures from the outset with a formal open reduction. Unless there is a displaced volar fragment (C2.2), the approach will be dorsal. Once the appropriate exposure has been accomplished (see Surgical Approaches) under tourniquet control, the fracture sites and surrounding hematoma are visualized. Gentle debridement of the hematoma and irrigation with saline or lactated Ringer's solution is performed until the fracture edges are clearly revealed. A blunt elevator (e.g., Freer) may be used to manipulate gently the apposed fragments until they may be repositioned into anatomic position. During this portion of the procedure, the intraarticular fracture plane often may be separated enough to permit a rather clear view of a good portion of the articular surface and to allow evacuation of any loose fragments that may be trapped within the joint. As each fragment is reduced, it should be secured with K-wires, either provisionally or permanently. If the plan is to utilize a plate for permanent fixation, then the K-wires must be placed so that they do not interfere with plate placement. This can be done by positioning them a bit more peripherally than the margins of the planned plate, that is, placing them at the distal dorsal articular margin and aiming them proximally and volarly so that they penetrate the volar radial cortex proximal to the fracture site. The K-wires may also be placed from radial to ulnar and vice versa. Once the provisional fixation is completed, a transverse capsulotomy may be created in the dorsal capsule to provide visualization of the reduced articular surface. A blunt curved elevator may be inserted also to palpate the articular surface where it is out of sight for the presence of any residual stepoffs. If the reduction is unsatisfactory, then the involved K-wires should be extracted and the reduction reperformed. Do not forget that dorsally angulated fractures are usually supinated and require correction of the rotational deformity by pronation. (Volarly angulated fractures are usually pronated and may be reduced in part by supination.) If there is still a question as to adequacy of the reduction, radiographs should be obtained.

Once the provisional reduction and fixation are satisfactory, any necessary permanent implants are applied in cases where the K-wires are insufficient. Because of the frequency of extensor tenosynovitis after 3.5-mm plate application on the dorsal radial surface, we prefer not to use a dorsal plate of this type (whether a T-plate, L-plate, or DC plate) whenever possible. We use exclusively the newly available π-plate, which has a much lower profile, and thereby obviate the use of an external fixator, which delays postoperative wrist mobilization. Alternatively, if the K-wires maintain the anatomic reduction of the articular surface, then an external fixator may be used to maintain both radial length and any corrected angulation at the metaphyseal level. In the case of subgroup C2.3 fractures with diaphyseal involvement, external fixation may not prove stable enough, and a plate may be required.

The C3 fractures all have three or more articular components, and these fractures are rarely amenable to closed or limited open treatment. The open surgical approach is selected based on the direction of fragment displacement and therefore may be dorsal, volar, or combined. Once the surgical exposure is completed, the fracture site is prepared as described above for group C2. The fragments are debrided and manipulated with blunt instruments. The fracture planes may be separated to permit examination of the articular surfaces. The reconstruction begins with reduction and provisional (or permanent) K-wire fixation of the articular fragments. If a plate will be used (after considering the potential problems of tenosynovitis and weighing them against stability of the reconstruction), then the K-wires must be inserted outside the planned location of the plate to avoid interfering with its later placement. After fixation of the articular fragments, the articular surface is examined through a transverse dorsal capsulotomy and perhaps also by radiographs. Once any necessary corrections are made, any additional permanent fixation is placed. Small isolated fragments may be secured with lag screws (the diameter of the screw should be no more than one third of the diameter of the fragment to be secured), but larger comminuted regions may occasionally require plate fixation, both for neutralization and for buttressing.

The C3.1 fractures do not have metaphyseal or diaphyseal comminution; hence, they may be treated with K-wires to restore the joint surface and either additional K-wires to secure the distal construct to the proximal radial fragment or an external fixator to maintain length and position of the articular reconstruction (Table 20.4).

The C3.2 fractures likewise can have their articular components treated with K-wire fixation after an open reduction. However, because of the metaphyseal comminution, an external fixator will be required to maintain length. Bone graft should be applied to the metaphysis (Figs. 20.13 and 20.14).

TABLE 20.4. SUMMARY OF GROUP C3 OPERATIVE TACTICS

Fracture Subgroup	Fixation	Why
C3.1	K-wires (external fixation)	The reconstructed articular component can be secured to the metaphysis and diaphysis by K-wires
C3.2	K-wires (external fixation)	Metaphyseal comminution requires more than K-wires to secure articular component to diaphysis
C3.3	Plate	Diaphyseal comminution

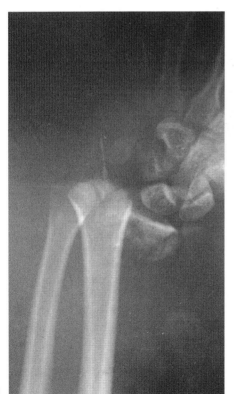
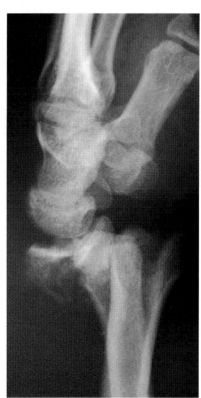
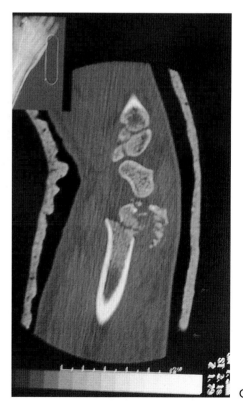

FIGURE 20.13. Example of a type III compression fracture (C3.2) treated with a dorsal buttress plate. Posteroanterior **(A)** and lateral **(B)** radiographs of the distal radius of a 20-year-old man who suffered a very high-energy vehicular injury to his dominant left wrist. There is complete dorsal and radial displacement of the comminuted fracture. **C:** Sagittal CT slice through the distal radius and scaphoid, when moving from right to left. The degree of metaphyseal comminution is much more apparent on this view than on the lateral plain film. *(continued on next page)*

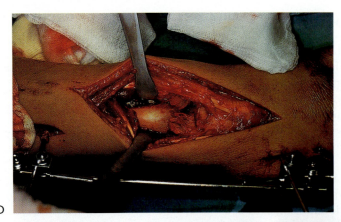

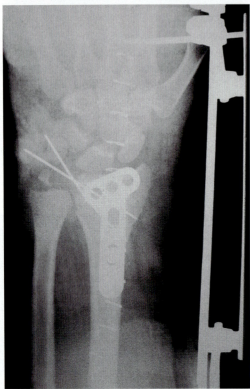

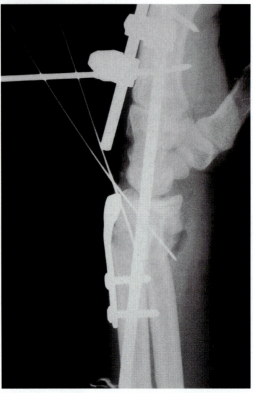

FIGURE 20.13. *(continued)* **D:** Clinical appearance of the dorsal radius after an exposure between the third and fourth compartments. The intraoperative external fixator is seen **(bottom),** and the metaphyseal comminution is seen distal to the white portion of the diaphysis. Posteroanterior **(E)** and lateral **(F)** radiographs after open reduction and placement of a dorsal buttress plate, K-wires, and a cancellous bone graft.

The C3.3 fractures involve additional diaphyseal comminution, and the extent of this factor may determine whether external fixation can provide adequate stability or if plating is necessary (Fig. 20.15).

Heretofore the plates available for fixation were bulky enough that it was not uncommon to have to remove them after fracture healing because of irritation of the overlying extensor tendons. Therefore, in many cases we elected to utilize the K-wires as permanent fixation devices because their profiles could be kept acceptably low and out of the way. Of course when significant dorsal buttressing was needed, there was no alternative to a contoured T- or L-plate. Now there are smaller titanium implants such as the π-plate, which was designed precisely for these situations (90) (Fig. 20.16).

The name of the plate derives from its shape, which resembles the Greek letter π. The plate has a limited contact design, and it sits around Lister's tubercle and permits both the securing of multiple fragments as well as buttressing against dorsal displacement. The four arms of the plate can each be shortened as necessary to accommodate a variety of fracture patterns, using 2.7-mm screws. The distal row of purchase holes is designed for the placement either of 2.4-mm screws or of secured 1.8 mm pins that give the plate many of the performance features of a blade plate. All screws and pins are recessed into the plate (Fig. 20.17). Because of its low profile, it is anticipated that there will be many fewer problems with postoperative extensor tenosynovitis.

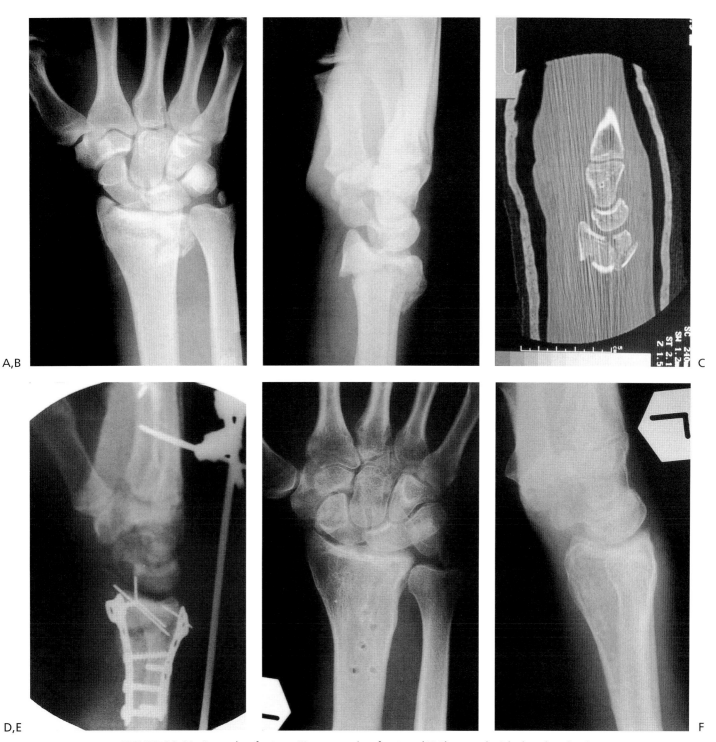

FIGURE 20.14. Example of a type III compression fracture (C3.2) treated with dorsal and volar buttress plates. Posteroanterior **(A)** and lateral **(B)** radiographs of the distal radius of a 20-year-old man who was involved in a high-energy vehicular accident and suffered this injury along with a perilunate fracture-dislocation of the opposite wrist and bilateral hemopneumothoraces. The lateral view **(B)** shows both dorsal and volar displacement of the distal radius fragments. **C:** Computed tomography slice showing, from bottom to top, the metaphyseal and intraarticular comminution of the distal radius, the lunate, the capitate, and the third metacarpal. **D:** Intraoperative fluoroscopic image (lateral view) demonstrates the intraoperative use of an external fixator, the dorsal and volar buttress plates, and K-wires used to reconstruct the isolated articular fragments. Iliac bone graft was also utilized. Posteroanterior **(E)** and lateral **(F)** views demonstrating the anatomic result 1 year after surgery, following removal of the hardware. (From Lipton HA, Wollstein R. Operative treatment of intraarticular distal radial fractures. *Clin Orthop* 1996;327: 110–124, with permission.)

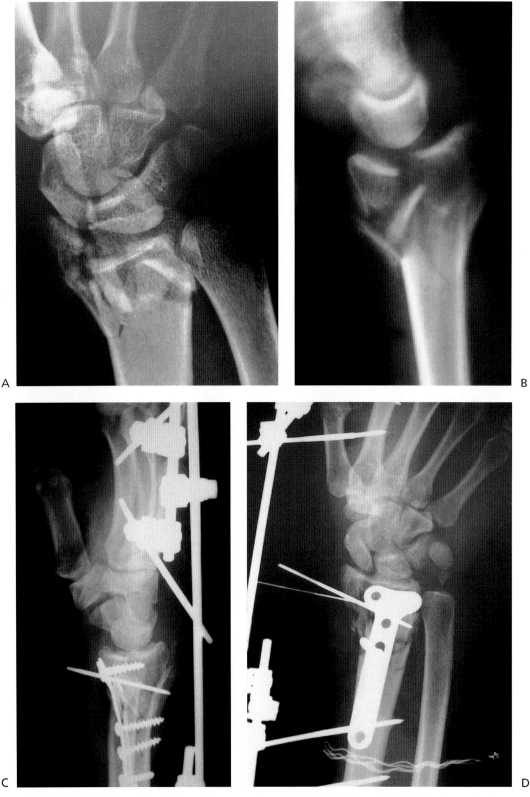

FIGURE 20.15. Example of a type III compression fracture (C3.3) treated with K-wires, a volar plate, bone graft, and an external fixator. **A:** Posteroanterior radiograph of the distal radius of a 35-year-old woman who fell from a standing position. Extreme articular comminution is seen. **B:** Lateral tomogram through the radius, lunate, and capitate highlights the articular disruption. Lateral **(C)** and anteroposterior **(D)** intraoperative views show the restoration of the articular surface; the volar plate, which buttresses and neutralizes a number of fragments; K-wires, used for isolated articular fragments; and the external fixator, which served as an intraoperative distractor and was continued for 5 weeks postoperatively because of the severe comminution. (From Lipton HA, Wollstein R. Operative treatment of intraarticular distal radial fractures. Clin Orthop 1996;327:110–124, with permission.)

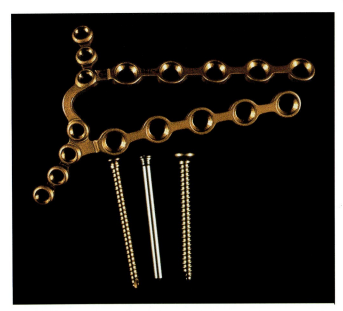

FIGURE 20.16. The π-plate. The four-limbed π-plate is oriented with the distal portion to the left and the radial portion to the bottom. Below the plate can be seen, from left to right, a 2.4-mm screw for insertion in the juxtaarticular band, a 1.8-mm pin, which secures to the juxtaarticular band via proximal threads for buttressing, and a 2.7-mm screw for insertion into one of the axial arms.

Fernandez Type IV Avulsion Fracture and Radiocarpal Dislocation

The Fernandez type IV injury is defined by a complete radiocarpal dislocation along with small avulsed fragments from the distal radius that remain attached to the intact radiocarpal ligaments. In the Comprehensive Classification, subgroup B2.3 addresses the dorsally directed injuries of this nature, but that classification system does not deal with the possible volarly or radially displaced fracture-dislocations. Although this entire category of injury is relatively rare in comparison to the other four Fernandez types, the dislocation component may be in any direction (Fig. 20.18).

Even in cases where the dislocation can be reduced by closed means, involving longitudinal traction and possibly rotation of the wrist and hand, we advocate an operative approach. The presenting deformity from the injury is usually so great that stretching, tearing, or occlusion of neurovascular structures is not uncommon. A dorsal fracture-dislocation, for example, might be associated with signs of median or ulnar nerve compromise, and arterial supply to the hand may be abnormal. Any of these conditions would necessitate exploration of those structures via an extensile volar approach. There may be signs of elevated compartmental pressures requiring fasciotomies. Furthermore, because the osseous component is comprised of small avulsed fragments of bone that may not be in continuity with each other, the site of the separation of the carpus from the residual radius is a combination of torn ligamentous insertions and osteochondral fracture beds. If the radiocarpal ligamentous mechanism (e.g., volar for the dorsal fracture-dislocations) is not repaired or reconstructed, then wrist function will be severely comprised by instability and/or subluxation later. To aid in all these aspects we begin by applying an external fixator to maintain gross alignment and mild distraction of the wrist. This will facilitate exposure of the capsular and ligamentous structures and permit

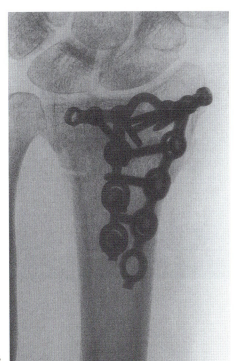
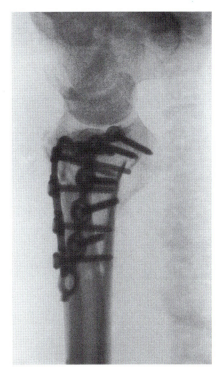

FIGURE 20.17. Clinical application of the π-plate. Posteroanterior **(A)** and lateral **(B)** views of a distal radius whose type III (group C3) fracture has been fixed with a π-plate.

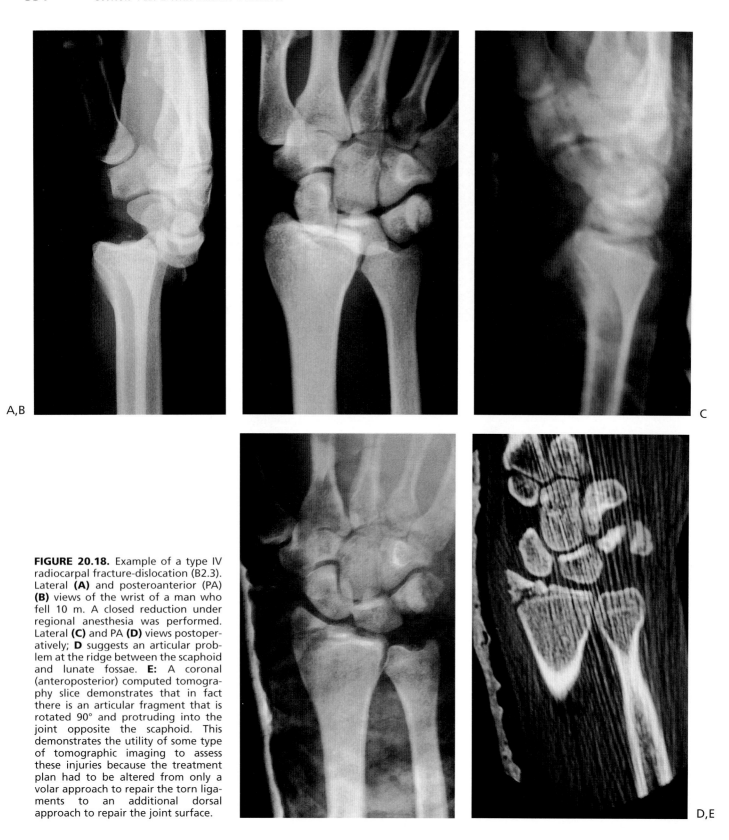

FIGURE 20.18. Example of a type IV radiocarpal fracture-dislocation (B2.3). Lateral **(A)** and posteroanterior (PA) **(B)** views of the wrist of a man who fell 10 m. A closed reduction under regional anesthesia was performed. Lateral **(C)** and PA **(D)** views postoperatively; **D** suggests an articular problem at the ridge between the scaphoid and lunate fossae. **E:** A coronal (anteroposterior) computed tomography slice demonstrates that in fact there is an articular fragment that is rotated 90° and protruding into the joint opposite the scaphoid. This demonstrates the utility of some type of tomographic imaging to assess these injuries because the treatment plan had to be altered from only a volar approach to repair the torn ligaments to an additional dorsal approach to repair the joint surface.

more complete visualization of the articular spaces through the rents in the ligamentous mechanism.

With an extensile volar approach, both the carpal and ulnar tunnels are released, and the median and ulnar nerves are explored. If there is a question of arterial injury, the ulnar artery is examined within the ulnar tunnel as well as distally to the superficial arch and proximally to a region of relatively uninjured investing tissues. The radial artery should also be explored if it is questionable. After the flexor tendons are retracted laterally, the disrupted volar capsular structures and the joint spaces are examined. Any hematoma or loose tissue is removed, and the carpal interosseous ligaments (scapholunate, lunatotriquetral) are inspected. If torn, these ligaments are repaired with intraosseous sutures, small suture anchors, or other appropriate means. Heavy nonabsorbable sutures are placed in the disrupted volar capsule in preparation for later repair. Attention is now directed to fixation of all reparable avulsion fragments, which should not be removed from their ligamentous attachments because the healing of an avulsion fracture may be more successful than reinsertion of an avulsed ligament. If the bony fragments are of adequate size, small lag screws may be used. Otherwise, K-wires and intraosseous wire sutures can stabilize these fragments. Once the osseous repair is complete, the capsular repair is finalized by tying the previously placed stay sutures through a residual cuff of soft tissue at their original attachments or through drill holes in the distal radius. Suture anchors may also prove useful in such circumstances.

If there are dorsal avulsion fractures, or if the dislocation was volarward, then the surgical approach is through an extensile dorsal incision. Occasionally the dorsal metaphysis is comminuted by impaction, and a buttress plate, supplemented by bone graft, may be required. Because of the gross instability that characterizes most of these injuries, fixation of ulnar styloid fractures and DRUJ instability may be necessary. The external fixator is generally left in place for 6 to 8 weeks in order to permit satisfactory healing of the ligamentous reconstructions.

Fernandez Type V Complex Fractures

These fractures are complex quite simply because they involve more than just the distal radius fracture. They do not correlate precisely with the Comprehensive Classification, although in general they reflect the C3.3 fracture pattern. They are made complex by any of a number of factors, both osseous and soft tissue. There may be a significant loss of bone and/or soft tissue, as with a gunshot injury or explosive blast. The distal radius fracture may be associated with a more extensive injury to the radius itself, including diaphyseal fractures, radial head fractures, and bipolar injuries. There may be adjacent carpal injuries, most commonly a fracture of the scaphoid (Fig. 20.19).

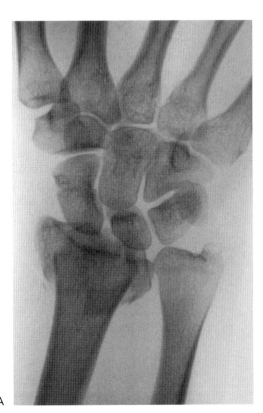 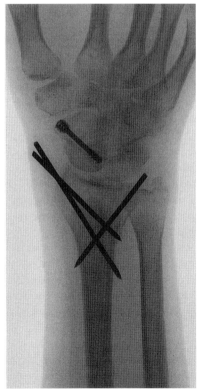

FIGURE 20.19. Example of a Fernandez type V complex fracture. **A:** Preoperative posteroanterior view of a comminuted intraarticular distal radius fracture (subgroup C1.2) with an associated scaphoid fracture. **B:** Postoperative view showing internal fixation of the scaphoid with a Herbert screw and of the distal radius with K-wires.

Because this category of injury is usually the result of very high energy, there is no limit to the extent of additional damage that may occur adjacent to the distal radius. The general paradigm for treatment remains the same, however. Soft tissue evaluation, including neurovascular and coverage problems, is paramount. Bony injuries that individually might not warrant operative intervention and internal fixation, when taken collectively, demand it. This is because of the greater propensity to displacement or inadequate porsitioning by nonoperative means when multiple levels are involved.

Postoperative Treatment

Finger, elbow, and shoulder motion exercises are begun immediately in all cases. Active finger extension and flexion are encouraged on awakening in the recovery room, and graduated formal elbow and shoulder activity is begun by the first postoperative day. Many cases fixed with percutaneous K-wires that are not protected with an external fixator (e.g., group C1) will have a sugar-tongs splint that restricts forearm rotation or a short arm volar wrist splint for the initial postoperative period, and therefore wrist motion is not begun during this period. At 2 weeks the sutures may be removed and immobilization continued with either a short arm or Muenster-type cast or with a well-molded thermoplastic splint. Care must be taken to avoid any pressure over protruding K-wires, and the casts must be windowed or the splints contoured to allow local pin care. At 5 to 6 weeks the cast (if present) may be removed, and active wrist exercises may be begun, using a removable thermoplastic splint between therapy sessions. The K-wires are generally removed at 7 to 8 weeks, as determined by the appearance of followup radiographs, which are obtained at 1, 2, 3, 6, and 8 weeks. The earliest postoperative films are to ensure that no loss of reduction or fixation has occurred, and the later ones are to assess bony healing.

When the articular fixation is rigid, and if the patient's condition permits, active wrist exercises may begin as early as 3 to 5 days after surgery. This situation may occur for many noncomminuted type B fractures as well as for group C1 and C2 fractures that have been fixed rigidly using an appropriate plate. In such circumstances a thermoplastic splint is used for support between therapy sessions.

If an external fixator is used either to protect the articular reconstruction or to maintain length in the case of metaphyseal comminution (e.g., groups C2 and C3), it usually may be removed at 3 to 4 weeks, or at 5 to 6 weeks, respectively. A removable thermoplastic splint is then applied, and wrist mobilization is begun in the time frames described above.

In cases of severe articular injury, continuous passive motion (CPM) devices have been helpful. When it is elected, there must be careful coordination between the surgical and hand therapy teams to ensure that no excessive forces are placed on the wrist.

Prevention of Complications

With compulsive attention to detail, many complications can be prevented. Thorough irrigation of the wound with copious amounts of saline or lactated Ringer's solution at several stages of the procedure, particularly just before closure, can help reduce the incidence of infection. Devices left protruding through the skin, such as K-wires or external fixator pins, should be dressed sterilely in a fashion that permits local pin care.

Swelling that may lead to a compressive neuropathy (e.g., acute carpal tunnel syndrome) or even to a compartment syndrome is always of concern when dealing with fractures of the distal radius. Hemostasis must be achieved thoroughly, and loupe magnification during operative dissection is very helpful in this regard, as is examining the wound after tourniquet release and before closure. Suction drains are appropriate in cases of severe comminution or soft tissue injury and in cases that require more complicated dissections, they are usually left in place for 24 to 48 hours. It is imperative that compressive dressings be avoided, and to this end it may be useful to use combinations of splints rather than fully circular casts as the initial rigid dressing. Close monitoring of any edema in the fingers or elsewhere in the extremity is necessary to ensure that the limb is being elevated appropriately and that the dressing has not become constrictive.

The incidence of reflex sympathetic dystrophy, or sympathetic-maintained pain, may be reduced by adhering to protocols that limit postoperative swelling and maximize early mobilization. Sympathetic blockade is effective should the syndrome appear. If there is any evidence of median nerve compression in patients who appear to be developing this complication, then electrodiagnostic testing and even carpal tunnel pressure measurements should be considered. If the findings confirm compression of the median nerve, surgical release is indicated (77).

Nonunions are quite unusual, but malunions may result if the reduction is inadequate or is subsequently lost but not diagnosed in a timely fashion. Although osteotomy can correct may cases of malunion, the surgical difficulty involved is usually much greater than that required to obtain the reduction initially.

The use of external fixation can lead to specific complications that may severely compromise the end result (47,91,92). Oversdistraction may encourage delayed or nonunion, and it may stretch the extensor tendons and limit finger flexion, producing a characteristic clawing of the fingers (37,91). The open technique of pin insertion is suggested as a way of minimizing injury to the adjacent nerves, vessels, and tendons.

Tendon injury may result either from the fracture itself or from the implants used to treat it. Ruptures of both flexor and extensor tendons may occur, and although the most commonly reported rupture associated with distal radius fractures is that of the EPL, even that is a relatively rare occurrence (4,77). Open exposure for placement of percutaneous K-wires and external fixator pins can prevent inadvertent skewering of nearby extensor tendons that may weaken them and lead to rupture.

Tenosynovitis, however, is not so unusual, especially involving the extensor tendons overlying a plate. This is one of the reasons to consider avoiding the use of a dorsal plate in fixing Fernandez type III (Comprehensive type C) fractures or to use a lower-profile plate that may produce less irritation of the overlying structures (77,90).

EDITORS' COMMENTS

Because of the unsatisfactory long-term results with articular fractures of the distal radius, the impetus for more acceptable articular alignment in all fractures has been significantly enhanced. The distal radius fractures have probably been at the forefront in demonstrating that a joint will not tolerate malalignment of articular segments without major loss of function. The segments of a comminuted articular fracture must be realigned with each other, and the entire surface must be aligned to the extremity. The former determines the life of the joint; the latter determines the ability to transfer loads. There is less and less place for percutaneous and partially open approaches in the treatment of distal fractures. The ideal surgical approach to comminuted fractures of the distal radius in our hands is a transverse incision, about a centimeter or two proximal to the articular surface of the radius. This dorsal incision allows retraction of the skin and visualization of the entire articular surface between extensor tendons.

It is important to visualize key support ligaments but to release less crucial ligaments as necessary for visualization, as a poorly aligned distal radius articular surface will soon have little use for ligament support. The extensor retinaculum is maintained for all compartments across the distal radius, just proximal to the articular surface. Proximal retraction of the incision allows direct visualization of fractures within the distal 6 cm of the radius. This incision allows a direct approach to die-punch fractures through the dorsal ulnar aspect of the radius. Radial styloid segments are easily dealt with as well. Central depression fractures can be elevated and either osteopore or autogenous bone graft added to support them. Pins running parallel to and immediately beneath the articular surface serve as support beams on which to rebuild comminuted articular surfaces. This approach in combination with an external fixator allows manipulation of multiple fragments of articular surface. There is the added advantage of an intact extensor retinaculum, usually at least 1 cm wide, just proximal to the articular surface. Because one can both directly visualize the articular surface through the joint and manipulate the fracture pieces within the radius, even difficult volar segments can be corrected through this dorsal approach. These fractures can be handled with an external fixator, multiple pinning, and bone-grafting techniques without the need for plates. Plates, though much improved recently (T, L, DC), add significant soft tissue insult. Some surgeons prefer them for volar fracture support.

Prolonged immobilization is seldom necessary. Usually at $4^1/_2$ weeks the external fixator may be removed and simple short arm splinting used for highly unstable fractures for an additional week or two. We have found that with pins and external fixation, osteopore or "coral bone" is successful. It fills space. It is not as strong in terms of physical support of fragments but rapidly incorporates and restores metaphyseal support. Maximum initial immobilization is important. Fragment "healing" is accomplished by 3 weeks, and sufficient strength is added by 6 weeks in difficult situations and by $4^1/_2$ weeks in more stable fractures.

REFERENCES

1. Alffram PA, Bauer GCH. Epidemiology of fractures of the forearm. A biomechanical investigation of bone strength. *J Bone Joint Surg Am* 1962;44:105–114.
2. Bengner U, Johnell O. Increasing incidence of forearm fractures. A comparison of epidemiologic patterns 25 years apart. *Acta Orthop Scand* 1985;56:158–160.
3. Altissimi M, Antenucci R, Fiacco C, et al. Longterm results of conservative treatment of fractures of the distal radius. *Clin Orthop* 1986;206:202.
4. Cooney WP III, Dobyns JH, Linscheid RL. Complications of Colles' fractures. *J Bone Joint Surg Am* 1980;62:613–618.
5. Frykman G. Fracture of the distal radius including sequelae: shoulder–hand–finger syndrome, disturbance in the distal radioulnar joint and impairment of nerve function. A clinical and experimental study. *Acta Orthop Scand [Suppl]* 1967;108:1–155.
6. Gartland JJ, Werley CW. Evaluation of healed Colles' fractures. *J Bone Joint Surg Am* 1951;33:895–907.
7. Golden GN. Treatment and prognosis of Colles' fracture. *Lancet* 1963;1:511–514.
8. Herndon JH. Distal radius fractures: Nonsurgical treatment options. *Instruct Course Lect* 1993;42:67–72.
9. Hollingsworth R, Morris J. The importance of the ulnar side of the wrist in fractures of the distal end of the radius. *Injury* 1976;7:263–266.
10. Kazuki K, Kusunoki M, Yamada J, et al. Cineradiographic study of wrist motion after fracture of the distal radius. *J Hand Surg [Am]* 1993;18:41–46.
11. Knirk JL, Jupiter JB. Intra-articular fractures of the distal end of the radius in young adults. *J Bone Joint Surg Am* 1986;68:647–659.
12. Kozin SH, Wood MB. Early soft-tissue complications after distal radius fractures. *Instruct Course Lect* 1993;42:89–98.
13. Kozin SH, Wood MB. Early soft-tissue complications after fractures of the distal part of the radius. *J Bone Joint Surg Am* 1993;75:144–153.

14. Seitz WH Jr. External fixation of distal radius fractures: Indications and technical principles. *Orthop Clin North Am* 1993;24:255–264.
15. Szabo RM. Comminuted distal radius fractures. *Orthop Clin North Am* 1992;23:1–6.
16. Short WH, Palmer AK, Werner FW, et al. A biomechanical study of distal radius fractures. *J Hand Surg [Am]* 1987;12:529–534.
17. Taleisnik J, Watson HK. Midcarpal instability caused by malunited fractures of the distal radius. *J Hand Surg [Am]* 1984;9:350–357.
18. Isani A, Melone CP Jr. Classification and management of intraarticular fractures of the distal radius. *Hand Clin* 1988;4:349–360.
19. Jupiter JB, Masem M. Reconstruction of post-traumatic deformity of the distal radius and ulna. *Hand Clin* 1988;4:377–390.
20. Sarmiento A, Pratt GW, Berry NC, et al. Colles fractures: Functional bracing in supination. *J Bone Joint Surg Am* 1975;57:311–317.
21. Sarmiento A, Zagorski JB, Sinclair WF. Functional bracing of Colles' fractures: A prospective study of immobilization in supination vs. pronation. *Clin Orthop* 1980;146:175–183.
22. Van Der Linden W, Ericson R. Colles' fracture: How should its displacement be measured and how should it be immobilized? *J Bone Joint Surg Am* 1981;63:1285–1291.
23. Weber ER. A rational approach for the recognition and treatment of Colles' fracture. *Hand Clin* 1987;3:13–21.
24. Zemel NP. The prevention and treatment of complications from fractures of the distal radius and ulna. *Hand Clin* 1987;3:1–11.
25. Ark J, Jupiter JB. The rationale for precise management of distal radius fractures. *Orthop Clin North Am* 1993;24:205–210.
26. Clancey GJ. Percutaneous Kirschner-wire fixation of Colles fractures. *J Bone Joint Surg Am* 1984;66:1008–1014.
27. Hastings H, Leibovic SJ. Indications and techniques of open reduction: Internal fixation of distal radius fractures. *Orthop Clin North Am* 1993;24:309–326.
28. Jupiter JB. Current concepts review: Fractures of the distal end of the radius. *J Bone Joint Surg Am* 1991;73:461–469.
29. Keating JF, Court-Brown CM, McQueen MM. Internal fixation of volar-displaced distal radius fractures. *J Bone Joint Surg Br* 1994;76:401–405.
30. Leibovic SJ, Geissler WB. Treatment of complex intra-articular distal radius fractures. *Orthop Clin North Am* 1994;25:685–706.
31. Louis DS. Barton's and Smith's fractures. *Hand Clin* 1988;4:399–402.
32. Melone CP Jr. Articular fractures of the distal radius. *Orthop Clin North Am* 1984;15:217–236.
33. Melone CP Jr. Open treatment for displaced articular fractures of the distal radius. *Clin Orthop* 1986;202:103–111.
34. Melone CP Jr. Distal radius fractures: Patterns of articular fragmentation. *Orthop Clin North Am* 1993;24:239–253.
35. Pattee GA, Thompson GH. Anterior and posterior marginal fracture-dislocations of the distal radius. *Clin Orthop* 1988;231:183–195.
36. Szabo RM, Weber SC. Comminuted intraarticular fractures of the distal radius. *Clin Orthop* 19;230:39–48.
37. Agee JM. External fixation: Technical advances based upon multiplanar ligamentotaxis. *Orthop Clin North Am* 1993;24:265–274.
38. Bishay M, Aguilera X, Grant J, et al. The results of external fixation of the radius in the treatment of comminuted intraarticular fractures of the distal end. *J Hand Surg [Br]* 1994;19:378–383.
39. Braun RM, Gellman H. Dorsal pin placement and external fixation for correction of dorsal tilt in fractures of the distal radius. *J Hand Surg [Am]* 1994;19:653–655.
40. Edwards GS. Intra-articular fractures of the distal part of the radius treated with the small AO external fixator. *J Bone Joint Surg Am* 1991;73:1241–1250.
41. Fernandez DL. Technique and results of external fixation of complex carpal injuries. *Hand Clin* 1993;4:625–637.
42. Jakim I, Pieterse HS, Sweet MBE. External fixation for intraarticular fractures of the distal radius. *J Bone Joint Surg Br* 1991;73:302–306.
43. Leung KS, Shen, WY, Tsang HK, et al. An effective treatment of comminuted fractures of the distal radius. *J Hand Surg [Am]* 1990;15:11–17.
44. Nakata RY, Chand Y, Matiko JD, Frykman GK, Wood VE. External fixators for wrist fractures: A biomechanical and clinical study. *J Hand Surg [Am]* 1985;10:845–851.
45. Putnam MD, Walsh TM IV. External fixation for open fractures of the upper extremity. *Hand Clin* 1993;4:613–623.
46. Raskin KB, Melone CP Jr. Unstable articular fractures of the distal radius: Comparative techniques of ligamentotaxis. *Orthop Clin North Am* 1993;24:275–286.
47. Sanders RA, Keppel FL, Waldrop JI. External fixation of distal radial fractures: Results and complications. *J Hand Surg [Am]* 1991;16:385–391.
48. Schuind F, Donkerwolcke M, Rasquin C, Burny F. External fixation of fractures of the distal radius: A study of 225 cases. *J Hand Surg [Am]* 1989;14:404–407.
49. Seitz WH Jr. Complications and problems in the management of distal radius fractures. *Hand Clin* 1994;10:117–123.
50. Seitz WH Jr, Putnam MD, Dick HM. Limited open surgical approach for external fixation of distal radius fractures. *J Hand Surg [Am]* 1990;15:288–293.
51. Simpson NS, Wilkinson R, Barbenel JC, Kinninmonth AW. External fixation of the distal radius: A biomechanical study. *J Hand Surg [Br]* 1994;19:188–192.
52. Suso S, Combalia A, Segur JM, et al. Comminuted intra-articular fractures of the distal end of the radius treated with the Hoffmann external fixator. *J Trauma* 1993;35:61–66.
53. Carrozzella J, Stern PJ. Treatment of comminuted distal radius fractures with pins and plaster. *Hand Clin* 1988;4:391–397.
54. Clyburn TA. Dynamic external fixation for comminuted intraarticular fractures of the distal end of the radius. *J Bone Joint Surg Am* 1987;69:248–254.
55. Cooney WP III, Linscheid RL, Dobyns JH. External pin fixation for unstable Colles' fractures. *J Bone Joint Surg Am* 1979;61:840–845.
56. Pennig DW. Dynamic external fixation of distal radius fractures. *Hand Clin* 1993;4:587–602.
57. Sommerkamp TG, Seeman M, Silliman J, et al. Dynamic external fixation of unstable fractures of the distal part of the radius: A prospective, randomized comparison with static external fixation. *J Bone Joint Surg Am* 1994;76:1149–1161.
58. Agee JM. Distal radius fractures: Multiplanar ligamentotaxis. *Hand Clin* 1993;4:577–585.
59. Bartosh RA, Saldana MJ. Intraarticular fractures of the distal radius: A cadaveric study to determine if ligamentotaxis restores radiopalmar tilt. *J Hand Surg [Am]* 1990;15:18–21.
60. Habernek H, Weinstabl R, Fialka C, et al. Unstable distal radius fractures treated by modified Kirschner wire pinning: anatomic considerations, technique, and results. *J Trauma* 1994;36:83–88.
61. Rayhack JM. The history and evolution of percutaneous pinning of displaced distal radius fractures. *Orthop Clin North Am* 1993;24:287–300.
62. Seitz WH Jr, Froimson AI, Leb R, et al. Augmented external fixation of unstable distal radius fractures. *J Hand Surg [Am]* 1991;16:1010–1016.
63. Axelrod T, Paley D, Green J, et al. Limited open reduction of the lunate facet in comminuted intra-articular fractures of the distal radius. *J Hand Surg [Am]* 1988;13:372–377.

64. Geissler WB, Fernandez DL. Percutaneous and limited open reduction of the articular surface of the distal radius. *J Orthop Trauma* 1991;5:255–264.
65. Axelrod TS, McMurtry RY. Open reduction and internal fixation of comminuted intraarticular fractures of the distal radius. *J Hand Surg [Am]* 1990;15:1–11.
66. Bradway JK, Amadio PC, Cooney WP. Open reduction and internal fixation of displaced, comminuted intra-articular fractures of the distal end of the radius. *J Bone Joint Surg Am* 1989; 71:839–847.
67. Fernandez DL, Geissler WB. Treatment of displaced articular fractures of the radius. *J Hand Surg [Am]* 1991;16:375–384.
68. Jupiter JB, Fernandez DL, Toh C-L, et al. Operative treatment of volar intra-articular fractures of the distal end of the radius. *J Bone Joint Surg Am* 1996;78:1817–1828.
69. Jupiter JB, Lipton HA. Operative treatment of intraarticular fractures of the distal radius. *Clin Orthop* 1993;292:48–61.
70. Missakian ML, Cooney WP, Amadio PC, et al. Open reduction and internal fixation for distal radius fractures. *J Hand Surg [Am]* 1992;17:745–755.
71. Trumble TE, Schmitt SR, Vedder NB. Factors affecting functional outcome of displaced intra-articular distal radius fractures. *J Hand Surg [Am]* 1994;19:325–340.
72. Aro HT, Koivunen T. Minor axial shortening of the radius affects outcome of Colles' fracture treatment. *J Hand Surg [Am]* 1991; 16:392–398.
73. Fernandez DL. Fractures of the distal radius: Operative treatment. *Instruct Course Lect* 1993;42:73–88.
74. Fernandez DL. Radial osteotomy and Bowers arthroplasty for malunited fractures of the distal end of the radius. *J Bone Joint Surg Am* 1988;70:1538–1551.
75. Linscheid RL. Kinematic considerations of the wrist. *Clin Orthop* 1986;202:27–39.
76. Posner MA, Ambrose L. Malunited Colles' fractures: Correction with a biplanar closing wedge osteotomy. *J Hand Surg [Am]* 1991; 16:1017–1026.
77. Fernandez DL, Jupiter JB. *Fractures of the distal radius. A practical approach to management.* New York: Springer-Verlag, 1996.
78. Johnston GHF, Friedman L, Kriegler JC. Computerized tomographic evaluation of acute distal radius fractures. *J Hand Surg [Am]* 1992;17:738–744.
79. Metz VM, Gilula LA. Imaging techniques for distal radius fractures and related injuries. *Orthop Clin North Am* 1993;24:217–228.
80. Pruitt DL, Gilula LA, Manske PR, et al. Computed tomography scanning with image reconstruction in evaluation of distal radius fractures. *J Hand Surg [Am]* 1994;19:720–727.
81. Friberg S, Lundstrom B. Radiographic measurements of the radiocarpal joint in normal adults. *Acta Radiol Diagn* 1976;17: 249.
82. Mann FA, Wilson AJ, Gilula LA. Radiographic evaluation of the wrist. What does the hand surgeon want to know? *Radiology* 1992;184:15–24.
83. Rubinovitch RM, Rennie WR. Colles fracture end results in relation to radiographic parameters. *Can J Surg* 1983;26:361.
84. DiBenedetto MR, Lubbers LM, Ruff ME, et al. Quantification of error in measurement of radial inclination angle and radiocarpal distance. *J Hand Surg [Am]* 1991;16:399–400.
85. Cooney WP, Agee JM, Hastings H, et al. Symposium: Management of intraarticular fractures of the distal radius. *Contemp Orthop* 1990;21:71–104.
86. Mueller ME, Nazarian S, Koch P. *AO classification of fractures.* Berlin: Springer-Verlag, 1987.
87. Mueller ME, Nazarian S, Koch P, et al. *The comprehensive classification of fractures of long bones.* New York: Springer, 1990.
88. Fernandez DL. Malunion of the distal radius: Current approach to management. *Instruct Course Lect* 1993;42:99–113.
89. Scheck M. Long-term follow-up of treatment of comminuted fractures of the distal end of the radius by transfixation with Kirschner wires and cast. *J Bone Joint Surg Am* 1962;44:337–351.
90. Ring D, Jupiter JB. Dorsal fixation of the distal radius using the π plate. *Atlas Hand Clin* 1997;2:25–44.
91. Kaempffe FA, Wheeler DR, Peimer CA, et al. Severe fractures of the distal radius: Effect of amount and duration of external fixator distraction on outcome. *J Hand Surg [Am]* 1993;18:33–41.
92. Weber SC, Szabo RM. Severely comminuted distal radial fracture as an unsolved problem: Complications associated with external fixation and pins and plaster techniques. *J Hand Surg [Am]* 1986;11:157–165.

RECONSTRUCTION OF SECONDARY CARPAL PROBLEMS FOLLOWING DISTAL RADIUS FRACTURE

BRIAN FINGADO
SCOTT W. WOLFE

Fractures of the distal radius represent one-sixth of all fractures evaluated in emergency rooms (1), occurring at a rate of 2.7 per 1,000 individuals per year (2). Colles treated distal radius fractures by reduction and application of tin splints and reported "perfect freedom in all [its] motions... completely exempt from pain" (3). This degree of success has not been echoed by modern literature. Cooney et al. reported complications following fracture of the distal radius as high as 31% (4). Persistent neuropathy was the most frequent complication, representing 25% of complications, with malunion and secondary carpal dysfunction close behind at 17% and 21%, respectively. The precise mechanism by which the latter complications manifest themselves is still a point of speculation and contention.

Secondary carpal dysfunction can arise directly from concomitant carpal ligament injury or indirectly from abnormal carpal posture or carpal mechanics that result from malunion.

PRIMARY CARPAL INSTABILITY ASSOCIATED WITH FRACTURES OF THE DISTAL RADIUS

Early writings on fractures of the distal radius suggested that the energy imparted by the injury was entirely dissipated by fracture of the bone, and the ligamentous structures were spared injury (5). Over the past three decades, a sizable body of literature has amassed to the contrary (4,6–19).

Retrospective reviews of initial injury films revealed that 0.9% to 30.6% of individuals met radiographic criteria for acute carpal instability following distal radius fracture

B. Fingado: Holy Cross Orthopaedics, Fort Lauderdale, Florida 33308.
S.W. Wolfe: Department of Orthopaedics, Yale University School of Medicine, and Department of Orthopaedics and Rehabilitation, Yale New Haven Hospital, New Haven, Connecticut 06520.

(4,10,13,18). Scapholunate diastasis and dorsal intercalated segment instability (DISI) were by far the most common patterns observed in these radiographic studies (4,6,10,12, 13,18). Instability patterns of volar intercalated segment instability (VISI) and ulnar carpal translocation were much less frequent. Somewhat disconcerting is the fact that for most of these studies, clear radiographic criteria for instability were present on initial injury films, and treatment of the fracture was rendered without regard for the associated ligamentous injury.

With the increased use of arthroscopy in assisting the treatment of fractures of the distal radius, reports of associated soft tissue injuries demonstrate a greater incidence than previously appreciated (20). In a report by Geissler et al., arthroscopic evaluation of 40 patients was performed when closed treatment failed to achieve adequate reduction; these authors observed tears of the triangular fibrocartilage complex (TFCC) in 43%, of the scapholunate interosseous ligament (SLIL) in 30%, and of the lunotriquetral interosseous ligament in 15% (11). Although these arthroscopic findings are somewhat alarming, they represent evaluation of only more severe fractures and those intraarticular fractures not amenable to closed reduction (11,15,16,20).

The mechanism of injury (a fall on the outstretched hand) was remarkably constant across those studies that reported it and did not vary for those fractures with and without associated ligament injury (6,7,9,12,13,18). Although there did not appear to be a disproportionate number of ligament injuries associated with higher-energy mechanisms such as motor vehicle collisions or falls from a significant height, several confounding variables make conclusions concerning exact mechanism of injury somewhat speculative. It is safe to conclude that regardless of injury mechanism, the amount of energy absorbed at the fracture site will directly parallel the degree of comminution and displacement, and the treating physician must be vigilant in recognition and treatment of associated ligament injuries.

Acute Associated Scapholunate Interosseous Ligament Injury

Diagnosis

Whether or not associated with a distal radius fracture, scapholunate dissociation is by far the most commonly reported acute carpal ligamentous injury in radiographic studies (4,6,9,10,13,18) and a close second to TFCC injuries in the arthroscopic literature (11,15,16). Complete or partial SLIL tears were visualized arthroscopically in as many as 44% of individuals with Frykman III to VIII fractures (16). These associated injuries are usually overlooked by plain radiographs because of the subtlety of initial presentation and the tendency to prioritize treatment of the acute fracture.

Although the SLIL has been demonstrated to have a failure strength nearly twice that of the radiocarpal ligaments (21,22), and elastic properties that permit 50% to 100% elongation before failure (21,22), the ultimate failure load of the SLIL is well within the energy imparted to the wrist in a fall on an outstretched hand. Scapholunate diastasis represented only the first stage in Mayfield's classification of perilunate instability and was demonstrated to arise from energy transmitted to the scapholunate joint with the wrist in an extended, ulnarly deviated position (23).

Complete scapholunate ligament disruption in the setting of acute distal radius fracture may be diagnosed by demonstrating scapholunate diastasis and/or increased lunate dorsal tilt on radiographs (Fig. 21.1). Neither complete nor partial tears can be ruled out on initial radiographs, however, as SLIL injury alone may be insufficient to cause acute carpal malalignment, and additional ligament attenuation and abnormal carpal posture may develop in the weeks and months following injury (10,24). A scapholunate ligament injury should be suspected in fractures associated with a markedly displaced radial styloid component or a deeply impacted lunate die-punch fragment. Diagnosis with a triple-injection arthrogram is somewhat impractical in the acute setting, and arthroscopic or open visualization of all involved structures is readily accomplished at the time of operative treatment of the fracture (20).

Leibovic and Geissler described a diagnostic classification system for arthroscopically assisted distal radial fracture treatment (14). In their scheme, grade I ligament injury shows attenuation or hemorrhage of the ligament as seen from the radiocarpal joint, but without incongruity of the carpal alignment seen in the midcarpal space. Grade II arthroscopic findings included attenuation or hemorrhage of the interosseous ligament as seen from the radiocarpal joint and incongruity or stepoff of the carpal space with a slight gap (less than the width of an arthroscopic probe) between carpal bones. The findings in a grade III injury include incongruity and stepoff of carpal alignment seen in both the radiocarpal and midcarpal space, so that a probe may be passed through the gap between carpal bones. The most severe injuries (grade IV) demonstrate incongruity of carpal alignment form both the radiocarpal and midcarpal views, with gross instability noted with manipulation and a gap sufficient to allow passage of a 2.7-mm arthroscope.

The natural history of untreated, or missed diagnosis, of scapholunate dissociation has been well described clinically

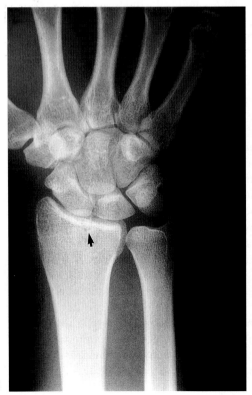
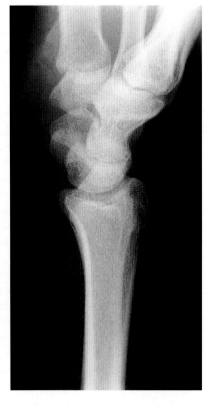

FIGURE 21.1. Radial styloid fracture. **A:** Nondisplaced radial styloid fracture exiting at scapholunate joint without evidence of increased scapholunate interval. **B:** Lateral view of the wrist reveals increased scapholunate angle, suggesting scapholunate interosseous ligament disruption.

A,B

and radiographically (25) (see Chapter 32). Ultimately, degenerative changes ensue, first at the radial styloid and subsequently at the radiocarpal and pancarpal joints [scapholunate advanced collapse (SLAC) wrist] (25).

Treatment

Management of simultaneous distal radius fracture and acute scapholunate ligament injury is predicated on the recognition of the ligament injury as well as the type and severity of the distal radius fracture. Successful management of either one is often contingent on the other. Nonanatomic alignment of the healed distal radius fracture may aggravate scapholunate instability or may result in secondary carpal instability (nondissociative DISI or dorsal carpal subluxation) and/or radiocarpal arthrosis (26–30). Conversely, the presence of a scapholunate ligament disruption may alter the planned management of the fracture, as certain positions of closed reduction or external fixation may exacerbate diastasis (23).

Whether the fracture is internally stabilized or neutralized with an external fixator, precise restoration of articular congruency and normal volar tilt is critical to decrease stress on the injured SLIL ligament and secondary stabilizers. One caveat should be reinforced with regard to external fixation of these injuries: the fixator must not be used with excessive distraction, as this may exacerbate diastasis and prolong or prevent healing of the ligament (6).

In preparing a treatment plan for combined ligamentous and bony injuries, the surgeon must define (a) whether the ligament injury is complete or partial, and (b) whether the ligament injury is acute or chronic. The latter is usually decided based on a history of a previous severe wrist injury or fall and a history of wrist clicking or pain with activities. In the absence of wide diastasis or lunate dorsal tilt, the extent and chronicity of an injury can be definitively determined by arthroscopy or direct visualization (31).

Closed reduction and cast management of simultaneous distal radius fracture and complete scapholunate dissociation has been reported by several authors (6,9,12,18), but with variable results. In the largest of these reports, Tang reported poor results from closed reduction and casting in 20 patients who demonstrated a 3.5-mm diastasis at the time of injury and lunate dorsal tilt (18). In follow-up of this group at 1 year, all demonstrated an increased scapholunate gap (3.8 ± 0.4 mm), none of the 20 had resumed regular employment or "normal use of the hand," 18 of the 20 demonstrated weakness of grip (60% of the contralateral hand), and all had limited range of motion. Eight of these same individuals went on to have surgical intervention, with all eight demonstrating complete disruption of both the SLIL and radioscapholunate ligament. Although overwhelming clinical evidence is lacking, closed reduction is likely counterproductive to the management of acute complete scapholunate ligament injury, as it tends to exacerbate scapholunate dissociation (23). In fact, without regard to distal radius fracture, Green proposed "that it is virtually impossible to consistently maintain a satisfactory reduction in a cast alone" in treating scapholunate dissociation (32).

Treatment of acute complete SLIL injuries in which adequate closed reduction is not possible, or those associated with marked lunate dorsal tilt, have been successfully addressed with open ligament repair and K-wire stabilization by many authors (29,32–40). Some have advocated augmentation of scapholunate ligament repair with a tendon graft (39,40), particularly if there are concerns about the integrity of the acute repair. Others have advocated a Blatt capsulodesis (41) to reinforce the ligament repair and to act as a check rein to limit scaphoid volar flexion (32,33,37,38).

Acute Associated Triangular Fibrocartilage Complex Injuries

Diagnosis

As noted earlier, injuries to the TFCC were the most common soft tissue injury reported during arthroscopic evaluation of intraarticular distal radius fractures, occurring in 43% to 55% of patients (11,15). In the report by Geissler et al., 47% were peripheral tears, 24% were central tears, and 29% avulsed from the radius (11). Actual instability of the distal radioulnar joint (DRUJ) was documented in fewer than half of the patients. Age-related perforations in the TFCC have been observed in approximately 50% of those between the ages of 40 and 60 and may be associated with rupture of the lunotriquetral ligament and chondromalacia of the ulnar head and lunate (42–44). These findings must be considered when evaluating the TFCC arthroscopically following an acute distal radius fracture in a mature patient.

The distal dorsal and palmar radioulnar ligaments, with their insertion into the base of the ulnar styloid, appear to be the structures imparting the greatest resistance to subluxation of the ulna (44–49). Additionally, proximal (or deep) portions of the radioulnar ligaments and the proximal portion of the DRUJ capsule contribute to the stability of the DRUJ (50,51). It should be noted that these more proximal radioulnar ligaments have a separate insertion into the foveal portion of the ulnar head, not the base of the ulnar styloid. The interosseous membrane, too, imparts some measure of stability to the DRUJ (50,52,53).

Ulnar styloid fractures have been noted by several authors to represent a potentially destabilizing injury to the DRUJ (50,54–59). This certainly follows from the fact that the primary stabilizing components of the TFCC, the distal dorsal and palmar radioulnar ligaments, insert at its base. Kleinman and others (50,60–62) have proposed that it is the location and displacement of the styloid fracture that should alert the treating physician to the possibility of a destabilizing injury. In particular, fractures through the proximal one-third of the styloid, representing disruption of the insertion of the distal radioulnar ligaments, are more likely to render the DRUJ unstable. In contrast, middle one-third and, even more so, distal one-third fractures of the ulnar styloid are much less likely to result in instability (50). The ulnar styloid fracture associated with a significantly displaced distal radius fracture (>20° dorsal angulation and 5 mm of shortening) is also strongly suggestive of a destabilizing TFCC avulsion fracture.

Treatment

Conservative management of nondestabilizing ulnar styloid fractures—closed reduction and immobilization (limitation of forearm rotation)—has been demonstrated to be sufficient (54). In the event these fractures progress to painful nonunion, their simple excision provides symptomatic relief without destabilizing the DRUJ (63,64).

Treatment of destabilizing injuries of the DRUJ in the face of distal radius fracture remains an area of debate. The practice of placing the DRUJ in extremes of pronation or supination for immobilization is now generally discouraged, as it may lead to motion-limiting contractures of the joint capsule (65). When operative intervention is indicated for the distal radius fracture, the stability of the DRUJ is generally assessed intraoperatively (50). Persistent instability may be treated by supplementing distal radial fixation with two 0.062-in. Kirschner wires across the DRUJ (50). More formal arthroscopic or open repair of the TFCC and/or ulnar styloid fracture at the time of distal radius fixation is advocated by some authors for instability (53,54). Clear clinical benefit to this added intervention is lacking (53,66), provided closed reduction and pinning provide a congruous joint and adequate fixation. Inability to achieve closed reduction necessitates arthroscopic evaluation and arthroscopic or open management (67). Instability following healed distal radius fracture may still be addressed with open reduction and internal fixation of the ulnar styloid fracture or arthroscopic or open reattachment of the TFCC up to 3 months out from injury (54).

Acute Associated Lunotriquetral Injuries

Diagnosis

As mentioned earlier, acute lunotriquetral ligament injury is less frequently seen with distal radius fracture than one of the TFCC or scapholunate ligament injuries. In those reports using plain radiographs for diagnosis, only two patients were demonstrated to have this combination of injuries (7,13). Partial or complete triquetrolunate ligament disruption was more commonly diagnosed with arthroscopic evaluation of intraarticular fractures, ranging from 7% to 24% in several studies (14–17). No clear distinction regarding ulnar variance and the possibility of preexisting tears was made in any of these studies. As pointed out in several biomechanical studies (68,69), additional disruption of the palmar arcuate ligament and/or the dorsal radiocarpal ligaments is necessary to produce VISI, and this pattern is seldom seen acutely.

Treatment

Management of these injuries is not unlike that of a combined scapholunate injury and distal radius fracture. Anatomic reduction of the articular surface and restoration of radial tilt and inclination are paramount to reduce stress on the injured capsular and interosseous ligaments. Restoration of neutral ulnar variance is critical to reduce stress on the lunotriquetral joint, and failure to adequately address this issue will likely lead to disappointing results (32,33,70). Injuries of the TFCC should be diagnosed and treated so as not to confound results of treatment of the lunotriquetral injury (32,33,38).

Partial or complete tears of the lunotriquetral ligament can be managed closed or by arthroscopically assisted debridement (partial) or pinning (complete) provided there is no associated volar instability (33,71,72). Because of the limited motion at the normal TL joint, some authors favor primary lunotriquetral arthrodesis (32,72–76). Complete tears with acute volar instability cannot be managed by lunotriquetral ligament repair or arthrodesis alone because of the associated midcarpal instability. When associated with a distal radius fracture, pinning of the malrotated carpus in the reduced position for 6 to 8 weeks is the preferred initial treatment. Should this initial management prove inadequate, direct ligament repair with reconstruction or imbrication of the dorsal radiotriquetral ligament and the volar space of Poirier is necessary to address all components of the injury (33,38,71). If limited intercarpal arthrodesis is deemed necessary, it should be done as a secondary procedure and will require a complete "four-corner" or CHTL fusion.

Authors' Preferred Treatment

The use of arthroscopy in acute treatment of distal radius fractures has focused our attention on a relatively high incidence of concomitant carpal ligament and TFCC injuries. Although profound disability may be expected from an untreated complete scapholunate ligament rupture, the need for primary treatment of each of these injuries has not been systematically investigated. Certainly many partial tears of interosseous and intracapsular ligaments will heal in the 6- to 8-week period of immobilization used for treatment of the fracture.

A high index of suspicion of serious ligament injury is warranted for fractures with a large radial styloid component, particularly when the fracture line exits at the scapholunate joint (Fig. 21.2). Similarly, lunate die-punch impaction injuries have resulted from transmission of high axial loads from the carpus to the lunate fossa, and the shear forces across the scapholunate joint may be sufficient to disrupt the interosseous ligament.

For those physiologically young patients with suspected interosseous ligament injuries, arthroscopic inspection is carried out within 5 to 7 days of the injury. Earlier intervention is not warranted, as clot and active bleeding will obscure adequate visualization of the ligamentous structures. If external fixation is to be used to neutralize the fracture, it is applied initially. The fixator can then be used to distract the radiocarpal joint for arthroscopy.

If abnormal motion of the carpus is diagnosed by manual manipulation, two percutaneous pins are driven across

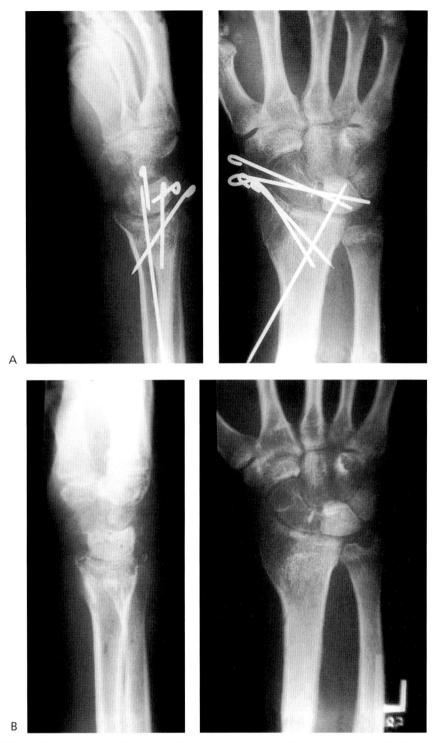

FIGURE 21.2. Radial styloid fracture. **A:** Patient at 6 weeks following closed reduction and pinning of a transstyloid perilunate fracture dislocation. Note early radioopacity of the lunate. **B:** Patient at 3 months following pinning. Note sclerotic changes of lunate, albeit without collapse or scapholunate diastasis.

the unstable joint under fluoroscopic guidance. The pins are left in place throughout the period of immobilization for the associated fracture (usually 6 weeks), and range-of-motion exercises are initiated. Gentle strengthening is begun at 8 weeks postinjury, and return to full activities generally allowed within 3 to 4 months postoperatively.

Complete tears of the SLIL with diastasis or associated lunate dorsal tilt are fortunately quite rare with these injuries. The injury should be treated with open reconstruction and transosseous reattachment of the ruptured ligament, using the technique described by Lavernia and Taleisnik (37). The ligament is usually avulsed from the scaphoid and reattached

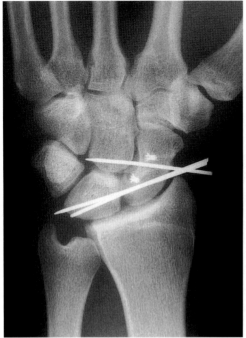 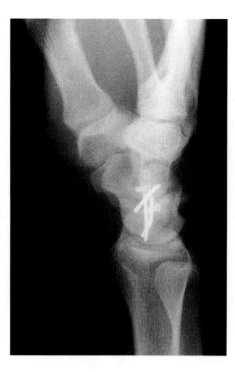

FIGURE 21.3. Repair of the scapholunate interosseous ligament (SLIL). **A:** Anteroposterior view of wrist following direct SLIL repair augmented with capsulodesis. Scapholunate joint is transfixed with two Kirschner wires for translational and rotational control. Transfixion of the scaphoid and capitate maintain capitolunate angle. **B:** Lateral view demonstrates reduced capitolunate and scapholunate joints.

into a bony trough. The important stout dorsal SLIL portion is replaced into position with a bone anchor, and the torn and attenuated dorsal capsule is imbricated at closure using bone anchors in the scaphoid or dorsal lip of the distal radius. Crossed Kirschner wires are introduced across the scapholunate and the scaphocapitate articulations (Fig. 21.3). The wires are removed at 8 weeks postoperatively, and gentle strengthening is begun at 12 weeks.

In the individual with chronic scapholunate dissociation and an acute distal radius fracture, the fracture is treated without regard for the chronic carpal changes, and reconstruction of the unstable carpus is addressed later as necessary.

Ulnar-sided ligamentous injuries are approached less aggressively. Complete lunotriquetral disruptions are pinned percutaneously for 4 to 6 weeks unless associated with a VISI deformity. Because the results for ligament reconstruction for acute or chronic VISI are mixed, no attempt is made to repair damaged structures operatively (74). The lunate is realigned and pinned in neutral position using a transstyloid or transcapitate 0.062-in. K-wire, and the lunatotriquetral joint is pinned with two parallel 0.045 K-wires for 6 weeks.

When treating combined transstyloid, perilunate injuries involving massive disruption of the intercarpal and intracapsular ligaments, palmar and dorsal approaches to the injured ligaments are recommended (77). An attempt is made to repair the important palmar radiocarpal and dorsal scapholunate disruptions, and multiple K-wires are introduced to stabilize the fractured and disrupted articulations (Fig. 21.2). The styloid wires are removed at 6 weeks when healing is evident, and intercarpal wires are sequentially removed at 8 weeks.

Ulnar styloid fractures are treated nonoperatively unless they are associated with distal radioulnar instability. Stability of the DRUJ is assessed at the conclusion of internal or external fixation, and, if unstable, the joint is pinned in supination using two 0.062 K-wires placed approximately 2 cm proximal to the DRUJ. No attempt is made acutely to

FIGURE 21.4. Arthroscopic repair of the triangular fibrocartilage complex (TFCC) following distal radius fracture. **A:** Arthroscopic view of the TFCC. The TFCC is detached from the ulnar styloid (US). **B:** Probe is used to evaluate the attachment of the TFCC to the radius (R); in this case, it is well attached. **C:** Arthroscopic repair of peripheral TFCC tears. 1, With the wrist distracted, establish arthroscopic portals to identify and trim the margins of the tear. Make a 1.5-cm incision over the extensor carpi ulnaris (ECU) tendon centered over the distal end of the ulna. 2, Insert the suture hook needle through the floor of the tendon sheath. Advance it from proximal to distal through the TFCC articular disc, 1–2 mm from the torn dorsal edge. 3, Insert the suture retriever through the floor of the ECU tendon sheath distal to the articular disc. Deploy the wire loop and place it over the needle tip; advance the suture into the joint. 4, Withdraw both instruments from the dorsal capsule, thereby delivering both suture ends outside the joint. Repeat this suturing procedure as necessary to span the tear. 5, Rotate the forearm to close the tear. Tie the sutures snugly over the floor of the ECU tendon sheath. (From Corso SJ, Savoie FH, Geissler WB, et al. Arthroscopic repair of peripheral avulsions of the triangular fibrocartilage of the wrist: a multicenter study. *Arthroscopy* 1997;13:78–84, with permission.) **D:** Nonabsorbable suture has been passed through the floor of the ECU sheath, grabbing the ulnarmost aspect of the TFCC. The suture is pulled taut, drawing the periphery of the TFCC to the base of the ulnar styloid.

repair the dorsal or palmar radioulnar ligaments. The TFCC avulsion, with or without associated ulnar styloid fracture, is insufficient to cause DRUJ instability without associated radioulnar ligament injury. If rigidly immobilized in the reduced position, the radioulnar ligaments can be expected to heal without the additional capsular scarring expected from surgical repair. Large peripheral tears of the TFCC may be managed arthroscopically with two or three percutaneous sutures tied through a limited incision in the extensor carpi ulnaris (ECU) sheath (Fig. 21.4). Flap or

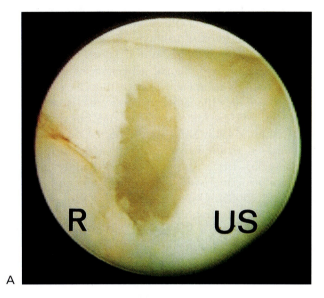

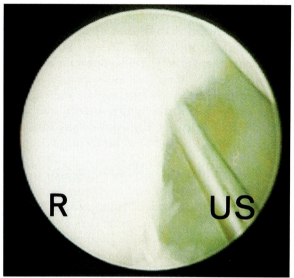

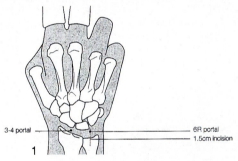

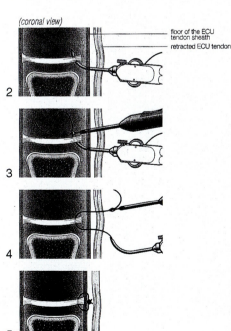

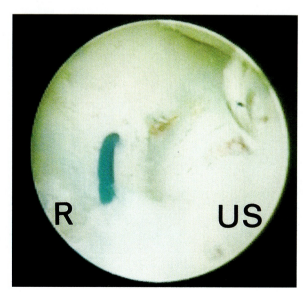

central tears of the triangular fibrocartilage are debrided to smooth edges.

SECONDARY CARPAL INSTABILITY ASSOCIATED WITH MALUNIONS OF THE DISTAL RADIUS

Normal carpal mechanics is dependent on the orientation of the articulating joint surfaces. Should orientation of one component change significantly, it follows that the mechanics of the joint must, by some increment, change as well. Secondary or compensatory changes may be imparted to neighboring joints distal to the injury site. Because malunion of distal radius fractures may involve more than one plane, alterations in normal joint mechanics may be multiplanar (Fig. 21.5).

Plain posteroanterior (PA) and lateral radiographs are the most common objective method used to evaluate the normal and abnormal alignment of the distal radius articular surface. Numerous descriptive radiographic parameters of the distal end of the radius have been described, most notably palmar tilt, radial inclination, and radial length (78–85). Palmar tilt refers to the orientation of the distal radius articular surface in the sagittal plane and is referenced by a line drawn perpendicular to the long axis of the radius. In normal individuals this averages 11° (range −2° to +28°) (86). The orientation of the distal radial articular surface in the coronal plane is referred to as radial inclination and is measured with respect to a reference line perpendicular to the long axis of the radius. This normally averages 23° (range 16°–30°) (86). Ulnar variance (or radial length) is a relative measurement of the most proximal aspect of the radial articular surface to the distal articular surface of the ulna and is usually neutral (−1.42 mm to +1.96 mm) (100) (Fig. 21.6).

There is considerable debate as to which components of distal radius fracture malunion are responsible for poor outcomes. As the articulations of the distal radius are many, so too become the potential generators of pain when these relationships are altered. Many authors have noted that it is often not only the radiocarpal joint that is affected by malunion, but the ulnocarpal and midcarpal joints as well (4,26,60,87–90). Some have reported that loss of normal radial length and radial inclination are most responsible for the pain, decreased strength, and diminished motion so often associated with malunion of fractures of the distal radius (79–85). Others contend that loss of the normal palmar tilt of the distal radius is the source of these symptoms (78). Although it would be convenient if one particular component of the malunion were responsible for poor outcomes, it would also be overly simplistic, as the surgeon is rarely faced with a malunion in a single plane.

For the purpose of discussion, we address each component of distal radius fracture malunion as it pertains to the carpus individually. With regard to treatment, however, the problems should be addressed simultaneously.

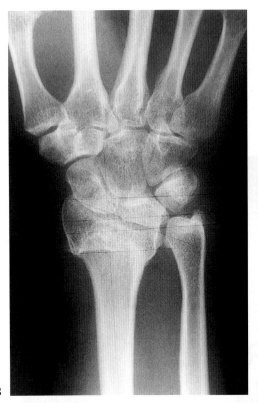
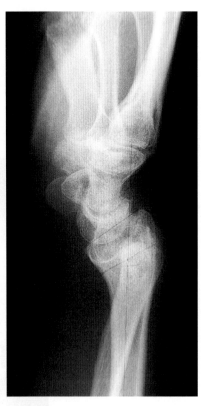

FIGURE 21.5. Pronation of the distal radial fragment with malunion. **A:** Anteroposterior view of malunited distal radius fracture. Loss of both radial length and inclination is seen. **B:** Lateral radiograph shows malunion with excessive palmar angulation.

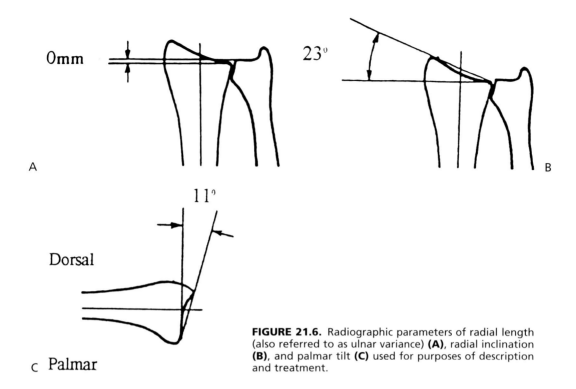

FIGURE 21.6. Radiographic parameters of radial length (also referred to as ulnar variance) **(A)**, radial inclination **(B)**, and palmar tilt **(C)** used for purposes of description and treatment.

Problems Associated with Loss of Normal Palmar Tilt

There is no consensus concerning the threshold for symptoms following dorsal malunion. Furrier et al. felt that symptoms begin to develop with 10° to 20° of dorsal angulation (90). Jenkins et al. did not demonstrate significant decreases in grip strength and endurance until at least 20° of dorsal angulation had occurred (88–90). Taleisnik and Watson observed symptomatic midcarpal instability between 10° and 30° of dorsal angulation (26). Dorsal subluxation of the entire carpus has been reported in individuals with much greater degree of dorsal angulation, on the order of 30° to 35° or more (92,93).

Instability Secondary to Malunion with Dorsal Angulation

Two different instability patterns have been attributed to malunion with significant dorsal angulation: adaptive or nondissociative DISI, and dorsal carpal subluxation. Instability can explain weakness, poor endurance to repetitive tasks, limited range of motion secondary to guarding, and reactive synovitis as is commonly seen in patients with dorsal malunion.

Midcarpal Instability

Compensatory, or adaptive realignment of the proximal carpal row (94) has been referred to as a "nondissociative" or CIND pattern of instability (94–96), and has been supported by the response of this malalignment to correction of the distal radius abnormality without directly addressing the intercarpal ligaments (27,92,97,98).

Taleisnik and Watson reported a group of patients who developed a dynamic instability of the midcarpal joint several months following a dorsally malunited distal radius fracture (26). These individuals could reproduce a characteristic painful and palpable snap in moving the wrist into ulnar deviation while the forearm was pronated. In full ulnar deviation, after voluntarily subluxation, lateral radiographs revealed that the normal palmar translation of the lunate had not occurred, and the longitudinal axis of the capitate had displaced dorsal to the long axis of the radius. An element of increased ligamentous laxity was thought to predispose certain individuals with dorsal malangulation to midcarpal subluxation. Complete resolution of symptoms was achieved by correction of the radial malunion.

Dorsal Carpal Subluxation

In a dorsal subluxation instability pattern, the collinear orientation of the capitate and lunate remains normal, but the orientation of the entire carpus becomes dorsal to the long axis of the radius. Watson and Castle (98) proposed a mechanism by which this deformity appears and progresses in the significantly dorsally angulated distal radius. The dorsal lip of the distal radius is normally a bony constraint to dorsal translation of the carpus and is effectively eliminated by severe loss of palmar tilt. With loss of normal palmar inclination, axial loads are directed away from the stronger palmar intracapsular ligaments and toward the weaker dorsal radiocarpal ligaments, which attenuate over time (98). The entire carpus subluxates dorsally from the radial articular surface, and ligamentous restraints are insufficient to prevent its progression (Fig. 21.7).

Problems Associated with Excessive Palmar Tilt

In palmar malangulation, the carpus adapts to the abnormally aligned articular surface by increasing lunate palmar angulation and capitolunate angle, thus effecting a nondissociative VISI pattern. The excessively palmarflexed distal radius also results in relative dorsal subluxation of the distal ulna (99). Consequently, patients tend to report limitation of dorsiflexion and supination.

Loading studies of excessive volar inclination show similar patterns to those seen with excessive dorsal tilt (60). It follows that excessive volarflexion malunion should also be considered a prearthritic condition.

Problems Associated with Loss of Radial Inclination

Because radial inclination is seldom seen in isolation, there are few studies reporting its specific role without a concomitant sagittal plane deformity or loss of radial length (79–83).

Limitation of ulnar deviation and loss of grip strength are common (89,100). The cosmetic defect of marked radial deviation is not inconsequential.

Loading studies (60) demonstrated only minimal changes in scaphoid and lunate contact areas with complete loss of radial inclination. This suggests that loss of radial inclination, in itself, poses little risk for early radiocarpal arthrosis.

Problems Associated with Loss of Radial Length

Many contend that radial shortening is the single most disabling component of distal radius fracture malunion (79–85). This likely represents more of an acknowledgment of the significant incidence of ulnar-sided wrist pain following loss of radial length. The role that radial shortening plays on radiocarpal or midcarpal kinematics is less well understood.

Load changes to the radius and ulna following minimal radial shortening are substantial. Palmer demonstrated that load to the ulna could be increased from 5% of the load across the wrist to 40% with a shift from −2 mm ulnar variance to +2.5 mm ulnar variance (i.e., radial shortening of 4.5 mm) (101). Positive ulnar variance is a known risk factor for degenerative and traumatic central tears of the triangular fibrocartilage (92). In contrast, scaphoid and lunate contacts were minimally affected by radial shortening.

Ulnar Impaction

Ulnar impaction is defined as abutment of the ulnar head against the structures of the TFCC and ulnar carpus. Persistent impaction results in degeneration of the TFCC, chondromalacia of the lunate or ulnar head, and attrition of the lunotriquetral ligament (102). Clinically this presents as

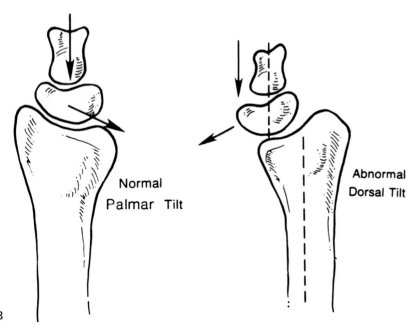

FIGURE 21.7. Dorsal carpal subluxation. **A:** Normal wrist. Dorsal lip acts as a block to dorsal subluxation of the carpus. **B:** Malunited wrist with dorsal angulation; bony impediment to dorsal subluxation is lost. (From Watson HK, Castle TH. Trapezoidal osteotomy of the distal radius for unacceptable articular angulation after Colles' fracture. *J Hand Surg [Am]* 1988;13:837–843, with permission.) **Editors' Notes:** *The main ligaments of the wrist are arranged to maintain the carpals upslope both dorsally and radially. With reversal of the normal volar tilt, there are no adequate upslope ligaments. The proximal row will flex and extend with radial and ulnar deviation, but normal downslope or volar migration, particularly in power grip, will not occur, displacing the capitate dorsally and setting up a cantilever situation with midcarpal overload.*

ulnar-sided wrist pain, particularly with rotational or ulnar deviation loading, and mechanical symptoms of clicking or crepitation localized to the TFCC (54). Characteristic radiographic findings are positive ulnar variance and occasionally sclerotic or cystic changes in the lunate or triquetrum. Anatomic studies have demonstrated changes in thickness of the TFCC articular disc that correlate directly with the degree of ulnar variance, and this may play a role in the threshold for symptomatic impaction in different individuals (103). The role of surgical intervention for this condition was first reported in 1941 by Milch (104), who developed an ulna-shortening osteotomy to prevent ulnocarpal contact.

Distal Radioulnar Joint Arthrosis

Degeneration of the DRUJ can result from persistent traumatic intraarticular incongruity and/or instability of the radioulnar joint (30). Clinical examination may help to localize crepitation to the DRUJ, particularly with compression of the radius and ulna in the forearm (102). Radiographs may show sclerosis or incongruity of the sigmoid notch. Significant arthritis of the joint would require joint resection or arthrodesis at the time of correction of the radial malunion.

TREATMENT OF THE SYMPTOMATIC DISTAL RADIUS MALUNION

Attempt at conservative management is warranted in low-demand or older individuals regardless of radiographic parameters (98). Physical therapy may adequately address issues of weakness and decreased range of motion.

Surgical Indications

Indications for surgical correction of the radial deformity in the physiologically young and active patient include significant loss of forearm rotation, radiocarpal pain or instability, ulnar-sided pain from impaction or DRUJ arthrosis, and persistent weakness secondary to abnormal carpal mechanics (93). McMurtry et al. detailed additional indications, including pain and disability for a minimum of 1 year, articular incongruity of more than 3 mm, dorsal tilt exceeding 20°, and radial shortening of more than 3 mm (105). The radiographic parameters outlined by McMurtry et al. lack consensus in the literature, with some authors noting symptoms associated with as little as 10° of dorsal angulation (26,106). Several studies have demonstrated that up to 5 mm of shortening is often well tolerated without other deformity (56,60,87,99). Knirk and Jupiter reported late radiocarpal arthrosis in 95% of patients with intraarticular incongruity of 2 mm or more (30). Many authors now advocate earlier intervention, citing less arduous surgery and less long-term disability (97,107). Fernandez suggests that surgery be performed when soft tissues have recovered from the initial injury and maximum benefit from physical therapy for range of motion has been achieved (92).

Contraindications to surgery include deficient bone stock, local infection, poor compliance, advanced age, poor systemic health, excessive apprehension, "illness behaviors," motivation by secondary gain, advanced degenerative changes in the radiocarpal or intercarpal joints, or fixed carpal malalignments (92,105).

Appreciation for and attention to the ulnar side of the wrist in malunions of the distal radius are imperative. Several series of distal radial malunions and their treatment report the need to perform an ulnar-sided procedure in upward of 50% of patients (92,97–99,108). Three conditions are commonly recognized with malunion of the distal radius: ulnar impaction, instability of the DRUJ, and arthrosis of the DRUJ.

Surgical Techniques

As follows with most complex problems in orthopedics, a plethora of solutions have been offered to address the malunited distal radius. The principles, however, are held in common: restoration of palmar tilt and radial inclination with attention to relative ulnar length and the reconstruction of the DRUJ.

The Radial Side

Closing Wedge Osteotomy

Dorsal tilt and radial inclination may be addressed simultaneously through a "biplanar" resection of dorsal and ulnar metaphyseal bone of the radius (93). The problem of relative ulnar length (radial shortening), which would be compounded by this technique, is treated with primary distal ulnar resection. This is controversial, as several authors cite loss of ulnar support and grip strength following distal ulnar resection in the younger active patient (97,99,103,109,110). An attractive feature of this technique is its lack of need for bone graft.

Technique

Correction of the abnormal dorsal angulation and loss of radial inclination are approached via a lateral incision carried down to the periosteum through the first dorsal compartment. Subperiosteal dissection is performed to facilitate placement of two volar-to-dorsal Kirschner wires: one perpendicular to the long axis of the radius and the second distal at an angle slightly greater than the measured angle of dorsal malunion. Using the Kirschner wires as guides, a volar-ulnar wedge of bone is resected. The exact amount of bone was determined by preoperative PA and lateral radiographs such that both palmar tilt and radial inclination are restored with reapproximation of the cut surfaces. Osteotomy is secured with two or three Kirschner wires.

Because the radius had been shortened, a distal ulnar procedure became necessary. The authors of this technique performed primary resection to the level of the distal radial flare via incision following the course of the ECU tendon. The distal ulna is then stabilized with a flap of the extensor retinaculum.

Postoperatively, the wrist is immobilized in slight extension. Finger motion is begun immediately with wrist motion beginning at the time of radiographic healing.

Opening Wedge Osteotomy

The principle of opening wedge osteotomy has been described since the early 1930s (111–113) as a treatment alternative to the Darrach (114) procedure for malunited distal radius fractures. Since these early reports, clinical support has continued to amass in the literature (87,92,97,98,108,115–118). The rationale behind opening wedge osteotomy is that all three deformities (loss of palmar tilt, loss of radial inclination, and loss of radial length) may be addressed simultaneously. Several authors have shown convincingly that opening wedge osteotomy can restore sufficient length to relieve the symptomatic ulnocarpal impaction in all but the most severely shortened malunions (>10 mm–12 mm) (97,108).

In Fernandez' review of 20 patients with dorsal malunion treated with opening wedge osteotomy, iliac crest bone grafting, and T-buttress plating, clinical improvement was significant at an average follow-up of 3.6 years (87). Palmar tilt was improved from an average of −34° (range −22° to −55°) preoperatively to −5° to +7° postoperatively. Radial inclination and radial length demonstrated notable improvements of an average of approximately +7° and increased length, averaging nearly 7 mm, respectively. Motion also demonstrated improvement in the dorsiflexion and palmarflexion arc to near that of the contralateral wrist. Preoperative pronation and supination were noted by the author to be particularly restricted in patients with radial shortening greater than 12 mm. Nine of 10 of these patients had normal pronation and supination at follow-up. Grip strength also improved greatly after osteotomy, increasing from 40% to 83% of that of the contralateral wrist after surgery in those with extraarticular fractures. Those patients who failed to improve, 5 of 20, had unrecognized carpal collapse, residual ulna subluxation, or early carpal arthrosis. The authors concluded that the patient most likely to benefit from this procedure is the younger high-demand patient with an extraarticular dorsally angulated malunion who has regained 70% of wrist motion and has no degenerative changes of the radiocarpal joints.

Ladd and Huene treated six patients with extraarticular fractures that healed with symptomatic dorsal angulation who were treated with slight modifications to the Fernandez technique (97). Their results echo those reported by Fernandez, with significant improvements in radial inclination (average of 16°) and palmar tilt (average of 24°). These authors did not report dramatic improvements in radial length, averaging 2 mm. The Mayo Clinic wrist score (119) for these patients averaged 85 or greater for this group of patients at a minimum follow-up of 1 year.

Brown and Bell treated seven individuals with dorsally angulated malunion of the distal radius with dorsal opening wedge osteotomy similar to that of Fernandez and reported significant improvements in both motion and pain scores (108). These authors corrected palmar tilt an average of 33° and suggest that the amount of correction may have as significant an influence on clinical outcome as the absolute value of final palmar tilt.

Fernandez reviewed five patients with palmarly angulated malunions treated with palmar opening wedge osteotomy, iliac crest bone grafting, and T-buttress plating followed for a minimum of 2 years (87). Palmar tilt averaged 32° (range 20°–40°), with loss of radial inclination averaging 5.6° (range 0°–10°) and loss of radial length averaging 8 mm (range 3 mm–15 mm) preoperatively. Clinical evaluation showed dorsiflexion, supination, and grip strength to be most profoundly affected. Follow-up showed significant improvement in all parameters. A Darrach procedure was required on the two patients with the most limited supination. Radiographically all were restored to a more normal palmar tilt (average +5.2°, range 0° to +9°). Osteotomy restored normal DRUJ congruity in three of five wrists.

Brown and Bell reported on four patients treated with palmar opening wedge osteotomy and bone grafting with 20-month average follow-up (108). Radiographic results were reported, with significant improvement in palmar angulation to a more anatomic average of +10° (range +5°–18°); however, all other parameters were grouped with those of the dorsally angulated malunions.

Dorsal Malunion

Technique

The preoperative plan for needed correction is based on anteroposterior (AP) and lateral x-rays with the forearm in neutral rotation to facilitate accurate measurement of all three radiographic parameters. Necessity for an ulnar procedure should be anticipated (see section on distal ulnar procedures below) and planned accordingly.

Approach to the dorsally angulated malunion of the distal radius is made through a dorsal 7 cm incision centered over Lister's tubercle. Deep dissection is carried through the extensor retinaculum in the third dorsal compartment. Subperiosteal reflection of the remaining dorsal compartments is performed. If a 3.5-mm T-plate is planned for fixation, Lister's tubercle is removed with an osteotome to allow the plate to sit flush. If fixation with Kirschner wires or a 2.7-mm condylar plate is planned, Lister's tubercle may be preserved (92).

The osteotomy site should be planned at approximately 2.5 cm from the joint surface to permit sufficient distal bone for screw purchase. Two stout Kirschner wires are then placed in a dorsal-to-palmar direction: one approximately 4 cm proximal to joint surface perpendicular to the long axis of the radius and a second distal to the planned osteotomy site at an angle 5° in excess of the measured abnormal dorsal angulation in the sagittal plane. Proper placement of this distal wire can be made easier by inserting a fine Kirschner wire by hand through the dorsal joint capsule to mark the angulation of the distal articular surface. Osteotomy is then performed in a plane parallel to the joint line with an oscillating saw or osteotome with care not to disrupt the palmar periosteum. The osteotomy site is then opened by distracting the Kirschner wires until they are parallel, thus recreating the desired 5° to 10° of palmar tilt. These wires may then be temporarily fixed by employing a small external fixator bar. The additional distraction usually required on the radial side of the osteotomy to restore radial inclination can be accomplished with a lamina spreader or by introduction of another Kirschner wire in the distal fragment to act as a joystick. Because there is often a supination component to the distal fragment with malunion, the additional distal wire may help to facilitate derotation as well.

Corticocancellous bone graft is harvested from the iliac crest and fashioned to exactly fit the newly created defect. The shape of this graft is that of a trapezoid when viewed from the cortical surface, as the defect created is greater on the radial aspect of the osteotomy than on the ulnar aspect. Viewed from the side, the graft appears as a triangle. If it has been determined that indications exist for distal ulna excision, the distal ulna may be substituted for iliac crest as the graft material.

Once matched to the defect, the graft is inserted and secured with a 3.5-mm T-plate. It is important to precontour the plate to the bone surface such that it does not apply an additional volar translatory force to the distal fragment. Initially, the plate is affixed with two proximal and two distal screws and stability is assessed. If the complex remains unstable, an additional screw is added proximally and distally. Should this fail to achieve the desired level of rigidity, an oblique lag screw may be placed through the radial styloid through the graft to the proximal fragment.

A slip of the extensor retinaculum is then threaded under the extensor tendons and secured over the plate to help prevent irritation or wear by the plate. The remainder of the extensor retinaculum is then reapproximated (Z-lengthening may be required).

The postoperative course must be tailored to the individual patient. In general, immobilization is maintained until the skin and soft tissues have healed (approximately 2 weeks), at which time active exercises are begun under supervision. Lifting is begun when radiographic healing is confirmed, with return to manual work generally by 8 to 10 weeks. Fernandez routinely removes the dorsal plate at 3 months after surgery (103).

Palmar Malunion

Technique

A 7-cm incision is made and deepened in the interval between flexor carpi radialis and the radial artery. The pronator quadratus is reflected ulnarly in a subperiosteal flap, exposing the malunion. A diaphyseal Kirschner wire is placed perpendicular to the long axis of the radius, well proximal to the osteotomy site. A second pin is placed distal to the planned osteotomy at an angle offset 10° from the articular surface to compensate for normal palmar angulation. Osteotomy is completed parallel to the distal pin such that the dorsal periosteum is not disrupted. Wires are then distracted until the sagittal plane is corrected. The radial aspect is then further distracted (again with a lamina spreader or an additional wire) to recreate radial inclination as necessary. Corticocancellous graft is harvested from the iliac crest and fashioned for an exact fit.

The graft is placed and secured with a volar precontoured 3.5-mm T-buttress plate. Palmarly angulated malunions are noted to have a high incidence of pronation deformity to the distal fragment that must be simultaneously corrected. The postoperative course is identical to that of a dorsal opening wedge osteotomy.

Trapezoidal Osteotomy

Watson and Castle describe the use of a locally harvested (dorsal distal radius), trapezoidally shaped corticocancellous bone graft in conjunction with a dorsal wedge opening osteotomy for correction of dorsal malunions of the distal radius (98). Benefits of this technique over a standard opening wedge osteotomy include elimination of iliac donor site morbidity, simplicity of Kirschner wire fixation, and avoidance of disruption of the extensor retinaculum. Highlights of the technique are summarized below.

Watson and Castle reported their results of 15 patients managed with a trapezoidal dorsal opening wedge osteotomy utilizing local bone graft and Kirschner wire fixation with a minimum 18-month follow-up (98). Radiographic parameters demonstrated improvement: palmar tilt was increased from an average of −18.8° (range −5° to −35°) to +12.4° (range +4°–30°); radial inclination was increased to an average of 17.8°; and, although exact length was not described, only one of 15 patients required an ulnar shortening osteotomy for inadequate radial length following osteotomy. There was only one poor result in the group owing to nonunion, with 8 excellent and 3 good results using the Fernandez criteria (87).

Technique

The approach is made via a transverse 4-cm incision located 3 cm proximal to the radial styloid. Deep dissection is carried out subperiosteally at the proximal edge of the extensor retinaculum to expose the planned osteotomy which is to be centered 1 to 1.5 cm proximal to the articular surface. Kirschner wires are then placed, one proximal to the osteotomy and perpendicular to the radial shaft, the other distal to the planned osteotomy and parallel to the joint surface. Osteotomy is performed parallel to the distal wire with care not to disrupt the palmar periosteum. Palmar angulation is then restored via rotation of the distal wire such that it is 10° palmarly angulated in reference to the proximal pin. The radial aspect of the osteotomy will require additional distraction to restore radial inclination.

Local corticocancellous graft is then harvested from the proximal border of the osteotomy site such that the broad radial aspect of the graft is oriented at the osteotomy (Fig. 21.8). The narrower ulnar aspect of the trapezoid to be harvested is the most proximal aspect of the graft. The planned graft is outlined with several small cortical perforations made with a Kirschner wire. Cortical cuts are completed with a small straight osteotome ($^{3}/_{16}$-in.), and the graft is removed.

The graft is rotated 90° and inserted in the defect of the osteotomy. The graft is then "caged" by one or two Kirschner wires such that they penetrate the cortex of the proximal and distal radial fragments while running dorsal

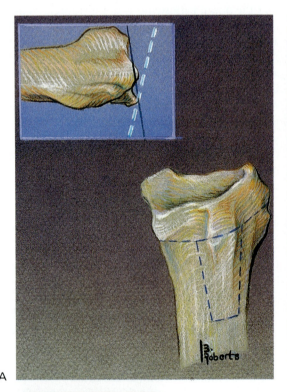
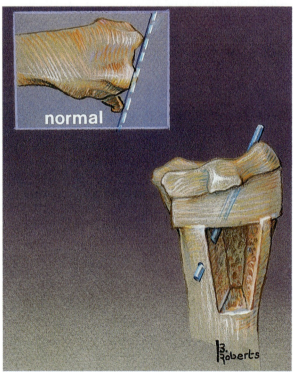
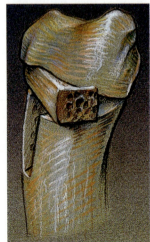

FIGURE 21.8. Technique of the trapezoidal osteotomy as described by Watson and Castle. **A:** Anteroposterior view of osteotomy site and graft harvest site. **B:** Anteroposterior view after harvesting of the trapezoidal corticocancellous graft from the distal radius, its 90° rotation, insertion, and K-wire fixation. Note that the graft is shaped such that it corrects the deformity in all three planes. **C:** Lateral view demonstrating that opening of the osteotomy site corrects the sagittal plane deformity. (From Watson HK, Castle TH. Trapezoidal osteotomy of the distal radius for unacceptable articular angulation after Colles' fracture. *J Hand Surg [Am]* 1988;13:837–843, with permission.)

to the corticocancellous graft. Wires are cut off below the skin for later removal in the office.

Postoperative course involves immobilization in a long arm splint at 90° of elbow flexion, neutral forearm rotation, and slight wrist extension for 5 to 7 days. This is converted to a long arm cast for 3 weeks. Watson prefers including the thumb, index, and long fingers in the long arm cast. A short arm cast is placed at 4 weeks postoperatively for an additional 2 weeks. The Kirschner wires are removed when healing is apparent (usually at 6 weeks), and motion is begun.

The Ulnar Side

Resection of the Distal Ulna (Darrach)

Resection of the distal ulna, first advocated by Darrach as a primary management for symptomatic malunion of the distal radius in 1913 (114), is still promoted by several authors as a primary treatment in the elderly patient (87,92,104, 109,110). In the low-demand, physiologically elderly patient with poor bone stock, the Darrach procedure is an excellent procedure for pain control (87,92). It is useful as an adjunct to corrective distal radial osteotomy in the higher-demand patient with distal radial malunion (93). In the event a more conservative subtotal resection has failed because of pain or persistent instability, the Darrach procedure is used as a salvage procedure (92,102).

Darrach originally described resection of the distal 25 mm of the ulna for symptomatic ulnar-sided wrist pain (114). Multiple modifications of the procedure have been proposed over the years and have been reviewed by Dingman (120). Considerable controversy exists concerning the importance of the ulnar styloid, preservation of the periosteal sheath, angle of the osteotomy, and the amount of bone resected (120). Dingman found the amount of distal ulna resected to be the single most significant factor in heralding a good result. Dingman suggested that the resection be limited to the ulna corresponding to the sigmoid notch, a recommendation echoed by many (50,54,121). Dingman also advocated preservation of a periosteal sleeve, which has become a routine part of the modern Darrach procedure (50,54,121–124).

Commonly cited complications of the Darrach procedure include grip weakness and instability of the ulnar stump (114,123); however, these criticisms are not universally borne out in the literature. Ulnar translation of the carpus has been reported following the Darrach procedure, but only in patients with rheumatoid arthritis (54,124). Reporting on the use of distal ulna resection in 62 patients for posttraumatic ulnar-sided wrist pain or loss of motion, Hartz and Beckenbaugh showed increases in grip strength (43% of contralateral wrist preoperatively to 79% postoperatively) without a single case of ulnar instability (122). Tulipan et al. reported similar increases in grip strength (60% of contralateral wrist preoperatively to 84% postoperatively) in 33 patients, with only one patient demonstrating instability of the distal ulna (preoperative diagnosis not disclosed) (121).

Technique

A 3- to 4-cm incision is made dorsally over the DRUJ in an oblique line from the base of the lunate distally to a point proximal to the sigmoid notch on the medial border of the ulna (50). Blunt dissection is carried down to the retinaculum, and an ulnar-based rectangle is raised. Dissection is continued down between the fifth and sixth dorsal compartments to the level of the dorsal capsule of the DRUJ. The capsule is incised just proximal to the distal dorsal radioulnar ligament and is carried along the ulna to a point just proximal to the flare as a single, full-thickness capsule and periosteal layer. The distal ulna is then further exposed subperiosteally to facilitate an osteotomy cut just proximal to the DRUJ articulation. An oscillating saw is employed for the bony cut. The distal ulnar fragment is then rotated distally to allow full subperiosteal–subtriangular fibrocartilage removal of the ulnar head and styloid. The capsule and periosteum are closed in a multilayered fashion.

The postoperative course begins with immobilization in compressive, bulky long arm splint with the elbow flexed 90° and the forearm in full supination. At 3 weeks, the patient is placed in a long arm posterior splint that may be removed for active elbow and forearm exercises. A strengthening program is initiated at 6 weeks.

Resection of the Distal Radioulnar Joint

The popularity of partial resection or limited resection of the distal ulna is borne of the dissatisfaction with the Darrach procedure in the higher-demand individual. The benefits offered by resection of the painful DRUJ while retaining the attachments of the TFCC and radioulnar ligaments are that the potentially destabilizing effects of an overzealous ulna resection are avoided (55,99). Bowers has advocated hemiresection–interposition arthroplasty as a substitution of a less painful instability in symptomatic DRUJ instability that may improve function (55). Watson et al. discuss the use of matched ulnar resection for the patient with residual limitation of the pronation–supination arc following distal radial osteotomy (125). If a pronation–supination arc of 100°, described as that necessary for normal activities of daily living, is not appreciated intraoperatively at completion of radial osteotomy, these authors augment the osteotomy with matched resection (126).

Hemiresection Interposition Arthroplasty of the Distal Radioulnar Joint (Bowers)

In 1985, Bowers described a technique for decompression of the DRUJ while maintaining the ulnar attachments of the TFCC (109). This technique employs the use of soft tissue interposition to prevent ulnar impaction into the radius and, in cases with minimal excess ulnar length, acts to prevent ulnocarpal impaction with power grip. A contraindication to the procedure is a deficient or irreparable TFCC (54).

Fernandez reported on the use of the hemiresection interposition arthroplasty in 15 patients undergoing corrective osteotomy for distal radial malunion (99). Thirteen of the 15 patients had no pain localized to the DRUJ. The remaining two patients experienced mild pain with extremes of active pronation and supination. Grip strength was noted to improve in all patients; however, it is difficult to separate the relative effects of the simultaneous corrective radial osteotomy.

Technique

A dorsal approach is made to the DRUJ between the fifth and sixth dorsal compartments beginning 5 cm proximal to the ulnar head and carried distally and dorsally over the ulnar shaft to the level of the midcarpus. Blunt dissection is employed to prevent damage to the dorsal branches of the ulnar nerve to the level of the extensor retinaculum. The proximal, ulnar one-half of the extensor retinaculum is reflected radially on a base inserting between the fourth and fifth extensor compartments. The extensor digiti minimi tendon is then retracted to expose the dorsal capsule of the DRUJ. The dorsal capsule is then incised along its radial aspect, leaving only a 1-mm radial margin for later repair, to the level of the dorsal radioulnar ligaments. The dorsal capsule is reflected ulnarly, exposing the ulnar head. The sigmoid notch and TFCC may be inspected using either a lamina spreader or small probe. Should additional exposure be deemed necessary, the remaining portion of the extensor retinaculum may be released in line with the extensor digiti minimi tendon and reflected ulnarly on a base inserting into the fibrous tunnel of the ECU tendon. Subperiosteal dissection of the sixth dorsal compartment from the distal ulna will also improve visualization of the ulnar head.

Resection of the articular surface and subchondral bone is performed, using small osteotomes and rongeurs. Diligent inspection and removal of osteophytes follows. Any remaining synovial tissue is then removed, and debridement or repair of the TFCC is performed as needed.

Examination for stylocarpal impaction is performed by compressing the radius and ulna together and ulnarly deviating the wrist. Any degree of impaction obligates ulnar shortening. The need for shortening can usually be anticipated in cases exceeding 2 mm positive ulnar variance. Shortening osteotomy can be performed distally through the metaphyseal region of the ulna and fixed with compressive interosseous wiring. A more formal diaphyseal shortening osteotomy with plating is another alternative.

Interpositional material, using the palmaris longus, a portion of the ECU tendon, or flexor carpi ulnaris tendon, is harvested and shaped to approximate the size and shape of the resected ulnar dome. This material is packed into the resection defect and secured to the dorsal and volar capsule of the DRUJ.

Stability of the ECU tendon is assessed for evidence of palmar subluxation or instability within the sixth dorsal compartment. Should either condition exist, the ECU tendon may be stabilized by creating a sling from the radially based flap of extensor retinaculum. The retinacular flap is woven under the ECU tendon and reflected back to the interval between the fourth and fifth extensor compartments where is it sewn in place. If the ECU tendon is stable, it is returned to its original position and secured by reattachment of the distal ulnar based retinacular flap to its original position.

The postoperative course is predicated by associated procedures. For those not requiring radial osteotomy or shortening, a short arm bulky dressing with plaster reinforcement is applied. Finger motion is begun immediately and forearm rotation is left to the patient's comfort. Two weeks after surgery, this is converted to a wrist splint to allow unrestricted motion. When a shortening osteotomy is performed, the patient is protected in an above elbow plaster splint. This is converted to a short arm cast with an interosseous mold at two weeks. The cast is removed by the sixth postoperative week and motion begun. An orthoplast protective splint is recommended for 8 to 12 weeks for those individuals in whom shortening was performed in the diaphyseal region of the ulna.

Matched Resection of the Distal Radioulnar Joint (Watson et al.)

In 1986, Watson et al. reported a technique of "matched resection" of the DRUJ (125). This technique resects the radial aspect of the distal ulna in a smooth convex curve to match the convex medial metaphysis of the radius while maintaining the full length of the ulna and ulnar attachments of the TFCC medially. The theory behind this resection is to provide a wide resection of the DRUJ and lateral ulna to prevent any impingement of the radius by the ulna through a full range of motion.

The authors of the technique report on 44 wrists with an average 6.5-year follow-up and demonstrate the technique to be reliable for pain relief and maintenance of motion. In this cohort, pronation and supination averaged 80° and 88°, respectively. Pain relief was complete in 30, with the remaining 14 only mildly symptomatic.

Technique

Approach to the DRUJ is through a dorsal 3-cm transverse incision just proximal to the joint. Careful blunt dissection is carried down to the level of the dorsal joint capsule and ulnar periosteum, protecting the dorsal branches of the ulnar nerve. The dorsal capsule is sharply incised just proximal to the dorsal radioulnar joint. The entire 270° arc of the ulna that contacts the radius (from full pronation to full supination) is resected in a fashion so as to "match" the medial surface of the radius in all three planes. To insure adequate resection, this resection should be carried out for the distal 4.5 cm of the ulna.

The wrist is then put through a full range of motion to evaluate for ulnar impingement on the radius or ulnocarpal impaction of the ulnar styloid. Should ulnar impingement persist, a more aggressive matched resection must be performed. If ulnocarpal impaction presents, a subperiosteal resection is performed of the distal styloid sufficient to prevent impaction. The resection of the styloid is performed such that a cuff of periosteum and the ulnar ligaments remain in continuity.

The patient is placed in a compressive dressing for 1 week. Motion is begun at 1 week unless contraindicated by associated procedures.

Ulnar Shortening Osteotomy (Milch)

Milch in 1941 (104) refined the shortening osteotomy of the distal ulna to what he described as the "cuff resection of the ulna" as a primary treatment of malunion of the distal radius associated with significant loss of radial length. The indication for the ulnar shortening osteotomy as a single procedure in the case of distal radial malunion with significant ulnocarpal impaction is the malunion with shortening but without significant (<10°) dorsal angulation (92,104). Additional requirements for successful implementation of the procedure include a functional TFCC, lack of arthrosis of the sigmoid notch and ulnar head, and that joint congruity must not be compromised by the change in ulnar length (56).

The ulnar shortening osteotomy has several indications in the management of distal radial malunions as a secondary procedure. The shortening procedure may be used as a single procedure on the ulnar side in the situation in which radial osteotomy failed to gain sufficient length to prevent ulnocarpal impingement (97). Ladd and Huene believe that a maximum of 4 mm of radial length is all that can be expected from a radial osteotomy alone, necessitating an additional ulnar leveling procedure in cases where preoperative radial shortening exceeded this distance (97). In contrast, Fernandez did not feel the ulnar length necessitated surgical attention until radial shortening exceeded 12 mm (87). The decision to proceed to ulnar shortening osteotomy may be an intraoperative judgment based on exam and/or radiographic evaluation after completion of the radial osteotomy.

When faced with significant degenerative changes of the DRUJ, ulnar-shortening osteotomy retains a role in the prevention of stylocarpal impaction (54,92,98) following resection of the DRUJ. The degree to which the ulnar styloid is "positive" may influence the need for formal ulnar shortening versus less aggressive management. Bowers reported that minimal excess of ulnar styloid length may be amenable to augmentation of the partial DRUJ resection with soft tissue interposition (54). This may displace the styloid sufficiently medially to prevent contact with the carpus. Watson et al. describe simply removing a "minimal amount" of the distal ulna to prevent impaction based on an intraoperative exam following matched ulna resection (125).

Milch described shortening of the ulna through a transverse diaphyseal osteotomy (104). Fixation at the osteotomy site was done with interosseous wiring. Although many modifications to the original procedure have evolved as a result of improved methods of fixation and understanding of fracture healing, the principle of unloading the ulnocarpal joint while leaving the TFCC, ulnocarpal ligaments, and distal radioulnar articulation remains intact.

Although the use of an ulnar shortening osteotomy simultaneously with corrective osteotomy of distal radial malunions has been reported (97,108), the number of patients is small, and differentiation of a postoperative result from that achieved by the radial osteotomy is difficult at best.

Plate Fixation

Technique. A direct approach is made to the osteotomy site, the junction of the middle and distal third of the ulnar diaphysis, along the subcutaneous border (102). The incision must be of sufficient length to insert a seven-hole 3.5-mm dynamic compression plate. Periosteal stripping is held to a minimum. A compression plate is loosely attached with a single screw distal to the volar shaft of the ulna, then rotated away to allow access to the planned osteotomy site. An oblique osteotomy is located such that a lag screw may be placed through the plate and across the osteotomy site when complete. The amount of bone to be resected is determined based on preoperative radiographs when performed as a single procedure; when it is performed in conjunction with a radial osteotomy, fluoroscopy is required. A partial cut is made with an oscillating saw, and a free saw blade is inserted to act as a cutting guide. Care is taken to orient the osteotomy such that the proximal fragment is trapped by the overlying plate. The second cut is completed so that the net ulnar variance is negative 1 to 2 mm. The first cut is completed, and a dynamic compression plate applied. As the plate is applied, compression at the osteotomy site is achieved by tightening the initial distal screw and placing a proximal screw in compression mode. A lag screw is then placed through the plate for additional compression at the osteotomy site. The remainder of the screws are placed in neutral.

A compressive sugar-tongs dressing is applied. This is later converted to a Muenster cast for 2 to 4 weeks. The arm is protected with a forearm gauntlet orthosis for two more weeks. The plate is removed at 1 to 2 years, and the arm is protected in a short arm cast for 6 weeks.

Arthrodesis of the Distal Radioulnar Joint with Proximal Pseudarthrosis (Sauvé-Kapandji)

Sauvé and Kapandji (127) introduced arthrodesis of the DRUJ in 1936 with creation of a proximal pseudarthrosis to maintain pronation and supination as a method to address arthrosis of the DRUJ (54,92,97,128). Like the limited ulnar resection, this technique retains the attachments of the TFCC and bony support of the ulnar carpus (127) with the added benefit of preserving the fibrous support system of the extensor carpi ulnar tendon (128). The added theoretical benefit of this procedure is that proximal migration of the distal ulnar fragment not only helps prevent ulnocarpal impaction but also acts to tighten the ulnocarpal complex (102,128). The Sauvé-Kapandji procedure may be complicated with postoperative instability of the proximal ulnar stump, particularly in those individuals with previous DRUJ instability (109,128).

Taleisnik reviewed his experience with the Sauvé-Kapandji procedure in 37 patients (40 wrists) followed for a minimum of 1 year (128). He differentiated those in whom the procedure had been performed for osteoarthritis and posttraumatic arthritis from those with rheumatoid arthritis. Of the 23 patients treated for arthritis, in a relatively young group averaging 32 years of age (range, 19–57 years), most demonstrated dramatic improvements in grip strength, motion, and pain relief. Of this group, four patients presented with malunion of the distal radius, three of whom had corrective osteotomy in addition to the Sauvé-Kapandji procedure. All three had marked improvement in pronation–supination, with two of the three also having significant increases in grip strength. Seven of the 40 wrists reported symptoms attributed to proximal ulna stump instability: three (all rheumatoid) responded to prolonged immobilization, and three of the remaining four (two rheumatoid and two posttraumatic) responded to reoperation.

Technique

Approach is made via a 6- to 7-cm longitudinal dorsal incision made over the interval between the fifth and sixth dorsal compartments from a point just distal to the ulnar prominence. Blunt dissection to the level of the retinaculum follows, and the retinaculum is then opened through the fifth dorsal compartment. This approach preserves the restraining fibrous structures of the ECU.

The periosteum of the ulnar shaft is now exposed, and the periosteum of the intended ulnar resection is excised. The resection is based approximately 1 to 2 mm proximal to the border of the articular cartilage of the ulnar head flare, with a 12- to 15-mm gap desired following correction for potential radioulnar length inequality. Taleisnik described the use of a towel clip to grasp the distal ulnar fragment to assist with manipulation and as a marker of correct rotational orientation to the radius (128). The osteotomy is performed transversely with an osteotome or oscillating saw in a line tangential to the proximal margin of the flare of the ulnar head; additional resection may be required if the ulnar head is recessed. The towel clip is then used to rotate the ulnar head to expose the articular surfaces of the ulnar head and sigmoid notch. Cartilage is removed to the level of cancellous bone. Bone graft is obtained from the resected ulnar shaft and packed into the fusion site. The ulnar head is reduced to the denuded sigmoid notch, with particular attention to length and rotational orientation, and transfixed with two Kirschner wires (0.54 or 0.045 in.). These wires are placed such that their distal ends are palpable on the lateral aspect of the wrist; the medial aspects of the wires are cut flush to the cortex. Cannulated or standard compression screws may be substituted for wires as preferred.

The proximal ulnar stump is then addressed by stabilization with the pronator quadratus. The pronator quadratus is divided from the ulnar shaft and transferred to a dorsal position over the distal aspect of the proximal ulnar stump. It is secured by transosseous sutures to the dorsal distal ulnar stump.

Immobilization is with a short arm or sugar-tongs splint for 3 weeks. One or both Kirschner wires are left in place until fused radiographic healing is evident (generally 6–8 weeks).

Authors' Preferred Technique

The most common reason for consultation following treatment of a distal radius fracture in the elderly population is ulnocarpal abutment secondary to loss of radial length. Poor bone quality and attendant dorsal comminution lead to radial settling in the majority of patients over the age of 65 in fractures treated by plaster immobilization (78). Generally speaking, radioulnar disparity of 5 mm or less is well tolerated. Posttraumatic positive ulnar variance in excess of 5 mm, even when associated with good restitution of radial inclination and palmar tilt, can lead to a painful loss of ulnar deviation and supination.

In the physiologically older population with a relatively low-demand wrist and symptomatic ulnocarpal abutment, isolated Darrach excision of the distal ulna is preferred. The ulna is resected at a level 1 cm proximal to the lesser sigmoid notch, and the resection is performed obliquely toward the ulnar styloid (Fig. 21.9). The sharp edges are smoothed with a rongeur, particularly on the dorsal and radial borders. Special care is given during closure to tightly close the periosteal sheath with imbricating nonabsorbable braided polyester while the ulna is held in the reduced position, and the patient is immobilized for 2 weeks in supination in a sugar-tongs splint. Gentle mobilization is begun thereafter, and few require structured physical therapy to restore rotation or wrist motion. Mild complaints of distal ulnar motion usually persist for 6 to 8 weeks but are not generally painful and do not restrict activity.

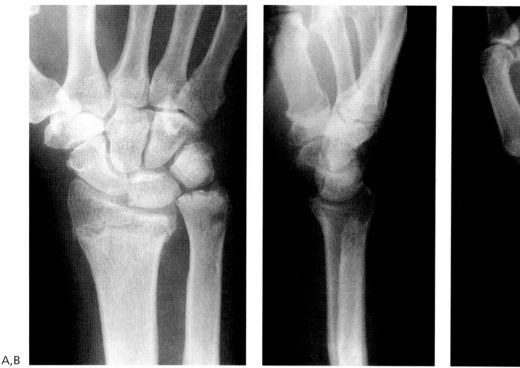
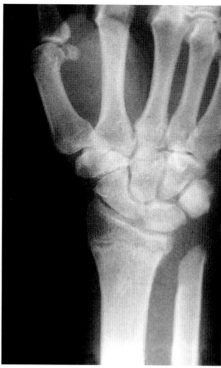

FIGURE 21.9. Isolated Darrach procedure for ulnar impaction secondary to radial shortening. **A:** Malunion with significant radial shortening. **B,C:** Anteroposterior and lateral views following the Darrach procedure: note that sagittal plane deformity is minimal. There is no dorsal subluxation of the distal ulnar stump.

In patients with combined loss of radial length and palmar tilt, simultaneous correction of radial alignment and reconstruction of the DRUJ are necessary to prevent radioulnar instability. Isolated Darrach resection in the face of an uncorrected radial malunion can lead to painful instability and is the basis of many failed Darrach resections in the literature (129). The choice of distal radial osteotomy technique is related to the extent of correction necessary. The trapezoidal osteotomy is a creative and attractive use of local bone graft to correct deformity but should be restricted to corrections of 35° or less in the sagittal plane (Fig. 21.10). Corrections in excess of this amount, particularly with multiplanar deformities or marked radial shortening, are best suited to iliac bone (Fig. 21.11). A fixator construct is then applied to hold the correction rigidly during graft measurement and acquisition. The graft is sculpted for fit and placed into the defect. A plate is contoured and applied in standard fashion, and the fixator is removed. Distal radioulnar reconstruction is carried out, and postoperative care is predicated on the stability of the construct and the care of the DRUJ.

Rupture or attenuation of the extensor pollicis longus tendon is occasionally noted as a complication following distal radius fracture (4). We prefer direct repair of a clearly ruptured tendon or transfer of the extensor indicis proprius tendon for attenuated tendon stumps to be sufficient in most instances.

At the time of distal radial realignment osteotomy, a decision can best be made concerning the type of reconstruction for the DRUJ. Whether an isolated DRUJ resection is performed, the distal ulna removed, or the ulna shortened depends to a great extent on the quality and congruency of the articular cartilage at the time of correction. In general, an attempt is made to salvage the DRUJ by joint-leveling procedures in younger, more active patients without traumatic incongruity of the DRUJ surface. When sufficient length cannot be gained by distal radial realignment alone, concomitant ulnar shortening may be performed. If the DRUJ must be resected or matched, or hemiresection arthroplasty maintains the ulnar-sided ligamentous tethers to the carpus, it is preferable when there is no risk of impaction of the ulnar styloid with the lunate or triquetrum. Resecting the ulnar styloid during a hemiresection or matched ulnar arthroplasty essentially converts the procedure to a conservative Darrach excision and is the procedure of choice in the face of persistent ulnar impaction with concomitant DRUJ arthrosis.

On occasion, restriction of rotation by radial malunion can cause secondary arthrofibrosis of the radioulnar joint. Despite full correction of radial malangulation, DRUJ rotation may continue to lag. Complete capsulolysis of the DRUJ, with preservation of the dorsal and palmar radioulnar ligaments as described by Kleinman, will

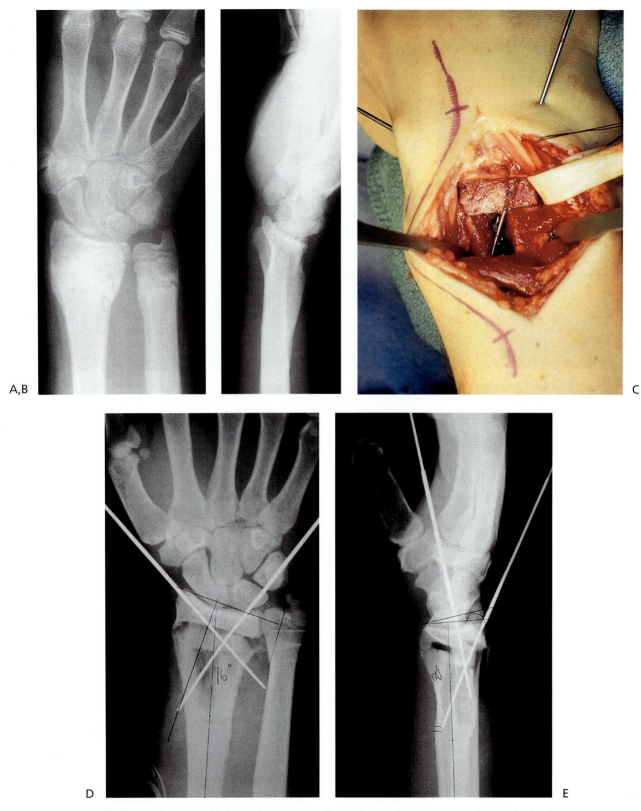

FIGURE 21.10. Trapezoidal osteotomy—operative series. **A:** Preoperative anteroposterior (AP) with loss of radial inclination but minimal loss of radial length. **B:** Lateral view shows dorsally angulated malunion. **C:** Trapezoidal graft has been harvested from the radius, placed into the osteotomy site, and fixed with Kirschner wires dorsal to the cortical surface of the graft. **D,E:** Intraoperative AP and lateral views are obtained to confirm correction in all three planes.

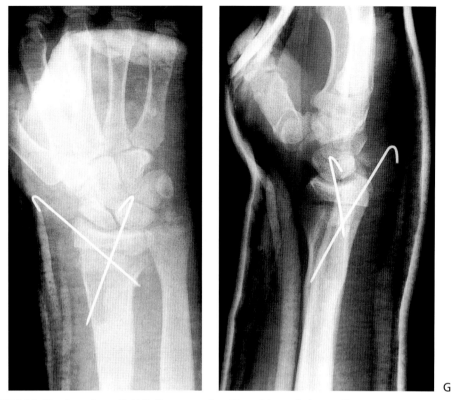

F G

FIGURE 21.10. *(continued)* F,G: Postoperative AP and lateral view. **Editors' Notes:** *In C, picture a transverse incision here instead of the longitudinal incision. The incision would be centered half-way between the articular surface of the radius distally and the most proximal aspect of the graft donor site proximally. The entire extensor retinaculum is then maintained in place over the distal segment of radius.*

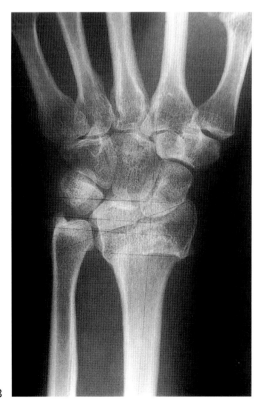
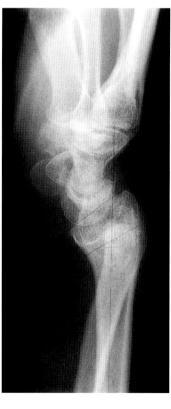

A,B

FIGURE 21.11. Opening wedge osteotomy for palmarly angulated malunion. **A,B:** Anteroposterior (AP) and lateral views showing loss of length and radial inclination and excessive palmar tilt.

(continued on next page)

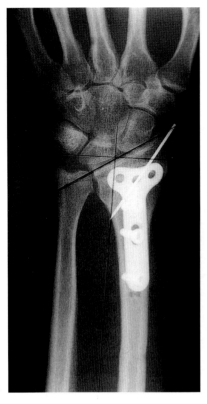
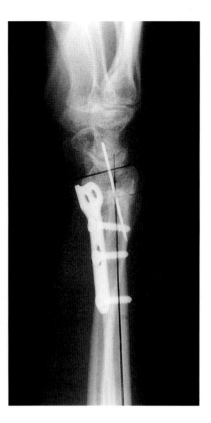

FIGURE 21.11. *(continued)* **C,D:** Postoperative AP and lateral images showing correction of length, radial inclination, and a more normal palmar tilt.

predictably restore rotation through a congruent and stable articulation (50,65). The distal radius reconstruction must be of sufficient stability to tolerate immediate postoperative rotation exercises for this procedure to be maximally effective.

Salvage Following Malunion of Fractures of the Distal Radius

As described earlier in this chapter, malunion of the distal radius in many instances should be considered a prearthritic condition. It follows that the long-term results of these malunions are manifest as arthrosis of the radiocarpal joint, midcarpal joint, or DRUJ. These conditions represent contraindications to reconstructive osteotomy (87,92,98), forcing the treating physician to consider salvage options for posttraumatic osteoarthritis. These options follow the same rationale for treatment as osteoarthritic changes not necessarily associated with distal radial malunion.

EDITORS' COMMENTS

Our comments here are restricted to secondary carpal problems, excluding the triangular fibrocartilage, the ulnar impaction syndrome, and/or dislocation of the distal ulna. The philosophy in an acute injury is a matter of priorities. The first priority in any articular fracture is the cartilage. It does not matter how well the ligamentous tear or potential carpal instability was handled if the distal radial articular surface is left with a step, unacceptable fragment, or sloping or articular malalignment. As with any acute orthopedic injury, once circulation adequacy is determined, the focus must be on articular cartilage and joint preservation.

In trauma of the wrist, the smaller carpal bones with the smaller radius of curvature act as ball-peen hammers against the articular surface of the radius. Once that surface is adequately reestablished, the surgeon may look to the ligamentous tears and potential carpal instability problems. There is no place for closed reduction or percutaneous pinning in these injuries. The morbidity of open operation over arthroscopy is not to be considered when weighed against the eventual wrist one can achieve under direct visualization. The key to preventing secondary carpal problems is anatomic realignment of the radius articular surface (Editors' Figs. 21.1–21.3). This is far more important than suturing of ligaments or other ligament repair techniques and enhancements. If the carpals are anatomically realigned and adequately immobilized, ligaments that have been acutely torn stand a reasonable chance of healing. Twenty-five percent of the asymptomatic normal adult population has some tearing of the SLIL; thus, an asymptomatic wrist may be achieved with less than total healing of all ligaments. Preexisting ligament tears have undergone involution and

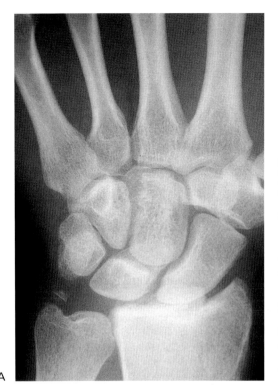
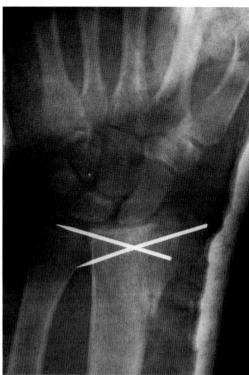

EDITORS' FIGURE 21.1. A: There is a large step in the articular surface of the radius. This will produce symptoms and early destruction of the radial scaphoid joint. The radial fragment is depressed without rotation. **B:** Without articular tilting, a straight osteotomy is sufficient. The fragment is moved directly distally until the step is corrected and the alignment with the scaphoid is normal.

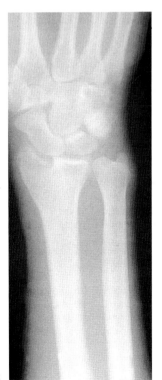
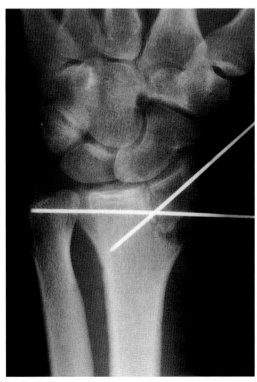

EDITORS' FIGURE 21.2. A: This step in the articular surface is similar to that in Editors' Fig. 21.1A. The radial fragment has rotated and requires that the ulnar aspect of the depressed segment be raised further than the radial styloid. **B:** In this case, a curved osteotomy is formed, creating a rotation plane, and as the fragment is elevated, it is also rerotated to reestablish a normal articular surface.

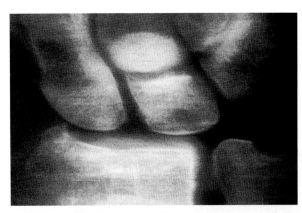

EDITORS' FIGURE 21.3. Secondary to a step in the articular surface, an operation had been performed, removing the styloid. Tomograms demonstrate that the entire step was not removed, and the small remnant of the articular step persists, producing a painful, symptomatic wrist. Simple resection of the elevated remnant of the radial fragment was sufficient to produce an asymptomatic wrist.

resorption of the ligaments and will not heal with reduction and immobilization. Acutely torn ligaments can and will repair themselves with long (8 weeks) immobilization, so long as reduction is anatomic. If attempts at ligament repair will interfere with the adequacy of articular alignment and reduction of the radius, then they are best ignored. There are adequate solutions for carpal instability on a secondary basis. There are only salvage procedures for loss of the articular cartilage.

Secondary carpal problems can exist without intercarpal ligamentous tear as a result of distal radial articular alignment. This secondary carpal overload from a dorsal articularly tilted radius is not "midcarpal instability." We have previously published the effect of a dorsally tilted radius on the carpals and erroneously called this a form of midcarpal instability. This phenomenon is better termed carpal overload following malaligned distal radius.

In ulnar deviation, the proximal row dorsiflexes and translates volarly or down the slope of the normal radius articular surface. This maintains a centralization of the capitate over the radius when seen from a lateral view. If the radial articular surface is tiled dorsally, then power grip produces the dorsiflexion of the proximal row, but downslope has now become upslope, and the volar carpal translation cannot occur. The dorsiflexion of the proximal row then carries the capitate and the hand dorsal to the long axis of the radius. This produces an overload of the dorsal ligamentous structures between the proximal and distal carpal rows as well as an impingement phenomenon between the volar lip of the lunate and the volar surface of the capitate. This produces symptomatic midcarpal overload. Trapezoidal osteotomy of the radius is a simple effective procedure to solve this problem. Through a transverse dorsal incision, a trapezoid-shaped graft is taken from the radius proximal to the corrective osteotomy. The graft is turned 90° and holds the opening wedge osteotomy in place (see Chapter 72).

REFERENCES

1. Hollingsworth R, Morris J. The importance of the ulnar side of the wrist in fractures of the distal end of the radius. *Injury* 1976;7:263–267.
2. Larsen CF, Lauritsen J. Epidemiology of acute wrist trauma. *Int J Epidemiol* 1993;22:911–916.
3. Colles A. On the fracture of the carpal extremity of the radius. *Edinburgh Med Surg J* 1814;10:182–186.
4. Cooney WP, Dobyns JH, Linscheid RL. Complications of Colles' fractures. *J Bone Joint Surg Am* 1980;62:613–619.
5. De Palma AF. Comminuted fractures of the distal end of the radius treated by ulnar pinning. *J Bone Joint Surg Am* 1952;34:651–662.
6. Mudgal CS, Jones WA. Scapholunate diastasis: A component of fractures of the distal radius. *J Hand Surg [Br]* 1990;15:503–505.
7. Brown IW. Volar intercalary carpal instability following a seemingly innocent wrist fracture. *J Hand Surg [Br]* 1987;12:54–56.
8. Jones WA. Beware the sprained wrist. The incidence and diagnosis of scapholunate instability. *J Bone Joint Surg Br* 1988;70:293–297.
9. Biyani A, Sharma JC. An unusual pattern of radiocarpal injury: brief report. *J Bone Joint Surg Br* 1989;71:139.
10. Rosenthal DI, Schwartz M, Phillips WC, et al. Fracture of the radius with instability of the wrist. *Am J Roentgenol* 1983;141:113–116.
11. Geissler WB, Freedland AE, Savoie FH, et al. Carpal instability associated with displaced intra-articular distal radius fractures. *Orthop Trans* 1993;17:1065.
12. King RJ. Scapholunate diastasis associated with a Barton fracture treated by manipulation, or Terry-Thomas and the wine waiter. *J R Soc Med* 1983;76:421–423.
13. Tang J. Carpal instability associated with fracture of the distal radius: incidence, influencing factors and pathomechanics. *Chin Med J* 1992;105:758–765.
14. Leibovic SJ, Geissler WB. Treatment of complex intra-articular distal radius fractures. *Orthop Clin North Am* 1994;25:685–706.
15. Hanker GJ. *Wrist arthroscopy in distal radius fractures.* Paper presented at the American Academy of Orthopaedic Surgeons Annual Meeting, Washington, DC, 1992.
16. Kolkin L. *Wrist arthroscopy.* Paper presented at the American Academy of Orthopaedic Surgeons Annual Meeting, Washington, DC, 1992.
17. Geissler WB, Fernandez DL. Percutaneous and limited open reduction of the articular surface of the distal radius. *J Orthop Trauma* 1991;5:255–264.
18. Tang J, Shi D, Gu Y, et al. Can cast immobilization successfully treat scapholunate dissociation associated with distal radius fracture? *J Hand Surg [Am]* 1996;21:583–590.
19. Berger RA, Amadio PC. Predicting palmar radio-carpal ligament disruption in fractures of the distal articular surface of the radius involving the palmar cortex. *J Hand Surg [Br]* 1994;19:108–113.
20. Wolfe SW, Easterling KJ, Yoo HH. Arthroscopic-assisted reduction of distal radius fractures. *Arthroscopy* 1995;11:706–714.
21. Mayfield JK, Johnson RP, Kilcoyne RF. The ligaments of the

human wrist and their functional significance. *Anat Rec* 1976; 186:417–428.
22. Logan SE, Nowak MD, Gould PL, et al. Biomechanical behavior of the scapholunate ligament. *Biomed Sci Instrum* 1986;22: 81–85.
23. Mayfield JK, Johnson RP, Kilcoyne RK. Carpal dislocations: pathomechanics and progressive perilunar instability. *J Hand Surg [Am]* 1980;5:226–241.
24. Wolfe SW, Katz LD, Crisco JJ. Radiographic progression to dorsal intercalated segment instability. *Orthopaedics* 1996;19: 691–695.
25. Watson HK, Ballet FL. The SLAC wrist: scapholunate advanced collapse pattern of degenerative arthritis. *J Hand Surg [Am]* 1984;9:358–365.
26. Taleisnik J, Watson HK. Midcarpal instability caused by malunited fractures of the distal radius. *J Hand Surg [Am]* 1984;9:350–357.
27. Linscheid RL, Dobyns JH, Beabout JW, et al. Traumatic instability of the wrist. *J Bone Joint Surg Am* 1972;54:1612–1632.
28. Sakai K, Doi K, Ihara K, et al. *Carpal alignment after fractures of the distal radius (abstract).* Paper presented at the International Symposium of the Wrist, Nagoya, Japan, March 6–8, 1991.
29. Dobyns JH, Linscheid RL, Chao EYS. Traumatic instability of the wrist. *AAOS Instr Course Lect* 1975;24:182.
30. Knirk JL, Jupiter JB. Intra-articular fractures of the distal end of the radius in young adults. *J Bone Joint Surg Am* 1986;68: 647–659.
31. Weiss AP, Akelman E, Lambiase R. Comparision of the findings of triple injection cinearthrography of the wrist and those of arthroscopy. *J Bone Joint Surg Am* 1996;78:348–356.
32. Green DP. Carpal dislocations and instabilities. In: Green DP, ed. *Operative hand surgery, 3rd ed.* 1993;861–928.
33. Ruby LK. Carpal instability. *J Bone Joint Surg Am* 1995;77: 476–487.
34. Linscheid RL, Dobyns JH. Athletic injuries of the wrist. *Clin Orthop* 1985;198:141–151.
35. O'Brien ET. Acute fractures and dislocations of the carpus. *Orthop Clin North Am* 1984;15:237–258.
36. Taleisnik J. Scapholunate dissociation. In: Strickland JW, Steichen JB, eds. *Difficult problems in hand surgery.* St Louis: CV Mosby, 1982;341–348.
37. Lavernia CJ, Cohen M, Taleisnik J. Treatment of scapholunate dissociations by ligamentous repair and capsulodesis. *J Hand Surg [Am]* 1992;17:354–359.
38. Goldner JL. Treatment of carpal instability without joint fusion—current assessment (editorial). *J Hand Surg [Am]* 1982; 7:325–326.
39. Bendar JM, Osterman AL. Carpal instability: evaluation and treatment. *J Am Acad Orthop Surg* 1993;1:10–17.
40. Linscheid RL. Scapholunate ligamentous instabilities (dissociations, subdislocations, dislocations). *Ann Chir Main* 1984;3: 323–330.
41. Blatt G. Capsulodesis in reconstructive hand surgery: dorsal capsulodesis for the unstable scaphoid and volar capsulodesis following excision of the distal ulna. *Hand Clin* 1987;3: 81–102.
42. Mikic ZD. Age changes in the triangular fibrocartilage of the wrist joint. *J Anat* 1978;126:367–384.
43. Viegas SF, Ballantyne G. Attritional lesions of the wrist joint. *J Hand Surg [Am]* 1987;12:1025–1029.
44. Palmer AK, Werner FW. The triangular fibrocartilage complex of the wrist: anatomy and function. *J Hand Surg [Am]* 1981;6: 153–172.
45. Palmer AK, Werner FW. Biomechanics of the distal radioulnar joint. *Clin Orthop* 1984;187:26–35.
46. Schuind F, An KN, Berglund L, et al. The distal radioulnar ligaments: a biomechanical study. *J Hand Surg [Am]* 1991;16: 1106–1114.
47. af Ekenstam FW, Hagert CG. Anatomical studies on the geometry and stability of the distal radioulnar joint. *Scand J Plast Reconstr Surg* 1985;19:17–25.
48. af Ekenstam FW, Palmer AK, Glisson RR. The load on the radius and ulna in different positions of the wrist and forearm: A cadaver study. *Acta Orthop Scand* 1984;55:363.
49. Bowers WH. Instability of the radioulnar articulation. *Hand Clin* 1991;7:311–327.
50. Kleinman WB, Graham TJ. Distal ulnar injury and dysfunction. In: Peimer CA, ed. *Surgery of the hand and upper extremity.* New York: McGraw-Hill, 1996;667–709.
51. Hagert CG. Distal radius fracture and the distal radioulnar joint—anatomical considerations. *Handchir Mikrochir Plast Chir* 1994;26:22–26.
52. Viegas SF, Pogue DJ, Patterson RM, et al. Effects of radioulnar instability on the radiocarpal joint: a biomechanical study. *J Hand Surg [Am]* 1990;15:728–732.
53. Rabinowitz RS, Light TR, Havey RM, et al. The role of the interosseous membrane and triangular fibrocartilage complex in forearm stability. *J Hand Surg [Am]* 1994;19:385–393.
54. Bowers WH. The distal radioulnar joint. In: Green DP, ed. *Operative hand surgery, 3rd ed.* New York: Churchill Livingstone, 1993;973–1019.
55. Bowers WH. The distal radioulnar joint. In: Green DP, ed. *Operative hand surgery, 2nd ed.* New York: Churchill Livingstone, 1988;957–989.
56. Jupiter JB, Masem M. Reconstruction of post-traumatic deformity of the distal radius and ulna. *Hand Clin* 1988;4:377–390.
57. Berger RA, Blair WF, El-Khoury GY. Arthrotomography of the wrist: The triangular fibrocartilage complex. *Clin Orthop* 1983;172:257–264.
58. Hagert GC. Functional aspects on the distal radioulnar joint. *J Hand Surg* 1979;4:585.
59. Paley D, McMurtry RY, Murray JF. Dorsal dislocation of the ulnar styloid and extensor carpi ulnaris tendon into the distal radioulnar joint: The empty sulcus sign. *J Hand Surg [Am]* 1987;12:1029–1032.
60. Pogue DJ, Viegas SF, Patterson RM, et al. Effects of distal radius malunion on wrist joint mechanics. *J Hand Surg [Am]* 1990;15: 721–727.
61. Mikic ZD. Treatment of acute injuries of the triangular fibrocartilage complex associated with distal radioulnar joint instability. *J Hand Surg [Am]* 1995;20:319–323.
62. Adams BD, Holley KA. Strains in the articular disk of the triangular fibrocartilage complex. *J Hand Surg [Am]* 1993;18: 919–925.
63. Burgess RC, Watson HK. Hypertrophic ulnar styloid nonunions. *Clin Orthop* 1988;228:215–217.
64. Maffulli N, Fixsen JA. Painful hypertrophic non-union of the ulna styloid process. *J Hand Surg [Br]* 1990;15:355–357.
65. Kleinman WB, Graham TJ. *The DRUJ capsule: Clinical anatomy and role in post traumatic limitation of forearm rotation.* Paper presented at the 50th Annual Meeting of the American Society for Surgery of the Hand, San Francisco, Sept 13–16, 1995.
66. af Ekenstam F, Jakobsson OP, Wadin K. Repair of the triangular ligament in Colles' fracture: No effect in a prospective randomized study. *Acta Orthop Scand* 1989;60:393–396.
67. Palmer AK. Triangular fibrocartilage disorders: Injury patterns and treatment. *Arthroscopy* 1990;6:125–132.
68. Viegas SF, Patterson RM, Peterson PD, et al. Ulnar-sided perilunate instability: an anatomic and biomechanical study. *J Hand Surg [Am]* 1990;15:268–278.
69. Trumble TE, Bour C, Smith RJ, et al. Kinematics of the ulnar

carpus related to the volar intercalated segmental instability pattern. *J Hand Surg [Am]* 1990;15:384–392.
70. Johnson RP, Carrera GF. Chronic capitolunate instability. *J Bone Joint Surg Am* 1986;68:1164–1176.
71. Ruch DS, Poehling GG. Arthroscopic management of partial scapholunate and lunotriquetral injuries of the wrist. *J Hand Surg [Am]* 1996;21:412–417.
72. Weiss AP, Sachar K, Glowcki KA. Arthroscopic debridement alone for intercarpal ligament tears. *J Hand Surg [Am]* 1997;22:344–349.
73. Alexander CE, Lichtman DM. Ulnar carpal instabilities *Orthop Clin North Am* 1984;15:307–320.
74. Pin PG, Young VL, Gilula LA, et al. Management of chronic lunotriquetral ligament tears. *J Hand Surg [Am]* 1989;14:77–83.
75. Nelson DL, Pruitt DL, Manske PR, et al. *Lunotriquetral arthrodesis.* Paper presented at the 45th Annual Meeting, American Society for Surgery of the Hand, Toronto, September, 1990.
76. Wolfe SW. Kinematics of the scaphoid shift test. *J Hand Surg [Am]* 1997;22:801–806.
77. Sotereanos DG, Mitsioni GJ, Giannakopoulos PN, et al. Perilunate dislocation and fracture dislocation: A critical analysis of the volar-dorsal approach. *J Hand Surg [Am]* 1997;22:49–56.
78. Gartland JJ Jr, Werley CW. Evaluation of healed Colles' fractures. *J Bone Joint Surg Am* 1951;33:895–907.
79. Green DP. Pins and plaster treatment of comminuted fractures of the distal end of the radius. *J Bone Joint Surg Am* 1975;57:304–310.
80. Cassebaum WH. Colles' fractures. A study of end results. *JAMA* 1950;143:963–965.
81. Linstrom A. Fractures of the distal end of the radius. A clinical and statistical study of end results. *Acta Orthop Scand [Suppl]* 1959;41:66–69.
82. Ashtrom JP. Treatment of Colles' fractures by posterior splint immobilization. *Orthop Rev* 1982;11:147.
83. Aro HT, Koivunen T. Minor axial shortening of the radius affects outcome of Colles' fracture treatment. *J Hand Surg [Am]* 1991;16:392–398.
84. Stewart HD, Innes AR, Burke FD. Factors affecting the outcome of Colles' fracture: An anatomical and functional study. *Injury* 1985;16:289–295.
85. Villar RN, Marsh D, Rushton N, et al. Three years after Colles' fracture: a prospective review. *J Bone Joint Surg Br* 1987;69:635–638.
86. Sarmiento A, Pratt GW, Berry NC, et al. Colles' fracture: Functional bracing in supination. *J Bone Joint Surg Am* 1975;57:311–317.
87. Fernandez DL. Correction of post-traumatic wrist deformity in adults by osteotomy, bone-grafting, and internal fixation. *J Bone Joint Surg Am* 1982;64:1164–1178.
88. Bickerstaff DR, Bell MJ. Carpal malalignment in Colles' fractures. *J Hand Surg [Br]* 1989;14:155–160.
89. Jenkins NH, Mintowt-Czyz WJ. Malunion and dysfunction in Colles' fracture. *J Hand Surg [Br]* 1988;13:291–293.
90. Melone CP. Articular fractures of the distal radius. *Orthop Clin North Am* 1984;15:217–236.
91. Martini AK. Die sekundare Arthrose des Handgelenkes bei der in Fehlstellung verheilten und nicht korrigierten distalen Radiusfraktur. *Akt Traumatol* 1986;16:143–148.
92. Fernandez DL. Malunion of the distal radius: current approach to management. *Instr Course Lect* 1993;42:99–113.
93. Posner MA, Ambrose L. Malunited Colles' fractures: correction with a biplanar closing wedge osteotomy. *J Hand Surg [Am]* 1991;16:1017–1026.
94. Larsen CF, Amadio PC, Gilula LA, et al. Analysis of carpal instability: I. Description of the scheme. *J Hand Surg [Am]* 1995;20:757–764.
95. Amadio P. Classification of carpal instabilities: A clinical and anatomic primer. *Clin Anat* 1991;4:1–12.
96. Wright TW, Dobyns JH, Linscheid RL, et al. Carpal instability non-dissociative. *J Hand Surg [Br]* 1994;19:763–773.
97. Ladd AL, Huene DS. Reconstructive osteotomy for malunion of the distal radius. *Clin Orthop* 1996;327:158–171.
98. Watson HK, Castle TH. Trapezoidal osteotomy of the distal radius for unacceptable articular angulation after Colles' fracture. *J Hand Surg [Am]* 1988;13:837–843.
99. Fernandez DL. Radial osteotomy and Bowers arthroplasty for malunited fractures of the distal end of the radius. *J Bone Joint Surg Am* 1988;70:1538–1550.
100. Lamoreaux L, Hoffer MM. The effect of wrist deviation on grip and pinch strength. *Clin Orthop* 1995;314:152–155.
101. Palmer AK, Werner FW. Biomechanics of the distal radioulnar joint. *Clin Orthop* 1984;187:26–35.
102. Friedman SL, Plamer AK. The ulnar impaction syndrome. *Hand Clin* 1991;7:295–310.
103. Palmer AK, Glisson RR, Werner FW. Relationship between ulnar variance and triangular fibrocartilage complex thickness. *J Hand Surg [Am]* 1984;9:681–682.
104. Milch H. Cuff resection of the ulna for malunited Colles fracture. *J Bone Joint Surg* 1941;23:311–313.
105. McMurtry RY, Axelrod T, Paley D. Distal radial osteotomy. *Orthopedics* 1989;12:149–155.
106. Fourrier P, Bardy A, Roche G, et al. Approche d'une definition du cal vicieux du poignet. *Int Orthop* 1981;4:299–305.
107. Jupiter JB, Ruder J, Roth DA. Computer-generated bone models in the planning of osteotomy of multidirectional distal radius malunions. *J Hand Surg [Am]* 1992;17:406–415.
108. Brown JN, Bell MJ. Distal radial osteotomy for malunion of wrist fractures in young patients. *J Hand Surg [Br]* 1994;19:589–593.
109. Bowers WH. Distal radioulnar joint arthroplasty: the hemiresection–interposition technique. *J Hand Surg [Am]* 1985;10:169–178.
110. Darrow JC Jr, Linscheid RL, Dobyns JH, et al. Distal ulnar recession for disorders of the distal radioulnar joint. *J Hand Surg [Am]* 1985;10:482–491.
111. Campbell WC. Malunited Colles' fracture. *JAMA* 1937;109:1105–1108.
112. Ghormley RK, Morz RJ. Fractures of the wrist: a review of one-hundred seventy-six cases. *Surg Gynecol Obstet* 1932;55:377–381.
113. Durman DC. An operation for correction of deformities of the wrist following fracture. *J Bone Joint Surg* 1935;17:1014–1016.
114. Darrach W. Partial excision of lower shaft of the ulna for deformity following Colles' fracture. *Ann Surg* 1913;57:764–765.
115. Hobart MH, Kraft GL. Malunited Colles' fracture. *Am J Surg* 1941;53:55–60.
116. Speed JS, Knight RA. Treatment of malunited Colles' fractures. *J Bone Joint Surg* 1945;27:361–367.
117. Fernandez DL, Albrecht HU, Saxer U. Die Korrekturosteotomie am distalen Radius bei posttraumatischer Fehlstellung. *Arch Orthop Unfallchir* 1970;90:199–211.
118. Bora FW, Ostermann AL, Zielinski CJ. Osteotomy of the distal radius with a biplanar iliac bone graft for malunion. *Bull Hosp Joint Dis Orthop Inst* 1984;44:122–131.
119. Cooney WP, Bussey R, Dobyns JH, et al. Difficult wrist fractures. *Clin Orthop* 1987;214:136–147.
120. Dingman PVC. Resection of the distal end of the ulna (Darrach operation). An end result study of twenty-four cases. *J Bone Joint Surg Am* 1952;34:893–900.
121. Tulipan DJ, Eaton RG, Eberhart RE. The Darrach procedure defended: Technique redefined and long-term follow-up (abstract). *J Hand Surg [Am]* 1990;15:828.

122. Hartz CR, Beckenbaugh RD. Long-term results of resection of the distal ulna for post-traumatic conditions. *J Trauma* 1979; 19:219–226.
123. Boyd HB, Stone MM. Resection of the distal end of the ulna *J Bone Joint Surg* 1944;23:313–321.
124. Rowland SA. Stabilization of the ulnar side of the rheumatoid wrist following radiocarpal arthroplasty and resection of the distal ulna. *Orthop Trans* 1982;6:474.
125. Watson HK, Ryu J, Burgess RC. Matched distal ulnar resection. *J Hand Surg [Am]* 1986;11:812–817.
126. Morrey BF, Askew LJ, An KN, et al. A biomechanical study of the normal functional elbow motion. *J Bone Joint Surg Am* 1986;63:872–877.
127. Sauvé L, Kapandji M. Nouvelle technique de traitment chirurgical des luxations recidivantes isolees de l'extremite inferieure du cubitus. *J Chir* 1936;47:589–594.
128. Taleisnik J. The Suavé-Kapandji procedure. *Clin Orthop* 1992; 275:110–123.
129. Bieber EJ, Linscheid RL, Dobyns, JH, et al. Failed distal ulna resections. *J Hand Surg [Am]* 1988;13:193–200.

22

MANAGEMENT OF THE PAINFUL DISTAL RADIOULNAR JOINT

JOSEPH E. IMBRIGLIA
JOHN W. CLIFFORD

The uniquely human trait of complex hand function is dependent to a large degree on the ability to position the hand in space. The wrist is particularly well adapted to help perform this task. The important functions of pronation and supination are accomplished by a complex interaction among elbow, forearm, and wrist. The distal radioulnar joint (DRUJ) represents the terminal portion of this complex interaction. It is often the site of pathology affecting function or the site where more proximal pathology is manifest. Over recent years, our understanding of this articulation, its basic anatomy and mechanics, and the problems affecting it have become better understood (1–6). Despite this, many questions still remain concerning management of the painful DRUJ. This chapter attempts to give the reader a better understanding of this joint, including its structure and function, pathology, diagnostic modalities, and treatment options.

ANATOMY

The DRUJ is a space separate and distinct from the radiocarpal joint. It is enclosed by a joint capsule on its dorsal and volar aspects and separated from the radiocarpal joint distally by the triangular fibrocartilage complex (TFCC). The articulation of the joint is between the sigmoid notch of the radius and the ulnar head. This basic arrangement allows rotation of the radius around the ulna. The development of this function from an evolutionary standpoint is an interesting topic and one that has been the subject of several papers (7–9). Examination of the wrist articulation in the progression from primitive primates to *Homo sapiens* shows a gradual shortening of the ulna, with the formation of a soft tissue envelope that excludes the distal ulna from the radiocarpal joint. This soft tissue envelope represents the TFCC in man and allows the formation of a separate, diarthrodial DRUJ. In fact, man is the only species in which complete separation of these joints occurs. The evolution of a separate DRUJ parallels species reliance on forearm pronation–supination. In earlier primates, debate continues as to whether the evolutionary impetus for pronation–supination was brachiating locomotion in tree monkeys or knuckle walking.

Thus, the evolutionary process has left man with a joint that is well suited to efficient forearm rotation. Both bony architecture and soft tissue components combine to provide function and stability to this joint. As mentioned, the joint itself is diarthrodial, composed of the distal radius sigmoid notch and the ulnar head. Hyaline cartilage covers approximately 90° to 135° of the ulnar head cylinder. The proximal–distal length of the ulnar head articular surface varies from 5 to 8 mm. The sigmoid notch is concave and varies in dorsovolar width from 1 to 1.5 cm. Articular cartilage covers an arc of 47° to 80° (10). The radii of curvature of these two components differ, with the ulnar head radius 1 cm and the sigmoid notch radius 1.5 mm. This difference affects motion at this joint, which is addressed shortly.

Important soft tissue components consist of the DRUJ capsule and the TFCC. Other extrinsic components that play a lesser part in DRUJ function and stability include the extensor carpi ulnaris (ECU) and its sheath, the interosseous membrane, the extensor retinaculum, and the pronator quadratus (11–13).

The role of the DRUJ capsule has recently been addressed by Kleinman and Graham (Fig. 22.1) (14). They note that the proximal portion is stout and may have some contribution to DRUJ stability. The more distal dorsal and volar aspects are more redundant and pliable. This redundancy is felt to be important in allowing DRUJ motion,

---

J. E. Imbriglia: Department of Orthopaedics, Western Pennsylvania Hand Center, Pittsburgh, Pennsylvania 15212.

J. W. Clifford: Department of Orthopaedics, Kaiser Santa Teresa Community Hospital, San Jose, California 95119.

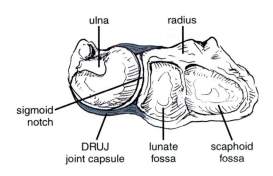

FIGURE 22.1. Capsule of the distal radioulnar joint.

and contracture associated with carpal pathology may cause limitation of motion.

The primary stabilizer of the DRUJ is the TFCC (Fig. 22.2), as shown by Palmer and Werner (15). The components of the TFCC, as defined by Palmer, include the articular disc, the dorsal and palmar radioulnar ligaments, the meniscus homolog, and the ECU sheath. Also important, and included by many in discussions of the TFCC, are the ulnotriquetral and ulnolunate ligaments. The TFCC is discussed in detail in Chapter 38, but a basic understanding is required in a discussion of the DRUJ. The articular disc arises from the ulnar margin of the radius and inserts into the fovea of the ulna and the base of the ulnar styloid. The dorsal and palmar margins, or limbi, of the disc constitute the dorsal and palmar radioulnar ligaments. These ligaments are the most important to DRUJ stability.

The central portion of the disc acts as a load-bearing component, serving to accept compressive loads from the carpus to the ulna. Its importance and pathologic states are discussed in Chapter 38. The ulnolunate and ulnotriquetral ligaments arise from the palmar margin of the articular disc and insert onto the lunate and triquetrum, respectively. They serve to suspend the distal ulna and ulnar carpus from the distal radius and resist volar-ulnar displacement of the carpus.

Other secondary stabilizers include the distal aspect of the interosseous membrane and, as dynamic components, the pronator quadratus and ECU.

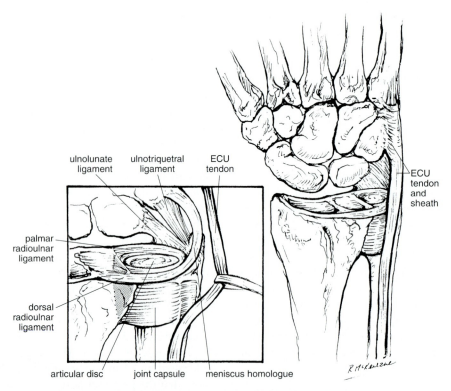

FIGURE 22.2. Triangular fibrocartilage complex. Components include the articular disc, dorsal and palmar radioulnar ligaments, meniscus homolog, ulnolunate and ulnotriquetral ligaments, and the extensor carpi ulnaris (ECU) tendon and its sheath. **Editors' Notes:** *We use the term ulnar sling mechanism to include all of the above structures excluding the ECU tendon but including its sheath and the capsule of the distal radioulnar joint.*

BIOMECHANICS

An understanding of motion and function of the DRUJ requires consideration of the forearm as a whole. Rotation involves motion at the proximal radioulnar joint and DRUJ, with the relationships of these two separate articulations maintained by the length, curvature and angulation of the forearm bones. The relationship of the forearm bones is further maintained and defined by the interosseous membrane. The radius and carpus rotate around a fixed ulna. This relationship has been compared to that of a bucket and handle. The bucket (ulna) and handle (radius and carpus) are connected at two points, the proximal radioulnar joint (PRUJ) and the DRUJ. Alteration of the bucket, handle, or either articulation results in incongruous motion of the handle.

With such an analogy, one can see that the DRUJ must be viewed in relation to the rest of the forearm rotational components. An axis of rotation for the forearm is defined by a line drawn between the radial head and the medial aspect of the ulnar head distally (16). There is slight variation of this axis depending on forearm position.

It is important to note that motion at the DRUJ is not purely rotational. Because of the different radii of curvature of the sigmoid notch and ulnar head, a translational component occurs in the dorsovolar plane as rotation occurs (17). This is also facilitated by some inherent laxity in the supporting ligamentous system. In neutral rotation, it is possible to translate the ulna approximately 3 mm dorsally and 5 mm volarly (18). This translational component dictates variable articular contact in different positions of rotation. In the midrange, 60° to 80° of the ulnar head is in contact with the sigmoid notch; however, at the extremes of rotation, less than 10° may be in contact (17). This underscores the inherent instability of the bony architecture and thus stresses the importance of ligamentous supporting structures in maintaining joint congruity.

As mentioned, the dorsal and palmar radioulnar ligaments are the most important stabilizers of the DRUJ. Controversy exists as to the constraining component in different positions of rotation. af Ekenstam and Hagert (5,17) interpreted data from cadaveric studies to show that the palmar radioulnar ligament (PRUL) had increased tension in pronation, and the dorsal radioulnar ligament (DRUL) in supination. Schuind (19), on the other hand, showed increased DRUL tension in pronation and increased PRUL tension in supination (Fig. 22.3). Hagert (20) has recently addressed the two opposing viewpoints by explaining that different portions of the TFCC were examined in these two studies, with the superficial portion behaving as Schuind described and the deep portion behaving as Hagert described. The importance of understanding normal physiologic stabilizers has implications in our understanding of pathologic states and in recognizing which components are damaged in various instability conditions.

Additional motion occurs at the DRUJ in an axial direction as the forearm rotates. Ulnar variance can change as much as 2 mm from full supination to full pronation. The ulna will be relatively more positive in full pronation.

Weiler (21) and King (22) have examined the axis of rotation of the DRUJ. Because of multiaxial motions, this axis does not fall at a fixed point but, rather, describes a locus of points called a centrode. In normal wrists, this centrode is a tightly grouped locus near the medial portion of the ulnar head. Weiler has shown that disease states such as rheumatoid arthritis cause much greater variability in the centrode.

DIAGNOSIS OF DISTAL RADIOULNAR JOINT PROBLEMS

Because the DRUJ is characterized by complex anatomy, complex mechanics, and interrelations with other forearm articulations and motions, evaluation of DRUJ problems is often difficult. These problems should be approached in a systematic fashion, with a thorough understanding of underlying anatomy, normal and pathologic states, and differential diagnoses. Armed with this knowledge and an expanding armamentarium of diagnostic tests, a clinician now can more readily diagnose problems that historically posed many dilemmas. The diagnosis of DRUJ disorders must be considered in the spectrum of ulnar-sided wrist pain. Therefore, a proper evaluation must address other closely related anatomic structures on the ulnar side of the wrist.

History

A thorough history can help to direct further examination and diagnostic studies. It is important to ascertain whether a problem is acute or chronic in nature, whether there is a history of trauma, and, if possible, the mechanism of that trauma. Also, the movements or activities that produce symptoms should be considered. Symptoms of acute inflammation may be present, as in calcific tendinitis or inflammatory arthropathies. Finally, consideration should be made for the patient's degree of daily activity and vocational or recreational demands, especially in considering treatment options.

Examination

General inspection of the involved hand should include attention to evidence of disuse, atrophy, or guarding. Areas of swelling should be noted. Range of motion of the wrist should be recorded, including flexion, extension, radial–ulnar deviation, and pronation–supination. Grip strength should also be measured and recorded.

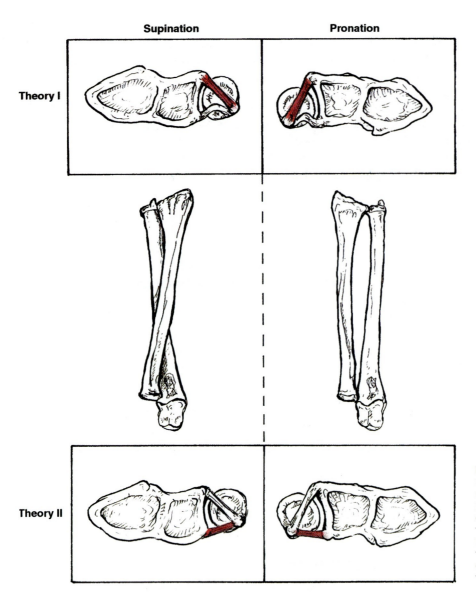

FIGURE 22.3. Diagram showing the dorsal radioulnar ligament (DRUL) and palmar radioulnar ligament (PRUL) in different positions of pronation and supination. Two different theories are represented, with the **top** diagrams showing the DRUL taut in pronation and the PRUL taut in supination. The **bottom** diagrams represent the opposing view of the PRUL taut in pronation and the DRUL taut in supination.

Palpation and provacative maneuvers should be performed with the patient seated at a table opposite the examiner, the elbow flexed to 90° on the table, and the fingers pointing toward the ceiling. The wrist should be at neutral rotation. Knowledge of underlying anatomy is crucial in attempting to elicit tenderness and understand its origin. Because so many anatomic structures are contained in such a small region, precise palpation using the eraser of a pencil can be helpful. Important structures to palpate are the ECU and flexor carpi ulnaris (FCU) tendons, the DRUJ, the TFCC, the lunotriquetral (LT) ligament, the ulnocarpal ligaments, and the pisotriquetral joint.

Provocative Maneuvers

Specific maneuvers, used in conjunction with information from the history and physical examination up to this point, can help to confirm a diagnosis. Compression or gentle ballotment of the DRUJ can elicit pain in the face of arthritic changes. Compression is best applied at the forearm proximal to the wrist to avoid confusion from aggravation of other tender areas. Stability of the DRUJ should be assessed in neutral, pronation, and supination. In neutral, there should be slight laxity of the joint. This should be compared to the contralateral side. The "piano key" sign is also useful to asses DRUJ stability. This sign is elicited by resting the palm flat on the table and pressing the hypothenar eminence into the table using the entire arm. The ulna will move from dorsal to volar. Again, it must be stressed that comparison is necessary, as some movement at the DRUJ is seen in most individuals performing this maneuver.

Provocative maneuvers are also useful for other areas on the ulnar side of the wrist. Pain reproduced with ulnar deviation is suspicious for ulnar impaction syndrome. Pisotriquetral pain can be reproduced by shearing or grinding the pisiform against the triquetrum. LT pain or instability can be reproduced using the shuck test of Reagan et al. (23). In this maneuver, the examiner grasps the pisotriquetral portion of the carpus with the thumb and index of one hand while the other hand stabilizes the forearm and radial carpus. The pisotriquetral unit is then translated dorsovolarly. Excessive mobility or pain is suspicious for LT pathology. Similarly, Kleinman (24) described a shear test of the LT joint, utilizing differential pressure on the lunate dorsally and the pisotriquetral region volarly.

Finally, stability of the ECU can be tested by ulnar-deviating the wrist and rotating from full pronation to full supination. Subluxation or dislocation of the ECU can be reproduced with this maneuver.

Diagnostic Modalities

A variety of imaging studies and diagnostic tools exist for use with the wrist and DRUJ. A judicious use of these studies is necessary, directed by findings from the history and physical exam.

Radiographs

Basic diagnostic studies for most cases should include a lateral and an anteroposterior (AP) radiograph in neutral rotation. The AP should be taken with the shoulder abducted to 90°. In this orientation, the ulnar styloid will be seen in full profile on the medial aspect of the ulna. This view allows good visualization of bony architecture and gives a good standard for comparing ulnar variance. Occasionally, with DRUJ instability, diastasis of the joint may be seen on the AP view. This finding can be accentuated with a clenched-fist view. The lateral view can be helpful for determining DRUJ subluxation or dislocation, but it needs to be an absolutely true lateral in neutral rotation. Small variations in x-ray positioning can lead to an erroneous diagnosis of subluxation (26).

Computed Tomography Scanning

Computed tomography (CT) scanning is a valuable tool for evaluating congruity of the DRUJ (27). The ability to obtain cross-sectional imaging of the DRUJ allows good visualization of articular relationships. However, the translational component of DRUJ motion can make it difficult to define normal parameters of articular congruity. Subluxation or dislocation that occurs in neutral can more easily be detected, especially with comparison scans of the opposite extremity. Mino and colleagues (25,26) described a method for detecting subluxation at neutral using lines tangential to the dorsal and palmar borders of the radius. In normal subjects, the ulnar head should fall between these lines. Other methods have been described using epicenter or congruity data to evaluate instability in pronation–supination. Pirela-Cruz and associates (18) described a method of CT stress views. They determined that normal stressed translation at neutral rotation was 2.8 mm dorsal and 5.4 mm volar, or a side-to-side difference of less than 3 mm.

Arthrography

With the advent of other imaging techniques and the increasing utility of diagnostic arthroscopy, arthrography is less frequently used for diagnostic purposes in the wrist. Arthrography can be useful in diagnosing TFCC and intercarpal ligament tears. However, consideration must be made for its invasive nature. Also, dye communication between compartments can be seen in normal wrists, especially in older patients (28).

Magnetic Resonance Imaging

Improvement in the quality of magentic resonance imaging of the wrist has led to an increased utilization of this technique. It is particularly useful for tears of the TFCC, but can also be useful for detecting chondral defects or injuries, ganglia or masses, and occult fractures. Comparison with arthrography in diagnosing TFCC tears has revealed similar accuracy with both techniques, with a sensitivity near 80% and specificity of nearly 100% (29,30). The expense of this test, however, should preclude its use as a screening tool in the wrist. Its utilization should be in well-defined situations where it will direct diagnosis and/or treatment.

Bone Scan

This is a sensitive but nonspecific test for detecting wrist pathology. It is useful when workup of a painful wrist has not provided a clear diagnosis. It can often confirm the existence of pathology and may direct diagnosis to a particular area of the wrist. Three-phase scanning should be utilized. It has a 95% sensitivity and a 96% specificity in separating pathologic from nonpathologic wrists (31). Early and intermediate scanning can detect ligament or soft tissue injury, and delayed scanning is useful in detecting bone and joint problems.

Arthroscopy

The expanding familiarity with arthroscopy of the wrist has led to more emphasis on the technique as a diagnostic tool. Several reports indicate good correlation of arthroscopic findings with arthrogram and MRI (29,32,33). In addition, arthroscopy provides the ability to treat pathology at the time of diagnosis. Specifically, its use in the DRUJ is in its ability to diagnose and treat lesions of the TFCC. Central tears and perforations can be debrided with good results. Treatment of peripheral detachments can be performed, and refinements in this technique are currently being developed. Arthroscopy of the DRUJ itself is a more difficult procedure and is less frequently utilized. The technique of DRUJ arthroscopy has been reported (34). Its utility is mainly in diagnosis of chondral lesions or wear. Synovectomy and treatment of proximal TFCC lesions may be performed, but instrumentation in this tight joint is difficult.

DISORDERS OF THE DISTAL RADIOULNAR JOINT

Problems at the DRUJ can be divided into broad categories that aid in consideration of diagnosis and treatment. Problems may be acute or chronic, with bone or soft tissue involvement. Often, there is overlap between conditions, with bone or soft tissue injury coexisting or an undiagnosed acute injury leading to a chronic condition. Table 22.1 provides an overview of problems seen at the DRUJ. It will serve as an outline for the following discussion.

Acute Problems

Soft Tissue

Triangular Fibrocartilage Complex Tear Without Instability

These injuries are discussed more fully in the section on the TFCC. Tears without associated instability are usually the result of a fall on the outstretched hand with an associated rotational component or are the result of a torsional mechanism. They are usually central or radial tears and respond well to arthroscopic debridement (35).

Triangular Fibrocartilage Complex Tear With Instability

Subluxation or Dislocation of the Distal Radioulnar Joint. These entities actually represent a spectrum of injuries to the DRUJ soft tissue stabilizing components. As previously stated, Palmer and Werner demonstrated the TFCC to be the most important stabilizer of the DRUJ (3). Thus, differing degrees of injury to the TFCC will result in a spectrum from minor instability to subluxation to frank dislocation. Kihara (36), using a cadaver model, showed that complete dislocation could occur only if several stabilizing structures were cut (the dorsal and palmar radioulnar ligaments, the pronator quadratus and distal IOM, and the entire IOM).

Those TFCC tears resulting in minor instability or subluxation are usually caused by peripheral detachment. Acutely, a trial of immobilization is warranted for these injuries. Open or arthroscopic repair may be performed if conservative measures fail.

Frank dislocation can occur palmarly or dorsally. This nomenclature refers to the direction of prominence of the ulna; however, in actuality it is the radius and carpus that dislocate from the fixed ulna. Dorsal dislocations most often result from a hyperpronation injury, usually associated with a fall (37,38). A direct blow to the radius or ulna may also produce this injury. The clinical presentation is that of a prominent ulnar head dorsally, with a forearm locked in pronation. Treatment is by closed reduction, accomplished by direct pressure on the ulnar head combined with forearm supination. This is followed by 4 to 6 weeks of immobilization with the forearm in neutral to supination. Volar dislocations (Fig. 22.4) usually result from a fall in hypersupination. The diagnosis is not as obvious as with dorsal dislocations, as the ulnar head will be somewhat obscured by volar soft tissues. The forearm will usually be locked in supination. Reduction is performed with direct volar-ulnar pressure and forearm pronation. Postreduction treatment consists of 4 to 6 weeks of forearm immobilization in neutral to pronation.

Failure to obtain adequate closed reduction or persistent instability following immobilization warrants open reduction with extraction of interposed soft tissue and repair of stabilizing structures (11).

Bone

Intraarticular Fractures

Sigmoid Notch and Ulnar Head. These fractures present the problem of joint incongruity with the potential for late posttraumatic degenerative changes. To assure the best possible result, congruent reduction of the articular surfaces is nec-

TABLE 22.1. PROBLEMS SEEN AT THE DISTAL RADIOULNAR JOINT

I. Acute problems
   A. Soft tissue injury
      1. TFCC tear without instability
      2. TFCC tear with instability
      3. DRUJ dislocation: ulna dorsal/volar
   B. Bone injury
      1. Intraarticular: Sigmoid notch/ulnar head
      2. Extraarticular
         a. Ulnar styloid
         b. Distal radius
         c. Ulnar shaft
         d. Radial shaft (Galeazzi)
         e. Radial head (Essex-Lopresti)
II. Chronic problems
   A. Soft tissue
      1. Chronic instability
      2. Ulnar impaction
   B. Bone
      1. DRUJ DJD
      2. Ulnar styloid nonunion, with/without instability
      3. Distal radius malunion
      4. Ulna/radius shaft malunion
      5. Chronic radius migration after radial head excision
      6. Growth disturbances

DJD, degenerative joint disease; DRUJ, distal radioulnar joint; TFCC, triangular fibrocartilage complex.

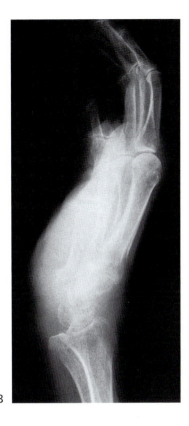
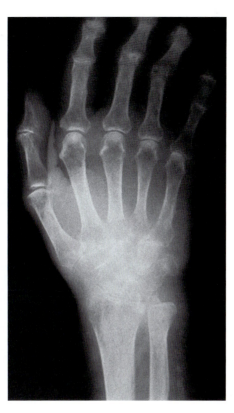

FIGURE 22.4. A: Lateral x-ray of a volar distal radioulnar joint (DRUJ) dislocation. This elderly woman was immobilized in supination for a hand infection, which led to dislocation of her DRUJ with her forearm locked in supination. **B:** Note the extreme radial position of her ulnar styloid on anteroposterior view.

essary. Unfortunately, these injuries often occur in high-energy trauma with other associated wrist fractures and are often overlooked in treatment. As many hand surgeons will attest, the DRUJ often is the site of long-term painful sequelae following wrist fractures (see Fig. 22.21). Because of this, more focus should be placed on the DRUJ in initial management and treatment. If necessary, tomograms or CT scans can be used to evaluate articular fragments and plan treatment accordingly. Accurate articular reduction can then be performed using plates, screws, K-wires, and/or external fixation.

Extraarticular Fractures

Ulnar Styloid. These fractures can occur as isolated entities or in association with distal radius or other wrist fractures. They occur as one of two types: a fracture at the styloid tip or at the styloid base (Fig. 22.5). Because of the attachment of the TFCC at the styloid base, fractures at this site are often associated with instability of the DRUJ. Treatment of styloid tip fractures is generally symptomatic, with a splint or cast used for pain relief. Nondisplaced fractures at the styloid base can be treated with cast immobilization. A short arm cast with slight ulnar deviation will usually suffice (11). Displaced fractures at the styloid base are often associated with distal radius fractures (Fig. 22.6) (39). Usually, reduction of the styloid will occur with reduction of the radius, and treatment will then be as for a nondisplaced fracture. For fractures that remain significantly displaced, or that demonstrate significant DRUJ instability following reduction, open reduction

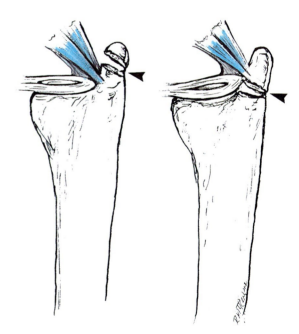

FIGURE 22.5. A: Ulnar styloid fracture at its tip. The triangular fibrocartilage complex (TFCC) remains attached at its base. **B:** Styloid fracture at its base, with accompanying TFCC separation. **Editors' Notes:** *Independent of its ligament attachments, an ulnar styloid that is separated by 3 to 5 mm or more from the ulna will be asymptomatic. If there is 1 mm or less between the styloid fragment and the parent bone, then symptoms occur, osteophytes will form, and a painful reactive process ensures. Styloidectomy will be necessary.*

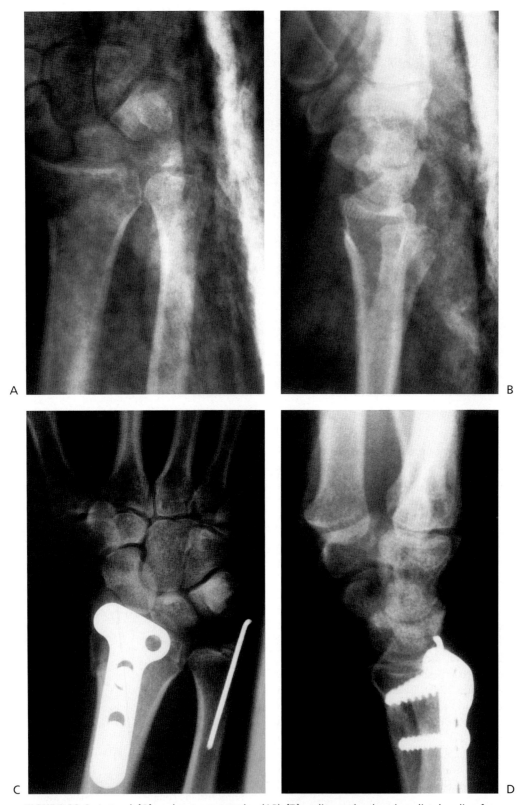

FIGURE 22.6. Lateral **(A)** and anteroposterior (AP) **(B)** radiographs showing distal radius fracture with displaced ulnar styloid fracture at its base. The distal ulna is diplaced. The triangular fibrocartilage complex is attched to the large styloid fragment, maintaining its relation with the radius. Lateral **(C)** and AP **(D)** radiographs following open reduction with internal fixation (ORIF) of the distal radius. The styloid remained displaced with an unstable distal ulna. This was treated by ORIF of the styloid fragment.

with internal fixation (ORIF) is indicated. K-wire and/or tension-band techniques can be used with good results (11).

A bony lunula is an anatomic variant and can be confused with a styloid fracture. The triquetrum secondarum or triangulare can be present distal to the ulnar styloid. It is usually seen bilaterally and is not associated with trauma.

Distal Radius. In addition to possible intraarticular involvement of the sigmoid notch, there are potential effects on DRUJ mechanics caused by extraarticular displacement of the distal radius. Treatment of distal radius fractures must address acute dislocations and subluxations of the DRUJ. This can happen because of the dorsal or volar displacement of the radius fragment. For complete dislocation of the DRUJ to occur, an injury to the TFCC must also occur. Restoration of alignment of the radius using rigid immobilization or fixation should be performed, with special attention paid to DRUJ relationships. Although TFCC repair is not usually required for good long-term results, consideration should be made for preserving DRUJ reduction in the unstable joint in the postoperative or postreduction period. This would include pinning the DRUJ or immobilizing forearm rotation with the DRUJ reduced.

In evaluating reduction of distal radius fractures, recent laboratory and clinical studies have helped define acceptable parameters (40–43). These parameters were developed to attempt to identify displacement patterns that lead to long-term disability. It is difficult to assign definitive values that correlate with good function, especially when dealing with a wide spectrum of patients with varying functional demands. It is also sometimes difficult to identify what component of wrist function is affected by malreduction. Radiocarpal, ulnocarpal, and DRUJ functions are at risk for alteration. Generally, values associated with poor function are greater than 20° dorsal angulation, radial inclination less than 10°, and radial translation greater than 2 mm. Shortening greater than 6 mm has also been correlated with poor results (44). In fact, a cadaver study by Adams (45) found that radial shortening had the greatest effect on DRUJ kinematics. Loss of radial inclination and dorsal angulation caused intermediate alterations, and dorsal displacement caused minimal changes.

Treatment of distal radius fractures requires attention to many details. The DRUJ is often neglected in addressing these problematic fractures. Cooney (46) has shown that DRUJ arthritis is more common than radiocarpal arthritis in long-term follow-up of distal radius fractures.

Ulnar Shaft. Fractures of either forearm bone proximal to the DRUJ have the potential to adversely affect DRUJ function with malunion. Ulna fractures are typically treated less aggressively than radius fractures. However, it is important to note that any angulation of the ulna proximally will amplify displacement distally. This displacement may affect DRUJ congruity and mechanics, with the potential for immediate and long-term effects (see Fig. 22.22). General guidelines for displacement necessitating reduction have been given as displacement greater than 50% of bone diameter or angulation greater than 10° (47). However, little is known regarding acceptable displacement for good long-term DRUJ function (14).

Radial Shaft (Galeazzi Fracture). Radial shaft fractures also have the potential to affect the DRUJ in the short and long term. An isolated fracture at the diaphysis of the distal third of the radius has special significance. This often (but not always) signifies an associated disruption of the DRUJ. This fracture was first reported in 1822 by Sir Astley Cooper (48). It has several eponymns, including the Galeazzi fracture (49), the reverse Monteggia fracture (50), the Piedmont fracture (51), and the "fracture of necessity" (52). The mechanism of injury is usually an axial load on the dorsiflexed/pronated wrist. This mechanism causes a propagation of forces to the DRUJ, with a resultant tear of the TFCC. Deforming forces elucidated by Hughston (53,54) then serve to displace the DRUJ. Sarmiento and Latta (55) have stated that injuries caused by direct blows to the radius are less likely to have associated DRUJ disruption.

Moore (56) has described four radiographic criteria for DRUJ disruption: (a) ulnar styloid fracture at its base, (b) widening of the DRUJ joint space on an AP view, (c) dislocation of the radius relative to the ulna on a lateral view, and (d) shortening of the radius by more than 5 mm. Definitive assesment, however, is made on a clinical basis. This assessment is after stabilization of the radius, which for this fracture implies ORIF.

Campbell's pseudonym "fracture of necessity" (52) implies the need for operative treatment of this injury. Hughston (53,54) reported a 92% failure rate for closed reduction and immobilization. Accurate ORIF with anatomic realignment should restore the DRUJ relationships. In a true Galeazzi fracture, DRUJ instability will persist and should be addressed with long arm casting in supination for 6 weeks or pinning of the DRUJ for 6 weeks. Open treatment of the TFCC is not required unless displacement of a styloid fracture or joint dislocation persists after anatomic radius fixation.

Radial Head (Essex-Lopresti Lesion). A fracture of the radial head caused by axial loading with associated longitudinal instability is known as the Essex-Lopresti lesion (Fig. 22.7). This instability results from injury to the interosseous membrane or TFCC combined with loss of proximal osseous support. First described in 1931 by Brockman (57), its name is derived from Essex-Lopresti's classic description in 1951 (58). This name implies an acute injury and should be distinguished from chronic radius migration following radial head excision (59). The actual incidence of acute injury to the interosseous membrane and TFCC with radial head fracture is unknown. Initial evaluation of the forearm and wrist is often incomplete in studies

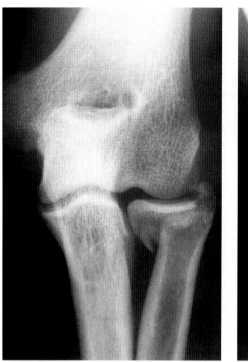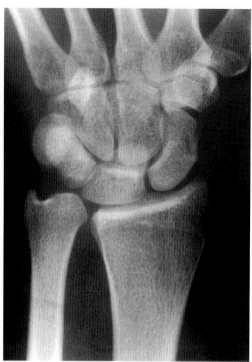

FIGURE 22.7. Essex-Lopresti injury showing radial head fracture and proximal migration of the radius. This patient complained of wrist pain in addition to elbow pain at initial presentation.

examining proximal migration. Also, the incidence of acute proximal migration of the radius after radial head resection is uncertain. Some studies estimate an incidence from 20% to 90% (60). However, these studies are unclear on when the migration occurred (i.e., short- or long-term).

For acute migration to occur, the primary longitudinal stabilizers of the forearm must be injured. Studies by Hotchkiss et al. (61) and Rabinowitz et al. (62) have shown that these are the radial head, the central portion of the IOM and the TFCC. Rabinowitz has shown that 7 mm of proximal translation under axial load can occur with radial head excision alone. More than 7 mm can occur if the IOM and TFCC are also deficient.

Treatment of the Essex-Lopresti injury is often difficult. If any forearm or wrist symptoms coexist with a radial head fracture, every attempt should be made to preserve the radial head. This requires ORIF with pins, screws, and/or plates. If this is not possible, a silastic or metallic implant should be placed, with consideration of pinning the DRUJ for 4 to 6 weeks for added longitudinal stability. There are problems with the long-term use of implants (silicone synovitis, dislocation, fragmentation) and questions regarding their efficacy. Some advocate limited (12–24 months) use of the implants while soft tissue healing occurs (14). Questions remain, however, regarding the ability of the IOM to heal. Knight (63) described a case of proximal translation occuring soon after the removal of a metallic prosthesis. Others (64,65) have reported documented proximal migration even with a silicone prosthesis in place. Metallic heads may provide more rigidity and resistance to translation, but not enough data are currently available concerning the long-term efficacy of metallic implants.

Because of the problems associated with proximal migration of the radius following radial head fracture and excision, it should be stressed that a high index of suspicion for distal injury should be maintained, and if possible, the radial head should be preserved.

Chronic Problems

Soft Tissue

Chronic Instability

This problem occurs because of chronic insufficiency of the TFCC and distal soft tissue restraints. It is often difficult to diagnose, but careful attention to history, physical exam, and diagnostic workup will help. If diagnosed early enough, TFCC repair or distal soft tissue reconstruction can be considered. As Bowers states (11), this should not be attempted if radius–ulna malunion exists or if degenerative joint disease (DJD) is present.

Some success has been reported with debridement and reattachment of the TFCC to the ulnar styloid (66). Bach (67) combined this technique with a strip of distally based ECU tendon woven through the radius and ulna. Many procedures have been described that attempt to recreate the

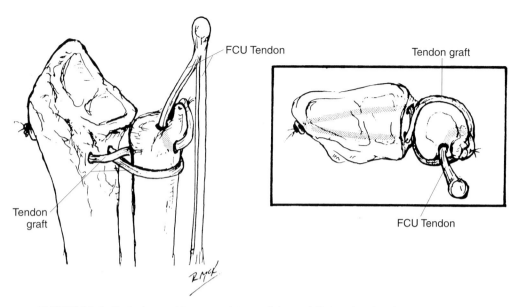

FIGURE 22.8. Technique of Boyes and Bunnell for stabilizing the distal radioulnar joint.

soft tissue stabilizing components of the DRUJ. These include procedures that attempt to recreate an ulnocarpal tether, a radioulnar sling, or both. Some of the more frequently cited reconstructive procedures can be briefly described. The Boyes-Bunnel reconstruction (68) uses a tendon graft sling from radius to ulna and a distally based strip of FCU to stabilize the distal ulna (Fig. 22.8). Fulkerson and Watson (69) described a sling procedure using a graft passed through a drill hole in the distal radius (Fig. 22.9). Hui and Linscheid (70) reported on the use of the FCU as an ulnar tether, attempting to recreate the volar ulnocarpal ligaments. Johnston-Jones and Sanders (71) presented a method to recreate the dorsal and volar radioulnar ligaments using a tendon graft.

Peterson and Adams (72), in a biomechanical study, found that none of these procedures restored normal stability. The radioulnar sling procedures, however, were stronger than the ulnocarpal procedures.

Other methods described do not try to recreate normal anatomic restraints. Rather, they substitute for them or augment them. Johnson (73) used a transfer of the pronator quadratus to act as a dynamic stabilizer, preventing dorsal

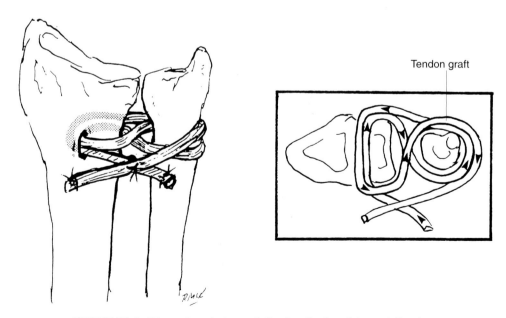

FIGURE 22.9. Watson's technique of distal radioulnar joint stabilization.

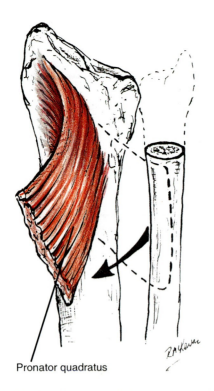

FIGURE 22.10. Dorsal transfer of the pronator quadratus to act as a dynamic stabilizer of distal ulna.

subluxation (Fig. 22.10). This procedure has been combined with tendon-stabilizing procedures to provide additional stability (see Fig. 22.14). Imbriglia and Matthews (74) and Short and Palmer (75) combine hemiresection of the distal ulna with stabilization procedures to address chronic subluxation or dislocation. Other procedures combine resection of the distal ulna with various stabilizing techniques. These techniques may be used in the arthritic or nonarthritic joint. They are further discussed later in this chapter.

The wide variety of procedures available to address chronic instability of the DRUJ tells us that no one procedure is completely effective in relieving pain and restoring function. Treatment must be tailored to individual patient symptoms and expectations, using available techniques of reconstruction.

Ulnar Impaction Syndrome

This problem is included here in a brief discussion. It stems primarily from distal ulna impingement on the ulnar carpus with damage to the intervening TFCC. Treatment is conservative in the early stages, with judicious use of nonsteroidal antiinflammatory drugs (NSAIDS) and splinting and/or casting. If this fails to relieve symptoms, operative intervention is undertaken to either debride the TFCC, shorten the ulna, or both (Fig. 22.11). This is further discussed in Chapter 39.

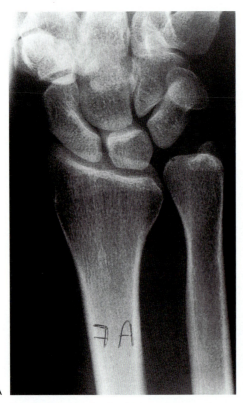
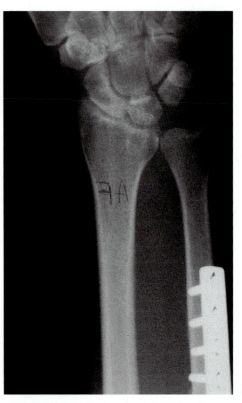

FIGURE 22.11. A: Significant ulna-positive wrist with impaction. **B:** Patient treated with ulnar shortening osteotomy.

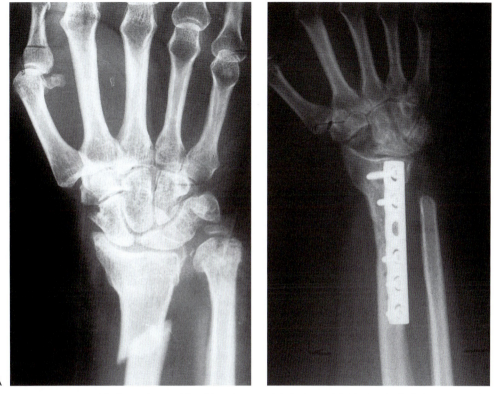

FIGURE 22.12. Elderly patient with old wrist/carpal injuries. Old injuries include intraarticular ulnar head fracture with degenerative joint disease. **A:** Patient also now has acute radius fracture. **B:** Patient had acute radius plating. Later reconsruction included intercarpal fusion and distal ulna resection.

Bone

Distal Radioulnar Joint Arthritis

Many of the problems discussed above may lead to incongruity at the DRUJ with the secondary development of degenerative arthritis. Treatment is then aimed at pain relief, either through conservative measures or operative techniques. Failing conservative treatment, several operative procedures are available.

Complete resection of the distal ulna, known as the Darrach procedure, is probably the oldest technique still in widespread use today (Figs. 22.1, 22.12, and 22.13). Darrach first presented the procedure in 1912, though others had previously described it (11). Numerous reports testify to good results using this technique (76–78). However, others point to problems related to residual ulnar instability, radioulnar impingement, ulnocarpal translation, and damage to surrounding tissues secondary to instability (76,79). This may be especially true of the younger posttraumatic patient (80). These problems may be reduced if care is taken to resect minimal bone and perform careful repair of surrounding soft tissues. Tulipan (78) reported 91% good to excellent 4-year follow-up in 30 patients when these principles were followed.

Many procedures have been described to manage the painful, unstable distal ulna following resection. Some are extensions of procedures to stabilize the intact distal ulna. Goldner (81) and Tsai (82) described the use of one-half of the ECU to tenodese the distal ulna stump. Kleinman and Greenburg (83) combined an ECU tenodesis with a dorsal transfer of the pronator quadratus (Fig. 22.14). Breen and Jupiter (84) described a tenodesis using one-half

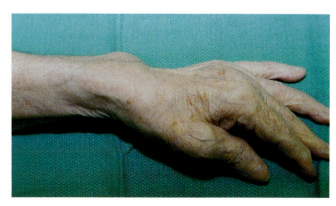

FIGURE 22.13. Clinical appearance of dorsally subluxed distal radioulnar joint in a patient with rheumatoid arthritis.

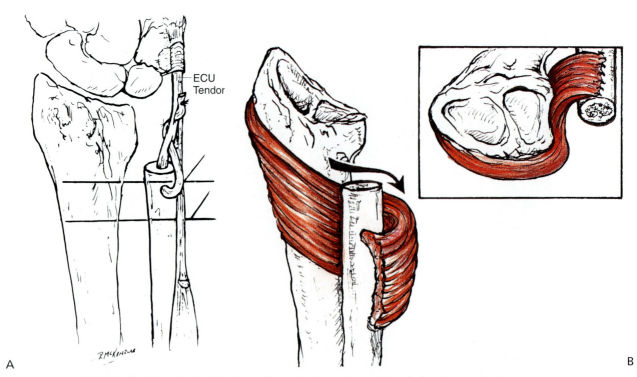

FIGURE 22.14. A,B: Stabilization of distal ulna with a strip of distally based extensor carpi ulnaris (ECU). Kleinman and Greenburg describe the combination of ECU stabilization with transfer of the pronator quadratus (Fig. 22.10). **Editors' Notes:** *In the short post-Darrach ulna, winging and radial impingement are both symptomatic problems. It is nearly impossible to solve this with ligament or tendon procedures. The only reliable solution is a step-cut lengthening of the ulna where the distal segment is brought to the level of the articular surface of the radius. This is combined with a matched shaping of the distal osteotomy segment.*

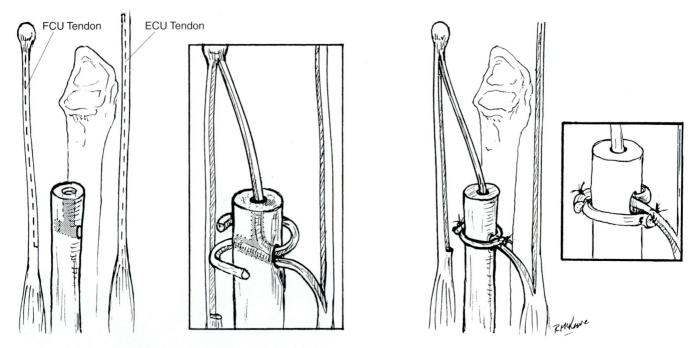

FIGURE 22.15. Stabilization of distal ulna as described by Breen and Jupiter. *ECU,* extensor carpi ulnaris; *FCU,* flexor carpi ulnaris.

of a proximally based ECU tendon and one-half of a distally based FCU tendon (Fig. 22.15). This technique can be used to salvage the failed Darrach or be combined with a Darrach for primary symptomatic degenerative instability. An isolated stabilization of the ulna stump using one-half of the FCU has also been described (Fig. 22.16) (71).

Although all of these procedures can provide some improvement in stability and symptoms, a certain subset of patients with Darrach procedures will have continued disabling problems. This can be a difficult group to manage. They tend to have multiple operations with little improvement in symptoms (79). Continued shortenings of the ulna do not tend to help. A final solution may be a radioulnar fusion as described by Carroll and Imbriglia (Figs. 22.1, 22.17, and 22.18) (85).

Dingman (86), in 1952, reported that the most successful Darrach procedures tended to have less bone resection or regenerated bone within their periosteal sleeve. This success is likely a result of retention or recreation of soft tissue stabilizers. In an attempt to preserve soft tissue stabilizers, hemiresection techniques have been developed (Fig. 22.19). These techniques resect only the articular portion of the ulnar head, leaving the styloid and TFCC attachment intact. Bowers (87)

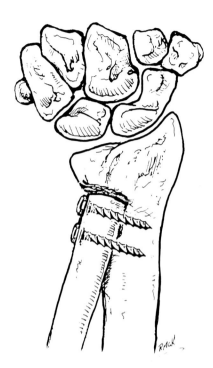

FIGURE 22.17. Diagram of distal radioulnar fusion.

used interposition material to prevent radioulnar impingement. He states that an intact or reconstructible TFCC is a prerequisite to provide stability. Watson et al. (88) use a matched hemiresection technique, which resects more bone on the proximal-radial aspect of the ulna in an attempt to

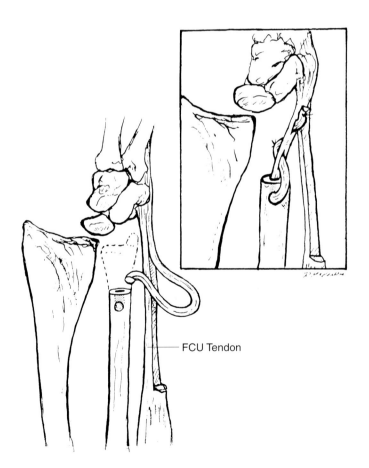

FIGURE 22.16. Stabilization of distal ulna using a strip of distally based flexor carpi ulnaris (FCU) tendon.

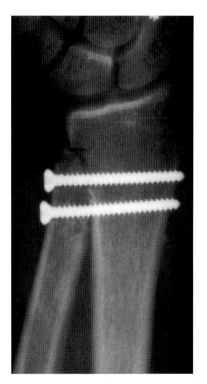

FIGURE 22.18. Radiograph of distal radioulnar fusion.

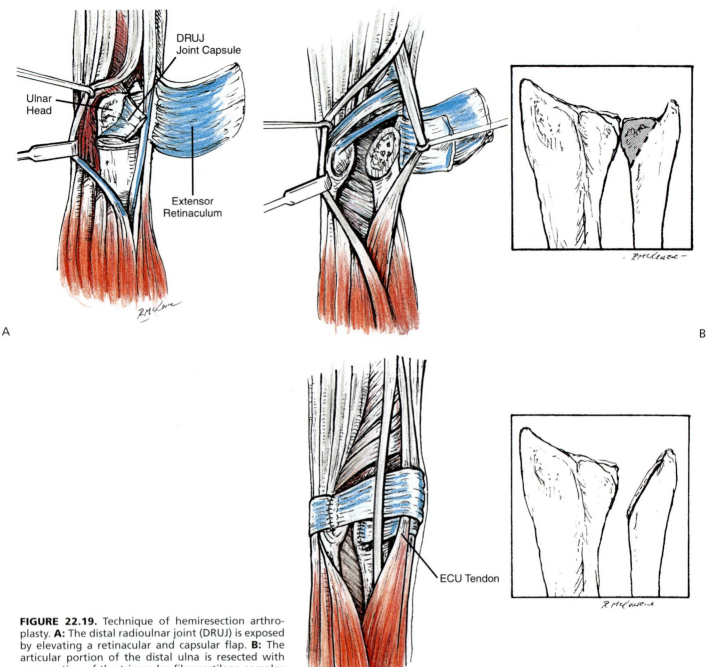

FIGURE 22.19. Technique of hemiresection arthroplasty. **A:** The distal radioulnar joint (DRUJ) is exposed by elevating a retinacular and capsular flap. **B:** The articular portion of the distal ulna is resected with preservation of the triangular fibrocartilage complex attachment. **C:** The DRUJ capsule is used as interposition material, and the retinaculum is repaired.

match the contour of the radius. These authors use no interposition material. A potential problem with either technique is migration of the radius and ulna together, creating radioulnar impingement and/or ulnocarpal impingement. Interposition may help to prevent this problem. Bowers (11) reviewed the results of 152 hemiresection–interposition procedures and found 76% to be pain-free and 24% with mild pain. Two percent required reoperation for ulnocarpal impingement.

Another procedure that can be used for either arthritis or chronic instability is the Sauvé-Kapandji or fusion–pseudoarthrosis technique (Fig. 22.20). In this procedure, the radius and ulna are fused at the DRUJ, and a pseudoarthrosis is created by resecting a portion of ulna proximally. This retains a load-bearing seat for the ulnar carpus. An intact TFCC is necessary to transmit axial load. Ulnocarpal impingement can also be addressed by fusing the ulnar head in a more proximal position. The potential exists for either instability of the proximal stump or reformation of bone, causing limited motion. For this reason, the recommended technique is to resect no more

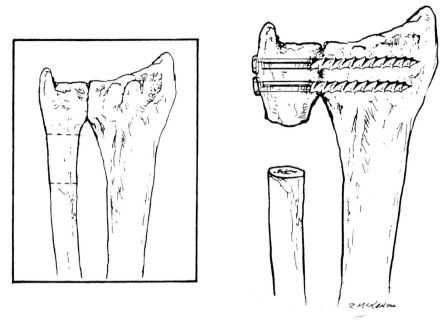

FIGURE 22.20. Sauvé-Kapandji technique.

than 1 cm of proximal ulna in a subperiosteal fashion to retain the soft tissue attachments. The periosteum or pronator quadratus can then be reflected over the raw bone ends to prevent bony regrowth. The pronator may also provide stability to the proximal stump.

Many advocate this procedure for osteoarthritis, posttraumatic arthritis, and rheumatoid arthritis (89,90). Theoretically, the preserved distal ulna provides more stable carpal-forearm motion, benefitting the younger, more vigorous population. Its utility in rheumatoid arthritis is to prevent ulnar drift of the carpus when the radiocarpal ligaments are deficient.

Ulnar Styloid Nonunion

The majority of ulnar styloid nonunions will be asymptomatic. Rarely, either nonunion site pain or DRUJ instability will require operative intervention. Hauk et al. (91) noted that only 32 cases requiring operative intervention had been reported in the English literature. They presented an additional 20. Their nonunions were classified as type I, not associated with clinical DRUJ instability, and type II, associated with clinical DRUJ instability. Type I fractures generally occur at the styloid tip, whereas type II occur at the base (see Fig. 22.5). Type I were treated with excision of the fragment, but type II were treated with either ORIF or excision combined with TFCC stabilization. The authors reported excellent results using this classification and treatment scheme.

Distal Radius Malunion

As mentioned in the section on acute fractures, it is often difficult to ascertain which malreductions and subsequent malunions of distal radius fractures will become symptomatic. If recognized early enough, based on gross displacement or high patient demand, a malunion can be addressed by distal radius osteotomy (92). If this is done before significant DRUJ chondromalacia occurs secondary to incongruity, the DRUJ articulation may be preserved. In the low-demand or elderly patient with DRUJ symptoms, more predictable good results can be obtained with osteotomy combined with Darrach or hemiresection (93). A malunion associated only with loss of radial height can more easily be dealt with by an ulnar shortening osteotomy (94). Finally, intraarticular DRUJ fracture or chronic incongruity with DJD should be treated by one of the salvage procedures described for arthritis of the DRUJ (Fig. 22.21).

Ulna or Radius Shaft Malunion

If DRUJ problems present following ulna or radius shaft malunions, consideration must be made for addressing the malunion before the DRUJ (11). These malunions can result in longitudinal, angular, or rotational problems at the DRUJ. This, in turn, will lead to ulnocarpal impaction, incongruity, or instability symptoms. Proper treatment will require careful preoperative planning using x-ray, tomograms, or CT scans. If established DRUJ arthritis is present, a joint salvage procedure will be necessary (Fig. 22.22).

Chronic Radius Migration After Radial Head Excision

Migration of the radius may occur late following radial head excision, even with no evidence of acute IOM or DRUJ injury (95,96). Although some report that if migration occurs, it will happen within 2 years (97), we have seen cases present as late as 15 years following radial head excision (Fig. 22.23).

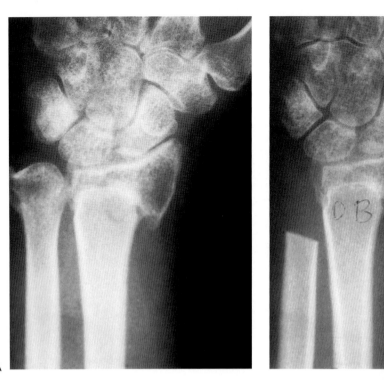

FIGURE 22.21. A: Elderly patient with old distal radius fracture and sigmoid notch involvement. **B:** Symptoms were isolated to the distal radioulnar joint, and treatment was by the Darrach procedure. **Editors' Notes:** Darrach felt strongly that no more than ³/₄ in. should be excised from the distal ulna in the normal adult. The two problems that must be taken into consideration when resecting the distal ulna are winging of the ulna and impingement of the ulna against the radius. With a sharp corner as noted here, impingement is a high probability, particularly with the shortened ulna. The ideal solution is to maintain the length of the ulna out to the level of the articular surface of the radius but to cut it away in a sloping fashion, much like an eccentrically sharpened pencil, to prevent sharp corner impingement of the radius (see Chapter 59).

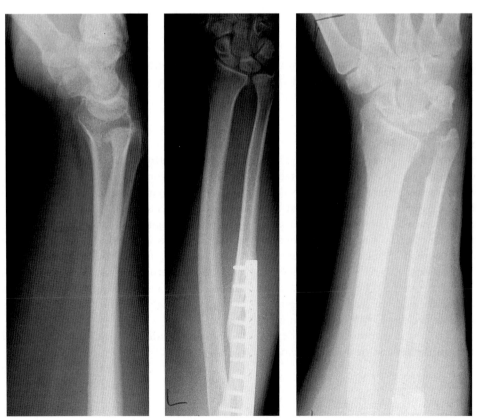

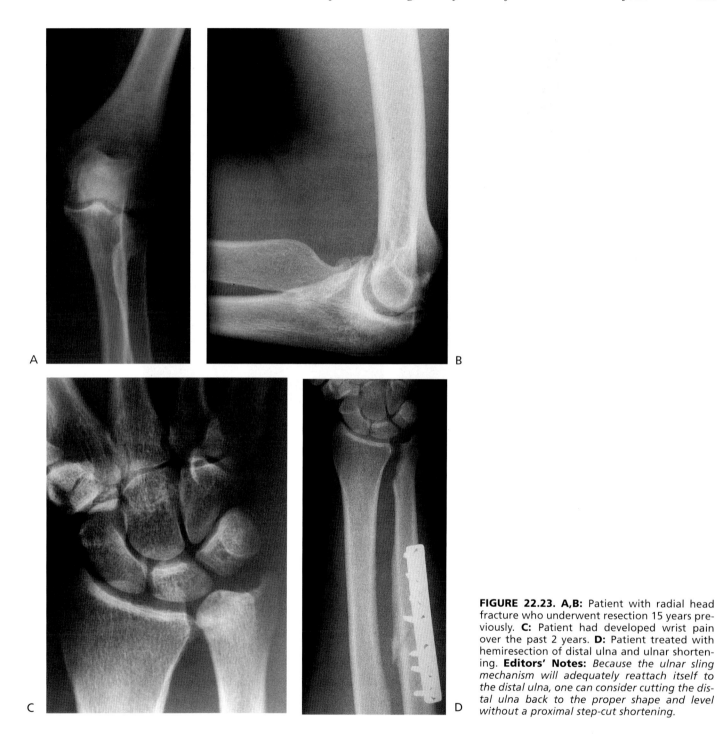

FIGURE 22.23. A,B: Patient with radial head fracture who underwent resection 15 years previously. **C:** Patient had developed wrist pain over the past 2 years. **D:** Patient treated with hemiresection of distal ulna and ulnar shortening. **Editors' Notes:** *Because the ulnar sling mechanism will adequately reattach itself to the distal ulna, one can consider cutting the distal ulna back to the proper shape and level without a proximal step-cut shortening.*

FIGURE 22.22. Lateral **(A)** and anteroposterior **(B)** radiographs of ulnar shaft fracture treated by open reduction with internal fixation. Patient had residual incongruity of his distal radioulnar joint with development of degenerative joint disease. **C:** Patient was later treated with hemiresection arthroplasty.

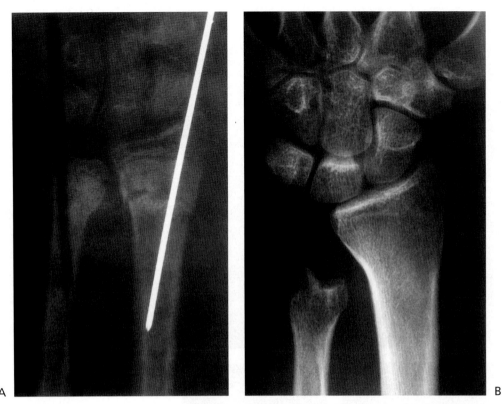

FIGURE 22.24. A: X-ray of a 7-year-old girl with distal radius and ulna fracture. **B:** Patient went on to develop distal ulna growth arrest and complete dissociation of the distal radioulnar joint by age 16.

Salvage of the proximally migrated radius is difficult. Attempts to address ulnocarpal impingement with ulnar shortening, Darrach, hemiresection, or Sauvé-Kapandji procedures tend to have mixed results, with continued migration leading to recurrence of symptoms (65). These procedures may be very helpful for symptom relief, but the patient and surgeon should be aware that it may be only a temporary solution. Consideration can be made for a shortening or DRUJ procedure to be combined with placement of a radial head prosthesis, even if more proximal bone needs to be resected (11). In the face of continued symptoms following reconstruction, salvage can be performed by radioulnar fusion (85) in an attempt to preserve painless wrist flexion–extension.

Growth Disturbances

Involvement of the DRUJ with growth disturbances can occur through either posttraumatic growth arrest or congenital disorders. Growth arrest can follow distal radius or ulna fractures, though it is rare (Fig. 22.24) (98). The DRUJ is always involved in Madelung's deformity. Conservative treatment is usually warranted, but operative treatment is sometimes needed in particularly symptomatic cases. It is difficult to predict how these procedures will fare in the face of continued growth around the DRUJ. Procedures described include radius osteotomy, ulnar shortening or angular osteotomy, epiphysiodesis, the Sauvé-Kapandji procedure, hemiresection, and the Darrach procedure (99,100).

EDITORS' COMMENTS

Phylogenetically, the ulna exists, and the wrist must deal with it. As the hand and wrist have increased their non–weight-bearing functional capacity, evolution has steadily downplayed the role of the distal ulna. The ulna must have a cartilage joint for the rotation motion of the radius. The ulna must be kept from displacing from the radius (winging), yet it must not interfere with wrist function. *The ulna needs the wrist; the wrist does not need the ulna.* Any series of wrist x-rays will demonstrate the incidence of ulnas that are so short, they can play no support role. Indeed, a neutral variant or positive variant ulna can be demonstrated to take load on its distal end. That load must be seen as incidental. In fact, if the distal ulna does take significant load over time, the patient is subject to destruction of the proximal articular cartilage on the lunate secondary to shear loading and the clinical entity of ulnar impaction syndrome. In full pronation, most of the distal ulnar articular surface can be palpated with the examining finger and clearly is not playing a significant carpal support role.

We begin, then, with an anatomy wherein the wrist would be better off if the ulna were not there at all. Because there is a DRUJ as part of the forearm rotation mechanism, the distal end of the ulna must be supported and held in place. This is accomplished by the dorsal and volar radius–ulnar ligaments, and, unfortunately, the soft tissue fill-in between these ligaments has created a triangular structure with the name and accompanying mystique of triangular fibrocartilage. Clinically, this should be simply thought of as the two ligaments that run to the rotation pivot point on the distal end of the ulna to maintain its stability. There are lax radius–ulnar capsular structures that enclose the synovial joint but play little role in stabilizing the ulna, except at the maximum of supination and pronation. The interosseous membrane is an important component of the stability between the radius and ulna.

There is a proximal pistoning phenomenon of the radius under load. Sudden high loads on the hand will cause a proximal migration of the radius with cartilage compression. The ulna does not take part in this pistoning. Momentary positive ulnar variance with use has in most people worn away this central portion of the triangular fibrocartilage with age.

No matter how thick the triangular fibrocartilage, it will transmit only light loading. As loads increase, this collagen compresses. As loads continue to increase, the cartilage also compresses, and the bone structures take 100% of the load. These loads primarily traverse the scaphoid, lunate, and radius. The ulnolunate and ulnotriquetral ligaments are misnomers in that these are really part of the ulnar sling mechanism depending on the radius for support. Stability of the carpals is not dependent on the distal ulna, nor is carpal instability caused by loss of the ulna.

Symptoms of the distal ulna will lie in three categories: (a) symptoms from synovitis in the DRUJ and rotation activities of the forearm; (b) symptoms from an excessively long ulna, the result of either patient ontogeny or because of shortening of the radius—these symptoms will occur with ulnar deviation, and tenderness will localize to the ulnar-lunate-triquetrum area; and (c) symptoms involving winging, that is, a laxity or loss of control of the distal ulna. This includes subluxations and dislocations.

The first clinical maneuver in the examination of the wrist involves passive pronation and passive supination produced in midforearm. This rotation will load the DRUJ and all structures up to and including the triangular fibrocartilage but will produce no load distal to the articular surface of the radius and triangular fibrocartilage. This one simple exam tends to incriminate or eliminate the DRUJ. The second step in the examination would be direct compression of the DRUJ in various degrees of supination and pronation. This is particularly useful if the problem lies with the articular relationship between the radius and ulna. Impaction of the articular surfaces with rotation will often elicit a cartilage fracture fragment in the form of a symptomatic catch or snap. Determination of distal ulna laxity is best done with the wrist in neutral. With the patient's elbow resting on the table, the distal ulna is grasped between thumb and forefinger and taken through a volar-dorsal displacement. This is then compared to the opposite side.

The clinical examination now leaves the DRUJ per se and begins to look at parajoint problems such as a nonunion fragment of the styloid, ulnar impaction syndrome, triquetral lunate instability, triquetral impaction ligament tear (TILT) syndrome, extensor carpi ulnaris synovitis, and other components of the ulnar side of the wrist discussed elsewhere.

Clinical examination is backed up by the x-rays taken in full supination, full pronation, and neutral. Tomography or CT will demonstrate ulna dislocation. Arthrography again plays no significant role; MRI and bone scan are not indicated. Arthroscopy is also not indicated, as an open approach is necessary if the clinical picture warrants repair.

If the ulna is dislocating and there is good cartilage in the joint, then the distal ulna must be stabilized. This requires reinsertion of the dorsal and volar radioulnar ligaments. This reinsertion must occur at the approximate rotational pivot point in the distal end of the ulna.

The patient is operated on under suitable anesthesia. A transverse incision is carried out at the level of the articular surface of the radius. Dissection is carried deep distal to the extensor retinaculum (Editors' Fig. 22.1). The extensor digiti quinti minimi is isolated, retracted, and maintained in its tunnel. A transverse incision is made in the capsule just distal to the triangular fibrocartilage level. The ruptured ligament, be it dorsal radioulnar, volar radioulnar, or both, is isolated and prepared for insertion into the distal end of the ulna. The pivot point of the ulna lies at the base of the ulnar styloid and is centered on the shaft of the ulna. A small hole is drilled, and rotation of the radius demonstrates the center of this point of rotation. The hole is then enlarged, correcting any centering errors, to accept the ends of the ligaments. Two drill holes are placed in the outer cortex of the ulna. A heavy 0 vicryl suture is passed down the pivot drill hole and out through the two lateral cortex holes. The tightest possible position of the DRUJ is

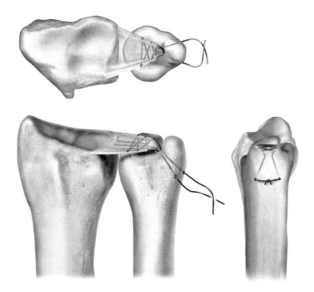

EDITORS' FIGURE 22.1. The distal radioulnar joint has adequate cartilage but is dislocated or significantly hypermobile, so restabilization of the ulna to the radius is indicated. The dorsal and volar radioulnar ligaments typically tear out from their insertion on the ulna. A drill hole is placed in the pivot point of the distal ulna, meaning at the center of rotation when seen from distally. A Bunnell-type suture can be placed in the ulnar-most aspect of the dorsal and volar radioulnar ligaments. Large 0 vicryl or 0 prolene stitches are used to secure the ligaments into the defect in the end of the ulna. The suture ends are passed out through two small cortical holes on the ulnar aspect of the ulna and tied over that cortex. The distal radius and ulna are cross-pinned to each other for 8 weeks of immobilization. The pin may be removed in 6 weeks.

Through a transverse incision, the dorsal sensory branch of the ulnar nerve is identified and retracted (Editors' Fig. 22.2). The operation is then performed extraperiosteally, leaving fat, areolar tissue, and the pronator quadratus in place. A ¼-in. drill hole is made in the radius in an anteroposterior direction at the level of the ulnar neck. A long free tendon graft is obtained and wrapped around the ulna as demonstrated. Separate sling components prevent volar, dorsal, and lateral subluxation of the ulna. A Kirschner wire is then inserted proximal to the anastomosis to hold the radius and ulna stationary in neutral rotation. After 6 weeks, immobilization is discontinued, and gentle range-of-motion exercises are begun.

Statistically, the most common problem with the DRUJ will occur post-Colles' fracture. Shortening during healing and a change in sulcus articular angulation leave no adequate seat for the ulna. The larger problem is the shortening of the radius. The stabilizing ligaments for the distal ulna must rupture during Colles' fracture displacement. On occasion, a fracture of the distal radius will displace directly without major dorsiflexion at the instant of achieved, and the sutures are tied over the lateral cortex of the ulna. The tight position of the DRUJ is usually in midneutral position. A small Steinmann pin or a 0.062 K-wire is then used to run from the ulna into the radius. The pin should be angled proximal to distal, usually from the ulna proximal into the radius distally. The angled pin is important because a pin that is perpendicular to the long axis of the forearm bones will allow the radius and ulna to distract from one another. One or two angled pins across both forearm bones will keep the load off the repair.

A bulk dressing with long arm splinting above the elbow is applied. Supination–pronation must be prevented to unload the transforearm pins. At 2 to 4 days postoperatively, the bulk dressing is removed, and a long arm cast is applied. The thumb and fingers may be free as long as the plaster is molded against the metacarpals. The forearm pins may be removed at 6 weeks, and the long arm splint maintained for an additional 2 weeks. We feel that probably 8 weeks of immobilization is appropriate for this repair. In a young person with an open epiphysis and major symptoms from a dislocating ulna, one might consider a tendon sling mechanism.

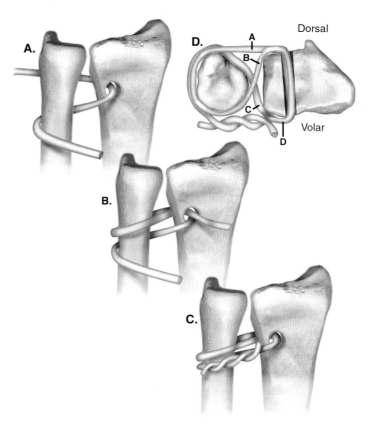

EDITORS' FIGURE 22.2. The tendon is woven through the radius (**A**), around the ulna, and back through the radius (**B**). It is woven into itself and sutured (**C**). Rotation is permitted between the radius and ulna. Segments *DA* and *DC* prevent ulnar separation; *DB* prevents volar migration of the ulna (**D**).

impact. The ulna may go with the distal fragment, thus preserving all DRUJ support.

Following Colles' fracture, patients frequently demonstrate stiffness and pain in the wrist. The majority of cases arise from the distal radioulnar malalignment, with or without ulnar impaction. A very effective approach for these people is to place them on a Dystrophile program for 2 to 3 weeks and then proceed with matched ulnar arthroplasty. This produces a rapid diminution of symptoms, typically an increase in flexion–extension motion in the wrist, as well as restoration of full supination–pronation. If the patient returns to significant load activities after several months, the potential is there for a midcarpal overload, secondary to dorsal articular tilt of the distal radius. This is amenable to a trapezoidal osteotomy in the future.

In solving the problems of the unsalvageable DRUJ, one has to deal with impingement between the ulna and radius and winging. If these two problems can be solved, the clinical result is satisfactory. There is no place for a Sauvé-Kapandji procedure, as the ulna needs the wrist, but the wrist does not need the ulna. One might make the point that in severe rheumatoid arthritis, resection of the distal ulna will allow ulnar translation of the carpals off the radius, but this is no longer a "wrist" and is best handled as discussed in Chapter 41. The problem of impingement is best solved by matching the shape of the ulna throughout supination, neutral, and pronation to the shape of the radius. This often requires resection of the flare of the fossa on the radius, particularly the dorsal flare. If the ulna is left at the level of the distal radial articular surface, the ulnar sling mechanism will, without surgical repair, reattach itself to the distal ulna and prevent winging, as described in Chapter 59. If the patient has had a Darrach procedure, and winging and impingement are a problem, the best solution is a step-cut lengthening of the ulna up to the level of the distal radial articular surface plane and matched shaping of this elongated portion of the distal ulna. The distal radius occasionally can have a high degree of curvature toward the ulnar side at the metaphyseal level. This can produce some impingement following matched ulnar arthroplasty. At reoperation, under these conditions, the radius is reshaped, the dorsal and volar interosseous nerves are transected, and the ulnar aspect of the pronator quadratus is brought up to meet a flap of dorsal fascia.

If the ulna is cut off transversely as in the Darrach, leaving a sharp corner, no amount of soft tissue interposition will serve to prevent the ulna from impinging on the radius and eventually producing symptoms. It is, therefore, a fallacy to assume that any amount of soft tissue can act over the long haul as a preventer of the impingement phenomenon. Also, no amount of tendon wrapping will hold the ulna away from the radius. The extensor carpi ulnaris anatomy is such that it can not act to prevent the ulna from striking the radius. The contact phenomenon must be solved by shaping the ulna so that a long broad surface rather than a sharp corner exists. The hemiresection interposition arthroplasty is more effective if one trims the hemiresection so that there are no sharp edges from full supination to full pronation.

The degenerative arthritis that occurs in the DRUJ begins at the proximal portion of the joint and gradually destroys the articular cartilage in a circumferential fashion moving distally. We have successfully utilized a form of modified arthroplasty on these cases, using a longitudinal incision because the potential for matched ulnar arthroplasty in the future is real. The proximal destroyed segment of articular surface of the ulna is removed, leaving the full circumference of normal cartilage distally. Dental rongeurs are used to excise bone in a circumferential manner. Occasionally, some resection of the proximal sulcus joint of the radius is carried out as well. A bulk surgical dressing is applied for 48 hours, then reduced to a small dressing. Supination–pronation is allowed from the time of surgery.

The postfracture radial head should be preserved at all costs. Even a small segment of radial head will have adequate articular cartilage for the impaction loads of the radius. As there is minimal tendency to shear loading, this small articular surface should be maintained. Once the radial head has been excised, proximal migration of the hand and radius result in ulnar impaction syndrome and dislocation at the DRUJ. The only repeatedly reliable procedure is the silicone radial head implant combined with a matched ulnar arthroplasty. There are those with very inelastic tight ligaments who may very well get along with the radial head resection without surgery. However, anyone with any significant load requirements will most likely require repair.

REFERENCES

1. Vesely DG. The distal radioulnar joint. *Clin Orthop* 1967;51:75.
2. Taleisnik J. Symposium on distal ulna injuries. *Contemp Orthop* 1983;7:81–116.
3. Palmer AK, Werner FW. Biomechanics of the distal radioulnar joint. *Clin Orthop* 1984;187:26–35.
4. Nathan R, Schneider LH. Classification of distal radioulnar joint disorders. *Hand Clin* 1991;7:239–248.
5. af Ekenstam F, Palmer AK, Glisson RR. The load on the radius and ulna in different positions of the wrist and forearm. A cadaver study. *Acta Orthop Scand* 1984;55:363–365.
6. Palmer AK, Werner FW, Murphy DJ, et al. Functional wrist motion. A biomechanical study. *J Hand Surg [Am]* 1985;10:39–46.
7. Lewis OJ. Evolutionary change in the primate wrist and inferior radioulnar joints. *Anat Rec* 1965;151:275.
8. Lewis OJ. The hominoid wrist joint. *Am J Phys Anthropol* 1969;30:251–267.

9. Almquist EE. Evolution of the distal radioulnar joint. *Clin Orthop* 1992;275:5–13.
10. Chidgley LK. The distal radioulnar joint: Problems and solutions. *J Am Acad Orthop Surg* 1995;3:95–109.
11. Bowers WH. Distal radioulnar joint. In: Green D, ed. *Operative hand surgery, 3rd ed.* New York: Churchill Livingstone, 1993; 973–1019.
12. Hotchkiss RN, et al. An anatomic and mechanical study of the interosseous membrane of the forearm: Pathomechanics of proximal migration of the radius. *J Hand Surg [Am]* 1989;14: 256–261.
13. Palmer AK. The distal radioulnar joint. *Orthop Clin North Am* 1984;15:321–330.
14. Kleinman WB, Graham TJ. Distal ulnar injury and dysfunction. In: Peimer CA, ed. *Surgery of the hand and upper extremity, 1st ed.* New York: McGraw-Hill, 1996;667–709.
15. Palmer AK, Werner FW, Glisson RR, et al. Partial excision of the triangular fibrocartilage complex. *J Hand Surg [Am]* 1988; 13:391–394.
16. Hagert CG. The distal radioulnar joint in relation to the whole forearm. *Clin Orthop* 1992;275:56–64.
17. af Ekenstam F, Hagert CG. Anatomical studies on the geometry and stability of the distal radioulnar joint. *Scand J Plast Reconstr Surg* 1985;19:17–25.
18. Pirela-Cruz MA, Goll SR, Klug M, et al. Stress computed tomography analysis of the distal radioulnar joint: A diagnostic tool for determining translational motion. *J Hand Surg [Am]* 1991;16:75–82.
19. Schuind F, An KN, Berglund L, et al. The distal radioulnar ligaments. A biomechanical study. *J Hand Surg [Am]* 1991;16: 1106–1114.
20. Hagert CG. Distal radius fracture and the distal radioulnar joint; anatomical considerations. *Handchir Mikrochir Plast Chir* 1994; 26:22–26.
21. Weiler PJ, Bogoch ER. Kinematics of the distal radioulnar joint in rheumatoid arthritis: An *in vivo* study using centrode analysis. *J Hand Surg [Am]* 1995;20:937–943.
22. King GJ, McMurtry RY, Rubenstein JD, et al. Kinematics of the distal radioulnar joint. *J Hand Surg [Am]* 1986;11:798–804.
23. Reagan DS, Linscheid RL, Dobyns JH. Lunotriquetral sprains. *J Hand Surg [Am]* 1984;9:502–514.
24. Kleinman WB. Physical examination of lunatotriquetral joint. *Am Soc Surg Hand Corr Newsl* 1985:51.
25. Mino DE, Palmer AK, Levinsohn EM. Radiography and computed tomography in the diagnosis of incongruity of the distal radioulnar joint. *J Bone Joint Surg Am* 1985;67:247–252.
26. Mino DE, Palmer AK, Levinsohn EM. The role of radiography and computerized tomography in the diagnosis of subluxation and dislocation of the distal radioulnar joint. *J Hand Surg [Am]* 1983;8:23–31.
27. Wechsler RJ, Wehbe MA, Rifkin MD, et al. Computed tomography diagnosis of distal radioulnar subluxation. *Skel Radiol* 1987;16:1–5.
28. Viegas SF, Ballantyne G. Attritional lesions of the wrist joint. *J Hand Surg [Am]* 1987;12:1025–1029.
29. Zlatin MB, Chao PC, Osterman AL, et al. Chronic wrist pain: Evaluation with high-resolution MR imaging. *Radiology* 1989; 173:723–729.
30. Golimbu CN, Firooznia H, Melone CP Jr, et al. Tears of the triangular fibrocartilage of the wrist: MR imaging. *Radiology* 1989; 173:731–733.
31. Burk DL, Karasick D, Wechsler FJ. Imaging of the distal radioulnar joint. *Hand Clin* 1991;7:263–275.
32. Mikic ZD. Detailed anatomy of the articular disk of the distal radioulnar joint. *Clin Orthop* 1989;245:123–132.
33. Pederzini L, Luchetti R, Soragni O, et al. Evaluation of the triangular fibrocartilage complex tears by arthroscopy, arthrography and magnetic resonance imaging. *Arthroscopy* 1992;8: 191–197.
34. Whipple TL. Arthroscopy of the distal radioulnar joint. *Hand Clin* 1994;10:589–592.
35. Osterman AL. Arthroscopic debridement of triangular fibrocartilage complex tears. *Arthroscpy* 1990;6:120–124.
36. Kihara H, Short WH, Werner FW, et al. The stabilizing mechanism of the distal radioulnar joint during pronation and supination. *J Hand Surg [Am]* 1995;20:930–936.
37. Alexander AH. Bilateral traumatic dislocation of the distal radioulnar joint, ulna dorsal: Case report and review of the literature. *Clin Orthop* 1977;129:238–244.
38. Snook GA, Chrisman OD, Wilson TC, et al. Subluxation of the distal radioulnar joint by hyperpronation. *J Bone Joint Surg [Am]* 1969:51:1315–1323.
39. Bacorn RW, Kurtzke JF. Colles fracture: a study of two thousand cases from the New York State Workmen's Compensation Board. *J Bone Joint Surg Am* 1953;35:643.
40. Lidstrom A. Fractures of the distal radius. A clinical and statistical study of end results. *Acta Orthop Scand* 1959;41:1–18.
41. Mcqueen M, Caspers J. Colles fracture: Does the anatomic result affect the final function? *J Bone Joint Surg Br* 1988;70:649–651.
42. Porter M, Stockey I. Fractures of the distal radius. Intermediate and end results in relation to radiologic parameters. *Clin Orthop* 1987;220:241–252.
43. Rubinovich RM, Rennie WR. Colles fracture: End results in relation to radiologic parameters. *Can J Surg* 1983;26:361–363.
44. Jupiter JB, Masem M. Reconstruction of post-traumatic deformity of the distal radius and ulna. *Hand Clin* 1988;4:377–390.
45. Adams BD. Effects of radial deformity on distal radioulnar joint mechanics. *J Hand Surg [Am]* 1993;18:492–498.
46. Cooney WP, Dobyns JH, Linscheid RL. Complications of Colles' fractures. *J Bone Joint Surg Am* 1980;62:613–619.
47. Dymond IWD. The treatment of isolated fractures of the distal ulna. *J Bone Joint Surg Br* 1984;66:408–410.
48. Mikic DJ. Galeazzi fracture-dislocations. *J Bone Joint Surg Am* 1975;57:1071–1080.
49. Galeazzi R. Uber ein besonderes Syndrom bei Verlrtzunger im Bereick der Unter Armknochen. *Arch Orthop Unfallchir* 1934;35: 557.
50. Valande M. Luxation en arriere du cubitus avec fracture de la deaphyse radiale. *Bull Mem Soc Nat Chir* 1967;55:75.
51. Kellam FK, Jupiter JB. Diaphyseal fractures of the forearm. In: Browner BD, ed. *Skeletal trauma*. Philadelphia: WB Saunders, 1992.
52. Anderson LD. Fractures of the shafts of the radius and ulna. In: Rockwood CA Jr, Green DP, eds. *Fractures in adults, 2nd ed.* Philadelphia: JB Lippincott, 1984;550–556.
53. Hughston JC. Fractures of the forearm. Anatomical considerations. *J Bone Joint Surg Am* 1962;44:1664.
54. Hughston JC. Fracture of the distal radial shaft. Mistakes in management. *J Bone Joint Surg Am* 1957;39:249.
55. Sarmiento A, Latta LJ. *Closed functional treatment of fractures.* New York: Springer, 1981;426.
56. Moore EM, Klein JP, Patzakin MJ, et al. Results of compression-plating of closed Galeazzi fractures. *J Bone Joint Surg Am* 1985; 67:1015–1021.
57. Brockman EP. Two cases of instability of the wrist joint following excision of the head of the radius. *Proc R Soc Med* 1930;24:904.
58. Essex-Lopresti P. Fractures of the radial head with distal radioulnar dislocation. *J Bone Joint Surg Br* 1951;33:244.
59. Aulicino PL, Siegel JL. Acute injuries of the distal radioulnar joint. *Hand Clin* 1991;7:283–293.
60. Hotchkiss RN. Displaced fractures of the radial head: Internal fixation or excision? *J Am Acad Orthop Surg* 1997;5:1–10.

61. Hotchkiss RN, An KN, Sowa DT, et al. An anatomic and mechanical study of the interosseous membrane of the forearm: Pathomechanics of proximal migration of the radius. *J Hand Surg [Am]* 1989;14:256–261.
62. Rabinowitz RS, Light TR, Havey RM, et al. The role of the interosseous membrane and triangular fibrocartilage complex in forearm stability. *J Hand Surg [Am]* 1994;19:385–393.
63. Knight DJ, Rymalzewski LA, Amis AA, et al. Primary replacement of the fractured radial head with a metal prosthesis. *J Bone Joint Surg Br* 1993;75:572–576.
64. Mackay I, Fitzgerald B, Miller JH. Silastic replacement of the head of the radius in trauma. *J Bone Joint Surg Br* 1979;61:494–497.
65. Sowa DT, Hotchkiss RN, Weiland AJ. Symptomatic proximal translation of the radius following radial head resection. *Clin Orthop* 1995;317:106–113.
66. Hermansdorfer JD, Kleinman WB. Management of chronic peripheral tears of the triangular fibrocartilage complex. *J Hand Surg [Am]* 1991;16:340–346.
67. Bach AW. *Correction of chronic distal radioulnar joint instability by combined ligamentous repair and ECU tendodesis.* Paper presented at the 48th Annual Meeting of the American Society for Surgery of the Hand, Kansas City, KS, September 29–Oct 2, 1993.
68. Boyes JH. *Bunnell's surgery of the hand, 5th ed.* Philadelphia: JB Lippincott, 1970;299–303.
69. Fulkerson JP, Watson HK. Congenital anterior subluxation of the distal ulna: A case report. *Clin Orthop* 1978;131:179–182.
70. Hui FC, Linscheid RL. Ulnotriquetral augmentation tenodesis. A reconstructive procedure for dorsal subluxation of the distal radioulnar joint. *J Hand Surg [Am]* 1982;7:230–236.
71. Johnston-Jones K, Sanders WE. *Posttraumatic radioulnar instability: Treatment by anatomic reconstruction of the volar and dorsal radioulnar ligaments.* Paper presented at the 50th annual meeting of the ASSH, San Francisco, CA, September 1995.
72. Petersen MS, Adams BD. Biomechanical evaluation of distal radioulnar reconstructions. *J Hand Surg [Am]* 1993;18:328–334.
73. Johnson RK. Stabilization of the distal ulna by transfer of the pronator quadratus origin. *Clin Orthop* 1992;275:130–132.
74. Imbriglia JE, Matthews D. Treatment of chronic post-traumatic dorsal subluxation of the distal ulna by hemiresection–interposition arthroplasty. *J Hand Surg [Am]* 1993;18:899–907.
75. Short WH, Palmer AK. Dorsal dislocation of the ulna. In: Blair WE, ed. *Techniques in hand surgery.* Baltimore: Williams & Wilkins, 1996;367–373.
76. Hartz CR, Beckenbaugh RD. Long-term results of resection of the distal ulna for post-traumatic conditions. *J Trauma* 1979;19:219–226.
77. McKee MD, Richards RR. *Dynamic radioulnar impingement following the Darrach procedure: A long term followup study.* Paper presented at the 45th annual meeting of the ASSH, Toronto, September 1990.
78. Tulipan DJ, Eaton RG, Eberhart RE. The Darrach procedure defended. Technique redefined and long-term follow-up. *J Hand Surg [Am]* 1991;16:438–444.
79. Beiber EJ, Linscheid RL, Dobyns JH, et al. Failed distal ulna resections. *J Hand Surg [Am]* 1988;13:193–200.
80. Darrow JC, Linscheid RL, Dobyns JH, et al. Distal ulna recession for disorders of the distal radioulnar joint. *J Hand Surg [Am]* 1985;10:482–491.
81. Goldner JL, Hayes MG. Stabilization of the remaining ulna using one half of the extensor carpi ulnaris tendon after resection of the distal ulna. *Orthop Trans* 1979;3:330.
82. Tsai TM, Shimizu H, Adkins P. A modified extensor carpi ulnaris tenodesis with the Darrach procedure. *J Hand Surg [Am]* 1993;18:697–702.
83. Kleinman WB, Greenburg JA. Salvage of the failed Darrach procedure. *J Hand Surg [Am]* 1995;20:951–958.
84. Breen TF, Jupiter JB. Extensor carpi ulnaris and flexor carpi ulnaris tenodesis of the unstable distal ulna. *J Hand Surg [Am]* 1989;14:612–617.
85. Carroll RE, Imbriglia JE. Distal radioulnar arthrodesis. *Orthop Trans* 1979;3:269.
86. Dingman PVC. Resection of the distal end of the ulna (Darrach operation). An end result study of twenty-four cases. *J Bone Joint Surg Am* 1952;34:893.
87. Bowers WH. Distal radioulnar joint arthroplasty. Current concepts. *Clin Orthop* 1992;275:104–109.
88. Watson HK, Ryu JY, Burgess RC. Matched distal ulna resection. *J Hand Surg [Am]* 1986;11:812–817.
89. Sanders RA, Frederick HA, Hontas RB. The Sauve-Kapandji procedure: A salvage operation for the distal radioulnar joint. *J Hand Surg [Am]* 1991;16:1125–1129.
90. Vincent KA, Szabo RM, Agee JM. The Sauve Kapandji procedure for reconstruction of the rheumatoid distal radioulnar joint. *J Hand Surg [Am]* 1993;18:978–983.
91. Hauck RM, Skahen J III, Palmer AK. Classification and treatment of ulnar styloid nonunion. *J Hand Surg [Am]* 1996;21:418–422.
92. Watson HK, Castle T. Tapezoidal osteotomy of the distal radius for unacceptable articular angulation after Colles' fracture. *J Hand Surg [Am]* 1988;13:837–843.
93. Fernandez DL, Jupiter JB. *Fractures of the distal radius.* New York: Springer, 1996.
94. Milch H. Cuff resection of the ulna for malunited Colles' fracture. *J Bone Joint Surg* 1941;23:311.
95. Coleman DA, Blair WF, Shurr D. Resection of the radial head for fracture of the radial head: Long term follow up of seventeen cases. *J Bone Joint Surg Am* 1987;69:385–392.
96. Taylor TK, O'Connor BT. The effect upon the inferior radioulnar joint of excision of the head of the radius in adults. *J Bone Joint Surg Br* 1964;46:83.
97. Morrisey RT, Nalebuff EA. Dislocation of the distal radioulnar joint: Anatomy and clues to prompt diagnosis. *Clin Orthop* 1979;144:154–158.
98. Buterbaugh GA, Palmer AK. Fractures and dislocations of the distal radioulnar joint. *Hand Clin* 1988;4:361–375.
99. White GM, Weiland AJ. Madelung's deformity: Treatment by osteotomy of the radius and Lauenstein procedure. *J Hand Surg [Am]* 1987;12:202–204.
100. Vickers DW. Epiphysiolysis. *Curr Orthop* 1989;3:41.

23

KIENBÖCK'S DISEASE

OVERVIEW AND CLASSIFICATION

ROBERT C. KRAMER
DAVID M. LICHTMAN

Kienböck's disease is a disorder characterized by sclerosis and collapse of the carpal lunate secondary to avascular necrosis (1–3). It is seen most often in the third to fifth decades and has a 2:1 male-to-female predominance. It occurs more often in a dominant versus nondominant wrist and in a patient apt to engage in manual labor (1,2). The disease is characterized by the insidious onset of dorsal wrist pain followed by a variable amount of swelling, tenderness, and stiffness. The purpose of this chapter is to provide an overview of the etiology of the disease and to review its natural history. We then discuss the staging of this entity and our treatment algorithm based on disease stage.

VASCULAR ANATOMY

The vascular anatomy of the lunate consists of an extraosseous system and an intraosseous system (4,5). The extraosseous blood supply consists of both dorsal and volar components. The dorsal blood supply arises from vessels on the middorsum of the carpus fed by branches of the radial artery and the dorsal branch of the anterior interosseous artery (4) (Fig. 23.1). These enter the bone through foramina in the dorsal, nonarticular surface of the bone. The extraosseous volar component consists of sources from the ulnar artery, the radial artery, the volar branch of the anterior interosseous artery, and a recurrent branch from the deep palmar arch (4) (Fig. 23.2). The main branches to the lunate can arise from any of these sources but are often from the ulnar and anterior interosseous arteries. One to two nutrient vessels enter the lunate through foramina in the nonarticular volar pole.

Gelberman et al. (4,6,7) demonstrated the intraosseous vascular anatomy of the lunate. Based on the entry point of vessels into the the lunate, they noted a "Y" pattern in 59% of specimens, an "I" pattern in 31%, and an "X" pattern in 10% (Fig. 23.3). The authors also noted that the proximal region of the lunate, adjacent to the radial articular surface, was relatively avascular.

Panagis and Gelberman (6) further studied the intraosseous vascular anatomy of cadaveric carpal bones and identified three distinct groups. Group I bones had a major portion supplied by a single vessel. Incuded in this group were the scaphoid (proximal pole), the capitate (head), and 20% of the lunates in this series. This was considered the "at-risk" group. Group II bones demonstrated a dual supply without intraosseous anastomosis. Included here were the trapezoid and hamate. Group III bones posessed two nutrient arteries via nonarticular surfaces, consistent anastomoses, and no large area dependent on a single vessle. Included were the trapezium, triquetrum, pisiform, and 80% of the lunates in their series. Additionally, the authors stated, in a larger sample of 60 lunates studied in their laboratory, the group I pattern was noted in only 7% of the specimens. They theorize that these lunates might be susceptible to Kienböck's disease; however, it is important to realize that none of the specimens studied by any of these authors had Kienböck's disease, so the vascular anatomy of a susceptible lunate may possibly differ from any of those previously described.

R. C. Kramer: Beaumont Bone and Joint Institute, Beaumont, Texas 77707.

D. M. Lichtman: Department of Surgery, Uniformed Services University of the Health Sciences, Bethesda, Maryland 20814; and Department of Orthopedic Surgery, The University of Texas Southwestern Medical Center at Dallas, Dallas, Texas 75235.

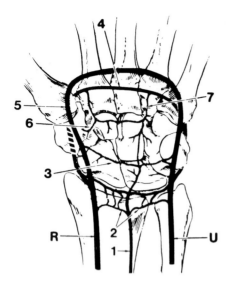

FIGURE 23.1. The palmar arterial blood supply of the wrist. *R*, radial artery; *U*, ulnar artery; *1*, volar branch, anterior interosseous artery; *2*, palmar radiocarpal arch; *3*, palmar intercarpal arch; *4*, deep palmar arch; *5*, superficial palmar arch; *6*, radial recurrent artery; *7*, ulnar recurrent artery. (From Williams CS, Gelberman RH. Vascularity of the lunate: anatomic studies and implications for the development of osteonecrosis. *Hand Clin* 1993;9:385–390, with permission.)

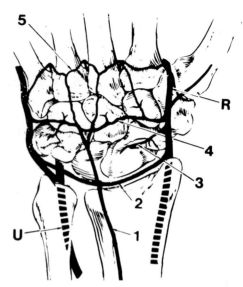

FIGURE 23.2. The dorsal arterial supply of the wrist. *R*, radial artery; *U*, ulnar artery; *1*, dorsal branch, anterior interosseous artery; *2*, dorsal radiocarpal arch; *3*, branch to the dorsal ridge of the scaphoid; *4*, dorsal intercarpal arch; *5*, dorsal basal metacarpal arch. (From Williams CS, Gelberman RH. Vascularity of the lunate: anatomic studies and implications for the development of osteonecrosis. *Hand Clin* 1993;9:385–390, with permission.)

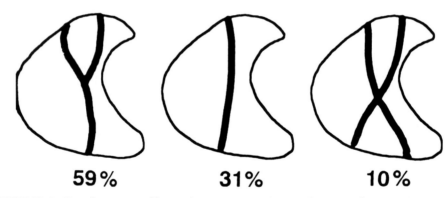

FIGURE 23.3. Noted patterns of lunate intraosseous anastomosis: Y, I, and X patterns and their respective rates of occurrence. (From Williams CS, Gelberman RH. Vascularity of the lunate: anatomic studies and implications for the development of osteonecrosis. *Hand Clin* 1993;9:385–390, with permission.)

ETIOLOGY

Early Reports

Collapse of the carpal lunate was first described in 1843 by Peste (8). There was no x-ray technology available at that time, and it was described from anatomic specimens only. Peste believed that it was caused by acute trauma. Kienböck (3) later theorized that the disease occurred secondary to repeated strains, contusions, and subluxations resulting in loss of blood supply to the lunate. Avascular necrosis was first identified histologically as a pathologic entity in Kienböck's disease by Baum (9) in 1913.

Load

Uneven loading across the radiocarpal joint as a cause of Kienböck's disease has been entertained since Húlten (10) first recognized the association of ulnar negative variance with collapse of the lunate (Fig. 23.4). He reported a 78% incidence of ulnar negative variance in patients with Kienböck's disease, whereas he noted a 23% incidence in the normal population. This relationship has been confirmed by additional studies; Gelberman et al. (11) also noted a statistically significant association between negative ulnar variance and Kienböck's disease. However, they pointed out

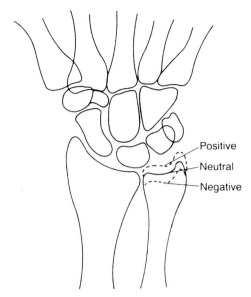

FIGURE 23.4. Schematic representation of ulnar variance. Neutral variance occurs when the carpal surfaces of the ulna and the radius are equal. If the ulna is shorter than the radius, negative ulnar variance exists; if the ulna is longer than the radius, positive ulnar variance exists. (From Alexander AH, Lichtman DM. Kienböck's disease. In: Lichtman DM, ed. *The wrist and its disorders*, 1st ed. Philadelphia: WB Saunders, 1991;329–343, with permission.)

that African-Americans have more positive ulnar variance and a lower incidence of Kienböck's disease than Caucasians.

Scientific support that uneven load across the carpus predisposes to Kienböck's disease can be found in the biomechanical studies of Palmar and Werner (12,13). They observed, in a normal wrist, that the radiocarpal joint supports 81.6% of the total transmitted load, whereas approximately 18.4% of the total load occurs in the ulnocarpal joint. With 2.5-mm ulnar shortening (from zero variance), the radiocarpal load increases to 96% compared to only 4% within the ulnocarpal joint. This suggests a radial shift of the normal load distribution with ulnar negative variance and supports uneven load as an etiology of Kienböck's disease.

Kienböck's disease is known to occur in the face of ulnar positive variance as well as ulnar neutral variance (1,2,14). Clearly, not all patients with ulnar negative variance develop Kienböck's disease. In fact, D'Hoore (15) measured ulnar variance in 125 normal wrists and 52 with Kienböck's disease. He found no statistical difference in ulnar variance between the age- and sex-matched control group and the group with Kienböck's disease. Kristensen (16) attributed the minus variant to formation of subchondral bone in the distal radius in response to the collapsing lunate. Nakamura et al. (17) noted that ulnar variance, in normal wrists, increases with age and is lower in men. Although loading patterns may be associated with the development of Kienböck's disease, there have been no clear-cut studies to demonstrate uneven loading patterns as the specific cause of Kienböck's disease.

Trauma

Several authors have hypothesized acute trauma as the etiology for Kienböck's disease. Peste (8) was the first on record to hold this opinion. Later, Marek (18), who described a single volar blood supply to the lunate, stated that lunatomalacia was likely a result of a hyperextension injury to the wrist with disruption of the volar blood supply. Lee (5), in 1963, noted Kienböck's disease in association with a horizontal fracture to the lunate and thought the etiology to be interruption of the blood supply secondary to trauma. Beckenbaugh et al. (19) also found lines suggestive of fracture in 82% of their patients. Gelberman et al. agree with the above authors and have written that lunates with a single-vessel blood supply (group I) are at risk for avascular necrosis after fracture (6).

On the other hand, Cave (20) noted only 1 of 12 of his patients with perilunate dislocations to have Kienböck's disease. Ståhl (21) noted only four patients with Kienböck's disease out of 187 patients with single fracture lines through the lunate. Even Kienböck himself, in 1910, stated that this disorder was more likely the result of chronic, repeated injuries than one single episode of trauma to the lunate (3).

Venous Congestion and Vascular Insult

Venous congestion was considered by Ficat and Arlet (22) as the etiology of avascular necrosis of the femoral head. Schiltenwolf et al. (23) noted higher venous pressure in necrotic lunates than in viable lunates. Jensen (24) studied the intraosseous pressure in 10 patients with Kienböck's disease and noted the pressure in the lunate to be significantly higher than the pressure obtained from the radial styloid or the capitate. These studies support venous congestion, as opposed to arterial insufficiency, as the precipitating event in avascular necrosis.

Conclusions

The exact etiology of Kienböck's disease remains unknown but is very likely a combination of the above theories. Recent studies support the idea that repetitive trauma with compression fracture of the lunate may cause vascular interruption leading to Kienböck's disease (4,7). Biomechanical studies support an abnormality of radiocarpal loading patterns leading to Kienböck's disease (12,13,25–27). We believe that repetitive loading or acute trauma to a "lunate at risk" (one that harbors a predisposing vascular anomaly) is the cause in most cases.

HISTORY, PHYSICAL EXAM, AND IMAGING

Early on, the patient with Kienböck's disease will note the insidious onset of dorsal wrist pain and mild to moderate swelling about the dorsum of the wrist (1,2). Later, severe pain, crepitation, and stiffness may ensue. The diagnosis of Kienböck's disease is made radiographically (1,2,28). The lunate may display a fracture but most characteristically will show increased density in the early stages, and fragmentation and collapse in the later stages (28,29). Youm (30) described the carpal height ratio to measure progressive collapse of the lunate radiographically (Fig. 23.5). The distance between the distal radius and the base of the third metacarpal is the differential variable, whereas the length of the third metacarpal is the fixed variable. This ratio normally is 0.54 ± 0.03 and will decrease with progressive lunate collapse. Another tool for radiographic assessment is the Ståhl index (21,31) (Fig. 23.6). This is obtained by dividing the length of the transverse axis of the lunate by the length of the vertical axis. The average value for a normal wrist is approximately 50%. This too will decrease with increasing lunate collapse.

In addition to plain radiographs, the diagnosis of Kienböck's disease may be aided by scintigraphy, tomography (trispiral or computed), or magnetic resonance imaging (MRI) (28). Bone scintigraphy using ^{99m}Tc-labeled phosphate compounds is a nonspecific but sensitive modality for the detection of metabolic bone abnormalities (28). It is

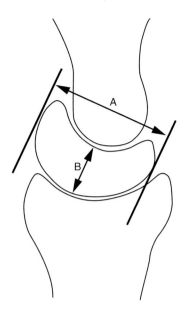

FIGURE 23.6. Ståhl index: *B* (transverse axis of the lunate) divided by *A* (vertical axis of the lunate). This value averages 50% in normal wrists. (From Miura H, Uchida Y, Ugioka Y. Radial closing wedge osteotomy for Kienböck's disease. *J Hand Surg [Am]* 1996;21:1029–1034, with permission.)

useful as a screening test in suspected Kienböck's disease and is less expensive than MRI. A "hot" lunate would suggest the diagnosis.

Tomography, either trispiral or computed techniques, is excellent for the detection of fractures not readily visible on plain radiographs (28,32). Many authors recommend the use of coronal computed tomography (CT) in the diagnosis of Kienböck's disease (28,33). Friedman et al. (33) reported on 12 patients with Kienböck's disease. In this series, the diagnosis was made on the basis of coronal CT in two patients, and three patients were noted to have fractured lunates not discernible on plain radiographs.

MRI is emerging as the imaging modality of choice for the early diagnosis of avascular necrosis (28,34). Coronal T1-weighted imaging nicely delineates the carpus. Cancellous bone gives a bright (high-intensity) signal as a result of its fatty marrow. As dead bone replaces the healthy, fatty tissue, signal intensity decreases. In spin-echo or gradient-echo (T2-weighted) images, the marrow is of intermediate to low intensity.

With avascular necrosis, T1-weighted images demonstrate the low signal of the necrotic bone in sharp contrast to the bright signal of the normal surrounding bone (28,34). T2-weighted imaging is not as reliable in the prediction of avascular necrosis. In a study by Desser et al. (35), the authors demonstrated a 17% false-negative rate in the diagnosis of avascular necrosis using T2-weighted images. Imaeda et al. (36) attempted to establish new criteria for the diagnosis, staging, and prognosis of Kienböck's disease using MRI signal characteristics. The authors agreed that a focal

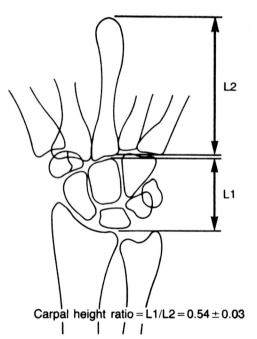

FIGURE 23.5. Carpal height ratio: *L1* (carpal height) divided by *L2* (third metacarpal length). In normals, this equals 0.054 ± 0.03. (From Youm Y, McMurtry RY, Flatt AE. Kinematics of the wrist, part I—an experimental study of radial–ulnar deviation and flexion–extension. *J Bone Joint Surg Am* 1978;60:423–431, with permission.)

loss of signal on T1 is an indication of the the presence of the disorder. Additionally, they note, on T2-weighted images, increased signal intensity of the lunate or a decreased signal containing a high spot indicated a better prognosis.

The differential diagnosis of Kienböck's disease includes inflammatory arthropathy, posttraumatic arthritis, fracture, carpal instability (acute or chronic), ulnocarpal impaction syndrome, and posttraumatic ischemia (1,2). White and Omer (37) described posttraumatic ischemia of the lunate following fracture-dislocation or dislocation of the carpus. They noted that increased radiodensity of the lunate may last between 5 and 32 months. One needs to be aware of this posibility when treating the acutely traumatized wrist.

STAGING

Ståhl (21) classified Kienböck's disease in 1947 based on roentgenographic charcteristics and pathologic observations. One of us (D.M.L.) modified this classification in 1977 based on clinical and x-ray findings to facilitate preoperative staging. Four stages were described.

Stage I

Stage I is characterized by an absence of radiographic findings with the exceptional possibility of a compression fracture (Fig. 23.7). T1-weighted MRI will demonstrate decreased or absent signal within the lunate. Bone scan will also be abnormal in this stage (see prior discussion). Clinically, the patient will describe intermittent dorsal, central wrist pain and may note swelling and loss of grip strength. These symptoms are caused by an acute synovitis.

Stage II

Stage II is characterized by increased radiodensity of the lunate (Fig. 23.8). There is no carpal collapse, therefore, the carpal height ratio and Ståhl index will be normal. This stage is easily recognized radiographically; therefore, MRI is unnecessary. Clinically, the patient will report persistent wrist pain and swelling caused by persistent synovitis. Grip strength is decreased, and stiffness may be present.

Stage IIIA

This stage is characterized by collapse of the lunate and a decrease in the carpal height ratio (Fig. 23.9). The collapse generally starts radially, and the lunate is noted to elongate on the lateral projection. The scapholunate relationship is maintained. At first, this stage is indistinguishable from stage II disease, but if collapse continues, the wrist becomes progressively more stiff.

Stage IIIB

Stage IIIB is characterized by advanced collapse of the lunate and carpal instability (Fig. 23.9). There is now fixed

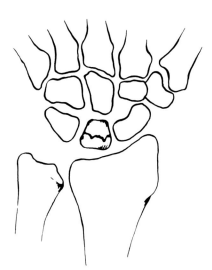

FIGURE 23.7. Stage I of Kienböck's disease: normal radiographically with the exception of a possible fracture. (From Lichtman DM, Alexander AH, Mack GR, et al. Kienböck's disease—update on silicone replacement arthroplasty. *J Hand Surg* 1982;7: 343–347, with permission.) **Editors' Notes:** *If the lunate is overloaded without adequate recovery time, a magnetic resonance image may demonstrate edema in the cancellous bone of the lunate. This is a common phenomenon, seldom seen as a clinical problem and probably represents a pre-Kienböck's state. This is much more common than recognized and is typically followed by full recovery with the patient's normal activity and rest patterns.*

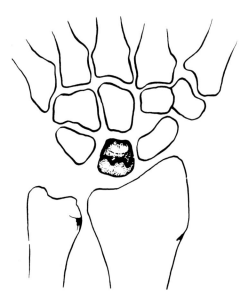

FIGURE 23.8. Stage II of Kienböck's disease: radiographs demonstrate increased density of the lunate relative to the remaining carpus. Collapse has not occurred. (From Lichtman DM, Alexander AH, Mack GR, et al. Kienböck's disease—update on silicone replacement arthroplasty. *J Hand Surg [Am]* 1982;7:343–347, with permission.)

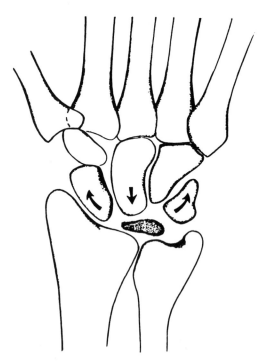

FIGURE 23.9. Stage III of Kienböck's disease: fragmentation and collapse. Stage IIIa: without fixed rotation of the scaphoid. Stage IIIb: fixed rotation of the scaphoid and a dorsal intercalated segment instability deformity are present. (From Lichtman DM, Alexander AH, Mack GR, et al. Kienböck's disease—update on silicone replacement arthroplasty. *J Hand Surg [Am]* 1982;7: 343–347, with permission.) **Editors' Notes:** *As the capitate approaches the radius in collapsed Kienböck's, rotary subluxation of the scaphoid becomes a symptomatic component. Fusing the scaphoid to the trapezoid will totally unload the lunate, if not collapsed, and will carry the loads around the lunate if collapse has occurred.*

rotatory subluxation (flexion) of the scaphoid as noted by the appearance of a cortical ring sign. The triquetrum may displace medially; there may be a static dorsal intercalated sement instability (DISI) or volar intercalated segment instability (VISI) pattern, and the lunate will appear elongated on lateral wrist radiographs. Clinically, the patient notes weakness, chronic pain, swelling, stiffness, and occasional "clunking." Synovitis is not as active as in the earlier stages of the disorder.

Stage IV

This stage is characterized by generalized degenerative changes within the carpus combined with fixed rotatory scaphoid subluxation and lunate collapse (Fig. 23.10). As with other end-stage forms of wrist degeneration, the patient may be markedly symptomatic, or the process may "burn out." Usually, symptoms are aggravated by active use of the wrist and are relieved by rest, splinting, and antiinflammatory medication.

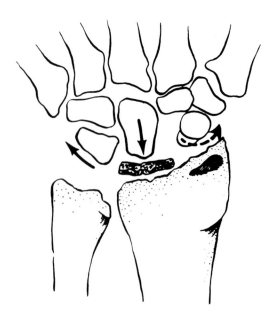

FIGURE 23.10. Stage IV of Kienböck's disease: fragmentation, collapse, and pancarpal arthritis representing end-stage disease. (From Lichtman DM, Alexander AH, Mack GR, et al. Kienböck's disease—update on silicone replacement arthroplasty. *J Hand Surg [Am]* 1982;7:343–347, with permission.)

TREATMENT

The treatment of Kienböck's disease is even more varied than the theories of its etiology. We discuss immobilization, direct and indirect revascularization techniques, arthroplasty, wrist denervation, and, finally, salvage procedures.

Immobilization

Cast or Splint

Cast immobilization as a treatment for Kienböck's disease is not a new treatment. Ståhl (21) was a noted advocate, and Lichtman et al. (38) in 1977 reviewed a series of 22 unstaged patients treated with a cast or splint. They noted 17 patients with progressive collapse and 19 patients with an unsatisfactory result. The authors felt that cast immobilization was insufficient to neutralize forces across the wrist. They now recommend its use only in the earliest stages of the disorder.

External Fixation

Lichtman et al. (14) recommended consideration of external fixation as a method to neutralize forces across the radiocarpal joint. The authors also advise the use of an external fixator following a vascular implantation procedure

(39). A possible indication is for immobilization of the wrist in stage I.

Direct Revascularization

Pronator Quadratus Pedicle Graft

In 1983, Braun (40) reported on eight patients with an average of 7 years of follow-up who underwent pronator quadratus pedicle grafting to the lunate for "no significant collapse." Braun noted seven patients with good results. In our own experience (unpublished), we noted the need to acutely flex the wrist to obtain proper positioning of the graft. This has led us to abandon use of the procedure.

Pisiform Transfer

Erbs and Böhm (41), in 1984, reported on 32 patients who underwent pisiform transfer (Fig. 23.11) for Kienböck's disease. In this series, all patients had an average of 5 years of follow-up. They reported all patients with good results and specifically noted that 14 patients with advanced stages of the disease were symptom-free at last follow-up.

Vascular Implantation

Vascular implantation techniques for avascular necrosis of carpal bones began, experimentally, back in the early 1970s when Hori and colleagues (42) implanted vascular bundles into avascular bone in canines in an attempt to regain vascularization. The principle behind vascular implantation lies in the observation that a significant amount of microcirculation exists in a vascular bundle. This intimate vascular network between an artery and a vein, when transplanted into bone, stimulates the proliferation of capillaries from within the vascular bundle. Yajima (43) noted vascular anastomoses between implanted vascular bundles and preexisting vessels by 3 weeks. The stage is then set for an acceleration of creeping substitution and new bone formation.

Saldana et al. (44) studied revascularization of avascular rat femoral heads. The femoral heads were drilled through and through and placed in the rat's opposite thigh. The ipsilateral femoral artery was lengthened with a graft and reanastomosed after being passed through the transplanted femoral head. Histologically, the authors noted neovascularization and new bone formation in the previously avascular femoral heads.

The Hori procedure (42,45) (Fig. 23.12) is a direct implantation of the second or third metacarpal artery and vein into the lunate. The authors report on 51 cases with an average of 2 years of follow-up. They note that 72.5% in their series had a disappearance of sclerosis radiographically, 19.6% had an increase in changes consistent with

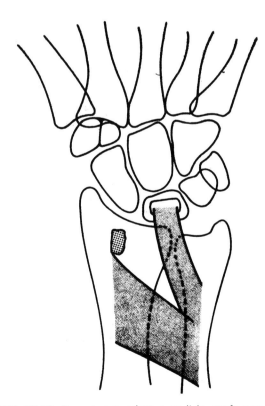

FIGURE 23.11. Pronator quadratus pedicle graft procedure. (From Alexander AH, Lichtman DM: Kienböck's disease. In: Lichtman DM, ed. *The wrist and its disorders, 1st ed.* Philadelphia: WB Saunders, 1991;329–343, with permission.)

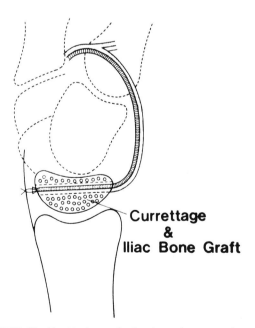

FIGURE 23.12. The Hori vascular implantation procedure. (From Tamai S, Yajima H, Ono H. Revascularization procedures in the treatment of Kienböck's disease. *Hand Clin* 1993;9:455–466, with permission.)

osteoarthritis, and 9.8% went on to fragmentation of the lunate. No patient in this series underwent wrist arthrodesis.

Indirect Revascularization (Decompressive Procedures)

Trumble et al. (47) studied the biomechanics of joint-leveling procedures using whole-arm cadaveric specimens in which they performed radial shortening and ulnar lengthening osteotomies as well as triscaphe and capitohamate arthrodeses. Using strain guages, the authors found radial shortening, ulnar lengthening, and triscaphe fusion to be successful in unloading the lunate. The capitohamate fusion was found to be ineffective, and triscaphe fusion was noted to significantly reduce range of motion.

Werner et al. (13), in a cadaveric study, performed radial shortening osteotomy or ulnar lengthening osteotomy in cadaver wrists. They noted that 2 mm of shortening or lengthening was optimum and that either procedure decreased the radiocarpal load by 70%.

Horii et al. (27), using a computer model, attempted to predict total force transmission through the radiolunate joint after either radial shortening or ulnar lengthening of 4 mm, intercarpal fusion, or capitate shortening. Intercarpal fusion reduced the radiolunate force by only 15% as compared to a 45% reduction after 4 mm of radial shortening or ulnar lengthening. Capitate shortening was also noted to reduce radiolunate load, but it was associated with a dramatic overload of the scaphotrapezial and triquetrohamate joints.

Generally, all decompressive procedures unload the lunate and allow revascularization to occur in the presence of reduced load. Osteotomies appear to have an advantage over intercarpal arthrodeses in terms of preservation of motion.

Joint-Leveling Procedures

Radial Shortening Osteotomy

In 1928, Húlten (10) studied the relationship of the distal radius and ulna in normal individuals and patients with Kienböck's disease. He noted that 78% of his patients with Kienböck's had negative ulnar variance compared to only 23% in his control group. He noted no ulnar positive variants in his series. This observation led Húlten to believe that a short ulna left the lunate "susceptible" to the development of vascular insufficiency. He later proposed radial shortening as a treatment for this condition (48).

Weiss (49) performed a metaanalysis of 121 patients with an average of 4 years of follow-up who underwent radial shortening osteotomy for Kienböck's disease. He noted 85% good or excellent results. However, shortening by more than 4 mm has been implicated as a cause of ulnar-sided wrist pain secondary to ulnocarpal impaction (50).

Ulnar Lengthening Osteotomy

Persson (51) is credited with being the first to propose ulnar lengthening as a treatment for Kienböck's disease. His suggestion that this osteotomy would redistribute radiocarpal load has been verified in numerous biomechanical studies (12,13,25–27).

The Mayo Clinic (52) reported on 64 patients with 24 months of average follow-up, all having undergone ulnar lengthening osteotomy for Kienböck's disease with an iliac crest autograft. The average size of the autograft was 4.1 mm. They noted 14% delayed or nonunion with 8% ulnocarpal impaction syndrome. Lunate density was unchanged or improved in 88%.

Radial Closing Wedge Osteotomy

Werner and Palmer (13) performed medial closing and lateral opening and closing wedge osteotomies on cadaveric radii (Fig. 23.13). Each was stabilized with an external fixator and axially loaded. Pressure-sensitive film data demonstrated that lateral opening or medial closing wedge osteotomy angulated from 4° to 8° significantly reduced pressure on the radiolunate fossa. The authors noted the opposite effect with lateral radial closing wedge osteotomies. In contrast, Tsunoda et al. (53) noted that the lateral radial closing wedge osteotomy increased the radial translation of the lunate. The authors believe that this increases the area of distribution of axial load through the lunate by increasing its contact area with the radius. Miura et al. (31) reported on 26 patients who underwent lateral radial closing wedge osteotomy for Kienböck's disease with 4.5 years of average follow-up. They note 73% good or excellent results, with better results in earlier stages.

Intercarpal Arthrodesis

As with joint-leveling procedures, the role of intercarpal arthrodesis is to biomechanically unload the lunate to permit revascularization. Moreover, intercarpal arthrodesis has the advantage of stabilizing the midcarpal joint and, therefore, can be used to recreate stability in the later stages of the disorder.

Scaphotrapeziotrapezoid

Light (54), in a cadaveric model, noted that a scaphotrapeziotrapezoid (STT) arthrodesis in neutral or with the wrist in slight dorsiflexion decreases the lunate load. Watson (55,56) studied 16 patients with an average of 20.5 months of follow-up undergoing STT arthrodesis for Kienböck's disease. Eight patients in this series were treated with triscaphe arthrodesis alone, and five patients were treated with triscaphe arthrodesis together with silicone replace-

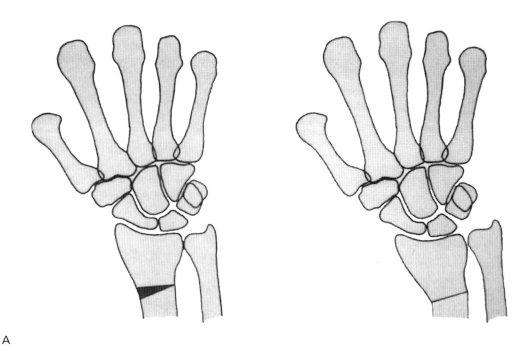

FIGURE 23.13. A,B: Radial closing wedge osteotomy. (From Miura H, Uchida Y, Sugioka Y. Radial closing wedge osteotomy for Kienböck's disease. *J Hand Surg [Am]* 1996;21:1029–1034, with permission.)

ment arthroplasty. Three patients in this series were treated with triscaphe arthrodesis after receiving a silicone replacement arthroplasty elsewhere. Relief of pain was noted to be satisfactory in all 16 patients. These authors noted no nonunions or surgical infections and concluded that triscaphe arthrodesis, without the additional use of an implant, may suffice to bear the wrist load and can be used to preserve the lunate in Kienböck's disease.

Scaphocapitate

Horii (27) studied scaphocapitate fusions in a laboratory. Using a rigid-body spring model, she noted that scaphocapitate fusion unloaded the radial lunate fossa by 12%. Sennwald et al. (57) reported on 11 patients having undergone scaphocapitate fusion for Kienböck's disease with an average of 36 months of follow-up. They noted 10 patients with complete pain relief and nine patients were able to return to work.

Capitohamate Fusion with Capitate Shortening Osteotomy

This procedure (Fig. 23.14) was conceived of as an extension to the capitohamate fusion described by Chuinard and Zeman (58). Capitate shortening alone has been shown to reduce radiolunate load, but it is also associated with a dramatic overload of the scaphotrapezial and triquetrohamate joints (27). Although the capitate has been shown to have a

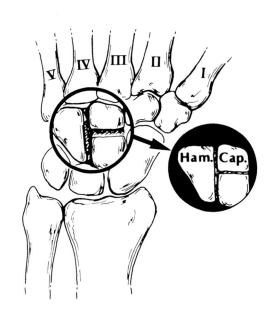

FIGURE 23.14. Capitate shortening with capitohamate arthrodesis procedure. (From Almquist EE. Capitate shortening in the treatment of Kienböck's disease. *Hand Clin* 1993;9: 505–512, with permission.)

single intraosseous blood supply (6), the nutrient vessel enters into the head at the articular margin (59). The osteotomy is performed just distal to this margin, thus preserving the blood supply. Almquist (59) reported on capitate shortening with capitohamate fusion and noted a prompt dramatic relief of symptoms with 83% of patients demonstrating revascularization on MRI. We believe that capitate shortening osteotomy, without capitohamate arthrodesis, is a reasonable alternative for stages II to IIIB with an ulnar positive variance.

Other Arthrodeses

Graner et al. (60), in 1966, described two separate limited intercarpal arthrodeses for Kienböck's disease. The first is a scapholunatocapitotriquetral fusion for Kienböck's without significant collapse. The second is a lunate excision combined with a capitate osteotomy and proximal displacement of the hemicapitate with interposition bone graft. The latter is reserved for advanced Kienböck's disease. The authors report on 27 cases and state that only two had persistent pain, and one had a slight weakness in grip.

We know of no biomechanical studies evaluating either of these arthrodeses and have had little experience with their use. One possible indication of the proximal displacement osteotomy is as a salvage procedure to retain radiocarpal motion.

Arthroplasty

Silicone

Lichtman et al. (38), in 1977, reported on 38 patients undergoing silicone replacement arthroplasty for Kienböck's disease with an average of 27 months of follow-up. Of the 20 patients in their series operated on before collapse of the lunate, 70% had satisfactory results. The same authors reported on 16 additional patients in 1982 (29). Seventy-five percent in this series had satisfactory results. The authors attribute their improving results to better implant materials. In 1990, Alexander et al. (61) reported on 10 patients from the same series with a minimum of 5 years of average follow-up. In this follow-up, only 50% had satisfactory results, and 30% had evidence of particulate synovitis. The authors now warn that the continued use of silicone replacement arthroplasty for Kienböck's disease is not warranted. These findings confirm those of other investigators (62,63).

Titanium

Swanson et al. (64) report on 24 patients with 8 years of average follow-up who underwent titanium lunate arthroplasty for Kienböck's disease. One patient in this series was revised to a total wrist fusion at 18 months. The authors noted no bony reaction to the titanium arthroplasty.

Excision/Fascial Interposition Arthroplasty

Eaton (65) reported on fascial interposition arthroplasty for late stages of Kienböck's disease using the fascia lata as the interposition material and recommended combination with an intercarpal fusion. Partecke and Buck-Gramcko (66), in 1985, reported on 38 patients who had undergone excision of the lunate with fascial interposition arthroplasty with 11 years average follow-up. All procedures were combined with a partial wrist denervation. These authors report 67% with good or excellent results.

Kato et al. (67), in 1986, compared results of interposition with silicone or with a coiled palmaris longus tendon after excisional arthroplasty in 32 patients with Kienböck's disease. Nineteen had silicone interposition arthroplasty, and the remainder underwent arthroplasty with a coiled palmaris longus tendon. Follow-up averaged 6 years, 4 months. The authors noted good clinical results after both procedures in patients with early lunate collapse. Additionally, they noted that silicone arthroplasty was more effective at preventing collapse than the coiled tendon. The coiled palmaris longus tendon interposition was associated with a better clinical result in their patients with advanced lunate collapse. In another series (68), lunate excision with coiled palmaris longus tendon interposition combined with triscaphe arthrodesis was performed in 15 patients with Kienböck's disease. Average follow-up was 57 months. Twelve patients were rated as satisfactory. All of the unsatisfactory patients in this series demonstrated progressive osteoarthritic changes at the radioscaphoid joint. Two of these (both stage IIIB) eventually underwent total wrist arthroplasty.

Wrist Denervation

Reports of wrist denervation began appearing in the literature in 1966 when Wilhelm (69) first reported its use as a method to "interrupt the signal to the brain." He reported, as an indication, painful restriction of wrist motion. Buck-Gramcko (70) reported a series of patients treated with wrist denervation for Kienböck's disease. Forty-seven patients were treated with wrist denervation combined with other techniques for Kienböck's disease. Seventy-six percent of patients in this series had no complaints, and 88% were reported as "remarkably satisfied." Fourteen patients underwent wrist denervation as the sole treatment for Kienböck's disease. He reports on this series with an average of 6.5 years of follow-up. Multiple points of denervation were performed. Three patients were noted to have complete relief of pain, and six patients were noted to have pain only with heavy labor.

Salvage Procedures

Proximal Row Carpectomy

Proximal row carpectomy was introduced by Stamm (71) in 1944 as a "reconstructive" procedure. He likens this procedure to the substitution of a ball and socket joint for the complicated link joint mechanism of the wrist. Culp et al. (72), in a multicenter study, reviewed proximal row carpectomy in 20 patients, some with Kienböck's disease, with a mean follow-up of 3.5 years. The authors note 15% loss of motion and 22% improvement in grip strength. The procedure failed in all rheumatoids in their series.

Begley and Engber (73) reported on 14 patients with an average of 3 years of follow-up treated with proximal row carpectomy for stage III Kienböck's disease. The authors note that all patients in their series had less pain and demonstrated 72% average grip strength as compared to the nonoperated side. All patients in their series returned to work.

Total Wrist Fusion

There have been no reports in the literature of total wrist fusion specifically as a treatment for Kienböck's disease. Authors having written about this subject reserve wrist fusion for advanced stages of Kienböck's disease or as a secondary reconstructive procedure. Reports of nonunion rates using the AO/ASIF wrist fusion plate and instrumentation have ranged from 0% to 4% (74).

AUTHORS' PREFERRED TREATMENT ALGORITHM

Stage I

No controlled studies of stage I patients have been performed to determine whether immobilization alone can halt progression of the disease. In transient ischemia (55), immobilization is the treatment of choice. After 3 months of immobilization, we begin aggressive management as in stage II. Because cast immobilization does not completely eliminate the transmitted load across the carpus, an external fixator can be considered in lieu of circular plaster.

Stage II/IIIA

In ulnar neutral or ulnar negative variance Kienböck's disease, we recommend radial shortening osteotomy (75). This adequately unloads the lunate as evidenced in several biomechanical studies (13,25,26,47). We prefer this to ulnar lengthening because it avoids the need for an additional bone graft. We do not recommend shortening beyond 1 to 2 mm, as excessive shortening has been associated with iatrogenic ulnocarpal impaction.

The details of our technique have been published elsewhere (75), but briefly, we expose the distal one-third of the radius through a palmar approach. A seven- or eight-hole dynamic compression plate (DCP) is placed over the radius to mark the level of the osteotomy. The plate is affixed to bone while marking the osteotomy, then removed for execution of the osteotomy. The amount of bone removed is determined by the ulnar variance noted in neutral variance preoperative wrist radiographs. The osteotomy is performed in an oblique fashion to facilitate interfragmentary compression. The plate is then affixed to the radius incorporating the interfragmentary lag screw (Fig. 23.15).

In ulnar positive variance, we recommend vascular implantation. We have experience with the Hori procedure (42) and have published a modification thereof (45). Briefly, the dorsal second metacarpal artery and vein are exposed and dissected free; 4-0 nylon is placed as a ligature, and the vessels are divided distally. A 1.0×0.5 cm dorsal corticocancellous graft is harvested from the dorsal distal radius, and a central hole is drilled through the graft with a 0.045-in. Kirschner wire. A window is created in the dorsal, nonarticular portion of the lunate, and avascular bone is removed with a curette. Next, the vascular bundle is placed into the hole made in the distal radius bone graft and secured with 4-0 nylon. The bone graft with the vascular bundle is placed into the lunate defect. Postoperative immobilization is accomplished with an external fixator (Fig. 23.16).

Stage IIIB

In stage IIIB Kienböck's disease, there is fixed rotatory subluxation of the scaphoid combined with proximal migration of the capitate (Fig. 23.17). For this, we recommend scaphocapitate or triscaphe fusion, as either of these procedures allows reduction of the scaphoid, stabilization of the midcarpal joint, and unloading of the lunate fossa. Triscaphe fusion is especially indicated when evidence of triscaphe arthritis exists. We use Watson's standard technique for triscaphe arthrodesis (55,56). We excise the lunate only when it is fragmented and causing a marked synovitis. We do not replace it with anything.

Stage IV

In stage IV Kienböck's disease, there is pancarpal arthritis as well as fixed rotatory subluxation of the scaphoid and proximal migration of the capitate in the face of lunate collapse (Fig. 23.18). As for any degenerative joint disorder, conservative therapy is indicated before recommending an operation. For those patients requiring surgery, we usually recommend proximal row carpectomy for older patients with a more sedentary life style and perform a total wrist fusion on younger patients who place active demands on their wrists. The decision between arthrodesis or arthroplasty also depends on individual requirements for radiocarpal motion based on occupation and avocational factors. Our standard technique for proximal row carpectomy has been published elsewhere (39). For total wrist arthrodesis, we now favor use of the AO/ASIF plates. There is no place for total wrist arthroplasty in the treatment of stage IV Kienböck's disease.

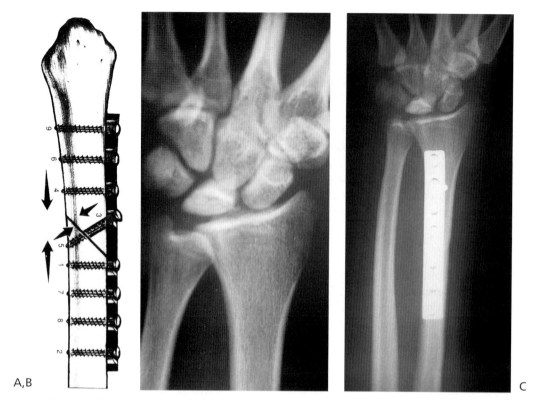

FIGURE 23.15. A: Radial shortening osteotomy procedure. (From Alexander CE, Alexander AH, Lichtman DM. Radial shortening in Kienböck's disease. In: Gelberman RH, ed. *Master techniques in orthopaedic surgery: The wrist.* New York: Raven Press, 1994;373–384, with permission.) **B:** Stage II Kienböck's disease with negative ulnar variance. **C:** The same patient soon after radial shortening osteotomy.

Conclusions

Kienböck's disease is a relatively uncommon wrist disorder whose exact etiology remains elusive. Nevertheless, technological advances in wrist surgery have made many treatment options available to the surgeon. Treatment needs to be tailored to the presenting stage of the disorder as well as the anatomic ulnar variance of the wrist. With this approach, good to excellent results can be expected.

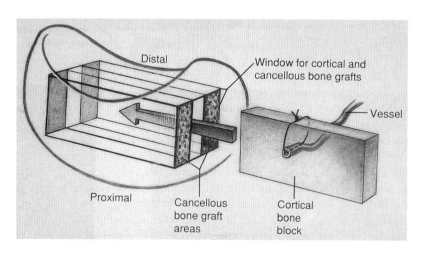

FIGURE 23.16. Second dorsal metacarpal artery implantation procedure (modified from Hori). (From Lichtman DM, Ross GR. Revascularization of the lunate in Kienböck's disease. In: Gelberman RH, ed. *Master techniques in orthopaedic surgery: The wrist.* New York: Raven Press, 1994;363–372, with permission.)

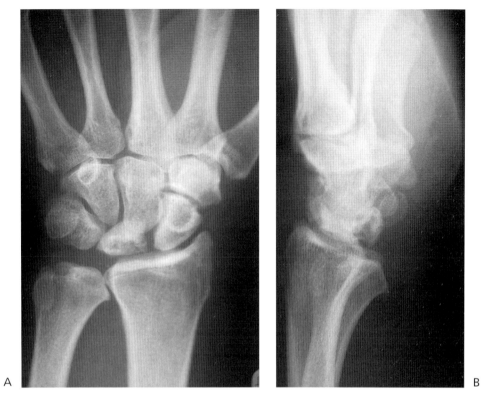

FIGURE 23.17. Posteroanterior **(A)** and lateral **(B)** radiographs of stage IIIB Kienböck's disease. (Courtesy of David H. Hildreth, M.D.)

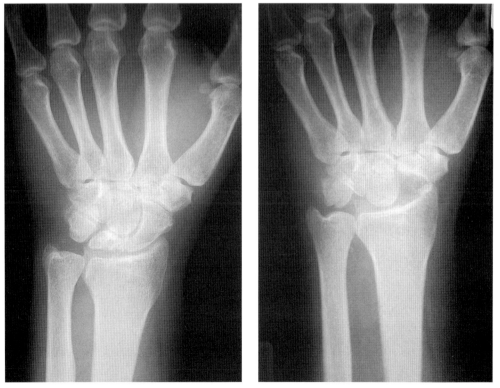

FIGURE 23.18. Pre- **(A)** and postoperative (proximal row carpectomy) **(B)** radiographs of stage IV Kienböck's disease.

REFERENCES

1. Alexander AH, Lichtman DM. Kienböck's disease. *Orthop Clin North Am* 1986;17:461–472.
2. Alexander AH, Lichtman DM. Kienböck's disease. In: Lichtman DM, ed. *The wrist and its disorders, 1st ed.* Philadelphia: WB Saunders, 1991;329–343.
3. Kienböck R. Uber traumatische Malazie des Mondbeinsund ihre Folgezustande: Entartungsformen und Kompressionfrakturen. *Fortschr Gebiete Roengtgenstr* 1910;16:78–103.
4. Gelberman RH, Bauman TD, Menon J, et al. The vascularity of the lunate bone and Kienböck's disease. *J Hand Surg [Am]* 1980;5:272–278.
5. Lee M. The intraosseous arterial pattern of the carpal lunate bone and its relation to avascular necrosis. *Acta Orthop Scand* 1963;33:43–55.
6. Panagis JS, Gelberman RH, Taleisnik J, et al. The arterial anatomy of the human carpus. Part II: The intraosseous vascularity. *J Hand Surg [Am]* 1983;8:375–382.
7. Williams CS, Gelberman RH. Vascularity of the lunate: anatomic studies and implications for the development of osteonecrosis. *Hand Clin* 1993;9:385–390.
8. Peste JL. Discussion. *Bull Soc Anat Paris* 1843;18:169–170.
9. Baum. Uber die traumatische Affektion des Os Lunatum und Naviculare carpi. *Beitr Z Klin Chir* 1913;87:568.
10. Húlten O. Uber anatomisch variationender Handgelenkknochen. *Acta Radiol Scand* 1928;9:155–168.
11. Gelberman RH, Salamon PB, Jurist JM, et al. Ulnar variance in Kienböck's disease. *J Bone Joint Surg Am* 1975;57:674–676.
12. Palmer AK, Werner FW. Biomechanics of the distal radioulnar joint. *Clin Orthop* 1984;187:26–35.
13. Werner FW, Palmer AK. Biomechanical evaluation of operative procedures to treat Kienböck's disease. *Hand Clin* 1993;9:431–444.
14. Lichtman DM, Roure AR. External fixation for the treatment of Kienböck's disease. *Hand Clin* 1993;9:691–697.
15. D'Hoore K, De Smet L, Verellen K, et al. Negative ulnar variance is not a risk factor for Kienböck's disease. *J Hand Surg [Am]* 1994;19:229–231.
16. Kristensen SS, Soballe K. Kienböck's disease—the influence of arthrosis on ulnar variance measurements. *J Hand Surg [Br]* 1987;12:301–305.
17. Nakamura R, Tanaka Y, Imaeda T, et al. The influence of age and sex on ulnar variance. *J Hand Surg [Br]* 1991;16:84–88.
18. Marek RM. Avascular necrosis of the carpal lunate. *Clin Orthop* 1957;10:96–107.
19. Beckenbaugh RD, Shives TC, Dobyns JH, et al. The natural history of Kienböck's disease and consideration of lunate fractures. *Clin Orthop* 1980;149:98–106.
20. Cave EF. Kienböck's disease of the lunate. *J Bone Joint Surg* 1939;21:858–866.
21. Ståhl F. On lunatomalacia (Kienböck's disease), a clinical and roentgenological study, especially on its pathogenesis and the late results of immobilization treatment. *Acta Chir Scand [Suppl]* 1947;126:1–133.
22. Ficat RP, Arlet J. Ischemia and necrosis of bone. In: Hungerford DS, ed. *Bone and circulation.* Baltimore: Williams & Wilkins, 1980;1–182.
23. Schiltenwolf M, Martini AK, Mau HK, et al. Further investigations of the intraosseous pressure characteristics in necrotic lunates (Kienböck's disease). *J Hand Surg [Am]* 1996;21:754–758.
24. Jensen CH. Intraosseous pressure in Kienböck's disease. *J Hand Surg [Am]* 1993;18:355–359.
25. An KN. The effect of force transmission on the carpus after procedures used to treat Kienböck's disease. *Hand Clin* 1993;9:445–454.
26. Coe MR, Trumble TE. Biomechanical comparison of methods used to treat Kienböck's disease. *Hand Clin* 1993;9:417–430.
27. Horii E, Garcia-Elias M, An KN, et al. Effect of force transmission across the carpus in procedures used to treat Kienböck's disease. *J Hand Surg [Am]* 1990;15:393–400.
28. Szabo RM, Greenspan A. Diagnosis and clinical findings of Kienböck's disease. *Hand Clin* 1993;9:399–408.
29. Lichtman DM, Alexander AH, Mack GR, et al. Kienböck's disease—update on silicone replacement arthroplasty. *J Hand Surg [Am]* 1982;7:343–347.
30. Youm Y, McMurtry RY, Flatt AE. Kinematics of the the wrist, part I—an experimental study of radial–ulnar deviation and flexion–extension. *J Bone Joint Surg Am* 1978;60:423–431.
31. Miura H, Uchida Y, Sugioka Y. Radial closing wedge osteotomy for Kienböck's disease. *J Hand Surg [Am]* 1996;21:1029–1034.
32. Posner MA, Greenspan A. Trispiral tomography for the evaluation of wrist problems. *J Hand Surg [Am]* 1988;13:175–181.
33. Friedman L, Yong HK, Johnson GH. The use of coronal computed tomography in the evaluation of Kienböck's disease. *Clin Radiol* 1991;44:56–59.
34. Jackson MD, Barry DT, Geiringer SR. Magnetic resonance imaging of avascular necrosis of the lunate. *Arch Phys Med Rehabil* 1990;71:510–513.
35. Desser TS, McCarthy S, Trumble T. Scaphoid fractures and Kienböck's disease of the lunate: MR imaging with histopathologic correlation. *Magn Reson Imaging* 1990;8:357–361.
36. Imaeda T, Nakamura R, Miura T, et al. Magnetic resonance imaging in Kienböck's disease. *J Hand Surg [Br]* 1992;17:9–12.
37. White RE, Omer GE. Transient vascular compromise of the lunate after fracture-dislocation or dislocation of the carpus. *J Hand Surg [Am]* 1984;9:181–184.
38. Lichtman DM, Mack GR, MacDonald RI, et al. Kienböck's disease: the role of silicone replacement arthroplasty. *J Bone Joint Surg Am* 1977;59:899–908.
39. Lichtman DM, Degnan GG. Proximal row carpectomy. In: Blair W, ed. *Techniques in hand surgery.* Baltimore: Williams & Wilkins, 1996;961–966.
40. Braun R. *The pronator pedicle bone grafting in the forearm and proximal carpal row.* Paper presented at the 38th Annnual Meeting of the Americal Society for Surgery of the Hand, March 1983.
41. Erbs G, Böhm E. Langzeitergebnisse der Os Pisiformeverlagerung bei Mondbeinnkrose. *Handchir Mikrochir Plast Chir* 1984;16:85–89.
42. Hori Y, Tamai S, Okuda H, et al. Blood vessel transplantation to bone. *J Hand Surg [Am]* 1979;4:23–33.
43. Yajima H, Tamai S. *Treatment of Kienböck's disease with vascular bundle implantation.* Paper presented at the 65th Meeting of the Japanese Orthopaedic Association, Fukuoka, 1992, p. S259.
44. Saldana MJ, Niebauer JJ, Brown R, et al. Microsurgical revascularization of ischemic rat femoral heads. *J Hand Surg [Am]* 1990;15:309–315.
45. Lichtman DM, Ross GR. Revascularization of the lunate in Kienböck's disease. In: Gelberman RH, ed. *Master techniques in orthopaedic surgery, the wrist.* New York: Raven Press, 1994;363–372.
46. Deleted in proof.
47. Trumble T, Glisson RR, Seaber AV, et al. A biomechanical comparison of the methods for treating Kienböck's disease. *J Hand Surg [Am]* 1986;11:88–93.
48. Torosian CM, Lichtman DM. Current trends in Kienböck's disease: an historical perspective. In: Vastamaki M, ed. *Current trends in hand surgery.* Amsterdam: Elsevier, 1995;99–107.
49. Weiss A-PC. Radial shortening. *Hand Clin* 1993;9:475–482.

50. Nakamura R, Imaeda T, Miura T. Radial shortening for Kienböck's disease: factors affecting the operative result. *J Hand Surg [Br]* 1990;15:40–45.
51. Persson M. Causal treatment of lunatomalacia. Further experiences of operative ulna lengthening. *Acta Chir Scand* 1950;100:531–544.
52. Quenzer DE, Linscheid RL. Ulnar lengthening procedures. *Hand Clin* 1993;9:467–474.
53. Tsunoda K, Nakamura R, Watanabe K, et al. Changes in carpal alignment following radial osteotomy for Kienböck's disease. *J Hand Surg [Br]* 1993;18:289–293.
54. Light T, Wehner J, Patwardhan AG. Load-bearing characteristics of the wrist with intercarpal arthrodesis. *J Rehab Res Dev* 1989;26:247.
55. Watson HK, Fink JA, Monacelli DM. Use of triscaphe fusion in the treatment of Kienböck's disease. *Hand Clin* 1993;9:493–499.
56. Watson HK, Ryu J, DiBella MB. An approach to Kienböck's disease: triscaphe arthrodesis. *J Hand Surg [Am]* 1985;10:179–187.
57. Sennwald GR, Ufenast H. Scaphocapitate arthrodesis for the treatment of Kienböck's disease. *J Hand Surg [Am]* 1995;20:506–510.
58. Chuinard RG, Zeman SC. Kienböck's disease: an analysis and rationale for treatment by capitate–hamate fusion. *Orthop Trans* 1980;4:18.
59. Almquist EE. Capitate shortening in the treatment of Kienböck's disease. *Hand Clin* 1993;9:505–512.
60. Graner O, Lopes EI, Carvalho BC, et al. Arthrodesis of the carpal bones in the treatment of Kienböck's disease, painful ununited fractures of the navicular and lunate bones with avascular necrosis, and old fracture-dislocations of the carpal bones. *J Bone Joint Surg Am* 1966;48:767–774.
61. Alexander AH, Turner MA, Alexander CE, et al. Lunate silicone replacement arthroplasty in Kienböck's disease: a long term follow-up. *J Hand Surg [Am]* 1990;15:401–407.
62. Carter PR, Benton LJ, Dysert PA. Silicone rubber carpal implants: a study of the incidence of late osseous complications. *J Hand Surg [Am]* 1986;11:639–644.
63. Peimer CA, Medige J, Eckert BS, et al. Reactive synovitis after silicone arthroplasty. *J Hand Surg [Am]* 1986;11:624–638.
64. Swanson AB, Swanson GdG. Implant resection arthroplasty in the treatment of Kienböck's disease. *Hand Clin* 1993;9:483–492.
65. Eaton RG. Excision and fascial interposition arthroplasty in the treatment of Kienböck's disease. *Hand Clin* 1993;9:513–516.
66. Partecke BD, Buck-Gramcko D. Technique and results of tendon interposition—arthroplasty of the lunate and scaphoid bone. *Handchir Mikrochir Plast Chir* 1985;17:211–218.
67. Kato H, Usui M, Minami A. Long-term results of Kienböck's disease treated by excisional arthroplasty with a silicone implant or coiled palmaris longus tendon. *J Hand Surg [Am]* 1986;11:645–653.
68. Minami A, Kimura T, Suzuki K. Long-term results of Kienböck's disease treated by triscaphe arthrodesis and excisional arthroplasty with a coiled palmaris longus tendon. *J Hand Surg [Am]* 1994;19:219–228.
69. Wilhelm A. Die Gelenkdenervation und ihre anatomischen Grundlagen. Ein nees Behandlungsprinzip in der Handchirurgie. *Hefte Unfallheilkd* 1966;86:1–109.
70. Buck-Gramcko D. Wrist denervation procedures in the treatment of Kienböck's disease. *Hand Clin* 1993;9:517–520.
71. Stamm TT. Excision of the proximal row of the carpus. *Proc R Soc Med* 1944;57:74–75.
72. Culp RW, McGuigan FX, Turner MA, et al. Proximal row carpectomy: a multicenter study. *J Hand Surg [Am]* 1993;18:19–25.
73. Begley BW, Engber WD. Proximal row carpectomy in advanced Kienböck's disease. *J Hand Surg [Am]* 1994;19:1016–1018.
74. Lin HH, Stern PJ. "Salvage" procedures in the treatment of Kienböck's disease: proximal row carpectomy and total wrist arthrodesis. *Hand Clin* 1993;9:521–526.
75. Alexander CE, Alexander AH, Lichtman DM. Radial shortening in Kienböck's disease. In: Gelberman RH, ed. *Master techniques in orthopaedic surgery, vol 24: the wrist.* New York: Raven Press, 1994;373–384.

THEORY AND ETIOLOGY OF KIENBÖCK'S DISEASE

H. KIRK WATSON
JEFFREY WEINZWEIG

The exact etiology of Kienböck's disease is unknown. What we present here is our working hypothesis of the etiology of Kienböck's disease.

FAULT PLATE HYPOTHESIS

The factors influencing lunate necrosis are multiple, and a combination of them must be present for the condition to develop (1). These factors are related to unusual stress on the lunate over a period of time (Fig. 24.1). They may be arbitrarily grouped as extrinsic factors, which are not features of the lunate itself but act on the lunate; or intrinsic anatomic features of the lunate that either render it unsuitable for load handling or contribute to its failure under load. The result of a combination of these factors is the formation of multiple plates or faults within the substance of the lunate. These fault plates are comparable to geologic faults and form in response to elastic deformation occurring in the trabeculae secondary to loading. The plates thus formed may be very small or very large. They may be localized to one area of the lunate or diffusely distributed throughout the bone. They may be short-lived or semipermanent. Enough of them in crucial areas forming more rapidly than repair can occur can eventually wall off and interfere with blood supply to areas within the lunate, resulting in bone necrosis (Fig. 24.2). The anatomy of specific blood vessels per se probably plays little or no role. It is probable that carpal trabecular overload is very common. The lunate and proximal scaphoid pole take the greatest load to the radius. A more common use of magnetic resonance imaging (MRI) is in demonstrating edema in trabecular areas of otherwise normal bones. Rest or activity change allows recovery of these "pre-Kienböck's" changes. It requires a prolonged unremitting load to carry these changes all the way to Kienböck's disease.

EXTRINSIC FACTORS

Capitate

The radius of curvature of the proximal lunate on the radius is large, and the bone is broadly and well supported. However, the radius of curvature of the capitate in the distal lunate fossa is quite small. This concentrates loads coming proximally through the capitate into a relatively small area, and loads here tend to spread the lunate (2). In a lunate with weakened internal structure secondary to bone cell death, the lunate will fail, usually producing palmar and dorsal segments. This fracture is probably a terminal event (3), not an etiologic one. Lunate fractures are the result of Kienböck's disease, not the cause. The capitate, however, is the chief pile driver in the engine of destruction resulting in Kienböck's disease (Figs. 24.3 and 24.4).

Lunate Loading

The tendency for the proximal pole of the scaphoid to displace dorsally under significant in-line loading probably protects the scaphoid. The lunate, however, cannot escape the small head of the capitate, and the loads are concentrated through the lunate even in extreme wrist flexion or extension. The lunate acts as a keystone (4), prevented from displacement by its attachments to the scaphoid and triquetrum (2). Proximally directed forces from the hand tend to center in the lunate, much as the keystone of an arch takes load at the apex of the convexity. Avascular necrosis of the scaphoid may represent multifactorial overload and fault plate formation in a scaphoid identical to Kienböck's

---

H. K. Watson: Connecticut Combined Hand Surgery Fellowship, Hartford Hospital, and Connecticut Children's Medical Center, Hartford, Connecticut 06106; Department of Orthopaedics, University of Connecticut School of Medicine, Farmington, Connecticut 06032; Department of Orthopedics, Rehabilitation, and Plastic Surgery, Yale University School of Medicine, New Haven, Connecticut 06520.

J. Weinzweig: Department of Plastic Surgery, Brown University School of Medicine, Rhode Island Hospital, and Hasbro Children's Hospital, Providence, Rhode Island 02905.

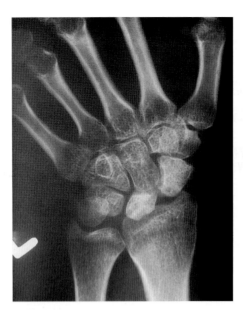
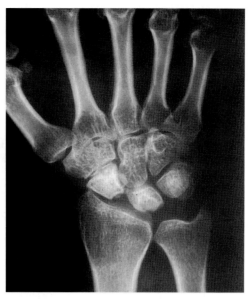

FIGURE 24.1. Unremitting loads on the wrist without adequate rest or recovery time can result in avascular necrosis of the scaphoid and lunate bilaterally.

disease but is less common because the scaphoid can more easily share loads with its ligaments (Fig. 24.5). In a sense, this is the scaphoid's salvation but clearly also is its downfall in terms of instability problems.

Ulnar Variance

This is one of the most commonly cited factors in lunate loading. Although the ulna is not necessary for wrist function, there are positions and activities when it may support the ulnar half of the lunate. If the ulna is short, there may be circumstances when loads in the lunate cannot be dissipated except through the ulnar edge of the radial articular surface. The lunate may be specifically overloaded by that ulnar radial ridge, which acts as a fulcrum localizing loads sufficiently to produce fault plates. There are numerous studies to support this mechanism (5–9). Additionally, there are reports of Kienböck's disease associated with ulna positive variance (10). Here, the mechanism may be an impaction phenomenon from the ulna; either results in formation of fault plates. Interestingly, however, the lunate seldom fractures into radial and ulnar segments over this ulnarmost edge of the radius. After necrosis, the capitate is responsible for fracturing the lunate into palmar and dorsal segments. This means that fault plates may be produced by changes in the lunate–ulna relationship, but loads are not sufficiently concentrated by lack of ulnar support to fracture the lunate along the ulnar edge of the radius. This gross fracture of the lunate would also be a terminal event separate from the overloads within the lunate that produce shear injuries to the trabeculae, resulting in the fault plates (e.g., the resultant dead bone fractures).

Load Type

The loads applied are etiologic (11). Intermittent, high-impact loads such as jack-hammering seem obvious culprits, but any heavy hand activity will suffice. Nonimpact, high-torque loads are magnified in the carpal bones by wrist flexion and extension. A mentally deficient patient who rocks incessantly on his hands falls into this factor

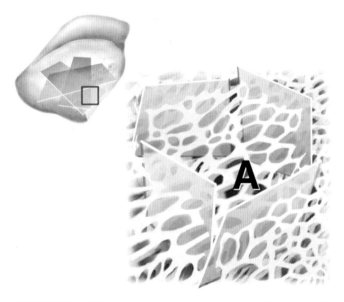

FIGURE 24.2. The four rectangular plates are diagrammatic fault plates of variable size and shape. Their presence tends to interrupt the trabeculae and blood supply, gradually isolating area A. Any additional interruption of the trabecular pattern and vascular availability to A will result in necrosis in that area.

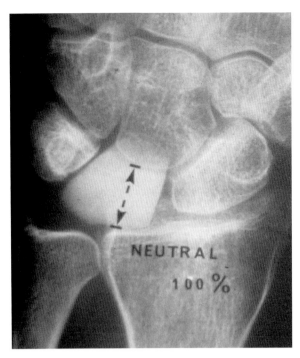 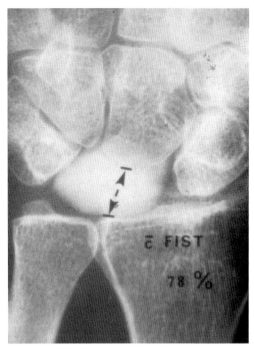

FIGURE 24.3. Collapse of the lunate allows the capitate to approach the radius. This drives the scaphoid into rotary subluxation as seen here on the right side. A silicone implant lunate was placed in this patient. The wrist on the **left** is relaxed; a dynamic full fist view is seen on the **right**. The capitate drives toward the radius, collapsing the silicone implant. Note the significant foreshortening and rotary subluxation of the scaphoid. *Arrows* indicate lunate height in each cardiograph.

group as much as the hard laborer. There is also a possible relationship between Kienböck's disease and the use of vibratory tools (12,13). This may be caused by a direct vascular insult but more probably is secondary to vibratory fatigue loading of the trabeculae, resulting in fault plates.

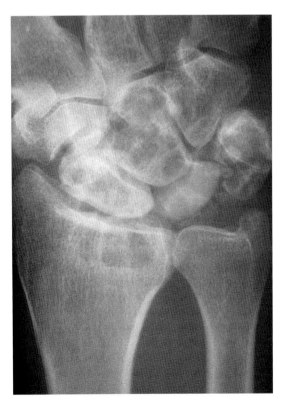

FIGURE 24.4. There is no place for silicone carpal replacement in the armamentarium of the wrist surgeon. Particulate synovitis produces a panligamentous destruction that allows ulnar translation of the entire carpus as well as a significant bone destruction component, typically resulting in the need for arthrodesis of the wrist.

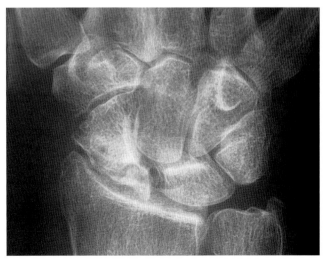

FIGURE 24.5. Preiser's disease—avascular necrosis of the scaphoid—is a rarer entity but follows the same clinical pattern as Kienböck's disease.

Instability

Scapholunate dissociation, with subsequent destabilization of the lunate, has been reported to be associated with Kienböck's disease (14,15). It is possible that instability is an extrinsic factor. The rotating scaphoid easily escapes to the dorsum of the capitate, leaving the lunate to take the load. The lunate then remains loaded even at maximal wrist displacement positions (2,16). The rotation of the scaphoid typically associated with Kienböck's disease is secondary to the lunate collapse and probably not causative, however (17,18).

INTRINSIC ANATOMIC FACTORS

Lunate Spherical Shape

The lunate is more spherical than most of the other loaded carpal bones and thus more dependent on trabecular than cortical support. For the same cortical thickness in similar-sized bones, the more spherical the bone, the more it will depend on trabecular support to prevent collapse under load.

Cortical Load

The lunate is physiologically ballottable. If one could actually measure the change in shape of the lunate under heavy load, one would see a bulging, particularly of the palmar and dorsal cortices and a compression of the distal cortex toward the proximal cortex. This compressive tendency of the luante dictates a degree of deformation within its substance. The elasticity and strength of the cortical walls will determine the "collapsability" of any given lunate under any given load (19). Clearly, if "collapsability" exceeds certain limits, trabecular faults will occur along shear planes within the lunate.

Type V and D Lunates

Kauer's work notwithstanding (20), there are significant numbers (23%) of lunates that are thinner palmarly than dorsally (type V as opposed to the classic type D) when viewed on lateral projection (21). The wedge shape may play a role by preventing either dorsal or palmar lunate displacement (escape) at the maximum dorsiflexion load position of the lunate. Either V- or D-type lunates may be etiologic factors in the creation of fault plates.

Anatomy of the Trabeculae

There are x-ray variations in lunate trabecular anatomy between individuals (22). Some x-rays demonstrate coarse, heavy, well-spaced trabeculae, and others demonstrate a fine-grain homogeneous trabecular appearance. One or the other may be more prone to elastic deformation and fault plate formation. A simple comparison of the trabecular type in normal wrists versus wrists with Kienböck's disease might be worthwhile.

Position and Type of Trabeculae

The ossification center position and architectural alignment of bone within the lunate may predispose to a decreased load tolerance. The quality and morphology of osteoid and mineralization may play a role in fault plate susceptibility.

Vascular Anatomy of the Lunate

The vascular anatomy of the lunate has often been cited as the cause of Kienböck's disease (4,7,23). This seems obvious, but one has to make the transition from blood supply to bone death in a manner that fits the clinical appearance of Kienböck's disease. The only theory that seems to allow for all known components is the multifactorial load creation of fault plates, which eventually wall off and interfere with capillary-level blood supply (24). It may be that the relative paucity of blood supply is a factor, as in the lunate with a single nutrient vessel, but how this produces Kienböck's disease remains obscure. What may be important, however, is the plane in which the vessels lie. If, for instance, the major vessels lie in a palmar-to-dorsal axis, the formation of sagittal fault plates would tend to devascularize across these planes, resulting in necrosis (23). There may be a particular vascular anatomy that plays a major role in etiology, but it is our impression that this is not the case.

ONSET OF KIENBÖCK'S DISEASE

Kienböck's disease presents in various forms. The changes in the lunate may be very localized or diffuse. With progression, the lunate may fracture into two pieces or crumble into granules or produce an osteochondral fracture from one surface. The cartilage is not primarily involved in the pathogenesis and remains relatively healthy. Bone death occurs over time. Often, a symptomatic wrist will demonstrate normal x-rays, with the diagnosis evident only on MRI (25). The degree of loading of the wrist appears to be important, and changes in the lunate are cumulative.

A typical scenario is a lunate with several of the intrinsic anatomic features noted above, predisposing the lunate to elastic deformation of trabeculae. Intratrabecular microfaults occur and heal but leave certain changes along the plane of injury. With repeated injuries along the same plane and resultant rupture of capillary systems, there develops a physiologic fault plate with increased resistance to normal blood flow (26).

Additional fault plates may form in other areas of the lunate. This phenomenon is probably present in most of our carpal bones, but time and the avoidance of similar overload injuries preclude development of multiple plates. Areas in the lunate reach a critical state in which either a small section or much of the bone becomes relatively walled off by multiple fault plates, and further "normal" injuries can no longer heal efffectively because the capillary blood supply is inadequate. This portion of bone then dies, providing a significant fault area further limiting vascular access.

Changing one or more of the etiologic factors can halt progression, and the necrosed areas walled off by fault plates can probably heal. Collapsed areas, however, remain deformed.

Most cases of Kienböck's disease develop, then, as the result of a long process of insult that is multifactorial in etiology, producing overload within the substance of the bone. In a susceptible lunate, miniplanes of injury result in relatively avascular fault plates, gradually sectioning off areas in the lunate. Healing in these small areas cannot occur quickly enough if the abnormal loads and demand continue, ultimately resulting in areas of cell death.

Management of Kienböck's Disease

Our approach to Kienböck's disease, based on this hypothesis, means that, first and foremost, anything that will allow the physiologic fault plates to heal or resolve is the primary treatment of choice. It is probable that simple splinting that prevents full dorsiflexion and palmar flexion would significantly relieve loading, as the loads on the lunate are much greater in flexion and extension than in neutral. If collapse is early or mild, then some way of diverting load around the lunate until it is healed is indicated. There have been several reports of temporary pinning of the scaphotrapeziotrapezoid (STT) or triscaphe joint; this permits transfer of load from the capitate to the scaphoid and around the lunate. This temporary load detour allows the lunate to heal and probably function adequately even with slight deformity. As collapse and deformity increase, we believe a permanent detour of loads around the lunate is indicated, and our approach to this has been the triscaphe arthrodesis (27,28) (Fig. 24.6). With a healed triscaphe fusion and loads that travel from capitate to scaphoid to radius, thus avoiding the lunate, even multifragmented collapsed lunates may be left in place. They are surprisingly asymptomatic. Even the most comminuted lunates do not seem to produce symptoms in most cases. Large fragments of lunate displaced volarly may produce carpal tunnel complaints. It has been our long-time practice to fuse the triscaphe joint and leave the lunate alone, regardless of its x-ray appearance. From that approach, we find that approximately 28% of collapsed

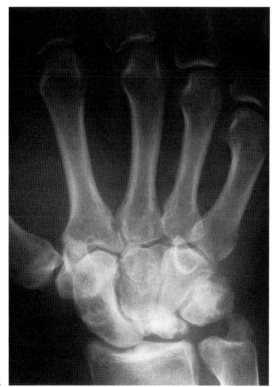
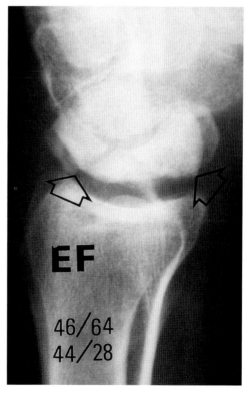

FIGURE 24.6. A: Triscaphe arthrodesis has been accomplished for severe collapsed Kienböck's disease in an engineer who performs manual house construction. **B:** The capitate has no support from the fractured lunate with fragments lying volarly and dorsally (*arrows*). The scaphoid is clearly taking all of the load for this wrist with excellent ranges of motion noted on the lateral view (46° of dorsiflexion; 64°; 44° of ulnar deviation; and 28° of radial deviation).

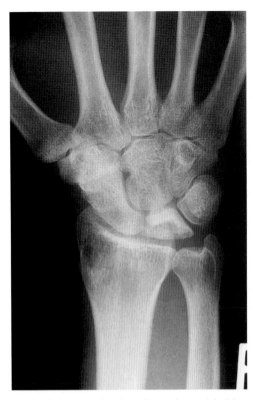

FIGURE 24.7. Even completely collapsed crumbled lunates are typically asymptomatic with good load ability following triscaphe limited wrist arthrodesis. However, lunates with osteochondral fragments as seen here frequently are painful, with postoperative symptoms apparently arising from the osteochondral fragment segment itself.

lunates continue to be symptomatic or to have significant range-of-motion restrictions requiring lunate excision within 2 years of the triscaphe arthrodesis. In reviewing these patients, it appears that it is not the comminuted, displaced lunate that produces the problem as much as it is the osteochondral fractures, often with minimal displacement. The osteochondral fractures with disease involving one area of the periphery of the lunate appear to directly produce symptoms; it is these lunates that are painful that typically require excision (Fig. 24.7).

Lunates heal following triscaphe limited wrist arthrodesis. It may be that the osteotomy procedures of the radius or ulna provide a time period in the operative and postoperative stages that allows the fault plates to heal. This may, indeed, be the effective treatment component, with or without removing one of the etiologic extrinsic factors of Kienböck's disease (e.g., radius–ulna alignment change). It is our contention, and our approach, that external splinting, immobilization, and protection of the lunate form the first line of defense, particularly in the case of undisplaced lunates in stage I or II of Kienböck's disease. With minimal collapse and displacement, particularly in young patients, a temporary detour of loads may be the best approach, such as pinning of the triscaphe joint. With more advanced collapse, STT limited wrist arthrodesis is a permanent solution to Kienböck's disease (Fig. 24.8).

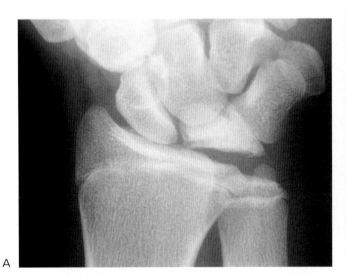
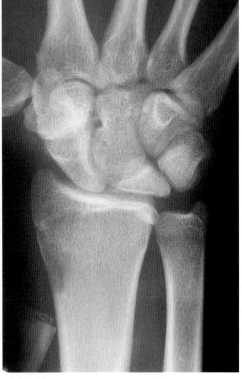

FIGURE 24.8. A: A young patient with open epiphyses presented with stage IIIB Kienböck's disease. **B:** Following treatment with a triscaphe limited wrist arthrodesis, the lunate has healed, but in a deformed configuration requiring that loads be transferred via the scaphoid permanently.

By contrast, proximal row carpectomy (PRC) is always a salvage procedure resulting in a less adequate solution. Both PRC and wrist fusion should be viewed in the same light. If there is normal cartilage on a joint through which the loads can be directed, then that will be a far superior wrist.

REFERENCES

1. Watson HK, Guidera PM. Aetiology of Kienböck's disease. *J Hand Surg [Br]* 1997;22:5–7.
2. Armistead RB, Linsheid RL, Dobyns JH, et al. Ulnar lengthening in the treatment of Kienböck's disease. *J Bone Joint Surg Am* 1982;64:170–178.
3. Beckenbaugh RD, Shives TC, Dobyns JH, et al. Kienböck's disease: the natural history of Kienböck's disease and consideration of lunate fractures. *Clin Orthop* 1980;149:98–106.
4. Marek FM. Avascular necrosis of the carpal lunate. *Clin Orthop* 1957;10:96–107.
5. Axelsson R. Behandling av lunatomalaci. In: *Elanders Boktrycker.* Goteborg, Sweden: Aktiebolag, 1971.
6. Chen WS, Shih CH. Ulnar variance and Kienböck's disease. *Clin Orthop* 1990;255:124–127.
7. Gelberman RH, Bauman TD, Menon J, et al. The vascularity of the lunate bone and Kienböck's disease. *J Hand Surg [Am]* 1980;5:272–278.
8. Hultén O. Über anatomische Variationen der Handgelenkknochen. *Acta Radiol* 1928;9:155–168.
9. Stahl S, Reis ND. Traumatic ulnar variance in Kienböck's disease. *J Hand Surg [Am]* 1986;11:95–97.
10. Nakamura R, Tanaka Y, Imaeda T, et al. The influence of age and sex on ulnar variance. *J Hand Surg [Br]* 1991;16:84–88.
11. Joji S, Mizuseki T, Katayama S, et al. Etiology of Kienböck's disease based on a study of the condition among patients of cerebral palsy. *J Hand Surg [Br]* 1993;18:294–298.
12. Gemme G, Saraste H. Bone and joint pathology in workers using handheld vibrating tools. An overview. *Scand J Work Environ Health* 1987;13:290–300.
13. Letz R, Cherniack MG, Gerr F, et al. A cross sectional epidemiological survey of shipyard workers exposed to hand–arm vibration. *Br J Indust Med* 1992;49:53–62.
14. Bourne MH, Linscheid RL, Dobyns JH. Concomitant scapholunate dissociation and Kienböck's disease. *J Hand Surg [Am]* 1991;16:460–464.
15. Cope JR. Rotary subluxation of the scaphoid. *Clin Radiol* 1984;35:495–501.
16. Kashiwagi D, Fukiwara A, Inoue T, et al. An experimental and clinical study of lunatomalacia. *Orthop Trans* 1977;1:7–12.
17. Watson HK, Fink J, Monacelli D. Use of triscaphe fusion in the treatment of Kienböck's disease. *Hand Clin* 1993;9:493–499.
18. Watson HK, Ryu J, Dibella A. An approach to Kienböck's disease: triscaphe arthrodesis. *J Hand Surg [Am]* 1985;10:179–187.
19. Koebke J, Fehrmann P, Mockenhaupt J. Stress on the normal and pathologic wrist joint. *Handchir Mikrochir Plast Chir* 1989;21:127–133.
20. Kauer J. Functional anatomy of the wrist. *Clin Orthop* 1980;149:9–20.
21. Watson HK, Yasuda M, Guidera PM. Lateral lunate morphology: An x-ray study. *J Hand Surg [Am]* 1996;21:759–763.
22. Antuna-Zapico JM. *Malacia of the semilunar bone.* Doctoral thesis, Universidad de Valladolid, Industrias y Editrial Sever Cuesta, Valladolid, Spain, 1966.
23. Williams CS, Gelberman RH. Vascularity of the lunate. Anatomic studies and implications for the development of osteonecrosis. *Hand Clin* 1993;9:391–398.
24. Goldsmith R. Kienböck's disease of the semilunar bone. *Ann Surg* 1925;81:857–862.
25. Desser TS, McCarthy S, Trumble T. Scaphoid fractures and Kienböck's disease of the lunate: MR imaging with histopathologic correlation. *Mag Res Imag* 1990;8:357–361.
26. Jensen CH. Intraosseous pressure in Kienböck's disease. *J Hand Surg [Am]* 1993;18:355–359.
27. Watson HK, Weinzweig J. Intercarpal arthrodesis. In: Green DP, Hotchkiss RN, Pederson WC, eds. *Operative hand surgery, 4th ed.* New York: Churchill Livingstone, 1999;108–130.
28. Watson HK, Weinzweig J. Treatment of Kienböck's disease with triscaphe arthrodesis. In: Vastamaki M, Vilkki S, Goransson H, et al, eds. *Proceedings of the 6th Congress of the International Federation of Societies for Surgery of the Hand.* Bologna, Italy: Monduzzi Editore, 1995;347–349.

25

LUNATE REVASCULARIZATION

HIROSHI YAJIMA

In 1843, Peste (1) first described collapse of the carpal lunate in anatomic specimens. However, this diagnosis did not gain popularity until 1910. Since Kienböck (2) described posttraumatic osteomalacia of the lunate in 1910, numerous authors have reported on Kienböck's disease. Despite continued efforts by various authors, the cause of Kienböck's disease is still unclear, and its treatment is controversial. In 1928, Hulten (3) made the association between ulnar variance and lunatomalacia. He reported a 78% incidence of ulnar negative variance in 23 patients with lunatomalacia compared with only 23% in 400 normal persons. He speculated that the increased shear forces on the lunate might be a contributing factor in the development of avascular necrosis of the lunate. Since this description, numerous authors have confirmed the increased incidence of ulnar-minus variance in Kienböck's disease (4–6). Based on their studies, joint-leveling procedures (radial shortening and ulnar lengthening) have been performed as the most popular operations for Kienböck's disease at numerous hospitals. However, there seem to be some racial differences with respect to the occurrence of ulnar variance. For example, as shown in Table 25.1, according to recent data, the average ratio of the ulnar-minus variance in patients with Kienböck's disease was only 22% in 136 patients from four hand centers in Japan (7–10), contrasting with Hulten's 78% in Austria reported in 1928 (3) and Lichtman's 65% in the United States reported in 1977 (11).

On the other hand, the revascularization procedure is one of the representative operations for Kienböck's disease (Table 25.2). Although the actual cause of the vascular impairment is still unclear, avascular necrosis of the lunate is an essential change in this disorder. Therefore, lunate revascularization is a logical treatment of Kienböck's disease. Hori and his colleagues (12), in our clinic, initiated vascular bundle implantation into bone in canines in 1970 to revascularize and revitalize necrotic bone. Since 1975, we have treated Kienböck's disease by promoting bone revitalization with vascular bundle implantation into the necrotic lunate, based on their experiments (13–15). Hori et al. reported successfully treating eight of nine patients with Kienböck's disease in 1979 (12). Moreover, in 1992, Yajima et al. (16) applied this technique in combination with scaphotrapeziotrapezoid (STT) arthrodesis for 21 patients with Kienböck's disease. Tamai et al. (17) reported a large series (51 patients) of vascular bundle implantations for the treatment of Kienböck's disease in 1993.

In 1983, Braun (18) described a method of taking a small piece of volar radial bone, still attached to the pronator quadratus muscle, which was then grafted to the avascular lunate. In 1984, Chacha (19) reported in detail the operative procedure of the pronator quadratus muscle pedicle bone graft. There were some problems with regard to the vascularity of the grafted bone after transfer. On the other hand, vascularized bone grafts using vessel pedicles with nutrient or periosteal vessels have been problem-free with regard to osseous vascularity. It is also easier to transfer a vascularized bone using a vessel pedicle rather than a muscle pedicle. Many reports of vascularized bone grafts to the carpus were for the purpose of treating scaphoid nonunions. Of course, some of these procedures can be applied for treating Kienböck's disease. In 1987, Kuhlmann et al. (20) reported the use of a vascularized bone graft pedicled on the volar carpal artery.

The 1,2-intercompartmental supraretinacular artery was first described in 1983 by Zaidemberg et al. (21) as a consistent ascending irrigating branch of the radial artery that supplied nutrient arteries to the dorsal distal radius. They also described a method of taking a small piece of radial bone (dorsoradial aspect of the distal radius), still attached to the 1,2-intercompartmental supraretinacular vessel, and grafting it to a scaphoid nonunion. Following this, Sheetz et al. (22) suggested that the modified 1,2-intercompartmental supraretinacular graft could be used for Kienböck's disease. They also described how the fourth extensor compartment artery graft based on retrograde flow from the intercarpal arch might be a useful donor for vascularized bone grafts. In 1991, Pagliei et al. (23) reported the anatomic basis of pedicled bone grafts attached to the anterior interosseous artery.

H. Yajima: Department of Orthopaedic Surgery, Nara Medical University, Kashihara, Nara 634-8522, Japan.

TABLE 25.1. INCIDENCE OF ULNAR MINUS VARIANCE IN JAPANESE PATIENTS WITH KIENBÖCK'S DISEASE

	Number	Plus Variance	Null Variance	Minus Variance
Ahsoh et al. (7)	20	4 (20%)	12 (60%)	4 (20%)
Minami et al. (8)	15	5 (33%)	7 (47%)	3 (20%)
Nakamura et al. (9)	50	22 (44%)	15 (30%)	13 (26%)
Yajima et al. (10)	51	7 (14%)	34 (67%)	10 (20%)
Total	136	38 (28%)	68 (50%)	30 (22%)

In 1992, Pierer et al. (24) described the detailed vascular anatomy of the second metacarpal bone and its use as a vascularized pedicled bone graft.

Transfer of the pisiform bone as a treatment of Kienböck's disease was first reported by Beck (25) in 1971. He reported a case of successful treatment transferring the pisiform bone on a vascular pedicle into the excavated lunate bone. In 1982, Saffar (26) reported a new technique for replacing the whole lunate by the pisiform, together with its vascular supply, while keeping it attached to the flexor carpi ulnaris. This procesure is not actually classified as a lunate revascularization procedure.

Some representative procedures that have been reported for lunate revascularization are now described.

TABLE 25.2. SURGICAL PROCEDURES FOR THE TREATMENT OF KIENBÖCK'S DISEASE

1. Load-altering procedures
    a. Joint-leveling procedures
        Radial shortening
        Ulnar lengthening
        Radial wedge osteotomy
    b. Intercarpal arthrodesis
        STT arthrodesis
        Scaphoid–capitate arthrodesis
        Capitate–hamate arthrodesis with capitate shortening
2. Revascularization procedures
    Vascular bundle implantation
    Vascularized bone graft
    Muscle pedicled bone graft
3. Replacement/resection arthroplasty
    a. Artificial lunate replacement
        Silicone lunate replacement
        Metal lunate replacement
    b. Soft tissue replacement
        Dorsal flap arthroplasty
        Tendon roll replacement
    c. Proximal row carpectomy
4. Wrist arthrodesis
    Radiolunate arthrodesis
    Total wrist arthrodesis
5. Wrist denervation procedure

STT, scaphotrapeziotrapezoid.

VASCULAR BUNDLE IMPLANTATION

Principles of Vascular Bundle Implantation

Vascular bundle implantation is the most representative method for lunate revascularization. Hori and his colleagues (12) started the experimental study on vascular bundle implantation using dogs and reported their results and clinical applications in 1979. Before this, there had been some reports of vessel transplantation into bones. However, only arteries had been transplanted into intact bones in all of these experiments (27–29). When an artery was transplanted into an isolated bone segment, all vessels thrombosed in Hori's experiment (12). He suspected the cause of vessel thrombosis to be the absence of an efferent tract. The vascular bundle consists of an artery, vein, and some attached fascia. Thrombosis does not occur in the vascular bundle because of the existence of microcirculation between the artery and vein. It is easy to understand that the vascular bundle is a minimal unit of circulation, otherwise described as a very narrow fascia flap.

The main principle supporting the implantation of a vascular bundle into bone is the significant amount of microcirculation existing in the vascular bundle. When contrast medium was injected into the artery of an isolated vascular bundle during microangiography, the injected medium flowed back from the vein immediately, and an intimate vascular network between the artery and vein could be observed (12) (Fig. 25.1).

There are two effects of vascular bundle implantation (30). One is vascular proliferation from the implanted vascular bundle. The proliferation of capillaries and fibloblasts around the implanted vascular bundle provides osteocytes and osteoblasts, which lead to rapid absorption of necrotic bone and simultaneous new bone formation and remodel-

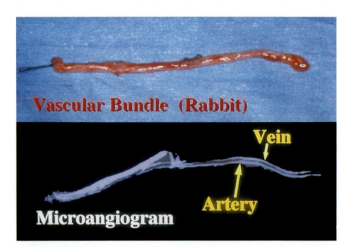

FIGURE 25.1. The isolated vascular bundle in a rabbit and its microangiogram. The contrast media injected into the artery flowed back via the vein.

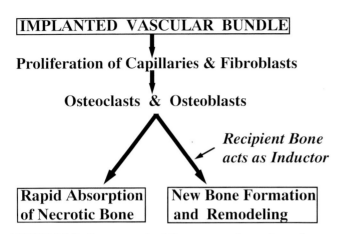

FIGURE 25.2. Our concept of the process of new bone formation after vascular bundle implantation.

ing, with accelerated creeping substitution. Figure 25.2 illustrates our concept of the revascularization procedure for the treatment of bone necrosis. This vascular proliferation was observed more conspicuously when implantation was into an isolated bone than when it was into an intact bone (31) (Fig. 25.3). However, it takes a long time for new bone formation to occur.

The other effect is a vascular connection with the preexisting vessels. It is difficult to make an ischemic model, so we performed an experimental study using a model in which a vascular bundle implants into an intact bone. When a vascular bundle was implanted into an intact bone, capillary proliferation proceeded from the vascular bundle within 1 week, and, thereafter, the vascular bundle and the preexisting vessels were anastomosed. Complete anastomosis between the implanted vascular bundle and the preexisting vessels was achieved by 3 weeks after surgery (30). This phenomenon of vascular connection is similar to that with a pedicled flap, which can also be detached at its pedicle within 3 weeks in clinical cases. In the latter case, vascular connection between the vessels of the transplanted flap and recipient vessels was completed by 3 weeks after the transfer.

The lunate without collapse in the early stage of Kienböck's disease is not totally avascular. One curetted specimen from the lunate at surgery revealed the central part of the lunate to be necrotic although its cortical side was viable (17). In my opinion, in the early stage of Kienböck's disease some vessels remain in the lunate. When a vascular bundle is implanted into a lunate, vascular connection proceeds quickly. Thereafter, revascularization soon occurs. Therefore, only a vascular bundle implantation is necessary for patients with the early stage of Kienböck's disease. On the other hand, for the patients with the advanced stage (completely necrosed lunate), the necrotic bone marrow should be curetted, and an iliac cancellous bone graft should be packed into the cavity. Some biomechanical procedures that reduce vertical stress on the lunate are useful until new bone formation and remodeling occur (16,17).

Operative Technique

Vascular Bundle Implantation

Before surgery, the pulse of the second dorsal metacarpal artery is examined with a Doppler ultrasound stethoscope. When the condition of the second dorsal metacarpal artery cannot be confirmed clearly, the third dorsal metacarpal artery and vein are used as an implanted vascular bundle. With a tourniquet on the upper arm and the patient under general anesthesia, a lazy curved longitudinal incision from the wrist joint to the second digital space is made on the dorsum of the hand. Under an operating microscope or binocular loupes, the second dorsal metacarpal artery and vein are atraumatically isolated as a vascular bundle with some attached fascia (Figs. 25.4–25.6). The vascular bundle end at the dorsal digital web space level is ligated using an absorbable suture and cut (Fig. 25.7). The vascular bundle is kept wet with 10% lidocaine (Xylocaine) until the recipient bed is prepared. The joint capsule is incised to expose the lunate bone. A drill hole is then made on the dorsal

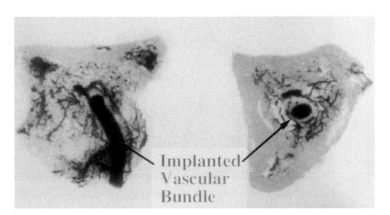

FIGURE 25.3. Microangiograms of cross sections of the isolated tibia segment 5 weeks after vascular bundle implantation, showing vascular proliferation from the implanted vascular bundle.

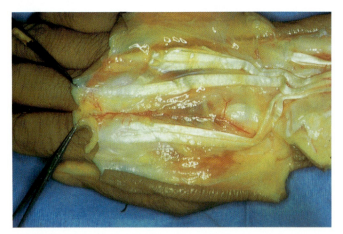

FIGURE 25.4. Batson's compound-injected specimen showing second dorsal metacarpal artery of a fresh cadaver hand.

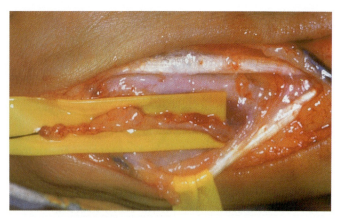

FIGURE 25.6. An elevated vascular bundle.

aspect of the lunate at the border between bone and cartilage.

For stage I and stage II (Lichtman's classification) (32) cases, only vascular bundle implantation into the lunate is performed, without curettage and bone graft. Another small transverse incision is made on the volar aspect of the wrist, and the joint capsule is exposed, retracting the median nerve and flexor tendons. An 18-gauge injection needle is inserted from the dorsal drill hole into the volar joint capsule, and then a 21-gauge needle is introduced from the volar aspect into the dorsal drill hole. The ligature suture of the vascular bundle is passed through this needle and pulled out volarly and is used to implant the vascular bundle into the lunate (Figs. 25.8 and 25.9). The ligature suture is firmly secured on the volar capsule (Fig. 25.10).

For stage III or early stage IV disease, saucerization of the necrotic bone is necessary. With a Surgi-Airtome power drill (Zimmer, Warsaw, IN), the necrotic bone marrow in the lunate is removed to create a lunate shell. Small iliac bone chips are then packed into the cavity so as to expand the collapsed lunate. A drill hole is then made again in the grafted bone, and the vascular bundle implantation is performed in the same manner as described previously. After release of the tourniquet, the pulsation of the implanted vascular bundle can be observed under magnification (Fig. 25.11). The skin is closed with 4-0 nylon sutures, followed by cast immobilization from the metacarpophalangeal (MP) joints to above the elbow.

The cast is removed 1 month after surgery, and range-of-motion exercise for the wrist joint is commenced using a dynamic splint. Thereafter, radiographic evaluations of the lunate bone are performed once a month at the outpatient clinic. Patients generally return to work 3 to 6 months postoperatively, wearing a dorsal splint on the wrist to protect against hyperextension.

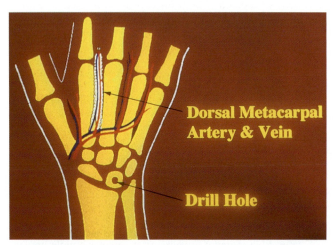

FIGURE 25.5. A schematic diagram of an elevated vascular bundle consisting of the second dorsal metacarpal artery and vein.

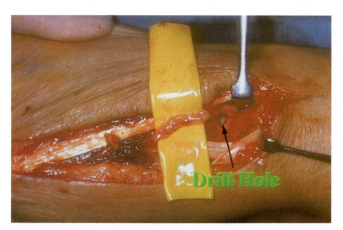

FIGURE 25.7. The vascular bundle is folded back toward the lunate.

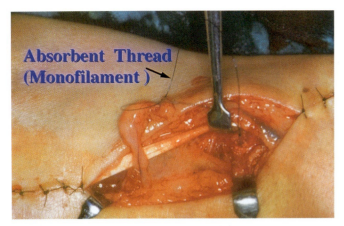

FIGURE 25.8. Introduction of the vascular bundle into the hole of the lunate.

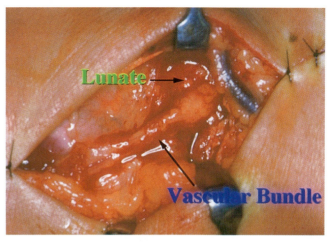

FIGURE 25.11. Pulsation of the implanted vascular bundle can be seen after release of the tourniquet.

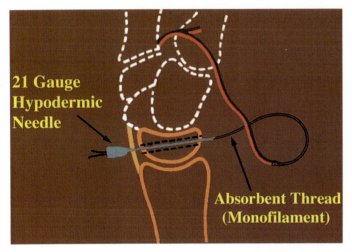

FIGURE 25.9. Introduction of the vascular bundle into the hole of the lunate (diagram).

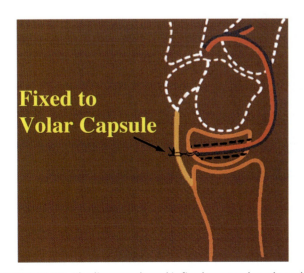

FIGURE 25.10. The ligature thread is firmly secured on the volar capsule.

Combination Procedures of Vascular Bundle Implantation

Because some patients showed progression of lunate collapse following this procedure, we attempted to use an external skeletal fixation device to apply a distraction force on the lunate in eight cases to increase or maintain its vertical height after the vascular bundle implantation with cancellous bone graft. A distraction apparatus was applied for approximately 2 to 3 months postoperatively. This method improved the operative results in cases of advanced Kienböck's disease. However, some cases still showed a decreased vertical height of the lunate after removal of the external skeletal fixation device (17). This unfavorable result may be attributed to (a) the long periods often necessary to produce bone formation by vascular bundle implantation, and (b) application of an external fixation device, which cannot permanently correct the carpal malalignment. Bearing this in mind, we recently attempted the combined use of vascular bundle implantation with STT arthrodesis as reported by Watson et al. (33). This combined surgical procedure is indicated for patients with stage IIIb Kienböck's disease (16,34). However, STT arthrodesis results in limitation of the postoperative arc of wrist flexion and extension (Fig. 25.12). We believe a permanent STT arthrodesis is unnecessary in the early stage of Kienböck's disease. Therefore, we attempted a temporary internal fixation of the STT joint using wires along with the vascular bundle implantation to retain wrist motion (16,34,35). In this technique, the STT joint was temporarily fixed with Kirschner wires in a position of slight dorsiflexion of the scaphoid to decompress the lunate. The wires were withdrawn 4 to 6 months later (Fig. 25.13). This procedure is indicated for patients with stage II and IIIa Kienböck's disease.

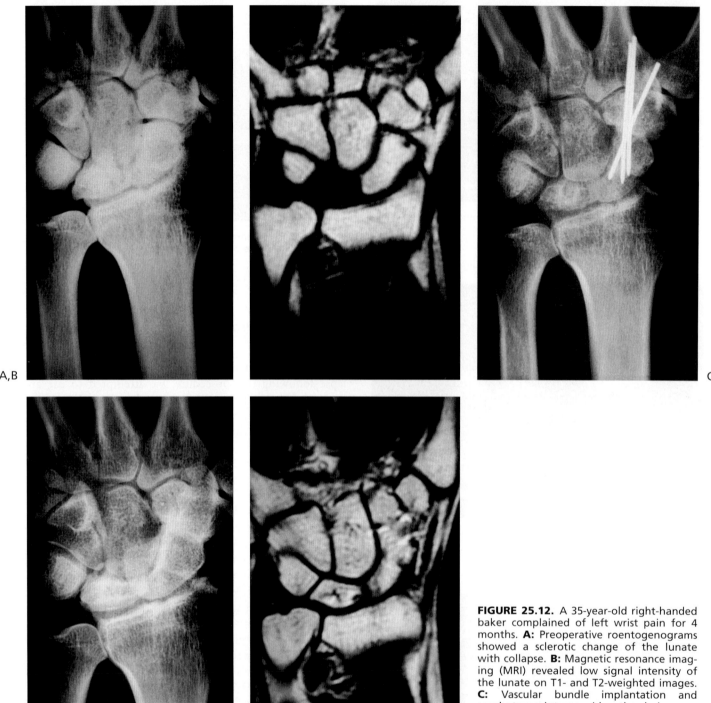

FIGURE 25.12. A 35-year-old right-handed baker complained of left wrist pain for 4 months. **A:** Preoperative roentogenograms showed a sclerotic change of the lunate with collapse. **B:** Magnetic resonance imaging (MRI) revealed low signal intensity of the lunate on T1- and T2-weighted images. **C:** Vascular bundle implantation and scaphotrapeziotrapezoid arthrodesis were performed. **D:** Twenty-four-month postoperative roentogenograms showed improvement of the bone architecture without further collapse. **E:** Postoperative MRI showed increased signal intensity of the lunate.

Scaphotrapeziotrapezoid Arthrodesis with Vascular Bundle Implantation

With a tourniquet on the upper arm and the patient under general anesthesia, a lazy curved longitudinal incision was made on the dorsum of the hand from the wrist joint to the second digital space. First, the implanted vascular bundle was elevated as mentioned above. Following the elevation of the vascular bundle, STT arthrodesis was performed. The operative technique for STT arthrodesis was similar to Watson's procedure (33). We believe that a partial radial styloidectomy for prevention of radial styloid impingement should be performed (36). Watson et al. (33) harvested cancellous bone for the bone graft from the distal radius. We harvested bone graft from the iliac crest because cancellous bone was grafted to both the STT joint and the lunate; and the amount of cancellous bone from the distal radius was insufficient. Following STT arthrodesis, the previously elevated vascular bundle was implanted into the lunate as mentioned above.

A bulky dressing with a long-arm cast was applied. One week postoperatively, the bulky dressing and sutures were removed, and a long arm thumb–spica cast was applied. Three weeks after surgery, the long arm cast was replaced with a short arm thumb–spica cast. Six to seven weeks after surgery, the cast was removed, and physical therapy for full range of wrist motion was begun. When x-rays demonstrated that arthrodesis was achieved, all wires were

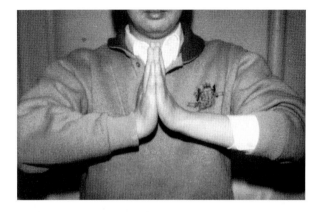
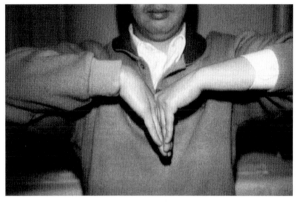

FIGURE 25.12. *(continued)* **F:** However, postoperative flexion and extension were slightly limited.

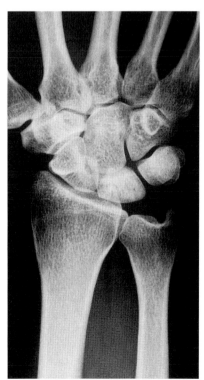
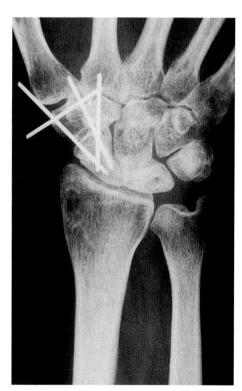
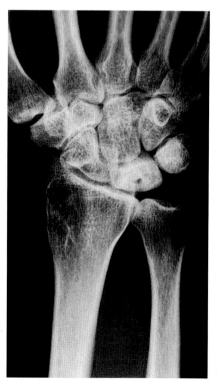

FIGURE 25.13. A 46-year-old right-handed woman who worked in a factory complained of right wrist pain. **A:** Preoperative roentgenograms showed a sclerotic change of the lunate without marked collapse. **B:** Vascular bundle implantation and temporary scaphotrapeziotrapezoid fixation were performed. **C:** Sixty-eight-month postoperative roentgenograms showed an increase of the radiodensity around the implanted vascular bundle, which suggested bone remodeling by means of vascular bundle implantation and cancellous bone grafting. The vertical height of the lunate was preserved even after removal of the wires.

removed (usually 2 to 3 months postoperatively). After removal of the wires, lifting and holding of lightweight objects (e.g., a full cup, a plate of food) were allowed.

Temporary Scaphotrapeziotrapezoid Fixation with Vascular Bundle Implantation

Following vascular bundle implantation, a 0.045-in. diameter Kirschner wire was inserted from the dorsal aspect of the scaphoid to the trapezium in the position of slight dorsiflexion (an increase of 10° to 20° relative to its preoperative resting position) of the scaphoid to lessen the vertical stress on the lunate. Fixation of the scaphoid in the position of excessive dorsiflexion may substantially lessen the stress on the lunate; however, it results in significant limitation of wrist motion. Another Kirschner wire was inserted from the dorsal aspect of the trapezoid to the scaphoid. A third Kirschner wire was inserted from the trapezium to the trapezoid. In the more recent cases of this series, two Kirschner wires were inserted from the trapezoid to the scaphoid, and one Kirschner wire was inserted from the scaphoid to the trapezium. We now believe that fixation between the trapezium and trapezoid in this procedure is unnecessary. After checking wrist motion to ensure that no wire had crossed the radiocarpal joint, all wires were clipped off beneath the skin. The wound was closed, and a bulky dressing with a long-arm cast was applied. One week postoperatively the bulky dressing and sutures were removed, and a short arm cast was applied. This remained for 3 to 4 weeks, allowing the soft tissue to heal and the connection between the implanted vascular bundle and the lunate to occur. For the first month after removal of the cast, exercise consisted of free flexion and extension with a little rotation. No splints or supports were used after removal of the cast. For the second month, non–weight-bearing wrist isometric exercises were performed. Throughout this time, no holding, grasping, or lifting were allowed. Three months postoperatively, lifting and holding of lightweight objects (e.g., a full cup, a plate of food) were allowed. After removal of all wires, the patient had full normal wrist strength and function. When monthly x-rays demonstrated diminished density of the lunate or improved trabecular structures of the lunate, all wires were removed. This usually occurred at 4 to 6 months postoperatively.

Indication of Vascular Bundle Implantation

In stage I or II (Lichtman's classification), before collapse of the lunate has occurred, it is theoretically possible for the lunate to regain its blood supply without significant alteration of wrist anatomy. Therefore, vascular bundle implantation is well indicated for these stages (Table 25.3). For stage III, saucerization of the necrotized bone and cancellous bone grafting should be performed before vascular bundle implantation. In addition, temporary STT fixation is added for stage IIIa and STT arthrodesis for stage IIIb. There is no indication for revascularization surgery for stage IV disease, nor is it indicated for stage III patients with lunate fragmentation. For such cases, the lunate should be resected and replaced with an artificial lunate or tendon roll. (These indications of vascular bundle implantation are similar to those of other revascularization procedures that we describe later.)

TABLE 25.3. PREFERRED TREATMENT APPROACH TO KIENBÖCK'S DISEASE

Classification[a]	Additional Factors[b]	Treatment
Stage I		Immobilization
		Revascularization
Stage II	Plus, null	Revascularization + temporary STT fixation
	Minus	Leveling procedures
Stage IIIa	Plus, null	Revascularization + temporary STT fixation
	Minus	Leveling procedures
Stage IIIb	Frag (+)[c]	Revascularization + STT arthrodesis
	Frag (–)	Tendon roll + temporary STT fixation
Stage IV	OA (+)	Tendon roll + temporary STT fixation
	OA (++)	Wrist arthrodesis

[a]Classification from Lichtman DM, Degnan GD. Staging and its use in the determination of treatment modalities for Kienböck's disease. *Hand Clin* 1993;9:409–416.
[b]Plus, null, minus: ulnar variance.
[c]Frag, lunate fragmentation.
OA, osteoarthritis; STT, scaphotrapeziotrapezoid.

PRONATOR QUADRATUS MUSCLE PEDICLE BONE GRAFT

The pronator quadratus muscle is a flat muscle that stretches across the distal one-third of the forearm. The blood supply of this muscle comes from the anterior interosseous artery. When a small segment of volar radial bone is elevated with its attached pronator quadratus muscle, its blood supply comes from the attached muscle as well as the anterior interosseous artery (Fig. 25.14).

This procedure is performed through a volar approach. The flexor tendons and median nerve are retracted toward the ulnar side to expose the pronator quadratus muscle. A fine osteotome is used to harvest corticocancellous bone from the volar side of the radial styloid process. Care is taken to avoid detaching the pronator quadratus from the harvested bone block. The pronator quadratus muscle is then split toward the ulna to secure a pedicle 20 mm in width. Leung et al. (37) advocated that great care be given to the anterior interosseous artery, which is attached to the undersurface of the muscle, during subsequent maneuvers when the pedicled graft was rotated to its destination. The joint capsule is incised to expose the lunate. A hole is made

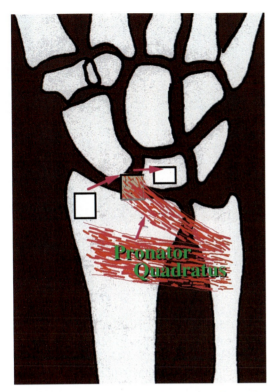

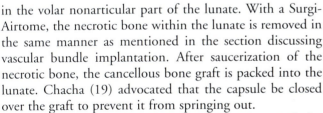

FIGURE 25.14. The pronator quadratus muscle pedicle bone graft is harvested from the distal radius and transferred to the lunate after saucerization of the necrotic bone.

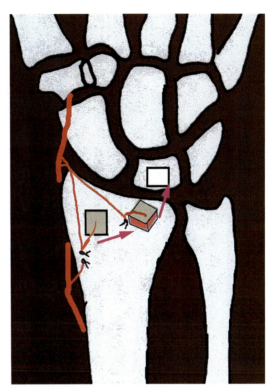

FIGURE 25.15. Vascularized bone graft based on the 1,2 intercompartmental supraretinacular artery and its branch to the second extensor compartment.

in the volar nonarticular part of the lunate. With a Surgi-Airtome, the necrotic bone within the lunate is removed in the same manner as mentioned in the section discussing vascular bundle implantation. After saucerization of the necrotic bone, the cancellous bone graft is packed into the lunate. Chacha (19) advocated that the capsule be closed over the graft to prevent it from springing out.

This procedure is indicated for stage IIIa and stage IIIb disease. Some additional procedures for reducing vertical stress on the lunate (i.e., external skeletal device or temporary STT fixation) are recommended until bone union is achieved.

VASCULARIZED PEDICULAR BONE GRAFT

Donor bone for vascularized bone grafts for Kienböck's disease can be harvested from the radius, ulna, and metacarpal bone. In 1995, Sheetz et al. (22) reported the extra- and interosseous blood supply of the distal radius and ulna systematically. They recommended a graft based on the 1,2-intercompartmental supraretinacular artery and its branch to the second extensor compartment (a modification of the Zaidemberg et al. technique) and a graft based on fourth extensor compartment artery with retrograde flow through the fifth extensor compartment artery from the dorsal intercarpal arch (Figs. 25.15 and 25.16). Some vascularized

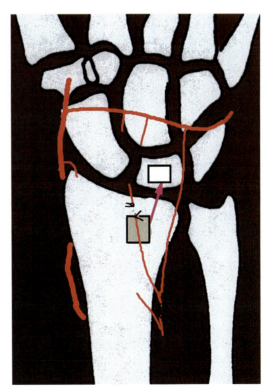

FIGURE 25.16. Vascularized bone graft based on fourth extensor compartment artery with reverse flow through the fifth extensor compartment artery from the dorsal intercarpal arch.

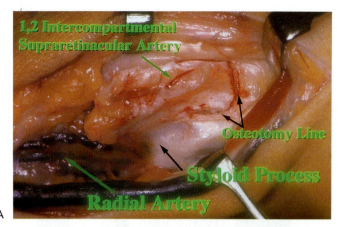 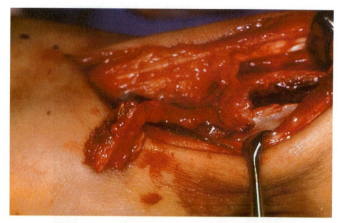

FIGURE 25.17. A: The 1,2 intercompartmental supraretinacular artery, described as the ascending irrigating branch of the radial artery by Zaidemberg et al., is identified as overlying the distal radius. **B:** Harvested vascularized bone graft on its vascular pedicle.

bone grafts can be taken from the palmar radius. However, Sheetz et al. (22) reported that palmar bone grafts had limited usefulness, in part because their harvest and placement required significant dissection of important radiocarpal ligaments. Among these possibilities, the vascularized bone graft based on the 1,2-intercompartmental supraretinacular artery is recommended because of its technical ease.

A dorsal approach is used for exposure, and an oblique incision on the radiodorsal aspect of the wrist joint is made. Care must be taken to avoid injury to the dorsal branch of the radial nerve. The extensor retinaculum is exposed and divided. The extensor pollicis brevis and abductor polilcis longus tendons are retracted volarly, and the extensor carpi radialis and extensor communis tendons are reflected ulnarly. The 1,2-intercompartmental supraretinacular artery, described as the ascending irrigating branch of the radial artery by Zaidemberg et al. (21), is then easily identified as overlying the distal radius (Fig. 25.17A). It originates proximally from the radial artery approximately 50 mm proximal to the radiocarpal joint. It runs superficial to the extensor retinaculum at the 1,2-intercompartmental septum and sends nutrient vessels through the retinaculum to enter cortical bone (Fig. 25.17A). In 56% of the specimens in the anatomic study by Sheetz et al. (22), the 1,2-intercompartmental supraretinacular had a branch that originated proximal to the extensor retinaculum and proceeded onto the floor of the second extensor compartment. This branch was generally a single large nutrient artery that usually penetrated cancellous bone (Figs. 25.15 and 25.17B). A vascularized bone graft is designed that centers this perfusing periosteal blood vessel over the bone to be harvested. With the original procedure of Zaidemberg et al. (21), the graft cannot be transposed to the lunate in some cases because its arc of rotation is short. Sheetz et al. (22) recommended modifying the Zaidemberg et al. technique to include the proximal branch of the artery to the floor of the second compartment for Kienböck's disease. This modification improves the medullary blood supply and increases the graft's potential arc of rotation. After the vascularized bone graft is obtained from the radius, a hole is made on the dorsal aspect of the lunate at the border between bone and cartilage (Fig. 25.15). Thereafter, the operative procedure is the same as that of the muscle pedicle bone graft. Procedures to reduce vertical stress on the lunate (e.g., external fixation device or temporary STT fixation) should be combined until bone union is achieved. This procedure is indicated for stage IIIa and stage IIIb in the same manner as the muscle pedicle bone graft.

EDITORS' COMMENTS

If our theories of Kienböck's disease are correct, then areas form in the cancellous portions of all bones secondary to loads that are too heavy, too great, or too prolonged for recovery. Operating in the vicinity of such a bone to produce a vascular response, followed by the requisite immobilization period, may provide the chief benefits in conditions such as Kienböck's disease. It would not be terribly important, therefore, whether the ulna was lengthened or shortened or whether the radius was lengthened, shortened, or tilted in any one direction. The benefits would derive from the procedure itself, not from any changes in anatomy. If patients returned to their preoperative activity levels at the full load capacities and for the same durations, over time one would expect recurrence of increased fault plates and cancellous abnormality leading to necrosis. For this reason, with any significant collapse, we would prefer a procedure that permanently carries the load around the lunate such as the triscaphe limited wrist arthrodesis procedure.

> More frequent use of magnetic resonance imaging is demonstrating edematous change in the lunate that is probably "pre-Kienböck's." Overload occurs in the cancellous bone, and continued insult reaches a point at which edema forms in response to repeated minor trabecular interruptions. Without rest, the process may on rare occasion progress to bone death (Kienböck's). "Pre-Kienböck's" is probably very common and occurs in many carpals in addition to the lunate.

REFERENCES

1. Peste JL. Discussion. *Bull Soc Anat Paris* 1843;18:169–170.
2. Kienböck R. Uber traumatishe Malazie des Mondbeins und ihre Folgezustande: Entrtungsformen und Kompressions Fracturen. *Fortschr Röntgenstr* 1910;16:77–103.
3. Hulten O. Uber anatomische Variationen der Handgelenkknochen. *Acta Radiol Scand* 1928;9:155–168.
4. Almquist EE. Kienböck's disease. *Hand Clin* 1987;3:141–148.
5. Nakamura R, Imaeda T, Miura T. Radial shortening for Kienböck's disease: Factors affecting the operative results. *J Hand Surg [Br]* 1990;15:40–45.
6. Sundberg SB, Linscheid RL. Kienböck's disease—results of treatment with ulnar lengthening. *Clin Orthop* 1984;187:43–51.
7. Ahsoh K, Masumi S, Uchida K. *Clinical evaluation of the wedge osteotomy of the radius for Kienböck's disease.* Paper presented at the 65th Meeting of the Japanese Orthopedic Association, Fukuoka, 1992, p. S256 (Japanese).
8. Minami A, Takahara M, Kimura C, et al. *Triscaphe arthrodesis in the treatment of Kienböck's disease.* Paper presented at the 65th Meeting of the Japanese Orthopedic Association, Fukuoka, 1992, p. S258 (Japanese).
9. Nakamura R, Horii E, Watanabe K, et al. *Radial shortening and radial wedge osteotomy for Kienböck's disease.* Paper presented at the 65th Meeting of the Japanese Orthopedic Association, Fukuoka, 1992, p. S257 (Japanese).
10. Yajima H, Tamai S. *Treatment of Kienböck's disease with vascular bundle implantation.* Paper presented at the 65th Meeting of the Japanese Orthopedic Association, Fukuoka, 1992, p. S259 (Japanese).
11. Lichtman DM, Mack GR, MacDonald RI, et al. Kienböck's disease: The role of silicone replacement arthroplasty. *J Bone Joint Surg Am* 1977;59:899–908.
12. Hori Y, Tamai S, Okuda H, et al. Blood vessel transplantation to bone. *J Hand Surg [Am]* 1979;4:23–33.
13. Yajima H, Tamai S, Miumoto S, et al. Vascular bundle transplantation for Kienböck's disease. *Orthop Traum Surg* 1987;30:69–77 (Japanese).
14. Yajima H, Tamai S, Mizumoto S, et al. Treatment of Kienböck's disease with vascular bundle implantation: Experimental and clinical studies. *J Jpn Soc Surg Hand* 1987;4:332–336 (Japanese).
15. Tamai S, Hori Y, Fujiwara H. Treatment of avascular necrosis of lunate and other bones by vascular bundle transplantation. In: Urbaniak JR, ed. *Microsurgery for major limb reconstruction.* St. Louis: CV Mosby, 1987;209–219.
16. Yajima H, Tamai S, Mizumoto S, et al. Treatment of Kienböck's disease with vascular bundle implantation and triscaphe arthrodesis. In: Nakamura R, Linscheid RL, Miura T, eds. *Wrist disorders.* Tokyo: Springer-Verlag, 1992;101–109.
17. Tamai S, Yajima H, Ono H. Revascularization procedures in the treatment of Kienböck's disease. *Hand Clin* 1993;9:455–466.
18. Braun RM. Proximal pedicle bone grafting in the forearm and proximal carpal row. *Orthop Trans* 1983;7:35.
19. Chacha PB. Vascularized pedicular bone grafts. *Int Orthop (SICOT)* 1984;8:117–138.
20. Kuhlmann IN, Mimoun M, Boabighi A, et al. Vascularized bone graft pedicled on the volar carpal artery for non-union of the scaphoid. *J Hand Surg [Br]* 1987;12:203–210.
21. Zaidemberg C, Siebert JW, Angrigiani C. A new vascularized bone graft for scaphoid nonunion. *J Hand Surg [Am]* 1991;16:474–478.
22. Sheetz KK, Bishop A, Berger RA. The arterial blood supply of the distal radius and ulna and its potential use in vascularized pedicled bone grafts. *J Hand Surg [Am]* 1995;20:902–914.
23. Pagliei A, Brunelli F, Gilbert A. Anterior interosseous artery: anatomic basis of pedicled bone-grafts. *Surg Radiol Anat* 1991;13:152–154.
24. Pierer G, Steffen J, Hoflehner H. The vascular supply of the second metacarpal bone: anatomic basis for a new vascularized bone graft in hand surgery. *Surg Radiol Anat* 1992;14:103–112.
25. Beck E. Die Verpflanzung des Os pisiforme am Gefasstiel zur Behandlung der Lunatummalazie. *Handchirurgie* 1971;3:64–67.
26. Saffar P. Remplacement du semi-lunaire par le pisiforme. *Ann Chir Main* 1982;1:276–279.
27. Woodhouse CF. The transplantation of patent arteries to bone. *J Int Coll Surg* 1963;39:437–446.
28. Dickerson RC, Duthie RB. The diversion of arterial blood flow to bone. *J Bone Joint Surg Am* 1963;45:356–364.
29. Boyd RJ, Ault LL. An experimental study of vascular implantation into femoral head. *Surg Gynecol Obstet* 1965;121:1009–1014.
30. Yajima H, Tamai S, Mizumoto S, et al. Experimental study on a secondary living bone graft by vascular bundle transplantation. *Jpn J Plast Reconstr Surg* 1987;30:171–181 (Japanese).
31. Yajima H, Tamai S, Mizumoto S, et al. Experimental study on a secondary living bone graft—method of creating new donor by vascular bundle implantation to isolated bone. *J Jpn Orthop Assoc* 1989;63:539–548 (Japanese).
32. Lichtman DM, Degnan GD. Staging and its use in the determination of treatment modalities for Kienböck's disease. *Hand Clin* 1993;9;409–416.
33. Watson HK, Ryu J, DiBella A. An approach to Kienböck's disease: Triscaphe arthrodesis. *J Hand Surg [Am]* 1985;10:179–187.
34. Yajima H, Tamai S, Inada Y, et al. Treatment of Kienböck's disease with vascular bundle implantation and triscaphe arthrodesis. *J Jpn Soc Surg Hand* 1990;7:747–750 (Japanese).
35. Yajima H, Ono H, Tamai S. Temporary internal fixation of the scaphotrapezio-trapezoidal joint for the treatment of Kienböck's disease: A preliminary study. *J Hand Surg [Am]* 1998;23:402–410.
36. Rogers WD, Watson HK. Radial styloid impingement after triscaphe arthrodesis. *J Hand Surg [Am]* 1989;14:297–301.
37. Leung PC, Hung LK. Use of pronator quadratus bone flap in bony reconstruction around the wrist. *J Hand Surg [Am]* 1990;15:637–640.

THE PATHOGENESIS OF CARPAL LIGAMENT INSTABILITY

JACK K. MAYFIELD

Although Claudius Galen knew of the carpal bones in A.D. 138 to 201, it was not until the Renaissance (A.D. 1300–1600) that a more complete awareness of the carpus developed. It was at this time that artistic drawings of the carpus emerged (1). Since then, our understanding of the carpus and carpal instability has grown immensely. Now, as a result of many years of extensive research, carpal instability as a result of carpal ligament injury is a widely accepted phenomenon. Various persistent malalignment patterns have been described as a result of a spectrum of ligamentous injury.

Even though many scientists were aware of the individual carpal bones, it was not until 1943 that Gilford and associates described carpal instability (2). They describe the carpus as a link mechanism, with the scaphoid serving as the link between the proximal and the distal carpal rows. A disturbance of this connecting rod (the scaphoid) led to longitudinal carpal collapse. Fisk (3) later described this same phenomenon of intercarpal instability as a "concertina deformity." This longitudinal collapse of the carpus is well recognized on a lateral roentgenogram, and the associated scaphoid instability has been described by various authors, using terms such as scaphoid subluxation and rotational subluxation, among others (4–14).

Linscheid and associates (15) later described a frequently observed posttraumatic intercarpal instability collapse deformity. Their classification was based primarily on the capitolunate angle seen on lateral roentgenogram. They described two basic patterns: dorsal intercalated segment instability (DISI) deformity and volar intercalated segment instability (VISI) deformity. They found that these collapse deformities of the carpus were directly caused by the loss of various ligamentous restraints.

Attention in the literature has been focused principally on describing patterns of radiocarpal instability (perilunate and scapholunate instabilities). Lichtman and co-workers (12,16,17) described the phenomenon of midcarpal instability and the implications of ulnar carpal instability patterns. Now, much attention has been focused on injuries of specific ligaments and associated instability patterns. Johnson and colleagues (18) described chronic capitolunate instability as a result of volar radiocapitate ligament (RCL) damage and resultant ligamentous laxity. He advocated a specific surgical reconstruction of the damaged palmar ligaments. We now know that wrist arthroscopy can play a valuable role in describing and understanding the subtleties of these ligament injuries (19–22).

Kauer (4) thoroughly described the mechanism of the carpal joint. The intricate and complex movement of the carpal bones is governed by the longitudinal and transverse linkage, the bone contours and joint contacts, and by ligamentous interconnections.

The pathomechanics of carpal injuries has been a subject of considerable controversy. Although some authors have suggested that hyperflexion is an important mechanism (2,3), many authors consider hyperextension to be the major mechanical factor leading to these injuries (3,14, 15,23–28). Most authors have been impressed with the wide spectrum of injuries that involve the carpus. It would seem unlikely that a single planar mechanism such as hyperextension could account for such a variety of fractures and dislocations of the carpus. For these reasons, investigators have looked for additional mechanisms.

Tanz (14) suggested that a rotational component might be important in perilunar dislocations. He considered lunate dislocations a result of compression, dorsiflexion, ulnar deviation, and pronation. He thought that perilunate dislocations were a result of the same mechanics, with the exception that supination, rather than pronation, of the hand is involved.

Explanations of the mechanism of scaphoid fractures have also been controversial. Fisk suggested that extension

---

J. K. Mayfield: Department of Biological, Chemical, and Materials Engineering, Arizona State University; Department of Orthopaedic Surgery, St. Luke's Hospital, Phoenix, Arizona, and St. Luke's Hospital Medical Building, Phoenix, Arizona 85006.

and ulnar deviation were the principal mechanical components (3). Squire (29) was convinced that forced radial deviation would fracture the scaphoid over the tip of the radial styloid. Verdan and Narakis showed that pronation and supination cause shearing forces at the scaphoid waist (30), implying that a rotational load would create shear stress in the scaphoid, leading to fracture, as suggested by Gilford and colleagues (2). Experimental investigations (11,27,31) have shown that the scaphoid can be fractured in cadaver specimens by hyperextension and ulnar deviation.

Perilunate fracture-dislocations are more frequent than perilunate dislocations at a ratio of two to one (32). In addition to scaphoid fractures and perilunate dislocations, other associated injuries are frequent. Many authors have noted the association of radial and ulnar styloid fractures with carpal injuries (5,7,32–34). The association of triquetral fractures with scaphoid fractures has been reported by Bartone and Grieco (35) and Borgeskov (36).

Because it has been difficult to implicate a single planar mechanism as the cause of the many types of carpal injuries and resultant instability patterns, investigations have focused on a three-dimensional mechanical concept to explain the pathogenesis of these perplexing injuries (3,23,37).

As our knowledge of carpal instability increases, we recognize that the role of the wrist ligaments in the development of this condition is very important. In order to understand the multitude of instability patterns that can develop with various combinations and degrees of ligamentous damage, a fundamental knowledge of wrist anatomy and wrist ligament biomechanics is essential.

WRIST LIGAMENT ANATOMY

The intimate relationship between the carpal bones and the distal radius and ulna is maintained in all planes of motion by a complex arrangement of ligaments (Fig. 26.1). Three types of ligaments are present across the wrist joint: (a) intercarpal, (b) capsular, and (c) intracapsular (30,38,39). The wrist ligaments may be thought of as extrinsic ligaments (radiocarpal) or intrinsic ligaments (intercarpal). An extrinsic ligament connects the radius to one or more carpal bones. An intrinsic ligament interconnects one carpal bone to another. Biomechanical studies (40) have shown that the palmar extrinsic ligaments are more numerous and stronger than dorsal extrinsic radiocarpal ligaments and thus more important clinically. In addition, the scapholunate and lunotriquetral ligaments are the most important intrinsic ligaments both mechanically and clinically.

The dorsal radiocarpal ligament is a thickening of the dorsal wrist capsule (2,38,41–43). It originates from the dorsal edge of the radial styloid process, passes obliquely across the dorsal surface of the lunate, to which it is also attached, and terminates in the dorsal aspect of the triquetrum. Taleisnik (30) describes this ligament as a broad

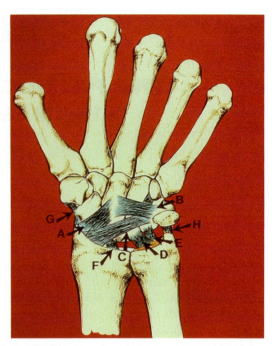

FIGURE 26.1. The palmar (volar) and collateral ligaments of the wrist. Volar ligaments: *A*, radiocapitate; *B*, capitotriquetral; *C*, radiotriquetral; *D*, ulnoulnate; *E*, ulnotriquetral; *F*, radioscaphoid. Collateral ligaments: *G*, radial collateral ligament; *H*, ulnar collateral ligament.

ligament that has three portions: a radioscaphoid, a radiolunate, and a radiotriquetral portion. It connects the dorsal aspect of the distal radius with the dorsal aspects of the proximal carpal row (Fig. 26.2).

The main functional ligaments of the wrist joint are palmar and intracapsular (13,30,38–40,44–48). In a functional sense, the complex intercarpal motion in radial and ulnar deviation and in dorsiflexion and palmar flexion is dependent on the specific arrangement and integrity of these palmar intracapsular ligaments.

The palmar radiocarpal ligament (lig. radiocarpeum palmare) is a large, thick intracapsular ligament seen only after the capsule is meticulously dissected from the palmar aspect of the wrist or after the wrist joint is opened dorsally and the wrist is palmarly flexed (Fig. 26.3) (39,44). This ligament is divided into three separate and discrete parts, the first connecting the radius with the capitate, the second connecting the radius with the triquetrum, and the third connecting the distal radius to the proximal scaphoid. The RCL (pars radiocapitate), the smaller and weaker of the first two, originates from the palmar aspect of the radial styloid process, traverses a groove in the waist of the scaphoid, and terminates in the center of the palmar aspect of the capitate body (Fig. 26.1). Other authors have described this ligament as the palmar radioscaphocapitate ligament (30,48). The palmar radiotriquetral ligament (RTL) (pars radiotriquetral) is the second portion and is thick and tendinous in appearance and is the

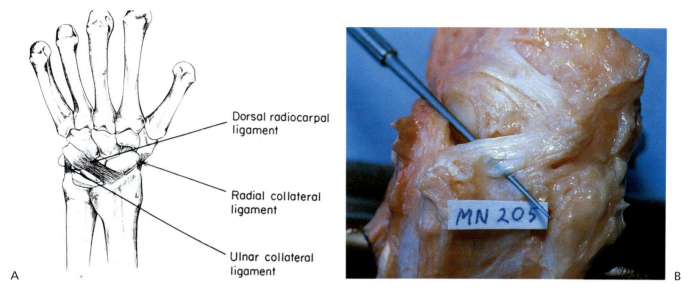

FIGURE 26.2. A: The dorsal radiocarpal and collateral ligaments of the wrist (drawing). **B:** The dorsal radiocarpal ligament of the wrist in a fresh dissected specimen. The probe is under the ligament.

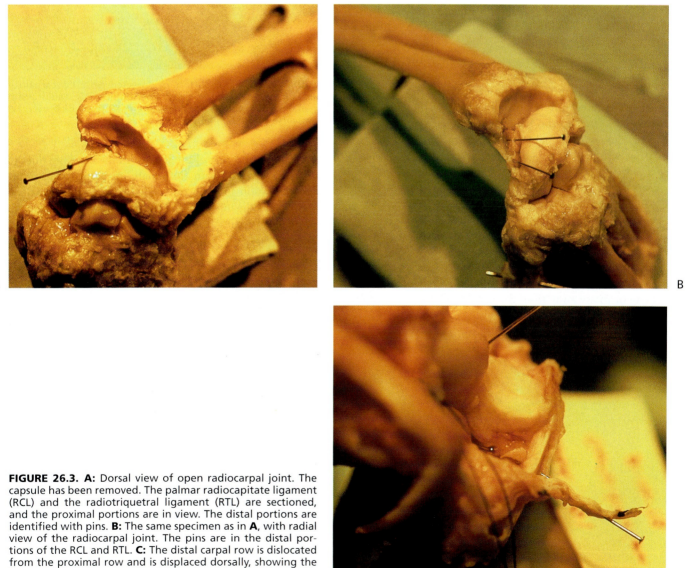

FIGURE 26.3. A: Dorsal view of open radiocarpal joint. The capsule has been removed. The palmar radiocapitate ligament (RCL) and the radiotriquetral ligament (RTL) are sectioned, and the proximal portions are in view. The distal portions are identified with pins. **B:** The same specimen as in **A**, with radial view of the radiocarpal joint. The pins are in the distal portions of the RCL and RTL. **C:** The distal carpal row is dislocated from the proximal row and is displaced dorsally, showing the lunate with the intracapsular RTL in view. Note the size of this ligament.

433

strongest of the palmar intracapsular extrinsic ligaments. It originates from the palmar aspect of the radial styloid process next to the RCL and, acting as a sling, passes under the lunate, to which it is also attached, and terminates on the palmar surface of the triquetrum (Fig. 26.3) (39,46,47). Berger et al. have described a short palmar radiolunate ligament that connects the palmar aspect of the radius with the palmar aspect of the lunate (Fig. 26.4) (49). It is intracapsular but extrasynovial. An additional intracapsular and palmar ligament described is the palmar scaphotriquetral ligament (50). In dissections of adult and fetal wrists, Zdravkovic and associates described this ligament as present between the capitate head and the palmar radioscaphocapitate ligament (50). It was thought to support the palmar aspect of the capitate head in dorsiflexion.

The separation of the RCL from the palmar RTL (the space of Poirier) over the palmar aspect of the capitolunate joint is evident in many specimens (Fig. 26.5) (39,46,51,52). The significance of this interligamentous space is evident when carpal motion is evaluated and after experimentally injured wrists are studied.

The scapholunate joint is connected by the intrinsic interosseous ligament and the third portion of the palmar radiocarpal ligament (pars radioscaphoid). This ligament actually originates from the palmar surface of the radial styloid process ulnar to the RTL and is directed vertically to terminate in the proximal palmar pole of the scaphoid (Fig. 26.6). It also has some small attachments to the palmar aspect of the lunate; hence, it has been described by other authors as the radioscapholunate ligament. The major portion of this ligament is separate from the interosseous ligament connecting the scaphoid to the lunate. The size of the radioscaphoid ligament (RSL) varies, but it is consistently present (30,39,53,54).

In the unloaded wrist, sectioning of the scapholunate interosseous ligament (SLIL) does not allow the scaphoid to separate or rotate away from the lunate (39,46). Only after

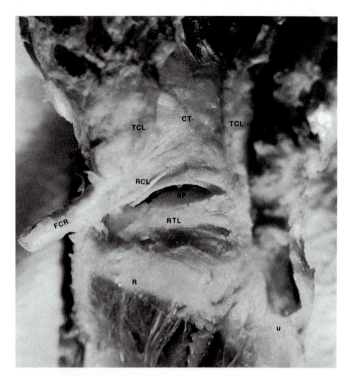

FIGURE 26.5. Palmar surface of dissected wrist. *CT*, carpal tunnel; *FCR*, flexor carpi radialis; *R*, volar radius; *RCL*, radiocapitate ligament; *RTL*, radiotriquetral ligament; *SP*, space of Poirier; *TCL*, transverse carpal ligament; *U*, volar ulna.

additional sectioning of the RSL from the scaphoid does the scaphoid separate from the lunate on palmar flexion and ulnar deviation (39). In the loaded wrist, sectioning of the interosseous ligament alone caused separation from the lunate plus proximal pole rotation of the scaphoid (24).

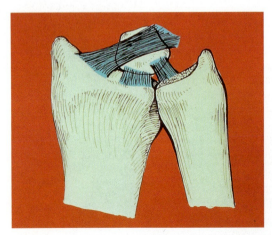

FIGURE 26.4. A drawing of the palmar ligament stabilizers of the lunate. From radial to ulnar: radiotriquetral, short radiolunate, ulnolunate.

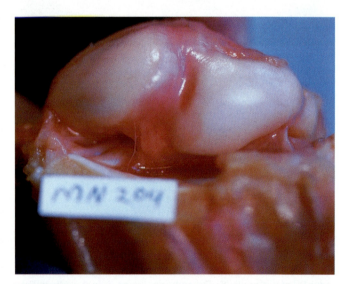

FIGURE 26.6. Intraarticular view of the proximal carpal row. The carpus is palmarflexed, showing the scaphoid and the lunate (from left to right). Note the large radioscaphoid ligament attached primarily to the proximal pole of the scaphoid. **Editors' Notes:** *It is this radial scaphoid ligament that Kauer believes provides blood supply to the proximal pole and explains the viability of small proximal pole segments in scaphoid nonunion.*

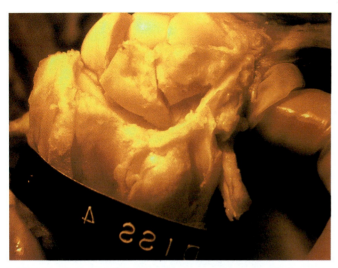

FIGURE 26.7. Dorsal intraarticular view of the ulnar side of the wrist. Note the ulnolunate and ulnotriquetral ligaments emanating from the palmar side of the triangular fibrocartilage complex.

A significant palmar intracapsular ligament, the capitotriquetral ligament (pars capitotriquetral), is evident only after the overlying capsule is dissected away. It is directed from the palmar surface of the center of the capitate body across the palmar surface of the hamate, to terminate in the palmar surface of the triquetrum (Fig. 26.1).

Ligamentous stabilization on the ulnar side of the wrist is provided by the ulnar collateral ligament and the intracapsular ulnocarpal ligament. This is a thick, discrete ligament that originates from the palmar aspect of the intraarticular triangular fibrocartilage complex (TFCC) (55) and separates in two directions, one to the lunate (pars ulnolunate) and the other to the triquetrum (pars ulnotriquetral) (Figs. 26.1 and 26.7).

The intrinsic ligaments of the proximal carpal row are the scapholunate and lunotriquetral interosseous ligaments, both of which are C-shaped in configuration; the open portion faces distally and joins the adjacent bones together peripherally at their proximal end. The intrinsic ligaments of the distal carpal bones are rarely injured and are not well described.

This descriptive analysis of the wrist ligaments forms a model that is useful in analyzing the function of the wrist joint. These ligaments form a complex of interacting units that control and direct carpal motion.

THE LIGAMENTOUS ANATOMY OF THE SCAPHOLUNATE JOINT

It has become clear that the scapholunate joint is the key joint connecting the proximal and distal carpal rows. Thus, the intrinsic ligamentous connections of this joint are of considerable significance. Complete ligamentous disruptions of this joint will disconnect the scaphoid from the proximal row, causing scapholunate insatiability and carpal collapse. Partial disruptions can lead to variable degrees of instability of this joint, which usually present as wrist pain. Therefore, an awareness of the ligamentous anatomy of this joint will be helpful.

Kauer (56) described the complex motion of the scapholunate joint in 1974. He noticed that the volar aspect of this joint was more mobile that the dorsal aspect. In dissections of 34 cadaver wrists, Nash and Mayfield (57) described the intricate ligamentous attachments of this joint. In their dissections, they found that the SLIL is triangular in cross section, occupying nearly one-third of the articular surface of this joint, and is peripherally attached at the joint (Figs. 26.8 and 26.9C). The fibers of the SLIL run in several directions. The fibers at the dorsum of the joint run transversely or perpendicular to the joint and form a thick bundle that is tendinous in appearance (57,58) and important to stability of this joint (Fig. 26.9A–C) (24). The fibers of the peripheral portion of the ligament run peripherally and obliquely along the arc of the joint from the scaphoid and are directed toward the lunate (Fig.

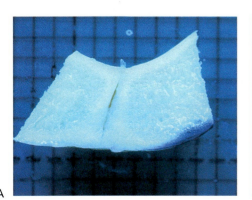 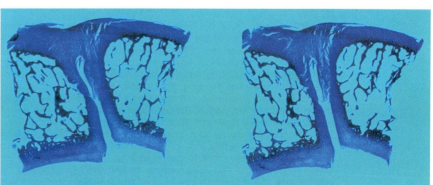

FIGURE 26.8. A: Coronally sectioned scapholunate complex. Note the triangular scapholunate interosseous ligament. **B:** Same specimen as **A** but decalcified. Note that this interosseous ligament covers about one-third of the articular surface of the joint.

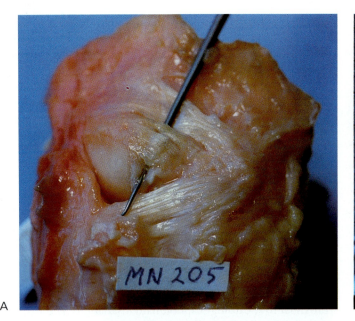
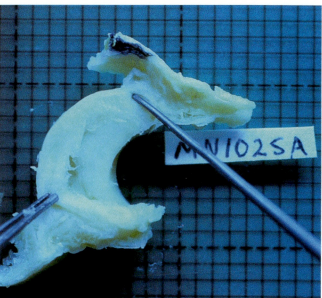
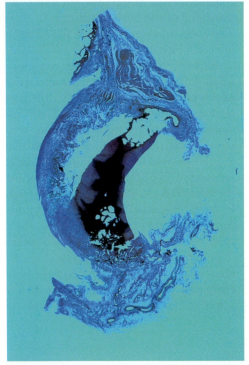
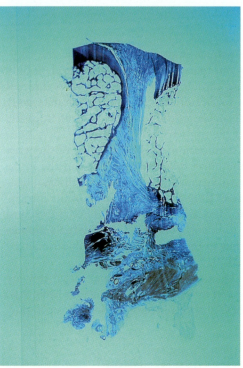

FIGURE 26.9. A: Dissected fresh specimen of the wrist, dorsal view. The probe is under the dorsal transverse portion of the scapholunate interosseous ligament. Note the size and thickness of the portion of this ligament (SLIL). **B:** A sagittal section through the scapholunate joint. Note the C-shape of the interosseous ligament and the amount of joint surface covered. However, some of the ligament is not connected intraarticularly (forceps are holding this ligament away from the articular surface). The probe is pointing to the dorsal transverse portion of this interosseous ligament. **C:** Histologic section of specimen in B. Note the dense collagenous fiber bundles in the dorsal transverse portion of the interosseous. Also note the peripheral direction of the peripheral portion of this ligament. **D:** Axial histologic section of the SLIL. Note the direction of the collagen fibers from dorsal to palmar. **Editors' Notes:** *The SLIL demonstrates some posttraumatic tearing in approximately 25% of the normal adult population. Dorsiflexion injuries rupture the volar aspect of the interosseous ligament. Healing is poorly accomplished, and subsequent trauma extends the ligament rupture. Dorsal wrist syndrome is the most common symptomatic wrist entity and represents overload of the scapholunate joint secondary to cumulative injuries to this ligament.*

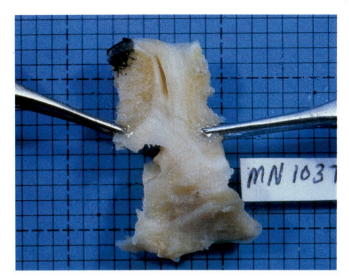

FIGURE 26.10. Axial section of the scapholunate joint showing the oblique direction of the palmar portion of the interosseous ligament running from scaphoid to lunate (the *black dot* is on the scaphoid).

Although there is some controversy whether the RSL is an actual ligament, it is consistently identified in adult and fetal wrist dissections (Fig. 26.6) (30,39,53,57). Lewis et al. describe this as a remnant of a mesenchymal septum that separated the radiocarpal and ulnocarpal joint cavities in fetal development (45). Berger and colleagues refer to this structure as a ligament that has a high degree of vascularity. Thus, this structure may function as a conduit for blood supply to the SLIL. This indicates that it probably has little direct mechanical effect on the behavior of the carpus (53,54). However, the location and direction of this structure does suggest that it may function as a check rein in extremes of dorsiflexion and palmar flexion in coordination with the more flexible volar aspect of the SLIL (Fig. 26.12).

It is interesting that the arrangement of the fibers of the SLIL are oriented in different directions in the three portions of this ligament. Rotationally, this arrangement of fibers in different directions controls a precise spatial mechanical motion between the scaphoid and lunate by way of a mechanical linkage system (Fig. 26.13). It is suggested by this author that the RSL plays a role in this linkage system.

26.9B–D). The volar portion of the ligament runs obliquely between the volar aspects of the lunate and the scaphoid (Fig. 26.10). The orientation of these fibers is such that they allow mobility of the volar aspect of the joint about a fixed dorsal axis (Fig. 26.11) (24,56,57). In addition to the three portions of the SLIL, the volar aspect of the proximal pole of the scaphoid and, to a lesser extent, the lunate are stabilized to the distal radius by the RSL (39,46), also called the radioscapholunate ligament because of its attachment to both the scaphoid and the lunate (Fig. 26.6) (30,53).

The scapholunate joint is hinged at the dorsum by the transverse portion of the interosseous ligament, allowing rotation between the scaphoid and lunate about a dorsal transverse axis (Fig. 26.13). In addition, the peripheral fibers (Fig. 26.9B–D) of this ligament, by their direction and loose nature, allow more volar motion of this joint about this dorsal axis, a fact noted by Kauer (44,56,58). This fact has significance because many carpal injuries are initiated by a hyperextension movement, causing the scaphoid to rotate dorsally with the lunate about this dorsal axis controlled by the transverse portion of the interosseous

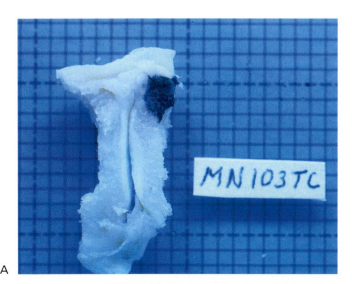
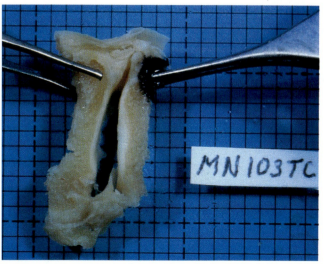

FIGURE 26.11. A: Axial section of the scapholunate joint (the *black dot* is on the scaphoid). The joint is approximated. **B:** Same specimen as **A** but with the lax palmar portion of the interosseous ligament pulled apart, opening the palmar portion of this joint.

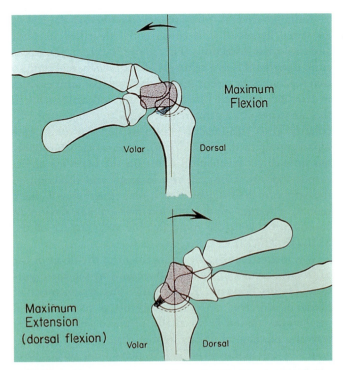

FIGURE 26.12. Lateral view of the wrist joint in palmar and dorsiflexion. Note that the radioscaphoid ligament controls scaphoid rotation.

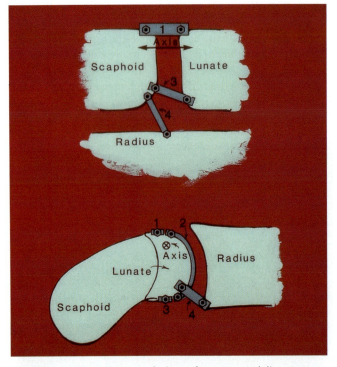

FIGURE 26.13. Artist's rendering of a proposed ligamentous mechanical linkage system of the scapholunate interosseous joint.

ligament. Because there is more volar mobility at this joint, some of the load can be dissipated because of the inherent elasticity of the volar aspect of the interosseous ligament. However, if forced extension occurs beyond the natural limits of this ligament, then failure of this ligament can begin to occur on the volar side of the joint (59). It is my opinion that some stage I perilunate instabilities (PLI) are early partial interosseus ligament tears on the volar side of this joint. Arthroscopically, this finding has been recognized by other authors (19,22).

SURGICAL RECONSTRUCTION OF THE SCAPHOLUNATE JOINT

From our understanding of the linkage mechanism inherently designed within the SLIL, it seems logical to reestablish the normal mechanics in any reconstructive surgical procedure designed to correct instability in this joint. Various reconstructive procedures have recently been utilized to stabilize this joint (60–63). Mayfield and House in 1980 (64) described an anatomic reconstruction of the SLIL and RSL (Fig. 26.14). This reconstruction was designed to restore the ligamentous linkage mechanism that was felt to be present at this joint. The ulnar half of the extensor carpi radialis brevis (ECRB) is stripped distally but left attached, and this tail is then divided. The first tail is passed under the capsular attachments of the capitolunate joint, through a dorsal interosseous tunnel in the lunate and scaphoid, and tightened and woven on itself. This portion reconstitutes the first or dorsal part of the interosseous ligament, maintains the dorsal axis of joint rotation, and corrects any existing diastasis. The passage of the tendon graft under the dorsal capitolunate capsule before entering the lunate corrects any residual dorsiflexion instability of the lunate when the system is tightened. A second tail of the ECRB is passed through a scaphoid tunnel, running obliquely in an ulnar direction to come out at the proximal inferior pole of the scaphoid in the area of the RSL insertion on the scaphoid. This is woven in the palmar RTL adjacent to the radius and not to bone in order to maintain some of the elastic aspects of this portion of the joint. The joint is transfixed with nonthreaded K-wires and immobilized in a thumb–spica cast for 6 weeks.

Nine young adults (mean age, 23 years) were treated surgically with this reconstruction because of chronic wrist pain as result of previous hyperextension injuries. All had moderate to severe wrist pain and restriction of activities or employment. The mean duration of symptoms was 2.3 years. Each patient underwent wrist joint evaluation preoperatively under fluoroscopy with stress applied. The stress views were taken during forced ulnar deviation and forced palmar flexion. Scapholunate instability or stage I PLI was documented in eight patients by radiographic criteria. At surgery, six patients had intact but elongated interosseous

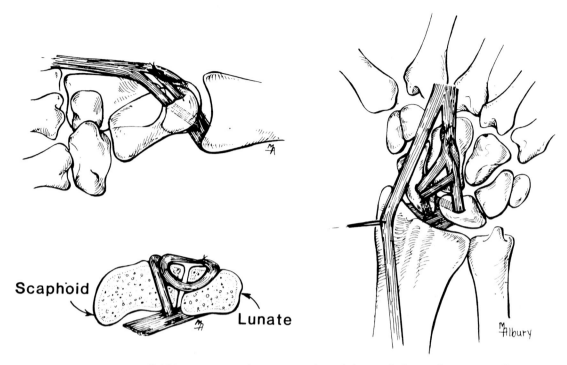

FIGURE 26.14. Mayfield-House anatomic reconstruction of the scapholunate interosseous ligament.

ligaments (partial failure), two patients had complete ligamentous failure, and one patient had only the peripheral and palmar portions of the interosseous ligament disrupted and one intact portion of the ligament. All had associated localized synovitis, and all had restoration of joint stability and normal anatomic alignment with this procedure. At a mean follow-up of 12.4 months, eight were back to their previous occupations, and six were known to be participating in sports (basketball, racquetball, skydiving, and cheerleading). Five had no wrist pain, and three had mild discomfort with forceful activities. Eight had maintained joint stability at follow-up as evidenced by normal joint alignment and approximation. All patients lost 30° to 40° of palmar flexion and/or extension. All were pleased with their result (Fig. 26.15).

THE DISTAL LIGAMENTOUS COMPLEX OF THE SCAPHOID

The distal ligamentous complex of the scaphoid has received little attention in the literature. In dissections of cadaver wrists, it is known that when the SLIL is sectioned, there is an inherent spring effect within the distal ligamentous tissue of the distal scaphoid, causing the proximal pole to displace dorsally in relation to the lunate. Drewniany et al. (65) studied the distal ligamentous complex of the scaphoid and trapezium anatomically and biomechanically. They described four components of a scaphotrapezial–trapezoidal ligament complex that stabilizes the distal pole of the scaphoid. Boabighi et al., in their biomechanical studies, found that the distal ligamentous complex was twice as strong as the SLIL. It was their conclusion from their studies that the distal ligament complex had to fail first before the SLIL failed *in vivo* (66). In contrast to Landsmeer (67), Mayfield (13,39,40,46,59), Kauer (56,58), and Ruby (24), they felt that the SLIL played no important role in normal wrist movement.

WRIST LIGAMENT BIOMECHANICS

To some extent, investigators have focused on the biomechanical properties of the wrist ligaments in recent years. These data have added to our more complete awareness of the exact process of failure during wrist injury. In order to understand the different patterns of injury that can occur in the different wrist ligaments, it is useful to have a better understanding of the biomechanics of the wrist ligaments themselves.

Wrist Ligament Histology

Kuhlman et al. (68) studied the histology of the wrist ligament collagenous structure. They found that the collagen fibers were grouped into (a) tendiniform bundles, (b) accordion-like bundles, and (c) dispersed bundles. The tendiniform bundles were formed by dense parallel fibers,

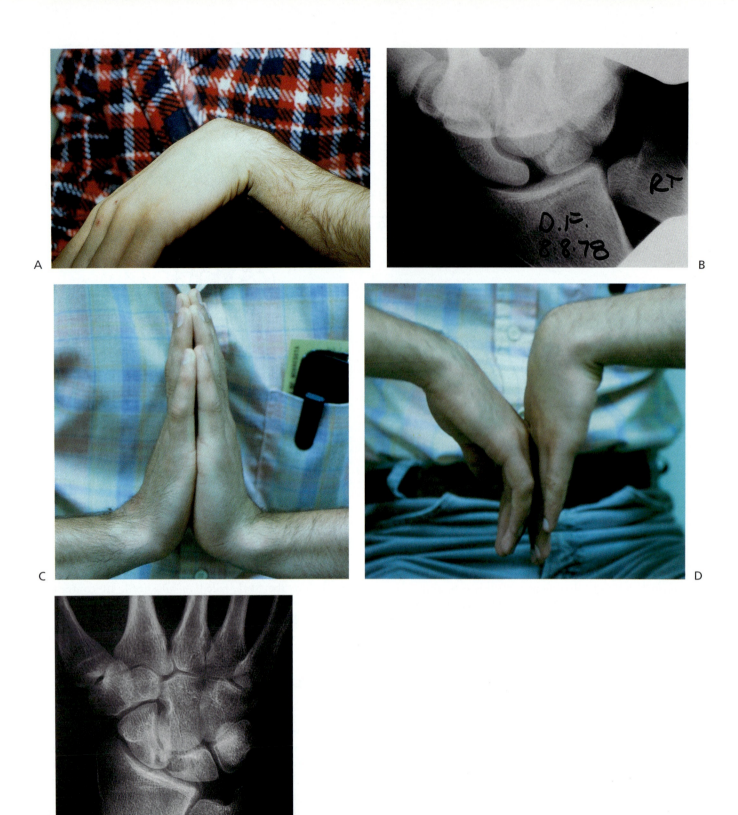

FIGURE 26.15. A: A 21-year-old man with a wrist injury. Note the dorsal dislocation of the proximal pole of the scaphoid on palmar flexion. **B:** Same patient with stress roentgenogram in stressed ulnar deviation. Note scapholunate diastasis. **C:** Same patient 11 months after anatomic reconstruction of the scapholunate interosseous ligament. Maximum dorsiflexion. **D:** Same patient, maximum palmar flexion. **E:** Wrist roentgenogram 14 months after surgery.

which are oriented in one direction. The accordion-like bundles were narrower than the tendiniform bundles and were composed of collagen fibers, also parallel but much more wavy. The dispersed bundles were thinner and dispersed in all planes, intermingled with numerous vessels with an abundant elastic network around and within the fibrils. In their biomechanical studies, they found that the ligaments with collagen fibers grouped in compact bundles withstood strains better. The length and amplitude of the waves of the collagen fibers and the diameter of the bundles at rest allowed an estimation of the resistance and the possibility of elongation in tension testing (68). The wrist ligaments consist of collagen fibers and interstitial connective tissue that is rich in fat, vessels, and elastic fibers (68). Nash and Mayfield (57) noted a relative abundance of elastic fibers in the RSL and less frequently in the SLIL. The presence of elastic fibers in the RSL has also been studied by Berger and associates (53). It was their conclusion from their research that elastic fibers were in the vascular structures of the ligament and not in the ligament itself (54). However, a recent study of the microvascular anatomy of the radioscapholunate ligament by Hixson (37) revealed no uptake of elastin stain by the vessels in the ligament. The presence of elastin in the SLIL and RSL lends itself to speculation concerning the mechanics of the scapholunate articulation because both of these ligaments have high strains at failure, and the RSL is biomechanically elastic with very low elastic modulus (40).

Boabighi and associates (66) indicated that ligaments are composed of collagen fibers and interstitial connective tissue. They noted two types of bundles: wavy and parallel, and intermingled. The ligaments of the distal ligamentous complex of the scaphoid consist of parallel regular, dense, wavy bundles. The scapholunate ligament is made of intermingled and dispersed fibers in its palmar part, forming a zone of weakness.

LIGAMENT BIOMECHANICS

Mayfield and Williams (40) studied the biomechanical properties of human carpal ligaments in 11 fresh or fresh-frozen human wrists. Ligament–bone–ligament complexes for each ligament of the wrist were dissected free. The lengths of all ligaments were measured, and their cross-sectional areas were measured using an area micrometer with a standardized blade pressure (28). The bony ends were mounted in aluminum cups, fixed to an 810 MTS materials-testing system, and tested in tension to failure with simultaneous graphic recording. Cinematography provided correlative data during ligament elongation and failure. A strain rate of 1 cm/s was utilized because a strain rate of 50% to 100% of ligament length per second most closely approximates the strain rate of a physiologic injury. The strain rate used for the SLIL was 1 mm/s because of its short length. The results of this study are very pertinent to a better understanding of the carpus.

Tensile Properties

The RCL and RTL were found to be approximately the same length (30 mm). The radioscaphoid was the shortest of all ligaments except for the SLIL, which averaged 5.7 mm in length. The dorsal radiocarpal ligament, which is the dorsal proximal carpal row stabilizer, was shorter than its mirror image, the RTL. The ulnar collateral ligament was over twice the length of the radial collateral ligament (40).

The *maximum force* required for failure of the volar RTL was the greatest required for any of the volar intracapsular ligaments. The dorsal radiocarpal ligament required a maximum force of 240 N to fail, which was the same as its mirror-image volar RTL. The average RCL failed at 170 N. The RSL was the weakest of all the volar ligaments, failing at 54 N. The SLIL was the strongest of all the ligaments tested in the wrist, failing at 359 N. Boabighi and colleagues (66) noted in their studies that the SLIL failed at 150 N. Of the two collateral ligaments, the radial collateral ligament failed with less force (70 N) (40).

The *stiffness* of the ligaments was also studied, and the SLIL was found to be the stiffest of all the wrist ligaments tested. The radiotriquetral was significantly stiffer than the radiocapitate at the 0.01 significance level (40).

The *elastic modulus* of the RSL was the lowest of the wrist ligaments, and the elastic modulus of the dorsal radiocarpal ligament was the highest. This suggests that the dorsal radiocarpal is the least elastic and the radioscaphoid is the most elastic of the carpal ligaments. The radial collateral ligament was more elastic than the ulnar collateral ligament (40).

Maximum stress, or tensile strength, is the maximum force per unit cross-sectional area. The dorsal radiocarpal ligament had the highest tensile strength of the wrist ligaments. This may explain why lunate dislocations are less frequent than perilunate injuries (40).

Maximum strain is the percent elongation at total failure. The two ligaments that elongated the most at failure were the RSL and the SLIL. The SLIL doubled its length before total failure, with a maximum strain of 225%. The RSL lost its continuity at 140% strain. The RCL, the distal carpal row stabilizer, had a maximum strain that was significantly greater than the RTL (40).

Distal Ligamentous Complex of the Scaphoid

Boabighi and associates (66) noted that the ligaments stabilizing the distal pole of the scaphoid were extensible but fragile. They have a Young's modulus varying between 50 and 25 N/mm^2. Their elongation before rupture varies from 70% to 100%. The ultimate load to failure for the lateral component of this complex was 180 N, and, for the medial component, 230 N.

Ulnar Carpal Ligamentous Complex

Palmer et al. (69) tested the TFCC and found that in the neutral position, the radius bore 60% of the total axial load, and the ulna 40%. Removal of the TFCC resulted in a redistribution of the axial load so that the radius transmitted 95% and the ulna 5%. Thus, the TFCC has an important role in axial force transmission from the carpus to the forearm. It also is important for stability of the distal radioulnar joint. The TFCC has three major functions: (a) it is a cushion for the ulnar carpus, carrying 20% of the axial load of the forearm, (b) it is the major stabilizer of the distal radioulnar joint, and (c) it is a stabilizer of the ulnar carpus.

FAILURE LOCATION AND MODE

The RCL failed proximally between the radial styloid and the scaphoid waist in 80% of fresh specimens (40) (Fig. 26.16). There were no avulsions.

The RTL failed distally more frequently than proximally, with 56% failing between the lunate and the triquetrum. (Fig. 26.17). Of the distal failures, four were ligament failures, and one was a triquetral avulsion.

There has been some controversy concerning the exact nature of the RTL. Other authors have indicated that this

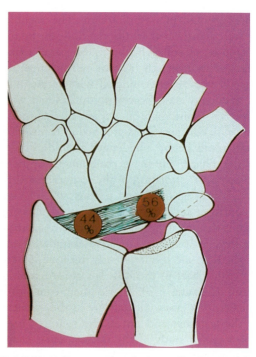

FIGURE 26.17. Failure mode of the radiotriquetral ligament (from 10 fresh specimens). Distal failure, 5 (ligament, 4; triquetral avulsion, 1); Proximal failure, 4 (ligament, 3; radial styloid avulsion, 1).

ligament is really two ligaments: the long radiolunate and the lunotriquetral ligaments. In my own extensive dissections in many wrists, it has been my opinion that this is truly one ligament from radius to triquetrum; hence, the term RTL. To test this hypothesis, we tested the strength of attachment of this ligament to the lunate. Most specimens

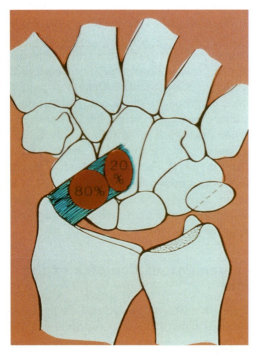

FIGURE 26.16. Failure mode of the radiocapitate ligament (from 10 fresh specimens). Distal failure, 2; Midligament failure, 8.

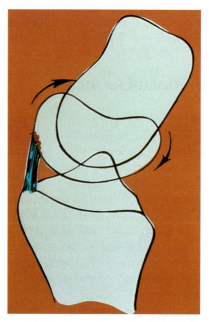

FIGURE 26.18. Insertional failure of the radiotriquetral ligament from the lunate. Mean force: 64.2 N. Range: 38.0–106.8 N.

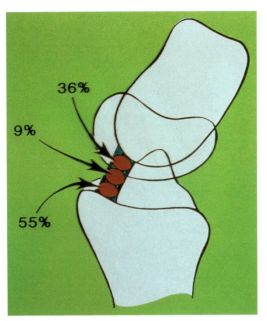

FIGURE 26.19. Failure mode of the radioscaphoid ligament (from 11 fresh specimens). Ligament failure, 11 (distal, 4; midligament, 1; proximal, 6).

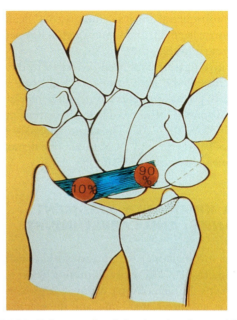

FIGURE 26.20. Failure mode of the dorsal radiocarpal ligament (from 10 fresh specimens). Distal failure, 9 (ligament 8; triquetral avulsion, 1).

(55%) experienced insertional failure (i.e., the ligament "pulled off" the lunate) with very low forces, averaging 64 N (Fig. 26.18). This fact suggests that this ligament traverses the palmar surface of the lunate, to which it has some attachment, but terminates in the triquetrum. If, indeed, this ligament is two ligaments, inserting and originating at the lunate, then it would seem that the failure mode would more likely be in the ligament itself or by avulsion. This weak attachment to the lunate may also explain the phenomenon of dorsiflexion instability of the lunate after hyperextension injuries.

The RSL failed in its substance in all specimens, the failures being equally divided between the proximal and distal ends (Fig. 26.19).

The dorsal radiocarpal ligament failed at its distal end in 90% of the specimens, eight in the ligament and one by triquetral avulsion (Fig. 26.20).

The SLIL rarely failed in its substance because of its remarkable stiffness and strength. In 56% of specimens, ligament failure occurred at 356 N, and in 44% of specimens, bone avulsion or cement failure occurred at 410 N (Fig. 26.21).

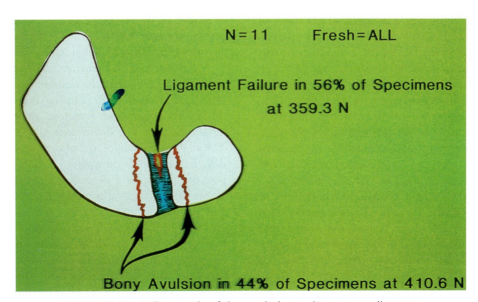

FIGURE 26.21. Failure mode of the scapholunate interosseous ligament.

The lunotriquetral intrinsic interosseous ligament and the ulnolunate ligament and ulnotriquetral ligament (UTL) were not tested in this study.

Other investigators have been interested in the mechanical properties of the wrist ligaments. Kuhlman et al. (68) noted that the wrist ligaments have Young's moduli ranging between 40 and 3 N/mm². Their elongation at rupture varies from 40% to 120%. The strain necessary to obtain rupture lies between 2 and 14 N/mm². The denser collagenous ligaments were stronger and less elastic.

CARPAL KINEMATICS, LIGAMENT MECHANICS, AND CARPAL INJURY

Numerous investigators have studied the kinematics of the carpus (46,70–81). The wrist joint functions with three parallel chains. In each of these chains, the proximal carpus functions as an intercalated bone, and the specific shape of the intercalated bone creates a simultaneous movement in the radiocarpal and the midcarpal joints (58).

In several studies using sonic digitalization, stereophotography, and magnetic tracking (72,74,76), the apex of carpal rotation in the anteroposterior (AP) plane has been shown to be in the center of the capitate or at the junction of the palmar radiocapitate and the capitotriquetral ligaments (Fig. 26.22) (39,74,81,82).

It is essential to integrate an understanding of ligament mechanics with carpal kinematics to fully appreciate the pathomechanics involved in carpal injuries. When the wrist moves from neutral position to maximum extension, the palmar ligaments become progressively more taut and achieve their maximum tautness in complete extension: 66% of the carpal motion in extension occurs in the radiocarpal joint, and 34% of carpal motion in extension occurs in the midcarpal joint (83). Likewise, as the palmar extrinsic ligaments become more taut, the degree of excursion of the carpus in radial and ulnar deviation becomes progressively smaller until maximum extension is reached. At this point, the taut palmar extrinsic ligaments lock the carpus in neutral position, preventing any radial or ulnar deviation. The same phenomenon occurs when the wrist is progressively flexed. In flexion, 60% of carpal motion is midcarpal, and 40% is radiocarpal (83). With progressive flexion the dorsal radiocarpal ligament locks the lunate in the radiolunate fossa, which prevents capitate movement in radial and ulnar deviation. Thus, the capitate is "centralized" in the AP plane in maximum flexion and extension (Fig. 26.23). In axial rotation, a progressive tightening of the ligamentous structures of the carpus is also seen when the wrist is moved into flexion and extension (Fig. 26.24). Rotational stability of the carpus should be considered in the treatment of carpal instabilities (84).

Movement of the wrist in radial deviation relaxes the palmar RCL. Movement of the wrist in ulnar deviation tight-

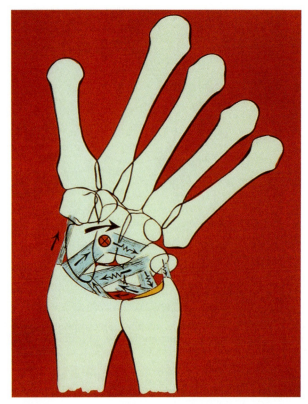

FIGURE 26.22. Ligament control of carpal kinematics in ulnar deviation. The *X* is the center of anteroposterior rotation in the center of the capitate.

ens the RCL and relaxes the palmar RTL (Fig. 26.22). When the wrist is progressively extended, an interligamentous space develops palmarly because of the separation of the RCL and RTL. This space overlies the capitolunate joint palmarly and is called the "space of Poirier" (39,46,52). This space is an inherently weak area on the palmar surface of the carpus. Even though individual ligaments influence carpal motion, complete carpal translation cannot occur without global ligament damage (85).

It has been shown anatomically (44,57,58) and kinematically (77,78) that the scapholunate joint has a dorsal axis of rotation (77,78). During impact loading over the thenar eminence, the scaphoid rotates dorsally on the lunate through this dorsal axis of the scapholunate joint. The anatomic arrangement of the fibers of the SLIL and the RSL in turn allows mobility of the palmar and proximal pole of the scaphoid (56,57). The ligamentous fiber orientation of this joint also allows separation of the scaphoid and the lunate at the palmar portion of this joint (Fig. 26.11). Mechanically, the scapholunate joint has a specialized design that enhances stability but also allows load dampening during excessive loads applied to the wrist in hyperextension and intercarpal supination.

The wrist functions as two carpal rows with the bones of the distal row tightly bound together and the bones of the

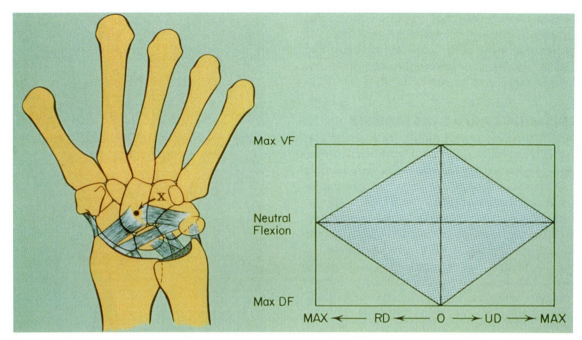

FIGURE 26.23. Capitate centralization in movement from flexion to extension from ligament control. X, center of anteroposterior rotation.

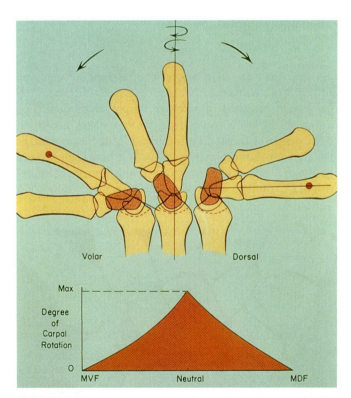

FIGURE 26.24. Ligament control of carpal rotation from flexion to extension.

proximal row more loosely bound together (86). The lunate and triquetrum are tightly connected anatomically by the interosseous ligament, as evidenced by close correlation of their screw axes of rotation with motion analysis (79). The greatest motion between the lunate and triquetrum occurs from 45° to 35° of flexion, whereas between the scaphoid and lunate the greatest motion is seen between 25° and 35° of extension (78). The lunate is the keystone in the proximal row about which the scaphoid and triquetrum move. The triquetrum is rigidly coupled to the lunate, and the scaphoid is loosely coupled to the lunate.

When the wrist is loaded axially, the load distribution across the radiocarpal joint is variable: 60% radioscaphoid and 40% radiolunate (87,88). The axial load distribution across the midcarpal joint is 23% scaphotrapeziotrapezoid, 28% scaphocapitate, 29% lunocapitate, and 20% triquetrohamate (89).

The following facts are useful in developing a mechanical concept of carpal injuries: (a) the proximal carpal row is stabilized to the distal forearm by five ligaments, whereas the distal carpal row is stabilized to the forearm by only one ligament (RCL); (b) the weakest ligaments of the wrist are on the radial side of the wrist; (c) the RCL is maximally taut in maximum extension and in ulnar deviation; (d) the space of Poirier is an inherently weak area over the palmar capitolunate joint; (e) the lunate is tightly connected to the radius by its palmar and dorsal ligaments; (f) the scaphoid is less coupled to the lunate by its interosseous ligament than is the triquetrum; (g) in hyperextension, the capitate is "centralized" in the AP plane and cannot move in radial and ulnar deviation, creating an "anvil effect" on the palmar RCL when radial deviation is forced; (h) axial loads are transmitted proportionally more across the radioscaphoid joint; and (i) the weakest link between the distal carpal row and the distal forearm is the palmar RCL.

MECHANISM OF CARPAL INSTABILITY

Carpal injuries represent a spectrum of bony and ligamentous damage. The names given to the various injuries only describe the resultant damage apparent on radiographs. Each injury is not a separate entity, but part of a continuum. The final injury is determined by (a) the type of three-dimensional loading, (b) the magnitude and duration of the forces involved, (c) the position of the hand at the time of impact, and (d) the biomechanical properties of the bones and ligaments. Laboratory reproduction of carpal injuries on fresh cadaver wrists has helped elucidate our understanding of these enigmatic injuries.

Carpal Dislocations

Thirty-two fresh embalmed cadaver wrists were loaded to failure using a gravity-dependent loading machine (46). The loading mechanism created hyperextension, ulnar deviation, and intercarpal supination. Thirteen dorsal perilunate dislocations were produced. All specimens had rupture of the RSL and SLIL. Scaphoid rotation was noted in six specimens. Two patterns of palmar ligamentous damage were noted. One pattern was represented by radiocapitate and radial collateral ligament failure and scapholunate failure (SLIL and RSL) with capitate and scaphoid dislocation and opening of the space of Poirier (Fig. 26.25). The other pattern with more severe ligamentous damage had similar findings, except that the RTL failure between the lunate and triquetrum was evident with lunotriquetral dislocation (Fig. 26.26).

Two lunate dislocations were also produced, and the pathomechanics were the same as the perilunate dislocations (extension, ulnar deviation, and intercarpal supination). Scaphoid rotation and scapholunate diastasis were noted in both specimens. The palmar ligamentous damage in the lunate dislocations was the same as that of the severe perilunate dislocation, but, in addition, there was failure of the dorsal radiocarpal ligament, which allowed palmar rotation of the lunate.

Scaphoid rotation was a direct result of progressive failure of the scapholunate ligamentous complex. Ligamentous failure began in the palmar aspect of the interosseous ligament and progressed dorsally.

Seven radial styloid fractures were produced by avulsion. Triquetral fractures were associated with perilunate and lunate dislocations in five specimens. The mechanism was by avulsion of either the RTL or the UTL.

All dislocations had varying degrees of perilunate instability. As the loading forces of extension, intercarpal supination, and ulnar deviation progressed, the scaphoid, capitate, and then the triquetrum were progressively dislocated by the lunate, creating progressive carpal instability. The degree of PLI has been divided into four stages, according to the degree of carpal dislocation and ligamentous damage that starts at the scapholunate joint and progresses around the lunate: stage I PLI, scaphoid dislocation or instability with SLIL and RSL injury; stage II PLI, capitate dislocation

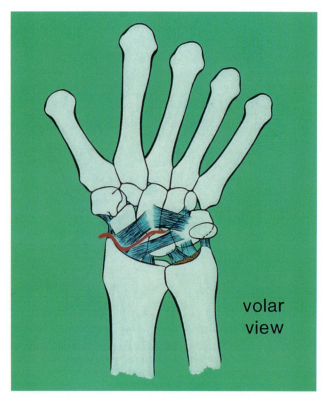

FIGURE 26.25. Palmar ligament damage in stage II perilunate instability.

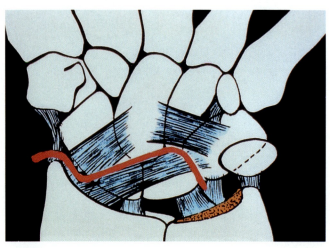

FIGURE 26.26. Palmar ligament damage in stage III perilunate instability.

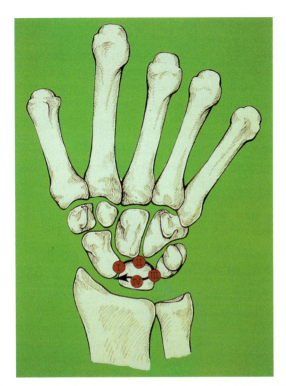

FIGURE 26.27. The four stages of perilunate instability (*I–IV*).

the lunate in carpal dislocations and fracture-dislocations. Fracture of the waist of the scaphoid is the most common injury to the carpal bones. Borgeskov (36) noted that there was an association of scaphoid fractures (71.2%) and triquetral fractures (20.4%) in carpal injuries. Seventy to eighty percent of scaphoid fractures occur at the waist, with the remainder occurring equally often at the proximal pole and at the tubercle (3,90). Displaced unstable fractures of the scaphoid associated with other carpal fractures and dislocations usually have a poor prognosis. This relationship between scaphoid fractures and perilunate dislocations is well known clinically (3,15,23,24,31,34,91–93). The degree of instability of the scaphoid fracture seems to be directly related to the degree of ligamentous damage and associated perilunate instability. Laboratory experiments by Johnson and colleagues (11,31) and Weber and Chao (27) have greatly aided our understanding of the pathomechanics of these fractures and fracture-dislocations.

Loading Studies

Twenty-nine fresh cadaver specimens were loaded with a hydraulic machine to create wrist extension, ulnar deviation, and intercarpal supination by Johnson et al. (31). The loading pressure plate was placed over the distal portion of the scaphoid with the wrist in maximum extension. Progressive loads were applied. Five scaphoid waist fractures, two proximal pole fractures, and six tuberosity fractures were produced. Five scaphoid fractures were associated with stage I PLI, and three associated with stage III PLI. Hyperextension and ulnar deviation were the primary mechanisms of the scaphoid waist fractures, with the dorsal aspect of the scaphoid engaging the dorsal rim of the radius, thereby creating an anvil effect and leading to fracture (Fig. 26.28).

Scaphoid waist fractures were described according to their stability. Type I were stable, not associated with signifi-

and opening of the space of Poirier; stage III PLI, triquetral dislocation and RTL failure; and stage IV PLI, radiocapitate ligament, RTL, and dorsal radiocarpal ligament failure with lunate dislocation (Fig. 26.27).

Scaphoid Fracture and Fracture-Dislocation

The scaphoid, as the connecting rod between the proximal and distal carpal rows, must either fracture or dislocate from

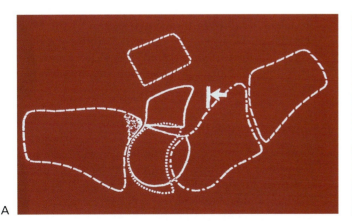 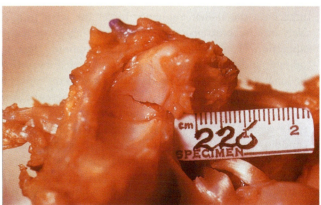

FIGURE 26.28. A: Scaphoid fracture by forced extension, fracturing over the dorsal rim of the distal radius. *Arrow,* load direction. (Courtesy of Roger Johnson, M.D. Milwaukee, WI). **B:** Experimental laboratory fracture of the scaphoid. Notice the fracture propagation starting on the palmar surface. (Courtesy of Roger Johnson, M.D., Milwaukee, WI).

cant ligamentous damage, and could not be displaced. Types II and III were unstable and associated with moderate to severe degrees of ligamentous damage and perilunate instability. The mechanism of fracture was hyperextension, with the scaphoid fracture beginning on the palmar side and progressing dorsally. The ligamentous damage and resultant perilunate instability were a direct result of the rotational component of intercarpal supination. This rotation of the scaphoid, distal carpal row, and triquetrum as a unit about the fixed lunate was also responsible for avulsion fracture of the triquetrum (avulsion of the RTL and UTL). The ligament failure started on the radial side of the carpus and progressed to the ulnar side of the carpus. Virtually all of the scaphoid fractures had some degree of SLIL failure, varying from a small tear palmarly to a complete disruption of the ligament.

Fractures of the proximal pole of the scaphoid were caused by subluxation of the scaphoid dorsally, before it was fractured over the dorsal rim of the radius. Scaphoid tuberosity fractures were caused by compression forces.

CARPAL INSTABILITY

Carpal instability is the resultant malalignment of the carpal bones under physiologic loads from ligamentous and bony injury that disrupts normal carpal equilibrium (94,95). The character of the final injury is determined by the type of three-dimensional loading, the magnitude and duration of the forces involved, the position of the hand at the time of impact, and the biomechanical properties of the bones and ligaments. Thus, a spectrum of injuries exist, depending on the resultant combinations of ligament disruptions and bony damage. Wrist arthroscopy has been invaluable in helping to delineate the exact ligamentous and bony damage (19–22).

Progressive Perilunar Instability

Impact on the thenar eminence forces the wrist progressively into hyperextension, ulnar deviation, and intercarpal supination (13,46). Progressively, the scaphoid, then the capitate, and finally the triquetrum are peeled away from the lunate, which is more rigidly connected to the radius by its ligamentous attachments. The injury progresses from scapholunate instability to the more severe lunate instability. In stage I PLI, the primary instability is limited to the scapholunate joint. In stage II PLI, there is also ligamentous damage at the capitolunate joint and opening of the space of Poirier. In stage III PLI, ligamentous damage at the triquetrolunate joint is added to the preceding injuries (Fig. 26.26) (46). Adolfsson (19) and Dautel (20) have documented arthroscopically the scapholunate ligament damage and associated instability in patients with chronic posttraumatic wrist pain. Stage I PLI has also been noted in patients with scaphoid fractures (91), distal radial fractures (96,97), and other injuries.

In stage IV PLI, dorsal disruption of the dorsal radiocarpal ligament allows the lunate to rotate palmarly on its palmar radiotriquetral and ulnolunate ligamentous hinge. In stage I and II PLI, spontaneous reduction of the capitolunate and triquetrolunate joints frequently occurs as the wrist recoils from injury. In this situation, persistent scapholunate diastasis may be the only manifestation of these more severe injuries. Experimental and clinical investigations (13,46) have also shown that the spectrum of carpal instability can also be associated with scaphoid and capitate fractures as well as avulsion fractures of the radial and ulnar styloid processes and of the triquetrum.

Scapholunate Instability

Scapholunate instability is the first stage in PLI and can be seen in the adult as well as the skeletally immature carpus (98). The scaphoid, as the connecting rod between the proximal and distal carpal rows, rotates dorsally on the lunate in hyperextension. If the loads applied in hyperextension exceed the physiologic limits of the SLIL and the radioscapholunate ligament, then ligament failure begins, starting on the palmar side of this joint. The first disruption occurs in the palmar aspect of the interosseous ligament and the radioscapholunate ligament (59). If the loading stops at this point, then clinically observable instability may not be evident, but microinstability of the scapholunate joint is present leading to wrist pain (Fig. 26.29). Arthroscopy can be very helpful in diagnosis in this situation. If hyperextension loading is combined with intercarpal supination, then the damage may progress to disrupt the dorsal portion of the interosseous ligament. Clinically detectable scapholunate instability would not be present. Stress roentgenograms may be helpful in diagnosis as well as arthroscopy. Disruption of normal carpal arcs may be present on radiographs (99). It is important to realize that the mechanics of injury of this joint may cause only partial failure of these ligaments, leading to ligament elongation with associated instability. This will be evident arthroscopically. The scaphoid will be subluxed on the lunate and can be reduced back onto the lunate by pulling on the thumb longitudinally (Fig. 26.30).

Capitolunate Instability

Complete disruption or partial failure with elongation of the palmar RCL in conjunction with ligament damage at the scapholunate joint is designated a stage II PLI. In stage II PLI, capitolunate and scapholunate instability are present. This will be evident clinically and on roentgenograms if joint dislocation is present. If spontaneous reduction occurs, then a dorsal displacement stress test as described by Johnson et al. (18) may be useful in diagnosis. If diagnosis

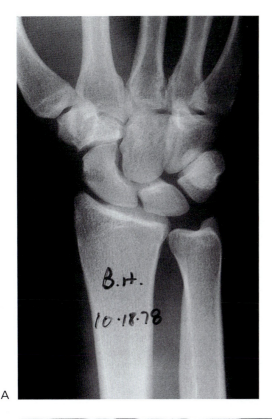
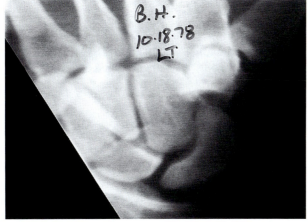
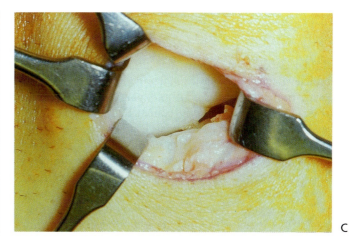

FIGURE 26.29. **A:** A 22-year-old man after an extension injury of the wrist. The patient complains of persistent radial wrist pain. The anteroposterior roentgenogram is normal. **B:** Roentgenogram in stress ulnar deviation. Note only minimal opening of the scapholunate joint and loss of the confluent line of the distal arc of the scapholunate joint. **C:** Intraoperative dorsal view of the scapholunate joint. Note the tear in only the palmar portion of the scapholunate interosseous ligament and rotatory displacement of the palmar portion of the scaphoid on the lunate in extension.

of capitolunate instability is not made acutely, chronic instability with chronic wrist pain can be problematic. Johnson and colleagues (18) brought attention to this chronic carpal instability pattern. They recommended a palmar ligamentous repair that closed the space of Poirier to restabilize the capitolunate joint. They tethered the RCL and RTL. In a series of 11 patients, the results were favorable (18).

Lunotriquetral Instability

It is known that lunotriquetral instability can be problematic (100). The diagnosis can be elusive, and the best treatment is not yet clear. Horii and colleagues (73) have demonstrated altered carpal kinematics after sectioning of the lunotriquetral ligaments, particularly the dorsal scaphotriquetral ligament and palmar RTL. A VISI pattern of carpal instability with palmar lunate rotation was evident. It was their conclusion that injuries to this joint loading to lunotriquetral dissociation can produce synovitis, joint wear, abnormal ligament tension, and wrist pain associated with clicking on the ulnar side of the wrist. These findings have been substantiated arthroscopically. Viegas and associates (101) in an anatomic and biomechanical study progressively sectioned the interosseous, palmar lunotriquetral, and dorsal radiocarpal ligaments at this joint

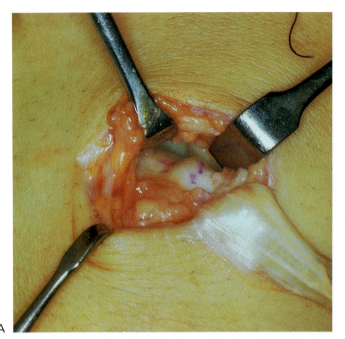 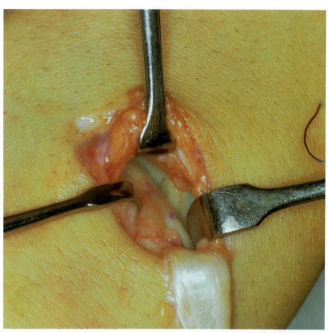

FIGURE 26.30. A: A 32-year-old man with chronic wrist pain after an extension injury. A dorsal intraoperative view of the scapholunate joint. The approximate joint edges of the scaphoid and lunate are marked. The hand is in normal position. Note the subluxed joint with a stepoff at the joint line with an intact interosseous ligament. **B:** The same patient as in **A**. Traction has been applied to the thumb. The scapholunate joint is reduced, indicating a stretched and partially failed interosseous ligament.

and then evaluated instability. For clinical and roentgenographic evidence of dynamic lunotriquetral instability to be present, both the interosseous and palmar lunotriquetral ligaments (distal portion of the palmar RTL) had to be disrupted. If the dorsal radiocarpal ligament between the lunate and the triquetrum is also disrupted, then static instability was evident. Experimentally (46) and clinically (102) it has been shown that fractures about the triquetrum represent avulsion fractures, indicating that these ligaments have been damaged. These fractures should be a clue that stage III PLI exists. Clinically, these findings of ligament damage have been substantiated arthroscopically. Zacitee et al. (103) arthroscopically described fraying of the UTL and ulnolunate ligament and signs of Palmer class 2D TFCC injury (104) as signs of longstanding triquetrolunate ligament rupture (103). Li and associates (75) studied the lunotriquetral joint by arthroscopically sectioning the lunotriquetral interosseous and palmar radiolunotriquetral ligaments in the laboratory. This altered the motion of this joint. They concluded that the lunotriquetral interosseous ligament stabilized the joint in ulnar deviation and the palmar radiolunotriquetral ligament stabilized the joint in extension. Most of the carpal instability patterns exist on the radial side of the carpus, but it is important to realize that the carpus is also suspended from the distal ulna. Wiesner and associates (105), in an experimental study, demonstrated that the ulnar ligamentous complex and TFCC take origin from the ulnar styloid and its base, as does the ulnar collateral ligament. The ulnar styloid plays a vital role in stabilizing the carpus to the forearm.

CONCLUSION

The wrist is an intriguing and complex joint, rich in mechanical design and function. We have learned much about this joint in the past several decades, and current research has developed significant momentum. We must pursue studies in ligament mechanics, pathomechanics of injury, and mechanical testing on the ulnar side of the wrist. In addition, further work needs to be done on clinical correlation of laboratory findings. This must be accomplished if adequate surgical reconstructive techniques are to be designed to solve many of the problems that continue to exist. We must strive toward this goal. The future for discovery within the wrist joint assuredly will be very exciting.

EDITORS' COMMENTS

The term "instability" has come under much scrutiny because it is more appropriate to describe an anatomic displacement. These anatomic displacements may or may not produce symptomatic dysfunction of a wrist. Carpal dysfunction more adequately describes the problem when speaking of a patient who has functional loss secondary to the inability to take load without producing synovitis. Synovitis occurs from overstretch of the synovium, shear loading, and abnormal cartilage contact. The anatomic displacements are clearly the disability, but the term instability is too deeply ingrained and will remain the defining term with modifiers to clarify the condition and severity.

Lunotriquetral instability describes the involved structures and implies a lack of alignment under load and a symptomatic result from that lack of alignment. The modifiers *dynamic* and *static* are also strictly misnomers and arose from a discussion between Julio Taleisnik and Kirk Watson in a taxi during a symposium hosted by Raoul Tubiana in Paris several decades ago. Dynamic instability has come to mean the condition of load intolerance, where the clinical exam makes the diagnosis but corroboration by x-ray studies is negative. Static instability describes a positive clinical exam with matching abnormal imaging.

According to a recent position statement from the International Federation of Societies of the Hand, a wrist joint should be considered clinically unstable only if it exhibits symptomatic dysfunction, is not able to bear loads, and exhibits abnormal kinematics during any portion of its arc of motion.

REFERENCES

1. Johnson RP. The evolution of carpal nomenclature: a short review. *J Hand Surg [Am]* 1990;15:834–838.
2. Gilford W, Bolton R, Lambriunidi C. The mechanism of the wrist joint. *Guy's Hosp Rep* 1943;92:52–59.
3. Fisk G. Carpal instability and the fractured scaphoid. *Ann R Coll Surg Engl* 1970;46:63–76.
4. Andrews FT. A dislocation of the carpal bones—the scaphoid and semilunar: report of a case. *Mich Med* 1932;31:269–271.
5. Campbell RD, Lance EM, Yeoh CB. Lunate and perilunar dislocations. *J Bone Joint Surg Br* 1964;46:55–72.
6. Campbell RD, Thompson RC, Lance EM, et al. Indications for open reduction of lunate and perilunate dislocations of the carpal bones. *J Bone Joint Surg Am* 1965;47:915–937.
7. Destot E. *Injuries of the wrist: a radiographic study.* New York: Paul B Koeker, 1926.
8. England JPS. Subluxation of the carpal scaphoid. *Proc R Soc Lond* 1970;63:581–582.
9. Green DP, O'Brian ET. Classification and management of carpal dislocations. *Clin Orthop* 1980;149:55–72.
10. Howard FM, Fahey T, Wojcik E. Rotatory subluxation of the navicular. *Clin Orthop* 1974;104:134–139.
11. Johnson RP. The acutely injured wrist and its residuals. *Clin Orthop* 1980;149:33–44.
12. Lichtman DM, Noble WH 3rd, Alexander CE. Dynamic triquetrolunate instability: case report. *J Hand Surg [Am]* 1984;9:185–188.
13. Mayfield JK. Mechanism of carpal injuries. *Clin Orthop* 1980;149:45–54.
14. Tanz SS. Rotational effect in lunar and perilunar dislocations. *Clin Orthop* 1968;57:147–152.
15. Linscheid RL, Dobyns JH, Beabout JW, et al. Traumatic instability of the wrist: diagnosis, classification, and pathomechanics. *J Bone Joint Surg Am* 1972;54:1612–1632.
16. Alexander CE, Lichtman DM. Ulnar carpal instabilities. *Orthop Clin North Am* 1984;15:307–320.
17. Lichtman DM, Schneider JR, Swafford AR, et al. Ulnar midcarpal instability—clinical and laboratory analysis. *J Hand Surg [Am]* 1981;6:515–523.
18. Johnson RP, Carrera GC. Chronic capitolunate instability. *J Bone Joint Surg Am* 1986;68:1164–1176.
19. Adolfsson L. Arthroscopic diagnosis of ligament lesions of the wrist. *J Hand Surg [Br]* 1993;18:65–69.
20. Dautel G, Goudot B, Merle M. Arthroscopic diagnosis of scapholunate instability in the absence of x-ray abnormalities. *J Hand Surg [Br]* 1993;18:213–218.
21. Rettig ME, Amadio PC. Wrist arthroscopy—indications and clinical applications. *J Hand Surg [Br]* 1994;19:774–777.
22. Ruch DS, Siegel D, Chabon SJ, et al. Arthroscopic categorization of intercarpal ligamentous injuries of the wrist. *Orthopedics* 1993;16:1051–1056.
23. Hill NA. Fractures and dislocations of the carpus. *Orthop Clin North Am* 1970;1:275–284.
24. Ruby LK, An KN, Lindsheid RL, et al. The effect of scapholunate ligament section on scapholunate motion. *J Hand Surg [Am]* 1987;12:5:767–770.
25. Verdan C, Narakas A. Fractures and pseudarthrosis of the scaphoid. *Surg Clin North Am* 1968;48:1083–1095.
26. Wagner CJ. Perilunar dislocations. *J Bone Joint Surg Am* 1956;38:1198.
27. Weber ER, Chao EY. An experimental approach to the mechanism of scaphoid waist fractures. *J Hand Surg* 1978;3:142.
28. Williams WJ, Erdman AG, Mayfield JK. Design and analysis of a ligament cross-sectional area micrometer. *Adv Bioeng Am Soc Mech Eng* 1980:50–52.
29. Squire M. Carpal mechanics and trauma. *J Bone Joint Surg Br* 1959;41:210.
30. Taleisnik J. The ligaments of the wrist. *J Hand Surg [Am]* 1976;1:110–118.
31. Johnson RP, Mayfield JK, Kilcoyne RF. Scaphoid fractures and fracture-dislocations—pathomechanics and perilunar instability. (Unpublished data, personal communication.)
32. Herzberg G, Comtet JJ, Linscheid RL, et al. Perilunate dislocations and fracture-dislocations: a multicenter study. *J Hand Surg [Am]* 1993;18:768–779.
33. Bonnin JG, Greening WP. Fracture of the triquetrum. *Br J Surg* 1943;31:278.
34. Wagner CJ. Fracture-dislocations of the wrist. *Clin Orthop* 1959;15:181.
35. Bartone NF, Grieco RV. Fractures of the triquetrum. *J Bone Joint Surg Am* 1956;38:3–53.
36. Borgeskov S, Christiansen B, Kjaer AM, et al. Fractures of the carpal bones. *Acta Orthop Scand* 1966;37:276–287.
37. Hixson ML, Stewart M. Microvascular anatomy of the radioscapholunate ligament of the wrist. *J Hand Surg [Am]* 1990;15:279–282.
38. Gardner EE, Gray J, O'Rahilly R. *Anatomy,* 3rd ed. Philadelphia: WB Saunders, 1969;160–163.
39. Mayfield JK, Johnson RP, Kilcoyne RK. The ligaments of the human wrist and their significance. *Anat Rec* 1976;186:417–428.
40. Mayfield JK, Williams WJ, Erdman AG, et al. Biomechanical properties of human carpal ligaments. *Orthop Trans* 1979;3:143.

41. Grant JCB. *An atlas of anatomy,* 5th ed. Baltimore: Williams & Wilkins, 1962; plates 90–94.
42. Gross CM. *Gray's anatomy of the human body,* 29th ed. Philadelphia: Lea & Febiger, 1973;333–336.
43. Schaeffer JPL. *Morris' human anatomy,* 11th ed. New York: McGraw-Hill, 1965;339–347.
44. Kauer JMG. The mechanism of the carpal joint. *Clin Orthop* 1986;202:16–26.
45. Lewis OJ, Hamshere RJ, Bucknill TM. The anatomy of the wrist joint. *J Anat* 1970;106:539–552.
46. Mayfield JK, Johnson RP, Kilcoyne RK. Carpal dislocations: pathomechanics and progressive perilunar instability. *J Hand Surg [Am]* 1980;5:226–241.
47. Mayfield JK. Wrist ligamentous anatomy and pathogenesis of carpal instability. *Orthop Clin North Am* 1984;15:209–216.
48. Taleisnik J. Wrist anatomy, function and injury. In: *American Academy of Orthopaedic Surgeons Instructional Course Lectures, vol XXVII.* St Louis: CV Mosby, 1978;61.
49. Berger RA, Landsmeer JMF. The palmar radiocarpal ligaments: a study of adult and fetal wrist joints. *J Hand Surg [Am]* 1990;15:847–854.
50. Zdravdovic V, Sennwald G, Fischer M, et al. The palmar wrist ligaments revisited, clinical relevance. *Ann Hand Surg* 1994;13:378–381.
51. Mayfield JK. Pathogenesis of wrist ligament instability. In: Lichtman DM, ed. *The wrist and its disorders.* Philadelphia: WB Saunders, 1988;53–73.
52. Poirier P, Charpy A. *Traité de l'anatomie humaine, tome I.* Paris: Masson et Cie, 1911;226–231.
53. Berger RA, Kauer JMG, Landsmeer JMF. Radioscapholunate ligament: a gross anatomic and histologic study of fetal and adult wrists. *J Hand Surg [Am]* 1991;16:350–353.
54. Berger RA, Blair WF. The radioscapholunate ligament: a gross and histologic description. *Anat Rec* 1984;210:393–405.
55. Palmer AK, Werner FW. The triangular fibrocartilage complex of the wrist. Anatomy and function. *J Hand Surg [Am]* 1981;6:153–162.
56. Kauer JMG. The interdependence of carpal articulation chains. *Acta Anat* 1974;88:481–501.
57. Nash D, Mayfield JK. The ligamentous anatomy of the scapholunate joint. (Unpublished data, personal communication.)
58. Kauer JMG. Functional anatomy of the wrist. *Clin Orthop* 1980;149:9–20.
59. Mayfield JK. Patterns of injury to carpal ligaments. A spectrum. *Clin Orthop* 1984;187:36–42.
60. Almquist EE, Bach AW, Sack JT, et al. Four-bone ligament reconstruction for treatment of chronic complete scapholunate separation. *J Hand Surg [Am]* 1991;16:322–327.
61. Brunelli GA, Brunelli GR. A new technique to correct carpal instability with scaphoid rotary subluxation: a preliminary report. *J Hand Surg [Am]* 1995;20:S82–S85.
62. Lavernia CJ, Cohen MS, Taleisnik J. Treatment of scapholunate dissociation by ligamentous repair and capsulodesis. *J Hand Surg [Am]* 1992;17:354–359.
63. Minami A, Kaneda K. Repair and/or reconstruction of scapholunate interosseous ligament in lunate and perilunate dislocations. *J Hand Surg [Am]* 1993;18:1099–1106.
64. Mayfield JK, House JH, Erdman AG. *The scapholunate joint— new insights into chronic instability and reconstruction.* Paper presented at the Proceedings of the American Society for Surgery of the Hand, Atlanta, GA, Feb 4–6, 1980.
65. Drewniany JJ, Palmar AK, Flatt AE. The scaphotrapezial ligament complex: an anatomic and biomechanical study. *J Hand Surg [Am]* 1985;10:492–498.
66. Boabighi A, Kuhlmann JN, Kenesi C. The distal ligamentous complex of the scaphoid and the scapholunate ligament. An anatomic, histologic and biomechanical study. *J Hand Surg [Br]* 1993;18:65–69.
67. Landsmeer JMF. Les coherences spatiales et équilibre spatial dans la région carpienne. *Acta Anat [Suppl]* 1968;70:1–84.
68. Kuhlman JN, Luboinski J, Laudet L, et al. Properties of the fibrous structures of the wrist. *J Hand Surg [Br]* 1990;15:335–341.
69. Palmer AK, Werner FW. Biomechanics of the distal radioulnar joint. *Clin Orthop* 1984;187:26–35.
70. Berger RA, Crowinshield RD, Flatt AE. The three-dimensional rotational behaviors of the carpal bones. *Clin Orthop* 1982;167:303–310.
71. DeLange A, Kauer JMG, Huiskes R. Kinematic behavior of the human wrist joint: a roentgenostereophotogrammetric analysis. *J Orthop Res* 1985;3:56–64.
72. Redman AG, Mayfield JK, Dorman R, et al. Kinematic and kinetic analysis of the human wrist by stereoscopic instrumentation. *Adv Bioeng Am Soc Mech Eng* 1978;79–82.
73. Horii E, Garcia-Elias M, An KN, et al. A kinematic study of the luno-triquetral dissociations. *J Hand Surg [Am]* 1991;16:355–362.
74. Jackson WT, Hefzky MS, Guo H. Determination of wrist kinematics using a magnetic tracking device. *Med Eng Phys* 1994;16:123–133.
75. Li G, Rowen B, Tokunaga D, et al. Carpal kinematics of lunotriquetral dissociations. *Biomed Sci Instrum* 1991;27:273–281.
76. Peterson JW, Robbin ML, Erdman AG, et al. Kinematic measurement of relative motion in the human wrist. *Adv Bioeng Am Soc Mech Eng* 1981:148–151.
77. Robbin ML, Erdman AG, Mayfield JK, et al. Kinematic measurement of relative motion in the human wrist. *Adv Bioeng Am Soc Mech Eng* 1981:159.
78. Sennwald GR, Zdravkovic V, Jacob HAC, et al. Kinematic analysis of relative motion within the proximal carpal row. *J Hand Surg* 1993;18:609–612.
79. Sennwald GR, Zdravkovic V, Kern HP, et al. Kinematics of the wrist and its ligaments. *J Hand Surg [Am]* 1993;18:805–814.
80. Wright RD. A detailed study of movement of the wrist joint. *J Anat* 1935;70:137.
81. Youngil Y, Flatt A. Kinematics of the wrist. *Clin Orthop* 1980;149:21–32.
82. Youm U, McMurtry RY, Flatt AE, et al. Kinematics of the wrist: an experimental study of radial–ulnar deviation and flexion–extension. *J Bone Joint Surg Am* 1978;60:423–431.
83. Sarrafian SK, Melamed JL, Goshgarian GM. Study of wrist motion in flexion and extension. *Clin Orthop* 1977;126:153–159.
84. Ritt MJ, Stuart PR, Berglund BS, et al. Rotational stability of the carpus relative to the forearm. *J Hand Surg [Am]* 1995;20:305–311.
85. Viegas SF, Patterson RM, Ward K. Extrinisic wrist ligaments in the pathomechanics of ulnar translation instability. *J Hand Surg [Am]* 1995;20:312–318.
86. Ruby LK, Cooney WP, An KN, et al. Relative motion of selected carpal bones: a kinematic analysis of the normal wrist. *J Hand Surg [Am]* 1988;13:1–10.
87. Viegas SF, Patterson R, Peterson P, et al. The effects of various load paths and different loads on the load transfer characteristics of the wrist. *J Hand Surg [Am]* 1989;14:458–465.
88. Weber ER. Concepts governing the rotational shift of the intercalated segment of the carpus. *Orthop Clin North Am* 1984;15:193–207.
89. Patterson R, Viegas SF. Biomechanics of the wrist. *J Hand Ther* 1995;8:97–105.
90. London PS. The broken scaphoid bone. *J Bone Joint Surg Br* 1961;43:237.

91. Braithwaite IJ, Jones WA. Scapholunate dissociation occurring with scaphoid fracture. *J Hand Surg [Br]* 1992;17:286–288.
92. Friedenberg ZB. Anatomic considerations in the treatment of carpal navicular fractures. *Am J Surg* 1949;78:379.
93. Mazet R, Hoal M. Fractures of the carpal navicular. *J Bone Joint Surg Am* 1963;45:82.
94. Taleisnik J. Post-traumatic carpal instability. *Clin Orthop* 1980;149:73–82.
95. Zdravkovic V, Jacob HAC, Sennwald GR. Physical equilibrium of the normal wrist and its relation to clinically defined "instability." *J Hand Surg [Br]* 1995;20:159–164.
96. Mudgal C, Hastings H. Scapholunate diastasis in fractures of the distal radius. Pathomechanics and treatment options. *J Hand Surg [Br]* 1993;18:725–729.
97. Tang JB. Carpal instability associated with fracture in the distal radius. *Chin J Surg* 1994;32:82–86.
98. Zimmerman NB, Weiland AJ. Scapholunate dissociation in the skeletally immature carpus. *J Hand Surg [Am]* 1990;15:701–705.
99. Peh WCG, Gilula LA. Normal disruption of carpal arcs. *J Hand Surg [Am]* 1996;21:561–566.
100. Reagan DS, Linscheid RL, Dobyns JH. Lunotriquetral sprains. *J Hand Surg [Am]* 1984;9:502–514.
101. Viegas SF, Patterson RM, Peterson PD, et al. Ulnar-sided perilunate instability: an anatomic and biomechanic study. *J Hand Surg [Am]* 1990;15:268–278.
102. Smith DS, Murray PM. Avulsion fractures of the volar aspect of triquetral bone of the wrist: a subtle sign of carpal ligament injury. *Am J Roentgenol* 1996;166:609–614.
103. Zacitee L, Demet L, Fabry G. Frayed ulnotriquetral and ulnolunate ligaments as an arthroscopic sign of longstanding triquetrolunate ligament rupture. *J Hand Surg [Br]* 1994;19:570–571.
104. Palmer AK. Triangular fibrocartilage complex lesions: a classification. *J Hand Surg [Am]* 1989;14:594–606.
105. Wiesner L, Rumelhart C, Pham E, et al. Experimentally induced ulnocarpal instability. *J Hand Surg [Br]* 1996;21:24–29.

27

DYNAMICS OF CARPAL INSTABILITY

WILLIAM B. KLEINMAN

Before embarking on the voyage that leads to understanding the dynamics of carpal instability, the student of wrist pathophysiology must first acquire an intimate knowledge of the fine details of carpal anatomy, including the complex of ligaments that link the bones of the wrist to each other and to the hand and forearm. Earlier chapters in this text have addressed much of the anatomy. In this chapter, I emphasize only those anatomic details that I believe must be clearly understood before the student of wrist pathophysiology can appreciate the subtle nuances of progressive carpal collapse.

The normal anteroposterior (AP) x-ray of the wrist in Fig. 27.1 is a good place to begin our journey. As we examine this x-ray, we must understand that the carpus is supported by an array of ligaments that act on the individual bones as struts and guy wires. In neutral hand–forearm position, these ligaments support the carpus with a great amount of stored-up potential energy. Under simple physiologic load, the three carpal bones of the proximal row "want to" collapse—either together or individually—into a physically and mechanically more stable position. If the ligamentous struts and guy wires that normally support the carpus are rendered incompetent by either injury or disease, the normal interrelationships among the bones and their articular surfaces will be lost; and if collapse were to occur, under the transcarpal load of the extrinsic wrist and finger flexor and extensor muscle–tendon units, kinetic energy would be dissipated, and the carpal bones would collapse into a more mechanically stable attitude. Unfortunately, the more mechanically stable posture of carpal collapse is physiologically incompatible with normal integrated carpal mechanics. Because the collapsed posture of carpal "instability" places a superphysiologic shear stress load on specific articular surfaces of the carpus (based on the particular mechanism of collapse), we continue to refer to this mechanically more stable attitude of the carpus as carpal instability.

The dynamics of carpal instability are fairly easy to understand if the reader visualizes the three-bone relationship that comprises the proximal row as being suspended as an intercalated segment between the hand and the forearm. I prefer to consider the distal carpal row (trapezium, trapezoid, capitate, and hamate) as "the hand," intimately attached to the metacarpals by the short intrinsic carpometacarpal ligaments (inherent ligamentous laxity of the fourth and fifth carpometacarpal joints should not be considered in understanding the fine nuances of carpal instability). The normal 15° and 40° arcs of flexion–extension at the fourth and fifth carpometacarpal joints, respectively, are not relevant in this discussion of the dynamics of carpal instability.

The proximal carpal row truly behaves as an intercalated segment—a free body in space, suspended (with all of its stored-up potential energy) in a position maintained between the hand and the forearm by the complex ligaments of the wrist (Fig. 27.2). The extrinsic palmar radiocarpal and disc–carpal (ulnocarpal) ligaments arise from the forearm and insert onto the palmar neck of the capitate after "touching down" on the proximal row. From the radius, the radioscaphocapitate ligament supports the radial side of the intercalated three-bone unit; from the triangular fibrocartilage and the fovea of the ulna, the deeper disc–lunate/disc–triquetral ligaments and the more superficial ulnocapitate ligament arise, respectively.

From the hand (i.e., the capitate and its intimately attached neighbors, the hamate, trapezoid, and trapezium), the arcuate ligament (also known as the V- or delta ligament) fans out from distal to proximal to form a suspensory sling for the three-bone unit comprising the proximal row. The medial limb of the arcuate ligament connects the capitate neck to the triquetrum along their palmar surfaces. The lateral limb functions similarly, connecting the palmar capitate to the scaphoid waist (Fig. 27.2). In this manner, the proximal row is anatomically suspended between the hand and the forearm. Figure 27.3 demonstrates a right hyperflexed cadaver wrist, viewed from a dorsal perspective. The probe in Fig. 27.3A rests among the extrinsic radiocarpal ligaments; the radioscaphocapitate and long radiolunate (radiolunatotriquetral) ligaments are to the left of the probe tip; the ligament of Testut and Kuenz (radioscaphoid–lunate) is to the right. Figure 27.3B shows the extrinsic disc–carpal lig-

---

W. B. Kleinman: Department of Orthopaedic Surgery, The Indiana Hand Center, Indiana University School of Medicine, Indianapolis, Indiana 46280.

Section X: Carpal Instability

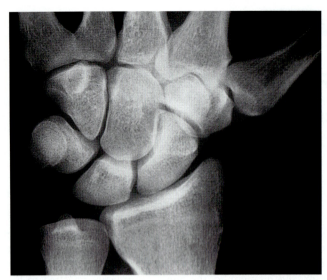

FIGURE 27.1. A plain anteroposterior x-ray of a normal adult wrist. Carpal alignment is maintained by a complex of extrinsic and intrinsic ligaments that hold the carpal interrelationships together with great amounts of stored-up potential energy and predisposition to collapse. If the restraining ligamentous struts and guy wires are rendered incompetent (by either injury or disease), the bones of the wrist will collapse into a more stable, but less physiologic, position. **Editors' Notes:** *Convenient terminology for the more stable, less physiologic position would be the neutral anatomy position. The normal anatomy position of any bone is maintained by its ligament support (normal anatomy). With a loss of the support mechanism from any cause, the bones will assume the position dictated entirely by their shape (neutral anatomy). Ulnar translation is the neutral anatomy position for the whole wrist. Flexion and supination of the scaphoid is its neutral anatomy position following scapholunate dissociation.*

aments of the triangular fibrocartilage complex (TFCC), supporting the intercalated proximal carpal row palmarly, from the medial side of the wrist.

The ligamentous "guy wires" that provide a coordinated mechanism for smooth kinematics among all intercarpal relationships during normal wrist motion are principally on the palmar side of the wrist (Fig. 27.2). Just as the radiotriquetral and scaphotriquetral (dorsal intercarpal) ligaments complete a dorsopalmar sling mechanism that anchors the carpus to the radius, the more important ligaments acting to maintain the intercalated proximal row segment in a precise position, suspended between the hand and the forearm, are concentrated on the palmar surface of the wrist. Their orientation from the center of the "hand" (the capitate) to the lateral and medial sides of the volar proximal row (the scaphoid and triquetrum, respectively) and from the forearm to the lateral and medial sides of the proximal row create a central area of the carpus relatively devoid of ligamentous support tissue. This space (Fig. 27.4) was described in 1911 by Poirier, and is still commonly referred to as "the space of Poirier" (1). It is through this particular area that most of the more common patterns of carpal collapse and resultant mechanical instability manifest themselves.

It would be a gross oversimplification of carpal mechanics to regard the entire three-bone proximal row relationship as a rigid free body in space, suspended between the hand and the forearm. Strong intrinsic intercarpal ligaments do hold the scaphoid and the triquetrum intimately to the lunate (Fig. 27.5), but an understanding of the fine details of anatomy of these three bones, and the anatomy of

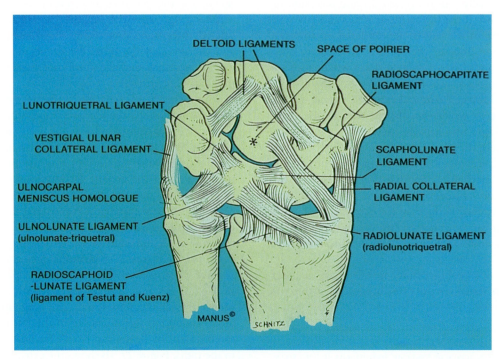

FIGURE 27.2. The schematic anatomy of the palmar extrinsic and intrinsic ligaments of the wrist.

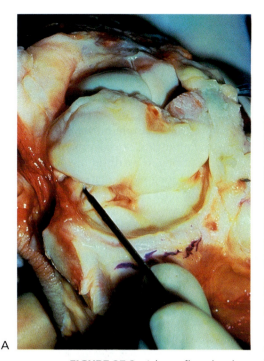
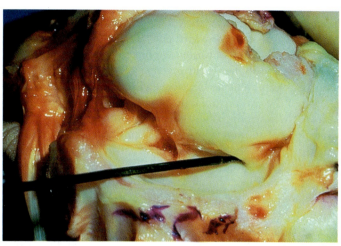

FIGURE 27.3. A hyperflexed cadaver right wrist viewed from the dorsum. **A:** The probe tip rests between the palmar radioscaphocapitate ligament to the left and the long radiolunate (radiolunatotriquetral) ligament to the right. **B:** The probe points to the extrinsic palmar disc–carpal ligaments, important in maintaining a normal mechanical relationship between the medial column of the carpus and the distal ulna.

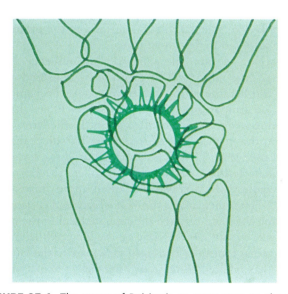

FIGURE 27.4. The space of Poirier is an open area on the palmar side of the carpus and is defined by the paucity of ligamentous support tissue that exists between the extrinsic and intrinsic ligaments of the medial and lateral sides of the wrist. It is through the space of Poirier that many wrist instability patterns manifest themselves.

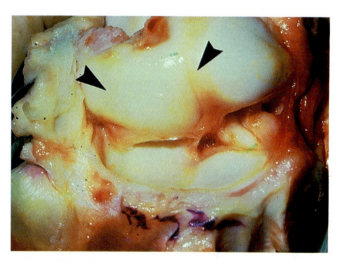

FIGURE 27.5. This cadaver dissection demonstrates the integrity of the dorsal scapholunate and lunotriquetral intrinsic ligaments. At first glance, it appears that the intimacy of these three bones allows the entire proximal carpal row to behave as a rigid body in space; the reality is that intricate kinematics take place among the three bones. Motion between the scaphoid and the lunate and between the lunate and the triquetrum is responsible in part for the normal fluid mechanics of the wrist. The *left arrow* points to the lunotriquetral ligament; the *right arrow* points to the scapholunate ligament.

the two intrinsic ligaments that function primarily to hold the three bones together, will help the student of carpal pathophysiology with a clear perspective of the events that lead to carpal instability.

Perhaps the most significant of these subtle details of anatomy is the difference in radius of curvature between the lunate and the proximal pole of the scaphoid. The radius of the proximal articular surface of the lunate is considerably greater than the radius of the proximal pole of the scaphoid (Fig. 27.6). These subtle but consistent architectural differences between the two bones (held together by a complicated interosseous scapholunate ligament) allow a different rate of rotation of the two proximal poles with wrist flexion and extension. These striking differences provide the foundation for reciprocal motion within the carpus and were first recognized in the laboratory and reported by Kauer (2–5). Kauer's careful anatomic dissections of the adult carpus not only clearly defined differences in rates of rotation but also provided the fine details of anatomy of the scapholunate ligament, which allows differential rotation while still providing stability. Particularly important was his desciption of the fundamental differences between the palmar and dorsal portions of this important structure.

The dorsal fibers of the ligament are thick, short, and relatively unyielding; the palmar fibers are loose, elastic, and less dense. The orientations of the individual fibers comprising these two segments of the ligament are responsible for allowing the scaphoid and the lunate to rotate at different rates in the flexion–extension arc. In extension, the short, dense fibers of the dorsal ligament support the relationship between these two bones intimately and tightly; the ratio of motion between the two bones in the extension arc is 1:1. In flexion, however, the two-bone relationship remains hinged dorsally, but loose palmarly, allowing the ratio of scaphoid rotation vs. lunate rotation to be 2:1 (Fig. 27.7). Berger et al. (6) further delineated the functional anatomy of the scapholunate ligament by dividing it into three components: dorsal, proximal, and palmar. Although not the strongest extrinsic or intrinsic ligament in the wrist (e.g., the long radiolunate portion of the radiolunatotriquetral ligament is much stronger) (2–8), the scapholunate interosseous ligament is of critical value in maintaining carpal alignment. Figure 27.8 is a true lateral x-ray of a normal wrist; the longitudinal axis of the third metacarpal and the longitudinal axis of the radius are collinear. The scaphoid is maintained at an attitude approximately 47° relative to the longitudinal axis of the hand–forearm unit. Physiologic load delivered to the distal pole of the scaphoid creates an internal force-couple; the principal axis along which load is delivered to the distal pole is more palmar than the axis along which this load is transferred to, and absorbed by, the elliptical scaphoid fossa of the radius. The force-couple within the scaphoid establishes a high propensity for the scaphoid to collapse into a more stable, but less physiologic, position under physiologic or superphysiologic loads. By anchoring the scaphoid to the lunate, the scapholunate interosseous ligament plays an integral role in neutralizing the propensity of the scaphoid to flex under load.

If separated from the palmarflexing influence of the scaphoid, the lunate will be predisposed to extend under load, also because of internal force-couple mechanics. In both the frontal and lateral planes, the lunate has an anatomic wedge-shaped configuration. In the lateral projection, the palmar pole of the lunate is "taller" than its dorsal pole (Fig. 27.9). The proximal articular surface of the lunate rests on a relatively flat, spherical fossa of the distal radius, which is palmarly tilted approximately 10° to 12°. The principal axis through which load is transmitted from the hand through the capitate head to the lunate is parallel to, but not the same as, the longitudinal principal axis that transmits load from the lunate to the forearm. Kauer has referred to these two parallel principal axes as "nonaxisymmetric" axes of rotation (2–5) (Fig. 27.10). By studying the three drawings in Fig. 27.10, the reader gains an appreciation of how nonaxisymmetric axes of rotation through the lunate create an internal force couple, albeit minor, relative to the force couple within the scaphoid (see above). With the palmar pole of the lunate "taller" than the dorsal pole, and with the support platform of the lunate fossa of the distal radius tilted palmarly 10° to 12°, if separated from the palmarflexing influence of the scaphoid, the lunate will naturally rotate into an extended posture. This rotation into a more mechanically (but less

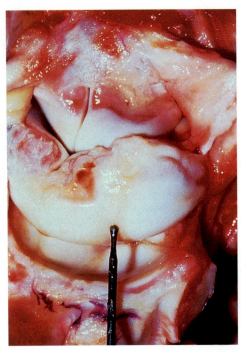

FIGURE 27.6. The proximal pole of the scaphoid and the proximal pole of the lunate have different radii of curvature.

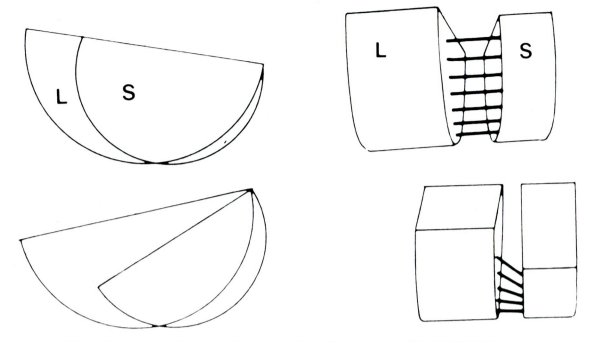

FIGURE 27.7. Because they are anchored dorsally by the short, dense fibers of the scapholunate ligament, the scaphoid and lunate will extend together in a ratio of 1:1; however, the loose, areolar palmar portion of the ligament will allow the different proximal pole radii of curvature to flex the scaphoid relative to the lunate in a ratio of 2:1. S, scaphoid; L, lunate.

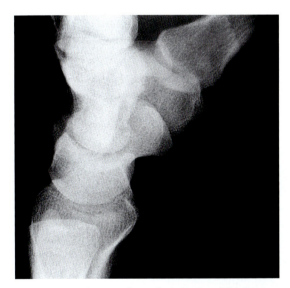

FIGURE 27.8. On the true lateral projection (third metacarpal and radius collinear), the longitudinal axis of the scaphoid is approximately 47°. Load is delivered to the distal pole of the scaphoid along an axis more palmar than the axis along which load is transmitted from the proximal pole of the scaphoid to the radius. This mechanical fact creates an internal force-couple with the body of the scaphoid and a constant tendency for this bone to flex out of its normal, resting 47° position, maintained by ligamentous struts and guy wires.

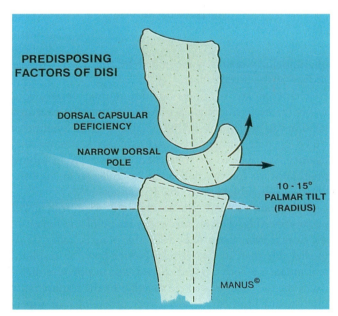

FIGURE 27.9. If the lunate is separated from the palmarflexing influence of the scaphoid, it will tend to extend. The narrower dorsal pole of the lunate, the paucity of dorsal capsular tissue, and the 10° to 15° palmar tilt of the radius are a few of the minor reasons this takes place; Fig. 27.10 emphasizes the major reason. **Editors' Notes:** *If a lunate is thinner volarly (V-type lunate), its neutral anatomy position would be just the reverse of this diagram.*

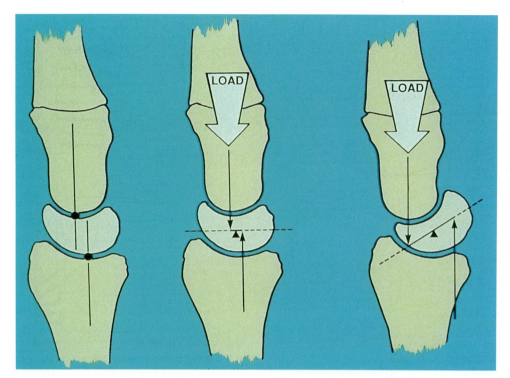

FIGURE 27.10. The radiocarpal and midcarpal axes of load-bearing through the lunate are parallel but not collinear; the distal axis is more dorsal than the proximal axis. This biomechanical fact sets up an internal force-couple within the lunate under load. If separated from the palmarflexing influence of the scaphoid, the lunate will tend to extend. This tendency to extend is neutralized by the integrity of the interosseous scapholunate ligament.

physiologic) position is facilitated by the tilted articular surface of the distal radius.

The complex of fibers of the normal interosseous scapholunate ligament anchor the two bones together in a relationship which, by definition, has a great amount of stored-up potential energy (2–10). If this key restraining ligament is ruptured or attenuated, there exists an inborn predisposition for the two bones to collapse in opposite directions, in a highly predictable manner.

If the reader observes the normal adult wrist from an AP perspective (Fig. 27.11), the wedge shape of the lunate in the frontal plane can also be seen; this bone is "taller" at its medial side than its lateral side. Notice how the scaphoid and lunate are both wedged-shaped, but in opposite directions; the two wedges are held together by the scapholunate interosseous ligament. Under either physiologic or superphysiologic load, the blunt bullet-shaped head of the capitate (in neutral position, located immediately distal to the scapholunate ligament) will tend to drive these two wedges apart, resulting in scapholunate instability or dissociation.

Linscheid and Dobyns, in their classic 1972 article on carpal instability, referred to the collapsed posture of the lunate (separated from the palmarflexing influence of the scaphoid) as "dorsiflexion intercalated instability" or DISI (10). If the reader clearly recognizes that the scaphoid and the triquetrum are intimately anchored to the lunate (the central keystone of the proximal carpal row), then he or she will understand that as the lunate moves, so moves the entire proximal row relative to the hand (the distal carpal row) and relative to the forearm (the radius and ulna) (7). This simple concept gives rise to the definition of reciprocal carpal motion. In wrist extension, the lunate extends

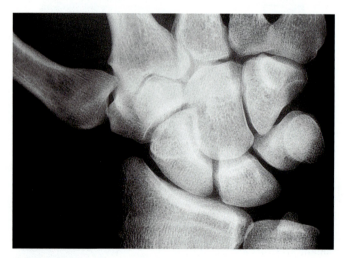

FIGURE 27.11. An anteroposterior x-ray of the adult wrist clearly reveals how the scaphoid and lunate are both wedge shaped, but in opposite directions. The medial edge of the lunate in the frontal plane is much "taller" than its lateral edge. Under load, there is a constant mechanical tendency for these two bones (wedges) to separate.

and shifts to the radius palmarly; the lunate simultaneously shifts to the capitate dorsally (4). In wrist flexion, the lunate shifts to the radius dorsally and to the capitate palmarly. This concept of reciprocal motion of the wrist simply means that in ulnar deviation of the wrist, the lunate shifts to the radius palmarly as well as to the capitate palmarly; in radial deviation, the lunate shifts to the radius dorsally and to the capitate dorsally.

To fully appreciate the dynamics of carpal instability, the reader of this chapter should understand the following: (a) lunate rotation will lead to simultaneous movement at both the radiocarpal and midcarpal levels; (b) the distal and proximal articular surfaces of the lunate have two nonaxisymmetric centers of rotation; (c) there is a consistent tendency of the lunate to rotate into extension if separated from the palmarflexing influence of the scaphoid; (d) physiologic movement of the lunate is dependent on the wedge shape of the lunate in both the lateral and frontal planes; and (e) there is a moving tendency of the scaphoid and lunate to separate from each other under load; therefore, the scapholunate interosseous ligament will always be tense (2–7,9,10).

With a clear appreciation of normal scaphoid and lunate mechanics as described in detail above, it is easy to understand how rupture or attenuation of the ligament that normally supports their relationship will always result in a scapholunate "gap." When we request the so-called "axial loading grip" AP x-ray in our patients with localized scapholunate tenderness following trauma, we hope to be able to demonstrate radiographically how scapholunate instability can manifest itself under load (Fig. 27.12). Complete loss of all ligamentous support between the scaphoid and lunate will result in classic scapholunate dissociation with rotary subluxation of the scaphoid (Fig. 27.13). As seen in this AP x-ray, if separated from the palmarflexing influence of the scaphoid, the lunate will rotate into extension (DISI collapse deformity). The internal force couples within both the scaphoid and the lunate are mechanically responsible for the final resting posture of these two bones following their pathologic dissociation from each other.

The lunate and the triquetrum are even more intimately attached to each other. In radial deviation, the triquetrum shifts 2 to 3 mm proximal (relative to the lunate); in ulnar deviation, the triquetrum shifts 2 to 3 mm distal (again, relative to the lunate). Otherwise, in flexion and extension of the wrist, the two bones move together in a ratio of 1:1.

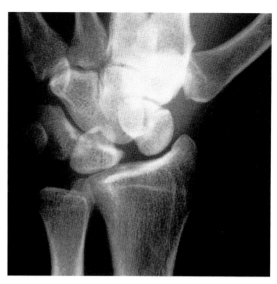

FIGURE 27.13. An anteroposterior x-ray of the wrist showing classic scapholunate dissociation with rotary subluxation of the scaphoid. Note the wide scapholunate diastasis, the triangular appearance of the extended lunate, and a "ring–pole" distance of the flexed scaphoid less than 7 mm.

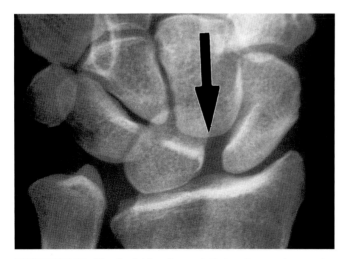

FIGURE 27.12. The "axial-loading grip" view is an anteroposterior (AP) x-ray taken with the patient's forearm in supination and the wrist centered on the cassette. The image is taken as the patient actively grips as tightly as possible, increasing the joint reaction force within the wrist and trying to drive the capitate head between the wedge-shaped scaphoid and lunate bones. In the presence of an incompetent scapholunate ligament (either ruptured or attenuated), the normal relationship of the scaphoid and lunate bones cannot be maintained under load; they will tend to separate. This x-ray demonstrates separation under the increased load of the "grip" view; the patient's resting AP x-ray was normal. The *arrow* represents axillary load, transmitted from the hand to the forearm.

CARPAL KINEMATICS

As the hand–forearm unit is brought into radial deviation, there are complicated but predictable mechanical changes that occur to the resting relationships among the carpal bones. As the distance between the "hand" (the trapezium and distal carpal row) and forearm (the radius) decreases in radial deviation, the joint reaction force on the distal and proximal poles of the scaphoid will increase; the scaphoid will be literally forced into an attitude more perpendicular to the plane of the palm. As the scaphoid flexes, the entire proximal carpal row will be dragged into flexion by (a) the palmarflexing influence of the scaphoid on the lunate (through the intact scapholunate ligament) and (b) through the influence of the lunate on the triquetrum [through the intact lunatotriquetral (LT) ligament]. With radial deviation, the entire medial aspect of the hand (the hamate) is mechanically disengaged from its relationship with the triquetrum along the helicoidal triquetrohamate interface. Notice how the trapezium and trapezoid ride dorsally and proximally onto the neck of the scaphoid and how the triquetrohamate helicoidal joint becomes disengaged. I prefer to call this latter position the "hamate-high" posture.

As the cadaver hand–forearm unit is moved into loaded ulnar deviation, a variety of changes occur. The hamate migrates into a "low" position, fully engaged along the helicoidal triquetrohamate interface. Active engagement of the triquetrohamate joint at the medial column of the wrist actually pushes the triquetrum into extension (Fig. 27.14). This process is both active and dynamic: as the triquetrum is extended in wrist ulnar deviation, the lunate is also extended by torquing force applied through the intact LT ligament. As separation between the hand (the trapezium and trapezoid) and the forearm increases in ulnar deviation, the scaphoid will be pulled into a more longitudinal attitude and extended with the lunate and the triquetrum. In ulnar deviation, the triquetrohamate helicoidal joint takes on a horizontal orientation, which is much more effective for load transmission, as the principal axis passes through the medial column of the wrist. It is instructive to compare the dynamics of medial column engagement and disengagement as the hand–forearm unit swings from radial to ulnar deviation. The differences between these two positions also reveal radiographically the dramatic change in the position of the lunate relative to the spherical lunate fossa of the radius. In ulnar deviation, the carpal-shift influence of the scaphoid on the lunate (through the intact scapholunate ligament) pulls the entire lunate onto the flat, spherical articular surface of the lunate fossa of the radius. There is essentially no lunate load being borne by the triangular fibrocartilage in this positon. The principal axis of load bearing passes from the hand through the medial head of the capitate, through the extended lunate, and into the forearm directly through the lunate fossa of the radius. In radial deviation, the scaphoid is driven into a relative perpendicular attitude as its proximal pole is guided ulnarly along the elliptical scaphoid fossa of the distal radius. This action displaces the flexing lunate medially, placing it much less squarely on the articular surface of the distal radius. As the entire proximal row pivots under the head of the capitate, the principal axis of load transmission across the wrist moves laterally, through the proximal pole of the scaphoid and through the elliptical scaphoid fossa of the distal radius.

Figure 27.15 is a schematic representation of the dynamics of radial and ulnar deviation of the wrist. In radial deviation, the medial column is completely disengaged and assumes a passive role in hand–forearm load transmission. Separation at the triquetrohamate joint occurs as the scaphoid simultaneously is actively driven into a flexed attitude. In ulnar deviation, the hamate drives the triquetrum (and the entire proximal row) into extension, as separation of the hand and the forearm affords the opportunity the scaphoid needs to be pulled up into a more longitudinal attitude. Note the changing position of the lunate relative to the lunate fossa of the radius.

Let us review the important factors that contribute to the anatomic and mechanical relationship between the scaphoid and the lunate: (a) the wedge shapes of these two bones, in both the frontal and sagittal planes; (b) the "stop-action" of the trapezium and trapezoid on the dorsal neck of the scaphoid, as the hand (the distal carpal row) moves closer to the forearm in wrist extension and/or radial deviation; (c) different radii of curvature of the proximal poles of the scaphoid and the lunate, resulting in proximal carpal row "shifts" relative to both the distal row and the radius; (d) dorsopalmar "shifts" between capitate and scaphoid, leading to changes in scaphoid orientation; and (e) widening and closing of the palmar aspect of the scapholunate cleft with flexion and extension, respectively (enabled by an interosseous ligament with long palmar and short dorsal components).

In sagittal projection, the longitudinal axis of the hand can be schematically visualized as a third metacarpal and capitate, intimately bonded by strong, unyielding car-

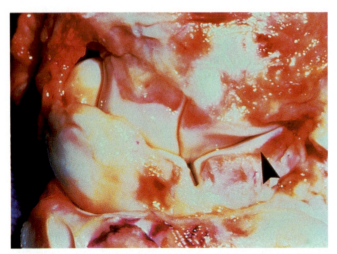

FIGURE 27.14. Active mediation of proximal-row extension by the medial column of the wrist, as the wrist ulnarly deviates, is dramatically demonstrated in this cadaver wrist. As the principal axis of load bearing moves ulnarly, the triquetrohamate joint is not only engaged, but the orientation of this helicoidal joint becomes horizontal and more suitable for transmission of load in the compression mode.

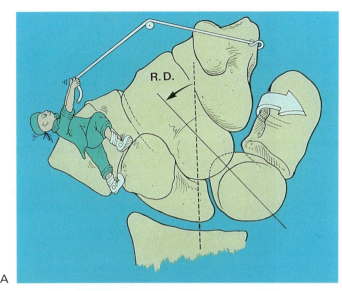
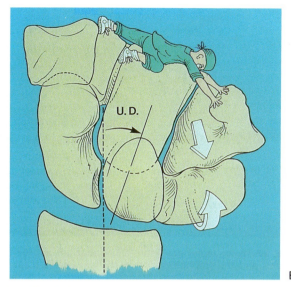

FIGURE 27.15. A: A schematic rendering of the wrist in radial deviation *(R.D.)* demonstrates the "hamate high" posture as the hamate is "pulled" into a disengaged relationship with the triquetrum. Concomitantly, the scaphoid is "pushed" into a perpendicular attitude as the trapezium (and the entire distal row) moves closer to the radius. **B:** In ulnar deviation *(U.D.)*, the hamate actively engages the triquetrum at the helicoidal joint, pushing the triquetrum into extension, while the separation of trapezium and radius along the lateral column allows the scaphoid to be "pulled up" into a longitudinal attitude. The lunate was pulled squarely onto the lunate fossa of the radius by the carpal shift.

pometacarpal ligaments (Fig. 27.16). The lunate (red) lies suspended between the capitate and the palmarly tilted articular surface of the radius. At rest, the lunate is maintained in neutral position, neither flexed nor extended. Figure 27.17 is essentially the same schematic, with the bony scaphoid and trapezium superimposed. The scaphoid is suspended at an attitude of approximately 47° in the "neutral" hand–forearm position. With radial deviation, the scaphoid is forced into a flexed attitude by an ever-closing space between the hand and the forearm. Through the palmarflexing influence of the scaphoid on the lunate, the lunate (red) will be pulled into flexion and displaced slightly dorsal on the articular surface of the radius (Fig. 27.18). As discussed above, if the lunate is separated from the palmarflexing influence of the scaphoid's internal force couple, it will move slightly more palmar on the spherical fossa of the radius and rotate into

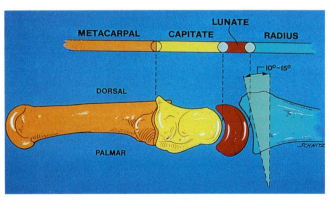

FIGURE 27.16. In neutral position, the longitudinal axes of the third metacarpal and the radius are collinear. The lunate *(red)* is supported in a "neutral" attitude, neither flexed nor extended.

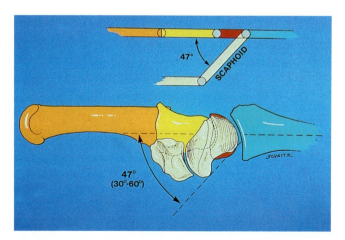

FIGURE 27.17. In this schematic, the scaphoid and trapezium have been superimposed over the lunate. The lunate is in neutral position; its natural tendency to extend is balanced perfectly by the palmarflexing influence of the scaphoid. Both bones transmit load through an internal force-couple mechanism acting in opposite directions. The neutralizing effect of the scaphoid on the lunate is through the intact scapholunate interosseous ligament.

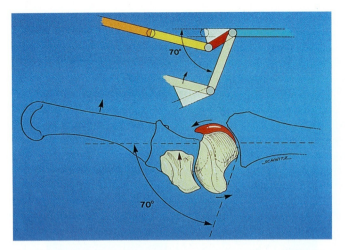

FIGURE 27.18. In radial deviation, the trapezium approaches the radius and the scaphoid is forced to flex. As the scaphoid flexes, it flexes the lunate (red) through the intact scapholunate ligament.

an extended attitude because of the nonaxisymmetric axes of rotation passing through the proximal and distal articular surfaces of the lunate (Fig. 27.19).

In 1981, Lichtman suggested that "the relationship of carpal bones might be thought of as a 'ring' with two mobile links permitting normal reciprocal motion between proximal and distal rows during radial and ulnar deviation" (11). This "carpal ring" concept not only suggests an anatomic link of the proximal row to the hand at both the lateral and medial sides of the carpus (Fig. 27.20), but is also consistent with a constantly changing principal axis of load transmission across the wrist, shifting from the radial side of the wrist in radial deviation to the ulnar side of the wrist in ulnar deviation. The "carpal ring" concept links the three-bone proximal row unit to the hand at the scaphotrapeziotrapezoid joint laterally and at the triquetrohamate joint medially. Load passes from the hand to the forearm in radial deviation through the lateral portion of this carpal

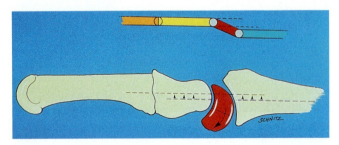

FIGURE 27.19. In this schematic, the lunate (red) has rotated into extension (dorsiflexion intercalated segment instability). If separated from the palmarflexing influences of the scaphoid, the nonaxisymmetric longitudinal axes of load bearing (radiolunate joint and midcarpal joint) establish an internal force couple, resulting in this predisposition to extend.

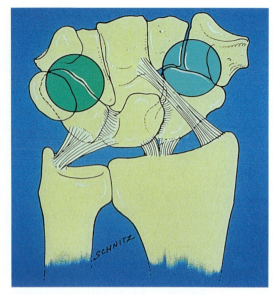

FIGURE 27.20. The "carpal ring" concept proposed by Lichtman in 1981 links the proximal carpal row to the "hand" (the distal row) at the triquetrohamate joint medially and at the scaphotrapeziotrapezoid joint laterally.

"link"; in ulnar deviation, load passes through the medial portion of the link (12).

The "carpal link" concept dovetails nicely with the columnar concept of carpal mechanics, first proposed by Navarro in 1921 (13) and revised by Taleisnik in 1976 and 1978 (14,15) (Fig. 27.21). Navarro's suggestions for undertanding carpal mechanics were based on his interpretation of anatomic relationships among carpal bones and the orientation of palmar support ligaments of the wrist. He divided the carpus into three "functional" columns: (a) the medial or rotational column, consisting of triquetrum and pisiform; (b) the central or flexion/extension column, consisting of capitate and lunate; and 3) the lateral or mobile column, consisting of scaphoid, trapezium, and trapezoid. Recognizing the intimate relationship of the trapezium and trapezoid to the hand, and appreciating the relative freedom of the distal pole of the scaphoid at the scaphotrapeziotrapezoid joint, Taleisnik modified Navarro's original ideas, producing a concept of medial and lateral carpal columns consisting of the triquetrum alone (the medial column) and the scaphoid alone (the lateral column) (Fig. 27.21).

The columnar concept of carpal kinematics is interesting in that almost a century ago, Navarro recognized that the manner in which load is transmitted from the hand to the forearm changes as the position of the hand–forearm relationship changes. We now clearly understand how the principal axis of load-bearing changes as the relationship between the hand and the forearm changes. The columnar concept of carpal mechanics and the carpal link concept are both clearly tied to the position changes of the principal axis as the orientation of the wrist changes in space.

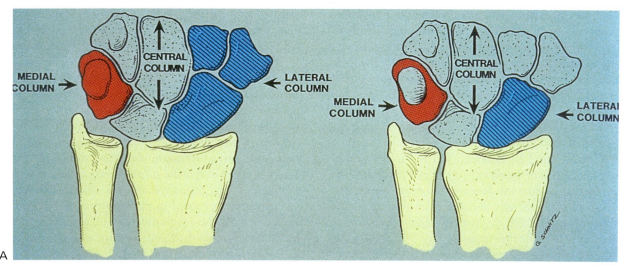

FIGURE 27.21. The columnar concept of carpal mechanics was first suggested by Navaro in 1921 **(A)** as a mobile lateral column (consisting of trapezium, trapezoid, and scaphoid), a central flexion–extension column (consisting of capitate and lunate), and a medial rotational column (consisting of the triquetrum and pisiform). **B:** Taleisnik revised Navarro's concept in 1976, based on a much more sophisticated understanding of carpal mechanics compiled over the intervening 55 years. In the Taleisnik model, the lateral column consists only of the scaphoid, and the medial column consists only of the triquetrum.

FAILURE OF THE SYSTEM

In the first part of this chapter, I attemped to explain normal carpal kinematics. The hand–forearm unit may seem, for all intents and purposes, to function as a ball-in-socket joint. The reality, though, is a great deal more complex. Ball-in-socket mechanics are actually small aggregate arcs of motion generated among each of the many articular surfaces that make up the carpus. These small additive arcs are precise and are guided by motor forces acting across the carpus, through the numerous ligamentous struts and guy wires discussed above. There are no muscle–tendon units that actually insert onto any of the carpal bones (the pisiform, although it appears to be the insertion of the pisiform, is actually a sesamoid bone suspended within the flexor carpi ulnaris on this tendon's pathway to insert at the base of the fifth metacarpal).

The carpal system fails either by the introduction of traumatic, destructive energy into the wrist or by the erosive effects of disease (e.g., rheumatoid arthritis). These two factors can promote carpal collapse by rupturing or attenuating intercarpal or radiocarpal ligaments, thus allowing dissipation of stored-up potential energy as the carpal bones collapse into a mechanically more stable, but less physiologic, attitude.

Carpal orientation is such that surface hyaline cartilage is always in compressive mode along the principal axis of load transmission. Within the limits of physiologic load, surface cartilage will thrive in compression (16–23). If the orientation of the carpus (with respect to load bearing) is changed by either injury or disease, then surface hyaline cartilage will be oriented to load transmission with a shear component. Although hyaline cartilage thrives in compression mode, it rapidly fails in shear (18). Microscopic shearing of the hyaline cartilage surface produces synovitis; enzymes released into the joint by the inflamed synovium create more cartilage destruction, which results in a vicious cycle of progressive degenerative change at those articular surfaces involved in pathomechanics.

The great majority of injuries to the wrist take place with the hand–forearm unit in extension (Fig. 27.22). The specific ligament failures that lead to pathophysiologic carpal instability always occur in tension. Under superphysiologic loads, ligamentous struts and guy wires that maintain

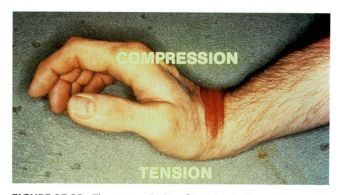

FIGURE 27.22. The vast majority of injuries to the wrist occur in extension, with tension forces established along the palmar aspect of the wrist and compression forces established along the dorsal aspect. Support ligaments of the wrist will fail in tension, but only under conditions of superphysiologic load.

normal carpal alignment may fail, leading to progressive carpal collapse. In addition to the common position of extension at the moment of impact load, if the hand–forearm unit is also in ulnar deviation, tensile forces will be propagated not only along the palmar aspect of the extended carpus but also along the radial border of the wrist. If the hand–forearm relationship is in radial deviation at the time of impact load, tensile forces will be propagated along the ulnar border of the wrist as well as the palmar border (Fig. 27.23). Whether ligament or bone will fail under pathophysiologic load will be based on the age of the patient, the patient's general health, the magnitude of the injury, the time action of load delivery, and the exact posture of the hand–forearm unit at the moment of injury. Two simple examples can help to further illustrate Fig. 27.23. (a) Visualize a 30-year-old healthy man running on the ice. He loses his footing; his feet slide out in front of him. In an effort to break his impending hard fall on the ice, he extends his outstretched hand behind him, thereby absorbing the entire load of his fall on his thenar eminence. Simultaneously, his wrist is driven by the hard ice into extension and ulnar deviation on a forearm that is being pronated by the momentum of the fall. The action of the pronating forearm on the fixed hand causes intercarpal supination. In this very common mechanism of injury, energy is delivered into the system radially and palmarly. The precise manner in which an energy vector is introduced into the system will result in specific tissue failure based on the four factors noted above.

Mayfield and Johnson (24), in their landmark 1980 cadaver study, referred to the predictable patterns of ligament and/or bone failure under the influence of this mechanism of injury as progressive perilunar dislocation. Their so-called "lesser arc" of injury finds the bolus of energy delivered into the radiocarpal relationship from the palmar-radial side (wrist extension, ulnar deviation, and intercarpal supination), through the scapholunate ligament, and along the path of least resistance into the space of Poirier. Damage may even be caused to the ligaments on the medial side of the wrist if the magnitude of injury and the degree of ulnar deviation of the hand–forearm unit is severe enough at the time of impact load (Fig. 27.24). Extension of the wrist beyond 95° at the time of impact, with less of an ulnar deviation component, will result in failure of the bony scaphoid rather than of the scapholunate ligament (25). Subtle changes in the position of the hand–forearm unit or in the energy level (or both) can result in a transscaphoid, transcapitate, or transhamate perilunar dislocation rather than the more purely ligamentous injury that results in scapholunate dissociation. In general, though, destructive energy introduced into the extended and ulnarly deviated

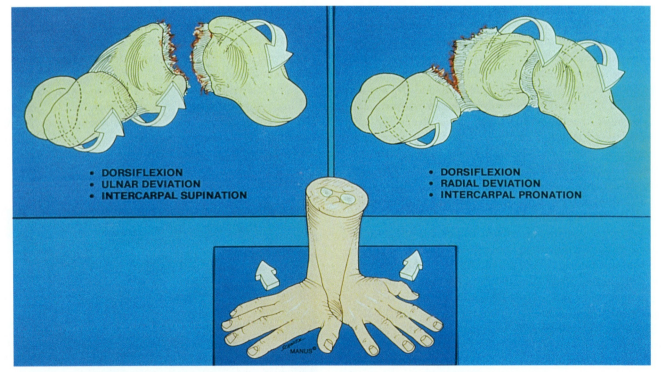

FIGURE 27.23. The position of the hand–forearm unit at the time of superphysiologic impact load is critical in determining which of the ligaments will fail. The addition of ulnar deviation to wrist extension will create tensile forces at the palmar and radial aspects of the wrist; damaging energy will enter the system from the palmar-radial border. If, however, the position of the hand–forearm unit is in radial deviation at the time of impact load, tensile forces will develop along the palmar and ulnar border, resulting in a completely different pattern of ligamentous damage.

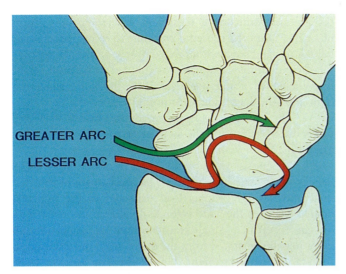

FIGURE 27.24. The age of this patient, the patient's general health, the precise position of the hand–forearm unit at the time of impact load, and the magnitude of superphysiologic energy delivered into the system by the mechanism of injury all determine the intracarpal pathway along which energy will be dissipated during injury. In Mayfield and Johnson's 1980 research (see text), two arcs of energy dissipation were described: a "greater arc" through bone and a "lesser arc" through ligamentous soft tissue.

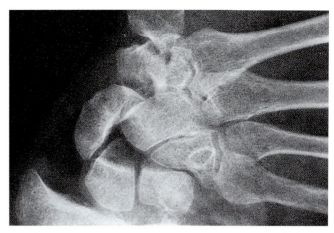

FIGURE 27.25. This reproduction of the original Mayfield and Johnson cadaver work on progressive perilunar instability clearly and dramatically demonstrates by x-ray how much ulnar deviation and extension are required in hand–forearm orientation to result in a stage I injury, the most minor in their classification of perilunar instability. The energy bolus enters the system along the palmar-radial border. It is sufficient to tear the radial collateral ligament and the long radiolunate ligament but will only partially injure the scapholunate interosseous ligament. (From Mayfield JK, Johnson RP, Kilcoyne RK. Carpal dislocations: pathomechanics and progressive perilunar instability. *J Hand Surg [Am]* 1980;5:226–241, with permission.)

wrist will injure the relationship between the scaphoid and lunate, most commonly at the scapholunate ligament.

Returning to Fig. 27.23, let us consider a second illustrative example. The same healthy 30-year-old in example 1 is now driving a car at 55 miles per hour with his hands securely on the steering wheel at the 10 o'clock and 2 o'clock positions. He is struck suddenly by another vehicle in the left front quarterpanel when the second car runs a red light. The steering wheel of the first car is violently spun to the right, as the driver grasps the steering wheel tightly, sensing the impending impact. The rotating wheel pulls his wrist severely (and instantly) into extension and radial deviation. In this scenario, the energy of injury will enter the radially deviated wrist through the tensile ulnar side, injuring the medial aspect of the carpus. Viegas et al. (26) have suggested a predictable pattern of injury based on this simple mechanism, which they refer to as "progressive ulnar-sided perilunate instability." Simply stated, superphysiologic loads delivered into the wrist in extension and radial deviation can result in destabilizing injuries to the relationship between the lunate and triquetrum.

Mayfield and Johnson (24) separated progressive perilunar instability into four stages, based on how much energy of injury would be delivered into the system. Their stage I injury is represented by Fig. 27.25, borrowed from their original published article. At the moment of impact load, there is a substantial extension and ulnar deviation attitude to the hand–forearm unit. A bolus of energy enters the system along the palmar-radial aspect of the wrist, tearing the extrinsic radiocarpal ligaments, but of insufficient magnitude to completely tear the scapholunate interosseous ligament. Schematically, stage I progressive perilunar instability is represented by Fig. 27.26; the radial collateral, the radioscaphocapitate, and a portion of the scapholunate ligaments have been injured. Because of its size and strength, the strong radiolunatotriquetral (i.e., long radiolunate) ligament deflects the energy of injury distally, into the substance of the scapholunate ligament, following a path of least resistance on its way to the space of Poirier (1). In a stage I injury there is not enough energy available to completely rupture the entire scapholunate ligament.

As reconstructive wrist surgeons, we must first and foremost be clinical anatomists. If the surgeon understands clearly the topographic and deep anatomy of the wrist, he or she can examine a patient with painful stage I progressive perilunar instability and elicit severe local tenderness by placing a palpating digit precisely on the dorsal scapholunate ligament. The patient's history of the mechanism of injury and a good physical examination are key elements in establishing a working diagnosis; because the scapholunate ligament has not been completely ruptured by the injury, plain, static x-rays (AP and true lateral) are frequently normal.

It is important for the student of wrist instability to appreciate that local tenderness precisely at the dorsal scapholunate ligament area can be attributable to basically four diagnoses: (a) scaphoid impaction syndrome; (b) occult dorsal carpal ganglion; (c) dorsal carpal impingement syndrome; and (d) dynamic scapholunate instability secondary to a partial interosseous scapholunate ligament sprain. The real charge to the reconstructive wrist surgeon

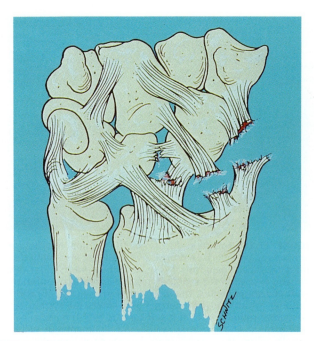

FIGURE 27.26. Diagrammatic representation of stage I progressive perilunar instability showing the residua of the injury: complete rupture of the radial collateral and radioscaphocapitate ligaments, but only partial remaining competency of the scapholunate interosseous ligament. The energy bolus has been deflected toward the space of Poirier by the strong, long radiolunate ligament but was insufficient to completely dissociate the scaphoid from the lunate.

is to sort out among these four diagnoses and to establish in the patient with chronic focal scapholunate pain and tenderness a definitive diagnosis. In order to accomplish this task, the surgeon has at his or her disposal a substantial diagnostic armamentarium, including provocative maneuvers and laboratory techniques. For example, establishing a definitive diagnosis of an occult dorsal carpal ganglion can be quite tricky; the typical patient presents with chronic pain, no particularly helpful history, and may be refractory to long-term conservative management (local steroid injections into the area, forearm-based thumb–spica splint immobilization, etc.); a high index of suspicion is necessary.

The definitive diagnosis of a true occult dorsal carpal ganglion (27,28) (no actual mass palpable on physical examination) can be made by ultrasound techniques (29–31) or by magnetic resonance imaging (MRI) (31–33). The former requires a fair degree of sophistication using the ultrasound equipment, but costs relatively little (unfortunately, the incidence of false negatives is quite high). The latter technique is much more sophisticated, has a much lower incidence of false negatives, but is considerably more costly. Diagnostic arthroscopy has also been advocated by some (34). My personal experience with diagnostic wrist arthroscopy for an occult dorsal carpal ganglion is that their usual location (at the more distal aspects of the dorsal interosseous scapholunate ligament) makes them very difficult to visualize with the 2.7-mm arthroscope, regardless of whether the 1,2-portal or the 3,4-portal is used. I continue to recommend to my fellows in hand surgery that they not rely on the arthroscope for their definitive diagnoses of this lesion because of the high incidence of false negatives. If the index of suspicion is high enough, diagnostic arthrotomy may be the best alternative. The interosseous ligament can be entirely inspected under direct vision, and the focus of myxoid degeneration or ganglionic fluid accumulation excised.

The diagnosis of scaphoid impaction syndrome relies heavily on the patient's history. The mechanism of injury is invariably a single impact load delivered to the hyperextended wrist. As the hand is forcefully driven into extension on the forearm, a small transchondral or osteochondral divot may be separated from the dorsal scaphoid adjacent to the scapholunate ligament. Unlike the low yield of bone scans encountered in attempting to diagnose occult dorsal carpal ganglion cysts, three-phase scintigraphy can be very effectively used to establish a definitive diagnosis of dorsal scaphoid impaction sydrome. MRI is of little value.

The last diagnosis to potentially confuse the picture of dynamic scapholunate dissociation is dorsal carpal impingement syndrome. The clinical presentation is usually in young athletes who spend a considerable amount of their training time creating extraordinary superphysiologic loads across the hyperextended hand–forearm unit. An excellent example of the "at-risk" athlete is the 17-year-old male gymnast with expertise in the pommel horse. These young men spend a great amount of time "squeezing" the synovium and dorsal capsule of the wrist between the hyperextended hand and the forearm. Over years of participation in the sport, the synovium will progressively thicken. Dorsal wrist pain may result when the athlete participates aggressively in those specific repetitive activities that initially caused the chronic synovial proliferation. The point of maximal tenderness in these patients is directly over the dorsal scapholunate ligament; this can become confusing with alternative diagnoses, such as dynamic scapholunate instability or occult scapholunate ganglion cyst.

The tissues overlying the scapholunate ligament in dorsal carpal impingement syndrome are usually thickened. The concentration of free nerve endings in the synovium and dorsal capsule make the "space-occupying" nature of this condition quite symptomatic for the patient. Once the wrist surgeon is comfortable with the working diagnosis, excisional biopsy of the hypertrophied synovial mass will result in cure.

Ruling out these other legitimate causes of chronic dorsal scapholunate tenderness leaves the clinician with the task (and responsibility) of making a definitive diagnosis of dynamic scapholunate instability after a partial traumatic tear of the interosseous scapholunate ligament.

It is important to remember that in stage I progressive perilunar instability (24), the clinician must search for signs of dynamic scapholunate instabilty; the energy bolus that created the injury was of insufficient magnitude to completely tear the scapholunate interosseous ligament. The definition of dynamic instability has been nicely carified over the past 10 years. The Nomenclature Committee of the International Wrist Investigators' Workshop (on which I have served for the last decade) has made a substantial effort to standardize the often-confusing terms used regularly in wrist research, both bench and clinical. Radiographically, standard AP and true lateral (the third metacarpal and the medullary canal of the radius collinear) x-rays of the wrist are normal in cases of true dynamic scapholunate instability, unless one of three things occurs: (a) a superphysiologic load is delivered across the hand–forearm relationship; (b) the position of the hand–forearm unit is altered to one of extreme ulnar deviation; or (c) the hand–forearm unit is moving as the x-ray is taken (e.g., in cases of cine- or videoradiography).

In the case of a normal wrist injured by the Mayfield and Johnson mechanism of grade I progressive perilunar instability described above, the relationship among all carpal bones on plain x-rays at rest is normal. As active axial-loading power grip is introduced to the system, and as the joint reaction force between the capitate (of the distal carpal row) and the scapholunate ligament (of the proximal carpal row) increases, the wedge shapes of the scaphoid and lunate bones (oriented in opposite directions, as discussed earlier in this chapter) will tend to separate (refer to Fig. 27.12).

THE USE OF PROVOCATIVE MANEUEVERS FOR ESTABLISHING THE DIAGNOSIS OF DYNAMIC SCAPHOLUNATE INSTABILITY

The diagnostic acumen of the clinician experienced in wrist pathology can be greatly enhanced by the use of provocative maneuvers in his or her physical examination of the wrist. One of the more useful techniques for delivering additional energy into the wrist for specific examination of the functional integrity of the scapholunate ligament was described by Watson in 1988 (35) and bears his name as the Watson maneuver; it is also referred to by some as the scaphoid shift test (36). The technique is performed relying on an intimate understanding of the fundamentals of normal carpal mechanics, as has been described in detail above (see also Fig. 27.14).

The examination is performed in the seated position, facing the patient across an examining table. With the patient's elbow on the table, and the forearm in neutral rotation (fingers toward the ceilng), the examiner's ipsilateral medial four fingers support the patient's dorsal radius (Fig. 27.27). The distal pulp of the examiner's thumb (same hand) is placed under the palmar aspect of the distal pole of the scaphoid. The examiner then uses his opposite examining hand to bring the patient's hand from ulnar deviation to radial deviation. The examiner expects the scaphoid to rotate from a longitudinal attitude to a perpendicular attitude relative to the plane of the palm (Fig. 27.28). If the palpating thumb will not allow this normal attitudinal change in the scaphoid to take place (simply by firmly pushing the thumb up under the scaphoid distal pole, as it is trying to flex), the kinetic energy being dissipated will be transferred from the distal pole of the scaphoid to its proximal pole. True lateral x-rays demonstrate that if the scapholunate ligament is competent, there should be neither pain nor "clunking instability" from the proximal pole. In the face of a partially damaged or an incompetent scapholunate ligament, a diagnosis of dynamic instability can be made by observing the behavior of the proximal pole of the scaphoid: as the wrist is passively radially deviated (with the examiner's thumb preventing rotation of the scaphoid into a flexed attitude), the proximal pole of the scaphoid will be lifted dorsally over the dorsal lip of the radius, creating pain and/or a palpable or audible "clunk" or "click." Findings must be interpreted based on a similarly performed Watson maneuver on the opposite, uninjured wrist. I have found this provocative maneuver for dynamic scapholunate instability to be of great value and teach my fellows in hand surgery to use it regularly and enthusiastically in their examination of the injured wrist.

As even more energy is delivered into the system by an injury of greater magnitude, the wrist will be stretched into severe ulnar deviation, extension, and intercarpal supination. There will now be enough energy to completely tear the scapholunate interosseous ligament and to separate the palmarflexing influence of the scaphoid from the lunate. This bolus of energy first tears through the radial collateral ligament; it then passes through the radioscaphocapitate ligament and is deflected distally by the very strong, palmar long radiolunate ligament (radiolunatotriquetral). The remaining energy bolus tears through the scapholunate ligament into the space of Poirier (1), where it dissipates in many directions. The damage that results eliminates the influence of the scaphoid and lunate on each other. Mayfield and Johnson described injuries of this magnitude as stage II progressive perilunar instability (24). The resultant static carpal collapse deformity is more commonly referred to as scapholunate dissociation with rotary subluxation of the scaphoid. With no restraining interosseous ligament left to neutralize the natural palmarflexing influence of the scaphoid under load, the scaphoid will collapse into a relative perpendicular attitude, allowing the LT unit to extend. The resultant DISI collapse deformity occurs secondary to the nonaxisymmetric axes of lunate load bearing described in detail above. When viewed schematically from the sagittal perspective, the bony scaphoid bridge linking the distal carpal row (i.e., the hand) and the proximal row has been lost, as the scaphoid collapses into a perpendicular attitude; the lunate rotates with the triquetrum into an extended posture.

The x-ray changes that occur with classic stage II progressive perilunar instability are widening of the scapholunate interval to greater than 2 mm (compared to the opposite, uninjured hand); a triangular appearance of the lunate, rotated into an extended posture; and a foreshortened

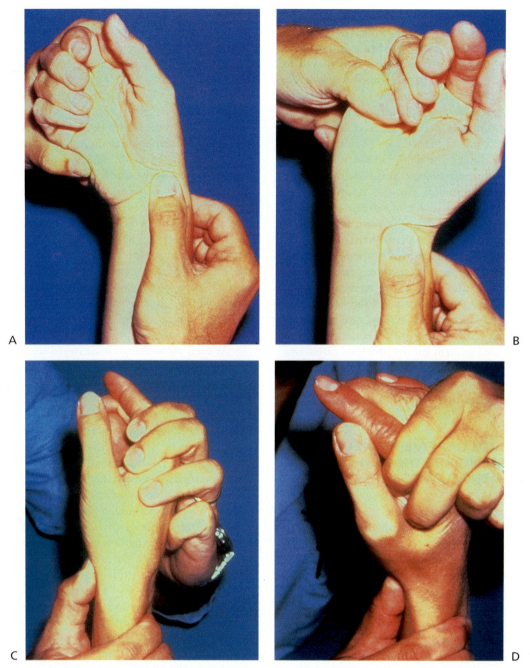

FIGURE 27.27. Frontal **(A,B)** and lateral **(C,D)** perspectives of the right wrist of a patient undergoing the Watson maneuver or scaphoid shift test. This provocative maneuver is performed to elicit signs of dynamic instability between the scaphoid and lunate in the presence of pain and tenderness in the scapholunate area.

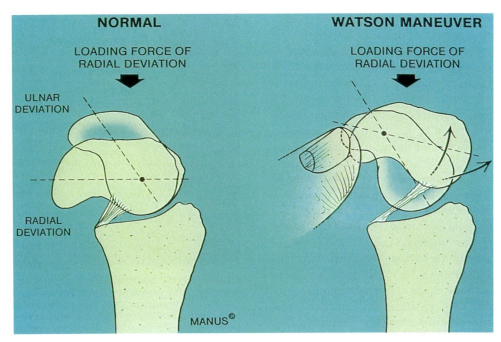

FIGURE 27.28. Normally, radial deviation of the wrist results in a physiologically flexed scaphoid as the trapezium approaches the radius (see text for normal biomechanics). The examiner performing the Watson maneuver tries to prevent normal scaphoid flexion with his thumb as the patient's hand–forearm unit is brought into radial deviation. In the face of dynamic scapholunate instability, energy during this maneuver will be transferred to the proximal pole of the scaphoid, which will then tend to lift out of its normal relationship to the elliptic fossa of the radius, producing a painful "click" or "clunk," relative to the opposite, uninjured side.

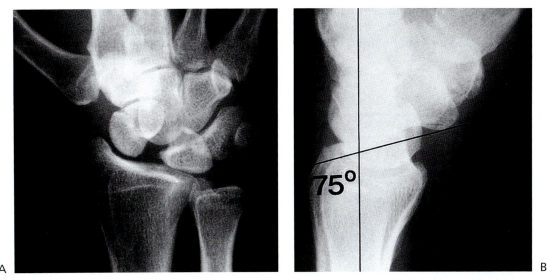

FIGURE 27.29. A,B: X-rays of the wrist showing classic scapholunate dissociation with rotary subluxation of the scaphoid. Note the dorsiflexion intercalated segment instability collapse posture of the lunate and the perpendicular attitude of the scaphoid. The scaphoradial angle is 75°; the scapholunate angle is approximately 110°.

scaphoid (Fig. 27.29). As the "ring" representing the distal pole of the scaphoid on the AP projection collapses into flexion, the distance between the "ring" and the proximal pole of the scaphoid will decrease to a value of less than 7 mm in an adult wrist (37–39).

Perhaps of greater value in making the diagnosis of classic scapholunate dissociation with rotary subluxation of the scaphoid is the true lateral projection; this x-ray will clearly demonstrate scaphoid collapse. In Fig. 27.29B, the scaphoid attitude is 75°, well outside the normal range of 30° to 60°, established in 1972 by Linscheid and Dobyns (10). The angle of the scaphoid relative to the longitudinal axis of the hand–forearm unit is measured by drawing the axis of the scaphoid, on lateral projection, through two points: the palmar surface of the proximal pole, and the palmar surface of the distal pole.

The normal lunate should appear in to be maintained in neutral position in lateral plain x-ray projection; it should be neither flexed nor extended when the hand–forearm unit is in neutral position. As I described above, with the assistance of schematic drawings, lunate rotation into extension can be predicted once its attachment to the scaphoid has been lost. The DISI collapsed posture of the independent lunate can be seen clearly on the true lateral x-ray in Fig. 27.29B. These lunate postural changes will take place whether disruption of the connecting link between the carpal rows is ligamentous (i.e., scapholunate dissociation) or bony (i.e., scaphoid fracture). If the bony scaphoid itself fails, the "link" will still be broken but will result now in lunate collapse into extension with the proximal pole of the fractured scaphoid. This pattern of collapse is still considered a carpal instability but is now associated with a bony rather than a ligamentous injury (Fig. 27.30). In either case, the carpus will collapse under load into a more stable, but less physiologic, position. Disrupting the "link" will allow stored-up potential energy to be dissipated as kinetic energy. Although technically more stable, load bearing through the principal axis of these new (collapsed) intercarpal relationships will create predictable shear forces on surface hyaline cartilage (16,18). The result, over years of pathophysiologic loading, is advanced degenerative change (40,41) (Fig. 27.31).

If even more pathologic energy forces the hand–forearm unit to the extreme of ulnar deviation and extension, tensile forces develop even medial to the head of the capitate. The mechanism of injury suggested by Mayfield and Johnson

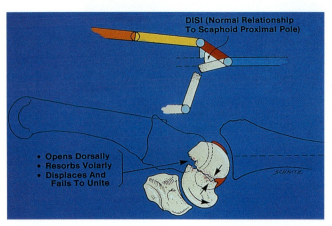

FIGURE 27.30. The scaphoid "links" the elements of the proximal carpal row to the elements of the distal carpal row. If either the scaphoid fractures or the scapholunate ligament ruptures, stored-up potential energy will be released as the proximal row collapses into a more stable, but less physiologic, attitude. In the diagram, after a displaced midwaist fracture of the scaphoid has occurred, the proximal pole will be dragged into extension by the lunate through the intact scapholunate ligament. As the lunate extends (nonaxisymmetric axes of rotation), the proximal pole of the scaphoid and the triquetrum will also extend.

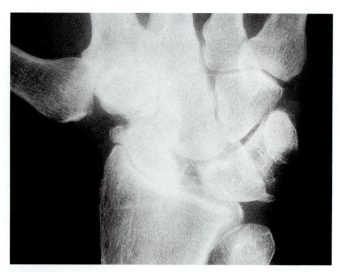

FIGURE 27.31. Scapholunate advanced collapse. This anteroposterior x-ray reveals the three major sites of severe degenerative change that occur over time in cases of untreated scapholunate dissociation with rotary subluxation of the scaphoid: radial styloid–scaphoid interface, proximal scaphoid pole–scaphoid fossa of the distal radius, and capitolunate joint.

from their cadaver work is simply the result of more energy being delivered into the system. This forces the axis of hand–forearm rotation further and further medial, even to an imaginary point outside the skin border of the medial wrist. In these injuries, the magnitude of the energy bolus is so great, and has to be delivered so rapidly, that ligamentous avulsion of bony carpal components may result. What portion of the triquetrum will fail will be based on the precise position of the hand–forearm unit at the time of impact load. A preponderance of ulnar deviation will lead to avulsion of the radial portion of the triquetrum by the radiolunatotriquetral ligament. More extension in the system will result in avulsion of the proximal portion of the triquetrum by the disc–triquetral portion of the TFCC.

If the magnitude of injury is even greater, the entire hand will be twisted from the forearm by an energy bolus great enough to tear first through the extrinsic palmar radiocarpal capsule, then through the scapholunate interosseous ligament into the space of Poirier (1), and then around the lunate through the LT ligament, sparing the palmar capsule attaching the body of the lunate to the radius (the radiolunate portion of the ligament of Testut and the short radiolunate ligament). This relatively common but catastrophic soft tissue injury to the wrist is referred to as a perilunate dislocation, the most frequent variation being the dorsal perilunate dislocation. This injury is incurred by severe wrist hyperextension, torquing intercarpal supination, and ulnar deviation. The dorsal perilunate dislocation results in the entire distal carpal row, the scaphoid and the triquetrum being dislocated dorsal to the lunate, while the lunate remains aligned with, and attached to, the radius. If the same mechanism of injury results in alignment of the capi-

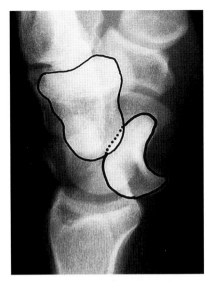

FIGURE 27.32. A lateral x-ray of the wrist demonstrating a palmar dislocation of the lunate. This injury represents the end stage of progressive perilunar instability of the wrist—the stage IV condition. Energy of extreme extension, ulnar deviation, and intercarpal supination results in pathologic tearing of all ligamentous tissue surrounding the lunate except the radiolunate limb of the ligament of Testut and the short radiolunate ligament.

tate and the radius, but with complete palmar dislocation of the lunate (Fig. 27.32), the final pathology is commonly referred to as a palmar dislocation of the lunate. In my personal experience, the majority of palmar lunate dislocations occur from failed attempts at closed reductions of dorsal perilunate dislocations.

PRIMARY INJURIES TO ULNAR-SIDED LIGAMENTS OF THE CARPUS

Earlier in this chapter, I described the significance of the hand–forearm position at the time of impact load in determining how pathologic energy enters the wrist system and how retaining ligaments of the carpus fail. In 1984, Reagan et al. (42) described what they believed was the pathophysiologic mechanism that resulted in injury to the LT ligament. As I mentioned above (and pointed out in my discussion of Fig. 27.23), radial deviation at the time of impact load is as critical to the development of LT injury as is wrist hyperextension. In a scholarly effort designed to quantify the degree of injury required to damage the main support ligaments of the medial column of the carpus, Viegas et al. (26) published their cadaveric load and motion studies in 1990. They proposed a progressive mechanism of injury leading to ulnar-sided perilunate instability. Their working hypothesis was that the ligamentous supports of the ulnar side of the wrist could be injured in a manner similar to that proposed by Mayfield et al., but obviously by a different mechanism.

By sectioning the LT interosseous ligaments of their cadavers, and subjecting the specimens to superphysiologic load, these investigators found increased motion between the lunate and the triquetrum under conditions of superphysiologic load but no evidence of either static of dynamic instability on x-ray. They referred to this as stage I progressive ulnar-sided perilunate instability. Laboratory sectioning of the interosseous LT ligament simulates a complete traumatic LT interosseous ligament rupture.

As a second stage of simulated progressive ulnar-sided perilunate instability, the authors sectioned not only the LT interosseous membrane but the palmar extrinsic terminal portion of the radiolunatotriquetral ligament as well. When these cadaver wrist specimens were loaded in a slightly flexed position, the authors were able to demonstrate a consistent dynamic palmarflexed (volar) intercalated segment instability (VISI) collapse deformity secondary to LT instability. These findings were particularly consistent if a palmar translational component was added to the load being placed on their specimens. Flexion of an intact scapholunate unit under load (with independent extension of the triquetrum) is consistent with a clinical diagnosis of dynamic LT instability. By anatomically sectioning the intrinsic LT interosseous membrane and the extrinsic palmar radiolunatotriquetral ligament, the authors were consistently able to simulate clinical dynamic LT instability.

Complete VISI collapse through the LT relationship can be achieved in the laboratory (using fresh, frozen cadaver specimens) only if the dorsal radiocarpal ligament is sectioned from the triquetrum (in addition to the divided interosseous LT membrane and the palmar radiolunatotriquetral ligament). If these three components are released from the triquetrum, this carpal bone will be rendered completely isolated from the lateral two elements of the proximal carpal row (the lunate and scaphoid). Under the palmarflexing influence of the scaphoid, the lunate will be dragged into a flexed attitude with the collapsing scaphoid. Figure 27.33 demonstrates an AP and true lateral x-ray of a 37-year-old man with classic static VISI carpal collapse secondary to a stage III LT injury. The following changes can be clearly observed: (a) a profoundly flexed resting attitude of the lunate; (b) the axis of the scaphoid almost perpendicular to the longitudinal axis of the hand–forearm unit; and (c) complete dissociation between the lunate and the triquetrum. As the lunate and scaphoid collapse together into flexion, the independent triquetrum extends.

The findings of Viegas et al. (26) were corroborated and published in 1989 by Horii et al. (43) from the Biomechanics Laboratory at the Mayo Clinic. These investigators found that "the essential lesion producing a static, palmarflexed intercalated segment instability (VISI) was division of the dorsal radiotriquetral and dorsal scaphotriquetral ligaments in association with the LT ligaments and interosseous membrane sectioning." Their sophisticated investigation techniques well documented the importance

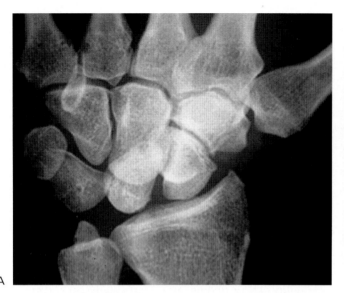 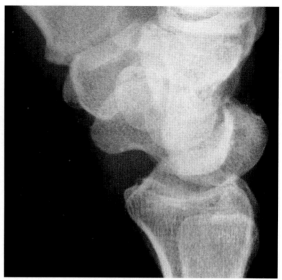

FIGURE 27.33. A: This anteroposterior x-ray of the carpus demonstrates stage III ulnar-sided perilunate instability or static lunatotriquetral (LT) dissociation. The scaphoid and lunate collapse into flexion together through the intact scapholunate ligament. The triquetrum extends, now independent of the lunate. **B:** Severe volar intercalated segment instability collapse deformity is demonstrated in the true lateral x-ray of static LT dissociation (stage III).

of complete palmar and dorsal separation of the triquetrum from the lunate in order to establish the pattern of static LT instability. The pathomechanics of static LT dissociation with VISI are defined by (a) the palmarflexing influence of the scaphoid as it pulls the lunate into flexion through the scapholunate interosseous membrane and (b) complete tearing of the dorsal extrinsic radiotriquetral ligament from the triquetrum in association with complete palmar LT ligament disruption.

DIAGNOSING LUNATOTRIQUETRAL INSTABILITY IN THE PRESENCE OF NORMAL PLAIN X-RAYS

Pain and tenderness within the medial aspect of the carpus and at the ulnocarpal area is an extremely common finding among patients following wrist trauma. Earlier in this chapter, I explained the importance of the patient's history in establishing a working diagnosis of wrist instability. Of even greater importance, however, is the clinician's ability to perform a skilled physical examination. Patients suffering from specific damage to the LT ligament will complain of topographic tenderness at the site of the LT ligament. It is incumbent on each of us as specialists in wrist pathophysiology to be able to determine the magnitude and specific site of injury to the wrist. Certainly, as I have shown in Fig. 27.33, if the patient has suffered a stage III lesion, the diagnosis will be easily confirmed by plain x-rays. Those patients who have local tenderness on palpation of the dorsal LT ligament but normal x-rays, require provocative maneuvers to help establish a definitive diagnosis. These maneuvers should be learned early and practiced regularly during the clinician's career as a wrist specialist.

More than a decade ago, I designed what I believe to be the most sensitive of these maneuvers and have referred to it consistently as the "shear test" (44–47). The mechanics of the technique are very specific to the LT joint; unlike other useful provocative maneuvers used to examine the LT relationship, there is no "spillover" into other areas of the ulnar side of the wrist, which might confuse the findings. Accuracy of the "shear test" depends only on the ability of the competent examiner to assure himself that no inflammation exists at the joint between the pisiform and the triquetrum.

The "shear test" for dynamic LT instability following injury is performed with the patient sitting at an examining table, opposite the examiner, with the elbow of the injured limb on the table; the fingers should be toward the ceiling, with the forearm maintained in neutral position (0° pronosupination). Neutral forearm rotation is the preferred examination position for all provocative maneuvers involving instability within the proximal carpal row. The examiner should then stabilize the patient's forearm by placing his opposite medial four fingers along the dorsal distal portion of the radius. His examining thumb is placed squarely on the palmar surface of the pisiform. The opposite examining thumb is placed on the dorsal body of the lunate; the specific site can be palpated by first finding

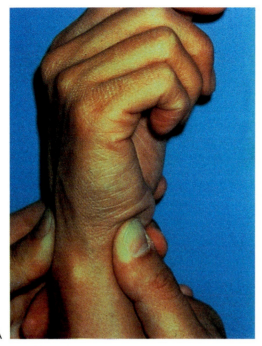 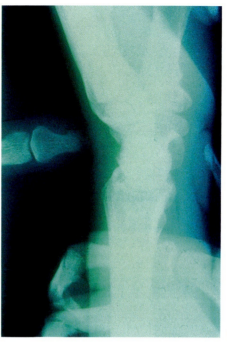

FIGURE 27.34. Clinical **(A)** and radiographic **(B)** examples of the "shear test" being properly performed. One of the examiner's thumbs compresses the pisotriquetral joint by direct palmar pressure on the pisiform; the contralateral thumb stabilizes the dorsal body of the lunate. Gently pushing the two examining thumbs together converts compression at the pisotriquetral joint to shear at the lunatotriquetral (LT) joint. If the "shear test" is properly administered, even the most minor of LT ligament injuries will be painful to the patient.

the distal medial corner of the dorsal radius, then moving the thumb distally onto the proximal row (Fig. 27.34). The thumb will fall directly onto the dorsal body of the lunate. The two examining thumbs are pushed toward each other, creating a shearing force across the LT joint (Fig. 27.35). Compression of the pisotriquetral joint is converted to shear at the LT joint, as long as the opposite thumb stabilizes the lunate.

The "shear test" is very specific for pathology at the LT joint. One of the most significant advantages of the maneuver is that the examiner has full control of how much energy will be delivered into the system. Even minor sprains of the LT ligament can be detected by subtle manipulation of the examiner's two thumbs. Energy can be literally titrated into the wrist. A positive "shear test" will be manifest as LT pain, not present when the maneuver is performed on the contralateral wrist for comparison. I prefer using the "shear test" for diagnosing dynamic instability of the LT joint because of its specificity and subtle nature.

The "shuck sign," described by Reagan et al. (42), is similar to the "shear test" described in detail above, but less subtle. A positive examination requires that a substantial amount of energy be delivered into the system by the examiner as he grasps the pisotriquetral unit with the thumb and index finger and rocks the unit back and forth in the AP plane, or "shucks" it (Fig. 27.36). The test is a bit less specific than the "shear test" because of energy spillover to tissues other than the LT ligament as the maneuver is performed. This provocative maneuver is also performed with the patient's elbow on the examining table, the forearm in neutral rotation, and the fingers

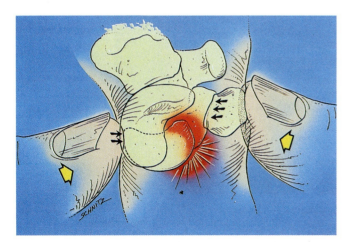

FIGURE 27.35. A diagrammatic representation of the "shear test." Pisotriquetral compression is converted to lunatotriquetral shear as long as the dorsal lunate is properly stabilized by the examiner's thumb.

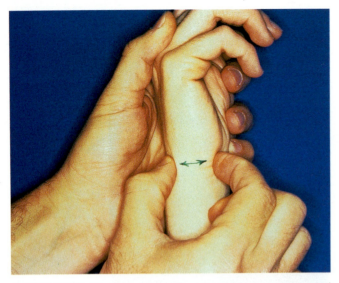

FIGURE 27.36. The "shuck" sign is a provocative maneuver used to examine the wrist for chronic posttraumatic lunatotriquetral (LT) instability. It is similar to the "shear test" but less subtle and much less for LT injury only. The pisotriquetral unit is literally rocked back and forth, or shucked, in the anteroposterior plane, thereby loading the LT ligament.

table, the forearm in neutral rotation, and the fingers toward the ceiling.

The third provocative maneuver I often use for examining the LT joint has been referred to by me and many of my colleagues as the "ballottement test." Figure 27.37 demonstrates the technique being performed, with the patient's wrist viewed from a dorsal and medial perspective. The forearm is maintained in neutral rotation (similiar to the provocative maneuvers described above), and the examiner's thumb is placed squarely on the medial border of the triquetrum. The examiner then pushes his thumb smartly against the triquetrum, which compresses the LT joint. If pathologic instability or inflammatory disease exists at the LT ligament, the patient will experience marked local pain.

Unfortunately, the ballottement test is not very specific for LT pathology. As the triquetrum is "ballotted," the energy delivered into the system not only creates a superphysiologic compression load at the LT joint (Fig. 27.38), but transmits load up the ≈22° angle of inclination of the radius to the scapholunate joint, and all along the extrinsic palmar radiocarpal ligaments. Unfortunately, lack of specificity of the "ballottement test" often results in confusion for the clinician, especially if wrist soft tissue other than the LT ligament have been damaged.

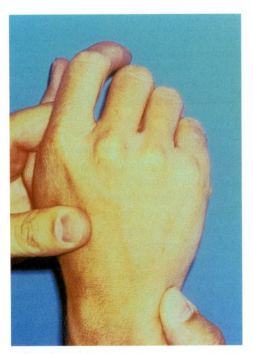 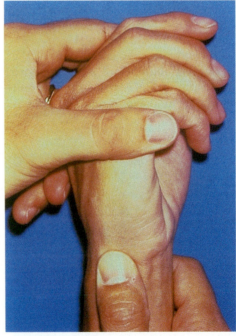

FIGURE 27.37. The "ballottement" examination for dynamic lunatotriquetral (LT) instability is the crudest of the three most commonly used provocative maneuvers but should be included in the wrist specialist's physical examination armamentarium. Energy is delivered by pushing, or "ballotting," the examining thumb against the medial border of the triquetrum. The purpose is to convert direct pressure placed on the medial border of the triquetrum to compression at the LT joint. Patients with inflammation at the LT joint will experience pain.

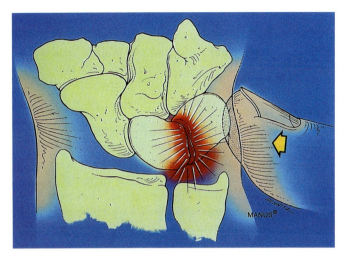

FIGURE 27.38. Unfortunately, the "ballottement" examination is the most nonspecific of the provocative maneuvers one should use to determine dynamic lunatotriquetral (LT) instability. Pushing the entire proximal carpal row up the angle of inclination of the distal radius will generate compression at the LT joint but will also put tension on a variety of extrinsic ligaments connecting the radius and ulna to the carpus. Incompetence or chronic inflammation of any of these injured tissues will result in pain outside the confines of the LT joint when the "ballottement" examination is performed.

INSTABILITY NOMENCLATURE

Major sections of this chapter have been devoted to understanding instability between the scaphoid and the lunate and between the lunate and the triquetrum. I have elected to focus most of my writing efforts on providing explanations that might facilitate the reader's understanding of how injuries (or disease processes) can alter the relationships among the three bones that comprise the proximal carpal row. These injuries, if severe enough, can have a profound effect on global carpal dynamics. Not only will patients afflicted by these changes have chronic wrist pain whenever involved in activities demanding superphysiologic loads across the carpus, but changes in bony carpal relationships will predispose the carpus to hyaline cartilage failure and degenerative arthritis.

Wright and his co-workers significantly influenced nomenclature relating to ligamentous damage within the carpus by their article on carpal instability nondislocations, published in 1994 (48). They used a system of carpal instability nomenclature that has only recently been adopted by the International Wrist Investigators' Workshop. I have served on the Nomenclature Committee of that organization for almost a decade and believe that this classification of ligamentous injury to the carpus makes understanding and describing carpal instability as easy as possible.

The authors refer to instability resulting from injury to the scapholunate or LT ligaments as *carpal instability disso-* *ciative* (CID) (48). Both scapholunate instability and LT instability fall into the CID category, regardless of whether the magnitude of injury results in either a static or dynamic change. Serious injury to either ligament will result in failure of the proximal row to function normally as a three-bone unit.

Carpal instability can also occur when there has been injury to neither the scapholunate nor the LT ligament. In these cases, the scaphoid, lunate, and triquetrum continue to interrelate normally as an intercalated proximal carpal row segment, suspended between the hand (the distal row) and the forearm. Traumatic instability can arise, however, either between the proximal row and the hand (the distal row) (11,48–52) or between the proximal row and the forearm (53). Carpal instability of this nature is referred to as *carpal instability nondissociative* (CIND) (48). Other common names for CIND between the proximal and distal rows are *midcarpal instability* (11), *capitolunate instability pattern* (50), *triquetrohamate instability,* and *ulnar-sided wrist instability,* to name a few (48,52). Other common names for CIND between the proximal row and the forearm are *radiocarpal instability* and *translational instability.* The advantage to the clinician of using the term CIND is that it emphasizes the integrity of the intercalated three-bone proximal row segment while signs of instability are still present elsewhere in the wrist.

The patient with classic midcarpal CIND presents with a history of chronic wrist pain, weakness, and a frequent, sudden, loud, and unpredictable "clunk" in the wrist. As the patient demonstrates to the clincian how he is able to generate this "clunk," he will clench his fist (to increase the load across the wrist) and move his wrist from radial deviation (with a small flexed attitude) to ulnar deviation (with a small extended attitude). As the hand–forearm unit approaches the ulnar deviation position, he will cause an audible and palpable "clunk," which can easily be heard across the examining room.

The radiographic hallmark of this type of CIND is a sagging, flexed posture of the entire proximal row, even though the longitudinal axes of the hand and forearm are lined up collinearly, in a neutral, resting position. This posture can be seen schematically in Fig. 27.39. Although the relationship among the scaphoid, lunate, and triquetrum remains entirely normal, the flexed attitude of the intercalated proximal row unit creates an unusual type of mechanical instability. If the hand–forearm unit remains in neutral position, and load across the wrist increases, then the "resting" flexed attitude of the proximal row will only increase.

In this type of CIND, the proximal row assumes an attitude expected only in normal radial deviation, even though the hand–forearm unit is in neutral position. The scaphoid is flexed, and the lunate and triquetrum flex through the palmarflexing influence of the scaphoid. Because the hand is ulnarly deviated, the proximal row does not move. Joint

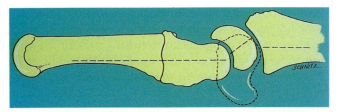

FIGURE 27.39. Schematic representation of midcarpal instability, the more common type of carpal instability nondissociative (CIND). With the hand–forearm unit in neutral position, the entire proximal carpal row "rests" in flexion (volar intercalated segment instability). This resting posture of the proximal row in midcarpal CIND presents as if the hand is in radial deviation relative to the forearm. The proximal row posture will remain unchanged as the wrist actively ulnarly deviates, until joint reaction forces at the malaligned midcarpal articular surfaces overcome the coefficient of friction, allowing the entire proximal row to instantly reduce against the articular surfaces of the bones of the distal row. This dynamic produces the so-called "catch-up clunk." Once the "clunk" is felt and heard, the helicoidal triquetrohamate joint is completely engaged, and the hand–forearm unit is in ulnar deviation.

reaction forces continue to increase across the midcarpal joint as the principal axis of load transmission through the wrist moves ulnarly toward the triquetrohamate joint. Because of the lack of fluid motion between the proximal and distal rows (in spite of ulnar deviation of the hand relative to the forearm), the joint reaction force increases until a critical load is reached along the helicoidal interface between the triquetrum and the hamate. At this critical point, the coefficient of friction preventing a smooth arc of proximal row motion is suddenly overcome. In a single instant, the entire proximal row "clunks" into a reduced posture, the attitude of which is the same as would be expected in normal ulnar deviation (see details above): (a) an extended triquetrum, completely engaged at the helicoidal triquetohamate joint; (b) an extended lunate; and (c) a longitudinally oriented scaphoid. This sudden reduction of the proximal row on the distal row is associated with a rather profound "clunk." Because this audible (and palpable) phenomenon is grossly delayed until a certain critical triquetrohamate load is generated in ulnar deviation, the entire mechanical process is referred to as a "catch-up clunk."

A consistent lesion responsible for midcarpal instability has not been identified. Hankin et al. suggested that injury to the palmar ligaments at the scaphotrapeziotrapezoid joint (including the lateral limb of the deltoid ligament) was responsible (53). Lichtman et al., however, have strongly suggested that the essential lesion is to the medial limb of the deltoid ligament (11) and have designed a frequently used surgical procedure to treat the problem. The precise details of the surgical reconstruction and its indictations and contraindications are beyond the scope of this chapter.

Another type of CIND (albeit rather rare) involves compromise to the main restraining palmar ligaments between the radius and the proximal carpal row (54). The major component involved is the long radiolunate ligament (see anatomic figures above). The carpus normally rests in balanced posture on a platform (the distal radius articular surface) that has a palmar tilt of approximately 10° to 12° and an angle of inclination of 20° to 25° (Fig. 27.1). Under load, injury- or disease-induced attenuation of the long radiolunate ligament will result in ulnar translation of the entire carpus down the angle in inclination of the radius to a more mechanically stable, but less physiologic, position. The fact that the entire proximal row collapses ulnarward as a unit defines this type of carpal instability as CIND as well.

In cultivating a general understanding of the dynamics of carpal instability, the reader should be aware that in extremely high-energy injuries, CID and CIND can coex-

TABLE 27.1. ORGANIZATION OF CARPAL INSTABILITIES

Severity	Direction	Location	Ligament Type	Acuity
Dynamic	DISI	Proximal	CID	Acute
Static	VISI	Distal	CIND	Subacute
Subluxation	Dorsal	Radial	CIC	Chronic
Dislocation	Palmar	Ulnar		
	Radial	Palmar		
	Ulnar	Midcarpal		
		Radiocarpal		
		Specific bone		
		Specific ligament		

CIC, carpal instability combined; CID, carpal instability dissociative; CIND, carpal instability nondissociative; DISI, dorsiflexion intercalated segment instability; VISI, palmarflexed (volar) intercalated segment instability.
Modified from Larsen CF, Amadio PC, Gilula LA, et al. Analysis of carpal instability: I. Description of the scene. J Hand Surg [Am] 1995;20:757–764; and from Hodge JC, Gilula LA, Larsen CF, et al. Analysis of carpal instability: II. Clinical applications J Hand Surg [Am] 1995;20:765–777.

ist. These rare injuries should be classified as *carpal instability combined* (CIC).

Amadio et al. have organized carpal instability into five basic categories in an effort to help the clinician accurately diagnose the responsible lesions and the resultant pattern of carpal collapse (55,56). Included among these categories are (a) the severity of the instability, (b) the direction in which the carpus collapses, (c) the anatomic location within the entire carpus in which the injury has occurred, (d) the type of ligament damage incurred (either CID, CIND, or CIC), and (e) the acuity of the injury. To facilitate the reader's understanding of this confusing subject, I have modified Amadio and his co-workers' ideas in Table 27.1.

SUMMARY

The carpal bones are maintained in normal alignment by ligamentous struts and guy wires, which hold them together with a great amount of stored-up potential energy and predisposition to collapse. If the restraining ligaments that hold normal anatomic intercarpal relationships are injured or rendered imcompetent in any way by disease, carpal bones will collapse relative to each other into more mechanically stable, but less physiologic, positions. The degree of collapse (as stored-up potential energy is converted to kinetic energy) is directly proportional to the magnitude of ligamentous damage. Each of the carpal bones of the intercalated proximal row, if isolated from the others, "wants" to collapse into a mechanically more stable position. Unfortunately, although the collapsed attitude may be more mechanically stable, it is also less physiologic. With continued motion and general use of the wrist, hyaline cartilage will slowly, but progressively, "melt away" under surface shear, leading to predictable patterns of degenerative arthritis, based on the type of instability.

If the three bones of the proximal row are maintained together as a free body in space and mechanically separated from the hand (the distal carpal row) by injury to either the medial or lateral limb of the deltoid ligament (see above), then under either physiologic or superphysiologic load, the entire proximal row will collapse into flexion, upsetting the synchronicity of normal carpal mechanics.

The pain and local tenderness that result from chronic dynamic or static carpal instability result first from abnormal loads being placed on damaged restraining ligaments. Abnormal alignment of carpal bones will irritate the joint lining and result in painful synovitis. As surface shear forces begin breaking down cartilage, the products of hyaline cartilage breakdown will cause even greater synovitis and pain. Eventually, the inflamed synovial tissue (and transudate of synovial fluid) will promote a more rapid cartilage breakdown. The result, as I have described above, is degenerative arthritis of the wrist with advanced carpal collapse.

EDITORS' COMMENTS

The wrist is unstable by design. The bones have a *normal anatomic position* and a *neutral anatomic position*. The neutral anatomic position is the position the bones would assume if not restrained. This position is based solely on the shape of the bones and is the position they will assume as inadequate or ruptured ligaments allow. The normal and neutral anatomic positions of the hip joint are the same. Some of the ligaments of the wrist are highly restricted, including short ligaments that will allow little or no play, such as the dorsal interosseous fibers of the scapholunate joint. Other ligaments, such as the radioscaphocapitate ligament, are more like spring lines on a boat; they are usually longer, and allow significant motion in certain planes, but restrict specific displacement.

The distal radius is sloped volarly and ulnarward, so major ligament restraints need only maintain the upslope position of the carpals. This frees the capsule from any major concern that the carpals will displace dorsally or radially. Hence, following a malunited Colles' fracture with a dorsally tipped articular surface, the wrist is prone to symptomatic capsular ligament overload, depending on the degree of patient activity. Ligaments exhibit large differences among individuals. Young girls have marked laxity, and x-ray studies can demonstrate major carpal displacements, yet these wrists transmit load without symptoms. Their cartilage is being loaded without shear and synovium is not being insulted by these displacements. The carpals are being adequately tethered in terms of unacceptable positions for load transfer. Similarly, an older man with tight ligaments may have complete rupture of key ligaments, but the remaining structures limit excursion to such an extent that synovium is not overstretched, cartilage is not abnormally loaded, and symptoms do not occur. The wrist that requires surgical attention may exhibit a spectrum of ligament injuries that produce symptoms with specific activities. Any patient may have successfully treated him- or herself by eliminating an activity, although the wrist anatomy is still deficient. Wrist injuries are cumulative, as ligaments heal poorly. Nearly 25% of the normal adult population demonstrates some difference in mobility unilaterally on scaphoid shift testing. It is only when sufficient attenuation or rupture has occurred that the patient develops symptoms that are only related to sufficient activity.

The most commonly damaged ligament system is the scapholunate interosseous ligament. The most common overload or trauma occurs in dorsiflexion of the wrist. This produces a significant spreading moment volarly between the scaphoid and lunate, enhanced by the capitate acting as an anvil, and the volar scapholunate system ruptures. Unfortunately, this ligament heals itself poorly. Subsequent trauma extends these volar tears until at some point there is an overload of the scapholunate joint with certain activities and a symptomatic wrist. The most common diagnosis of the wrist is *dorsal wrist syndrome*, which is a direct result of the inadequacy and susceptibility of the scapholunate ligament. It is probable that most static rotary subluxation of the scaphoid is the result of a terminal event superimposed on preexisting tears of the scapholunate system. Of course, a single significant injury is certainly capable of producing static rotary subluxation of the scaphoid, but this scenario probably occurs less frequently.

With modest scapholunate interruption, the scaphoid can displace under load. This is the most common etiology for wrist activity pain and postactivity ache. With severe loss of scapholunate interosseous support, the bones begin to assume their neutral anatomic position under lighter and lighter loads, eventually producing static malpositioning. The hamate–triquetral joint is one of the most lax and unsupported carpal relationships in the wrist. At surgery, a small nick in the dorsal capsule allowing air into the joint will let the hamate and triquetrum literally fall away from each other. There is almost never an indication for hamate–triquetral limited wrist arthrodeses, as rupture of the ligaments of this capsular system are tertiary or terminal events following rupture of a major portion of the radial-sided ligament systems. Thus, any tears of the hamate–triquetral ligament system are not responsible for instability patterns.

The capitate–lunate joint can become unstable. Although young girls can demonstrate complete dorsal dislocation of the capitate from the lunate fossa, when this occurs as a symptomatic phenomenon, usually in active patients in their thirties, it can require repair. We classify this as a homing instability, meaning that the carpals tend to reposition themselves toward normal, but have the ability to displace. A nonhoming instability applies to rotary subluxation of the scaphoid where increasing loss of ligament support results in increasing displacement of the scaphoid with no tendency to return to its home position. Homing instabilities respond to soft tissue procedures and ligament repairs. Reinforcement of the dorsal capsule between capitate and lunate is usually sufficient for a symptomatic wrist demonstrating this instability.

There are two major types of scaphoid instabilities: The classic type is loss of control of the proximal pole. The proximal pole separates from the lunate, escapes from the proximal capitate, and displaces dorsally while supinating. This escape of the proximal pole from beneath the capitate is the main symptomatic component. Another form of scaphoid ligament pathology occurs at the distal end of the scaphotrapeziotrapezoid (STT) or triscaphe joint. The plane of motion of the triscaphe joint is from radial dorsiflexion to ulnar volar flexion (the long axis of wrist motion). Loss of support results in lateral displacement of the distal pole of the scaphoid which shear loads the STT joint, resulting in the classic, isolated degenerative arthritis at this joint. Severe ligament injury at the distal end of the scaphoid results in flexion of the scaphoid in relation to the capitate, usually producing a severe volar intercalated segment instability (VISI) and is the cause of radial midcarpal instability (type III or IV). These wrists are significantly dysfunctional, and the patient can rarely escape surgery with modification of activities.

REFERENCES

1. Poirier P, Charpy A. *Traite de l'anatomie humaine, tome I.* Paris: Masson et Cie, 1911;226–231.
2. Kauer JMG. The interdependence of carpal articulation chains. *Acta Anat* 1974;88:481–501.
3. Kauer JMG. Functional anatomy of the wrist. *Clin Orthop* 1980;149:9–20.
4. Kauer JMG. The mechanism of the carpal joint. *Clin Orthop* 1986;202:16–26.
5. Kauer JMG. The carpal joint: anatomy and function. *Hand Clin* 1987;3:23–29.
6. Berger RA, Blair WF, Crowninshield RD, et al. The scapholunate ligament. *J Hand Surg [Am]* 1982;7:87–91.
7. Boabighi J, Kuhlmann N, Kenesi C. The distal ligamentous complex of the scaphoid and the scapho-lunate ligament: anatomic, histological and biomechanical study. *J Hand Surg [Br]* 1993;18:65–69.
8. Drewniany JJ, Palmer AK, Flatt AE. The scaphotrapezial ligament complex: an anatomic and biomechanical study. *J Hand Surg [Am]* 1985;10:492–498.
9. Linscheid RL, Dobyns JH, Beabout JW, et al. Traumatic instability of the wrist: diagnosis, classification, and pathomechanics. *J Bone Joint Surg [Am]* 1972;54:1612–1632.
10. Linscheid RL, Dobyns JH, Beckenbaugh RD, et al. Instability patterns of the wrist. *J Hand Surg [Am]* 1983;8:682–686.
11. Lichtman DM, Schneider JR, Swafford AR, et al. Ulnar midcarpal instability—clinical and laboratory analysis. *J Hand Surg [Am]* 1981;6:515–523.
12. Brown DE, Lichtman DM. Midcarpal instability. *Hand Clin* 1987;3:135–140.
13. Navarro A. Luxaciones del carpo *An Fac Med Montevideo* 1921;6:113.
14. Taleisnik J. The ligaments of the wrist. *J Hand Surg [Am]* 1976;1:110–118.
15. Taleisnik J. The wrist: anatomy, function, and injury. *Instr Course Lect* 1978;27:61–87.
16. Ateshian GA. A theoretical formulation for boundary friction in articular cartilage. *J Biomech Eng* 1997;119:81–86.
17. Suh JK. Dynamic unconfined compression of articular cartilage under a cyclic compressive load. *Biorheology* 1996;33:289–304.
18. Broom ND, Oloyede A, Flachsmann R, et al. Dynamic fracture

characteristics of the osteochondral junction undergoing shear deformation. *Med Eng Phys* 1996;18:396–404.
19. Kelly PA, O'Connor JJ. Transmission of rapidly applied loads through articular cartilage. Part 1: Uncracked cartilage. *Proc Inst Mech Eng [H]* 1996;210:27–37.
20. Kelly PA, O'Connor JJ. Transmission of rapidly applied loads through articular cartilage. Part 2: Cracked cartilage. *Proc Inst Mech Eng [H]* 1996;210:39–49.
21. Suh JK, Li Z, Woo SL. Dynamic behavior of a biphasic cartilage model under cyclic compressive loading. *J Biomech* 1995;28: 357–364.
22. Ateshian GA, Lai WM, Zhu WB, et al. An asymptotic solution for the contact of two biphasic cartilage layers. *J Biomech* 1994;27: 1347–1360.
23. Schwartz MH, Leo PH, Lewis JL. A microstructural model for the elastic response of articular cartilage. *J Biomech* 1994;27: 865–873.
24. Mayfield JK, Johnson RP, Kilcoyne RK. Carpal dislocations: pathomechanics and progressive perilunar instability. *J Hand Surg [Am]* 1980;5:226–241.
25. Weber ER, Chao EY. An experimental approach to the mechanism of scaphoid waist fractures. *J Hand Surg [Am]* 1978;3:142–148.
26. Viegas SF, Patterson RM, Peterson PD, et al. Ulnar-sided perilunate instability: an anatomic and biomechanic study. *J Hand Surg [Am]* 1990;15:268–278.
27. Steinberg B, Kleinman WB. Occult scapholunate ganglion: a cause of dorsal wrist pain. *J Hand Surg [Am]* 1999;24:225–231.
28. Sanders WE. The occult dorsal wrist ganglion. *J Hand Surg [Br]* 1985;10:257–260.
29. Bianchi S, Abdelwahab IF, Zwass A, et al. Ultrasonographic evaluation of wrist ganglia. *Skel Radiol* 1994;23:201–203.
30. Hoglund M, Tordai P, Muren C. Diagnosis of ganglions in the hand and wrist by sonography. *Acta Radiol* 1994;35:35–39.
31. Cardinal E, Buckwalter KA, Braunstein EM, et al. Occult dorsal carpal ganglion: comparison of US and MR imaging. *Radiology* 1994;193:259–262.
32. Miller TT, Potter HG, McCormack RR. Benign soft tissue masses of the wrist and hand: MRI appearance. *Skel Radiol* 1994;23: 327–332.
33. Vo P, Wright T, Hayden F, et al. Evaluating dorsal wrist pain: MRI diagnosis of occult dorsal wrist ganglion. *J Hand Surg [Am]* 1995; 20:667–670.
34. Viegas SF. Intraarticular ganglion of the dorsal interosseous scapholunate ligament: a case for arthroscopy. *Arthroscopy* 1986; 2:93–95.
35. Watson HK, Ashmead D, Makhlouf MV. Examination of the scaphoid. *J Hand Surg [Am]* 1988;13:657–660.
36. Wolfe SW, Gupta A, Crisco JJ. Kinematics of the scaphoid shift test. *J Hand Surg [Am]* 1997;22:801–806.
37. Bjelland JC, Bush JC. Secondary rotary subluxation of the carpal navicular. *Ariz Med* 1977;34:268–269.
38. Crittenden JJ, Jones DM, Santarelli AG. Bilateral rotational dislocation of the carpal navicular. *Radiology* 1970;94:629–630.
39. Thompson TC, Campbell RD, Arnold WD. Primary and secondary dislocations of the scaphoid bone. *J Bone Joint Surg Br* 1964;46:73–82.
40. Watson HK, Ballet FL. The SLAC wrist: scapholunate advanced collapse pattern of degenerative arthritis. *J Hand Surg [Am]* 1984; 9:358–365.
41. Viegas SF, Patterson RM, Hokanson JA, et al. Wrist anatomy: incidence, distribution, and correlation of anatomic variations, tears, and arthrosis. *J Hand Surg [Am]* 1993;18:463–475.
42. Reagan DS, Linscheid RL, Dobyns JH. Lunotriquetral sprains. *J Hand Surg [Am]* 1984;9:502–514.
43. Horii E, Garcia-Elias M, An KN, et al. A kinematic study of lunotriquetral dissociations. *J Hand Surg [Am]* 1991;16:355–362.
44. Kleinman WB. The shear test. *Am Soc Surg Hand Corr Newsl* 1985:51.
45. Green DP. Carpal dislocations and instabilities. In: Green DP, ed. *Operative hand surgery*, 3rd ed., New York: Churchill Livingstone, 1993;894–895.
46. Kleinman WB. Distal ulnar injury and dysfunction: part I. *Indiana Hand Center Newsl* 1995;2:7–17.
47. Schmidt CC, Kleinman WB. Lunotriquetral fusion. *Atlas Hand Clin* 1998;3:115–127.
48. Wright TW, Dobyns JH, Linscheid RL, et al. Carpal instability non-dissociative. *J Hand Surg [Br]* 1994;19:763–773.
49. Dobyns JH, Linscheid RL, Macksoud WS. Proximal carpal row instability—non-dissociative. *Orthop Trans* 1985;9:574.
50. Louis DS, Hankin FM, Greene TL, et al. Central carpal instability—capitate lunate instability pattern: diagnosis by dynamic displacement. *Orthopedics* 1984;7:1693–1696.
51. Schernberg F. L'instabilite medio-carpienne. *Ann Chir Main* 1984; 3:344–346.
52. Trumble TE, Bourg CJ, Smith RJ, et al. Kinematics of the ulnar carpus related to the volar intercalated segment instability pattern. *J Hand Surg [Am]* 1990;15:384–392.
53. Hankin FM, Amadio PC, Wojtys EM, et al. Carpal instability with volar flexion of the proximal row associated with injury to the scapho-trapezial ligament: report of two cases. *J Hand Surg [Br]* 1988;13:298–302.
54. Rayhack JM, Linscheid RL, Dobyns JH, et al. Post-traumatic ulnar translation of the carpus. *J Hand Surg [Am]* 1987;12:180–189.
55. Larsen CF, Amadio PC, Gilula LA, et al. Analysis of carpal instability: I. Description of the scheme. *J Hand Surg [Am]* 1995;20: 757–764.
56. Hodge JC, Gilula LA, Larsen CF, et al. Analysis of carpal instability: II. Clinical applications. *J Hand Surg [Am]* 1995;20:765–777.

28

DORSAL WRIST SYNDROME

PREDYNAMIC CARPAL INSTABILITY

JEFFREY WEINZWEIG
H. KIRK WATSON

The most vulnerable components of the wrist are certainly the scaphoid and its support mechanism. Scaphoid instability produces a sequence of events with resultant changes at the radiocarpal, scapholunate (SL), and triscaphe joints that range from wrist sprain and dorsal wrist syndrome (DWS) to a scapholunate advanced collapse (SLAC) wrist (Fig. 28.1). Periscaphoid ligament damage represents a spectrum of carpal instability with varying and progressive findings on physical examination, radiographic study, and intraoperative exploration (1,2).

The radial side of the wrist is responsible for the major load transfers across the wrist. Ganglia are a response to joint overload; almost all wrist ganglia have a periscaphoid origin. The radial wrist is well designed for motion but poorly designed for heavy and, in particular, sudden heavy loading at the positional extremes. The design makes the wrist far more susceptible to permanent and symptomatic injury than has been previously recognized. Injuries resulting in functional limitation occur as a spectrum from the common overload of the SL joint through ligament rupture to arthritis. Almost all of these events are periscaphoid in nature.

DORSAL WRIST SYNDROME

Acute wrist trauma, in the absence of an SL ligament tear, produces SL synovitis and some degree of internal ligamentous strain in its mildest form. A more substantial insult may result in pain on the dorsum of the wrist accompanied by significant SL synovitis with or without measurable ligamentous disruption (Fig. 28.2). This clinical entity, which we have termed *dorsal wrist syndrome*, is the most common manifestation of wrist pathology and is the result of overload and insult to the SL joint. In any clinical setting, this will be the most common diagnosis.

The clinical presentation of DWS is one of activity pain in the wrist, often not well localized, and associated with episodes of postactivity ache. The duration of postactivity ache indicates the severity of synovial insult produced by an activity. The patient may be asymptomatic except, for example, after playing racquetball, when postactivity ache may last for 2 days. This may be interpreted to mean that the wrist is capable of nearly all activity, but racquetball loads the scaphoid in such a way that the involved synovium is overstressed or torn, requiring 2 days to recover. The patient will usually avoid racquetball, and the DWS requires no treatment in this situation. The basic etiology is a scaphoid that can be abnormally displaced under certain conditions. This may be the patient's normal anatomy or represent some ligamentous injury.

DWS will typically respond to conservative treatment. When signs and symptoms are relatively constant within the first 3 months of onset, splinting, nonsteroidal antiinflammatory medication, and load avoidance are the treatments of choice. In the second 3 months of continued symptoms, full activity may be carried out without restriction; splinting is not indicated, but a steroid injection may help. After 6 months without evidence of improvement, surgery may be indicated.

DWS presents with the minimum findings of (a) tenderness dorsally over the SL joint and (b) a positive finger extension test (performed with the wrist flexed and load applied to the dorsum of the digits with the metacarpophalangeal joints extended) (3). These are the first two of five clinical findings used to diagnose rotary subluxation of the

J. Weinzweig: Department of Plastic Surgery, Brown University School of Medicine, Rhode Island Hospital, and Hasbro Children's Hospital, Providence, Rhode Island 02905.

H. K. Watson: Connecticut Combined Hand Surgery Fellowship, Hartford Hospital, and Connecticut Children's Medical Center, Hartford, Connecticut 06106; Department of Orthopaedics, University of Connecticut School of Medicine, Farmington, Connecticut 06032; Department of Orthopedics, Rehabilitation, and Plastic Surgery, Yale University School of Medicine, New Haven, Connecticut 06520.

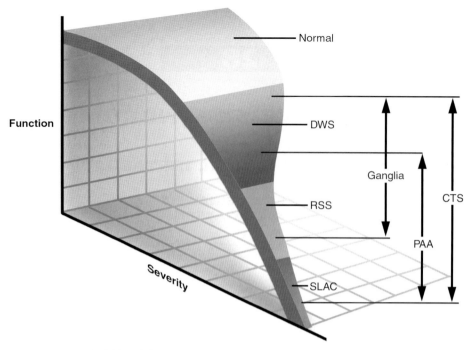

FIGURE 28.1. Scaphoid instability produces a sequence of events that create a spectrum of disorders ranging from wrist sprain and dorsal wrist syndrome (DWS) to rotary subluxation of the scaphoid (RSS) and a SLAC wrist. The findings of carpal tunnel syndrome (CTS), ganglia, and postactivity ache (PAA) are often indicators of more severe underlying wrist pathology. Note that the development of ganglia seems to require a more intact joint; ganglia are absent with major joint displacement and destruction.

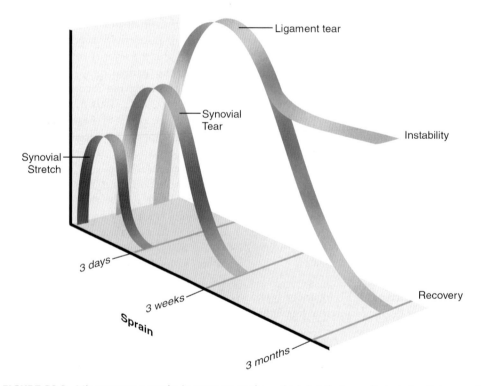

FIGURE 28.2. Minor trauma results in soreness to the wrist joint that usually lasts for 3 days and is the result of synovial stretching without hemarthrosis. More severe injury will produce some synovial tearing, possibly some hemarthrosis, and is typically completely resolved in 3 weeks, leaving no residual sequelae. A more severe wrist injury results in some capsular tearing along with synovial rupture and hemarthrosis and a major clinical injury response in the wrist. These injuries usually take 3 months to resolve and may result in some permanent loss of ligament support, often undetectable except under heavy load.

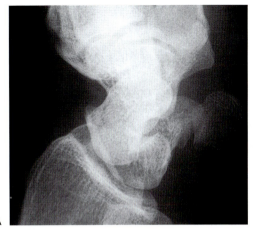 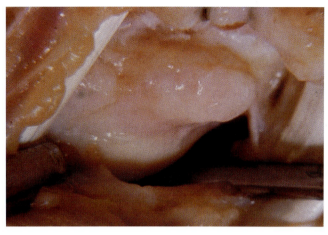

FIGURE 28.3. Dorsal bony ridging. **A:** An oblique x-ray of the wrist demonstrates the ridging that occurs on the dorsum of the scaphoid and lunate. **B:** This is the intraoperative view of that ridging.

scaphoid (RSS). The other three findings are (c) scaphoid articular–nonarticular tenderness (performed by palpating the radial aspect of the wrist just distal to the radial styloid with the wrist ulnarly deviated), (d) scaphotrapeziotrapezoid (STT) synovitis and tenderness, and (e) an abnormal scaphoid shift (4) (see Chapter 5).

Two hundred nine of 1,000 normal subjects examined demonstrated a unilateral abnormal scaphoid shift maneuver with hypermobility of the scaphoid and/or pain. This represents 21% of examined subjects and 10% of examined wrists (5). All wrists with bilateral hypermobile scaphoids were excluded; thus, nearly one in four of us has sustained enough scaphoid ligament insult to be clinically evident whether symptomatic or not. Tears of the SL interosseous ligament heal poorly if at all, and subsequent injuries produce more ligamentous interruption, which is also permanent. It is probable that most cases of RSS are a result of cumulative ligament tears rather than a single major injury. Often one sees a symptomatic RSS dated to an injury that, although significant, did not produce the expected major hemarthrosis and soft tissue reaction. This trauma represented a terminal event now allowing static scaphoid positioning. Radiographic examination of DWS is usually normal but may demonstrate osteophyte formation on the distal dorsal ridges of the scaphoid and lunate in the lateral projection with or without evidence of RSS (Fig. 28.3). DWS exists secondary to overload of a SL joint with preexisting predynamic RSS or from overload of a normal joint.

Surgical management of DWS involves exploration of the SL joint with attention directed at existing soft tissue synovitis overlying the SL joint, usually including the terminal carpal branch of the posterior interosseous nerve, evaluating the integrity of the SL ligament, removal of regular or occult ganglia, removal of the ridges on the scaphoid and lunate, and creation of cancellous surfaces for capsular adhesion.

This is accomplished through a dorsal transverse incision, approximately 3 cm in length, centered over the SL joint at the level of the radial styloid. The dorsal capsule is opened along the sheath of the extensor pollicis longus tendon, which is retracted radially. A soft tissue mass, consisting of thickened synovium and often containing ganglia, is invariably found between the third and fourth compartments and is excised to reveal the underlying SL joint. An occult ganglion is often identified on the dorsal SL ligamentous surface and excised (Fig. 28.4). Traction on the hand permits visualization and evaluation of the proximal portion of the SL interosseous ligament. Flexion of the distracted wrist and placement of a probe (joker)

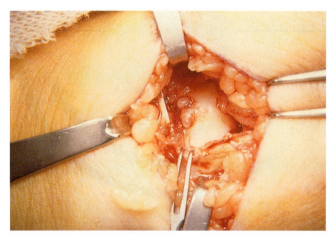

FIGURE 28.4. Two occult ganglia, identified within the scapholunate joint at the time of exploration for dorsal wrist syndrome, are excised.

within the radiocarpal joint between the scaphoid and lunate permits evaluation of the volar portion of the SL ligament.

The partially ruptured SL ligament is often bridged by repair tissue and a synovial layer that possess negligible intrinsic strength. This layer is readily separated by the probe, and the SL joint space is entered volarly. The probe is swept proximally and then dorsally, tracing the curve of the SL joint until intact ligamentous fibers are encountered. This process permits complete evaluation of the extent of ligamentous rupture. Bony ridging on the dorsum of the scaphoid and lunate, which is present in every case, is excised using a dental rongeur. A broad cancellous surface is thus created for capsular attachment on the dorsum of the scaphoid and lunate. If the surgeon wishes, then elevation of the fourth dorsal compartment tendons allows identification and transection of the terminal branch of the posterior interosseous nerve. We have not been able to identify any difference in postoperative status between transected and preserved nerves. The skin is then closed. The bulky dressing and splint applied intraoperatively are removed 3 days postoperatively, and the wrist is fully mobilized.

On the basis of intraoperative findings, we have classified SL interosseous ligament rupture into four distinct types: type 0, intact ligament; type I, ≤50% tear; type II, >50% tear but less than total disruption; and type III, complete tear (Fig. 28.5).

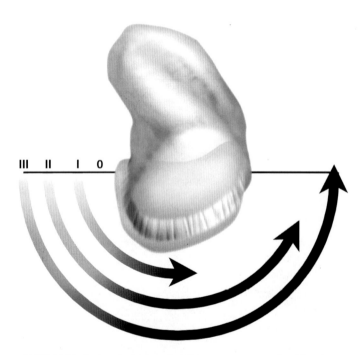

FIGURE 28.5. Scapholunate (SL) ligament rupture classification. Ligament ruptures usually commence volarly, extend proximally around the SL joint, then continue dorsally to complete the tear. Ligament tears are classified on the basis of the extent of the tear.

ROTARY SUBLUXATION OF THE SCAPHOID

RSS is *not* an all-or-none phenomenon where the patient has symptoms only when the SL angle exceeds 70°. We believe that RSS is far more common than previously thought and that degenerative periscaphoid disease may be the late result of undiagnosed predynamic or dynamic RSS. RSS is a well-recognized entity in which the SL articulation is disrupted and the wrist develops an instability pattern (6). It is classicly described as diastasis between the scaphoid and lunate with dorsal displacement and rotation of the proximal pole of the scaphoid. This produces a scaphoid with abnormal motion, which can subject the radius–scaphoid joint to abnormal stresses and subsequent destruction resulting in a SLAC wrist (7). A less common form of scaphoid instability allows lateral shear loads between the scaphoid, trapezium, and trapezoid, resulting in triscaphe and SL degenerative joint disease (DJD).

A spectrum of radiographic findings of RSS parallels the clinical findings of RSS. As scaphoid instability progresses, clinical findings become more severe, and radiographic findings more apparent. Our current classification describes five types of RSS: (I) predynamic, (II) dynamic, (III) static, (IV) degenerative, and (V) secondary.

Predynamic RSS (type I) is diagnosed when signs and symptoms of scaphoid instability exist in the absence of radiographic abnormalities. The patient usually presents with a history of wrist pain of at least 6 months that is worse with activity and is accompanied by a substantial postactivity ache that lasts from several hours to several days. The patient usually demonstrates decreased range of motion of the wrist, particularly of flexion, and all five clinical findings of RSS.

Dynamic RSS (type II) presents in a manner similar to predynamic RSS, but the diagnosis is supported by findings on stress radiographic views (e.g., clenched fist, radial or ulnar deviation). These findings include foreshortening of the scaphoid, overlapping of the scaphoid and capitate, and a ring sign [produced on posteroanterior (PA) view by overlapping of the proximal and distal poles of the scaphoid with scaphoid rotation]. Routine PA and lateral radiographs demonstrate no abnormalities. Clinical findings may or may not be more severe than in patients with predynamic RSS.

Static RSS (type III) is diagnosed based on findings on routine PA and lateral radiographs in the presence of clinical findings that are similar to those of predynamic and dynamic RSS, but more severe. There is usually a history of a significant injury. In addition to the radiographic findings of dynamic RSS, findings of SL dissociation, a widened SL joint, and an increased SL angle are also observed, with or without dorsal intercalated segment instability (DISI) of the lunate.

Note that type II and type III RSS are nearly the same phenomenon and are very close on the spectrum of wrist problems. They differ only in the type of x-ray necessary to demonstrate the instability. Type II exists because the International Wrist Investigators' Workshop has put forth this definition.

Degenerative RSS (type IV) is diagnosed on the basis of a history similar to those of types I to III but with symptoms that are usually more severe, their duration often longer, and the patient often older. Radiographic findings of degenerative changes at the radius–scaphoid or STT joints (i.e., triscaphe arthritis) are present (SLAC wrist). A triscaphe arthrodesis can be successfully performed despite a small area of DJD on the proximal scaphoid because this area is centered in the normal cartilage of the radius–scaphoid fossa. Secondary capitate–lunate joint changes occur.

Secondary RSS (type V) designates involvement of the scaphoid secondary to other carpal lesions such as a collapsed wrist from Kienböck's disease or nonunion of the scaphoid. Radiographic review of patients who had undergone triscaphe arthrodesis showed that 9% of patients demonstrated dynamic RSS (type II), 47% static RSS (type III), 14% degenerative RSS (type IV), and 30% secondary RSS (type V) (8). In addition, approximately 40% of patients with isolated triscaphe arthritis demonstrated static RSS. We believe isolated triscaphe arthritis is a secondary manifestation of RSS in which the distal pole of the scaphoid becomes unstable and the articular destruction of the triscaphe joint ensues. Approximately 1,000 triscaphe arthrodeses have been performed; in this group there has been no evidence of subsequent degenerative change of the radius–scaphoid joint or other intercarpal joints (9–11).

Wrist ganglia are a secondary manifestation of an underlying periscaphoid ligamentous injury (12–14). The severity of this injury will determine whether the wrist will develop symptomatic RSS in the future. On review of 174 patients who had undergone 177 triscaphe arthrodeses, it was noted that 17 (9.6%) patients had previously undergone wrist ganglion excision; 10 of these ganglia had been dorsal and seven volar. All 17 patients were treated for continuing or recurring wrist pain. The length of time between initial ganglion excision and referral was 35 months (range 6–130 months). All 17 patients had painful scaphoid shift maneuvers; 12 of these patients also demonstrated excessive mobility in comparison with the opposite wrist. Radiograph review demonstrated static RSS in six patients, isolated degenerative arthritis of the triscaphe joint in five patients, and evidence of avascular necrosis of the lunate in one patient. The remaining five patients had predynamic or dynamic RSS. Following triscaphe arthrodesis, all patients noted decreased pain and were able to stress the wrist with 75% to 80% of the flexion–extension of the contralateral normal wrist. These data support the concept of a spectrum of scaphoid instability in which the ganglion is a secondary manifestation of the underlying wrist pathology and joint overload.

DISCUSSION

Symptoms involving the SL joint dorsally are the most common manifestation of wrist overload with or without demonstrable ligamentous injury (Fig. 28.6). One in four (25%) adults demonstrates abnormal scaphoid mobility. Insults to the scaphoid restraint mechanism appear to be cumulative. Injuries appear to produce tears initially of the SL interosseous ligament system. These SL tears begin volarly and progress around the proximal pole of the SL joint to complete the tear distally on the dorsum (Fig. 28.7). The thin midproximal portion of the ligament system is typically torn when the more clinically relevant volar ligaments are ruptured. The dorsal ligament appears to rupture as the terminal traumatic event.

In dorsiflexion, the scaphoid and lunate tend to separate volarly with the capitate acting as a proximal driving wedge. Thus, with repeated injury, ligamentous attenuation and rupture occur volarly, followed by rupture of the midportion and, finally, with difficulty, the dorsal ligaments. Arthroscopically, the lesions are often unrecognized, being sealed over by repair tissue and synovium. A joker is introduced on open examination, and the scaphoid and lunate are pried apart. The repair tissue easily separates, but the intact ligaments cannot be ruptured by this maneuver. The subsequent requirement for triscaphe arthrodesis in 9.3% of patients with DWS appears to support the hypothesis that there is a progressive pattern of SL ligamentous tearing. The presence of ganglia in 60% of patients and carpal tunnel syndrome in 22% indicates that the conditions are

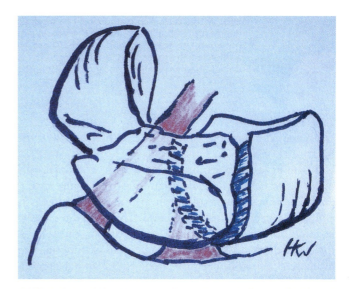

FIGURE 28.6. The diagrammatic outline of the scaphoid and lunate demonstrates the tightness of the interosseous ligament system compared to the extrinsic ligamentous system. The loads caused by trauma are dissipated first in tearing the scapholunate interosseous ligament system. Typically, tears begin volarly and, with subsequent trauma, extend around to the more dorsal fibers.

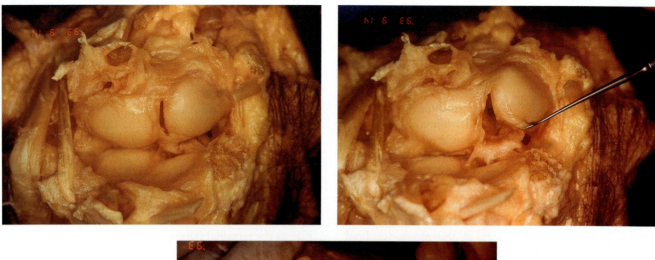

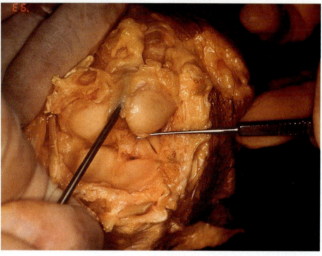

FIGURE 28.7. A: This cadaveric specimen demonstrates separation between the proximal aspect of the scaphoid and lunate. This is the weak part of the scapholunate interosseous system. **B:** On arthroscopy, the volar ligaments appear to be intact and would resist probe manipulation. However, with a reasonable amount of force, these volar structures separate easily; thus, they are not ligamentous at all, but primarily synovial closure. **C:** Intact ligaments are demonstrated dorsally between the scaphoid and lunate. These ligaments cannot be ruptured with full arm power applied to the joker. The fact that patients are symptomatic (dorsal wrist syndrome) with intact dorsal ligaments raises concerns for the adequacy of dorsal scapholunate interosseous ligament repairs.

associated with, and probably secondary to, overload of the SL joint (DWS).

SL joint exploration in patients with DWS permits direct assessment of ligamentous integrity, symptomatic dorsal ridge excision resulting in a form of capsuloplasty, and ganglionectomy when indicated. This procedure results in resolution of symptoms in 91% of patients with DWS; those patients with significant ligamentous disruption who ultimately require triscaphe arthrodesis (9.3%) have predynamic RSS of the scaphoid.

Thus, scaphoid instability should be viewed as a spectrum condition ranging from minor asymptomatic findings (seen in nearly 25% of normal adults) through symptomatic findings in patients with normal x-rays to abnormal instability on radiographs to degenerative change to, ultimately, a SLAC wrist (Fig. 28.8). Appropriate diagnosis and management of each of these wrist disorders are highly dependent on a keen understanding of normal periscaphoid anatomy as well as the anatomic derangements that occur within the wrist that predispose a given patient to subsequent degenerative changes. With that understanding, the appropriateness of conservative therapy, SL exploration and arthroplasty, ligament repair, triscaphe arthrodesis, or SLAC reconstruction in each case can be readily determined (15–17).

Chapter 28: Dorsal Wrist Syndrome   489

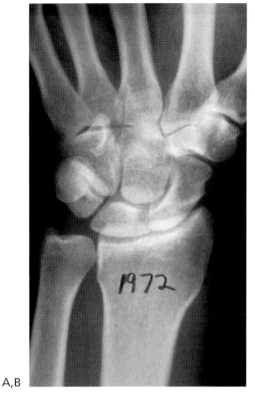
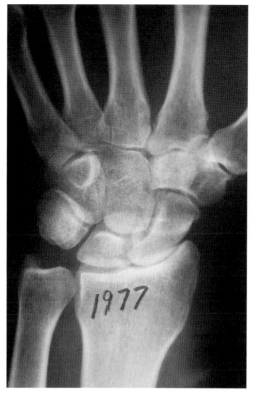
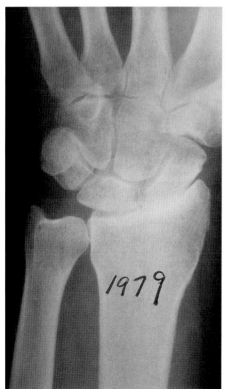
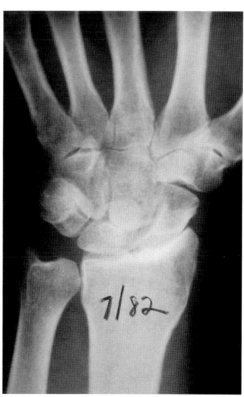
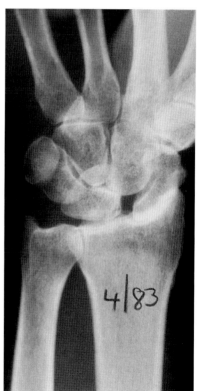

FIGURE 28.8. Dorsal wrist syndrome developed in this patient sometime prior to 1972 **(A)**. He was followed by an orthopedic surgeon with conservative therapy. Symptoms persisted, and by 1977, changes began to develop between the radius and scaphoid **(B)**. There were no demonstrable ligamentous tears. In 1979, the rotating scaphoid had destroyed the cartilage between the scaphoid and radius **(C)**. By 1982, the capitate was approaching the radius, and the scaphoid and lunate collapse pattern became more severe **(D)**. By 1983, there is a classic static rotary subluxation of the scaphoid, and SLAC wrist has occurred as the terminal event **(E)**. The clinical entity, dorsal wrist syndrome, is best recognized and treated before this disastrous sequence of events occurs.

REFERENCES

1. Watson HK, Weinzweig J, Zeppieri J. The natural progression of scaphoid instability. *Hand Clin* 1997;13:39–50.
2. Weinzweig J, Watson HK. Wrist sprain to SLAC wrist: a spectrum of carpal instability. In: Vastamaki M, ed. *Current trends in hand surgery.* Amsterdam: Elsevier Science, 1995;47–55.
3. Watson HK, Weinzweig J. Physical examination of the wrist. *Hand Clin* 1997;13:17–34.
4. Watson HK, Ashmead D, Makhlouf MV. Examination of the scaphoid. *J Hand Surg [Am]* 1988;13:657–660.
5. Watson HK, Ottoni L, Pitts EC, et al. Rotary subluxation of the scaphoid: A spectrum of instability. *J Hand Surg [Br]* 1993;18:62–64.
6. Linscheid RL, Dobyns JH, Beabout JW, et al. Traumatic instability of the wrist: Diagnosis, classification, and pathomechanics. *J Bone Joint Surg Am* 1972;54:1612–1632.
7. Kleinman WB, Steichen JB, Strickland JW. Management of chronic rotary subluxation of the scaphoid by scapho-trapezio-trapezoid arthrodesis. *J Hand Surg [Am]* 1982;7:125–136.
8. Watson HK, Ryu J, Akelman E. Limited triscaphoid intercarpal arthrodesis for rotary subluxation of the scaphoid. *J Bone Joint Surg Am* 1986;68:345–349.
9. Watson HK, Ballet FL. The SLAC wrist: Scapholunate advanced collapse pattern of degenerative arthritis. *J Hand Surg [Am]* 1984;9:358–365.
10. Watson HK, Hemptson RF. Limited wrist arthrodesis. Part I: The triscaphoid joint. *J Hand Surg [Am]* 1980;5:320–327.
11. Watson HK, Weinzweig J. Intercarpal arthrodesis. In: Green DP, Hotchkiss RN, Pederson WC, eds. *Operative hand surgery, 4th ed.* New York: Churchill Livingstone, 1998;108–130.
12. Angelides AC, Wallace PF. The dorsal ganglion of the wrist: its pathogenesis, gross anatomy, and surgical treatment. *J Hand Surg [Am]* 1976;1:228–235.
13. Carstam N, Eiken O, Andren L. Osteoarthritis of the trapezioscaphoid joint. *Acta Orthop Scand* 1968;39:354–358.
14. Watson HK, Rodgers WD, Ashmead D. Reevaluation of the cause of the wrist ganglion. *J Hand Surg [Am]* 1989;14:812–817.
15. Ashmead D 4th, Watson HK, Damon C, et al. Scapholunate advanced collapse wrist salvage. *J Hand Surg [Am]* 1994;19:741–750.
16. Rogers WD, Watson HK. Degenerative arthritis at the triscaphe joint. *J Hand Surg [Am]* 1990;15:232–235.
17. Watson HK, Brenner LH. Degenerative disorders of the wrist. *J Hand Surg [Am]* 1985;10:1002–1006.

29

LIGAMENTOUS REPAIR FOR SCAPHOLUNATE INSTABILITY AND DISSOCIATION

MARK S. COHEN
JULIO TALEISNIK

Dissociation between the carpal scaphoid and lunate is the most common pattern of wrist instability (1–3). Complete dissociation results in a palmar flexion attitude of the scaphoid and concomitant extension of the lunate. Because scapholunate dissociation leads to progressive degenerative arthritis of the wrist (2,4,5), reduction and internal fixation is the preferred method of treatment, particularly in the acute setting (6–10). The treatment of subacute and chronic scapholunate dissociation is more controversial.

We previously reported on the treatment of acute and subacute scapholunate dissociations with a direct ligamentous repair and a reconstructive capsular augmentation (11). The procedure was performed for documented dissociations with an adequate ligament still available for repair at the time of surgery, a reducible joint, and the absence of degenerative changes within the carpus. Although this procedure is best when performed early, the results were not found to be dependent on the interval between injury and surgical repair. This chapter reviews our current understanding of scapholunate dissociation and the methods utilized for soft tissue repair.

DIAGNOSIS

Scapholunate dissociation most commonly results from a dorsiflexion injury to the wrist. Experimentally, the pathogenesis has been identified as excessive dorsiflexion and ulnar deviation of the wrist with intercarpal supination (12). Patients typically recall a specific injury to their affected wrist. They present with complaints of dorsal and radial-sided wrist discomfort, loss of wrist motion, and weakness of grasp.

Examination commonly reveals tenderness, most specifically in the scapholunate interval, that can be palpated just distal and slightly ulnar to Lister's tubercle. The scaphoid shift maneuver reproduces their discomfort and usually reveals a hypermobile scaphoid, for it is now devoid of ligamentous attachment to the lunate (13). Plain films may reveal a flexed scaphoid and an extended lunate. A stress film, such as an anteroposterior (supinated) view in maximum ulnar deviation, will accentuate the diastasis between the scaphoid and lunate (Fig. 29.1). Additional studies can be obtained if required to make the diagnosis.

TREATMENT

Dissociation between the scaphoid and lunate will significantly alter articular contact areas and stress patterns within the carpus and lead to a progressive degenerative arthritis of the wrist (14,15). In the acute setting, open reduction and internal fixation is indicated to repair the ligament and reestablish integrity of the wrist ligaments (6–8,10). After the acute phase (arbitrarily defined as between 3 and 8 weeks after injury) (6,9,16–20), the ligaments are believed to heal poorly and to be no longer amenable to repair by direct suture.

Our experience, however, has shown that in the absence of degenerative disease and with an adequate ligament remaining as determined at surgery, soft tissue reconstruction can successfully stabilize the carpus long after the acute disruption. Although it is optimal to intervene soon after injury, we currently do not alter our surgical technique based on the time elapsed from the initial trauma. All scapholunate dissociations are treated similarly, with direct ligamentous repair and a capsular augmentation, if the appropriate conditions are satisfied.

M. S. Cohen: Hand and Elbow Program and Orthopaedic Education, Department of Orthopaedic Surgery, Rush-Presbyterian-St. Luke's Medical Center, Chicago, Illinois 60612.
J. Taleisnik: Division of Orthopaedics, Department of Surgery, University of California, Irvine, School of Medicine, Irvine, California 92717.

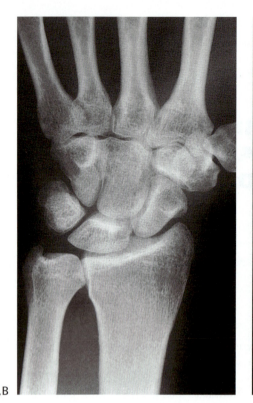
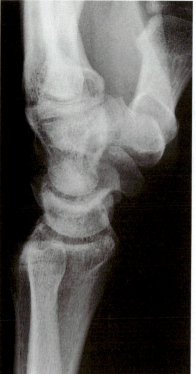
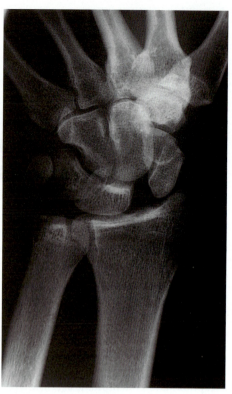

FIGURE 29.1. Posteroanterior **(A)** and lateral **(B)** roentgenograms of a patient with scapholunate dissociation. The dissociation is not seen on the frontal projection. On the lateral film there is very subtle flexion of the scaphoid and extension of the lunate. **C:** Anteroposterior (supinated film) in maximum ulnar deviation clearly delineates the dissociation between the scaphoid and lunate. Stress films are helpful to accentuate the gap in patients with this ligament disruption. (See Fig. 29.5 for treatment and results of this patient.)

SURGICAL TECHNIQUE

Under pneumatic tourniquet control, a dorsal longitudinal incision is centered over the scapholunate interval. The dorsal retinaculum is divided in line with the third compartment, and the extensor pollicus longus is retracted radially. The posterior interosseous nerve can be found on the radial floor of the third dorsal compartment. A neurectomy is performed because this nerve in part innervates the scapholunate ligament (21). The fourth dorsal compartment is subperiosteally reflected ulnarly to aid in the exposure, but its subsheath is not violated.

The wrist joint is exposed through a straight capsular incision. Care is taken not to elevate the radial capsular flap off the radius. Alternatively, the radial flap can be elevated in a subperiosteal fashion, but this will later need to be secured to the dorsal aspect of the distal radius to complete the capsulodesis. The dorsal and membranous portions of the scapholunate interosseous ligament are evaluated. The ligament is typically torn off the scaphoid (occasionally with a fragment of articular cartilage) but remains attached to the lunate (Fig. 29.2). However, it can avulse off the lunate and remain attached to the scaphoid. One can also occasionally observe central attenuation within the ligament proper. If there is little or no

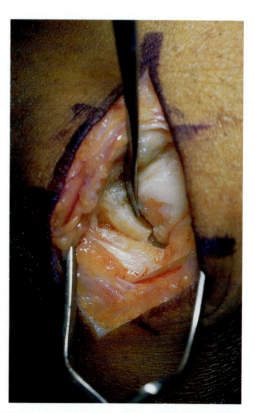

FIGURE 29.2. Intraoperative photograph of a patient with an acute scapholunate dissociation. The ligament has avulsed off the scaphoid with a rather large fragment of articular cartilage. The interosseous ligament is most commonly pulled off the scaphoid.

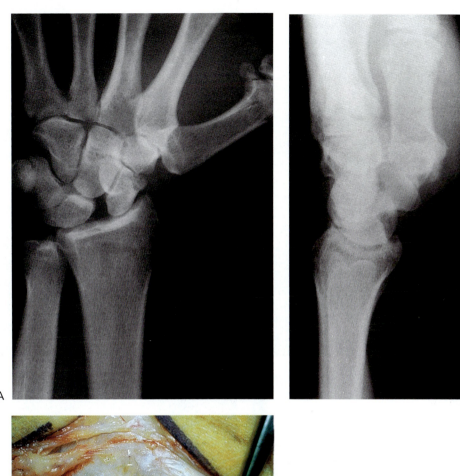
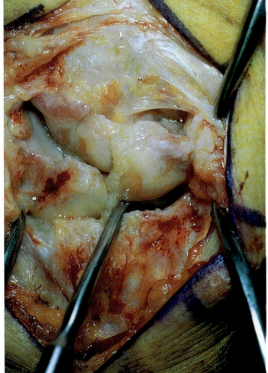

FIGURE 29.3. Anteroposterior **(A)** and lateral **(B)** roentgenograms of a patient with a scapholunate dissociation. The age of the ligament disruption was unknown, as he had several injuries to the affected wrist over many months. **C:** Intraoperative photograph demonstrates the dissociation with significant articular cartilage loss on the proximal pole of the scaphoid (freer elevator). Note the midcarpal arthrosis as well on the proximal aspect of the capitate and hamate (left). The presence or degree of arthritis cannot always be appreciated on preoperative roentgenograms. This constitutes a contraindication to a ligament or soft tissue repair.

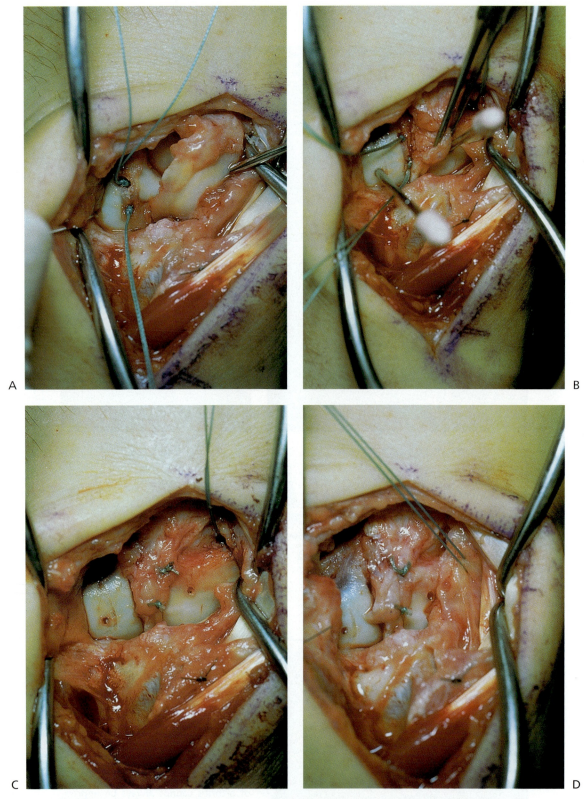

FIGURE 29.4. A: Intraoperative photograph of a patient with a scapholunate dissociation. The ligament in this case has pulled off the lunate while remaining attached to the scaphoid. Note the minianchors that have been placed in the lunate at the site of detachment. Kirschner wires are used as joysticks to manipulate the individual bones during reconstruction. **B:** The scapholunate dissociation has been reduced and secured with percutaneous Kirschner wires placed from the scaphoid into the lunate and from the scaphoid into the capitate. The "joysticks" have thus been rotated into view. Note the thick dorsal ligament (pickups) now in place for repair. **C:** The ligament has been secured to the lunate using a free needle. The Kirschner wire joysticks have been removed. Note the bone anchor that has been placed in the center of a trough created in the distal scaphoid. **D:** The sutures in the scaphoid are passed through the radial capsule, which is pulled under tension distally with the wrist in slight extension.

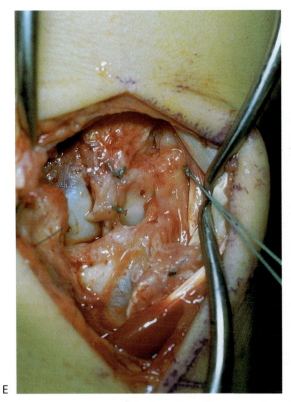 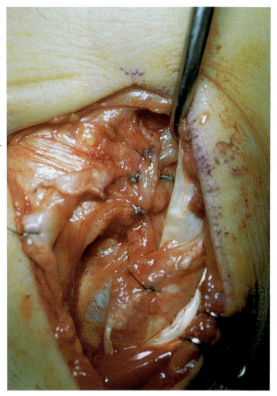

FIGURE 29.4. (continued) E: The sutures have been tied, completing the dorsal capsulodesis. **F:** The ulnar capsule is sutured in an overlapping fashion to reinforce the dorsal capsular augmentation. Note the extensor carpi radialis brevis running longitudinally along the radial aspect of the wound. This tendon often must be released and retracted radially to expose the radial capsule used in the capsulodesis. The extensor pollicus longus tendon is seen coursing obliquely at the most proximal and radial aspect of the wound. This will be relocated outside the extensor retinaculum at the completion of the procedure.

interosseous ligament remaining for repair, we prefer to stabilize the scaphoid by partial wrist arthrodesis between the scaphoid and trapezium–trapezoid or between the scaphoid and capitate (22–26).

The dorsal aspect of the proximal pole of the scaphoid and corresponding scaphoid facet of the distal radius are inspected for degenerative changes. If significant degeneration exists, one should perform a salvage-type operation (Chapters 32–34) (5,27,28). Advanced radioscaphoid arthritis is a contraindication to ligamentous repair. Loss of articular cartilage cannot always be appreciated on preoperative roentgenograms (Fig. 29.3). If only slight pointing at the radial styloid exists, a limited styloidectomy can be performed. Care is taken to protect the radial capsule during subperiosteal dissection in this setting.

If a repair and reconstruction are to be carried out, Kirschner wires are inserted in a dorsopalmar direction into the scaphoid and lunate to be used as joysticks. Because significant force may be required to reduce the diastasis, 0.062-in wires are utilized for this purpose. The scaphoid wire is placed in a slightly distal-to-proximal direction; the lunate pin is angled slightly from proximal to distal to facilitate subsequent rotation of the bones. A narrow trough is next created along the dorsal lunate or scaphoid with a burr or fine rongeur at the site of detachment. Although the repair was originally described utilizing drill holes and Keith needles, newer bone minianchors can be utilized to aid in the repair (Fig. 29.4). Two anchors can usually be placed within the trough.

The joint is next reduced using the Kirschner wires by extending the scaphoid and flexing the lunate. Occasionally, the bones will also have to be pulled together as well, supinating the scaphoid. In addition to flexion, the scaphoid pronates when it dissociates from the lunate (29,30). Once reduced (slight overreduction may be preferable), the bones are pinned with 0.045-in Kirschner wires directed from the scaphoid into the lunate and from the scaphoid into the capitate. The reduction is checked and verified under fluoroscopy. With the scapholunate joint reduced, the ligament is repaired to the trough using free needles and bone anchor sutures (Fig. 29.4). It is sometimes easier to place the sutures into the ligament before the final reduction and simply tie them once the joint is stabilized. An advantage of our original technique (11) is that it

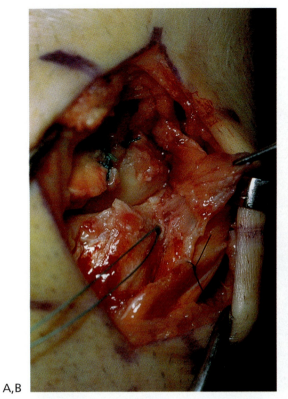
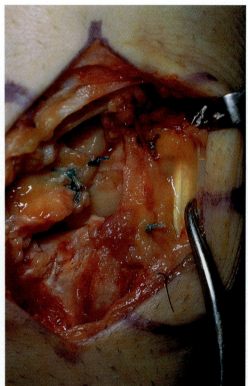

FIGURE 29.5. A: Intraoperative photograph of patient from Fig. 29.1 depicting an alternative method for completing the dorsal capsulodesis. The dorsal capsule is first secured to the distal scaphoid trough with a prolene pullout suture tied over a palmar bolster. **B:** Once fixed distally, the radial capsule can be pulled taut and fixed to the radius using a bone anchor. Tension on the capsulodesis is easily controlled in this manner. Postoperative posteroanterior **(C)** and lateral **(D)** films showing Kirschner wires utilized to maintain the reduction during the healing phase.

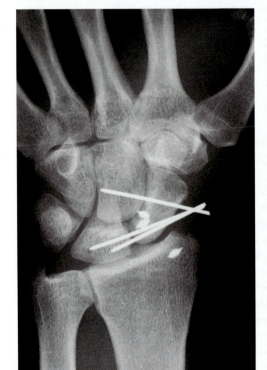
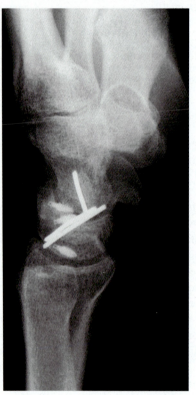
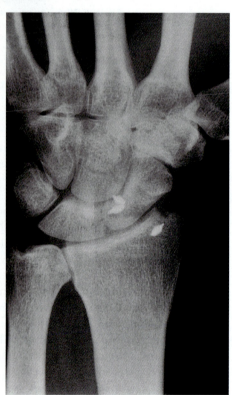

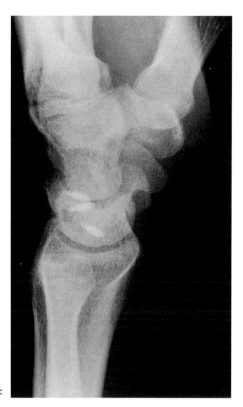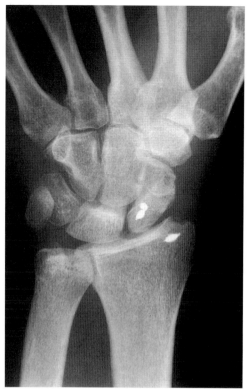

FIGURE 29.5. *(continued)* Final follow-up posteroanterior **(E)**, lateral **(F)**, and anteroposterior **(G)** stress views revealing a maintained reduction.

allowed access to the sutures securing the repair of the interosseous membrane when it was no longer visible under the dorsal rim of the radius following reduction. Although this advantage is lost when bone anchors are used, the ease of repair is much greater.

A dorsal capsular augmentation is performed next. Securing the radial capsule to the distal scaphoid provides a dorsal tether to resist subsequent scaphoid flexion (7). Although the capsulodesis was initially described using a palmar pullout suture, attachment of the radial capsule to the distal scaphoid can also be facilitated using a small bone anchor (Fig. 29.4). Care must be taken to create a trough in the dorsal aspect of the scaphoid distal to the midwaist. This improves the mechanical advantage of the capsulodesis. With the radial capsule pulled distally under tension, the capsule is secured down to the scaphoid trough using free needles and bone anchor sutures or with a pullout suture tied palmarly over a bolster. If the bone anchor is chosen, it is easiest to place it in the center of the trough before reduction and pinning of the dissociation.

Because it is occasionally difficult to push the thick dorsal capsular tissue down to the trough under tension using a bone anchor (if sutured too tightly, it will not reach, and if too loose, it will not provide an adequate dorsal tether), one can alternatively fix the distal capsule to the scaphoid first. This technique is utilized if it was chosen to perform a radial styloidectomy or if the radial capsule was subperiosteally dissected off the radius during exposure. In this way, the capsule can first be secured distally under minimal tension. This ensures that the capsule is directly secured to the cancellous trough created in the scaphoid. The radial capsule can then be pulled taught proximally and secured to the radius under tension using an additional bone anchor (Fig. 29.5).

One of us (M.S.C.) presently uses a modified technique to perform the dorsal capsulodesis. The radial capsular flap is simply imbricated in its midsection. Shortening the radial capsule itself tends to tether the scaphoid from a flexed posture. The ulnar capsular flap is then overlapped and secured to the radial capsule (Fig. 29.4). The extensor retinaculum is then approximated, leaving the extensor pollicus longus outside the retinaculum. A long arm compression dressing with splints is then applied.

The wrist is immobilized in a long arm cast for approximately 4 weeks, followed by a short arm cast for an additional 4 weeks. Eight weeks postoperatively, the Kirschner wires (and pullout suture) are removed. A gradual range-of-motion program is then started under occupational therapy guidance with interval splinting of the wrist for protection and support. Return of wrist motion is generally slow. Resisted exercises are not allowed until approximately 4 months postoperatively. Activities requiring wrist extension against vigorous resistance are not permitted until 6 months following surgery.

RESULTS

Our experience with this technique has remained satisfactory since we published our results in 1992 (11). We reported then on 21 patients treated for scapholunate dissociation using the aforementioned technique (11). The average time from injury to surgical repair was 17 months. Wrist motion at an average follow-up of 33 months was equal to that in the unaffected wrist in all planes except flexion ($p < 0.001$). This limitation is most likely related to the dorsal capsulodesis, which provides a tether limiting terminal scaphoid flexion. Thus, patients must be counseled on an expected loss of approximately 15° of wrist flexion following the repair. Fortunately, this is rarely a functional problem.

Using visual analog scales (31), both peak and general levels of pain were significantly improved at follow-up ($p < 0.001$). Roentgenographically, the scapholunate gap was reduced from a mean of 3.2 mm preoperatively to 1.9 mm at follow-up.

CONCLUSION

Scapholunate dissociation can be successfully treated by direct ligament repair and dorsal capsular augmentation. The rationale for soft tissue repair is based on the premise that restoration of the normal intracarpal relationships will halt degenerative changes while maximizing wrist motion and function. The dorsal capsulodesis provides a check rein to excessive palmar flexion of the scaphoid. This may limit terminal palmar flexion of the wrist, but it appears to functionally support the unstable scaphoid. Although surgical repair is best performed early, the described reconstruction can be performed regardless of the time since injury. Requirements include an adequate interosseous ligament identified at surgery and absent degenerative changes at the radioscaphoid articulation.

EDITORS' COMMENTS

Ligaments may be repaired early with open reduction and anatomic carpal immobilization. Ligaments quickly lose their ability to repair themselves and, when unrepaired, are resorbed by the body as inconsequential tissue. The major problems with ligament repair in the chronic state are the inability to repair the ligaments that are most responsible for the symptoms and the great difficulty in recognizing which combination of ligaments has produced any particular symptomatic state. As most wrist loaded ligament cutting studies have demonstrated, it takes multiple combinations of ligament transection to produce clinically recognizable entities. There are multiple ligament rupture combinations that will produce static and dynamic clinical entities.

Scapholunate dissociation is the most common ligament problem in the wrist. Approximately 25% of people in their forties will have some inadequacy of the scapholunate interosseous system. The symptomatic overload of the scapholunate joint termed *dorsal wrist syndrome* (DWS) is the most common wrist diagnosis. Dorsiflexion of the wrist causes a spreading moment between the volar scaphoid and lunate, resulting in tears that begin volarly, heal poorly, and are extended by subsequent trauma. Ligament support may reach a point where the abnormal motion of the scaphoid produces symptoms. Multiple lesser traumas are probably more at fault than single major injuries. It is our contention that dorsiflexion injuries supposedly producing static rotary subluxation of the scaphoid are most commonly terminal traumatic events, superimposed on some previous tears or attenuation of the interosseous ligament.

At surgery, with the diagnosis of DWS, these tears frequently extend half or two-thirds of the way from the most volar distal aspect, leaving intact the most dorsal fibers. Because these patients are coming to surgery with chronic symptoms, they demonstrate the fact that strong, normal dorsal ligaments between the scaphoid and lunate are not always adequate for the demands of any particular individual. This raises concerns for the efficacy of a dorsal ligamentous repair. To date, the repairs and capsuloplasties that claim success are all dorsal. There is no effective repair for the volar scapholunate interosseous ligaments. A prerequisite for ligament repair as herein described is the existence of "adequate remaining ligament." Following ligament repair, there is a tendency for persistence of the scapholunate gap. This gap may be considered abnormal if it measures greater than twice the normal cartilage space as determined by the other cartilage spaces for that wrist. The gap raises concern for future degenerative scapholunate advanced collapse (SLAC) changes. However, the success of these procedures relates more to the patient demands than to external or anatomic criteria. Many patients' activity levels are compatible with abnormal scaphoid mobility; witness asymptomatic positive scaphoid shifts in nearly one-quarter of all adults.

Degenerative arthritis occurs between the scaphoid and radius with scapholunate dissociation. Degenerative changes occur at the triscaphe joint with ligament ruptures at this joint. These two forms of joint destruction occur in a ratio of 4 to 1. Combinations of ligament damage can result in other forms or combinations of these two, all under the diagnosis of rotary subluxation of the scaphoid. Depending on patient demand level, successful ligament repairs are possible, and we are currently in a rapid state of development toward better procedures. If the wrist demands will be great (construction laborer, professional athlete, etc.), the only reliable procedure that improves with time and demonstrates little or no secondary degenerative arthritis is fusion of the triscaphe joint.

REFERENCES

1. Jones WA. Beware of the sprained wrist: the incidence and diagnosis of scapholunate instability. *J Bone Joint Surg Br* 1988;70:293–297.
2. Linscheid RL, Dobyns JH, Beabout JW, Bryan RS. Traumatic instability of the wrist. *J Bone Joint Surg Am* 1972;54:1612–1632.
3. Taleisnik J. Carpal instability: current concepts review. *J Bone Joint Surg Am* 1988;70:1262–1267.
4. Sebald S, Dobyns JA, Linscheid RL. The natural history of collapse deformities of the wrist. *Clin Orthop* 1974;104:104–108.
5. Watson HK, Ballet FL. The SLAC wrist: scapholunate advanced collapse pattern of degenerative arthritis. *J Hand Surg [Am]* 1984;9:358–365.
6. Beckenbaugh RD. Accurate evaluation and management of the painful wrist following injury: an approach to carpal instability. *Orthop Clin North Am* 1982;15:289–300.
7. Blatt G. Capsulodesis in reconstructive hand surgery: dorsal capsulodesis for the unstable scaphoid and volar capsulodesis following excision of the distal ulna. *Hand Clin* 1987;3:81–102.
8. Goldner JL. Treatment of carpal instability without joint fusion: current assessment. *J Hand Surg [Am]* 1982;7:325–326.
9. Kleinman WB. Management of chronic rotary subluxation of the scaphoid by scapho-trapezium-trapezoid arthrodesis. *Hand Clin* 1987;3:113–133.
10. Nathan R, Lester B, Melone CP. The acutely injured wrist: an anatomic basis for operative treatment. *Orthop Rev* 1987;6:80–95.
11. Lavernia CJ, Cohen MS, Taleisnik J. Treatment of scapholunate dissociation by ligamentous repair and capsulodesis. *J Hand Surg [Am]* 1992;17:354–359.
12. Mayfield JK, Johnson RP, Kilcoyne RK. Carpal dislocations: pathomechanics and progressive perilunar instability. *J Hand Surg [Am]* 1980;5:226–241.
13. Watson HK, Ashmead D, Makhlouf MV. Examination of the scaphoid bone. *J Hand Surg [Am]* 1988;13:657–660.
14. Burgess RD. The effect of rotatory subluxation of the scaphoid on radioscaphoid contact. *J Hand Surg [Am]* 1987;12:771–774.
15. Viegas SF, Tencer AF, Cantrell J, et al. Load transfer characteristics of the wrist. Part II. Perilunate instability. *J Hand Surg [Am]* 1987;12:978–985.
16. Dobyns JH, Linscheid RL, Chao EYS, et al. Traumatic instability of the wrist. *AAOS Instr Course Lect* 1975;24:182–199.
17. Howard FM, Fahey T, Wotcik E. Rotary subluxation of the navicular. *Clin Orthop* 1974;104:134–139.
18. Loeb TM, Urbaniak JR, Goldner JL. Traumatic carpal instability: putting the pieces together. *Orthop Trans* 1977;1:163.
19. Palmer AK, Dobyns JA, Linscheid RL. Management of post-traumatic instability of the wrist secondary to ligament rupture. *J Hand Surg [Am]* 1978;3:507–532.
20. Taleisnik J. Post-traumatic carpal instability. *Clin Orthop* 1980;149:73–82.
21. Berger RA, Blair WF, Crowinshield RD, et al. The scapholunate ligament. *J Hand Surg [Am]* 1982;7:87–91.
22. Eckenrode JF, Louis DS, Greene TL. Scaphoid-trapezium-trapezoid fusion in the treatment of chronic scapholunate instability. *J Hand Surg [Am]* 1986;11:493–502.
23. Kleinman WB. Long-term study of chronic scapholunate instability treated by scapho-trapezium-trapezoid arthrodesis. *J Hand Surg [Am]* 1989;14:429–445.
24. Peterson HA, Lipscomb PR. Intercarpal arthrodesis. *Arch Surg* 1967;95:127–134.
25. Watson HK, Black DM. Instabilities of the wrist. *Hand Clin* 1987;3:103–111.
26. Watson HK, Hempton RF. Limited wrist arthrodesis. I. The triscaphoid joint. *J Hand Surg [Am]* 1980;5:320–327.
27. Inglis AE, Jones EC. Proximal row carpectomy for diastasis of the proximal carpal row. *J Bone Joint Surg Am* 1977;59:460–463.
28. Neviaser RJ. On resection of the proximal carpal row. *Clin Orthop* 1986;202:12–15.
29. Kauer JMG. The mechanism of the carpal joint. *Clin Orthop* 1986;202:16–26.
30. Short WH, Werner FW, Fortino MD, et al. A dynamic biomechanical study of scapholunate ligament sectioning. *J Hand Surg [Am]* 1995;20:986–999.
31. Huskisson EC. Measurement of pain. *Lancet* 1974;2:1127–1131.

30

LUNOTRIQUETRAL JOINT INSTABILITY

NEAL HOCHWALD
MARTIN A. POSNER

Lunotriquetral (LT) instability is an unusual cause of wrist pain, making diagnosis and treatment difficult. The difficulty in making the diagnosis is compounded by the complexity of carpal kinematics and ligamentous support in the area. Understanding carpal anatomy and kinematics is therefore a vital prerequisite to diagnosis and treatment. Current concepts in the diagnosis and treatment of acute and chronic ligament injuries to the LT joint are discussed.

ANATOMY

Osseous Anatomy

In the traditional concept of wrist anatomy, the carpal bones are aligned in two transverse rows comprising two important joints, the radiocarpal and midcarpal. The scaphoid spans and stabilizes both carpal rows and functions to resist compressive forces (1).

In 1919, Navarro introduced the concept of the vertical or columnar carpus (2). He believed that the carpus was composed of three vertical columns: a central or flexion–extension column, formed by the lunate, capitate, and hamate; a lateral or mobile column, consisting of the scaphoid, trapezium, and trapezoid; and a medial or rotation column, comprising the triquetrum and pisiform. The triquetrum as the axis for carpal rotation was a concept also emphasized by Ghia in 1939. He noted that during wrist motions, dorsal and volar displacement was greatest for the scaphoid and least for the triquetrum (3).

In 1976, Taleisnik proposed two changes in Navarro's concept of wrist kinematics (4). He included the trapezium and trapezoid in the central column, which left the scaphoid as the only bone in the lateral coumn. The scaphoid continued to serve as an important midcarpal joint stabilizer. Taleisnik's second change was to eliminate the pisform from the medial column because it is not involved in wrist motions. The medial column, comprising only the triquetrum, functions as a pivot around which carpal rotation occurs.

In 1981, Lichtman proposed the *oval ring* concept, which eliminated the lunate from the rigid central column because of the considerable movement that normally occurs between it and the capitate during flexion and extension as well as during radial and ulnar deviations (5). In Lichtman's concept, the mobile scaphotrapezial joint and the rotary triquetrohamate joint are the key links that permit reciprocal movements between the proximal and distal carpal rows during radial and ulnar deviation. A disruption in the ring at any point results in abnormal movements or instability. When the disruption is at the triquetrohamate joint, the result is midcarpal instability, and when it occurs at the LT joint, instability at that joint (6).

Ligamentous Anatomy

The ligaments of the wrist are complex and are traditionally classified into two categories, extrinsic and intrinsic (7).

Extrinisic Ligaments

The extrinsic ligaments are divided into proximal and distal subcategories. The proximal ligaments connect the radius and ulna to the carpal bones, and the distal ligaments connect the carpal bones to the metacarpals.

There are four proximal volar ligaments that originate from the radius. Beginning laterally, they are the radioscaphocapitate (RSC) ligament, the long radiolunate ligament (also referred to as the volar radiolunotriquetral or volar radiotriquetral ligament), the radioscapholunate ligament, and the short radiolunate ligament. The RSC ligament begins proximally at the radial styloid, courses distally and ulnarly, and inserts into the pole of the scaphoid and capitate. At the waist of the scaphoid, most of its fibers contribute to the capsule of the midcarpal joint. Distally, its fibers curve around the lunate and merge with the distal fibers of the ulnocapitate and triquetrocapitate ligaments to

---

N. Hochwald: Department of Orthopedics, Huntington Hospital, Huntington, New York 11743.

M. A. Posner: Department of Orthopaedics, New York University School of Medicine; Hand Services, Hospital for Joint Diseases and Lenox Hill Hospital, New York, New York 10128.

form the arcuate ligament. The RSC ligament limits radiocarpal pronation and ulnocarpal translocation (8). The long radiolunate ligament originates from the scaphoid fossa of the distal radius and attaches to the volar horn of the lunate as well as further distally into the triquetrum. It prevents ulnar migration of the lunate without impeding its dorsal and volar flexion. The radioscapholunate ligament, which originates on the volar edge of the radius and inserts on the proximal volar borders of the scaphoid and lunate, restrains angulation of the lunate. The short radiolunate ligament begins at the level of the lunate fossa on the radius and attaches distally into the lunate.

The dorsal wrist capsule is not as important as the volar capsule. The main proximal dorsal ligament is the dorsal radiocarpal ligament, also referred to as the dorsal radiotriquetral or dorsal radiolunotriquetral ligament. It has a broad proximal attachment on the distal radius that extends ulnarly from Lister's tubercle to the sigmoid notch, and distally, it attaches to the dorsum of the lunate and triquetrum where it merges with fibers of the intrinsic dorsal LT interosseous ligament. The dorsal radiocarpal ligament restrains ulnar translocation of the carpus and ulnocarpal supination (9).

The extrinsic ligaments that begin at the distal ulna are the ulnolunate, ulnotriquetral, and ulnocapitate ligaments. All three connect the ulna, triangular fibrocartilage complex (TFCC), and carpus. They stabilize the ulnocarpal joint and are also partly responsible for guiding the movements of the lunate and triquetrum. The ulnolunate ligament attaches proximally to the volar radioulnar capsule and distally to the lunate and forms the volar joint capsule, ulnar to the lunate fossa. The ulnotriquetral ligament has dorsal and volar components that originate from the volar and dorsal radioulnar joint ligaments, respectively, and attach to the triquetrum. They form part of the volar and dorsal ulnocarpal joint capsule and function to constrain ulnocarpal supination. The ulnocapitate ligament arises from the fovea of the ulnar head proximally, merges distally with the fibers of the LT interosseous ligament, and then proceeds around the lunate to merge with fibers of the RSC ligament. The connection of the ulnocapitate ligament with the RSC ligament forms the arcuate ligament, which links the proximal and distal carpal rows. The ulnocapitate ligament supports the ulnocarpal joint capsule, and it may also reinforce the LT joint (9).

Intrinsic Ligaments

Intrinsic ligaments are all intercarpal and are categorized according to length: short, intermediate, and long. The intrinsic ligaments that span the midcarpal joint volarly and dorsally contribute indirectly to LT joint instability by providing stabilization to adjacent joints. The volar intrinsic ligaments are the scaphotrapezium–trapezoid, scaphocapitate, triquetrocapitate, and triquetrohamate ligaments.

Only the last two are involved in LT joint stability. The triquetrocapitate ligament attaches proximally to the radial aspect of the triquetrum and distally to the ulnar aspect of the capitate. It constitutes the ulnar half of the midcarpal joint capsule and contributes to midcarpal stability by constraining supination. The triquetrohamate ligament is a strong ligament that spans the triquetrum and hamate and also contributes to midcarpal stability.

The dorsal intrinsic midcarpal ligaments include the dorsal intercarpal and dorsal scaphotriquetral ligaments. The dorsal intercarpal ligament attaches proximally to the triquetrum and distally to the scaphoid. It crosses the midcarpal joint and limits midcarpal rotation. The dorsal scaphotriquetral ligament spans the proximal carpal row and midcarpal joint and reinforces stability provided by the scapholunate and LT ligaments. The LT ligament spans the interval between the lunate and the base of the pisiform facet of the triquetrum. It is strongly reinforced by the extrinsic ulnocarpal ligaments and to a lesser degree by the dorsal radiocarpal ligaments that lie directly over it. The membranous proximal portion of the LT ligament is composed of fibrocartilage and is less substantial than the thick collagen fibers of its volar and dorsal portions. The volar portion ensures that the lunate and triquetrum move together as a unit while the dorsal portion restrains flexion and extension of the lunate and triquetrum (10).

KINEMATICS

Appreciation of the functional role of the triquetrum is essential to understanding the mechanics of carpal motion. The triquetrum acts as a link between the distal carpal row and the lunate, to which it is firmly secured. The triquetrum is also important in maintaining the relative positions of the carpal rows during radial and ulnar deviation.

During radial deviation, the scaphoid flexes under the radial styloid to allow for radiocarpal shortening. The trapezium moves toward the radial styloid, and the triquetrum and lunate move together dorally as a unit, relative to the carpus. The triquetrum also rotates dorsally as a function of the configuration of the triquetral–hamate articulation (11). Concomitant rotation and movement of the lunate is largely related to its firm attachment to the triquetrum.

During ulnar deviation, the triquetrum moves volarly on the hamate, pulling the lunate with it. Weber considered the triquetrum to be "low" when it assumed a volar position in wrist extension and "high" when in a dorsal position (12). The triquetrum is stabilized by the LT, triquetrocapitate, dorsal intercarpal, and dorsal radiocarpal ligaments. These ligaments permit the fluid movements of the triquetrum on the hamate between its "low" and "high" positions. In addition, the LT and dorsal radiolunotriquetral ligaments permit the triquetrum to extend relative to the lunate, which occurs in wrist extension.

LUNOTRIQUETRAL INSTABILITY

The mechanism of injury to the LT joint is usually one of extreme wrist extension combined with rotation. This is a different mechanism from that which results in a perilunate dislocation. Although wrist extension occurs in both injuries, it is ulnar rather than radial deviation, and intercarpal pronation rather than supination, that results in a LT sprain (13).

Two patterns of LT instability have been identified by Dobyns: carpal instability nondissociative (CIND) and carpal instability dissociative (CID). In the CIND pattern, there is a loss of extrinsic ligamentous support, which results in proximal carpal row instability and a rotational deformity. Of the extrinsic ligaments, the volar radiocarpal ligaments are most commonly damaged, although recent studies have also implicated the dorsal radiocarpal ligament (14). The intrinsic ligaments remain intact. In the CID pattern, there is a loss of intrinsic ligamentous support and dissociation of the bones within the proximal carpal row. Complete disruption of the LT ligament results in some LT instability, although an actual gap between the bones is uncommon. However, motion between the two bones increases, and the triquetrum extends at its articulation with the hamate. The normal "low" or dorsiflexed position of the triquetrum on the hamate during ulnar deviation is no longer transmitted to the lunate, and it volarflexes because of its connection to the scaphoid.

In order to destabilize the LT joint sufficiently to cause either a static or dynamic pattern of instability, not only does the LT ligament have to be completely disrupted, but also the volar radiotriquetral and/or dorsal radiocarpal ligament. This was demonstrated in a study by Viegas using cadaveric wrists in which the LT, the volar radiotriquetral, and the dorsal radiocarpal ligaments were sequentially sectioned (15). When only the LT ligament was sectioned, a volar intercalated segment instability (VISI) deformity could not be detected by either direct visualization or radiographs. Sectioning the LT and volar radiotriquetral ligaments resulted in a dynamic VISI deformity, and when the dorsal radiocarpal ligament was also sectioned, a static VISI deformity occurred.

A similar study by Horii had slightly different results (16). As in the Viegas study, sectioning the LT ligament did not result in a static VISI deformity, but some instability of the LT joint was noted. Sectioning of the dorsal radiocarpal and dorsal scaphotriquetral ligaments caused a VISI pattern of instability. Horii concluded that the dorsal ligaments were the essential constraints to maintain normal carpal stability in the absence of the LT ligament.

In yet another study using cadaver wrists, Li showed that movement of the triquetrum during ulnar deviation signif-
icantly increased after arthroscopic sectioning of the LT ligament (17). He also found that the volar radiotriquetral ligament functioned as a stabilizer of the LT joint during wrist extension.

Diagnosis

An acute LT sprain results in ulnar-sided wrist pain, swelling, limitation of motion, and point tenderness over the injured joint. Grip strength may also be diminished. Testing for joint laxity is important to determine if there is any dissociation. This is carried out by first ballotting the joint and then subjecting it to shear stress. Shear stress is applied by grasping the triquetrum and pisiform between the thumb and index finger of one hand while stabilizing the lunate with the other hand (13). The triquetrum and pisiform are then pushed in a volar-to-dorsal direction (Fig. 30.1). Increased motion indicates instability, which is usually accompanied by pain at the joint and, frequently, a palpable or audible click.

Chronic LT instability is commonly manifested as pain and clicking of the ulnar side of the wrist with active extension and/or ulnar deviation for more than 6 months. The diagnosis is aided by positive ballottement and shear stress tests. Another useful diagnostic test is if pain is relieved following a local injection of an anesthetic into the joint. The differential diagnosis includes a tear of the TFCC, ulnar

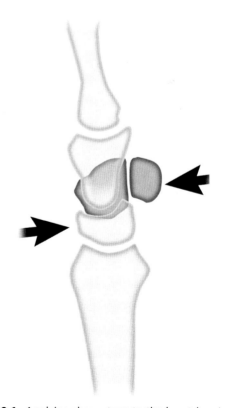

FIGURE 30.1. Applying shear stress to the lunotriquetral joint.

impaction syndrome, disruption of the distal radioulnar joint, subluxation of the extensor carpi ulnaris tendon, midcarpal instablity, and a triquetral fracture. With injury to the TFCC, there is pain with forearm pronation and supination, which differentiates it from an isolated LT tear. However, when pronation and supination are resisted, a twisting motion is transmitted to the carpal bones, and pain will usually occur when there are abnormal movements at the LT joint. The other conditions can be diagnosed by physical examination and imaging studies.

Diagnostic Imaging

Imaging studies are essential for evaluating any wrist injury, beginning with conventional radiographs. Radiographs required for suspected LT instability include a posterior–anterior view, anterior–posterior (supination) clenched-fist views in radial and ulnar deviation, an oblique view, and a lateral view. Frequently, all the views are normal when the tear is confined to the LT ligament. However, with more severe injuries, there is widening of the joint space because of a dissociation between the two carpal bones, overlapping of the lunate and triquetrum, and disruption of the normally smooth curve of the proximal carpal row as a result of proximal displacement of the triquetrum (Fig. 30.2). The lateral radiograph may show a VISI deformity. Consequently, the angle formed by the longitudinal axes of the triquetrum and lunate (LT angle) on this view, which normally averages +14°, will be reversed and measure less than 0° (average, −16°).

Arthrography can also be valuable for diagnosing LT tears (18), although abnormal communications between the radiocarpal and midcarpal joint have been demonstrated in 50% of normal subjects (19), and LT tears were noted in 55% of arthrograms in a study of cadaver wrists (20). Most normal arthrograms in asymptomatic subjects are thought to indicate degenerative ligamentous tears, which are common after the age of 40 (21). Localizing tenderness to the LT joint in a patient with wrist pain increases the specificity of a "positive" arthrogram. Arthrography should always be performed using fluoroscopy in order to document the precise area of joint leakage. Separate injections into the radiocarpal and midcarpal joints are recommended because the dye may leak in only one direction. Exercising the wrist before the injections is a useful provocative procedure to increase intraarticular pressure. In spite of all these maneuvers, a small number of false-negative arthrograms still occur. When arthrography is combined with cinearthrography, sensitivity is 93%, specificity 97%, and accuracy 96% (22).

Magnetic resonance imaging (MRI) is not as sensitive for evaluating LT ligament tears as it is for tears of the scapholunate ligament because the LT ligament is a less substantial ligament. In addition, the incidence of joint widening is lower for isolated LT tears than for similar injuries to the scapholunate ligament. The LT ligament normally has a low signal intensity on T1-weighted images. An intermediate signal density or the presence of excess fluid in the joint may indicate a torn ligament. Disruption of the LT ligament is frequently identified by its absence on T2-weighted coronal images (23). MRI has been shown to be 56% sensitive, 100% specific, and 80% accurate when compared to arthroscopy or arthrotomy (23,24). MRI and arthrography are frequently carried out together.

Arthroscopy is the gold standard for diagnosing LT ligament tears (25). The procedure permits insertion of a probe into the LT joint in order to evaluate integrity and to assess stability. The procedure also makes it possible to stress the joint under direct visualization. A large percentage of ligament tears are degenerative or attritional in origin, and studies using cadaveric wrists have shown that up to 62% of specimens have combined LT ligament and TFCC tears (20,26). The LT tears in these situations are secondary to ulnar impaction syndrome, which is the primary pathology.

If no LT dissociation or incongruity is seen on radiographs, dynamic instability must be considered, particularly when there is "clicking" or "snapping" with wrist movements. The instability in such cases can be documented only by motion imaging studies (videoradiography or cineradiography) (Fig. 30.3). In the lateral projection, the lunate is inclined volarly with the wrist in slight ulnar deviation. As the wrist is deviated further volarly, there is a snap-

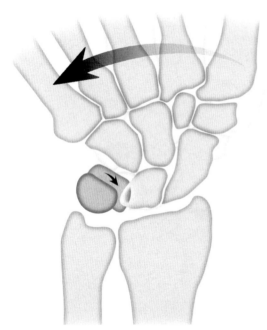

FIGURE 30.2. The normally smooth curve of the proximal carpal row is disrupted *(large arrow)*, and there is overlapping of the lunate and triquetrum *(small arrow)*. (Adapted from Alexander CE, Lichtman DM. Triquetrolunate and midcarpal instability. In: Lichtman DM, ed. *The wrist and its disorders*. Philadelphia: WB Saunders, 1988;274–285, with permission.)

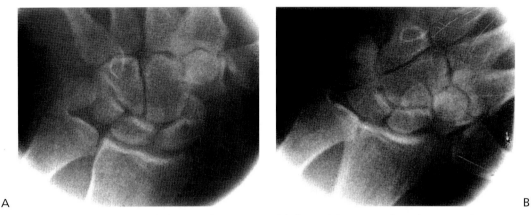

FIGURE 30.3. Patient with dynamic lunotriquetral (LT) instability. **A:** In ulnar deviation, the normal curvature of the proximal carpal row was maintained. **B:** However, with active radial deviation, there was and audible "click," and the LT joint was momentarily subluxated, resulting in incongruity (arrow) of the joint.

ping motion of the lunate manifested clinically by pain and an audible "click." A high index of suspicion is required to make the diagnosis of dynamic instability.

Treatment

The treatment of injuries to the LT joint is dependent on the extent and chronicity of the injury. For the acute isolated strain, if there is no dissociation of the joint, the wrist is splinted or casted for 6 weeks. Generally, the pain will resolve within a few months. However, the patient should be followed longer to ensure that there is no progression to a dissociation pattern or to a VISI deformity, indicative of LT instability. Although most patients never develop instability, wrist pain associated with "popping," "clicking," or "catching" can persist. In such cases, there is often a flap tear of the LT ligament or a chondral lesion of the triquetrum. Arthroscopic debridement of these lesions is usually beneficial (27,28). In debriding the ligament, it is important to debride only its central fibrocartilaginous portion to avoid producing iatrogenic instability.

Acute LT dissociation is a severe injury and frequently is a component of perilunate dissociation (29). However, in rare instances, the dissociation can occur as an isolated problem for which surgery is usualy indicated. The flexed position of the lunate is corrected, and the LT joint is pinned in its normal anatomic position with fine, nonthreaded Kirschner wires. The ligament is then repaired using nonabsorbable sutures, which are inserted into drill holes into either the lunate or triquetrum, depending on the bone from which the ligament avulsed. The wires are removed at 8 weeks, and active range-of-motion exercises are started.

Treatment for chronic instability, whether it is static or dynamic, includes direct repair or reinsertion of the ligament into bone, ligament reconstruction, or intercarpal arthrodesis. A direct repair is usually impossible after several weeks. Ligament reconstructions are performed using one-half of either the extensor carpi ulnaris or flexor carpi ulnaris tendon, which is passed through drill holes in the lunate and triquetrum. Reconstructing the ligament on both dorsal and volar aspects of the joint has been recommended, as has reinforcing the reconstructed ligament using a dorsal intermetacarpal ligament (14). When LT dissociation and VISI deformity are both present, and the deformity can still be reduced, similar ligament reconstructions can be attempted and should include reattachment of the extrinsic dorsal ligaments (dorsal radiotriquetral) to the triquetrum. The LT joint is then fixed with Kirschner wires for 6 to 8 weeks, followed by an additional 4 to 6 weeks of wrist splinting.

Arthrodesis of the LT joint is an alternative to ligament reconstruction and is the procedure we recommend because of its high predictability of success. Although a pseudoarthrosis rate of 57% has been reported, the operations in that series were performed without using an autogenous bone graft (30). When a bone graft is used, fusion rates exceed 80% (31,32), and in one study it was 100% (33). Postoperative wrist motion following LT fusions averages approximately 85% of normal. Pain relief varies considerably from study to study. In one study, only 1 of 14 patients had residual pain (31), whereas in another study, 77% of patients remained symptomatic (33). This disparity in results emphasizes the importance of careful patient selection and proper surgical technique using an autogenous bone graft. Patients with VISI deformities are not candidates for LT fusions because of the extent of ligamentous damage. In these patients, a four-bone fusion (lunate, capitate, hamate, and triquetrum) is a more effective procedure (34). Patients with LT ligament tears that accompany degenerative tears of the TFCC are also not candidates for a LT fusion. Frequently, these patients have chondromalacia of their lunate, triquetrum, and/or ulna head, which should be the focus of treatment, and not the LT

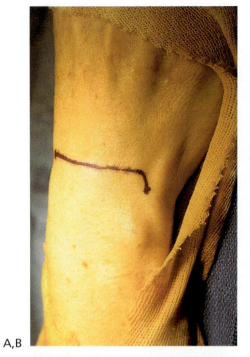
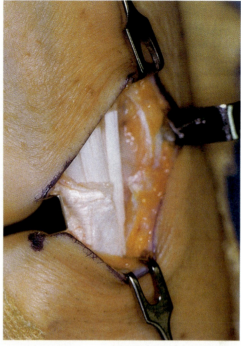
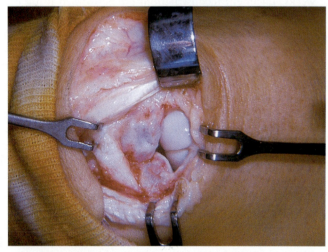
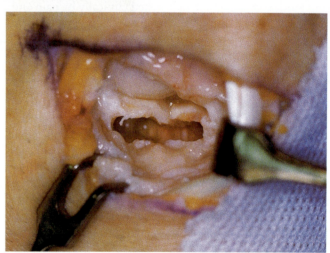
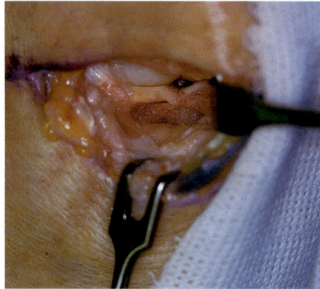
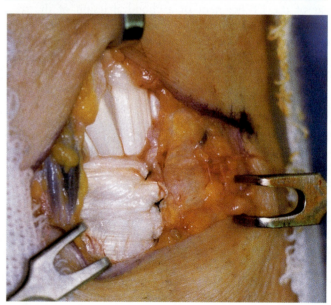

FIGURE 30.4. Technique for arthrodesis of the lunotriquetral (LT) joint in a patient with chronic instability. **A:** Surgical incision. **B:** Longitudinal incision in the extensor retinaculum over the fourth compartment. **C:** The LT ligament had completely eroded. **D:** Deep transverse trough across the LT joint. **E:** Cancellous iliac bone graft within the trough. **F:** The capsule and extensor retinaculum are repaired.

(Figure continues on next page.)

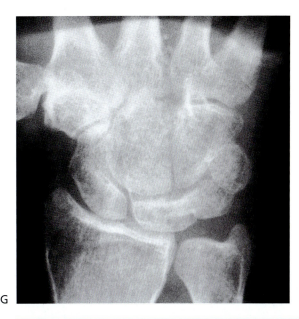

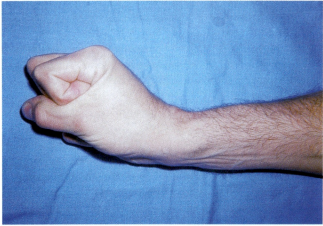
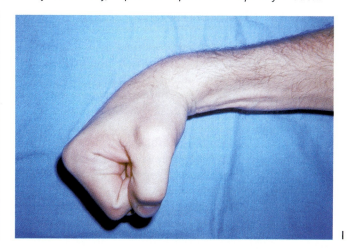

FIGURE 30.4. *(continued)* **G:** Final radiograph showing fusion of the LT joint. **H,I:** Postoperative wrist motion. **Editors' Notes:** *Limited wrist arthrodesis is often best accomplished by decorticating the entire two opposing surfaces, forming slight concavities of the cancellous bone on each side. This tends to centralize the graft and maintain external dimensions that match the normal shape and configuration of the bones involved. Cortical inlays tend to use a much smaller bone surface area. The cortex occupies space where healing cancellous bone could be, and cortex is not necessary for stability, as pins accomplish the temporary fixation.*

ligament tear, which is the secondary problem. When the problem is an ulna impaction syndrome, a distal radioulnar joint stabilization combined with ulna head resection is usually effective.

Arthrodesis of the LT joint is carried out via a transverse incision over the proximal carpal row (Fig. 30.4). If additional exposure is required, the ulnar end of the incision is carried proximally for a short distance (1–2 cm). The skin flaps are mobilized, and the extensor retinaculum is divided longitudinally over the fourth extensor compartment. The septum between the fourth and fifth compartments is also divided, which permits the tendons in the fourth compartment to be retracted radially and the extensor digiti quinti proprius tendon in the fifth compartment to be retracted ulnarly. The dorsal capsule is incised transversely, leaving a small proximal edge to facilitate later closure, and the distal portion of the capsule is elevated, exposing the LT joint. A deep transverse trough is then fashioned across the joint using a power burr. The bone graft we recommend is a corticocancellous graft from the ilium. It is fashioned to be slightly longer and deeper than the trough and is wedged into place. The cancellous portion of the graft is placed within the trough, and the cortical portion, from the thin outer table of the ilium, comprises the roof of the trough. In many cases, particularly those with dynamic instability where there is no dissociation, a cancellous graft is sufficient. Supplemental fixation with one or two Kirschner wires or a compression screw is required only in cases of gross joint instability. The capsule and extensor retinaculum are repaired, but not the septum between the tendon compartments. Postoperatively, the wrist is immobilized until the graft consolidates, which averages 10 to 12 weeks.

SUMMARY

Injury to the LT joint must be considered in the differential diagnosis of ulnar-sided wrist pain. The spectrum of injury can vary from an uncomplicated grade I or II sprain to a grade III sprain accompanied by joint instability. The diagnosis of these injuries requires a careful physical examination, localizing tenderness and any instability to the joint. Imaging studies are always necessary. Aside from conventional radiographs, arthrography and MRI are useful, and for difficult diagnostic problems, arthroscopy. Treatment depends on the severity and chronicity of symptoms and the disability they cause. Acute simple sprains can be treated with temporary wrist immobilization, but when there is joint instability, surgery is warranted. Chronic injuries can be treated effectively by arthroscopic debridement of the damaged portion of the ligament. For chronic instability, ligament reconstruction or LT arthrodesis is often required. Arthrodesis is the preferred operation because it has a high predictability of success to eliminate discomfort without significantly restricting wrist mobility.

EDITORS' COMMENTS

The lunate and triquetrum are united by a near syndesmosis. They may be considered to be almost a single bone in terms of wrist kinematics. Indeed, the most common congenital fusion is lunotriquetral, and it results in wrists that are essentially normal. The position of the scaphoid controls the position of the lunate and, therefore, the position of the triquetrum. Because of its length and distal extension, the scaphoid is controlled by positions of the wrist. Therefore, wrist position determines scaphoid position, lunate position, and triquetral position. If the lunate becomes detached from the scaphoid, the position of the lunate and triquetrum then depend on their neutral anatomy tendencies. Neutral anatomy is the position a bone would assume based entirely on its shape, independent of any ligamentous restraints. The classic lunate is described as thinner dorsally and thicker volarly. Its neutral anatomy position is, therefore, a dorsal intercalated segment instability (DISI), and, indeed, that is the common pattern with total scaphoid dissociation. In a radiographic study of lunate shape, however, nearly one-quarter of all lunates are thinner volarly than dorsally. Their neutral anatomy position is, therefore, VISI. If the scaphoid loses its external ligamentous support and flexes with an intact scapholunate interosseous system, it will carry the lunate and triquetrum into VISI, independent of lunate shape. The loads of the wrist will flex the unstable scaphoid and drive the lunate into VISI, forcing the thicker portion of the lunate beneath the capitate and wedging it away from the radius. If the lunate and scaphoid are detached from one another, the lunate and triquetrum are free to assume the neutral anatomy position of the lunate. A V-type lunate, or one that is thinner volarly and detached from the scaphoid, will produce the midcarpal instability picture of VISI with a scapholunate gap. Severe midcarpal instability with VISI deformity is primarily a scaphoid problem and must be dealt with from the radial side of the wrist, typically by fusion of the scaphoid–trapezium–trapezoid joint.

The triquetrum cannot control the position of the lunate. The triquetrum is a passive intercalated segment. The triquetral–hamate joint is the most lax intercarpal joint in the wrist. The triquetrum moves proximally and distally, and volarly and dorsally on the hamate. Making a small cut in the dorsal capsule of the triquetral–hamate joint at surgery for other reasons will demonstrate to the observer that this joint is terribly lax, without significant restraint, and that the hamate cannot control the position of the triquetrum through ligamentous attachment. The hamate influences the position of the triquetrum only by its proximal pressure on the articular surface. The flexion position of the triquetrum, therefore, is controlled by the lunate. Interosseous rupture and instability between the triquetrum and lunate are not responsible for midcarpal instability. Tears of the LT interosseous system are most common in the presence of a long ulna but can occur from a severe pronation injury. Patients frequently can get along adequately with tearing of the LT interosseous system as long as it is not unstable and is compatible with the patient's demands.

When the diagnosis is clearly ulnar wrist pathology with carpal involvement in a patient with significant persistent symptoms requiring repair, an open approach is indicated rather than arthroscopy. With the transverse open approach, all of the symptomatic components of the ulnar side of the wrist can be dealt with in a definitive fashion. If there is tearing of the proximalmost aspect of the LT interosseous ligament with intact volar and dorsal segments, surgery on the LT joint is seldom indicated. If there are changes in the proximal portion of the lunate toward the ulnar side and similar changes on the distal end of the ulna with attenuation of the central portion of the triangular fibrocartilage, then step-cut shortening of the ulna is indicated. The long ulna acts as a piston against the LT joint under heavy load, and step-cut shortening is usually all that is required even though there is fairly significant tearing between the lunate and triquetrum. If the LT interosseous system is completely torn and the lunate and triquetrum can be easily separated, then LT limited wrist arthrodesis is indicated (see Fig. 57.4). There is no place for LT interosseous ligament reconstruction. Tearing of components of the ulnar sling mechanism is seldom the cause of symptoms unless there is dislocation or subluxation of the distal ulna from the radius. Thus, repair of tears involving the ulnolunate and ulnotriquetral ligaments is rarely indicated.

REFERENCES

1. Green DP. Carpal dislocations and instabilities. In: Green DP, ed. *Operative hand surgery, 3rd ed.* New York: Churchill Livingstone, 1993;861–928.
2. Taleisnik J. Post-traumatic carpal instability. *Clin Orthop* 1980; 149:73–82.
3. Taleisnik J. Triquetrohamate and triquetrolunate instabilities. *Ann Chir Main* 1984;3:331–343.
4. Taleisnik J. Wrist: Anatomy, function and injury. *AAOS Instr Course Lect* 1978;:61–87.
5. Lichtman DM, Schneider JR, Swafford AR, et al. Ulnar midcarpal instability—clinical and laboratory analysis. *J Hand Surg* 1981;6:515–523.
6. Alexander CE, Lichtman DM. Triquetrolunate and midcarpal instability. In: Lichtman DM, ed. *The wrist and its disorders.* Philadelphia: WB Saunders, 1988;274–285.
7. Taleisnik J. The ligaments of the wrist. *J Hand Surg [Am]* 1976;1:110–118.
8. Viegas SF, Patterson RM, Ward K. Extrinsic wrist ligaments in the pathomechanics of ulnar translational instability. *J Hand Surg [Am]* 1995;20:312–318.
9. Berger RA. The ligaments of the wrist: A current overview of anatomy with considerations of their potential functions. *Hand Clin* 1997;13:63–82.
10. Ritt MG, Berger RA, Kauer JMG. The gross and histologic anatomy of the ligaments of the capitohamate joint. *J Hand Surg [Am]*, 1996;21:1022–1028.
11. Alexander CE, Lichtman DM. Ulnar carpal instabilities. *Orthop Clin North Am* 1984;15:307–320.
12. Weber ER. Biomechanical implications of scaphoid wrist fractures. *Clin Orthop* 1980;149:83–90.
13. Reagan DS, Linscheid RL, Dobyns JH. Lunotriquetral sprains. *J Hand Surg [Am]* 1984;9:502–514.
14. Cooney WP III, Linscheid RL, Dobyns JH. Carpal instability: Treatment of ligament injuries of the wrist. *AAOS Instr Course Lect* 1991;:33–44.
15. Viegas SF, Patterson RM, Peterson PD, et al. Ulnar-sided perilunate instability: An anatomic and biomechanic study. *J Hand Surg [Am]* 1990;15:268–278.
16. Horii E, Garcia-Elias M, An KN, et al. A kinematic study of lunotriquetral dissociations. *J Hand Surg [Am]* 1991;16:355–362.
17. Li G, Rowen B, Tokunaga D, et al. Carpal kinematics of lunotriquetral dissociations. *Bioimed Sci Instrum* 1991;27:273–281.
18. Palmer AK, Levinsohn EM, Kuzma GR. Arthrography of the wrist. *J Hand Surg [Am]* 1983;8:15–23.
19. Shigematsu S, Abe M, Onomura T, et al. Arthrography of the normal and posttraumatic wrist. *J Hand Surg [Am]* 1989;14:410–412.
20. Mrose HE, Rosenthal DI. Arthrography of the hand and wrist. *Hand Clin* 1991;7:201–217.
21. Viegas SF, Ballantyne G. Attritional lesions of the wrist joint. *J Hand Surg [Am]* 1987;12:1025–1029.
22. Weiss APC, Akelman E, Lambiase R. Comparison of the findings of triple injection cinearthrography of the wrist with those of arthroscopy. *J Bone Joint Surg Am* 1993;78:348–356.
23. Stoller DW. *Magnetic resonance imaging in orthopaedics and sports medicine.* Philadelphia: JB Lippincott, 1993;712–739.
24. Reicher MA, Kellerhouse LE. *MRI of the wrist and hand.* New York: Raven Press, 1990;69–85.
25. Cooney WP. Evaluation of chronic wrist pain by arthrography, arthroscopy, and arthrotomy. *J Hand Surg [Am]* 1993;18:815–822.
26. Viegas SF, Patterson RM, Hokanson JA, et al. Wrist anatomy: Incidence, distribution, and correlation of anatomic variations, tears, and arthrosis. *J Hand Surg [Am]* 1993;18:463–475.
27. Ruch DS, Poehling G. Arthroscopic management of partial scapholunate and lunotriquetral injuries of the wrist. *J Hand Surg [Am]* 1996;21:412–417.
28. Weiss AP, Sachar K, Glowacki KA. Arthroscopic debridement alone for intercarpal ligament tears. *J Hand Surg [Am]* 1997;22:344–349.
29. Kuhlman JN. Lunotriquetral dissociation. In: Buchler U, ed. *Wrist instability.* London: Martin Dunitz, 1996;147–154.
30. Sennwald GR, Fischer M, Mondi P. Lunotriquetral arthrodesis. *J Hand Surg [Br]* 1995;20:755–760.
31. Kirschenbaum D, Coyle MP, Leddy JP. Chronic lunotriquetral instability: Diagnosis and management. *J Hand Surg [Am]* 1993;18:1107–1112.
32. Nelson DL, Manske PR, Pruitt DL, et al. Lunotriquetral arthrodesis. *J Hand Surg [Am]* 1993;18:1113–1120.
33. Pin PG, Young VL, Gilula LA, et al. Management of chronic lunotriquetral ligament tears. *J Hand Surg [Am]* 1989;14:77–83.
34. Ambrose L, Posner MA. Lunate–triquetral and midcarpal instability. *Hand Clin* 1992;8:653–668.

MIDCARPAL INSTABILITY

ANDREW E. CAPUTO
H. KIRK WATSON
JEFFREY WEINZWEIG

Midcarpal instability (MCI) is a term securely fixed in wrist nomenclature. The problem is its application to many different pathologic conditions. The term is currently used to describe a symptomatic hyperflexed scaphoid, volar intercalated segment instability (VISI) when symptomatic, ulnar wrist pronation, subluxation of the capitate from the lunate [capitate–lunate instability pattern (CLIP)], overload symptoms from a dorsally tilted radius postfracture, triquetrolunate (TL) dissociation, and triquetrohamate (TH) dissociation. We have chosen to link the term *midcarpal instability* with the volarflexed lunate. This means that a volarflexed lunate or VISI position is a necessary component of any MCI. This proximal row volarflexion can occur on the ulnar or radial side. The lunate flexion is a product of several different components. The lunate can volarflex because it is attached to the scaphoid by the scapholunate interosseous ligaments, and the scaphoid hyperflexes. The lunate can flex secondary to its innate shape with detachment from the scaphoid or the triquetrum or both.

MCI occurs as type I, type II, type III, and type IV. Type I is a physiologic supination of the wrist originating on the ulnar side and is basically asymptomatic. Type II is the same supination phenomenon occurring on the ulnar side of the wrist, either with or without the patient's control, and is symptomatic. Type III is radial-sided MCI with involvement of the scaphoid with an intact scapholunate interosseous system. Type IV is radial-sided MCI involving the scaphoid with scapholunate dissociation.

RESEARCH MATERIAL

We have utilized a combination of the results from the world literature using the term *midcarpal instability* and the authors' experience with MCI. The series included for review were obtained from a Medline search for *midcarpal instability* and from the reference sections of related articles. These series were reviewed for diagnostic inclusion criteria, including exam and radiographs, types of treatment, and outcomes.

The authors' results were obtained from a consecutive series of patients who were treated with a triscaphe or scaphotrapeziotrapezoid (STT) fusion for type III and IV MCI. The diagnosis of radial MCI was given to patients who had rotary subluxation of the scaphoid (RSS) with VISI. In this study, the combinations of these two findings were used as the diagnostic criteria for radial MCI. The diagnosis of RSS was established by a combination of clinical signs including dorsal wrist tenderness, articular or nonarticular scaphoid tenderness, triscaphe synovitis, a positive resisted finger extension test, and a positive scaphoid shift maneuver with scaphoid subluxation. Patients with type III and IV MCI were all noted to have some degree of volar or pronation subluxation of the wrist. Some patients had a grossly obvious catch-up clunk. We described the catch-up clunk as the sign of the return of the carpal bones (not always a specific one) from a stressed position to a normal position. The return of the carpal bones to the normal position occurs after the release of the stress and makes a palpable, visible, and sometimes audible shift referred to as the clunk.

All patients had failed conservative treatment consisting of a combination of activity modification, intermittent wrist splinting, and oral antiinflammatory medication. Preoperative evaluation included assessment of mechanism of injury, activity-related pain, rest pain, wrist motion, grip strength, and pinch strength. Preoperative radiographs were evaluated

---

A. E. Caputo: Department of Orthopaedic Surgery, University of Connecticut Health Center, Farmington, Connecticut 06032; Department of Orthopaedic Surgery, Hartford Hospital and Connecticut Children's Medical Center, Hartford, Connecticut 06106.

H. K. Watson: Connecticut Combined Hand Surgery Fellowship, Hartford Hospital, and Connecticut Children's Medical Center, Hartford, Connecticut 06106; Department of Orthopaedics, University of Connecticut School of Medicine, Farmington, Connecticut 06032; Department of Orthopedics, Rehabilitation, and Plastic Surgery, Yale University School of Medicine, New Haven, Connecticut 06520.

J. Weinzweig: Department of Plastic Surgery, Brown University School of Medicine, Rhode Island Hospital, and Hasbro Children's Hospital, Providence, Rhode Island 02905.

for VISI, scapholunate gap, and scaphocapitate angle. We measured the scaphocapitate angle to objectively record the scaphoid flexion relative to the carpus. We based this angle on a longitudinal line central in the capitate relative to a line tangent to the proximal contours of the scaphoid (Fig. 31.1). Lunates were described as either V-type (thinner volarly), D-type (thinner dorsally), or N-type (neutral) (1). Radiographically, the integrity of the scapholunate joint was divided into MCI type III (no abnormal increase in scapholunate gap in static or loaded views) and MCI type IV (obvious increase in scapholunate gap in static or loaded views). A wrist was considered to be in VISI when the lunate was volarflexed as viewed on a lateral radiograph in neutral wrist position (2). Postoperative examination including pain assessment, wrist motion, grip strength, and radiographic analysis for union and possible related arthritis.

We found 37 patients (40 wrists) who met the inclusion criteria for the study. Of these, 31 patients (36 wrists) had appropriate radiographs for review. The average age was 35 years (range, 15–62 years). The involved wrist was dominant in 25 cases and nondominant in 11. A traumatic etiology was involved in 13 cases. Preoperatively, most had severe activity-related pain, and approximately half had severe rest pain.

Radiographically, all patients exhibited VISI with a volarflexed lunate. All patients also had significant scaphoid flexion with volar subluxation of the scaphoid relative to the trapezoid and trapezium. In other words, the proximal portion of the trapezoid and trapezium rested on the dorsal neck of the scaphoid. In actuality, this can be described as a dorsal subluxation of the triscaphe joint, which, because of the concertina collapse effect, is visualized grossly as volar subluxation of the hand relative to the forearm. The average preoperative scaphocapitate angle was 80°. Fifty-six percent of wrists (19/34) were type III with a radiographically normal scapholunate interval, and 44% (15/34) were type IV with an abnormally wide scapholunate interval. Approximately 56% of wrists (19/34) had V-type lunates, 35% (12/34) were N, and 9% (2/34) were D-type. Type V lunates were seen in 80% (12/15) of type III wrists compared to 37% (7/19) of type IV wrists.

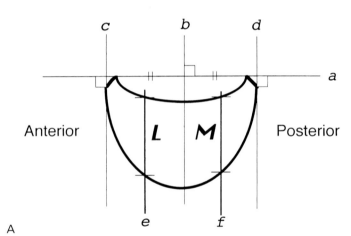

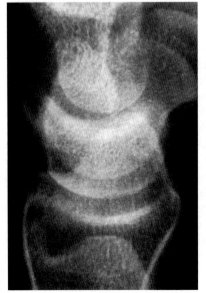
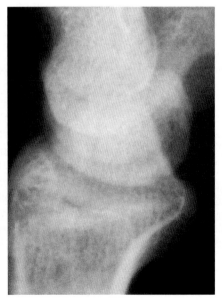
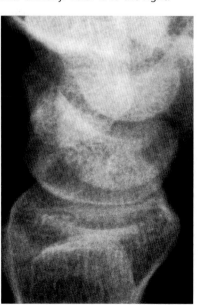

FIGURE 31.1. A: Lateral lunate morphology was determined by true lateral x-ray measurements. Volar and dorsal lines *L* and *M* were used to compare thickness. We recognize that these x-rays are produced by the entire width of the lunate. Recent anatomic studies, however, tend to confirm the fact that approximately 20% of lunates are thinner volarly, 5% to 10% are neutral or equal thickness dorsally and volarly, and nearly 75% are the classic, thinner dorsally, lunates. **B:** This is a neutral lunate, equal thickness volarly and dorsally. Volar is to the right. **C:** This is a D-type lunate, thinner dorsally, thicker volarly. Volar is to the right. **D:** This is a V-type lunate, which is clearly thinner volarly, thicker dorsally. Volar is to the right.

Time to surgery averaged 17 months (range, 2–84 months). All patients included in the study had failed conservative treatment and underwent a triscaphe fusion. Average follow-up was 3.1 years (range, 1–9 years). Preoperative activity-related pain was severe in 83% and moderate in 17%. Postoperative activity-related pain was moderate in 33%, mild in 39%, and not present in 27%. Preoperative rest pain was severe in 61%, moderate in 17%, mild in 11%, and not present in 11%. Postoperative rest pain was mild in 33% and not present in 67%. Postoperatively, no patients complained of, or had physical exam signs of, MCI including the catch-up clunk.

The ligaments of the proximal pole of the scaphoid can rupture, resulting in loss of radial-sided support. Scapholunate dissociation with or without radioscaphoid ligament rupture along with other supporting ligaments usually results in scaphoid hyperflexion and supination as the proximal pole climbs the dorsum of the capitate. This is a form of RSS probably best described as scapholunate dissociation type. Scaphoid hyperflexion and loss of radial carpal support can also occur as a result of rupture of the ligaments at the distal scaphoid or triscaphe joint. The distal pole of the scaphoid can shift laterally under load, causing shear loading of the triscaphe joint cartilage and resulting in eventual STT degenerative arthritis. In the more severe form, the scaphoid can hyperflex and the distal pole shift laterally, resulting in symptomatic loss of radial-side load transference. This rotary subluxation is best termed a distal scaphoid or triscaphe dissociation type of RSS. When the scaphoid is not attached to the lunate (scapholunate dissociation type RSS), the scaphoid hyperflexes and will not take load. This allows the lunate and proximal row to assume their neutral anatomy position. *Neutral anatomy* is the position dictated by the bone shape. If the lunate is thinner dorsally, then it will assume a dorsal intercalated segment instability (DISI) position (Fig. 31.2A). If the lunate is thinner volarly, then VISI will predominate (1) (Fig. 31.2C). The scaphoid in the triscaphe dissociation type of RSS is commonly not detached from the lunate at its proximal pole. The hyperflexing scaphoid now carries the proximal row with it into flexion (VISI), independent of the neutral anatomy position of the lunate (Fig. 31.2B).

For the purposes of this chapter, MCI types III and IV refer to patients with RSS and VISI. Based on the above discussion, if RSS occurs with triscaphe and scapholunate involvement, then MCI can exist with a D-type lunate and

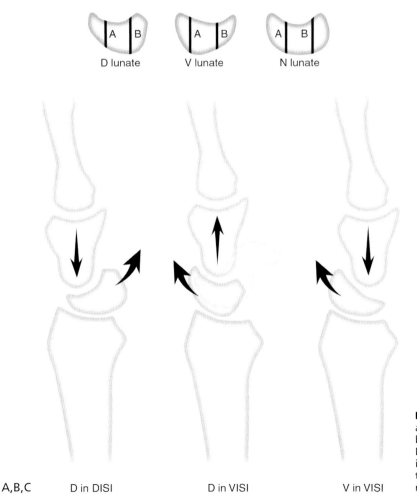

FIGURE 31.2. A: Standard D-type lunate with ruptured ligaments escaping into a dorsal intercalated segment instability (DISI) pattern as the capitate approaches the radius. **B:** D-type lunate being driven into volar intercalated segment instability (VISI) by an intact scapholunate interosseous system and a flexing scaphoid. **C:** V-type lunate going into its neutral anatomy position of VISI.

DISI. The reasons for clarifying the patients in this study as a unique group are based on their consistent clinical presentation with the volar subluxed wrist and catch-up clunk.

CATCH-UP CLUNK

One of us (H.K.W.) coined this phrase in the early 1980s to describe the audible, palpable clunk that occurs when a carpal or group of carpal bones catches up with the wrist position after being restrained in an untenable position. The maintenance of an untenable position is usually accomplished by the forearm musculature but can be imposed by a proximal load from the examiner or even the patient's opposite hand. A rotated scaphoid can be held in flexion as the hand is ulnarly deviated. The end of the untenable position is reached as the need for the scaphoid to extend demanded by wrist position equals the proximal load from the forearm holding the scaphoid flexed. Slight release of the forearm musculature will allow the scaphoid to catch up, accompanied by the clunk. In another example, the proximal load of the capitate can hold a lunate in VISI position. The wrist is ulnarly deviated until the need for the lunate to snap into the DISI position of full ulnar deviation exceeds the proximal load of the forearm musculature. The lunate will then catch up. The volume of the noise and the severity of the clunk are governed, therefore, by the amount of proximal load, whether active muscle or examiner induced. In some patients with MCI, their wrists rest in a severe volar-subluxed position that can be corrected to normal with active grip in ulnar deviation or passive axial load combined with dorsal translation or ulnar deviation.

WHAT IS NOT MIDCARPAL INSTABILITY?

Dorsal Radius Angulation Carpal Overload

In 1919 Jeanne and Mouchet described "dorsal luxation of the capitate" as a complication of malunited distal radius fracture. Linscheid (2) described a similar loss of alignment between the distal and proximal carpal rows as a result of distal radial malunion. Linscheid and Dobyns described "intercarpal collapse deformity" as a complication of Colles' fractures (2). Taleisnik and Watson described "midcarpal instability" caused by malunited fractures of the distal radius (3). Amadio and Botte have also reported on this "dynamic midcarpal instability" and its treatment by corrective osteotomy of the malunited distal radius (4). The condition is not to be related to the initial injury but instead to the repetitive overload of the midcarpal joint as a result of the reversal of the normal palmar tilt of the distal radius.

The wrist is structured to deal with all loads resulting in a volar ulnar force vector. Major upslope ligaments, such as the radioscaphocapitate, prevent downslope migration during load. If the radius is left in a dorsiflexion or, more rarely,

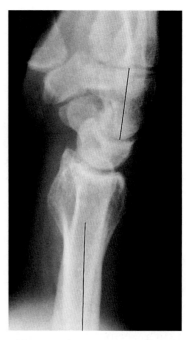

FIGURE 31.3. This x-ray demonstrates a dorsal articular tilt of the radius. Under these circumstances, the lunate will still assume a dorsal intercalated segment instability position in ulnar deviation power grip, but downslope volarly has now become upslope, producing a dorsal instead of volar displacement of the lunate. This cantilevers the capitate dorsal to the axial line of the radius, producing a synovial and capsular overload at the midcarpal joint dorsally and lunate impingement on the capitate volarly. This is not midcarpal instability.

a radially angled position, there are inadequate ligaments to prevent the wrist from shifting dorsally or radially under load. We erroneously published this condition as MCI (3). It is not. The problem is pain and synovitis with load because the capitate sits dorsal to the load line of the radius. Normally in ulnar deviation power grip, the lunate tilts dorsally (DISI) but shifts volarly, maintaining the capitate centered on the radius when seen from the lateral view. If the radius is tipped dorsally, however, the DISI positioning still occurs, but now downslope is upslope, and the lunate migrates dorsally, not volarly, under load. The distal carpal row and hand become cantilevered dorsally. The result is painful capsular and synovial stretching. This occurs primarily at the dorsal capsule between the capitate and lunate as well as between the radius and proximal carpal row. There is also a bone impingement component volarly between the capitate and lunate (Fig. 31.3). This is not MCI and is probably more appropriately termed "dorsal radius angulation carpal overload." Treatment is best achieved by radius osteotomy reestablishing volar ulnar articular angulation.

Capitate–Lunate Instability Pattern (CLIP Wrist)

White et al. described the CLIP wrist in 1984 as a specific type of carpal dissociation (5). By dynamic fluoroscopy, the capitate was found to dorsally sublux out of the lunate fossa with the application of traction, flexion, and scaphoid pressure by the examiner. All patients were treated successfully with rest and splinting. Louis et al. (6) described 11 patients with central carpal instability or a capitate lunate instability pattern. Ten patients were diagnosed with a dynamic traction displacement test under fluoroscopy. Ten became asymptomatic by activity modification.

Johnson and Carrera reported on 11 of 12 patients with chronic capitolunate instability who were treated with surgical reconstruction (7). They described a fluoroscopic dorsal displacement stress test and confirmed the dorsal subluxation of the capitate from the lunate fossa with an associated audible snap or click. They believed that the condition was caused by attenuation of the radiocapitate ligament as a result of prior trauma. Their surgical procedure involved obliterating the space of Poirier by tethering the central portion of the volar radiocapitate ligament to the radiotriquetral ligament.

Apergis reported 12 young women (14 wrists) with chronic wrist pain secondary to capitolunate instability who were treated with surgical reconstruction (8). The author believes that in these "delicate" wrists, the midcarpal laxity is secondary to involvement of both the radial and ulnar limbs of the volar V arcuate ligament. Therefore, surgical management consisted of ligamentous reefing of the whole palmar aspect of the midcarpal joint [radial, radioscaphocapitate and long radiolunate ligaments; ulnar, capitotriquetral and lunotriquetral (LT) ligaments and obliterating the space of Poirier] and the radiolunate joint when needed. The author also points out that dorsal displacement without apprehension is a normal finding in persons with lax joints.

Ono et al. presented five cases of dorsal capitolunate instability that were treated conservatively (9). The diagnosis in these patients was based on a positive dorsal capitate displacement test, which was considered positive if it reproduced "pain of presenting type."

In the CLIP wrist, the capitate displaces dorsally from the acetabulum of the lunate (Fig. 31.4). This can be produced with a provocative maneuver in most young girls and individuals with lax ligaments with dorsal displacement of the metacarpals while maintaining collinear hand and radius. Pathologically, the displacement will occur under load. Tennis is a common aggravating activity. This is not radial MCI but a subluxation phenomenon and angular deformity under load. It appears from the literature that most patients are treated successfully with temporary conservative treatment including activity modification. When this fails, dorsal capitate–lunate capsular reinforcement may be the appropriate treatment.

Lunotriquetral Dissociation

In their study of patients with LT instability, Reagan et al. noted that "sprain of the intercarpal region allows a snapping wrist syndrome, wherein the transition from the palmarflexed to the dorsiflexed position of the proximal row during the transition of the wrist from radial to ulnar deviation occurs dramatically and is associated with a visible, palpable, and audible movement" (10). VISI is often attributed to dissociation between the triquetrum and the lunate. A lunate that is not connected to the triquetrum has the predominant tendency to flex secondary to its connection to the scaphoid (10).

Horii et al. kinematically studied LT dissociation (11). The authors initially divided the LT ligaments and interosseous membrane but found it necessary to divide the dorsal radiotriquetral and dorsal scaphotriquetral ligaments to create a VISI pattern. In these cadaveric specimens, the authors were able to create an audible clunk through passive manipulation of the wrists. When the wrist was deviated from neutral to ulnar deviation under axial compression, the lunate abruptly rotated from a palmarflexed to a dorsiflexed position, producing an audible clunk that was enhanced by pushing the capitate palmarly. Lichtman created a similar phenomenon in an experimental study of ulnar MCI (12).

LT dissociation probably occurs most commonly secondarily to distal migration of the ulna with impaction loads on the triquetrum. Normally, a long ulna will, over time, destroy the proximal ulnar cartilage of the lunate. Heavy inline loads or impaction trauma, however, are taken by the

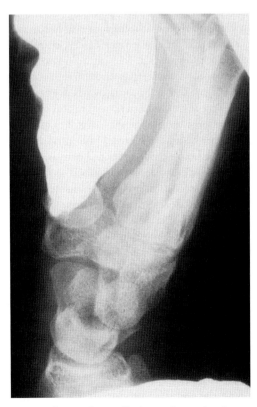

FIGURE 31.4. The capitate displaces from the lunate under load. The complaint was an inability to play tennis without a periodic, painful clunk. This is not midcarpal instability.

triquetrum, displacing it distally and rupturing the interosseous ligaments. Also, severe dorsiflexion and volarflexion injuries are capable of rupturing the entire LT interosseous ligament system as seen in both lunate and perilunate dislocations. Although LT instability may be part of a larger injury resulting in MCI in a fixed VISI or DISI positioning, it in itself is not MCI.

The treatment for injury to the LT ligaments involves decreasing the load to the joint. This can involve step-cut shortening of the ulna if there is any interosseous ligament remaining or if the patients' load requirements are not heavy. When complete interosseous ligament disruption is present and/or load requirements are significant, then LT limited wrist arthrodesis is indicated.

Triquetrohamate Instability

Lichtman et al. (12) discussed the ring concept of wrist stability and theorized that radial-sided injuries (scaphoid fracture, scapholunate dissociation, etc.) would result in scapholunate–capitate complex instabilities, and ulnar-sided injuries (triquetrohamate laxity) would result in MCI. The authors did not mention the possibility of MCI occurring through the radial side of the midcarpal joint, specifically the STT joint. The authors mentioned the possibility of these patients having an aggravation of an already lax wrist. They also noted that symptomatic MCI appears to be only a matter of degree or severity of "normal" hypermobile wrists.

In 1993, Lichtman et al. (13) described palmar midcarpal instability and the effectiveness of soft tissue reconstruction or limited midcarpal arthrodesis in 13 patients. All patients had painful clunking in the wrist with activity and no definitive incident of severe trauma before the onset of symptoms. Four of the patients had documented MCI in the contralateral wrist (painful in two patients). Patients created the clunk by active wrist radial deviation from a neutral position. The examiner also recreated the clunk by holding the patient's wrist in neutral position and forearm pronation with a palmarly directed force, axial load, and ulnar deviation. The test was positive if it recreated the painful clunk. All patients had a VISI pattern on plain radiographs and normal arthrograms. The clunk was recreated fluoroscopically, and no dissociative lesions were noted. Thirteen patients were treated surgically after failing conservative treatment. Six of the nine soft tissue reconstructions failed. The three successful procedures involved a distal advancement of the ulnar arm of the arcuate ligament combined with a dorsal capsulodesis. All six of the limited midcarpal arthrodeses (triquetrohamate fusion in three and triquetrohamate–capitolunate in three) were successful in relieving symptoms. The authors concluded that midcarpal arthrodesis is the surgical procedure of choice for palmar MCI. The authors also noted the similarity of the pathomechanics of what was described as MCI to what Taleisnik described as "laxness which is otherwise normal" occurring

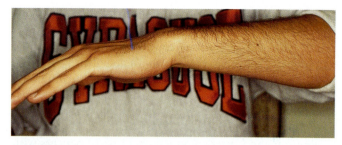

FIGURE 31.5. Volar intercalated segment instability deformity clinically mimics the silver fork deformity of a Colles' fracture with the volar displacement occurring more distally in the midcarpal plane.

during passive manipulation in asymptomatic individuals (14,15). Similarly, Linscheid et al. pointed out that congenital ligamentous laxity allows some patients to sublux the wrist into the VISI position (2).

Importantly, Garth has pointed out that a capitolunate fusion would stop all midcarpal motion and mask medial and lateral findings (16).

We feel that the TH interosseous ligaments are so lax in the normal state that rupture occurs only as a tertiary phenomenon following other significant ligamentous ruptures. Patients in our series likely have similar findings to those in the series of palmar MCI from Lichtman et al. (13) (Fig. 31.5). However, the discrepancy is in the site of pathology. Lichtman et al. (13) localize the pathology to the TH joint, whereas we localize the pathology to the radial side of the wrist or triscaphe joint. Treatment of this condition with a midcarpal fusion involving the capitolunate joint would obviously stop any midcarpal motion. In our series of patients, the signs and symptoms of MCI were successfully treated with a more limited intercarpal fusion of the triscaphe joint. The possibility of pathologic instability of the TH joint is lessened by the fact that isolated TH limited arthrodeses do not cure the pathologic movement. There is, therefore, no isolated condition that can be described as TH instability. TH limited wrist arthrodesis has almost no indication because even isolated destruction between the hamate and triquetrum, as from selective external damage (e.g., a bullet), is best handled by scapholunate advanced collapse (SLAC) reconstruction (capitate–lunate–hamate–triquetrum) limited wrist arthrodesis.

WHAT IS MIDCARPAL INSTABILITY?

MCI may be classified as type I, II, III, and IV. We are taking the position that the term MCI applies only when there is abnormal flexion or a VISI position of the proximal carpal row or the ability to produce this abnormal position. Instabilities of this nature can be classified as to whether they occur on the ulnar or radial side of the wrist.

Type I: Ulnar Midcarpal Instability

The ulnar side of the wrist can supinate either suddenly with activity or as produced by the patient, often with the help of the opposite hand. The distal carpal row displaces volarly on the proximal carpal row (Fig. 31.6). The scaphoid is not involved. Type I includes the physiologic condition that is similar to the swan-neck configuration that hyperlax people can achieve in their fingers. Typically, the patient will volarly depress the metacarpals with the opposite hand while maintaining collinear metacarpals and radius. The hand will return to normal with release. Rarely, the patients can collapse and supinate the ulnar side actively. This phenomenon can be produced in many young girls as a manifestation of ligament hypermobility. There is no synovitis and no postactivity ache unless the patient repeatedly displaces the wrist as a nervous habit or party trick. There is no involvement of the scaphoid or the radial side of the wrist. No treatment is needed.

Type II: Ulnar Micarpal Instability

Type II, ulnar MCI, occurs when the ulnar side of the wrist supinates under load and can be symptomatic. The patient often gets along for years with a wrist that is occasionaly annoying but seldom limits functional capacity. Loads are taken adequately on the radius and with no scaphoid involvement. These wrists run a spectrum from minimal symptoms adjacent to the type I, up to significant complaints in a wrist that displaces volarly on the ulnar side, flexing the proximal row with even light activities. The joint overload produces symptomatic synovitis. Patients may demonstrate a catch-up clunk. Treatment may be necessary. These wrists have been categorized previously as MCI amenable to ligamentous repair on the ulnar side. It is probable that these wrists represent those reported in the literature as successfully treated by ligament repair. There is no radial-sided involvement, obviating the need for treatment to the load-bearing capitate, scaphoid, and lunate.

Type III: Radial Midcarpal Instability

Radial MCI involves the radial side of the wrist and hyperflexibility of the scaphoid with proximal row flexion on the distal carpal row. In type III, the scaphoid–lunate interosseous ligaments are intact, and the proximal row is controlled by the flexion of the scaphoid, with rupture of the support mechanism at the STT joint. The scaphoid–capitate angle increases significantly in the displaced position

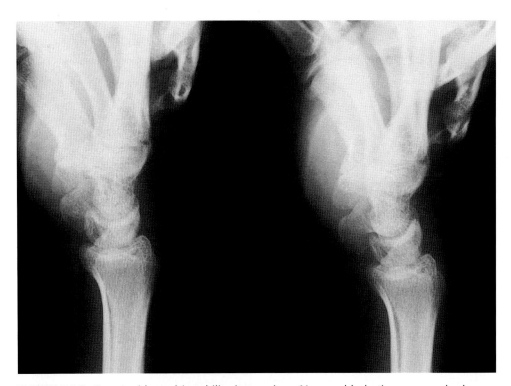

FIGURE 31.6. Type I midcarpal instability is seen in a 41-year-old plastic surgeon who has no symptoms and carries on all normal daily activities including athletics. The ulnar side of the wrist supinates and collapses into a volar intercalated segment instability (VISI) pattern, much more dramatic clinically than by x-ray. There is a visible, palpable clunk as the dislocation occurs and again as it returns to normal. The x-ray on the **right** demonstrates the "out" position. The lunate VISI is minimal, as there is no scapholunate dissociation and the scaphoid is maintaining alignment in the load-bearing radial side of the wrist.

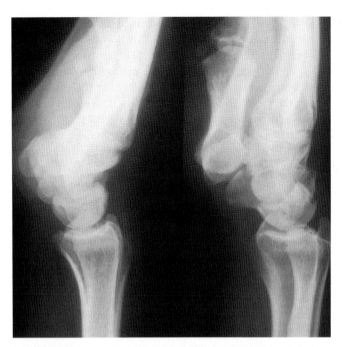

FIGURE 31.7. This 40-year-old tax collector has mild wrist symptoms using postage equipment. The wrist is normal at rest **(left)**. She can actively produce severe volar intercalated segment instability **(right)**. The scaphocapitate angle is 80°. There is no scapholunate dissociation. This is the mildest form of type III midcarpal instability.

(Fig. 31.7). These wrists can rest in a normal position and displace under load, or they may rest in the severe VISI position (Fig. 31.8). The scaphoid is involved in all cases. The loss of radial wrist support makes these wrists typically very symptomatic: even light loads are often not tolerated without resultant synovitis and postactivity ache. The patient can often control the collapse pattern actively by radial and ulnar deviation. A catch-up clunk is common.

Type IV: Radial Midcarpal Instability

This severest form of MCI is associated with complete scapholunate dissociation (Fig. 31.9). It is more often static and unreducible than type III. The scaphoid is in flexion with capitate–scaphoid angles over 80°. The lunate is detached from the scaphoid. The interesting part of this lesion is that a D-type lunate that is thinner dorsally, detached from the scaphoid, will assume its neutral anatomy position of DISI and not be included in MCI. If a V-type lunate that is thinner volarly is detached from the scaphoid, the neutral anatomy position of the lunate is severe VISI.

Types III and IV involve the scaphoid, produce significant functional limitation, and require treatment aimed at the scaphoid. Types III and IV represent the failures of ligamentous repairs aimed at the ulnar side of the wrist. Any solution must address the scaphoid rotation component in these forms of MCI (Fig. 31.10).

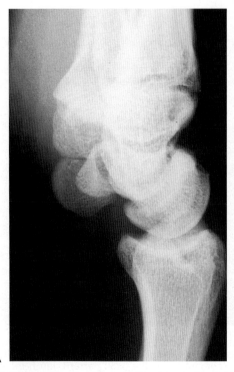 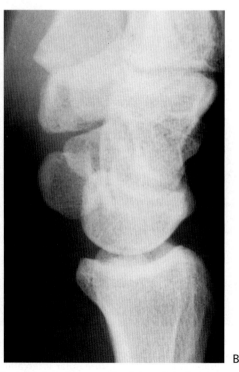

FIGURE 31.8. A: This type III midcarpal instability reflects a severe volar intercalated segment instability (VISI). There is no scapholunate dissociation, and the hyperflexed scaphoid is taking the proximal row into a VISI position with a D-type lunate. There is activity pain and a constant low-grade ache. **B:** The wrist can be passively corrected.

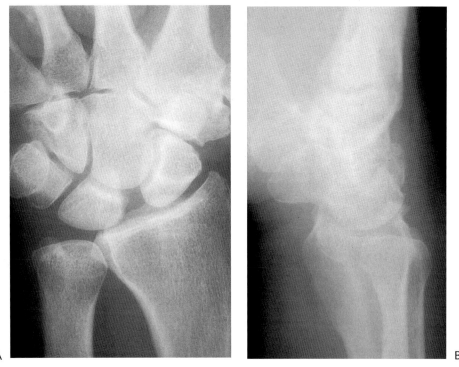

FIGURE 31.9. A: The scaphoid and lunate are completely dissociated. **B:** The scaphoid is flexed into a significant capitate–scaphoid angle. The lunate is thinner volarly, thicker dorsally, and has flexed to its neutral anatomy position of volar intercalated segment instability. This is a symptomatic wrist that will not tolerate load and requires a repair directed at the scaphoid.

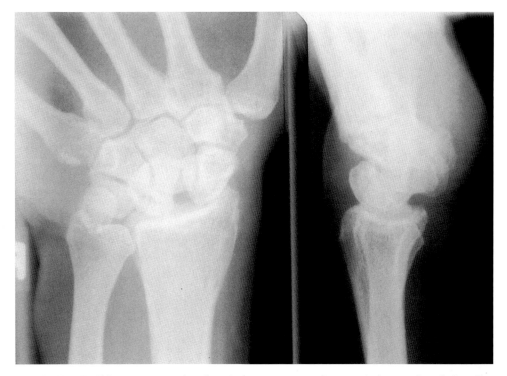

FIGURE 31.10. This posteroanterior view demonstrates complete scapholunate dissociation. The condition is longstanding with marked narrowing of the radius scaphoid joint. This is now a wrist with scapholunate advanced collapse secondary to severe midcarpal instability. The lateral image demonstrates a scaphocapitate angle exceeding 90°. A V-type lunate is in its neutral anatomic position with 52° of volar intercalated segment instability.

Historic terminology is preserved, and only a small shift in thinking is required to recognize that severe radial MCI has a scaphoid etiology.

REFERENCES

1. Watson HK, Yasuda M, Guidera PM. Lateral lunate morphology: an x-ray study. *J Hand Surg [Am]* 1996;21:759–763.
2. Linscheid RL, Dobyns JH, Beabout JW, et al. Traumatic instability of the wrist. Diagnosis, classification, and pathomechanics. *J Bone Joint Surg Am* 1972;54:1612–1632.
3. Taleisnik J, Watson HK. Midcarpal instability caused by malunited fractures of the distal radius. *J Hand Surg [Am]* 1984;9:350–357.
4. Amadio PC, Botte MJ. Treatment of malunion of the distal radius. *Hand Clin* 1987;3:541–561.
5. White SJ, Louis DS, Braunstein EM, et al. Capitate–lunate instability: recognition by manipulation under fluoroscopy. *Am J Roentgenol* 1984;143:361–364.
6. Louis DS, Hankin FM, Greene TL, et al. Central carpal instability—capitate lunate instability pattern: diagnosis by dynamic displacement. *Orthopedics* 1984;7:1693–1696.
7. Johnson RP, Carrera GF. Chronic capitolunate instability. *J Bone Joint Surg Am* 1986;68:1164–1176.
8. Apergis EP. The unstable capitolunate and radiolunate joints as a source of wrist pain in young women. *J Hand Surg [Br]* 1996;21:501–506.
9. Ono H, Gilula LA, Evanoff BA, et al. Midcarpal instability: is capitolunate instability pattern a clinical condition? *J Hand Surg [Br]* 1996;21:197–201.
10. Reagan DS, Linscheid RL, Dobyns JH. Lunotriquetral sprains. *J Hand Surg [Am]* 1984;9:502–514.
11. Horii E, Garcia-Elias M, An KN, et al. A kinematic study of lunotriquetral dissociations. *J Hand Surg [Am]* 1991;16:355–362.
12. Lichtman DM, Schneider JR, Swafford AR, et al. Ulnar midcarpal instability—clinical and laboratory analysis. *J Hand Surg [Am]* 1981;6:515–523.
13. Lichtman DM, Bruckner JD, Culp RW, et al. Palmar midcarpal instability: results of surgical reconstruction. *J Hand Surg [Am]* 1993;18:307–315.
14. Taleisnik J. Triquetrohamate and triquetrolunate instabilities (medial carpal instability). *Ann Chir Main* 1984;3:331–343.
15. Taleisnik J. Current concepts review. Carpal instability. *J Bone Joint Surg Am* 1988;70:1262–1268.
16. Garth WP Jr, Hofammann DY, Rooks MD. Volar intercalated segment instability secondary to medial carpal ligamental laxity. *Clin Orthop* 1985;201:94–105.

32

LIMITED WRIST ARTHRODESIS

JEFFREY WEINZWEIG
H. KIRK WATSON

Limited wrist arthrodesis is a proven method for treating specific carpal pathology that maximizes postoperative wrist motion, function, and strength while eliminating pain and instability. Also referred to as intercarpal arthrodesis, selective fusion of specific carpal units serves to address a diverse group of wrist disorders including degenerative disease of the wrist, rotary subluxation of the scaphoid (RSS), midcarpal instability, scaphoid nonunion, Kienböck's disease, carpal osteonecrosis, and congenital synchondrosis or partial fusion of various intercarpal joints (1–10).

This approach to the treatment of carpal pathology has evolved from principles that permit the transference of load from one carpal column to another, provide adaptation of preserved intercarpal mobility to compensate for motion pathways lost to fusion, and ensure prevention of subsequent degenerative change of other intercarpal joints.

This chapter defines the principles, indications, and outcomes for the commonly performed limited wrist arthrodeses. Specific operative techniques and technical modifications, including distal radius bone graft harvest, can be found in Section XVI.

WRIST MOTION

Numerous experimental models simulating intercarpal arthrodesis have been reported (11–16). However, it is impossible to predict the *in vivo* physiologic kinematics of the wrist and its response to injury simply from intercarpal arthrodesis of the cadaver carpus. The injured wrist is a complex, dynamic structure that undergoes significant change and adaptation as ligamentous and bony healing occur. In the normal wrist, adjacent carpal bones demonstrate motion limitations specific to a given intercarpal joint. However, when two or more carpal bones undergo fusion, a compensatory increase in motion occurs at the unfused joints, thereby maximizing total wrist motion. This adaptation of the carpus is not usually fully achieved until 9 to 12 months following limited wrist arthrodesis (17,18). Although the scaphoid–capitate and triscaphe [scaphotrapeziotrapezoid (STT)] fusions are mechanically similar in the cadaver, increasing motion of the capitate on the scaphoid in the triscaphe arthrodesis produces increased total wrist motion over the course of time. Fusions crossing the radiocarpal joint (e.g., radiolunate arthrodesis) result in the greatest loss of motion; those crossing the proximal and distal rows of the carpus or midcarpal joint [e.g., capitate–lunate–hamate–triquetral arthrodesis or scapholunate advanced collapse (SLAC) reconstruction] result in an intermediate loss of motion; and those within a single carpal row [e.g., lunotriquetral (LT) arthrodesis] result in the least loss of motion.

Gellman et al. (19) found that two-thirds of flexion occurs at the radiocarpal joint, and one-third occurs at the midcarpal joint, with slightly more extension occurring at the radiocarpal joint than at the midcarpal joint. Youm et al. (20,21), however, concluded that both the radiocarpal and midcarpal joints contribute to all phases of flexion and extension motion of the wrist.

Palmer et al. (22) have determined that the functional range of motion of the wrist is 5° flexion, 30° extension, 10° radial deviation, and 15° ulnar deviation. Almost all activities of daily living are completed within this range. These ranges of motion are all usually surpassed with each of the limited wrist arthrodeses with the exception of radioulnar deviation following radiocarpal fusions (1,9,17,18,23–25).

PRINCIPLES OF LIMITED WRIST ARTHRODESIS

Three principles have evolved that apply to limited wrist arthrodesis (1,5,8,24):

1. *Unaffected joints must be left unfused.* This is critical if maximal range of motion is to be maintained postoper-

---

J. Weinzweig: Department of Plastic Surgery, Brown University School of Medicine, Rhode Island Hospital, and Hasbro Children's Hospital, Providence, Rhode Island 02905.

H. K. Watson: Connecticut Combined Hand Surgery Fellowship, Hartford Hospital, and Connecticut Children's Medical Center, Hartford, Connecticut 06106; Department of Orthopaedics, University of Connecticut School of Medicine, Farmington, Connecticut 06032; Department of Orthopedics, Rehabilitation, and Plastic Surgery, Yale University School of Medicine, New Haven, Connecticut 06520.

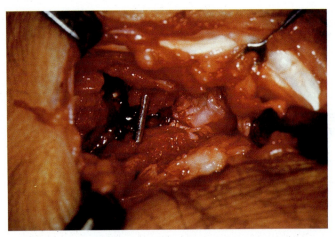

FIGURE 32.1. The basic principle of any limited wrist arthrodesis is to maintain the external dimensions of the fused unit. An inverted "T" is demonstrated here between the scaphoid proximally and the trapezium–trapezoid distally. That T shape is to be filled with cancellous bone graft. A pin has already transversed the trapezoid to the scaphoid, maintaining this open T-shaped area.

atively and forms the conceptual basis for selective limited wrist fusion. An exception to this principle is the inclusion of the hamate and triquetrum in SLAC wrist reconstruction in order to maximize the surface area for bone graft consolidation. Inclusion of these two carpal bones has no effect on the range of motion once the capitate–lunate joint is fused.

2. *The normal external dimensions of the carpal bones included in the arthrodesis must be preserved.* This is essential in order to maintain normal articulations with adjacent bones. Preservation of the external dimension of the triscaphe joint is accomplished with a temporary spacer during arthrodesis that is removed following pin placement (Fig. 32.1). In LT arthrodesis, the distal rim of cartilage on the adjacent surface of each bone is left intact. This is an important guide in maintaining reduction and alignment of the bones before fixation. SLAC reconstruction with fusion of the capitate, lunate, hamate, and triquetrum presents an exception to this principle. Although reduction of the lunate and correction of any dorsal intercalated segment instability (DISI) deformity is essential, maintenance of the original external dimensions of the four carpal bones is not. Some collapse of the capitate and hamate on the lunate and triquetrum is tolerated and has no effect on other joints; nor does this affect the range of motion ultimately achieved as load is transferred through the radiolunate joint.

3. *Bony fixation should include only those bones involved in the arthrodesis.* This permits any encountered stresses or loads to be dissipated by motion in the adjacent local joints. Inadvertent inclusion of adjoining bones during fixation will inhibit the motion of adjacent joints, thus increasing the amount of load transferred through the healing arthrodesis and potentially disrupting the fusion site.

TRISCAPHE ARTHRODESIS

Triscaphe arthrodesis is a fusion of the scaphoid, trapezium, and trapezoid bones and is often referred to as an STT fusion. A single bony unit is created with external dimensions identical to those of the three carpal bones before fusion (Fig. 32.2). Preservation of the external bony dimensions is necessary to prevent carpal collapse and excessive loading of the capitate. This would ultimately result in degenerative change and instability of the lunocapitate column followed by a SLAC wrist. The scaphoid should be fused in more flexion than in the normal configuration, however.

Indications for triscaphe arthrodesis include dynamic or static RSS, persistent symptomatic predynamic RSS with

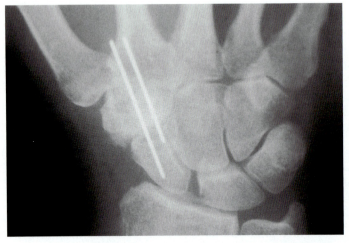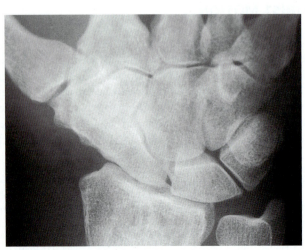

FIGURE 32.2. Triscaphe arthrodesis. **A:** Postoperative radiographic examination 6 weeks following triscaphe arthrodesis demonstrates typical pin placement and adequate bony consolidation. **B:** Three months following triscaphe fusion, the arthrodesis is radiographically solid.

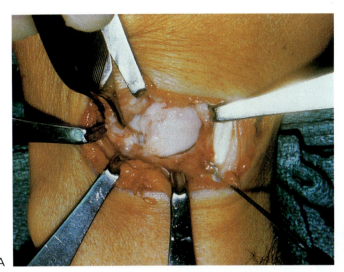
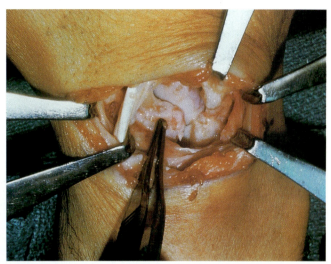

FIGURE 32.3. A: Complete rupture of the scapholunate interosseous system allows the proximal pole of the scaphoid to displace up onto the back of the capitate as the scaphoid flexes and supinates. When the wrist is opened, the proximal articular surface of the scaphoid faces the surgeon. **B:** A great deal of force is required to drive the scaphoid back to its alignment with the lunate. The capitate is seen distally. The scaphoid's mechanical disadvantage requires a reliable technique to maintain this position.

instability, degenerative disease of the triscaphe joint, nonunion of the scaphoid, Kienböck's disease, scapholunate (SL) dissociation (Fig. 32.3), traumatic dislocations, midcarpal instability, and congenital synchondrosis of the triscaphe joint (1,5,6,9,18,26–28). Triscaphe arthrodesis provides a stable radial column for load transfer across the wrist to the radius and permits the unloading of carpal units no longer capable of bearing load, such as the lunate in Kienböck's disease. In addition, it provides stability and strength to a wrist affected by the pathomechanics of RSS or midcarpal instability.

Triscaphe arthrodesis is contraindicated if significant degenerative change is found at the radioscaphoid joint (18,29). However, we have found an exception to this rule in professional athletes who require maximum functional capacity during their short but high-income years. Even with loss of nearly the entire proximal scaphoid pole cartilage, triscaphe arthrodesis places this degenerative area on normal radius cartilage in the center of the scaphoid fossa. This provides full-load, asymptomatic wrists with good motion until the radius cartilage is destroyed, usually 5 to 10 years following arthrodesis.

ROTARY SUBLUXATION OF THE SCAPHOID

RSS is a well-recognized entity in which the SL articulation is disrupted and the wrist develops a pattern of instability with loading (5,10,24,25). It is classically described as a diastasis between the scaphoid and lunate with dorsal displacement and rotation of the proximal pole of the scaphoid (Fig. 32.4). Disruption of the ligamentous

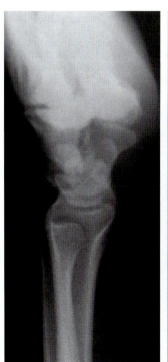
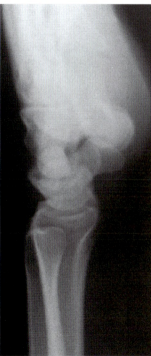

FIGURE 32.4. Lateral x-ray demonstrates rotary subluxation of the scaphoid on the right and a normal scapholunate (SL) angle on the left. A quick check of the SL angle can be accomplished by placing the lunate on the horizontal edge of the x-ray view much as a cereal bowl would sit on a table. The line along the volar scaphoid can then be estimated directly as it relates to the horizontal. An SL angle greater than 70° may be considered abnormal.

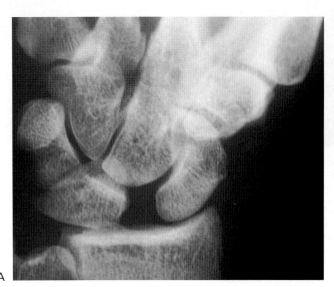
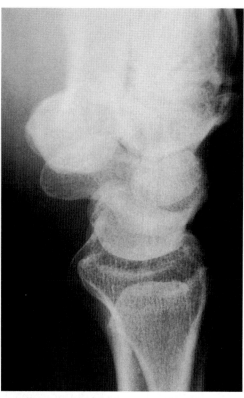

FIGURE 32.5. Static rotary subluxation of the scaphoid. **A:** Radiographic findings on the neutral posteroanterior view are foreshortening of the scaphoid, a positive ring sign, and an increased scapholunate (SL) gap. **B:** Radiographic findings on the neutral lateral view are an SL angle greater than 70° (90° in this case), with or without dorsal intercalated segment instability of the lunate (present in this case). Complete disruption of the SL interosseous system with some attenuation of extrinsic ligaments results in major displacement of the scaphoid, completely out from beneath the capitate, rendering it totally incapable of transmitting loads to the radius. This will result in destruction of the capitate–lunate joint cartilage (stage II scapholunate advanced collapse).

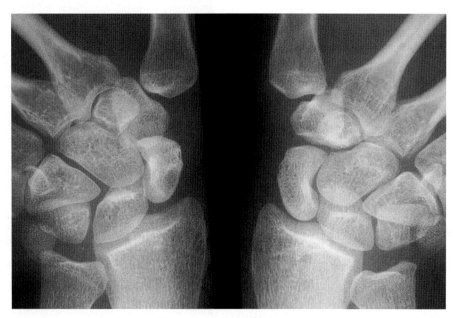

FIGURE 32.6. Ligament hypermobility, particularly in young girls, can produce x-rays with significant space and abnormal-appearing configurations that do not represent rotary subluxation of the scaphoid.

support of the proximal pole permits it to rotate dorsally while the distal pole rotates volarly, producing an increased SL angle on lateral radiographic examination with the scaphoid lying more perpendicular to the long axis of the forearm (Fig. 32.5). This produces a scaphoid with abnormal motion that can subject the radioscaphoid joint to abnormal loading stresses, eventually resulting in destruction of this joint and the development of a SLAC wrist. However, RSS must be distinguished from ligamentous hypermobility, which is often seen in young women and does not represent carpal pathology (Fig. 32.6).

However, RSS is not an all-or-none phenomenon in which the patient experiences symptoms only when the SL angle exceeds 70° and is far more common than previously thought. Degenerative periscaphoid disease may be the late result of undiagnosed predynamic or dynamic RSS. A less common form of scaphoid instability occurs secondary to lateral instability of the distal scaphoid with shear loading between the scaphoid and the trapezium and trapezoid. This results in isolated degenerative disease of the triscaphe joint. In its more serious form, it is the etiology of radial midcarpal instability, types I and II (30) (see Chapter 31).

PATHOMECHANICS

The susceptibility of the scaphoid to degenerative arthritic changes is based on its anatomy and position within the wrist (31). The articular surface of the distal radius is composed of two articular fossae, a radial fossa for the scaphoid and an ulnar fossa for the lunate. The fossa for the scaphoid is ovoid or elliptical in shape and narrows in a dorsal–volar plane as it approaches the radial styloid. The fossa for the lunate is spherical in shape; part of the sphere is composed of the most radial portion of the triangular fibrocartilage (Fig. 32.7). The proximal articular surface of the scaphoid resembles a simple teaspoon whose handle lies just dorsal and just radial to the position of the relaxed thumb. Flexion and extension occur with full articular contact of the spoon (scaphoid) in the elliptical fossa of the radius (25) (Fig. 32.8).

If the spoon handle is brought toward the little finger and flexed so that the handle is perpendicular to the long axis of the forearm, the contact surface of the spoon in the elliptical fossa is disrupted. When this occurs, the distal spoon surface (scaphoid) lies on the radial edges of the elliptical fossa (proximal spoon surface), and fairly rapid destruction between the scaphoid and radius occurs in these regions. Loss of radial load transfer results in shear loading of the capitate–lunate joint. Similar joint destruction secondary to shear loading resulting from articular surface curvature mismatch is seen between the capitate and radius following proximal row carpectomy (Fig. 32.9). With ligamentous attenuation and eventual separation of the proximal scaphoid and the lunate as a result of RSS, the capitate is driven off the radial edge of the lunate. Destruction occurs on both the capitate and lunate articular surfaces and is the culmination of the SLAC degenerative process.

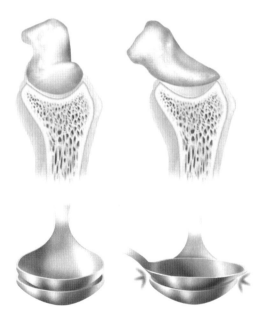

FIGURE 32.8. The radioscaphoid joint. The elliptic radioscaphoid joint is similar to two teaspoons. The contact surfaces of the proximal scaphoid and the elliptic fossa of the radius are analogous to spoons sitting congruently with even load distribution. When rotary subluxation of the scaphoid occurs, the distal "handle" moves from the plane of the thumb to a more volar position with respect to the forearm, and the spoon surfaces malalign. Instead of congruent loading, there is high-stress loading at the edges of the radius and the center of the proximal pole of the scaphoid. The bowls of the spoons are congruous as long as the handles remain collinear. When the upper spoon is rotated, they unseat. Destruction begins in the center of the scaphoid articular surface and on the periphery of the radial fossa, demonstrating early styloid tip sharpening advancing to complete destruction of the radioscaphoid joint. Secondarily, destruction occurs between the capitate–lunate and hamate–lunate joints.

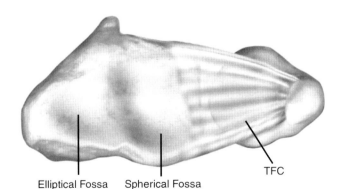

FIGURE 32.7. Distal radius and ulna anatomy. An end-on view of the distal radius and ulna demonstrates the elliptic scaphoid fossa and the spherical lunate fossa. The radial portion of the triangular fibrocartilage *(TFC)* contributes to the support mechanism for the lunate.

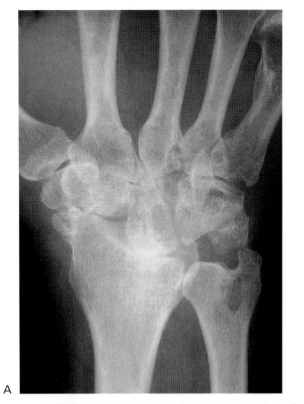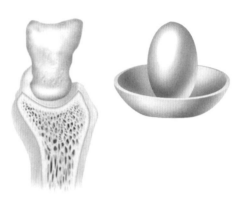

FIGURE 32.9. A,B: Proximal row carpectomies will almost always destroy the joint between the capitate and radius, as there is a significant difference in the radius of the curvature of the capitate versus the radius of curvature of the lunate fossa, not unlike placing an egg in a soup bowl.

This initially involves the radial portion of the radius–scaphoid joint beginning at the radial styloid (stage IA); subsequently, the remainder of the radius–scaphoid joint (stage IB), and finally the capitate–lunate joint (stage II), become involved. With carpal collapse and proximal migration of the capitate, the hamate is also driven proximally, and destruction of the lunate–hamate joint ensues. The proximal lunate articulation with the radius is spared even in the presence of volar intercalated segment instability (VISI) or DISI because of the sphericity of the joint, which maintains a preserved perpendicular cartilage-loading mechanism in contrast to the elliptic radius–scaphoid joint in the presence of all forms of radial-sided support loss (31).

Collapse of the radial column with RSS causes impingement of the trapezium and trapezoid on the neck of the scaphoid dorsally, at the articular–nonarticular (ANA) cartilage junction with hyperemia, synovitis, and significant cartilage change. Similar changes occur at the scaphoid–radial styloid joint. These changes are readily visualized intraoperatively even in patients with predynamic RSS (25).

CLASSIFICATION

The spectrum of radiographic findings in RSS parallels the clinical findings. As scaphoid instability progresses, clinical findings become more severe, and radiographic findings more apparent. Our current classification includes five types of RSS: I, predynamic; II, dynamic; III, static; IV, degenerative; and V, secondary (10,25).

Predynamic RSS (type I) is diagnosed when signs and symptoms of scaphoid instability exist in the absence of radiographic abnormalities (see Chapter 28). The patient usually presents with a history of wrist pain of at least 6 months that is worse with activity and is accompanied by a substantial postactivity ache, which lasts from several hours to several days. The patients usually demonstrate decreased range of motion of the wrist, particularly of flexion, and all five clinical findings of RSS (see below).

Dynamic RSS (type II) presents in a manner similar to predynamic RSS, but the diagnosis is supported by findings on stress radiographic views (e.g., clenched fist, radial or ulnar deviation). These findings include foreshortening of the scaphoid, overlapping of the scaphoid and capitate, and a ring sign [produced on posteroanterior (PA) view by overlapping of the proximal and distal poles of the scaphoid with scaphoid rotation]. Routine PA and lateral radiographs demonstrate no abnormalities. Clinical findings may or may not be more severe than in patients with predynamic RSS.

Static RSS (type III) is diagnosed on the basis of findings on routine PA and lateral radiographs in the presence of clinical findings that are similar to those of predynamic and dynamic

RSS but more severe. There is usually a history of a significant precedent injury. In addition to the radiographic findings of dynamic RSS, findings of SL dissociation, a widened SL joint, and an increased SL angle are also observed, with or without abnormal positioning of the lunate (e.g., DISI) (Fig. 32.5).

Note that type II and type III RSS are nearly the same phenomenon and are very close on the spectrum of wrist problems. They differ only in the type of x-ray necessary to demonstrate the instability.

Degenerative RSS (type IV) is diagnosed on the basis of a history similar to those of types I to III, but with symptoms that are usually more severe, their duration often longer, and the patient often older. Radiographic findings of degenerative changes at the radius–scaphoid joint (SLAC wrist) or STT joint (triscaphe arthritis) are present. A triscaphe arthrodesis can be successfully performed despite a small area of degenerative joint disease (DJD) on the proximal scaphoid because this area is centered in the normal cartilage of the radius–scaphoid fossa. Secondary capitate–lunate joint changes (midcarpal SLAC) may subsequently occur.

Secondary RSS (type V) designates involvement of the scaphoid secondary to other carpal lesions such as a collapsed wrist from Kienböck's disease or nonunion of the scaphoid.

Radiographic review of patients with positive x-ray findings who had undergone triscaphe arthrodesis showed that 9% of patients demonstrated dynamic RSS (type II), 47% static RSS (type III), 14% degenerative RSS (type IV), and 30% secondary RSS (type V) (10). In addition, approximately 40% of patients with isolated triscaphe arthritis demonstrated static RSS. We believe isolated triscaphe arthritis is a secondary manifestation of RSS in which the distal pole of the scaphoid becomes unstable and the articular destruction of the triscaphe joint ensues. Of approximately 1,000 triscaphe arthrodeses performed, there has been no evidence of subsequent degenerative change of the radioscaphoid joint or other intercarpal joints.

CLINICAL PRESENTATION

Patients with RSS present with various combinations of five consistent complaints: (a) activity pain; (b) postactivity pain; (c) activity modification; (d) carpal tunnel syndrome symptoms; and (e) wrist ganglia. All patients present with at least three of these historical findings; many patients present with all five.

Activity Pain

Activity pain is always the patient's chief complaint. It is usually localized to the radial aspect of the wrist but often radiates distally along the metacarpals or proximally along the forearm. The severity of pain is usually a direct reflection of the degree of scaphoid and periscaphoid pathology and can be exacerbated by both recreational and occupational activities. Patients with severe RSS may experience ulnar wrist pain as well. Patients with longstanding symptoms and prolonged conservative treatment, often for years, may have little or no synovitis radially. Their complaints are frequently ulnar-sided. It is worthwhile to return these patients to heavy work for a week or two, followed by reexamination. Conversely, their wrists can be loaded on a Baltimore Therapeutic Equipment (BTE) machine or by simple contrived heavy-load activities for 6 hours under supervision, followed by reexamination. This approach will clarify and usually shift the symptoms back to the periscaphoid region.

Postactivity Ache

The pathokinematics of a subluxing scaphoid will produce synovial stretch, tears, hemorrhage, and chronic inflammation. Postactivity ache is a manifestation of the degree of synovitis produced by an activity and can last from less than an hour to numerous days. It is a useful barometer with which to gauge the degree of joint insult.

Activity Modification

A patient's voluntary modification of activity level will vary with the degree of activity pain and postactivity ache and is usually representative of the severity of the carpal pathology.

Carpal Tunnel Syndrome Symptoms

Carpal tunnel symptomatology is a frequent early manifestation of RSS. Many patients who eventually require triscaphe arthrodesis will have already been treated for carpal tunnel syndrome, either conservatively or operatively, as the intercarpal synovitis commonly produces symptoms of median nerve compression. Dorsal wrist syndrome (DWS), the result of overload of the SL interosseous ligament with resultant SL synovitis, with or without ligamentous disruption, precedes RSS. We have observed an incidence of carpal tunnel syndrome in 26% of the first 76 patients surgically treated for DWS (10). That percentage has remained the same after treatment of over 500 such patients over an 18-year period (unpublished data, H. K. Watson and J. Weinzweig).

Wrist Ganglia

Wrist ganglia are a secondary manifestation of an underlying periscaphoid ligamentous injury (32). Both clinically palpable and occult dorsal wrist ganglia are associated with overload of the SL joint and are seen frequently in patients with DWS, predynamic RSS, and dynamic RSS. We have seen wrist ganglia in 60% of patients treated for DWS; 31% of these were occult ganglia; 29% were known ganglia (10).

Once complete SL ligament disruption has occurred, or carpal pathology has progressed to a SLAC wrist, ganglia are seen only rarely because the joint space is now widely separated and the pathoanatomy required to create a ganglion stalk no longer exists.

PHYSICAL EXAMINATION

Because the vast majority of carpal pathology originates on the radial aspect of the wrist, a systematic clinical examination consisting of five maneuvers has evolved (33). Each of these maneuvers is not necessarily diagnostic of a specific entity by itself, nor is it intended to be. However, a diagnosis can almost always be derived by coupling the entire picture of the patient's wrist mechanics and pathomechanics with the history, symptomatology, and radiographic examination. Prior to performing these maneuvers, wrist motion should be thoroughly assessed. In our experience, any loss of *passive flexion* consistently represents a sign of underlying organic carpal pathology. It is rare, for example, that a patient with Kienböck's disease, even stage I, will not present with some degree of loss of passive flexion.

Our radial wrist examination consists of the following five maneuvers (see also Chapter 5).

Dorsal Wrist Syndrome: Scapholunate Joint

Identification of the SL joint is facilitated by following the course of the third metacarpal proximally until the examiner's thumb falls into a recess. That recess lies over the capitate with the wrist in flexion. The SL articulation is readily palpable just proximal between the extensor carpi radialis brevis and the extensors of the fourth compartment. A normal joint will produce no pain with palpation. SL dissociation, Kienböck's disease, dorsal wrist syndrome, or other pathology involving the SL or radiolunate joints, or the lunate itself, will elicit pain with direct palpation.

Finger Extension Test

The increased mechanical advantage of carpal loading during the finger extension test (FET) produces a reliable indicator of carpal pathology. With the patient's wrist held passively in flexion, the examiner resists active finger extension. In patients with significant periscaphoid inflammatory change, radiocarpal or midcarpal instability, symptomatic RSS, or Kienböck's disease, the combined radiocarpal loading and pressure of the extensor tendons will cause considerable discomfort. In our experience, patients with these carpal disorders always demonstrate a positive FET. The FET has become a very reliable indicator of problems at the SL joint. Full-power finger extension against resistance (i.e., a negative FET) almost always rules out dorsal wrist syndrome, RSS, Kienböck's disease, midcarpal instability, SLAC, and carpal disease in general involving scaphocapitate, lunate, and radius articulations.

Articular–Nonarticular Junction of Scaphoid

The proximal pole of the scaphoid articulates with the radius within the radiocarpal joint. The articular surface of the proximal scaphoid continues distally toward a junctional point along the radial aspect where the cartilage changes from articular to nonarticular. With the wrist in radial deviation, that ANA junction is obscured by the radial styloid. With the wrist in ulnar deviation, the ANA junction is easily palpated just distal to the radial styloid. The ANA maneuver is performed with the examiner's index finger firmly palpating the radial aspect of the patient's wrist just distal to the radial styloid with the wrist initially in radial deviation, then in ulnar deviation. The normal asymptomatic wrist will demonstrate mild to moderate tenderness and discomfort at the ANA junction with direct palpation in almost every individual. However, the patient with periscaphoid synovitis, scaphoid instability, nonunion, or SLAC changes will experience severe pain with this maneuver. For purposes of comparison, it is useful to perform this maneuver as a bilateral examination.

Scaphotrapeziotrapezoid or Triscaphe Joint

Identification of the triscaphe joint is facilitated by following the course of the second metacarpal proximally until the examiner's thumb falls into a recess. That recess is the triscaphe joint. A normal joint will produce no pain with palpation. Any triscaphe synovitis, degenerative disease, or other pathology involving the joint or scaphoid will elicit pain with direct palpation.

Scaphoid Shift Maneuver

The scaphoid shift maneuver provides a qualitative assessment of scaphoid stability and periscaphoid synovitis when compared with the contralateral asymptomatic wrist (34). This exam, therefore, is meaningful only when performed bilaterally.

With the patient's forearm slightly pronated, the examiner grasps the wrist from the radial side, placing his thumb on the palmar prominence of the scaphoid while wrapping his fingers around the distal radius. This enables the thumb to push on the scaphoid with counterpressure provided by the fingers. The examiner's right thumb is used to examine the patient's right scaphoid; his left thumb is used to examine the left scaphoid. The examiner's other hand grasps the patient's hand at the metacarpal level to control wrist position. Starting in ulnar deviation and slight extension, the wrist is moved radially and slightly flexed with constant thumb pressure on the scaphoid.

When the wrist is in ulnar deviation, the scaphoid axis is extended and lies nearly in line with the long axis of the forearm. As the wrist deviates radially and flexes, the scaphoid also flexes and rotates to an orientation more nearly perpendicular to the forearm, and its distal pole becomes prominent on the palmar side of the wrist. The examiner's thumb pressure opposes this normal rotation and creates a subluxation stress, causing the scaphoid to shift in relation to the other bones of the carpus. With experience, the wrist can be placed in the position of maximum scaphoid mobility (slight ulnar deviation and wrist flexion), and the scaphoid positioned dorsally and volarly. This "scaphoid shift" may be subtle or dramatic. In a patient with rigid periscaphoid ligamentous support, only minimal shift is tolerated before the scaphoid continues to rotate normally, pushing the examiner's thumb out of the way. In patients with ligamentous laxity, the combined stresses of thumb pressure and normal motion of the adjacent carpus may be sufficient to force the scaphoid out of its elliptic fossa and up onto the dorsal rim of the radius. As thumb pressure is withdrawn, the scaphoid returns abruptly to its normal position, sometimes with a resounding "thunk."

The scaphoid may shift smoothly and painlessly or with a gritty sensation, or clicking, accompanied by pain. Grittiness suggests chondromalacia or loss of articular cartilage, and clicking or catching may indicate bony change sufficient to produce impingement. Pain is a significant finding, especially when it reproduces the patient's symptoms. Pain associated with unilateral hypermobility of the scaphoid is virtually diagnostic of rotary subluxation or scaphoid nonunion. A less well localized pain associated with normal or decreased mobility is encountered in patients with periscaphoid arthritis, whether of triscaphe or SLAC pattern.

Experience performing the scaphoid shift maneuver is essential to obtaining useful diagnostic information and distinguishing the normal wrist from the pathologic one. Two hundred nine of 1,000 normal asymptomatic subjects examined demonstrated a unilateral abnormal scaphoid shift maneuver with hypermobility of the scaphoid and/or pain (35). This represents 21% of examined subjects and 10% of examined wrists and makes the point that some degree of periscaphoid ligamentous injury is extremely common.

TREATMENT ALGORITHM

The preferred treatment for RSS secondary to an acute ligament injury is open reduction and internal fixation, usually with Kirschner wires. The most important goal of open reduction is to reestablish a normal scaphoid–lunate–capitate relationship under direct visualization. In order to maintain this reduction, pinning of these three bones is mandatory. Disruption of the ligamentous support mechanism across the radiocarpal joint may require pinning of the scaphoid and lunate to the radius as well. Direct ligamentous repair is also recommended when feasible. A long arm "Groucho Marx" cast (see below) is then applied for 4 weeks, after which a short arm cast is applied for an additional 4 to 6 weeks.

The results of open reduction are less satisfactory when performed more than 3 weeks following injury. These patients are then included in the group with chronic RSS who may require reconstruction. Ligamentous reconstruction of the SL joint as advocated by Taleisnik (36), with or without the dorsal capsulodesis described by Blatt (37), is commonly performed. We believe that triscaphe limited wrist arthrodesis is the procedure of choice for symptomatic chronic RSS (more than 3 weeks postinjury) (18,24). Liga-

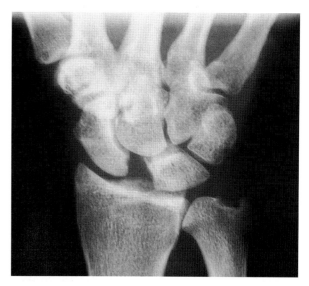

FIGURE 32.10. A 57-year-old surgeon is seen 4½ months after a Blatt capsulodesis for rotary subluxation of the scaphoid. The patient remains symptomatic and unable to operate. The degree of flexion of the scaphoid may be improved, but this wrist is functionless and at significant risk for degenerative arthritis and a scapholunate advanced collapse wrist.

mentous reconstruction in patients with chronic RSS is less likely to produce a satisfactory long-term result (Fig. 32.10).

Even normal ligaments cannot maintain the scaphoid in anatomic position if significant loading occurs. In stage IIIB Kienböck's disease, for example, collapse of the lunate produces a secondary RSS in the face of uninjured interosseous ligaments. It is difficult to imagine how ligamentous repairs can be sustained despite the significant mechanical disadvantage of the rotated scaphoid under active wrist loading, especially in the laborer or athlete. Triscaphe arthrodesis prevents abnormal cartilage loading and restores full power with minimal symptoms at the extremes of flexion and extension. This procedure results in motion equivalent to approximately 80% of the flexion–extension of the contralateral normal wrist and demonstrates no secondary DJD with time (5). These findings are based on results of approximately 1,000 triscaphe limited wrist arthrodeses, some dating back over 25 years.

Not every patient with RSS requires a triscaphe arthrodesis. On the other hand, patients with predynamic RSS who present with symptoms of more than 6 months' duration, including activity pain and postactivity ache, a decrease in passive wrist flexion, as well as several of the five physical findings of RSS, and rupture of the SL interosseous ligament at surgery may require limited wrist arthrodesis. Operative treatment is based on clinical and physical findings, not on the presence or absence of radiographic findings.

SCAPHOID NONUNION

Untreated scaphoid nonunion will progress to degenerative wrist disease, often culminating in a SLAC wrist, and,

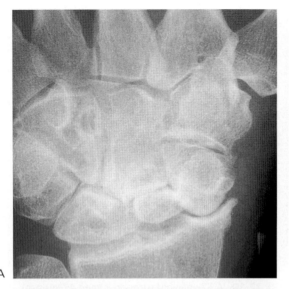
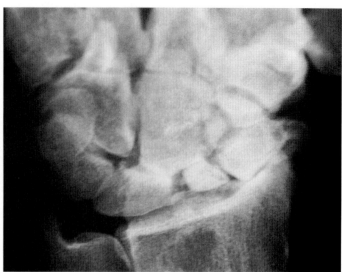
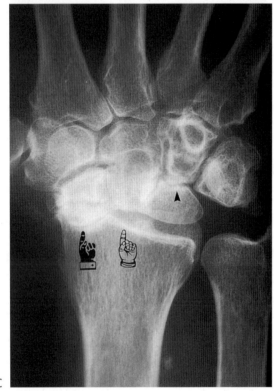

FIGURE 32.11. Scapholunate advanced collapse wrist secondary to scaphoid nonunion. **A:** Scaphoid nonunion deprives the wrist of scaphoid support. The distal fragment of the scaphoid nonunion rotates, destroying the radioscaphoid support. The proximal pole is treated as a small lunate, maintaining its articular surface with the radius but destroying its articular surface with the capitate. **B:** All scaphoid nonunions follow this pattern of isolated distal pole/radius destruction and secondary midcarpal (capitate–lunate) destruction. **C:** With chronicity, further midcarpal destruction involves both the capitate–lunate (*arrowhead*) and hamate–lunate joints; despite this, the radius–lunate is preserved. The *black hand* points to the destroyed distal scaphoid fragment-radius joint. The *white hand* points to the preserved proximal scaphoid fragment-radius joints.

therefore, should be treated early (Fig. 32.11). The treatment of choice for nonunion of the scaphoid in the absence of degenerative change is reduction of the bony fragments along with cancellous bone grafting (26,38,39).

There are three indications for triscaphe arthrodesis in the management of scaphoid nonunion:

1. When scaphoid fracture results in a very small proximal fragment, up to several millimeters in dimension, the pathology closely resembles an SL dissociation. Instead of a ligamentous tear between the scaphoid and lunate, the disruption is simply shifted radially, resulting in an avulsion of the proximal pole of the scaphoid. Without sufficient control of the proximal pole of the scaphoid, rotary subluxation of the distal fragment, the majority of the scaphoid in this case, often occurs. With this small proximal fragment, one may consider bone grafting the nonunion through a dorsal approach along with concomitant triscaphe arthrodesis. The small proximal pole will often develop a stable fibrous union, which, combined with scaphoid control by limited wrist arthrodesis, will produce an asymptomatic wrist. We would not argue with a two-stage approach in which the nonunion is treated and a triscaphe fusion is performed at a later date if necessary.
2. Occasionally the scaphoid nonunion is quite distal and results in malalignment of the triscaphe joint. Bone grafting the nonunion is frequently combined with triscaphe arthrodesis in these cases.
3. Scaphoid fracture can occur with simultaneous SL dissociation. In these cases, repairing the nonunion alone does not correct the RSS, which requires a concomitant triscaphe arthrodesis. Failed scaphoid nonunion surgery, perhaps even repeat failed grafting procedures, can be salvaged by fusing both fragments to the capitate.

KIENBÖCK'S DISEASE

Collapse of the lunate in Kienböck's disease permits proximal migration of the capitate. This overloads the radial wrist, dissociates the scaphoid and lunate, and drives the scaphoid into rotary subluxation. Many approaches have been described for the treatment of this wrist disorder. Currently, ulnar lengthening and radial shortening, with or without lunate revascularization procedures, are the most popular approaches (40–42). Proximal row carpectomy is often utilized as a salvage procedure (43). Our approach has been to perform a triscaphe arthrodesis without excising the lunate. This serves to unload the lunate, permitting it to revascularize over the course of time. Approximately 18% of our cases have required subsequent lunate removal within 2 years following triscaphe arthrodesis because of persistent pain and/or stiffness. These lunates frequently demonstrate osteochondral fractures and are not the displaced fractured lunates one might expect to be the most symptomatic.

In the past, many authors have advocated Silastic lunate arthroplasty. However, Silastic implants have no solid core and little capability to resist compression (6,27). Progressive compression with heavy loading causes overloading of adjacent joints. In addition, and more importantly, particulate synovitis caused by Silastic implants results in panligamentous destruction, often necessitating wrist fusion. For these reasons, we believe there is no indication for Silastic lunate or scaphoid implants in the wrist.

SCAPHOLUNATE DISSOCIATION

Rupture of the SL interosseous ligament results in dissociation of these carpal bones. The volar radioscapholunate ligament is probably more of an elastic vascular ligament than a restrictive supportive ligament and may not be torn in this process (44). The lunate subsequently assumes its neutral anatomic position of volar displacement and dorsiflexion. Neutral anatomy is the position a carpal bone will assume without ligamentous support, relying solely on its shape (45). Static RSS is usually present following SL dissociation and is the etiology of the associated symptomatology. If degenerative change is present in the radioscaphoid or capitate–lunate joints, then SLAC reconstruction is indicated.

In the case of partial or incomplete rupture of this interosseous ligament, the tear begins volarly and progresses around the proximal pole of the SL joint to complete the tear distally on the dorsum of the SL joint. On the basis of our experience of SL joint exploration during operative treatment of over 500 patients with DWS, we have classified SL ligament rupture into four groups: type 0, intact ligament; type I, ≤50% ligament tear extending to the mid-proximal point of the SL joint; type II, >50% ligament tear but less than 85%; and type III, complete ligament tear (25). In this group of patients, 50% demonstrated type 0 SL ligaments, 26% type I, 15% type II, and 9% type III (see Chapter 28).

Triscaphe arthrodesis corrects the RSS, provides a load transfer mechanism for the wrist, and relieves the symptoms but does not necessarily correct the associated DISI deformity of the lunate. However, because symptoms are related to scaphoid instability, which is corrected by triscaphe arthrodesis, any residual DISI may be ignored, as loads are now taken almost entirely by the scaphoid. Even with long-standing DISI or VISI, degenerative change between the lunate and radius in the spherical radiolunate fossa is almost nonexistent. Therefore, reducing the lunate during triscaphe arthrodesis is not necessary.

TRISCAPHE JOINT DISLOCATION

Dislocation of the triscaphe joint is relatively rare but can occur when the hand sustains a significant force directed along a radioulnar vector. The index and thumb metacarpals along with the trapezium and trapezoid dislocate from the scaphoid through the triscaphe joint. This four-bone dislocated unit is usually dorsally displaced. In cases in which complete dislocation has not occurred, the diagnosis is frequently overlooked. Stress radiographs and tomograms are usually needed to demonstrate the instability in this case. Our preferred treatment is realignment of the triscaphe joint and limited wrist arthrodesis.

MIDCARPAL INSTABILITY

Midcarpal instability is the result of pathologic changes in angulation between the proximal and distal carpal rows in which the proximal row assumes a VISI position and the distal row is angulated dorsally. Support of the midcarpal joint depends on the integrity of periscaphoid ligamentous attachments as well as the volar carpal ligaments traversing this joint. Because of this, midcarpal instability can occur as either a *radial* or *ulnar* process. With *radial midcarpal instability,* some degree of periscaphoid ligamentous rupture has occurred with resultant RSS. The SL interosseous ligament may or may not be torn, but distal scaphoid support is insufficient and allows the distal carpal row to collapse on the proximal carpal row. With *ulnar midcarpal instability,* the distal carpal row displaces volarly on the proximal carpal row, but the scaphoid is not involved (see Chapter 31).

Severe damage to the ligaments supporting the scaphoid can result in carpal collapse with either a resultant VISI or DISI deformity of the lunate. The incidence of midcarpal instability, however, is related not only to the disruption of a particular interosseous ligament on one side of the lunate or the other, but also to the inherent morphology of the lunate.

With disruption of the SL interosseous ligaments, the lunate typically assumes the classic position of dorsiflexion (DISI). This occurs as a result of the shape of the lunate and the biomechanics of the adjacent carpal bones. DISI occurs when the lunate is thinner dorsally than volarly on lateral projection, as described by Kauer (46,47). In this case, the capitate load forces the lunate volarly, with resultant dorsal angulation of the lunate. We refer to the position that a carpal bone assumes based solely on its anatomic shape as its neutral anatomic position.

Interestingly, in some cases of SL dissociation, the lunates migrate in the opposite direction: they shift dorsally and tilt volarly (VISI). This phenomenon, too, is related to the morphology of the lunate. Approximately 20% of lunates are thinner volarly than dorsally. Recent work of ours has demonstrated this anatomic variation radiographically (45) and in a cadaver study (J. Weinzweig et al., *unpublished data*). We refer to the lunate that is thinner volarly as type "V" for its neutral anatomic position of VISI; similarly, the lunate that is thinner dorsally is referred to as type "D" for its neutral anatomic position of DISI.

Our treatment of choice in cases of midcarpal instability in which the radiocarpal joint is preserved is a triscaphe arthrodesis. Review of all patients who had undergone triscaphe arthrodesis for SL dissociation revealed a subset of patients (17 cases) who had a VISI deformity. Interestingly, almost two-thirds of the patients with SL dissociation and a VISI lunate position demonstrated type V lunates. It appears that the type D lunate will tend to assume a DISI position and a type V lunate a VISI position, even in cases with no known ligamentous disruption.

DEGENERATIVE DISEASE OF THE TRISCAPHE JOINT

In its normal anatomic position, the scaphoid articulates with the radius at the radiocarpal joint and with the trapezium and trapezoid at the triscaphe joint. However, the scaphoid is poorly designed for its role within the carpus. As a result, approximately 95% of all degenerative disease of the wrist is periscaphoid in origin (10). Degenerative disease of the triscaphe joint is common and occurs primarily between the scaphotrapezium and scaphotrapezoid joints (Fig. 32.12). During surgery for predynamic RSS, the trapezium and trapezoid are frequently found to rest on the dorsal nonarticular portion of the distal scaphoid. Early degenerative changes are often seen in this region. Some cases of RSS produce degenerative disease limited to the triscaphe joint. Triscaphe arthrodesis is generally accepted as the procedure of choice for the management of degenerative disease of this joint (16,27).

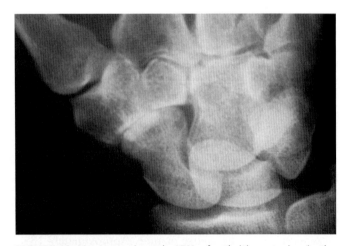

FIGURE 32.12. Approximately 15% of arthritis occurring in the wrist occurs among the scaphoid, trapezium, and trapezoid within the scaphotrapeziotrapezoid joint. The scapholunate interosseous ligaments are intact. Ligament damage at the distal scaphoid allows lateral displacement and shear loading, which destroys only the articular surfaces between the scaphoid and the trapezium and trapezoid.

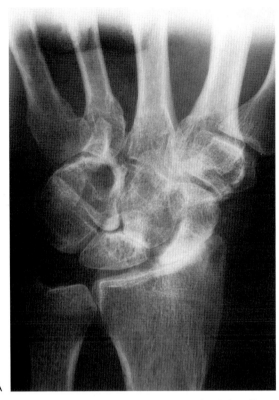 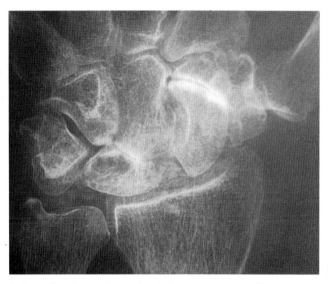

FIGURE 32.13. Degenerative joint disease of the wrist. **A:** Any loss of radial wrist support will result in scapholunate advanced collapse wrist. Here the rotary subluxation of the scaphoid has destroyed the cartilage between the radius and scaphoid with secondary capitate–lunate changes. **B:** Radial wrist support loss has occurred at the triscaphe joint with complete destruction of this joint, and again the secondary changes have occurred between capitate and lunate.

Review of more than 4,000 radiographs of the wrist yielded 210 films demonstrating degenerative arthritic change; the SLAC pattern of degenerative change was seen in 57%, triscaphe joint arthritis in 27%, and a combination of these in 15% (Fig. 32.13) (31).

CONGENITAL CARPAL SYNCHONDROSIS

Cavitation of a common cartilaginous precursor during the fourth to eighth weeks of intrauterine life results in the formation of individual carpal bones. Incomplete cavitation results in congenital carpal synchondrosis or incomplete separation of the carpal bones, which becomes radiographically apparent as the carpus ossifies (48). This is a forme fruste of carpal coalition and may lead to degenerative change at the site of coalition. This occurs most commonly at the LT joint (13), where the joint has the pathognomonic appearance of a "fluted champagne glass" (Fig. 32.14). It occurs because the distal portion of the joint usually has normal cartilage development, whereas normal joint development has been arrested proximally, predisposing it to DJD. The capitate–hamate joint is the next most commonly involved. Such anomalies occur rarely, are generally believed to be asymptomatic, and are usually discovered as incidental findings during radiographic evaluations for minor trauma.

Congenital synchondrosis of a joint can be recognized radiographically by the presence of bone where articular cartilage should be found (Fig. 32.15A). This unique radiographic finding is diagnostic of this interesting anomaly, in contradistinction to degenerative arthritis wherein the articular cartilage has developed and subsequently been worn away and the normal bony surfaces consequentially approach one another. A spectrum of synchondrosis exists ranging from partial to complete fusion, depending on the degree of formation of the articular cartilaginous elements (49).

We have recently described the finding of congenital synchondrosis of the STT joint (Fig. 32.15B), a type of carpal coalition not previously reported (28). Significant activity pain and postactivity ache, activity modification, loss of wrist motion, and all five clinical findings of periscaphoid pathology were present in one such case.

Exploration of the scaphoid and triscaphe joint revealed a joint largely devoid of cartilage along its dorsal and interosseous surfaces. A segment of normal cartilage (approximately 20%) existed on the volar aspect of the joint, between the distal scaphoid and proximal trapezium and trapezoid. The trapezium–trapezoid joint was also

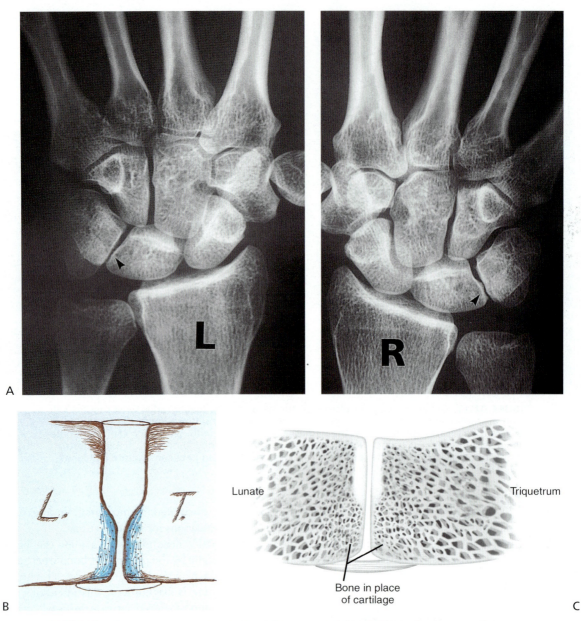

FIGURE 32.14. Congenital synchondrosis of the triquetral–lunate joint. **A:** Congenital incomplete development of the triquetral–lunate joint is not an uncommon source of wrist pain. The joint develops from distal to proximal, forming normal cartilage distally, then demonstrating bone where cartilage should be in the proximal portion of the articular surface. This phenomenon is pathognomonic of congenital incomplete joint development. Findings are typically bilateral. This patient demonstrates a typical bilateral fluted champagne glass appearance between the triquetrum and lunate (*arrows*). **B,C:** The incomplete development of the joint occurs proximally. Bone exists where cartilage should be, covered by thin, inadequate cartilage that typically wears out completely by the third decade, producing a highly localized degenerative arthritis. Instability, on the other hand, will produce degenerative joint disease of the entire joint surface. The fluted champagne glass appearance is present and is pathognomonic.

poorly developed proximally and devoid of cartilage, with a V-shaped notch between the bones distally. The remainder of the joint contained a thin, discolored, ineffective cartilaginous layer, typical of incomplete joint development. A triscaphe limited wrist arthrodesis provided painless wrist motion, restored grip strength, and permitted the patient to resume full participation in all activities.

SCAPHOLUNATE ADVANCED COLLAPSE

SLAC wrist is the most common pattern of degenerative disease of the wrist, accounting for 72% of all wrist arthritis (31). The most common etiology of SLAC is RSS followed by scaphoid nonunion. Other conditions that will produce SLAC degeneration include Preiser's disease, mid-

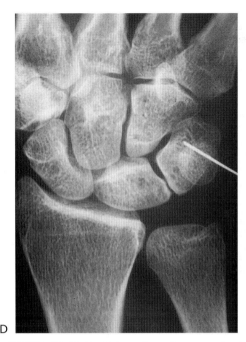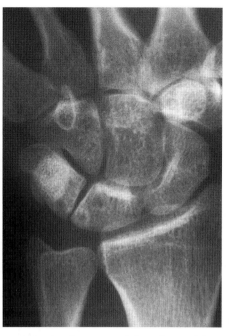

FIGURE 32.14. D: This patient demonstrates incomplete development of the triquetral–lunate joint with symptomatology necessitating arthrodesis. **E:** This patient with incomplete development of the triquetral–lunate joint has developed small degenerative cysts proximally in both bones.

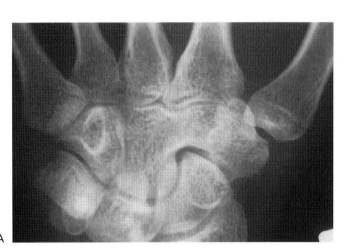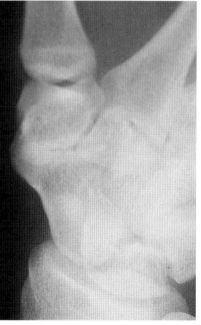

FIGURE 32.15. A: A congenital coalition is seen between the trapezoid and capitate. The opposite side demonstrated a painful partial coalition that required limited wrist arthrodesis. **B:** Congenital synchondrosis of the scaphotrapeziotrapezoid joint, a rare carpal coalition, is notably more severe on the radial aspect of the joint, where bony bridging between the scaphoid and trapezium is found. (From Weinzweig J, Watson HK, Herbert TJ, et al. Congenital synchondrosis of the scapho-trapezio-trapezoid joint. *J Hand Surg [Am]* 1997;22:74–77, with permission.)

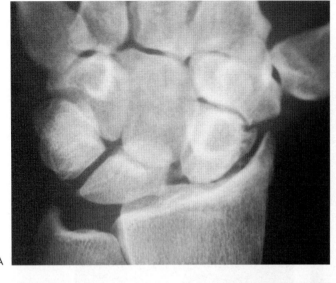
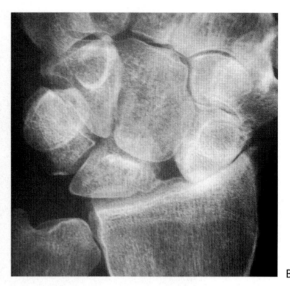
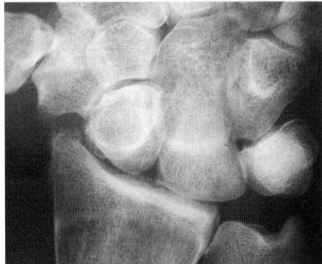

FIGURE 32.16. Stages of scapholunate advanced collapse (SLAC) wrist. **A:** SLAC changes are seen earliest at the radial aspect of the radius–scaphoid joint, beginning at the radial styloid (stage IA). **B:** Subsequently, the remainder of the radius–scaphoid joint is involved (stage IB). **C:** Finally, destruction of the capitate–lunate joint occurs (stage II). Isolated involvement of the capitate–lunate joint may also be seen and is referred to as midcarpal SLAC.

carpal instability, intraarticular fractures involving the radioscaphoid or capitate–lunate joints, and Kienböck's disease, tertiary to the secondary RSS.

Each of these etiologic factors involves the scaphoid, the weak link in the wrist with regard to degenerative disease. The specialized radioscaphoid joint is particularly susceptible. Any injury to the scaphoid or its support mechanism can produce a collapse pattern on the radial side of the wrist, ultimately leading to SLAC destruction, which occurs first between the radial styloid and the scaphoid (stage IA) (Fig. 32.16A). With progressive degenerative disease, complete destruction of the radioscaphoid joint occurs with collapse of the articular space (stage IB) (Fig. 32.16B). Once this collapse has occurred, whether it is secondary to scaphoid instability or scaphoradial in nature, the capitate–lunate joint is then unable to bear loads normally. The capitate drives off the radial or dorsal radial portion of the distal lunate articular surface, causing cartilage shear stress with eventual destruction of the capitate–lunate joint and resultant midcarpal SLAC (stage II) (Figs. 32.16C and 32.17).

The rationale for the SLAC wrist reconstruction lies in the radiolunate joint, which is highly resistant to degenerative change and is preserved at all stages of the SLAC sequence (Fig. 32.18). The articulation of the lunate with the radius is spherical in shape. The lunate can be moved volarly or dorsally, radially or ulnarly, and the proximal articular surface of the lunate will still be perpendicularly loaded. Even with significant displacement of the lunate into VISI or DISI, the radiolunate joint will be preserved. Thus, following SLAC reconstruction, both load transference and motion are dependent on the radiolunate joint. The key to successful SLAC reconstruction lies in satisfactorily correcting the DISI lunate position associated with the advanced collapse state (Fig. 32.19).

SLAC wrist reconstruction involves excision of the scaphoid and arthrodesis of the capitate, lunate, hamate, and

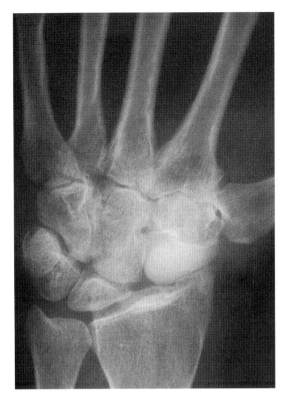 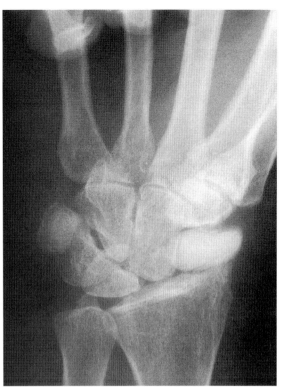

FIGURE 32.17. This patient presented with a silicone scaphoid and an excellent demonstration of how destruction occurs between the capitate and lunate. When the wrist is at rest **(left)**, the capitate sits squarely on the lunate. When the patient makes a fist **(right)**, the capitate drives off the radial side of the lunate with resultant shear loading of the cartilage. This shear loading rapidly destroys the capitate–lunate joint, resulting in the secondary stage of a scapholunate advanced collapse wrist.

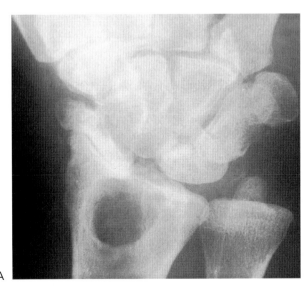 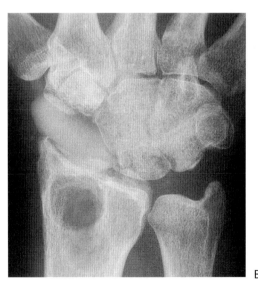

A B

FIGURE 32.18. A: Severe longstanding symptoms in a patient who refused total wrist fusion from multiple orthopedic surgeons. Note the normal radius–lunate joint typical of a scapholunate advanced collapse wrist. There is a large degenerative cyst which may be ignored, as loads will be taken by the normal trabeculae beneath the lunate. **B:** In the late 1970s, fusion of the capitate–lunate–hamate–triquetrum and silicone scaphoid replacement were performed. There is no place for silicone now, as particulate synovitis will occur even in wrists where the load is taken by the fusion. *Figure continues on next page.*

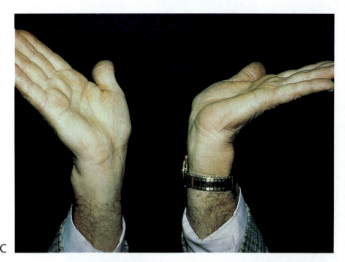
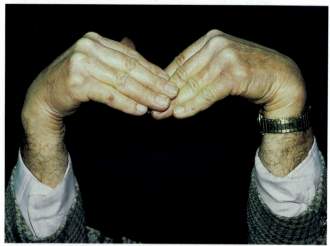

FIGURE 32.18. (continued) C,D: One year postoperatively, the right wrist was asymptomatic with full power and good motion.

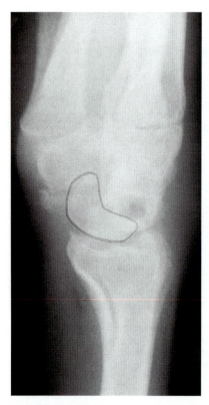

FIGURE 32.19. Lateral x-ray demonstrates an outlined lunate in dorsal intercalated segment instability (DISI) position with proximal migration of the capitate. In addition, a large cyst is noted in the proximal pole of the capitate. Failure to correct the DISI lunate resulted in persistent symptomatology following scapholunate advanced collapse wrist reconstruction.

triquetrum (Fig. 32.20). This procedure is also referred to as a "four-bone fusion." Patients who present with a SLAC wrist in conjunction with lunate or radiolunate pathology are *not* candidates for this type of reconstruction. Significant ulnar translation, which disrupts the concentric congruity of the radiolunate articulation and predictably leads to joint destruction, osteonecrosis of the lunate, as in Kienböck's disease, and preexisting radiolunate degenerative change, are absolute contraindications to SLAC wrist reconstruction (23). The salvage procedures under these conditions include proximal row carpectomy or wrist arthrodesis.

LUNOTRIQUETRAL ARTHRODESIS

Pathology arising from the LT joint is a known etiology of ulnar wrist pain (50–52). Indications for limited wrist arthrodesis of this articulation include LT joint instability, degenerative arthritis, and symptomatic congenital synchondrosis or incomplete separation of the lunate and triquetrum (Fig. 32.14). Patients with LT pathology usually experience pain from palpation directly over the LT joint or from shear loading of the joint by performing an LT ballottement test (33,53).

Although complete ligamentous disruption (static instability) is relatively rare, even small changes in LT kinematics will produce synovitis, degenerative change, and pain (54). Although patients with partial ligamentous injuries often have normal plain radiographs, stress views may demonstrate dynamic dissociation (55) or ulnar impaction syndrome (56). LT instability is often associated with ulnar positive variance, and secondary to ulnar impaction with resultant LT interosseous ligament disruption and joint dissociation. Partial LT ligament tears associated with low-grade instability may be managed by an ulnar shortening procedure alone, but significant symptomatic instability necessitates LT arthrodesis.

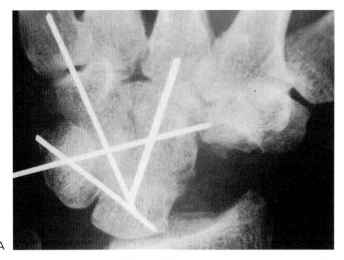 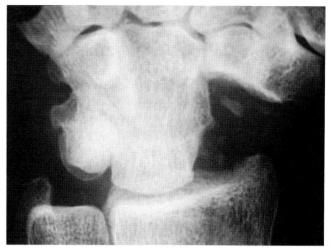

FIGURE 32.20. Scapholunate advanced collapse (SLAC) wrist reconstruction. **A:** Postoperative radiographic examination 6 weeks following SLAC reconstruction with limited wrist arthrodesis and scaphoid excision demonstrates typical pin placement and adequate bony consolidation. **B:** Six months following SLAC reconstruction, the arthrodesis is radiographically solid, and the radiolunate joint well preserved. Note the ulnar displacement of the capitate on the lunate, which tightens the radioscaphocapitate ligament and prevents ulnar translation.

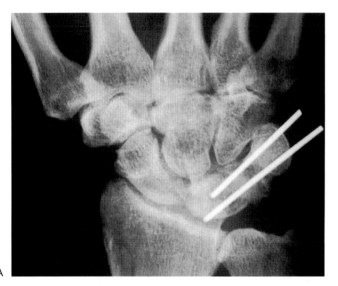 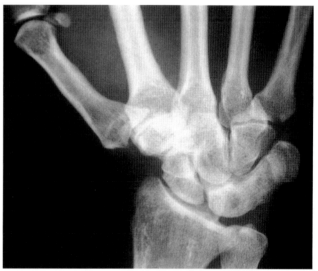

FIGURE 32.21. Lunotriquetral (LT) arthrodesis. **A:** Postoperative radiographic examination 6 weeks following LT arthrodesis demonstrates typical pin placement and bony consolidation. **B:** Three months following LT fusion, the arthrodesis is radiographically solid.

Radiographs will demonstrate positive findings in cases of static LT dissociation, advanced degenerative disease, and congenital synchondrosis of the joint (19). Radiographic findings associated with degenerative change secondary to congenital synchondrosis include joint narrowing with bony impingement, loss of cartilaginous space, and the presence of cystic changes (49). A consistent appearance in partial coalition of the LT joint is that of a "champagne flute." Most LT degenerative arthritis is secondary to congenital partial coalition. Radiographs of the contralateral wrist are recommended in these patients, as most demonstrate bilateral disease. The biconcave bone-grafting technique of LT arthrodesis results in 100% union with few complications, yielding functional wrists with minimal loss of wrist motion (Fig. 32.21; see Chapter 57).

CAPITATE–LUNATE ARTHRODESIS

Capitate–lunate arthrodesis is indicated only rarely in the case of articular fractures within this joint, isolated degenerative arthritis (midcarpal SLAC), or destruction of either of these articular surfaces secondary to various bony lesions (57). However, it is unusual to perform an isolated capitate–lunate arthrodesis because there is no additional resultant morbidity in terms of loss of wrist motion, strength, or durability by adding the hamate and triquetrum to the arthrodesis and performing a formal SLAC wrist reconstruction. In this reconstruction, the likelihood of successful fusion is significantly enhanced by increasing the total cancellous surface area at the fusion site.

TRIQUETRAL–HAMATE ARTHRODESIS

The articulation between the hamate and triquetrum allows a wide range of motion, with the triquetrum normally moving proximally and distally as well as volarly and dorsally in relation to the hamate. Before injury occurs to the ligaments of the triquetral-hamate joint, other more restricting and stabilizing intercarpal ligaments must rupture. Appropriate treatment is usually directed at those more significant coexisting midcarpal instabilities. Thus, there is rarely an indication for an isolated triquetral–hamate fusion.

SCAPHOID–LUNATE ARTHRODESIS

Although scaphoid–lunate limited wrist arthrodesis would seem an ideal approach to the management of SL dissociation, there are several important contraindications to arthrodesis of this joint. Perhaps the most obvious of these contraindications is the difficulty of achieving union by fusion of the relatively small articular surfaces of these two bones. Cancellous contact areas are inadequate, and, therefore, nonunion rates are predictably high. However, there are two additional compelling reasons to avoid this procedure. The first reason is that any joint fusion requires sufficient bone to carry the loads that cross it. The banana-shaped SL combination provides inadequate bony volume to carry the loads that this fusion would be required to bear and would result in carpal symptomatology. A second reason is that the scaphoid and lunate reside in two different fossae on the same bone. A ridge is always found between these fossae on the radius and is occasionally substantial. Fusing the scaphoid to the lunate would remove the small, but necessary, degree of motion between these bones and consequently result in decreased range of motion compared to the SLAC reconstruction and degenerative change of the radiocarpal joint.

SCAPHOID–CAPITATE ARTHRODESIS

Scaphoid–capitate arthrodesis and triscaphe arthrodesis are, in principle, two very different operations. The scaphoid–capitate fusion transmits load directly across the fusion site from capitate to scaphoid and then to the radius. With triscaphe arthrodesis, the loads are not transmitted primarily through the fusion site. In fact, most of the load passes from the capitate across normal cartilage to the scaphoid and again across normal cartilage to the radius. Arthrodesis of the triscaphe joint prevents the proximal pole of the scaphoid from displacing beneath the capitate under load, but the fusion does not carry the load. The normally small amount of motion between the capitate and scaphoid gradually increases and provides the significant difference of wrist motion between these two types of limited wrist arthrodeses.

RADIUS–LUNATE ARTHRODESIS

Destruction of the radiolunate joint and ulnar translation of the carpus are the only indications for radius–lunate arthrodesis (Fig. 32.22). The former usually occurs secondary to die-punch fractures involving the spherical lunate fossa on the distal radius. The latter may occur following trauma, infection, particulate synovitis, or inflammatory arthritis. Destruction of the capitate–lunate joint is an absolute contraindication to this procedure, as wrist motion is dependent on this midcarpal joint following radius–lunate arthrodesis. This procedure requires a sufficient distal radius bone graft to elevate the lunate and, thereby, prevent loss of carpal height (Fig. 32.23). Overcorrection of the position of the lunate on the radius by slightly excessive elevation is well tolerated by the wrist and, in fact, preferred; undercorrection of the lunate position with loss of carpal height will result in decreased wrist motion and wrist instability.

DISCUSSION

The complex anatomy of the carpus allows certain patterns of multiplanar motion to occur within the normal wrist. The scaphoid and lunate, for example, can be considered a mobile unit, albeit each with a different arc of motion, in flexion, extension, and radioulnar deviation. However, a limited wrist arthrodesis that incorporates the lunate into the fusion (e.g., SLAC reconstruction or radius–lunate arthrodesis) demonstrates significantly more motion between the scaphoid and fused lunate on cineradiography. The implication is that the normal patterns of intercarpal motion are modified by a variety of limited wrist arthrodeses. Intercarpal adaptations compensate for motion pathways lost as a result of fusion. The new planes of motion do not become completely manifest until maximal postoperative mobility has been achieved some 9 to 12 months later. Each particular intercarpal arthrodesis unit may result in increased motion between certain carpal bones, ultimately preserving a considerable amount of total wrist motion (17).

In the course of performing, and subsequently reviewing, more than 1,300 limited wrist arthrodeses, we have gleaned significant experience. The concepts of limited wrist arthrodesis presented have evolved based on this experience. Procedures have been modified, and indications more precisely defined. Twenty-nine of these cases involved the fusion of various combinations of carpal bones (e.g., capitate–hamate, capitate–lunate, scaphoid–capitate–lunate, scaphoid–trapezium–trapezoid–capitate) that have since been abandoned. However, the importance of these limited wrist arthrodeses in the evolution of the limited fusions currently most commonly performed (e.g., triscaphe, SLAC reconstruction, lunate–triquetrum) cannot be overstated. An understanding

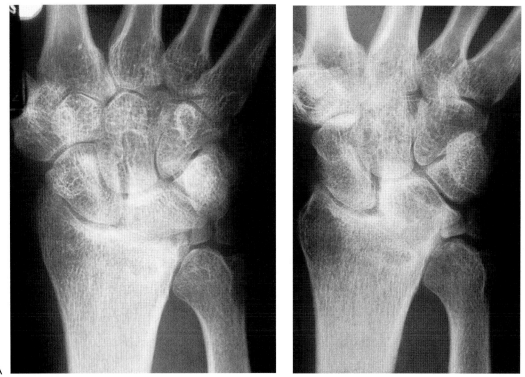

FIGURE 32.22. Radius–lunate arthrodesis. **A:** Isolated destruction of the radius–lunate joint is best treated by radius–lunate limited wrist arthrodesis. **B:** The principles of the procedure are to displace the lunate distally and maintain a transverse articular surface for the capitate.

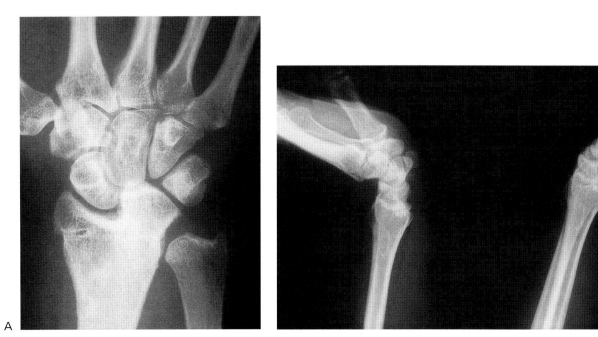

FIGURE 32.23. Radius–lunate arthrodesis. **A:** Posteroanterior x-ray demonstrates the radiolunate arthrodesis maintaining or accentuating the normal distance between radius and lunate. **B:** Lateral x-ray of this radiolunate fusion demonstrates the significant flexion–extension arc available with proper lunate positioning.

of the principles involved in load transfer through the carpus and the requirements necessary to preserve maximal wrist motion postoperatively is the direct outgrowth of the experience with these earlier fusions.

Complication rates for all types of intercarpal arthrodeses are remarkably low, and patient satisfaction is high. No pattern of secondary changes or degenerative arthritis has been seen. These procedures are effective and reliable techniques for treating a myriad of carpal pathologies; they maximize postoperative wrist motion, function, and strength while eliminating pain and instability.

REFERENCES

1. Ashmead D, Watson HK. SLAC wrist reconstruction. In: Gelberman R, ed. *The wrist*. New York: Raven Press, 1994;319–330.
2. Graner O, Lopes EI, Carvalho BC, et al. Arthrodesis of the carpal bones in the treatment of Kienböck's disease, painful ununited fractures of the navicular and lunate bones with avascular necrosis, and old fracture-dislocation of carpal bones. *J Bone Joint Surg Am* 1966;48:767–774.
3. Peterson HA, Lipscomb PR. Intercarpal arthrodesis. *Arch Surg* 1967;95:127–134.
4. Trumble T, Bour C, Smith R, et al. Intercarpal arthrodesis for static and dynamic volar intercalated segment instability. *J Hand Surg [Am]* 1988;13:396–402.
5. Watson HK, Ashmead D. Triscaphe fusion for chronic scapholunate instability. In: Gelberman R, ed. *The wrist*. New York: Raven Press, 1994;183–194.
6. Watson HK, Fink JA, Monacelli DM. Use of triscaphe fusion in the treatment of Kienböck's disease. *Hand Clin* 1993;9:493–499.
7. Watson HK, Weinzweig J. Intercarpal arthrodesis. In: Green DP, Hotchkiss RN, Pederson WC, eds. *Operative hand surgery, 4th ed.* New York: Churchill Livingstone, 1998;108–130.
8. Watson HK, Weinzweig J, Guidera P, et al. One thousand intercarpal arthrodeses. *J Hand Surg [Br]* 1999;24:320–330.
9. Watson HK, Weinzweig J. Treatment of Kienböck's disease with triscaphe arthrodesis. In: Vastamaki M, Vilkki S, Goransson H, et al, eds. *Proceedings of the 6th Congress of the International Federation of Societies for Surgery of the Hand*. Bologna: Monduzzi Editore, 1995;347–349.
10. Weinzweig J, Watson HK. Wrist sprain to SLAC wrist: A spectrum of carpal instability. In: Vastamaki M, ed. *Current trends in hand surgery*. Amsterdam: Elsevier Science Publishers, 1995;47–55.
11. Douglas DP, Peimer CA, Koniuch MP. Motion of the wrist after simulated limited intercarpal arthrodesis. An experimental study. *J Bone Joint Surg Am* 1987;69:1413–1418.
12. Garcia-Elias M, Cooney WP, An KN, et al. Wrist kinematics after limited intercarpal arthrodesis. *J Hand Surg [Am]* 1989;14:791–799.
13. Gross SC, Watson HK, Strickland JW, et al. Triquetral–lunate arthritis secondary to synostosis. *J Hand Surg [Am]* 1989;14:95–102.
14. Meyerdierks EM, Mosher JF, Werner FW. Limited wrist arthrodesis: A laboratory study. *J Hand Surg [Am]* 1987;12:526–529.
15. Palmer AK, Werner FW, Murphy D, et al. Functional wrist motion: A biomechanical study. *J Hand Surg [Am]* 1985;10:39–46.
16. Viegas SF, Patterson RM, Peterson PD, et al. Evaluation of the biomechanical efficacy of limited intercarpal fusions for the treatment of scapho-lunate dissociation. *J Hand Surg [Am]* 1990;15:120–128.
17. Watson HK, Goodman ML, Johnson TR. Limited wrist arthrodesis. Part II: Intercarpal and radiocarpal combinations. *J Hand Surg [Am]* 1981;6:223–232.
18. Watson HK, Hempton RE. Limited wrist arthrodesis. Part I: The triscaphoid joint. *J Hand Surg [Am]* 1980;5:320–327.
19. Gellman H, Kauffman D, Lenihan M, et al. An in vitro analysis of wrist motion: The effect of limited intercarpal arthrodesis and the contributions of the radiocarpal and midcarpal joints. *J Hand Surg [Am]* 1988;13:378–383.
20. Youm Y, Flatt AE. Kinematics of the wrist. *Clin Orthop* 1980;149:21–32.
21. Youm Y, McMurtry RY, Flatt AE, et al. Kinematics of the wrist. I. An experimental study of radial–ulnar deviation and flexion–extension. *J Bone Joint Surg Am* 1978;60:423–431.
22. Palmer AK, Dobyns JH, Linscheid RL. Management of post-traumatic instability of the wrist secondary to ligament rupture. *J Hand Surg [Am]* 1978;3:507–532.
23. Ashmead D, Watson HK, Damon C, et al. Scapholunate advanced collapse wrist salvage. *J Hand Surg [Am]* 1994;19:741–750.
24. Watson HK, Ryu J, Akelman E. Limited triscaphoid intercarpal arthrodesis for rotary subluxation of the scaphoid. *J Bone Joint Surg Am* 1986;68:345–349.
25. Watson HK, Weinzweig J, Zeppieri J. The natural progression of scaphoid instability. *Hand Clin* 1997;13:39–50.
26. Vender MI, Watson HK, Wiener BD, et al. Degenerative change in symptomatic scaphoid non-union. *J Hand Surg [Am]* 1987;12:514–519.
27. Watson HK, Ryu J, DiBella A. An approach to Kienböck's disease: Triscaphe arthrodesis. *J Hand Surg [Am]* 1985;10:179–187.
28. Weinzweig J, Watson HK, Herbert TJ, et al. Congenital synchondrosis of the scaphotrapezio-trapezoid joint. *J Hand Surg [Am]* 1997;22:74–77.
29. Rogers WD, Watson HK. Radial styloid impingement after triscaphe arthrodesis. *J Hand Surg [Am]* 1989;14:297–301.
30. Linscheid RL, Lirette R, Dobyns JH. L'arthrose degenerative scapho-trapezienne. In: Saffar P, ed. *La rhizarthrose. Monographies du Group d'Etude de la Main*. Paris: Expansion Scientifique Francaise, 1990:144–152.
31. Watson HK, Ballet FL. The SLAC wrist: scapholunate advanced collapse pattern of degenerative arthritis. *J Hand Surg [Am]* 1984;9:358–365.
32. Watson HK, Rogers WD, Ashmead D. Reevaluation of the cause of the wrist ganglion. *J Hand Surg [Am]* 1989;14:812–817.
33. Watson HK, Weinzweig J. Physical examination of the wrist. *Hand Clin* 1997;13:17–34.
34. Watson HK, Ashmead D, Makhlouf MV. Examination of the scaphoid. *J Hand Surg [Am]* 1988;13:657–660.
35. Watson HK, Ottoni L, Pitts EC, et al. Rotary subluxation of the scaphoid: A spectrum of instability. *J Hand Surg [Br]* 1993;18:62–64.
36. Taleisnik J. *The wrist*. New York: Churchill Livingstone, 1985;229–303.
37. Blatt G. Capsulodesis in reconstructive hand surgery. Dorsal capsulodesis for the unstable scaphoid and volar capsulodesis following excision of the distal ulna. *Hand Clin* 1987;3:81–102.
38. Cooney WP, Linscheid RL, Dobyns JH. Scaphoid fractures: Problems associated with nonunion and avascular necrosis. *Orthop Clin* 1984;15:381–391.
39. McGrath MH, Watson HK. Late results with local bone graft donor sites in hand surgery. *J Hand Surg [Am]* 1981;6:234–237.

40. Alexander CE, Alexander AH, Lichtman DM. Radial shortening in Kienböck's disease. In: Gelberman R, ed. *The wrist.* New York: Raven Press, 1994;373–382.
41. Lichtman DM, Ross G. Revascularization of the lunate in Kienböck's disease. In: Gelberman R, ed. *The wrist.* New York: Raven Press, 1994;363–372.
42. Quenzer DE, Linscheid RL. Ulnar lengthening procedures. *Hand Clin* 1993;9:467–475.
43. Lin HH, Stern PJ. "Salvage" procedures in the treatment of Kienböck's disease: Proximal row carpectomy and total wrist arthrodesis. *Hand Clin* 1993;9:521–526.
44. Berger RA, Kauer JMG, Landsmeer JMF. Radioscapholunate ligament: A gross anatomic and histologic study of fetal and adult wrists. *J Hand Surg [Am]* 1991;16:350–355.
45. Watson HK, Yasuda M, Guidera PM. Lateral lunate morphology: An x-ray study. *J Hand Surg [Am]* 1996;21:759–763.
46. Kauer J. Functional anatomy of the wrist. *Clin Orthop* 1980;149:9–20.
47. Kauer J. The mechanism of the carpal joint. *Clin Orthop* 1986;202:16–26.
48. Cockshott WP. Carpal fusions. *Am J Roentgenol* 1963;89:1260–1262.
49. Resnik C, Grizzard J, Simmons B, et al. Incomplete carpal coalition. *Am J Radiol* 1986;147:301–304.
50. Kirschenbaum D, Coyle M, Leddy J. Chronic lunotriquetral instability: Diagnosis and treatment. *J Hand Surg [Am]* 1993;18:1107–1112.
51. Lichtman DM, Noble WH, Alexander CE. Dynamic triquetrolunate instability: Case report. *J Hand Surg [Am]* 1984;9:185–188.
52. Pin P, Young V, Gilula L, et al. Management of chronic lunotriquetral ligament tears. *J Hand Surg [Am]* 1989;14:77–83.
53. Tubiana R, Thornine JM, Mackin E. *Examination of the hand and wrist.* Philadelphia: CV Mosby, 1995;185–197.
54. Horii E, Garcia-Elias M, An K, et al. A kinematic study of lunotriquetral dissociations. *J Hand Surg [Am]* 1991;16:355–362.
55. Viegas SF, Patterson RM, Peterson PD, et al. Ulnar-sided perilunate instability: an anatomic and biomechanical study. *J Hand Surg [Am]* 1990;15:268–278.
56. Friedman S, Palmer A. The ulnar impaction syndrome. *Hand Clin* 1991;7:295–310.
57. Kirschenbaum D, Schneider LH, Kirkpatrick WH, et al. Scaphoid excision and capitolunate arthrodesis for radioscaphoid arthritis. *J Hand Surg [Am]* 1993;18:780–785.

33

PROXIMAL ROW CARPECTOMY

ROBERT LEE WILSON
DOUGLAS M. HASSAN

HISTORICAL BACKGROUND

Proximal row carpectomy (PRC) was first reported in 1944 by Stamm (1). Stack also described a technique of PRC in 1948 (2), but he excised only the scaphoid and the lunate. Historically, the merit of PRC has been controversial. Criticism of this procedure has largely been based on anecdotal opinion. Thus, PRC has carried an undeserved reputation for poor results. However, all large series reporting PRC have shown favorable long-term results (3–11). Good pain relief with a functional range of motion and satisfactory grip strength should be the expected result.

Imbriglia et al. in 1990 performed a radiographic analysis of the curvature of the capitate and lunate (5). The radius of curvature of the capitate is about two thirds that of the lunate. Motion between the capitate and radius is translational. They postulated that this moving center of motion may help to dissipate the load on the lunate fossa (5). It may also explain the relatively long recovery period following a PRC.

Several authors have described PRC as a salvage procedure (12–14). However, Jorgensen has emphasized that a PRC "should not be thought of as a salvage procedure to be attempted when all else fails" (4). It is a logical first-line procedure when the indications are sound.

INDICATIONS AND CONTRAINDICATIONS

The options available to treat degenerative changes of the radiocarpal joint include limited fusion, total wrist fusion, soft tissue arthroplasty, implant arthroplasty, and resection of the proximal carpal row. Each option has its own advantages and disadvantages. The primary indication is pain refractory to conservative management. Improving grip strength and preserving range of motion are secondary goals. Whether these goals can be achieved depends on the patient's disease and the success of postoperative rehabilitation.

When patients present with a chronic degenerative wrist condition, an initial course of splinting, antiinflammatory drugs, and occasionally therapy is often the first therapeutic step. The surgeon must determine which procedure, if any, can be best matched to the needs of the patient. PRC can be considered for posttraumatic and avascular disorders of the proximal row with subsequent degenerative changes. To be successful, the head of the capitate and lunate fossa of the radius must be relatively free of degenerative changes. PRC preserves motion that would otherwise be lost by a limited or total wrist fusion.

Scapholunate Advanced Collapse

Chronic scapholunate instability is the most frequent cause of degenerative arthritis in the wrist joint. The pattern of scapholunate advanced collapse (SLAC) wrist progression is well documented by Watson and Ballet (15). Degenerative changes begin between the tip of the radial styloid and the scaphoid. Following this, the scaphoid fossa of the radius and the scaphoid are involved. Eventually the capitolunate joint is involved. However, the radiolunate articulation is almost always spared. The preserved lunate fossa makes a PRC an attractive option provided that extensive changes have not occurred in the proximal pole of the capitate.

Scaphoid Nonunion

Old nonunions of the scaphoid can develop a similar collapse pattern [scapholunate nonunion advanced collapse (SNAC)] with degenerative changes. A PRC can provide a satisfactory result in this situation. Scaphoid nonunions with very small proximal poles can also be considered for a PRC.

Kienböck's Disease

The management of Lichtman stages II and III Kienböck's disease remains controversial. Surgical options include

R. L. Wilson: Department of Surgery, University of Arizona, Tucson, Arizona 85719; and Phoenix Orthopedic Program, Maricopa Medical Center, Phoenix, Arizona 85004.

D. M. Hassan: Department of Surgery, St. Joseph's Medical Center, Tacoma, Washington 98405.

immobilization, intercarpal fusion, leveling osteotomies of the forearm bones, and revascularization procedures. A PRC has been advocated for Lichtman stage III Kienböck's disease by several authors (8,9,16,17). We recommend a PRC for stage IIIB disease and have found the other options mentioned above more applicable for earlier conditions including stage IIIA. A PRC can be considered for stage IV disease if the patient does not want a wrist fusion and only minimal or mild degenerative changes exist (3,7,12,17).

Carpal Dislocations and Fracture Dislocations

These injuries are occasionally missed and not recognized for weeks or even months. Chronic perilunate dislocations and fracture dislocations can be managed by open reduction on occasion, but often will require a wrist fusion or a PRC. Acute injuries can also be managed by a PRC (18). This is particularly useful for severe injuries with multiple fractures or serious articular cartilage damage. A PRC may also be indicated as a salvage procedure after a failed open reduction of a carpal fracture-dislocation.

Avascular Necrosis of the Scaphoid

Idiopathic or posttraumatic avascular necrosis of the scaphoid with or without collapse is another indication.

Neuromuscular Disease

Patients with severe flexion deformities of the wrist such as arthrogryposis or spastic paralysis may benefit from a PRC (19,20). Contractures may be so severe that tendon transfers alone will not allow satisfactory repositioning of the wrist. A PRC is performed in conjunction with tendon transfers, and prolonged splinting is required (19).

Salvage

PRC can be considered after a previous failed wrist procedure. Unsuccessful scapholunate ligament reconstruction, failed grafting for scaphoid nonunion and reactions to silicone implants of the scaphoid and lunate are potential indications (21). However, we agree with van Heest and House that the results of PRC are superior when performed as a primary procedure.

A PRC is contraindicated when significant degenerative changes involve the proximal pole of the capitate or the lunate fossa of the radius. This is assessed most commonly by preoperative x-rays and confirmed intraoperatively. Magnetic resonance imaging (MRI) or arthroscopy may also be used to evaluate the articular surface. Several authors have reported satisfactory results when mild degenerative changes exist (3,7,12,17). Imbriglia and coworkers feel that fibrillation of the cartilage or full-thickness cartilage lesions less than 3 mm in diameter are not contraindications (5). However, more recent studies favor a PRC only when there is no capitolunate arthritis (10,22).

Patient selection is also an important factor. If the patient is willing to sacrifice motion for a totally stable and pain-free wrist, partial or total wrist fusion should be considered. However, the requirements for heavy lifting alone should not be considered a contraindication (4,5,9). This is an often-mentioned and erroneous contraindication for PRC. The presence of rheumatoid arthritis should be considered a contraindication. The reported results are disappointing (8,13).

SURGICAL TECHNIQUE

Anesthesia for a PRC may be obtained using an axillary block or a general anesthetic. After a tourniquet is applied to the upper arm, a standard surgical prep and draping is carried out. Following exsanguination, the tourniquet pressure is elevated.

The landmarks are outlined on the dorsum of the wrist. Either a longitudinal or a transverse incision can be utilized. The longitudinal incision is more versatile. Depending on what is discovered at the time of operative exploration, it allows other surgical options to be performed, such as a

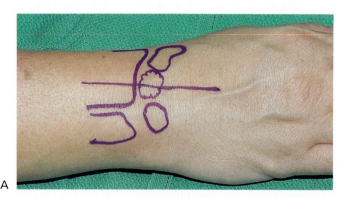 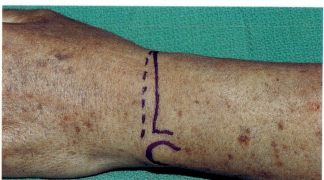

FIGURE 33.1. A: Longitudinal incision. **B:** Transverse incision *(dotted line)*.

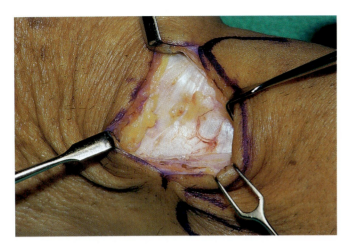

FIGURE 33.2. The retinaculum is exposed.

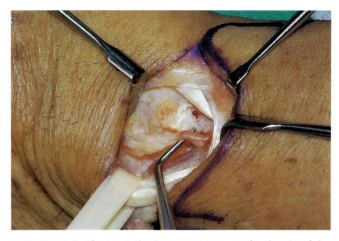

FIGURE 33.4. The posterior interosseous nerve (at the tip of the probe).

complete wrist arthrodesis. A transverse incision allows better visualization of the wrist medially and laterally and facilitates removal of the distal pole of the scaphoid and the radial styloid (Fig. 33.1).

The dissection is carried down to the retinaculum. The overlying soft tissues are raised, and care is taken to spare the branches of the superficial radial and ulnar nerves (Fig. 33.2).

The retinaculum and the extensor tendons may be approached several different ways. Our preferred technique is to incise the third compartment, allowing the extensor pollicis longus to be mobilized and retracted along with the radial wrist extensor tendons. The distal fascia that is confluent with the retinaculum is reflected ulnarward (Fig. 33.3).

The fourth extensor compartment is left intact but is opened on the radial side to demonstrate the posterior interosseous nerve. One to two centimeters of the nerve is resected; the proximal end of the nerve is sealed with bipolar cautery and injected with local anesthetic (Fig. 33.4).

Alternative techniques are to incise the retinaculum between the third and fourth compartments, leaving the proximal half to one-third intact. Another choice is to divide the retinaculum in a zig-zag fashion, the ulnar-based flap left proximally and the distal radially. When the retinaculum is subsequently repaired, it may be reapproximated with less tension so as to prevent restriction of extensor tendon gliding.

The capsule is incised transversely, leaving a cuff of soft tissue proximally for repair at the time of closure. A central incision creating a proximally based "T" flap is recommended by some authors. We prefer a distally based "U" flap, with the longitudinal limbs parallel to the second and fifth compartment tendons (Fig. 33.5). The capsule is sharply elevated from the carpals and retracted. Care should be taken to prevent any injury to the radial artery as it passes across the scaphoid (Fig. 33.6).

The wrist is explored to confirm the abnormalities that are anticipated and to check for ones that cannot be easily

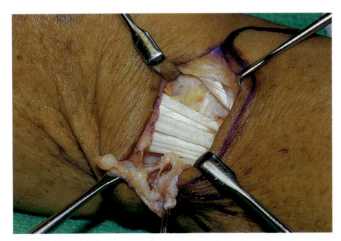

FIGURE 33.3. The distal fascia is reflected to expose the extensor tendons.

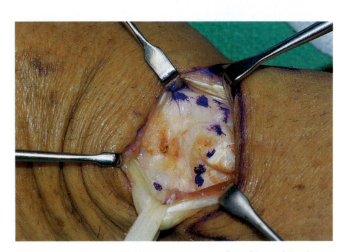

FIGURE 33.5. Distally based capsular flap *(dotted line)*.

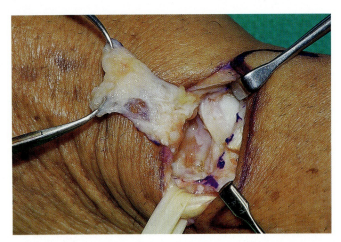

FIGURE 33.6. Elevation of the capsule, retracted with clamps.

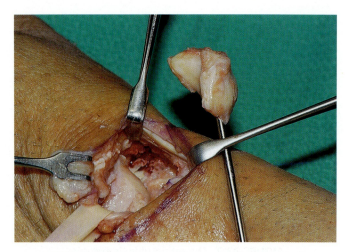

FIGURE 33.8. The scaphoid is removed in one piece.

determined with routine x-rays. These would include cartilage injuries on the articulating surfaces and trauma to the triangular fibrocartilage complex (Fig. 33.7). It is necessary to visualize the articular surface of the capitate and the lunate fossa of the radius. Cartilage abrasions on the periphery or mild wear such as fibrillations of the cartilage are not by themselves contraindications to a PRC.

The surgeon may elect the sequence for removal of the proximal carpal row. The triquetrum is the easiest bone to remove, and we prefer to begin on the ulnar side of the wrist and progress radially. With a scaphoid nonunion, the distal pole of the scaphoid can be difficult to remove (Fig. 33.8). Great care needs to be taken when excising the lunate (Fig. 33.9). It is important not to damage the articular surfaces of the capitate or the lunate fossa of the radius. Preservation of the volar ligaments is essential.

Whether the carpals are removed piecemeal or dissected out and removed intact is at the discretion of the surgeon. With the first technique, the bones are divided with an osteotome and removed with the rongeur. We prefer to insert a pin into each bone and use it as a joystick for reflecting the soft tissues and removing the bones intact. The joystick may be a threaded 0.062 Kirschner wire, a Knowles pin, or an AO external fixation pin attached to a T-handle with a chuck (Fig. 33.10). All three of the proximal row carpals are removed in sequence (Fig. 33.11). The pisiform is left in place.

The capitate articular surface and the radius are once again inspected (Fig. 33.12). The capitate is seated in the lunate fossa of the radius. Impingement between the trapezium and the radial styloid is evaluated. With radial deviation of the wrist, it should be possible to place one's little finger at the styloid tip and not be impacted by the trapezium. Should impaction occur, a styloidectomy will be necessary. Enough bone (5–15 mm) is resected with a saw, osteotome, or power burr (Fig. 33.13). It is important not to detach the volar radiocapitate ligament (Fig. 33.14). Long vertical oblique or transverse styloid excisions, as described by Siegel and Gelberman, may be detrimental (23).

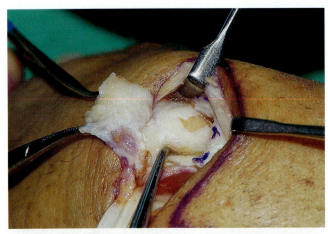

FIGURE 33.7. Full-thickness cartilage loss on the scaphoid with scapholunate interosseous ligament disruption (probe in the ligament defect).

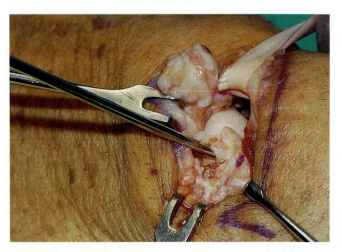

FIGURE 33.9. Pin in the lunate.

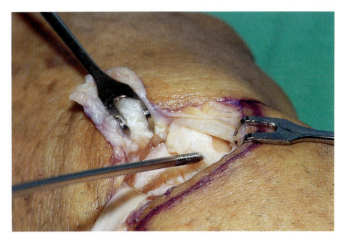

FIGURE 33.10. The threaded pin is inserted along the scaphoid axis.

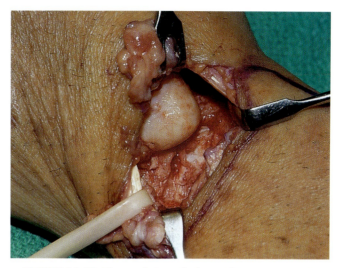

FIGURE 33.12. The capitate articular surface is inspected.

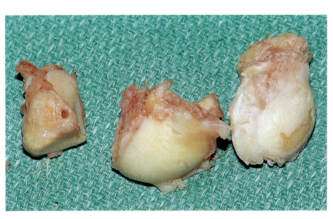

FIGURE 33.11. The proximal carpal row.

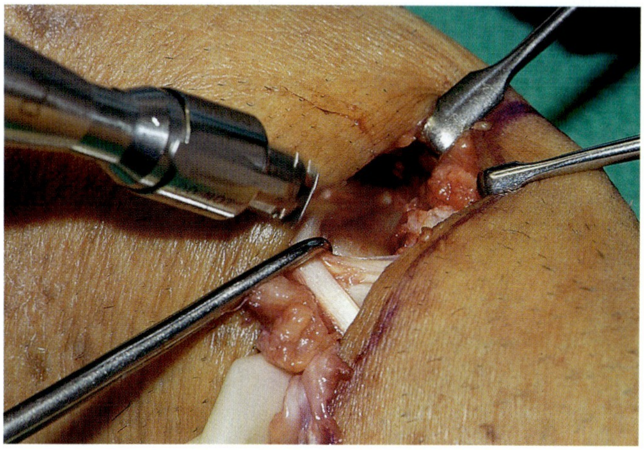

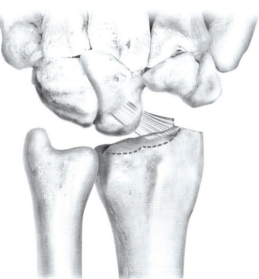

FIGURE 33.13. Styloidectomy is performed with a saw.

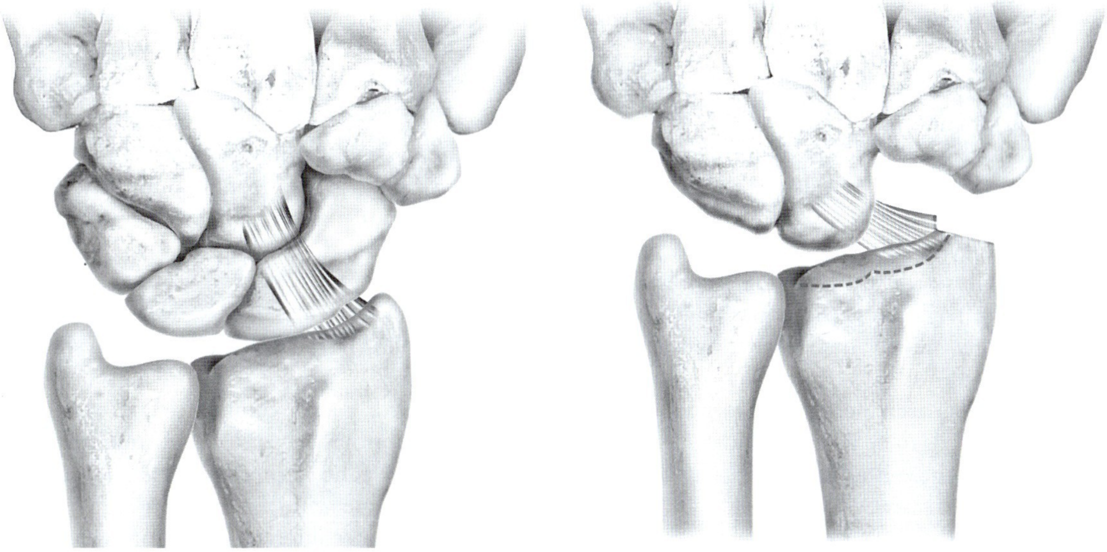

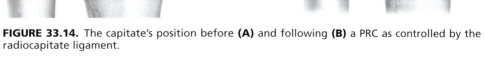

A   B

FIGURE 33.14. The capitate's position before **(A)** and following **(B)** a PRC as controlled by the radiocapitate ligament.

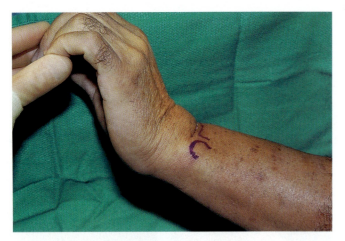

FIGURE 33.15. Wrist extension.

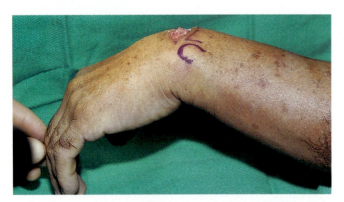

FIGURE 33.16. Wrist flexion.

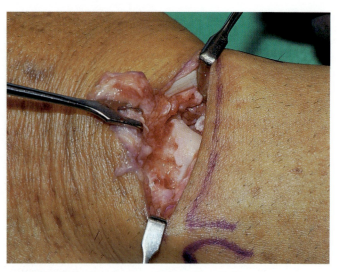

FIGURE 33.17. The capitate is seated in the lunate fossa of the radius.

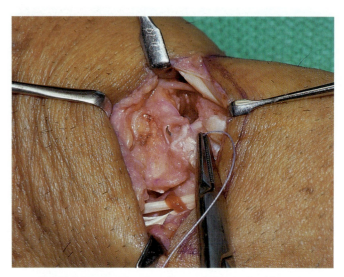

FIGURE 33.18. The dorsal capsule is repaired loosely.

Once the styloidectomy is complete, the capitate is seated in the lunate fossa. Motion and stability are assessed (Figs. 33.15 and 33.16). Pin fixation of the capitate to the radius is rarely indicated and should be used only if a problem with stability exists. It would be preferable to repair the volar ligaments to achieve stability rather than insert a wire. Should a wire be used, it must not pass through the lunate fossa of the radius or the articular surface of the capitate.

Hemostasis is achieved after the tourniquet is released. Any vessels that might produce a hematoma are ligated or cauterized. Following irrigation of the wound, the capsule is repaired, removing redundant tissue for a loose closure (Figs. 33.17 and 33.18).

If the retinaculum has been incised or disrupted with the surgical approach, it needs to be repaired. A drain should be temporarily inserted if there is any concern with hemostasis. A layered closure is carried out using a 3-0 or 4-0 absorbable material in the deeper tissues and a permanent suture for the skin.

The wrist is immobilized in neutral or slight extension with a bulky gauze dressing supplemented with anterior and posterior plaster splints. Patients are usually admitted overnight for pain control.

ALTERNATIVE SURGICAL TECHNIQUES

A PRC with partial capitate resection and dorsal capsular interposition has recently been presented by Salomon and Eaton (24). The authors remove the projecting proximal capitate in line with the articular surface of the hamate to create a broader interface for compressive forces within the wrist. A radial styloidectomy is not performed. A distally based dorsal flap of capsule is sutured to the volar wrist capsule, and a wire is placed across the reconstructed joint for 3 weeks. Motion is initiated at 4 weeks after surgery. A wrist motion arc of 94° is reported with significant improvement in grip and minimal pain. The authors observed that this PRC modification provided fewer complications than wrist fusion, either complete or partial.

The results of a distraction resection arthroplasty of the wrist were presented by Fitzgerald, Peimer, and Smith in 1989 (25). The authors utilized this technique for patients who had cartilage destruction of the capitate and/or lunate fossa of the radius. They believed that replacement arthroplasties of the wrist often failed because of loosening. The technique includes resection of the proximal capitate and hamate at the time of excision of the proximal row. The wrist is then distracted to create a gap of 2 cm. This space is maintained with three or more 0.062-in. Kirschner wires passed through the radius into the remaining carpus. The redundant capsule is interposed between the radius and the capitate, and the retinaculum is placed beneath the tendons to reinforce the capsular closure. The pins are removed at 6 to 8 weeks, and a splint is applied for 2 months for protection during the early rehabilitation. At follow-up 32 months postoperatively, the patients demonstrated 79° of motion in the flexion–extension arc with average grip strength two-thirds of that on the uninvolved side. Three of 14 wrists required an arthrodesis later because of failure.

The techniques mentioned expand the role for PRC and allow the patient to retain motion.

POSTOPERATIVE CARE AND REHABILITATION

Postoperatively, the extremity is kept elevated, and finger motion is encouraged. A moderate amount of postoperative edema can be expected. Before the patient is discharged, the dressings need to be inspected for drainage and constriction.

The recommended length of continuous postoperative immobilization varies between 17 and 42 days. We prefer to begin remobilization as soon as the wound is healed at 10 to 15 days, emphasizing gentle active assisted motion by the patient and passive motion by the hand therapist. The patient should also be started on isometric exercises. Once the pain subsides, a progressive resistive and strengthening program should follow. Patients may return to light manual tasks by 6 to 8 weeks and to heavier manual labor at 3 to 6 months. The postoperative rehabilitation is lengthy. It takes at least 6 months, and frequently up to 1 year, before the condition becomes stationary. The patients must continue to exercise, particularly to build up their strength and endurance.

RESULTS AND COMPLICATIONS

The first large series of patients with PRC was reported by Crabbe in 1964 (6). He reported on 20 cases done between 1943 and 1962. He described his results as 15 good, two fair, and three failures. The results were based on pain relief, subjective strength, and motion. The radial styloid was excised in 15 patients. However, five patients had good results with an intact styloid.

Jorgensen reported on 22 patients in 1969 (4). The diagnoses were avascular necrosis of the scaphoid, Kienböck's disease, and perilunate dislocation. The best results were for acute perilunate dislocations, with eight excellent, one good, and one fair. For avascular necrosis of the lunate and scaphoid, the results were six excellent, four good, and two fair. There were no poor outcomes in this study. Subjective weakness was reported by all patients. Objective weakness was demonstrated in all but 1 of 10 patients with grip strength measurements. Follow-up ranged from 3 to 19 years.

Inglis and Jones, in 1977, reviewed 12 patients following PRC (7). Six of these patients were followed for over 14 years. The diagnoses were Kienböck's disease, scaphoid fractures, scaphoid instability, and perilunate dislocations. Functional results were satisfactory in all patients. All had an arc of motion greater than 90°. All patients returned to their previous employment.

Neviaser reviewed 31 patients who underwent PRC for posttraumatic arthritis (3). They ranged in age from 19 to 64 years. Follow-up ranged from 2 to 12 years. Twenty-nine had satisfactory results, and there were two failures. Both failures were later converted to a wrist fusion. The average motion when compared to the opposite wrist was 68% extension, 57% flexion, 85% ulnar deviation, and 17% radial deviation. Grip strength was 90% to 100% compared to the opposite side. All affected wrists were on the dominant side. This represented a 10% to 20% loss of strength when hand dominance was accounted for. Twenty-eight patients returned to their previous employment. Several of these patients returned to heavy labor occupations. Imbriglia et al., in 1990, reported on 27 patients with an average follow-up of 4 years (5). Twenty-six patients achieved relief of their pain. However, two of these 26 patients required reoperation to excise the radial styloid. The one failure required wrist fusion. There were no other complications. The average arc of motion was 84°. This compares with an average arc of motion of 65° preoperatively. Grip strength was 80% when compared to the nondominant side. All but three patients were able to return to their previous employment.

Culp et al. reviewed 20 patients with an average follow-up of 3.5 years (8). The procedure failed in all three patients with rheumatoid arthritis. Their ages ranged from 20 to 86 years. The diagnoses for the nonrheumatoid patients were Kienböck's, scaphoid nonunion, carpal fracture-dislocation, and scapholunate dissociation. Nine of these patients had a radial styloidectomy. Radial deviation was slightly better in the group receiving styloidectomies. However, there were no other differences between the two groups. There was a modest decrease in motion relative to the preoperative values. Grip strength increased 22% above the preoperative measurements. A wrist function scale based on pain, motion, grip strength, and activities of daily living was used. The scores revealed 6% excellent, 35% good, 29% fair, and 30% poor results. However, 14 of the 17 nonrheumatoid patients subjectively considered the operation a success.

PRC for stage III Kienböck's was reviewed in a study by Begley and Engber (16). Fourteen patients were followed for an average of 3 years. Eleven patients had satisfactory pain relief. There was a modest improvement in average range of motion. When compared to the opposite side, the motion was 68% flexion, 68% extension, 77% ulnar deviation, and 52% radial deviation. The average grip strength increased from 16 kg to 38 kg after surgery. There were no early complications reported.

Tomaino et al. compared PRC to limited wrist fusion in SLAC wrists (10). They looked at 24 patients with an average follow-up of 5.5 years. Fifteen patients had PRC, and nine had a limited fusion. All except three in the PRC group achieved pain relief. Two of these three had capitolunate arthritic changes (stage III SLAC). Grip strengths were comparable for the two groups. They recommended limited wrist fusion for stage III SLAC wrist. The flexion–extension arc was 48% better for the proximal carpectomy group. Either procedure worked well for stage I and II SLAC wrists. In a second study, Tomaino et al. evaluated the long-term results in 23 patients with PRC (9). Twenty had satisfactory function and pain relief. They reported an average arc of motion of 74°. The average grip strength was 79% compared to the contralateral side. He corrected for hand dominance in assessing grip strength. Fifteen patients were followed for more than 15 years.

Krakauer et al. also compared PRC to limited wrist fusion (22). They drew similar conclusions to those of Tomaino et al. PRC was satisfactory for a stage II SLAC wrist. However, limited wrist fusion provided more reliable pain relief for stage III SLAC wrists.

Wyrick et al. compared PRC to four-corner intercarpal fusion for the treatment of SLAC wrists (11). Seventeen patients had four-corner fusion, and 11 wrists in 10 patients had PRC. There were three failures in the fusion group. Motion and grip strengths were significantly better in the PRC group. They did not mention the stage of SLAC wrist or whether this influenced the decision to perform PRC. The follow-up averaged 27 months.

Salomon and Eaton reported on 12 patients who underwent a modified PRC (24). The proximal row was removed along with the head of the capitate. A dorsal capsular flap was interposed between the capitate and the radius. Ten of these patients had significant capitolunate or radiolunate arthritis. Two had acute carpal articular damage with complex radiocarpal trauma. Eleven patients obtained satisfactory pain relief. The follow-up averaged 55 months. Motion and grip strengths were comparable to, or better than, those of previous studies on "traditional" PRC. They recommended this modified technique to expand the indications of PRC for involvement of the capitate or lunate fossa of the radius.

Several studies confirm that PRC provides pain relief and functional improvement. We were unable to find a single large study that substantiates its poor reputation historically. Satisfactory pain relief can be expected in over 90% of patients based on the recent literature (3–11,14). The average arc of flexion and extension is about 75° (3–5,7,9,10,16,22). This is about 60% to 65% of the contralateral side. Radial deviation may be limited to 0° to 10°, and ulnar deviation is usually around 20° to 30° (3,8–11,14). However, compared to limited wrist arthrodesis, PRC preserves more motion (3,10,11). Grip strength varies from 67% to 94% compared to the opposite side (3,5,8,10,14,16). Most studies in the literature do not control for hand dominance in assessing grip strength outcome. Contrary to popular belief, some heavy laborers are able to return to their original work. Imbriglia et al. found that 85% of these patients returned to their original job (5). Tomaino et al. reported similar results for 69% of heavy laborers (10).

These results for PRC do not seem to deteriorate with time. If failure occurs, it usually is evident early. Several reports confirm lasting results for more than 5 years (3,4, 7–10,12). PRC compares favorably with four-corner fusion and scaphoid excision for SLAC (10,11,22). Other studies also confirm favorable results with PRC for stage III and IV Kienböck's disease when compared to other treatment methods (16,17).

Complication rates for PRC are low. The main complication is failure to relieve pain. Instability can occur but is uncommon. This complication reinforces the importance of assessing the position of the capitate to assure that it sits in the lunate fossa. If there is concern about stability, the wrist joint should be pinned. However, in our experience, this is an uncommon occurrence.

EDITORS' COMMENTS

PRC is a salvage procedure wherein the proximal articular cartilage of the capitate is placed in the lunate fossa on the radius. The excision of the entire proximal row typically addresses any scarring or decreased range of motion secondary to tight capsular structures. There is admittedly some effective lengthening of all tendons across the wrist as the hand migrates proximally and now rests on the radius. It is one of the two salvage procedures for the human wrist; the other is arthrodesis of the wrist. Arthrodesis will produce the more powerful pain-free wrist, but all motion is absent. The PRC almost always develops degenerative arthritis between the capitate and lunate fossa on the radius even if there is normal cartilage on these two surfaces at the time of PRC. The problem here is that the radius of curvature of the capitate is so much smaller than the radius of curvature of the lunate fossa on the radius. This major incongruity cannot be overcome, and in any active person, this joint, which takes 100% of the load from the hand to the radius, destroys itself fairly rapidly. As degenerative symptoms develop, the patient will usually cut back activity to match the symptomatic level. These people appear to get along adequately, though not nearly as well as they would with other nonsalvage procedures. The question then is: Can a more functional wrist be established in ways short of these two salvage procedures?

In the most common form of degenerative change, there is loss of radial support via the scaphoid with concomitant degenerative arthritis. It matters not whether this is rotary subluxation of the scaphoid, scaphoid nonunion, or Preiser's disease; all will result in loss of scaphoid load transfer capability. This will be followed by shear loading at the capitate–lunate joint and the second stage of SLAC wrist. In the great majority of cases, the radius lunate fossa is almost never damaged. With severe malpositioning of the lunate, one might see peripheral osteophytes as in longstanding severe dorsal intercalated segment instability, but the central portion of the radius–lunate joint remains normal and can be used for reconstruction. The essence of the procedure is capitate–lunate fusion. Adding the hamate and triquetrum to the fusion enhances fusability and does not change eventual range of motion and is recommended (e.g., for SLAC reconstruction or four-corner fusion). The fact that the capitate–lunate joint is destroyed as SLAC wrist progresses means that there is no cartilage on the proximal capitate, and PRC is even less desirable. Given the option in a PRC of a proximal lunate articular surface on the capitate instead of the proximal capitate articular surface, the choice would be the lunate surface. This, of course, is precisely what is accomplished with SLAC wrist. Therefore, if the radius–lunate joint is normal, PRC is contraindicated under all circumstances, and the capitate should be fused to the lunate with the addition of the hamate and triquetrum for SLAC reconstruction. If the proximal lunate articular surface is destroyed with no cartilage between the radius and lunate, the procedure of choice is a radius–lunate limited wrist arthrodesis. The main loads are transferred then through the normal joint between the proximal capitate and the distal lunate. This again leaves a congruous normal joint for loads, and PRC is again contraindicated. In collapsed Kienböck's with destruction of the lunate and ulnar translation of the entire carpus, the choices become PRC or wrist arthrodesis. We feel this is the one place PRC salvage has an application.

PRC has been used to treat stiff wrists. Severe fibrotic contractures are better handled with resection of capsular structures maintaining a wrist on its normal cartilage surfaces and correcting contractures where the problem exists rather than producing the laxity of PRC and potential for degenerative change.

REFERENCES

1. Stamm TT. Excision of the proximal row of the carpus. *Proc R Soc Med* 1944;38:74–75.
2. Stack JK. End results of excision of the carpal bones. *Arch Surg* 1948;57:245–252.
3. Neviaser RJ. On resection of the proximal carpal row. *Clin Orthop* 1986;202:12–15.
4. Jorgensen EC. Proximal-row carpectomy. *J Bone Joint Surg Am* 1969;51:1104–1111.
5. Imbriglia JE, Broudy AS, Hagberg WC, et al. Proximal row carpectomy: clinical evaluation. *J Hand Surg [Am]* 1990;15:426–430.
6. Crabbe WA. Excision of the proximal row of the carpus. *J Bone Joint Surg [Br]* 1964;46:708–711.
7. Inglis AE, Jones EC. Proximal-row carpectomy for diseases of the proximal row. *J Bone Joint Surg Am* 1977;59:460–463.
8. Culp RW, McGuigan FX, Turner MA, et al. Proximal row carpectomy: a multicenter study. *J Hand Surg [Am]* 1993;18:19–25.
9. Tomaino MM, Delsignore J, Burton RI. Long-term results following proximal row carpectomy. *J Hand Surg [Am]* 1994;19:694–703.
10. Tomaino MM, Miller RJ, Cole I, et al. Scapholunate advanced collapse wrist: proximal row carpectomy or limited wrist arthrodesis with scaphoid excision? *J Hand Surg [Am]* 1994;19:134–142.
11. Wyrick JD, Stern PJ, Kiefhaber TR. Motion-preserving procedures in the treatment of scapholunate advances collapse. PRC versus four-corner fusion. *J Hand Surg [Am]* 1995;20:965–970.
12. Neviaser RJ. Proximal row carpectomy for posttraumatic disorders of the carpus. *J Hand Surg [Am]* 1983;8:301–305.
13. Ferlic DC, Clayton ML, Mills MF. Proximal row carpectomy: review of rheumatoid and nonrheumatoid wrists. *J Hand Surg [Am]* 1991;16:420–424.
14. Green DP. Proximal row carpectomy. *Hand Clin* 1987;3:163–168.
15. Watson HK, Ballet FL. The SLAC wrist: scapholunate advanced collapse pattern of degenerative arthritis. *J Hand Surg [Am]* 1984;9:358–365.
16. Begley BW, Engber WD. Proximal row carpectomy in advanced Kienböck's disease. *J Hand Surg [Am]* 1994;19:1016–1018.
17. Lin HH, Stern PJ. "Salvage" procedures in the treatment of Kienböck's disease. *Hand Clin* 1993;9:521–526.
18. Campbell RD, Thompson TC, Lance EM, et al. Indications for

open reduction of lunate and perilunate dislocations of the carpal bones. *J Bone Joint Surg Am* 1965;47:915–937.
19. Omer GE, Capen DA. Proximal row carpectomy with muscle transfers for spastic paralysis. *J Hand Surg [Am]* 1976;1:197–204.
20. Mennen U. Early corrective surgery of the wrist and elbow in arthrogryposis multiplex congenita. *J Hand Surg [Br]* 1993;18:304–307.
21. Van Heest AE, House JH. Proximal row carpectomy. In: Gelberman RH, ed. *The wrist: Masters techniques in orthopaedic surgery.* New York: Raven Press, 1991;331–334.
22. Krakauer JD, Bishop AT, Cooney WP. Surgical treatment of scapholunate advanced collapse. *J Hand Surg [Am]* 1994;19:751–759.
23. Siegel DB, Gelberman RH. Radial styloidectomy: An anatomical study with special reference to radiocarpal intercapsular ligamentous morphology. *J Hand Surg [Am]* 1991;16:40–44.
24. Salomon GD, Eaton RG. Proximal row carpectomy with partial capitate resection. *J Hand Surg [Am]* 1996;21:2–8.
25. Fitzgerald JP, Peimer CA, Smith RJ. Distraction resection arthroplasty of the wrist. *J Hand Surg [Am]* 1989;14:774–781.

TOTAL WRIST ARTHRODESIS

HILL HASTINGS II
MARTIN I. BOYER

Wrist arthrodesis is a well-established technique for the elimination of pain and the enhancement of function for the painful arthritic wrist. Arthrodesis of the radiocarpal, midcarpal, and third carpometacarpal (CMC) joints may relieve pain, correct deformity, and improve overall upper extremity function.

Many methods of radiocarpal arthrodesis have been developed over the past 100 years. Surgical approach, position of fusion, methods of fixation, degree and duration of immobilization, and source and type of bone graft have varied among different techniques. The goal of this chapter is to familiarize the reader with the historical literature and to present our modern concepts of wrist arthrodesis, including indications, complications, and rehabilitation.

INDICATIONS
Instability Patterns

The most common condition requiring wrist arthrodesis is arthrosis secondary to chronic scapholunate dissociation or scaphoid nonunion. In both conditions, arthrosis develops and progressively affects the styloscaphoid, radioscaphoid, and capitolunate joints, which may be reliably addressed by total wrist arthrodesis. Although other motion-preserving reconstructive procedures are available, diffuse arthrosis may be reliably addressed by total wrist arthrodesis. Should a pain-free stable wrist be necessary for manual labor, total wrist arthrodesis may be preferable to motion-preserving procedures.

Failed Scaphotrapeziotrapezoid or Capitolunate Fusion

Should limited intercarpal arthrodeses fail to allow the patient a sufficiently pain-free wrist to engage in heavy

H. Hastings II: The Indiana Hand Center, Indianapolis, Indiana 46260.
M. I. Boyer: Department of Orthopaedic Surgery, Washington University School of Medicine, St. Louis, Missouri 63110.

labor, then conversion to total wrist arthrodesis may be necessary. Limited intercarpal arthrodesis fails to achieve union and relief of pain in approximately 30% of cases (1). An initially successful limited intercarpal arthrodesis may develop progressive arthrosis with time, necessitating conversion to a total wrist arthrodesis.

Primary Degenerative Joint Disease

Degenerative arthrosis of the radiocarpal and midcarpal joints secondary to calcium pyrophosphate deposition disease (CPPD, or pseudogout) may be treated effectively with wrist arthrodesis. Often an accompanying attritional destabilizing tear of the scapholunate ligament with attendant scapholunate instability and scapholunate advanced collapse (SLAC) pattern arthrosis are not treatable by limited intercarpal arthrodesis because of an abnormality of the radioscaphoid or radiolunate articular cartilage as a result of the underlying disease process.

Preiser's Disease

Idiopathic avascular necrosis of the scaphoid may be addressed by midcarpal arthrodesis and scaphoid excision or by a vascularized pedicle bone graft from the dorsal distal radius. Should either of these procedures fail to provide pain-free motion and return to function, a total wrist arthrodesis may be undertaken.

Inflammatory Arthritis

Limited intercarpal arthrodesis is seldom advised except in early disease states, where radiolunate fusion may protect against progressive ulnar drift. Total joint fusion is advised for most cases of late diffuse wrist arthritis with ulnar translocation, volar displacement, and radiocarpal supination deformity.

In instances of poor quality bone, a single or double Steinman pin technique is advised. When multiple simultaneous procedures are planned, such as metacarpophalangeal joint replacements and interphalangeal joint fusion, the

Steinman pin technique allows all to be accomplished within a single tourniquet time.

Although Steinman pin fixation is technically easier, the position of fusion is necessarily in neutral, and irritation from the pin at the entry portal in the third metacarpal may be a problem. Conversely, although the position of arthrodesis may be adjusted with plate fixation, purchase of the screws in severely osteopenic bone may pose difficulties, especially for fixation into the third metacarpal.

In the early literature on wrist arthrodesis, tuberculous arthritis of the wrist was a frequent indication for arthrodesis. Recent series of compression plate arthrodeses of the wrist include few patients with arthrosis secondary to infection with either bacterial or mycobacterial organisms. The principles of treatment of bacterial infections necessarily differ from mycobacterial ones, as fusion may be obtained in the presence of mycobacterial infection but is unlikely in the presence of active bacterial infection.

Tumor

The third most common location for giant cell tumors of bone is in the distal radius. Treatment often requires resection of the entire distal radius including the radiocarpal articular surface. Reconstruction of the segmental osseous defect with an autogenous iliac crest or vascularized fibular graft may be undertaken, with radioscapholunate or total wrist arthrodesis as a stabilizing procedure.

Failed Total Wrist Arthroplasty

In the setting of infected, loose, or painful total wrist arthroplasty, the only procedure available to salvage hand function is total wrist arthrodesis. Interposition corticocancellous iliac crest bridge grafts may be required in order to maintain length.

Neurologic

Stabilization of the spastic wrist is sometimes required in patients with severe spastic flexion deformities of the wrist. This allows wrist flexor or extensor tendons to be used as transfers to motor finger or thumb motion. Combined with other procedures to address extrinsic and intrinsic flexor tendon, arthrodesis may also aid in overall hygiene of the hand.

Wrist arthrodesis in the setting of brachial plexus injury or combined major peripheral nerve palsy allows wrist flexor or extensor tendons to be used as transfers to finger or thumb motion.

Severe Unremitting Wrist Pain

In this setting, no etiology is found for the patient's wrist pain. Wrist arthrodesis may be the last resort in the surgical treatment of this pain.

CONTRAINDICATIONS

Active Infection

Active bacterial infection is a relative contraindication to wrist arthrodesis. Control of the infection by means of bone and soft tissue debridement, external skeletal stabilization, and administration of pathogen-specific antibiotics is carried out before definitive bone grafting and arthrodesis is attempted.

Inadequate Skin Coverage

In the setting of inadequate or unstable dorsal skin coverage, arthrodesis of the wrist through conventional dorsal approaches should not be undertaken. Local or free flap closure of the unstable or exposed area may be accomplished before or at the time of bone grafting and internal fixation.

Occupational Constraints on Wrist Arc of Motion

Limited arthrodesis may be preferable in patients with special occupational demands on wrist positioning and motion requirements, such as general surgeons, electricians, or mechanics. If arthrodesis is required, positions other than slight dorsiflexion and ulnar deviation may need consideration.

Tenodesis Requirement to Activate Tendon Transfer

Wrist motion may be required in certain groups of patients in order to activate digital and thumb flexion and extension by means of the tenodesis effect. Most commonly this is seen in tetraplegic patients who require wrist palmarflexion for digital extension and wrist dorsiflexion for digital flexion and pinch.

DEVELOPMENT OF HISTORIC TECHNIQUES OF WRIST ARTHRODESIS

Much of the early literature on wrist arthrodesis focused on fusion methods involving bone grafting without coincident internal fixation. These methods still have utility, as situations and patients exist in whom plate fixation is not possible. Arthrodeses carried out in Third World countries without the technical means to perform plate fixation in their operating rooms may be better performed by historical methods not involving compression plates and screws. External immobilization is necessarily utilized for extended periods postoperatively in these patients (up to 16 weeks, in some series).

A review of the historic literature on arthrodesis of the wrist before and after the era of compression plate fixation is presented. The differing opinions on the positioning of the arthrodesis, method of internal fixation and postoperative immobilization, donor site and type of bone graft, surgical approach, and inclusion or exclusion of the CMC joints in the arthrodesis are reviewed.

POSITION OF THE ARTHRODESIS

There is no single ideal position for wrist arthrodesis. Palmer has evaluated functional wrist motion in 10 normal subjects carrying out standard tasks and has shown that the "normal" functional range of wrist motion is through an arc of 30° extension, 5° flexion, and 25° of radioulnar deviation (2).

Ryu (3) has found that "the majority of hand placement and range of motion tasks . . . could be accomplished with 70 percent of maximal range of wrist motion," a range of 40° extension, 40° flexion, and 40° combined radioulnar deviation. Different jobs mandate the performance of set tasks in different modes of flexion or extension; the position of wrist arthrodesis must be adjusted to meet the needs of the individual patient.

Early publications have advocated fusing the wrist in positions of extension that have corresponded with the angle of flexion of the corticocancellous graft utilized. Scherb (4) has advocated fusing the wrist in a position of extension corresponding to the degree of extension of the proximal femoral corticocancellous graft. Similarly, Gill (5), Smith-Petersen (6), Colonna (7), Wickstrom (8), and Debeyre and Goutallier (9) have allowed the chosen type of corticocancellous bone graft to determine the degree of extension of the fusion.

Other authors have chosen to fuse the wrist in more precise degrees of extension, controlling this position with limited percutaneous fixation and, more frequently, external immobilization with long and short arm casts. Most authors have attempted to achieve an arthrodesis of between 10° and 15° of extension (10–13).

Others have advocated a greater degree of extension, presumably to increase mechanical advantage of the digital flexors in power grip. Positions of 20° (14–16) or greater (17) have been described.

The position of the arthrodesis in the coronal plane has been less well described for the techniques of wrist arthrodesis antedating rigid plate fixation. Most authors who have discussed radioulnar positioning of the arthrodesed wrist have supported a neutral position (15), a position of "slight" ulnar deviation (11), or a position of marked ulnar deviation (17).

Robinson and Kayfetz described, in a preliminary report, excision of the proximal carpal row and capitoradial fusion with a screw (17). They arthrodesed the wrist in 20° to 30° of extension and 20° of ulnar deviation in order to maximize grip strength. They felt that "unless definite deviation of the hand toward the ulnar side is given, the use of . . . tools which must be held in the hand and pointed away from the body such as hammers, screw drivers and fishing poles, is greatly interfered with."

The reported advantage of an arthrodesis that has not been stabilized by internal or percutaneous fixation devices is that positioning can be changed during the immediate postoperative period, in accordance with patient wishes (9). This technique may come at the price of a lower rate of fusion.

IMMOBILIZATION AND FIXATION OF THE ARTHRODESIS

Early techniques of wrist arthrodesis did not employ either percutaneous or internal fixation. After resection of cartilage and subchondral bone and bone grafting by any of a number of techniques, the wrist was immobilized by external casts (either long or short arm) for varying lengths of time.

Long arm casts with the elbow routinely at 90° were employed by multiple authors (5,7,10–12,16–21). Several of these authors changed the immobilization to below elbow at varying lengths of time postoperatively (10,12,17,21) and continued the immobilization until union of the arthrodesis had been demonstrated.

The use of internal screw fixation was proposed by Robinson and Kayfetz (17). Several authors routinely used Kirschner wires inserted percutaneously to enhance the stability of the arthrodesis construct (8,11,13,21). Details of insertion, duration of fixation, pin care, and sites transfixed were not uniformly described.

Rybka (22) advocated use of the Ilizarov technique, as it allowed adjustment to the positioning of the arthrodesis during the early postoperative phase. This technique was described for use in patients with rheumatoid arthritis.

BONE GRAFT SITE AND TYPE

The donor site and type of bone graft used for wrist arthrodesis is variable. Early authors have used donor sites such as the distal radius (5,8,13,19), proximal femur (4), distal ulna (6,14,16), iliac crest (9–12,15,21), and proximal tibia (18).

The types of grafts varied. All of the above donor sites have served as a supply of corticocancellous graft. The iliac crest and, when excised, the proximal carpal row (17) serve as ready supplies of cancellous bone chips for packing into the interstices of denuded radiocarpal, intercarpal, and sometimes CMC joint surfaces.

In addition to serving as a supply of osteogenic elements, the bone grafts were often employed as the method of internal fixation for the arthrodesis. This is appreciated in the methods that have used distal radial "turnabout grafts," shaped distal ulnar grafts, split rib grafts, proximal tibial grafts, and proximal femoral grafts as either "peg" grafts or "slot" grafts to bridge the radius, carpus, and often the third (and second) CMC joints. The corticocancellous graft supplies the internal support, whereas external cast immobilization provides some means of external immobilzation and additional safeguards on the frontal and coronal plane positioning of the arthrodesis.

Gill (5) advocated the use of a distal radial turnabout graft in which "a broad plate of bone" was harvested in the coronal plane from the dorsal distal radius then turned 180° to lie with the proximal end "driven into this (transverse) cleft in the . . . capitate." Smith-Petersen (6) believed that the "excised portion of the ulna, properly shaped, makes an efficient graft," embedded within slots cut into the distal radius and carpus. Colonna (7) felt that "the desired degree of cocked-up position of the wrist was easily achieved by the shape of the harvested rib graft, introduced into slots carved in the distal radius and the third metacarpal."

Some peculiar methods of bone grafting have been used in attempts to secure arthrodesis. Dubar (23) published in the French literature on the use of dog bone "hétéroplastique" xenografts. This paper was not solely on the topic of wrist arthrodesis. Little has been published in the English literature on the use of such grafts. Concern about both xenograft rejection phenomena and viral transmission mitigate against the use of such bone graft donors at present.

INCLUSION OF THE CARPOMETACARPAL JOINTS IN THE ARTHRODESIS

Controversy exists over the inclusion or exclusion of the third (and often the second) CMC joints in the fusion mass. Some authors encourage its inclusion in the fusion mass (7,8,11,14,18). They believe that inclusion of the CMC joints enhances the stability of the fusion mass and allows for a completely motion-free and pain-free state. Conversely, others have advocated sparing the third and second CMC joints (6,9,10,17). The reasoning employed by these authors is that a minimum amount of wrist motion is preserved, and this serves the patient functionally. In addition, the preserved CMC joint serves as a "shock absorber" for the hand in those employed in heavy labor activities. Seddon (14) felt that "the few degrees of motion remaining in these joints allow sufficient movement to absorb the shocks encountered in the course of every-day activity."

Other authors (24,25) have noted that subsequent degenerative changes may occur following a wrist arthrodesis that spares the second and third CMC joints. Even with modern methods of compression plate fixation of wrist arthrodesis, inclusion of the third CMC joint in the fusion mass remains a contentious issue.

SURGICAL APPROACH FOR ARTHRODESIS

The surgical approach for arthrodesis of the wrist may be radial (11), ulnar (6,14,16), or dorsal. Although most authors have favored a straight dorsal approach, either through the fourth dorsal compartment or through the interval between the third and fourth dorsal compartments, several authors have championed either radial or ulnar approaches to wrist arthrodesis.

The support for the ulnar approach derives from the fact that it avoids dorsal scarring and adherence of the digital extensor tendons, and it allows the wrist to be approached through the defect created after Darrach resection of the distal ulna.

In 1940, Smith-Petersen (6) proposed an ulnar approach to arthrodesis of the radiocarpal joint to obviate the complications of the dorsal approach. He combined this approach with a Darrach resection of the distal ulna, which he performed first to allow him access to the ulnar side of the radiocarpal and midcarpal joint. His was a report of technique only, without complications or results.

Seddon (14) supported the use of an ulnar approach to radiocarpal arthrodesis, first advocated by Smith-Petersen. He found that the wrist was slightly thickened after arthrodesis and that the lateral wrist was difficult to access from the medial side. The distal ulnar graft was also somewhat irregular.

Debeyre and Goutallier utilized a 3-mm–thick embedded iliac crest graft inserted from the distal radius to the third metacarpal (9). As in the work of Smith-Petersen and Seddon, an ulnar approach with resection of the head of the ulna was used. The authors described two cases that sustained a "lesion of the dorsal cutaneous branch of the ulnar nerve," a complication unmentioned in the previous two papers advocating the ulnar approach to the radiocarpus. The "improved pronation and supination as a result of the resection of the distal radio-ulnar joint" was seen as a key benefit of this approach.

Riordan advocated a radial approach to arthrodesis of the wrist because of complications of dorsal exposure such as extensor tendon adhesions and the technical difficulties encountered with the ulnar approach, most importantly the inability to access the lateral wrist from a medial approach (11). The interval between the first and second dorsal compartments was utilized, and a slot graft of corticocancellous iliac crest bone was utilized. The second and third CMC joints were routinely included, and the position of fusion was in 15° of dorsiflexion and slight ulnar deviation.

Not all dorsal approaches were uniform. Abbott reported an ambitious technique in 1942, involving the reflection of an osteocapsular flap from the distal radius and carpus (10). Cancellous strips and chips of bone harvested from the iliac crest are then placed on the denuded bone surfaces of the radiocarpal and midcarpal joints, and the flap is replaced over the joint surfaces packed with graft. The CMC joints are not included in the fusion.

Campbell described the *en bloc* resection of all radiocarpal and intercarpal joints to be fused, from a dorsal approach (21). An autogenous block graft of corticocancellous iliac crest bone was then placed in the defect created under "moderate pressure." This method was particularly successful in their series in those patients having giant cell tumors of the distal radius requiring massive bony resection.

PLATE FIXATION

Variations in the technique of wrist arthrodesis have continued despite the introduction of compression plate fixation. Although all methods below utilize compression plate fixation from the dorsal distal radius to the third (or rarely, the second) metacarpal introduced from a dorsal approach, the differences between techniques lie in the positioning of the arthrodesis, implants chosen for internal fixation, method of postoperative immobilization, donor site and type of bone graft, and inclusion or exclusion of the CMC joints in the arthrodesis.

Most authors support positioning the arthrodesis in some degree of extension. Most patients were fused between 10° and 15° of extension, although some authors have reported patients fused in neutral flexion–extension (26,27) and in as much as 25° of extension (28). The necessity of contouring the plate to the degree of extension desired by the patient must be emphasized. Occupational and recreational considerations must come into play in determining the optimal positioning of the fusion mass in the coronal plane.

The devices used for internal fixation have varied. Larsson used a "6 hole self-compression plate" (27), and Axelrod and Hastings (26,28) have used eight- to 10-hole 3.5-mm dynamic compression plates in a double-bend configuration (with a depression created in the plate for the carpal bones). Others have used T-plates (29,30). Several authors have used 3.5-mm plates as well, but with a single bend (25,31). Reports of the new Synthes wrist fusion plate are forthcoming, but the technique appears particularly promising, as the benefits of internal compression plate fixation are retained while many of the potential complications of plate irritation are eliminated as a result of the low profile of the plate over the distal metacarpal.

Most authors have used iliac crest cancellous graft packed in the interstices of the denuded chondral and subchondral bone surfaces of the joints to be fused. Occasional corticocancellous inlay grafts for both osteogenic and structural support have been employed.

The inclusion of the third CMC joint in the fusion remains a point of debate. Some authors advocate its fusion (25,26,30,31). Others disagree (1,28,29,32). If plate fixation is used, and the CMC joints are not fused in order to allow motion at these joints after arthrodesis, then the plate must be removed after fusion is demonstrated.

TECHNIQUE

With the hand aligned in neutral position, a straight incision is marked starting over the dorsal distal diaphysis of the radius, extending across Lister's tubercle, and ending distally between the midportion of the index and middle metacarpals (Fig. 34.1). The incision is carried through the skin and dermis. Usually, one or two crossing subcutaneous veins require division and ligation.

A thick skin and subcutaneous flap is elevated containing the dorsoradial veins and dorsal sensory branches of the radial nerve over to the first dorsal compartment. The third dorsal compartment is opened, and the extensor pollicis longus (EPL) tendon is reflected and transposed radially.

A straight incision is made along the dorsal radius just ulnar to the extensor carpi radialis brevis. Distally, this incision is continued longitudinally through the capsule down to the joint. The extensor tendons of the index and middle finger are retracted ulnarly. Most distally, the fascia is incised radial to the third metacarpal. The dorsal aspect of the third metacarpal is exposed without dissection around the margins of the metacarpal and without disturbance of the adjacent intrinsic musculature. The capsule and fourth dorsal compartment are reflected from the carpus ulnarly, and the capsule and second compartment are reflected radially.

AO wrist fusion employs one of three plates, chosen based on the reconstructive situation (Fig. 34.2). A long-bend plate is chosen for larger hands and wrists. A short-bend version is chosen for smaller hands and wrists as well as when fusion is accompanied by or follows proximal row carpectomy. Finally, a straight version plate is chosen in those unusual situations where reconstruction is required for segmental carpal loss. A straight version facilitates stabilization in cases of an interposition corticocancellous bone graft required for replacement of large carpal defects created by trauma or tumor. The long- and short-bend versions of the plate dictate and require removal of the dorsal distal radius. The design of the plate assumes the surgeon will remove a portion of the dorsal distal aspect of the radius. This is accomplished both to minimize the profile of the plate and to provide a source of cancellous bone graft. The dorsal distal radius is removed by serial osteotome cuts or shavings (Fig. 34.3). The dorsal aspect of the third CMC joint is removed with an osteotome to expose the underlying joint. The dorsal two-thirds of the third CMC joint is decorticated down to cancellous bone (Fig. 34.4).

Next, the dorsal carpus is decorticated, removing up to one-third of its anteroposterior diameter as multiple cancellous shavings, which can also be used as a source of bone graft. The intercarpal joints are decorticated, including, in all instances, the radioscaphoid, radiolunate, and capitolunate joints (Figs. 34.5 and 34.6). The ulnar midcarpal joints are decorticated in instances of rheumatoid disease and in those

Section XI: Osteoarthritis of the Wrist

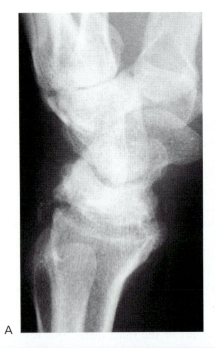
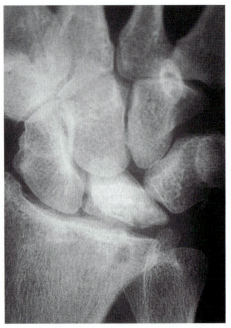
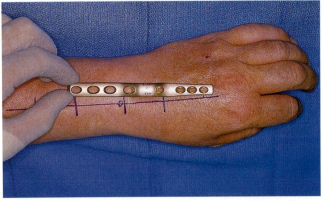

FIGURE 34.1. A: This 37-year-old male heavy laborer presents with painful radiolunate arthrosis secondary to a motorcycle accident sustained 4 years before. Wrist motion is painful with limited dorsiflexion of 35°, palmar flexion of 45°, and grip strength 70% of his comparison, dominant side. **B:** Preoperative anteroposterior radiograph. **C:** Straight incision with the wrist aligned in neutral position.

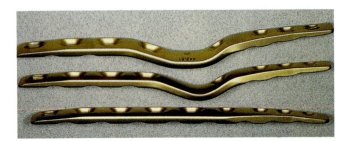

FIGURE 34.2. Three versions of AO wrist fusion plate.

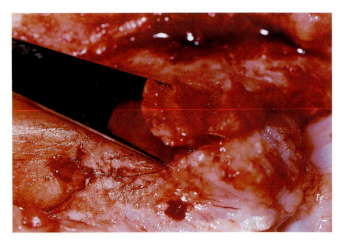

FIGURE 34.3. The removal of Lister's tubercle and dorsal distal radial metaphysis through serial osteotome cuts.

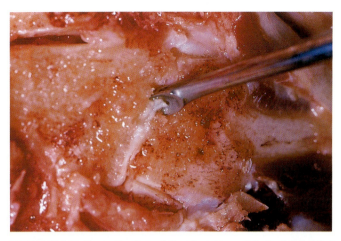

FIGURE 34.4. Decortication of the dorsal two-thirds of the third carpal–metacarpal joint.

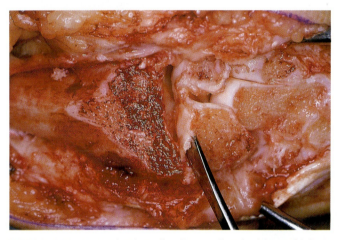

FIGURE 34.5. Decortication of radiocarpal and midcarpal joints.

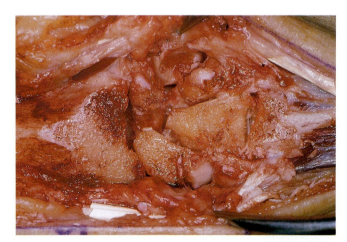

FIGURE 34.6. Final appearance after preparation of radial carpal, intercarpal, and third carpal–metacarpal joints.

situations where preoperative clinical and/or radiographic exam has shown degenerative ulnar midcarpal arthrosis.

The appropriate plate is positioned over the dorsal aspect of the third metacarpal. The site for the most distal screw hole is marked with a marking pen through the plate on the dorsal aspect of the third metacarpal. The plate is then removed to assure that the mark is centered between the ulnar and radial margins of the third metacarpal. This most distal hole is then drilled with a 2.0-mm drill, assuring that the drill passes directly dorsal to volar in the sagittal plane. Misdirected oblique drilling of the metacarpal will later position the plate out of the frontal plane. Proximal fixation of an obliquely positioned plate may then torque the third metacarpal and cause a rotational deformity. With the plate temporarily repositioned, the depth is measured, both cortices tapped with a 2.7-mm tap, and the appropriate length 2.7-mm screw is inserted.

The joints to be fused are packed with abundant cancellous bone graft (Fig. 34.7). The plate is then aligned along the third metacarpal, and the proximal two screw holes are filled with appropriate length 2.7-mm screws. The middle hole requires tapping of both cortices. The proximal metaphyseal hole requires tapping only of the dorsal cortex.

The hole overlying the capitate is then drilled with a 2.0-mm drill, depth measured, and an appropriate length untapped 2.7-mm screw inserted.

Finally, the plate is aligned over the dorsal aspect of the radius, the wrist manually compressed, and the second most distal hole in the radius secured with an appropriate length 3.5-mm screw. This screw is placed in compression mode by use of a compression LC-DCP drill guide, which positions the drill in the most proximal aspect of the screw hole. Both cortices are tapped, and an appropriate length 3.5-mm screw is placed. Correct digital rotational alignment is confirmed by composite flexion of the digits. Additional holes are then filled with appropriate length 3.5-mm screws (Fig. 34.8) after being predrilled with a 2.5-mm drill, having the depth measured, and tapping both cortices with a 3.5-mm cortical tap.

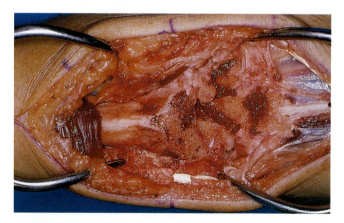

FIGURE 34.7. Packing of radiocarpal and midcarpal joints with cancellous bone.

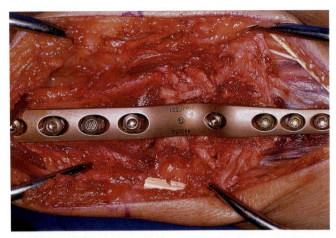

FIGURE 34.8. Completed fixation of the metacarpal and capitate with 2.7-mm screws and the radius with 3.5-mm screws.

Any additional bone graft material available is positioned about the dorsal aspect of the fusion surfaces. In most instances of central column fusion (radius, scaphoid, lunate, capitate, and third metacarpal), fusion can be reliably obtained by a regionally obtained bone graft. When ulnar midcarpal arthrodesis is required, or when the amount of autogenous bone graft is considered inadequate, additional bone is harvested from the olecranon or iliac crest. A small cortical window is made in the top of the crest

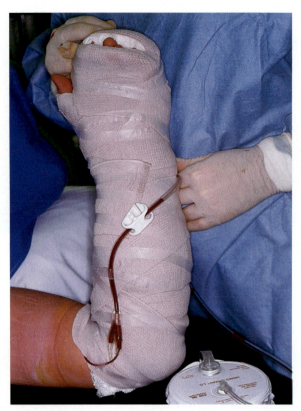

FIGURE 34.9. Application of short arm bulky dressing.

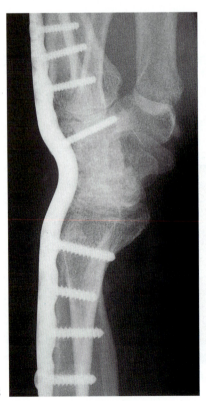
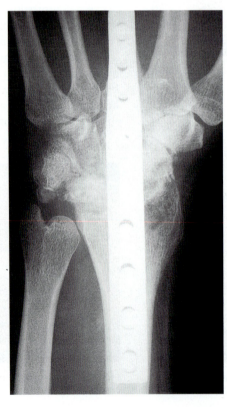

A,B

FIGURE 34.10. Postoperative lateral **(A)** and anteroposterior **(B)** radiographs.

without elevation of the abductors. A large curette is used to harvest cancellous bone from between the two tables of the iliac crest. The donor site is regionally infiltrated with long-acting local anesthetic and the fascia, subcutaneous tissue, and skin are closed. Additional cancellous bone may also be harvested from the distal radial metaphysis radial to the plate and 1 to 2 cm proximal to the radiocarpal joint.

The dorsal wrist capsule is closed with 3-0 braided nylon sutures. The EPL tendon is left transposed radially. The opened margins of this third dorsal compartment are sutured back together. A suction drain is brought out proximally and left within the subcutaneous space. The dermis is closed with resorbable 3-0 sutures, and the skin closed with 5-0 monofilament nylon or staples. A short arm, soft, bulky dressing is applied for light compression (Fig. 34.9). The digits may be left free for active range of motion, and elastic digital socks or wraps applied to prevent edema. More often, initial postoperative comfort is facilitated by incorporation of the digits within the initial dressing in safe position (metacarpophalangeal joint flexion and interphalangeal joint extension). A protective splint is not required unless the ulnar midcarpal joints have required fusion as well. The dressing is removed within 5 to 7 days of surgery to allow for unrestricted range of motion to the thumb through small digits. A small protective wrist splint is applied that does not support the fusion but serves as a reminder to the patient and other individuals that protection of the operation site is required. Light, functional activities of daily living are allowed within a 2-lb weight restriction. Postoperative radiographs confirm proper plate alignment and fixation (Fig. 34.10).

COMPLICATIONS

Pseudarthrosis at the Wrist or at the Carpometacarpal Joint

Many of the early published procedures to obtain wrist arthrodesis required prolonged cast immobilization in order to maintain wrist position and secure union. Pseudarthrosis was a frequent complication of these procedures, with frequency as high as 19% (33), often requiring a repeat fusion with supplemental bone grafting.

With the advent of modern compression plate fixation, the incidence of pseudarthrosis in a recently published series has decreased to 2% or less (26). This usually involves the third CMC joint. Secondary procedures for bone grafting and repeat internal fixation are required.

Carpal Tunnel Syndrome

Early published reports on techniques of wrist arthrodesis did not include median nerve compression in the carpal tunnel as being a postoperative complication of any importance. Recent reports of compression plate fixation have, however, emphasized carpal tunnel syndrome as being a frequent and major postoperative complication of wrist arthrodesis.

Rates as high as 25% of cases have been reported (30). Other authors report a lower incidence, with cases of postoperative carpal tunnel syndrome that have required surgical decompression (4 of 57 in Hastings' series) (26) and also cases that were managed without decompression of the carpal tunnel (26,30,33).

It has become common surgical practice among some to release the transverse carpal ligament at the time of wrist arthrodesis. Hastings feels that the prevalence of postoperative carpal tunnel syndrome merits special preoperative consideration during the evaluation of the patient but does not advocate routine carpal tunnel release.

Infection Requiring Either Antibiotic Treatment or Drainage

Wrist arthrodeses stabilized with percutaneous pins developed local infections around fixation pins in as many as 30% of cases, in one series (26). Superficial wound infections are listed as complications in multiple series of wrist arthrodeses done by a number of methods.

An infrequent yet devastating complication is deep infection requiring surgical drainage (28,30,33). These may be immediately postoperative or may occur as late as 4 years postarthrodesis (28). Compression plate removal is often mandated.

Hematoma Requiring Drainage and Split-Thickness Skin Grafting

Wrist arthrodesis by modern compression plate fixation methods involves the exposure of large areas of bleeding subchondral bone. Inadequate wound hemostasis and suction drainage postoperatively may result in hematoma formation and, if left undrained, results in superficial skin necrosis and wound dehiscence requiring a secondary coverage procedure (28). We feel suction drainage of the arthrodesis is mandated for the first postoperative day.

Neuroma: Ulnar Sensory or Sensory Branch of the Radial Nerve

In either the ulnar or radial approach to wrist arthrodesis, the risk of injury to the dorsal cutaneous branch of the ulnar (9) or the sensory branch of the radial nerve (11) is increased. In dorsal approaches to wrist arthrodesis, however, injury to cutaneous nerves is infrequent (25,26,28).

Plate or Hardware Irritation or Removal

Complaints of hardware irritation are frequent in those techniques of wrist arthrodesis not involving dorsal plate fixation and in those techniques involving the introduction of a thick plate over the dorsum of the third metacarpal, under the digital extensor tendons. In addition, techniques utilizing intramedullary Rush pin or Steinman pin fixation often result in skin irritation at the sites of pin introduction, often necessitating implant removal.

The presence of a thick dorsal fixation plate increases the likelihood of secondary surgery after successful arthrodesis in order to remove the implant (25,28–31). From 35% to 65% of patients require dorsal plate removal.

Extensor Tendon or Flexor Tendon Adherence

Tenosynovitis or adherence of the extensor or flexor tendons in dorsal approaches for wrist arthrodesis led several surgeons to advocate an ulnar or radial approach for arthrodesis, thus leaving the dorsal and volar surfaces unscarred (6,11,14,16).

Extensor tendinitis and adhesion are frequent complications of dorsal plate fixation, and early postoperative digital motion is mandatory to minimize these complications.

Distal Ulnar Instability

Stanley carried out 14 wrist arthrodeses in men with osteoarthritis of the wrist secondary to scapholunate instability, scaphoid nonunion, or distal radius fracture (34). Distal ulnar excision without soft tissue reconstruction was carried out in nine of these patients. Seven of these patients showed distal ulnar instability after excision, six of whom required further distal ulnar surgery. The authors recommended that simple excision of the distal ulna at the time of wrist arthrodesis be avoided.

Distal Ulnar Impingement (Ulnocarpal Abutment)

Distal ulnar impingement on the ulnar carpus may cause pain in patients undergoing wrist arthrodesis. Three patients, reviewed by Trumble, had arthrodeses for conditions in which the ulnocarpal distance had foreshortened: two for degenerative arthritis and silicone synovitis after lunate replacement for Kienböck's disease and one for degenerative arthritis after intraarticular distal radius fracture (35). Relief was obtained in all three by resection of either the triquetrum or the pisiform.

Five of 20 patients in Herbert's series complained of "ulnocarpal pain" without abutment being given as a specific diagnosis (30). One of these patients underwent capitohamate and triquetrolunate arthrodeses (as well as burying of a sensory radial nerve neuroma).

Hastings believes that ulnocarpal abutment is more likely to occur when the radius is aligned and plated to the second metacarpal than when aligned and plated to the third metacarpal (26).

Radius or Metacarpal Fracture

Wrist arthrodeses done by modern compression plating as well as Riordan block graft techniques may fracture after solid arthrodesis is achieved. Axelrod has reported a case of fracture of the radius through the proximal screw hole of a 3.5-mm dynamic compression plate 3 years after arthrodesis (28). This healed uneventfully after replating. Hastings has reported one case of a third metacarpal fracture. This was treated nonoperatively and went on to uneventful union. Green has reported two cases of fracture through the healed graft site 7 and 14 months after successful Riordan fusions (33). Both were treated nonoperatively.

Malunion

There is no optimal position for arthrodesis of the wrist. A malunion may thus be thought of as a fusion in a position either not desired by the surgeon (because of loss of fixation) or by the patient (with specific occupational or recreational demands).

Reflex Sympathetic Dystrophy

Reflex sympathetic dystrophy (RSD) is a particularly feared complication of wrist arthrodesis. In several large series of compression plate arthrodesis of the wrist (26,28,31), RSD has complicated the postoperative course of one patient in each. Goutallier reported one case of RSD in a series of 34 patients treated by an embedded iliac crest graft through a straight ulnar approach (9). One of these patients required a subsequent operative procedure for pain relief. No specific recommendations for the treatment of RSD have been given in any of the aforementioned series.

Intrinsic Tightness Requiring Release

This may be caused by postoperative swelling and fibrosis or by local trauma to the interossei around the third metacarpal. Although early digital range-of-motion exercises and postoperative therapy attempt to combat this problem (as well as metacarpophalangeal joint flexion contractures), operative release may be necessary to restore full digital extension. The avoidance of undue stripping of the interosseous muscles around the third metacarpal may prevent this complication.

Malrotation of the Arthrodesis

Oblique drilling of the metacarpal will position the plate out of the frontal plane. Subsequent plate fixation to the radius may torque the metacarpal into a rotational deformity (J.B. Steichen, personal communication, 1998, Indiana Hand Center, Indianapolis, Indiana).

Lateral Cutaneous Nerve and Thigh Irritation (Meralgia Paresthetica)

The lateral cutaneous nerve of the thigh (LCNT) emerges 2.5 cm medial to the anterior superior iliac spine and travels inferolaterally between the sartorius and tensor fascia lata muscles. It becomes superficial to the enveloping fascia of the anterior thigh musculature at a variable distance below the inguinal ligament.

If the iliac crest bone graft is harvested from an incision placed too anteriorly, irritation or injury to the LCNT may occur. This complication is rare, having been reported in only one patient (28). This patient, however, required excision of the LCNT neuroma and burying of the nerve in local muscle. Symptoms were unrelieved by the additional procedure.

Infection of the Iliac Crest Bone Graft Donor Site

Infection requiring surgical drainage may complicate the harvest of iliac crest bone graft. More commonly, only a superficial cellulitis is present, mandating treatment by oral or intravenous antibiotics.

Cellulitis and stitch abscess have been reported in several series (28,31), and deep infections requiring surgical drainage and/or bony debridement have been reported as well (2,25,26).

Fracture of the Iliac Crest Bone Graft Donor Site

Hastings reported one patient who sustained a fracture of the iliac crest after bone graft harvest (26), who subsequently developed a hernia that required surgical repair. Palmer (31) reported one patient who avulsed his anterior superior iliac spine after bone graft harvest. No further surgical treatment was required.

Wound Dehiscence

Axelrod has reported one patient whose iliac crest bone graft harvest wound dehisced (28). This required irrigation, debridement, and closure.

Iliac Crest Pain Possibly Related to Sacroiliac Joint Injury

A troublesome complication of iliac crest bone graft harvest is the development of postoperative iliac crest pain for which no cause can be found. Multiple series have described this (26,28,31,33). There is no operative or nonoperative treatment except for pain control. Osteomyelitis, fracture, and sacroiliac joint trauma should be ruled out.

REHABILITATION

Sutures or staples are removed at 10 to 14 days. A light compressive dressing or elastic bandage is applied with a molded short arm thermoplastic splint to remind the patient and others that only light use is permitted.

Light strengthening with putty is initiated at 4 weeks after surgery, and the splint is discontinued at 6 weeks. After further strengthening exercises, full unrestricted use is permitted at 10 to 12 weeks postoperatively.

Exercise instructions are given to the patient emphasizing active and passive metacarpophalangeal joint flexion and extension with the interphalangeal joints flexed, "blocking" exercises to the flexor digitorum superficialis and profundus tendons, active range of motion isolating the extensor indicis proprius and extensor digiti quinti proprius tendons, and passive stretching of the intrinsic tendons.

Scars are managed with lotion, scar retraction, and the use of either 50/50 elastomer or otoform. Ultrasound may be used postoperatively should extensor tendon adhesion be a problem. Ultrasound treatment is reserved for those patients not demonstrating adequate active digital extension or passive digital flexion with the previously mentioned treatments or with dynamic splinting.

EDITORS' COMMENTS

Total wrist arthrodesis is a salvage procedure and should be reserved as such. Even a small amount of wrist motion greatly facilitates functional capacity. Denying the patient that asset should mean that all alternatives have been exhausted. Total wrist arthrodesis is indicated if there are not articular surfaces on which to base wrist function. Even a small articular surface with cartilage that is properly loaded will last the patient's lifetime. A decrease in total available cartilage should not be a consideration for wrist fusion. In SLAC wrist reconstruction, the scaphoid is removed entirely, and all loads are taken between the lunate fossa of the radius and the lunate. The radius of curvature and position of this joint make it highly resistive to shear loading. The normally loaded cartilage, though it represents half of the normal wrist articular cartilage, will outlive the patient. Normally loaded cartilage is a living tissue that replaces itself, and even very small surfaces can repair and perpetuate so long as the loads are not excessive. Similarly, following a radius–lunate limited wrist arthrodesis, nearly the entire wrist load will be transferred to the capitate and the distal lunate, again sufficient for a lifetime of functional capacity. Reducing the total amount of cartilage is, therefore, not a consideration.

How that cartilage is loaded is a consideration. Our experience with limited wrist arthrodeses has produced a convincing mass of material, substantiating the fact that adequate painless, full-power motion with lifetime durability is the norm following limited wrist arthrodeses. If there is no adequate joint remaining between the scaphoid and radius and lunate and radius, there is still the potential for function in the capitate–lunate joint. If there is destruction of the radioscaphoid joint, the radiolunate joint, and the distal lunate articular surface, as with a severely collapsed Kienböck's, one might place the remaining capitate cartilage on the remnant articular surface of the lunate fossa, recognizing that almost all proximal row carpectomies go on to degenerative arthritis. Certain patients seem to get along with this salvage technique.

Wrist arthrodesis is probably best done excluding the index and middle CMC joints. With time and aging of the patient, they may or may not require inclusion of these joints if degenerative arthritis occurs from overload, but our experience is that they seldom require inclusion in the fusion and do provide some "give" to hand loads. Wrist arthrodesis is almost never indicated in paralysis situations. The wrist is the great compensator for decreased power and decreased range of motion in muscle–tendon units.

REFERENCES

1. Larsen C, Jacoby R, McCabe S. Nonunion rates of limited intercarpal arthrodesis: A meta-analysis of the literature. *J Hand Surg [Am]* 1997;22:66–73.
2. Palmer A, Werner F, Murphy D, et al. Functional wrist motion: A biomechanical study. *J Hand Surg [Am]* 1985;10:39–46.
3. Ryu J, Cooney W, Askew L, et al. Functional ranges of motion of the wrist joint. *J Hand Surg [Am]* 1991;16:409–419.
4. Scherb. Zur Versteifung des Hand- und Sprunggelenkes bei Lahmungen. *Verh Dtsch Orthop Ges* 1927;48.
5. Stein I. Gill turnabout radial graft for wrist arthrodesis. *Surg Gynecol Obstet* 1958;106:231–232.
6. Smith-Petersen M. A new approach to the wrist joint. *J Bone Joint Surg Am* 1940;22:122–124.
7. Colonna P. A method for fusion of the wrist. *South Med J* 1944;37:195–199.
8. Wickstrom J. Arthrodesis of the wrist: Modification and evaluation of the use of split rib grafts. *South Med J* 1954;47:968–972.
9. Debeyre J, Goutallier D. L'arthrodese du poignet par greffon iliaque intra-carpien. *Presse Med* 1970;78:1893–1894.
10. Abbott L, Saunders J, Bost F. Arthrodesis of the wrist with the use of grafts of cancellous bone. *J Bone Joint Surg Am* 1942;24:883–898.
11. Haddad R, Riordan D. Arthrodesis of the wrist: A surgical technique. *J Bone Joint Surg Am* 1967;49:950–954.
12. Rayan G. Wrist arthrodesis. *J Hand Surg [Am]* 1986;11:356–364.
13. Wood M. Wrist arthrodesis using a dorsal radial bone graft. *J Hand Surg [Am]* 1987;12:208–212.
14. Seddon H. Reconstructive surgery of the upper extremity, poliomyelitis. In: *Second International Poliomyelitis Congress*. Philadelphia: JB Lippincott, 1952.
15. Liebolt F. Surgical fusion of the wrist joint. *Surg Gynecol Obstet* 1938;66:1008–1023.
16. Mittal R, Jain N. Arthrodesis of the wrist by a new technique. *Int Orthop* 1991;14:213–216.
17. Robinson R, Kayfetz D. Arthrodesis of the wrist: Preliminary report of a new method. *J Bone Joint Surg Am* 1952;34:64–70.
18. Brittain H. *Architectural principles in arthrodesis*. Edinburgh: E and S Livingstone, 1952;145–160.
19. Stein I. Gill turnabout radial graft for wrist arthrodesis. *Surg Gynecol Obstet* 1958;106:231–232.
20. Salenius P. Arthrodesis of the carpal joint. *Acta Orthop Scand* 1966;37:288–296.
21. Campbell C, Keokarn T. Total and subtotal arthrodesis of the wrist. *J Bone Joint Surg Am* 1964;46:1520–1533.
22. Rybka V, Popelka S, Pech J, et al. Total arthrodesis of the wrist in rheumatoid arthritis. In: Simmen BR, ed. *The wrist in rheumatoid arthritis*. Basel: Karger, 1992;128–135.
23. Dubar L. Greffes osseuses heteroplastiques. *Bull Acad Med* 1897;38:459.
24. Louis D, Hankin F, Bowers W. Capitate–radius arthrodesis: an alternative method of radiocarpal arthrodesis. *J Hand Surg [Am]* 1984;9:365–369.
25. Bolano L, Green D. Wrist arthrodesis in post-traumatic arthritis: A comparison of two methods. *J Hand Surg [Am]* 1993;18:786–791.
26. Hastings H, Weiss A, Quenzer D, et al. Arthrodesis of the wrist for post-traumatic disorders. *J Bone Joint Surg Am* 1996;78:897–902.
27. Larsson S. Compression arthrodesis of the wrist: A consecutive series of 23 cases. *Clin Orthop* 1974;99:146–153.
28. O'Bierne J, Boyer M, Axelrod T. Wrist arthrodesis using a dynamic compressin plate. *J Bone Joint Surg Br* 1995;77:700–704.
29. Wright C, McMurtry R. AO arthrodesis in the hand. *J Hand Surg [Am]* 1983;9:932–935.
30. Field J, Herbert T, Prosser R. Total wrist fusion: A functional assessment. *J Hand Surg [Br]* 1996;21:429–433.
31. Sagerman S, Palmer A. Wrist arthrodesis using a dynamic compression plate. *J Hand Surg [Br]* 1996;21:437–441.
32. Nagy L, Buchler U. Advances in arthrodesis of the hand and wrist. *Curr Opin Orthop* 1994;5:51–61.
33. Clendenin M, Green D. Arthrodesis of the wrist: Complications and their management. *J Hand Surg [Am]* 1981;6:253–257.
34. Craigen M, Stanley J. Distal ulnar instability following wrist fusion in men. *J Hand Surg [Br]* 1995;20:155–158.
35. Trumble T, Easterling K, Smith R. Ulnocarpal abutment after wrist arthrodesis. *J Hand Surg [Am]* 1988;13:11–15.

35

THE CARPOMETACARPAL JOINT

N. GEORGE KASPARYAN
ANDREW J. WEILAND

The thumb trapeziometacarpal (TM) joint and the ulnar four carpometacarpal (CMC) articulations comprise the carpometacarpal joints of the hand. Injuries to these joints and the subsequent processes that result in articular degeneration differ markedly. The purpose of this chapter is to review the pathologic processes that occur in these joints secondary to trauma, overuse, or primary arthritides and their subsequent treatments (1–81). This chapter is separated into two sections, one involving the pathologic precesses of the second to the fifth CMC joints and one focusing on the specialized thumb CMC articulation.

ANATOMY

The distal carpal row mimics the construction of a stable "Roman arch" in the hand. This fixed transverse arch is best visualized on transverse images of computerized tomograms (Fig. 35.1), which demonstrate how each carpal bone of the distal row keys into its neighbor (1). This distal row of carpal bones, in association with the second and third metacarpals, constitutes the central fixed unit in the hand (2). The joints of the central fixed unit are further supported by powerful and stout interosseous ligaments, which add soft tissue support to the stable bony architecture. Around this central fixed unit, the thumb is allowed to rotate on the radial side of the hand, and, to a significantly smaller degree, the fourth and fifth metacarpals move on the ulnar side of the hand. The arch is supported by the volar soft tissue tension of the deep transverse carpal ligament. While the central fixed unit of the hand provides phenomenal stability, the basal joint complex of the thumb acts much as a universal (saddle) joint, allowing the thumb to encompass a broad arc of motion. This combination of rigidity and mobility in different CMC

N. G. Kasparyan: Section of Hand Surgery, Department of Orthopaedic Surgery, Lahey Clinic, Burlington, Massachusetts 01805.
A. J. Weiland: Department of Orthopaedic Surgery and Plastic Surgery, Cornell University Medical College, New York, New York 10021.

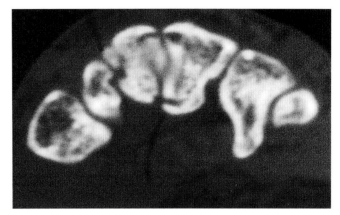

FIGURE 35.1. Transverse computerized tomography of the distal carpal row demonstrating the "Roman arch" construct of the distal carpal row.

joints allows for stable weight bearing on the hands as well as the ability to gently hold a glass (1,2).

The Second to Fifth Carpometacarpal Joints

Gunther (2) demonstrated in cadaver dissections that the central fixed unit complex allows no more than 1° of motion at the second ray and no more than 3° of motion at the third ray. This inherent stability arises from the wedge-shaped trapezoid and its articulation with the second metacarpal, whereas the third metacarpal with its dorsal styloid precess keys nicely into the distal pole of the capitate (1,2). This process on the third metacarpal can degenerate over time to form a painful carpal boss. Taut intermetacarpal ligaments between the second and third ray along with the capsular ligamentous structures between the capitate, trapezoid, and trapezium add greater stability. The extensor carpi radialis longus and brevis insert on the dorsoradial aspects of the second and third metacarpals, respectively. The flexor carpi radialis (FCR) inserts on the palmar aspect of the second metacarpal. Together, these three extrinsic insertions provide an added dynamic compressive stability on the radial-sided CMC articulations (1,2). The ulnar-sided metacarpals articulate with the hamate, which is saddle shaped at its distal articulation. This saddle shape of the hamate is separated into two separate facets, with the more radial one articulating with the base of the fourth metacarpal and the ulnar facet with the base of the fifth metacarpal. The interosseous ligaments between the bases of the fourth and fifth metacarpals are fairly stout. However, the fourth and fifth CMC joints are hypermobile as compared to the radial-sided articulations. Studies indicate that the fourth CMC joint moves between 8° and 10° in flexion–extension, whereas the more mobile fifth CMC joint moves anywhere from 15° to 30° in flexion–extension (1,2). The fifth CMC joint, because of its saddle-shaped ulnar facet, also allows a rotatory component of motion that facilitates subtle movements such as cupping the hand or opposition to the thumb. Extrinsic stability is provided to the ulnar side of the hand by the extensor and flexor carpi ulnaris insertions.

The Thumb Carpometacarpal Joint

The thumb CMC joint or basal articulation possesses a broad arc of motion. This freedom of motion comes at the expense of basal joint stability. The thumb CMC joint is comprised of a saddle-shaped articulation between the metacarpal base and the trapezium. The saddle allows for motion in the flexion–extension plane and the abduction–adduction plane. These principal movements can also accommodate axial rotation. Axial rotation, however, causes an incongruity of the saddle joint, focusing strong compressive forces at the perimeter of the articular cartilage. This peripheral focal compression is poorly tolerated by the basal joint and results in the process of degeneration. It is ironic that much of the elegant work of the thumb in axial rotation (opposition and fine pinch) is the principal initiator of instability and resultant articular erosion (2,3).

The volar beak ligament at the base of the thumb metacarpal is the strongest ligament stabilizing this joint. This ulnar-volar beak ligament arises from a groove just distal and ulnar to a tuberosity of the trapezium and inserts on the prominent volar beak of the first metacarpal. This beak ligament allows for the key tethering of the thumb basal joint. The capsule, combined with the confluent radial and dorsal ligaments, provides a minor component of stability to the thumb CMC joint (2,3). Extrinsic dynamic support is principally provided by the abductor pollicis longus tendon, inserting on the proximal aspect of the dorsoradial surface of the thumb metacarpal (2). Support is also provided to a lesser degree by the flexor pollicis brevis, abductor pollicis brevis, adductor pollicis, and opponens pollicis.

THE SECOND TO FIFTH CARPOMETACARPAL JOINTS

Chronic Sprains

Chronic sprains of the CMC joint, specifically of the second and third metacarpal articulations, are rather innocuous conditions. This group of disorders often go undiagnosed and result from injury that is insufficient to dislocate the joint, cause fracture, or result in carpal bossing. Typically, these are a result of minor trauma with minimal traumatic subluxation at the joint or repetitive microtrauma, which is cumulative and causes chronic synovitis within the joint. This condition is often misdiagnosed as various other disorders. The correct diagnosis can be made by awareness and maintaining a high index of suspicion in patients who present with a history of repetitive trauma (such as a jackhammer operator) or a single minor injury. Classically, the pain is difficult for the patient to localize. The pain may be felt in either the volar or dorsal aspect of the midpalm. Critical findings demonstrate minimal laxity of the joint and minimal to moderate tenderness. The diagnosis can often be made via a diagnostic injection of lidocaine into the joint, which usually relieves the pain (2,41).

Studies have indicated that complete resolution of this chronic problem can be obtained with arthrodesis of the CMC joint. The best results of this arthrodesis have been obtained by those investigators who have used a tricortical iliac crest bone graft in "hockey puck"-shaped fashion, similar to those used in anterior cervical fusion. The wedge of bone is placed within the joint space after the proximal and distal aspects of the articular cartilage are completely denuded. Temporary K-wire fixation is used for 8 to 10 weeks. A number of investigators have demonstrated excellent results with this technique, with no evidence of functional loss, complete resolution of pain, and return to nearly 100% grip strength as compared to the contralateral side. It is hypothesized that once fusion of these joints is obtained, chronic micromotion ceases within the joint, and the local synovitis resolves (2,41).

Posttraumatic Degenerative Arthritis

The spectrum of injury, from minor trauma resulting in chronic sprains of the second and third CMC joints to trauma resulting from higher energy, is a continuum that can eventually result in degenerative arthrosis. Numerous investigators have demonstrated that posttraumatic incongruity of the articular surface will result in cartilage degeneration and joint destruction. It remains unclear whether minimal-energy repetitive trauma may also result in a similar fate. The technique of arthrodesis for these injuries is identical to that for chronic sprain injuries that are recalcitrant to nonoperative management. Little has been published in the literature regarding arthrodesis of the more mobile fourth and fifth CMC joints. A number of surgeons have advocated primary arthrodesis of the markedly comminuted reverse Bennett's fracture or one in which the patient presents with an acute fracture with significant chronic osteoarthritis of the joint at the time of injury (1,2,41).

Figures 35.2 and 35.3 demonstrate the case of a 34-year-old mechanic who incurred a subtle injury secondary to an automobile engine falling on the dorsum of his nondominant hand, resulting in no evidence of fracture or fracture-dislocation on initial plain film views. The patient presented with chronic pain at the base of the second and third metacarpals 4 weeks after injury. Examination revealed point tenderness directly over the dorsal aspects of the second and third CMC joints without evidence of crepitance or subluxation. The computed tomography scan (Fig. 35.2) demonstrated evidence of posttraumatic arthrosis and periarticular degenerative cyst formation only 4 weeks postinjury. The patient had an arthrodesis (Fig. 35.3) using internal fixation augmented with iliac crest cancellous bone grafting with excellent results. He demonstrated complete resolution of pain within 6 weeks and returned to his prior employment in 8 weeks' time.

Carpal Boss

A carpal boss is a bony prominence that occurs on the dorsum of the third and, to a lesser degree, second CMC joints. The cause of carpal boss formation remains unclear. Reports in the literature indicate that just under 50% of individuals with a carpal boss present with pain. The bony prominence arises from the dorsal base of the metacarpal and on initial exam appears much like a type of osteophytic overgrowth of bone. However, on closer examination of the joint, sclerosis and articular damage of the joint are not readily apparent. Certain authors have surmised that carpal bossing may be caused by abnormalities of ossification at the base of the third or second metacarpal (2). Some investigators have also suggested that periostitis secondary to chronic microtrauma of the joint capsule may result in the laying down of new bone (1,2,42–45). The literature shows that individuals under 15 years of age rarely present with a carpal boss (1,2,42–45).

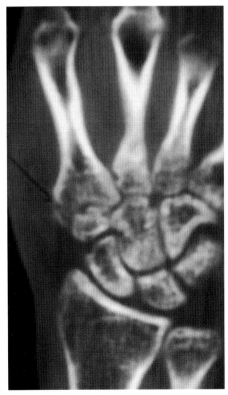
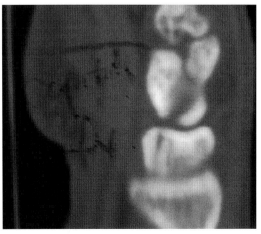

FIGURE 35.2. A: Coronal computerized tomographic image of a 34-year-old mechanic who had an automobile engine fall on his hand. The computed tomography (CT) scan demonstrates fracture and traumatic degeneration of the carpometacarpal joints of the second and third metacarpal articulations not appreciated on plain films. **B:** Sagittal CT of the same patient, demonstrating a fracture through the articular surface of the capitate at the capitate–third metacarpal articulation with traumatic degeneration.

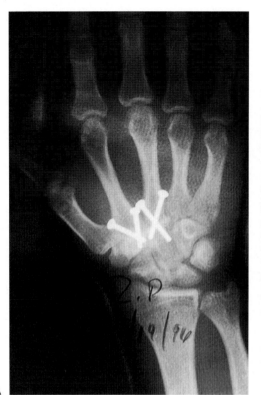
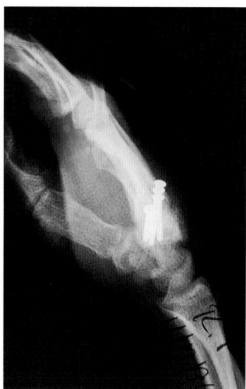

FIGURE 35.3. Anteroposterior **(A)** and lateral **(B)** plain films of the 34-year-old man shown in Fig. 35.2 who underwent arthrodesis of the second and third carpometacarpal joints for post-traumatic arthritis.

Indications for surgical excision of a carpal boss include significant pain secondary to activities of daily living. A certain amount of controversy surrounds the usefulness of surgical resection. Initial reports in the literature of resection demonstrated a high rate of recurrence and a long course of postoperative recovery from discomfort. In our experience, although the surgical technique of removing the bony overgrowth is quite simple, patients sometimes have significant discomfort at the surgical site for up to 3 months postoperatively. More recently, a series of 16 patients demonstrated good to excellent results when a sizable wedge resection of the involved portion of both the proximal and distal aspects of the joint was performed down to normal articular cartilage. A number of authors have reported on ganglion formation in conjunction with a carpal boss at the CMC joint. The formation of a ganglion in relation to a boss may complicate treatment of the boss and may necessitate resection of the ganglion and fusion of the joint in order to prevent recurrences (1,2,42–45).

Rheumatoid Arthritis

In general, rheumatoid arthritis involving the CMC joints is quite rare. The literature is sparse regarding this condition. Gunther (2) believes that the reason these joints rarely become deformed in rheumatoid arthritis is their strong interosseous ligaments and because the flexor and extensor tendons of the wrist insert at the bases of the metacarpals. This exerts a generalized compressive force on the joints as opposed to forces consistent with angular momentum. Gunther (2) has shown that these joints may be become problematic when the midcarpal or radiocarpal joints fuse spontaneously or are electively fused in the setting of end-stage rheumatoid arthritis. When this occurs, a new flexion and extension moment is applied to the nascent CMC joint, often resulting in transmitted pain and instability. Arthrodesis may be the only option for pain relief and stabilization (2).

THE THUMB

The human thumb has a wide range of motion at the TM articulation, with relatively little bony contact to the trapezium at any given point in time. This range of motion allows the fine motor skills of opposition, fingertip pinch, key pinch, and grasp, which we utilize on a daily basis (46–48). Flatt (47) likened the structure of the base of the thumb to that of a boom attached to the main mast of the second metacarpal shrouded by sheets of suspensory ligaments and muscle. By allowing an enormous range of motion, the thumb becomes susceptible to loosening and instability by violent injury or degenerative arthritis. Some individuals present at birth with markedly lax joints that continue to loosen over time secondary to no known pathologic precess. Injuries to the base of the thumb may result in catastrophic consequences with decreased hand function that often require complex reconstructive procedures to reestablish a useful working hand (46–48).

Trapeziometacarpal Instability

In the continuum of degenerative pathoanatomy at the thumb basal joint, the first stage usually presents with instability, with or without pain, and always without radiographic evidence of arthrosis. Eaton and Littler (58,59) first described the state of instability of the TM joint as being posttraumatic in men and idiopathic in women. Eaton and Glickel (3) later described this first and early stage of degeneration as one of painful synovitis, effusion, and hypermobility. Pain is exacerbated by activities involving forceful pinch. The articular surfaces are normal. Eaton and Littler (58) felt that the primary insult was a partial rupture or attrition of the volar beak ligament. Radiographs obtained in the AP plane with both thumbs pushing radially on one another in a stress view often demonstrate the instability. We concur with the thinking of Eaton and co-workers (3,58,59) that the initial treatment should include splinting and antiinflammatory medications for a period of 3 to 4 weeks, followed by tapering of the splint. If, after this initial treatment, the pain is recalcitrant to nonoperative measures, we concur with Eaton and co-workers and advocate a volar ligament reconstruction. Hypermobility alone without pain is not an indication for operative treatment. In those individuals with pain, we reconstruct the joint using a slight modification of the method described by Eaton and Littler (59).

Volar Ligament Reconstruction: Authors' Preferred Technique

Weiland Modification of Eaton and Littler's Technique

A Waggner approach is made along the subcutaneous radial border of the thumb metacarpal curving in an S-shaped fashion along the distal aspect of the wrist flexion crease. Care is taken during the subcutaneous dissection to protect the longitudinal branch of the dorsal sensory radial nerve and the palmar cutaneous branch of the median nerve. The superficial radial artery lies on the volar aspect of the approach and must be identified early. Once dissection is taken down to the thenar musculature, the thenar muscles are gently reflected from the metacarpal base and carpal attachments to the level of the FCR tendon. The FCR tendon can be identified at the level of the distal palmar crease.

Care is taken to preserve the maximum amount of TM joint capsule at this stage. An arthrotomy of the TM joint can be performed to ensure and confirm the quality of the articular surface of the joint. The most dorsal aspect of the incision exposes the dorsal radial aspect of the thumb metacarpal base and the extensor tendons. Dissection and mobilization of the dorsal sensory branch of the radial nerve in an ulnar direction, with the subcutaneous fat, is performed. With the dorsum of the thumb metacarpal base exposed and well visualized, the extensor pollicis brevis tendon is mobilized and retracted ulnarly. A longitudinal incision can be made in the periosteum in the middorsum of the thumb metacarpal, approximately 3 to 4 mm distal to the articular surface of the joint, as described by Eaton and Glickel (3). A No. 4 Hall burr is used to form a channel beginning perpendicular to the plane of the thumbnail directed to a point approximately 3 mm distal to the volar beak of the metacarpal. The soft tissues about the volar base are mobilized and protected during this procedure.

A passageway is made in this manner and cleared of bony debris. The FCR tendon is exposed through a series of 1-cm–long transverse incisions to the level of the musculotendinous junction of the FCR in the forearm. The peritenon is then split longitudinally on its superficial surface to facilitate passage of the mobilized tendon strip, beginning at the musculotendinous junction, about 8 cm proximal to the wrist. Fifty percent of the FCR is cut in cross section, divided, and split longitudinally and distally beneath the skin bridges until it emerges at the level of the wrist. It is freed to the proximal border of the trapezium or just distal to it by carefully incising the insertion of the transverse carpal ligament from the shelf of the trapezium. This brings the FCR tendon strip close to the hole made by the Hall burr at the metacarpal base. The free end of the tendon is then placed through this channel and pulled through with a small curved snap to the dorsal aspect of the metacarpal. The path of the tendon should be 3 mm distal to and parallel to the articular surface of the metacarpal. The tension of the ligament is set by stabilizing the thumb metacarpal in the functional position of abduction, extension, and mild pronation. Tension is then placed on the strip of tendon emerging from the metacarpal, kinks are removed, traction is relaxed, and a suture is placed through the reconstructed tendon and the dorsal periosteum of the metacarpal to set the final position. Eaton and Glickel (3) have shown that the ligament reconstruction should not be too tight; otherwise the rotation of the metacarpal–trapezium saddle joint will be restricted, and this may result in attrition of the peripheral joint cartilage during rotary motions of the thumb.

After tensioning of the ligament, the remaining tendon is routed under the abductor pollicis longus tendon as close to the metacarpal insertion as possible. Several 4-0 Tycron sutures are placed at this point to further secure the tendon. The free end of the tendon is passed volar to the FCR tendon just proximal to the trapezium. An additional suture may be placed here, and the tendon is redirected across the radial aspect of the joint to ensure further stability. If we are seeking further stability at this point, the terminal aspect of the tendon is anchored to the metacarpal by placing a mini-Mitek suture anchor into the dorsum of the metacarpal base. We use this technique routinely in basal joint arthroplasty and have found it to provide excellent terminal support to the reconfigured tendon.

Closure of the thenar musculature is performed anatomically, maintaining physiologic tension. The thumb abductor is advanced at the time of closure. We do not use K-wire fixation of the joint provisionally. The thumb is immobilized with a compressive dressing and thumb–spica splint, allowing full movement of the interphalangeal (IP) joint and leaving the ulnar four digits free and extending to the midforearm. Immobilization is continued for 4 to 5 weeks, and early motion is initiated thereafter. Pinch strengthening is begun 6 to 8 weeks postoperatively.

Trapeziometacarpal Osteoarthritis

The basal joints of the thumb, namely the TM joint and the scaphotrapezial joint, are markedly susceptible to degenerative arthritis. Exactly why degenerative arthritis has a predilection for these joints is poorly understood. The thumb CMC joint ranks only seventh among joints in the hand in the incidence and severity of osteoarthritis when radiographic criteria are used. A sampling of middle-aged individuals by Kelsey et al. (60) demonstrated that one out of six women demonstrated moderate to severe arthritic changes radiographically in the thumb TM joint. This joint was involved in 60% of the women examined. In men, the osteoarthritic disease of the TM joint was the sixth most common joint involved in the hand, occurring in 5% of the male population. It is logical to assume that osteoarthritis of the basal joints is secondary to frequent, cumulative, and heavy stresses. The large numbers of patients with this disease have prompted the creation of various surgical procedures for its reconstruction including arthrodesis (58, 61–66), ligament reconstruction (59,67,68), hemiarthroplasty (69,70), and trapezial resection, with or without interposition (71–76). As with any other malady for which numerous reconstructive procedures have been advocated, it may be presumptuous to assume that any one procedure to correct basal joint arthritis is a panacea for all types of pathoanatomy.

Eaton and co-workers (3,59) have elegantly categorized the different radiographic stages of basal joint osteoarthritis into four separate and distinct entities that they feel are an evolution of the disease process. Certain patients develop a severe arthritis radiographically that is accompanied by very little clinical distortion and function in the thumb. Other individuals with identical or less pronounced radiographic changes may develop severe angular deformities with dorsolateral subluxation of the base of the metacarpal on the trapezium, adduction of the metacarpal shaft, and hyperextension of the metacarpal phalangeal articulation. Many patients present in the sixth or seventh decade with significant pain and a marked bony prominence at the joint. There is often noticeable tenderness at the joint with pain produced by axial compression. Eaton et al. used radiographic criteria to aid in determining what surgical procedure should be performed in a specific patient (3,59). However, Eaton states that this must be tempered with an awareness of the patients' clinical findings and complaints. Each surgeon must be comfortable with the technique chosen and its outcome (3,59).

Stages of Basal Joint Arthritis

As described by Eaton and Littler (59) and later by Eaton and Glickel (3), staging of basal joint arthritis is as follows:

Stage I: Articular contours are normal. There may be a small amount of widening of the joint space. This joint space expansion may be secondary to effusion or ligamentous laxity of the TM joint. (The treatment of this stage has been outlined previously in the section on instability).

Stage II: There is slight narrowing of the TM joint. Minimal sclerotic changes of the subchondral bone are present. Joint debris does not exceed 2 mm in diameter in the form of loose bodies or osteophytes. The scaphotrapezial joint remains unaffected.

Stage III: There is marked narrowing or complete obliteration with cystic changes of the TM joint. Sclerotic bone with varying degrees of dorsal subluxation exists. Joint debris is greater than 2 mm in diameter. The scaphotrapezial joint remains normal.

Stage IV: Stage IV is identical to stage III in regard to the TM joint, with complete deterioration. Stage IV is characterized by arthritic changes of the scaphotrapezial joint.

The hallmark of the clinical presentation of basal joint arthritis is pain. The pain is generalized to the volar thenar aspect of thumb and palm. The discomfort is sometimes diffuse and poorly localized. There is frequently a visible prominence at the TM joint on the volar radial aspect of the thenar eminence. Patients classically present with a history of chronic repetitive activities that involve fine pinch or key pinch for a number of hours of each day. However, no evidence exists that these activities have a causal relationship to the development of basal joint arthritis. There is a predilection for individuals who have a history of "loose joints" and those who have the ability to place their thumb in trick positions.

On physical examination, patients may present with point tenderness directly over the TM joint. In stage III or stage IV disease, patients may present with classic crepitus, and the joint is increasingly painful when stressed or compressed axially. In earlier stages, patients may present with varying degrees of hypermobility, which in turn changes to marked stiffness and more bony deformity with time. During later stages of advanced degeneration, the Swanson grind test may be utilized to elicit exquisite pain. During the physical examination, care should be taken to differentiate between symptoms of stenosing tenosynovitis of the first dorsal extensor compartment (de Quervain's tendinitis) and trigger thumb, which may present in conjunction with basal joint arthritis. Each of these three separate entities can be readily diagnosed by a careful physical examination and radiographic evaluation. We have seen a number of cases in which patients present with all three separate pathologic processes. De Quervain's tenosynovitis can be carefully differentiated from the other two disorders by performing a Finklestein's test with the thumb hyperflexed into the palm, making a fist, with careful ulnar deviation applied to the wrist. A positive exam will be elicited by producing extreme pain directly over the radial styloid. Pain from a trigger thumb secondary to stenosis of the flexor pollicis longus tendon at the A1 pulley will often present with a thickened nodularity on the volar aspect of the thumb base and locking of the thumb in different positions. Pain specifically presents at the IP joint of the thumb. When all three of these entities occur simultaneously in one individual, they should be addressed at one operative sitting (2,3).

Radiographic evaluation should include standard posteroanterior (PA), lateral, and oblique views of the thumb (Fig. 35.4). Eaton and Glickel (3) advocate stress views of the thumb by having a PA projection of both TM joints with lateral, radial stress applied to one another by opposing the two thumbs on one film. Eaton and Glickel (3) feel that this stress view demonstrates the potential for a lateral shift of the metacarpal shaft off the saddle of the trapezium in a subluxatable joint. At the time of this writing, computerized tomography and MRI are not indicated and are unnecessary in the evaluation of osteoarthritis at the base of the thumb. These studies are not only costly but provide no further useful information (except on rare specific occasions) when compared to plain films in multiple views (2,3).

When a patient initially presents with basal joint arthritis, we usually advocate a course of nonoperative therapy involving antiinflammatory medications and a thumb–spica custom-molded splint for a period of 2 to 4 weeks. Patients who present with Eaton stage I or II disease clearly may benefit from conservative therapy for a longer period of time. Patients with stage III or IV disease may also benefit with partial relief of pain from a period of splinting while consideration for operative intervention is undertaken. If the deformity is severe and the patient is active and healthy, it may be reasonable to proceed with

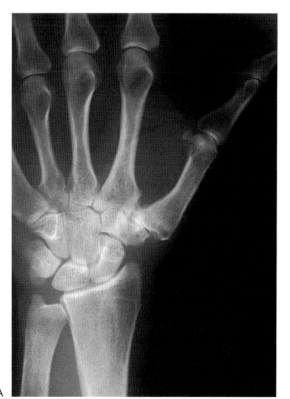
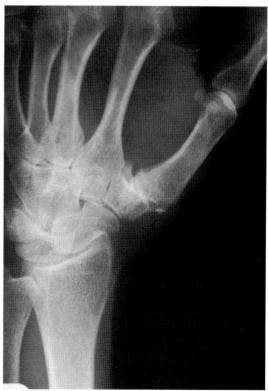

FIGURE 35.4. Anteroposterior **(A)** and oblique **(B)** views of 67-year-old woman with Eaton stage III trapeziometacarpal arthritis.

surgical correction after a brief period of splinting and nonsteriodal antiinflammatory drugs (NSAIDs). Patients with recurrent and persistent symptoms on a daily basis after routine daily activities are a clear indication for surgical reconstruction. Patients who cannot use NSAIDs secondary to the risk of gastrointestinal side effects may benefit from cortisone injections. Cortisone injections remain a viable option to palliate the patient with significant TM arthritis and articular cartilage degeneration. A cortisone injection is relatively easy to perform, and pain relief is usually quite excellent, but the duration of improvement in pain may be unpredictable (2,3). We favor the use of the soluble steroid Celestone. Our experience has indicated that Celestone, because of its high degree of water solubility, will not form particulate matter within the joint space.

The two main categories of surgical intervention include arthroplasty and arthrodesis. Throughout the history of basal joint resection arthroplasty, procedures can be separated into those that remove a portion of the metacarpal (69), those that remove a portion of the trapezium (74), and those that remove the entire trapezium (72,75). More specifically, those that involve excising the entire trapezium may leave an empty space (72), use a biological spacer (71), use a silastic implant (69,70), or use a metal implant.

Our preference in the treatment of stage I hypermobility and instability has been outlined in the previous section. There remains no consensus as to the superiority of any specific technique in resection arthroplasty. The bulk of resection arthroplasty procedures performed today in one form or another are based on the work of Eaton et al. in 1985 (74), Burton in 1973 (75), and Burton and Pellegrini in 1986 (76). Basal joint resection arthroplasty with ligament reconstruction performed by most hand surgeons in the world presently is based on some modification of these two techniques.

Ligament Reconstruction with Interposition Arthroplasty

Eaton and Littler first described their technique of ligament reconstruction in 1973 (58). Since that time, minor modifications of the technique have been made by Eaton and associates into the present form of resection arthroplasty with ligament reconstruction (3,73,74). The procedure is performed through the same Waggner incision with a volar approach to the TM joint as previously described in the instability section. The transverse arthrotomy of the TM joint is made to inspect the surfaces for articular degeneration. Simultaneously, an arthrotomy of the scaphotrapezial joint is performed with joint distraction and inspection. In this way, an evaluation of the articular cartilage of both joints can be made. If the scaphotrapezial joint is not involved with significant wear, resection arthroplasty of the TM joint can be performed alone (3,73,74).

When the status of both joints is ascertained, the base of the thumb metacarpal is trimmed perpendicular to the long axis. A gouge tract is then made in place in the thumb metacarpal. A wire is placed for subsequent passage of the strip of FCR tendon (3,73,74).

The FCR tendon is harvested at its musculotendinous junction and passed beneath skin bridges to the base of the thumb metacarpal. The proximal two-thirds of the released FCR is then transected and set aside for preparation of a tendon sandwich. The remaining free end is placed through the channel in the thumb metacarpal base to emerge on the dorsum and held with a hemostat. A K-wire is placed distally from the center of the base of the thumb metacarpal down the intramedullary canal emerging at the metacarpophalangeal (MP) joint dorsal to the proximal phalanx (3,73,74).

The free segment of FCR is folded in half and sutured with 3-0 plain chromic suture. The suture is then placed through the center of the folded tendon. Two long limbs of anchoring suture are passed through the joint with straight needles to emerge on the dorsum of the thumb web space. Traction is now placed on the tendon previously folded in half and doubled once again, creating four layers within the joint space and folded perpendicular to the axis of the thumb metacarpal. This creates a four-layer membrane of folded FCR interposed between the metacarpal base and the trapezium. The thumb metacarpal is then positioned in the optimal pronated-abducted alignment, and the previously placed Kirshner wire is passed across the FCR tendon sandwich into the trapezium and then into the proximal scaphoid. The correct tension is adjusted in the FCR stump passing through the medullary canal of the metacarpal by gentle traction to remove slack before it is fixed by suture to the metacarpal periosteum. The remaining free end is then passed beneath the insertion of the abductor pollicis longus tendon at the thumb base and secured with several nonabsorbable sutures. The TM joint capsule is closed with nonabsorbable sutures as completely as possible (3,73,74).

In stage IV basal joint arthritis with scaphotrapezial involvement, Eaton and co-workers recommend resection of both the proximal and distal facets of the trapezium with a section of FCR sandwich placed in the scaphotrapezial joints and tethered to surrounding capsular and periosteal tissues as an interposition arthroplasty (3,73,74). The hallmark of the Eaton-Littler reconstruction involves maintaining the overall height of the thumb basal joints by limited articular resection and tendon interposition with ligament reconstruction.

Plaster immobilization is utilized for 4 weeks followed by progressive mobilization. Eaton and co-workers advocate avoidance of early thumb metacarpal adduction and flexion, which they feel places undue stress on the reconstructed ligament leading to stretching of the volar restraints and a tendency for dorsal subluxation of the thumb metacarpal base.

Ligament Reconstruction–Tendon Interposition Arthroplasty

This procedure, first described by Burton in 1973 (75) and presented in a series of 25 procedures followed for an average of 2 years by Burton and Pellegrini in 1986, is a modification of the Eaton and Littler technique previously described. A segment of the FCR for ligament reconstruction is combined with trapezial excision and interposition. The distal one-half or entire trapezium is excised according to the extent of trapezial joint involvement and thumb web space contracture. A Waggner approach is made as previously described. The entire trapezium is removed if degenerative changes of the scaphotrapezial joint are noted on preoperative films. Care is taken not to injure the FCR tendon on trapezial resection. The base of the thumb metacarpal is then excised perpendicular to its long axis including the diseased articular surface. A hole is placed at the base of the radial cortex with a 6-mm gouge passing through the medullary canal into the trapezium fossa. The radial half of the distally based 12 cm of FCR tendon is harvested through a series of short transverse incisions in the forearm as described by Eaton and Littler (58). The FCR is split longitudinally to its insertion on the index metacarpal and passed into the dorsal radial wound through the trapezium fossa. Nonabsorbable sutures are placed in the deep capsule for subsequent use. The metacarpal is seated in an ulnar direction toward the fixed and stabilized fist position with a longitudinal K-wire. The free end of the FCR is passed into its intact distal insertion proximal to the base of the ulnar metacarpal cortex into the medullary canal and out the hole in the radial metacarpal cortex. The tendon slip is then pulled tight and sutured to the lateral periosteum of the metacarpal and then back to itself to resurface the base of the metacarpal. The terminal end of the tendon is now folded into an anchovy and sutured to itself and the deep palmar capsule with one of the previously placed sutures. The second deep suture is utilized to complete a two-layered pursestring lateral capsule closure over the interposition arthroplasty.

Burton and Pellegrini (76) feel that a critical component of this reconstruction involves the distal orientation of the tendon slip from the base of the thumb metacarpal to its intact insertion on the base of the index metacarpal, creating a supporting ligamentous sling beneath the ulnar cortex of the thumb metacarpal. This aids in prevention of proximal migration and radial subluxation of the thumb metacarpal. At the conclusion of the procedure, the extensor pollicis brevis is advanced proximally to a bony insertion on the metacarpal shaft in order to augment metacarpal abduction and eliminate the hyperextension force from the proximal phalanx at the metacarpal phalangeal joint. Burton and Pellegrini also augment their reconstruction with pinning of the joint.

Postoperatively, the patient is immobilized for 4 weeks, followed by pin removal and initiation of gentle range-of-motion exercises. Burton and Pellegrini, in their landmark work, demonstrated 92% patient satisfaction in terms of both pain relief and stability in the thumb (76). Ligament reconstruction and tendon interposition consistently improved pinch strength, increased grip strength and endurance, and restored the thumb web space. Proximal metacarpal migration averaged only 11% of the initial arthroplasty space versus nearly 50% loss of height as compared with silicone implants. Subluxation averaged only 7% of the width of the thumb metacarpal base relative to the scaphoid versus subluxation of 35% of the base of the implant with silicone arthroplasty (76). No deterioration of function or stability was noted over the average 2-year follow-up with a range of 1 to 4.5 years (76).

Authors' Preferred Technique: Resection Arthroplasty with Ligament Reconstruction

Our technique of basal joint arthroplasty involving trapezial resection and FCR ligament reconstruction is based primarily on modifications of the procedures described initially by Eaton and Littler (58) and later by Burton and Pellegrini (76). Recent experience at our institution has demonstrated that loss of metacarpal height does not occur with ligament reconstruction when the void left by trapezium resection is not filled with tendon or other interpositional material. Our technique utilizes a Waggner approach. The thenar musculature is carefully elevated from its origin on the dorsoradial aspect of the thumb metacarpal (Fig. 35.5). Great care is taken to insure maintenance of the TM joint capsule. Iden-

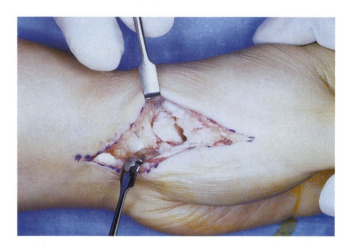

FIGURE 35.5. Surgical exposure of trapezium after elevation of thenar musculature and exposure of the joint capsule.

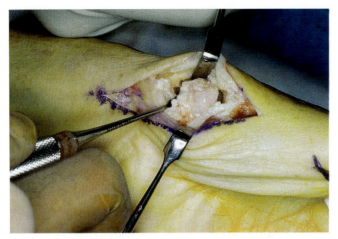

FIGURE 35.6. Subperiosteal dissection of the trapezium from surrounding ligamentous attachments before excision.

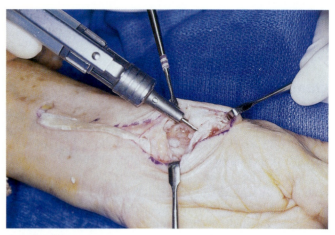

FIGURE 35.8. Demonstration of the Hall burr being utilized for preparation of the oblique burr hole through the metacarpal base and dorsum of the metacarpal. Note harvested flexor carpi radialis tendon in the field with distal attachment intact.

tification and protection of the dorsal sensory branch of the radial nerve and the superficial branch of the radial artery are performed (Fig. 35.6). The capsule is entered longitudinally, preserving both halves. Subperiosteal dissection of the soft tissues about the trapezium is performed. The trapezium is quartered with a sharp ½-in. osteotome and excised under direct vision with a small rongeur. Great care is taken in preserving the entire extent of the FCR beneath the resected trapezium. The radial one-half of the FCR tendon is harvested midway between the musculotendinous junction and the most distal junction of the FCR into the second metacarpal (Fig. 35.7). The FCR is harvested through a series of small incisions and advanced distally to the base of the second metacarpal. With a Hall burr, an oblique hole is made at the base of the metacarpal, and a second hole is made on the dorsal aspect of the thumb metacarpal 3 to 4 mm from the articular surface, providing a strong bridge of bone (Fig. 35.8). The two holes are easily connected. We utilize a Hall burr because it forms a smooth passageway without stripping the FCR substance. The FCR is woven through this hole through the thumb base and out the dorsal radial aspect of the metacarpal, brought beneath itself, and tensioned to an appropriate pronated abducted position of the thumb (Fig. 35.9). Once appropriate tension is attained, this weave of the FCR at the thumb base is sewn into place with two horizontal mattress sutures of 4-0

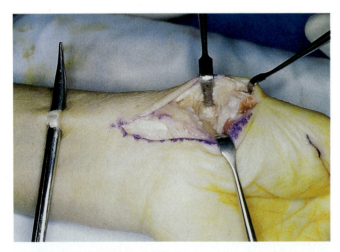

FIGURE 35.7. Exposure of the flexor carpi radialis (FCR) proximally before harvesting of the radial half of the FCR tendon down to the level of the base of the second metacarpal.

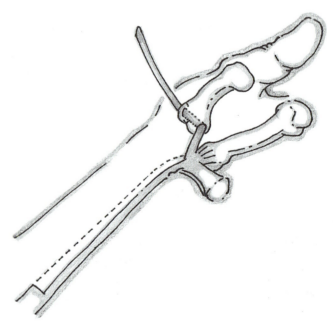

FIGURE 35.9. Demonstration of weaving of one-half of the flexor carpi radialis tendon through a drill hole at the base of the thumb metacarpal.

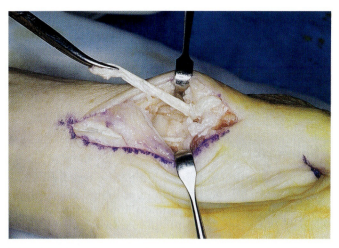

FIGURE 35.10. Weaving of harvested flexor carpi radialis through the base of the thumb metacarpal, out the dorsal burr hole, looped beneath itself (ulnarly), and fixed with 4.0 Tycron suture.

Tycron (Fig. 35.10). The remaining terminal end of the FCR is secured to the thumb metacarpal and anchored in using a mini-Mitek GII anchor suture with four arms of 3-0 Ethibond (Fig. 35.11). The tourniquet is deflated, and hemostasis is obtained. The capsule overlying the resected TM joint is closed with 3-0 Vicryl suture. A tendon interposition in the space left by trapezial resection is not performed. The abductor pollicis longus is advanced and sewn into place to the periosteum after the thenar musculature is reapproximated to the insertion with 3-0 Vicryl suture. Subcutaneous closure is performed with 3-0 Vicryl suture, and the skin is closed with nylon. The patient is placed in a thumb–spica splint for a period of 4 weeks, with gentle range-of-motion exercises started thereafter.

Silicone Arthroplasty

A brief mention of silicone arthroplasty must be made for the sake of completeness. Experience with silicone implant wear in the basal joint with resultant synovitis and significant bony changes has led many surgeons to abandon silicone implants in higher-demand patients with osteoarthritis in the TM joint. Amadio and colleagues (77) compared 25 consecutive Swanson arthroplasties with 25 resection arthroplasties to evaluate which procedure was better. By examining rates of complication, pain relief, motion, pinch strength, postoperative appearance, and patient satisfaction, it was concluded that there was no difference between the two. More recent studies, however, have demonstrated significant problems with instability, material wear, and cold flow and foreign body synovitis with silicone body implants. Our feeling is that silicone implants play no role in the reconstruction of the TM joint or the thumb in the setting of osteoarthritis. The principle use of silicone implants remains in the low-demand rheumatoid patient.

Arthrodesis

TM joint arthrodesis is indicated when degenerative changes are isolated to this joint and are clearly contraindicated in patients with pantrapezial arthritis. Arthrodesis, as an alternative to arthroplasty for basal joint arthritis, provides stability and increases strength. It has been criticized in the past for creating a predisposition for increased arthrosis in adjacent joints, significant limitation in range of motion, limitation in the ability to flatten the hand, the necessity for prolonged postoperative immobilization, compensatory hyperextension of the metacarpal phalangeal joint, and at times, nonunion. Numerous investigators have

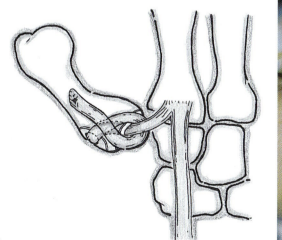
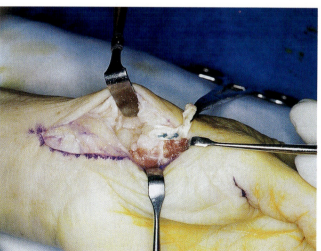

FIGURE 35.11. A: Application of mini-Mitek anchor suture to the dorsum of the thumb metacarpal, reinforcing the flexor carpi radialis (FCR) reconstruction. **B:** Final fixation of the terminal end of reconstructed FCR with Mitek suture anchor to the dorsum of the thumb metacarpal.

reported series of TM fusion with variable results (61–66). Bamberger et al. (61) published a series of 39 fusions performed in 37 patients. Pin fixation was utilized in 27 fusions, and staple fixation in 12. All 37 patients were bone grafted. They reported five delayed unions and three nonunions. Twenty-four of the 37 fusions were examined at an average 4-year follow-up. Of these, 11 had excellent results, seven good, five fair, and one poor. Grip and pinch were symmetric, and dexterity was reported to be better on the treated side. Bamberger et al. showed a 72% reduction in the adduction–abduction arc and a 61% reduction in the flexion–extension arc in the 24 patients evaluated at follow-up. According to the authors, subjective functional complaints were minimal despite the limitation of motion. Of the final 24 evaluated, only two patients were noted to have changes in the scaphotrapezial joint.

Positioning of the thumb metacarpal during arthrodesis of the TM joint has been considered critical in obtaining a functional fusion. Leach and Bolten (64) recommended 35° to 40° of palmar abduction and 10° to 15° of extension. This position was ascertained by making a fist with the thumb clasped over the middle phalanx of the index finger. The exact position of the thumb TM joint remains controversial in the setting of fusion. We feel that arthrodesis of the TM joint is indicated in the young male patient with significant posttraumatic basal joint arthritis without pantrapezial involvement. This patient will clearly require a stable, pain-free basal joint for functions of daily living and work-related activities with strength for an extended period of time. Arthrodesis may be favorable as compared to resection arthroplasty with ligament reconstruction for this limited patient population.

Arthroscopy

The use of arthroscopy in the treatment of the osteoarthritic thumb is in its infancy. Menon (78) recently published a series of 33 patients in which a partial resection of the trapezium was undertaken arthroscopically with the use of synthetic Gore-Tex graft or allograft fascia lata as the interposition. According to Menon (78), 87.8% of patients obtained pain relief. Average postoperative pinch strength was 11 lb. No ligament reconstruction was utilized by the author. Menon (78) reported no complications with the procedure involving the dorsal sensory branch of the radial nerve or the radial artery. Significantly more studies must be undertaken before arthroscopic techniques for treatment of degenerative arthritis of the TM joint is widely accepted.

Total Joint Arthroplasty

Braun (79) reported on a 10-year experience with a series of 50 patients in which he performed a cemented total joint arthroplasty of the thumb CMC joint. According to Braun, most patients demonstrated a full range of motion within 4 weeks of suture removal (6 weeks). Of these patients, five demonstrated loosening clinically or radiographically. Little has been published in the literature since this work regarding total TM joint arthroplasty. Success rates of trapezial resection arthroplasty with ligament reconstruction have been so good on a long-term basis that a 10% failure rate of total joint replacement in this setting is not warranted (79).

Rheumatoid Arthritis

Rheumatoid arthritis presents a different set of problems from osteoarthritis of the thumb basal joint. Much of our understanding of the rheumatoid thumb derives from the work of Millender, Nalebuff, and co-workers (80,81). In rheumatoid arthritis it is more commonly found that the IP and MP joints of the thumb are deformed by arthritis as well as the basal joint. When this is the case, arthrodesis of the TM joint is not an ideal option. Arthrodesis is an ideal form of reconstruction for the metacarpal–phalangeal joint of the rheumatoid thumb and may be the best single operation in the hand for the rheumatoid patient. Reconstruction of the basal joint, however, may be the most important of the three. In our experience, resection arthroplasty with ligament reconstruction of the basal joint is best performed with concomitant fusion of the MP or IP joints of the thumb when needed (80,81). We advocate identical reconstructive procedures for resection arthroplasty of the thumb as described in the osteoarthritic patient when the soft tissue and bony degeneration of the basal joint is minimal to moderate. Greater caution must be utilized in the placement of channels through the metacarpal base because of the increased fragility of the bony substance. Great care must be taken to avoid the cheese-cutter pull-through of a reconstructed FCR through the metacarpal base in porous bone.

Millender et al. (80) published a series of 21 thumbs in 19 patients utilizing the Swanson silicone prosthesis with mixed results. Two of these patients required reoperation, one for infection and one for failure to correct the deformity. In three patients, the prosthesis was reported to be malpositioned.

In cases of severe rheumatoid arthritis in which the soft tissues are markedly attenuated and the bone is extremely soft, ligament reconstruction tends to result in failure. In this scenario, we advocate a titanium basal joint implant. This implant restores some height to the basal joints and generally relieves pain.

Summary

The thumb CMC joints have developed to provide for a maximum of rotatory motion in the presence of ligamentous supports. In contrast, the CMC joints of the ulnar four rays provide greater stability while sacrificing motion. The stout ligaments of the second and third CMC joints, with their well-fitting bony edges, are well suited for withstanding longstanding longitudinal compression. Rarely, and under unusual circumstances, do degenerative or posttraumatic problems occur in these joints. Because of its more hypermobile nature, the thumb is clearly more susceptible to ligamentous instability and posttraumatic or chronic degenerative arthrosis of the CMC joint.

Therapeutic efforts for the ulnar four CMC joints must be focused on obtaining stable reconstructions, usually in the form of arthrodesis, whereas reconstructions of the thumb CMC joint in general should be focused on maintaining maximum motion while obtaining a painless reconstruction.

EDITORS' COMMENTS

The CMC joint is intolerant of even small articular steps. It must be remembered that this joint is probably the most common site of degenerative arthritis distal to the elbow. It is almost universally present to some degree in the elderly and is a major symptomatic clinical problem, most commonly in women in their 40s and 50s. Inline loading of this joint produces a lateral shear effect of the metacarpal on the trapezium. Cartilage does not tolerate shear loading, and even a very small step will speed the natural process of degeneration in this joint. With fracture, open reduction, direct visualization and anatomic realignment of the articular surfaces of this joint are mandatory. External fixators should not be necessary so long as there is continuity between a segment of cartilage surface and the shaft of the metacarpal. Surgery on this joint is facilitated by a transverse incision. Exposure is lost by a longitudinal limb running up the metacarpal. Significant capsular cutting must be carried out for adequate visualization. This may be done with some impunity so long as the ligamentous support to the smaller ulnar articular segment is not disturbed.

The mindset for the surgeon is important. Adequate visualization and anatomic reduction must be clearly in mind from the outset. If there is discontinuity with the shaft of the metacarpal and no way to place load on an unfractured portion of the articular surface, then a form of external fixation may be indicated. The two keys to this injury then are stability, maintained by the ligamentous support of the usually smaller ulnar fragment, and anatomic articular realignment. There is a rare injury to this joint that is not unlike the "five part" inline fractures at the base of the middle phalanx. Typically there is a central depressed segment and four segments of articular surface at the four points of the compass. Often one of the lateral fractures still has continuity with the shaft. Despite the appearance of the x-ray, which may lead the clinician to write the joint off, these articular surfaces can be adequately realigned. The depressed central segment can be brought down and pinned. Osteopore or similar nonautogenous bone may be packed behind the fragments. The joint can often be stabilized making use of the articular segment still in continuity with the shaft. If all five parts are free from the shaft, then external fixation is necessary.

Dislocations require immediate recognition and early reduction repair with prolonged immobilization. In chronic thumb CMC subluxation, there is little indication for secondary ligamentous repair. Extending the life of the joint in any worthwhile fashion is not likely.

Fractures of the trapezium involve the same high susceptibility to early degeneration at the thumb CMC joint and must be approached with the same exactitude. Open reduction, direct visualization, and internal fixation is the treatment of choice except for very small peripheral fractures not associated with instability.

There is an injury that should be mentioned in this context, and that is a dislocation of the index metacarpal, thumb metacarpal, trapezium, and trapezoid. The mechanism of injury is usually a crush of the hand in the lateral plane, that is, an impact from radial to ulnar that ruptures the ligaments between the bases of the index and middle metacarpals, continues proximally between the trapezoid and the capitate, and tears out through the less well restrained scaphotrapeziotrapezoid joint. These injuries are often unrecognized, and late diagnosis usually requires a triscaphe arthrodesis.

CMC dislocations with or without fracture of the finger metacarpals have the clinical advantage of being through joints with highly limited ranges of motion. This allows one to frequently treat these closed and conservatively with simple immobilization, returning later for definitive care if localized symptoms develop. This philosophy applies to the minimally displaced and articular fractures of particularly the index, middle, and ring metacarpals. Clearly a major dislocation or displaced fracture will require repair. An ongoing symptomatic joint can be arthrodesed with minimal loss of functional capacity.

The fifth CMC is somewhat different in that the loss of motion of this joint will hinder the ability to change the longitudinal arch of the hand. There is a saving feature in that even a small amount of articular cartilage on the base of the metacarpal resting on adequate articular cartilage of the hamate will provide a functional, painless, mobile metacarpal. Late treatment often can be accomplished by resection of the offending portion of the base of the fifth metacarpal. In one instance, a failed arthrodesis had been performed following a fracture dislocation of the fifth metacarpal-hamate joint. At surgery, there was a 5- to 6-mm disc of articular cartilage on the base of the fifth metacarpal that had not been removed during the attempted fusion. Bone was resected from the base of the metacarpal and the hamate, leaving the small disc of normally loaded articular cartilage; the patient has remained asymptomatic with normal motion for over 15 years. The articular disc on the base of the fifth metacarpal represented less than one-fourth of the articular surface.

Carpal boss is a form of highly localized degenerative arthritis involving typically the index and middle metacarpals, the capitate and trapezoid. Most often there is a congenital os involved that has remained asymptomatic over the patient's life, gradually producing and increasing cartilage destruction, highly localized to the dorsum of this four-bone complex. The most common configuration was found to be fusion of the os styloidium to the base of the middle metacarpal, overlying the capitate joint and, on occasion, the index and trapezoid bones. The onset of carpal boss, which can be traumatic in nature, usually serves as the instigating factor and then symptomatically does not resolve. Ganglia are frequently associated with a tender mass at the base of the index and middle metacarpals.

In addition to the Fusi counterrotation of the index and middle metacarpals, a reliable test is to malalign the index and middle metacarpals. This is accomplished by pressing dorsally on the volar plate of the middle metacarpal while volarly depressing the index metacarpal. The compliment is to reverse the two directions. This will cause rather acute pain if there is localized degenerative change and synovitis. On occasion, if the osteophytic prominence is significant dorsally, radial and ulnar deviation at the wrist can produce a snapping of the extensor communis and the extensor indicis proprius of the index finger over the bony mass. Any inflammation of the tendons is entirely secondary and not part of the etiology of the carpal boss. The treatment, of course, should be directed to the joint problem.

The first CMC joint is a specialized joint; resistance to trauma, damage, and arthritis is low. With degenerative arthritis, the decision to proceed beyond conservative means should be based entirely on the interference with the patient's quality of life. No other criteria play any significant role in determining the need for surgery. There are CMC joints with as much change and destruction, osteophytes, sclerosis, and cysts as one would find in any destroyed joint in the body, yet the patient seems to have minimal symptoms and minimal interference with functional activity. In contrast, minimal narrowing or some slight sharpening of the joint edges may be accompanied by years of unrelenting pain that interferes with activity as well as resting ache that can interfere with sleep. Cortisone is the biggest conservative gun and may be effective in cases in which there appears to be some remnant cartilage.

With the success of the tendon arthroplasty technique, our indications for CMC arthrodesis have dropped to a younger and younger age and for those in heavy manual employment. Because of the postfusion propensity for trapezium–scaphoid degenerative change, the late problem potential is probably worse than tendon arthroplasty. The principles behind the tendon arthroplasty are twofold: suspension of the base of the metacarpal with a portion of the FCR tendon and interposition of a collagen mass between metacarpal and scaphoid. It is important that the pivot point for the tendon be the most radial cortex of the thumb metacarpal. Inline loads will then tend to tuck the base of the metacarpal in, allowing abduction. The details of this procedure are included in Chapter 51.

Tendon arthroplasty has also been reliable in rheumatoid arthritis. Following surgery, there is no longer rheumatoid synovium available to destroy tissue, and the thumb metacarpal is suspended on the FCR tendon. Because of general panligamentous destruction, we feel that silicone implants are not indicated.

REFERENCES

1. Rawles JG. Dislocations and fracture-dislocations at the carpometacarpal joints of the finger. *Hand Clin* 1988;4:103–112.
2. Gunther SF. The carpometacarpal joints. *Orthop Clin North Am* 1984;15:259–277.
3. Eaton RG, Glickel SZ. Trapeziometacarpal osteoarthritis: Staging as a rationale for treatment. *Hand Clin* 1987;3:455–469.
4. Garcia-Elias M, Rossignani P, Cots M. Combined fracture of the hook of the hamate and palmar dislocation of the fifth carpometacarpal joint. *J Hand Surg [Br]* 1996;21:446–450.
5. Litner SA, Rettig AC. Isolated volar carpometacarpal dislocation of the fifth digit. *Am J Orthop* 1995;24:918–919.
6. Kogan MG, Ostrum RF. Concomitant carpometacarpal and metacarpophalangeal joint dislocations of the small finger. *Orthopedics* 1996;19:63–66.
7. Foster RJ. Stabilization of the ulnar carpometacarpal dislocations or fracture dislocations. *Clin Orthop* 1996;327:94–97.
8. Hanel DP. Primary fusion of fracture dislocations of central carpometacarpal joints. *Clin Orthop* 1996;327:85–93.
9. Yildiz M, Baki C, Sener M. Isolated dislocation of all five carpometacarpal joints. *J Hand Surg [Br]* 1995;20:606–608.
10. Pack DB, Grossman TW, Resnick CS, et al. Isolated volar dislocation of the index carpometacarpal joint: a unique injury. *Orthopedics* 1995;18:389–390.
11. Liaw Y, Kalnins G, Kirsh G, et al. Combined fourth and fifth metacarpal fracture and fifth carpometacarpal joint dislocation. *J Hand Surg [Br]* 1995;20:249–252.
12. Pai CH, Wei DC. Traumatic dislocations of the distal carpal row. *J Hand Surg [Br]* 1994;19:576–583.
13. Jebson PJ, Engber WD, Lange RH. Dislocation and fracture-dislocation of the carpometacarpal joints. *Orthop Rev* 1994;Feb (Suppl):19–28.
14. Hsu KY, Wu CC, Wang KC, et al. Simultaneous dislocation of the five carpometacarpal joints with concomitant fractures of the tuberosity of the trapezium and the hook of the hamate: case report. *J Trauma* 1993;35:479–483.

15. Mehara AK, Bahn S. Rotatory dislocation of the second carpometacarpal joint: case report. *J Trauma* 1993;34:464–466.
16. Gurland M. Carpometacarpal joint injuries of the fingers. *Hand Clin* 1992;8:733–744.
17. Van der lei B, Klasen HJ. Dorsal carpometacarpal dislocation of the index finger: a report of three cases and a review of the English-language literature. *J Trauma* 1992;32:789–793.
18. Takami H, Takahashi S, Hiraki S. Coronal fracture of the body of the hamate: case reports. *J Trauma* 1992;32:110–112.
19. Lawlis JF 3rd, Gunther SF. Carpometacarpal dislocations. Long term follow up. *J Bone Joint Surg Am* 1991;73:52–59.
20. Garcia-Elias M, Bishop AT, Dobyns JH, et al. Transcarpal carpometacarpal dislocations excluding the thumb. *J Hand Surg [Am]* 1990;15:531–540.
21. Fernyhough J, Trumble T. Late posttraumatic carpometacarpal dislocation of the ring and little finger. *J Orthop Trauma* 1990;4:200–203.
22. Carroll RE, Carlson E. Diagnosis and treatment of injury to the second and third carpometacarpal joints. *J Hand Surg [Am]* 1989;14:102–107.
23. Fayman M, Hugo B, de Wet H. Simultaneous dislocation of all five carpometacarpal joints. *Plast Reconstr Surg* 1988;82:151–154.
24. Ho PK, Choban SJ, Eshman SJ, et al. Complex dorsal dislocation of the second carpometacarpal joint. *J Hand Surg [Am]* 1987;12:1074–1076.
25. Cain JE Jr, Shepler TR, Wilson MR. Hamatometacarpal fracture-dislocation: classification and treatment. *J Hand Surg [Am]* 1987;12:762–767.
26. Henderson JJ, Arafa MA. Carpometacarpal dislocation. An easily missed diagnosis. *J Bone Joint Surg Br* 1987;69:212–214.
27. Berg EE, Murphy DF. Ulnopalmar dislocation of the fifth carpometacarpal joint—successful closed reduction: review of the literature and anatomic reevaluation. *J Hand Surg [Am]* 1986;11:521–525.
28. Oni OO, Mackenny RP. Multiple dislocations of the carpometacarpal joints. *J Hand Surg [Br]* 1986;11:47–48.
29. Mueller JJ. Carpometacarpal dislocations: report of five cases and review of the literature. *J Hand Surg [Am]* 1986;11:184–188.
30. Gunther SF, Bruno PD. Divergent dislocation of the carpometacarpal joints: a case report. *J Hand Surg [Am]* 1985;10:197–201.
31. Bergfield TG, Dupuy TE, Aulicino PL. Fracture-dislocations of all five carpometacarpal joints: a case report. *J Hand Surg [Am]* 1985;10:76–78.
32. Reznick SM, Greene TL, Roeser W. Simultaneous dislocation of the five carpometacarpal joints. *Clin Orthop* 1985;192:210–214.
33. Hartwig RH, Louis DS. Multiple carpometacarpal dislocations. A review of four cases. *J Bone Joint Surg Am* 1979;61:906–908.
34. Imbriglia JE. Chronic dorsal carpometacarpal dislocation of the index, middle, ring, and little finger: a case report. *J Hand Surg [Am]* 1979;4:343–345.
35. Lilling M, Weinberg H. The mechanism of dorsal fracture dislocation of the fifth carpometacarpal joint. *J Hand Surg [Am]* 1979;4:340–342.
36. Kleinman WB, Grantham SA. Multiple volar carpometacarpal joint dislocation. Case report of traumatic volar dislocation of the medial four carpometacarpal joints in a child and review of the literature. *J Hand Surg [Am]* 1978;3:377–382.
37. Gore DR. Carpometacarpal dislocation producing compression of the deep branch of the ulnar nerve. *J Bone Joint Surg Am* 1971;53:1387–1390.
38. Bora FW Jr, Didizian NH. The treatment of injuries to the carpometacarpal joint of the little finger. *J Bone Joint Surg Am* 1974;56:1459–1463.
39. Weiland AJ, Lister GD, Villareal-Rios A. Volar fracture-dislocations of the second and third carpometacarpal joints associated with acute carpal tunnel syndrome. *J Trauma* 1976;16:672–675.
40. Smith GR, Yang SS, Weiland AJ. Multiple carpometacarpal dislocations. A case report and review of treatment. *Am J Orthop* 1996;25:502–506.
41. Joseph RB, Linscheid RL, Dobyns JH, et al. Chronic sprains of the carpometacarpal joints. *J Hand Surg [Am]* 1981;6:172–180.
42. Artz TD, Posch JL. The carpometacarpal boss. *J Bone Joint Surg Am* 1973;55:747–752.
43. Carter RM. Carpal boss: a commonly overlooked deformity of the carpus. *J Bone Joint Surg [Am]* 1941;23:935–940.
44. Cuomo CB, Watson HK. The carpal boss: surgical treatment and etiologic considerations. *Plast Reconstr Surg* 1979;63:88–93.
45. Lamphier TA. Carpal bossing. *Arch Surg* 1960;81:1013–1015.
46. Kuczynski K. Carpometacarpal joint of the human thumb. *J Anat* 1974;118:119–125.
47. Flatt AE. *Care of minor hand injuries, 3rd ed.* St Louis: CV Mosby, 1972;3–5.
48. Pellegrini VD Jr. Fractures of the base of the thumb. *Hand Clin* 1988;4:87–102.
49. Bennett EH. On fracture of the metacarpal bone of the thumb. *Br Med J* 1886;3:12–18.
50. Green DP, O'Brien D. Fractures of the thumb metacarpal. *South Med J* 1972;65:807–814.
51. Foster R, Hastings H. Treatment of Bennett, Rolando, and vertical intraarticular trapezial fractures. *Clin Orthop* 1987;214:121–129.
52. Harvey F, Bye W. Bennett's fracture. *Hand* 1976;8:48–53.
53. Ruedi TP, Burri C, Pfeiffer KM. Stable internal fixation of fractures of the hand. *J Trauma* 1971;11:381–389.
54. Burton RI, Eaton RG. Common hand injuries in the athlete. *Orthop Clin North Am* 1973;4:809–838.
55. Rolando S. Fracteur de la base du premier metacarpien et principalementi sur une variete non encore decrite. *Presse Med* 1910;33:303.
56. Gelberman R, Vance R, Zakaib G. Fractures at the base of the thumb: Treatment with oblique traction. *J Bone Joint Surg Am* 1979;61:260–262.
57. Breen TF, Gelberman RH, Jupiter JB. Intraarticular fractures of the basilar joint of the thumb. *Hand Clin* 1988;4:491–501.
58. Eaton RG, Littler JW. A study of the basal joint of the thumb. Treatment of its disabilities by fusion. *J Bone Joint Surg Am* 1969;51:661–668.
59. Eaton RG, Littler JW. Ligament reconstruction for the painful thumb carpometacarpal joint. *J Bone Joint Surg Am* 1973;55:1655–1666.
60. Kelsey JL, Pastides H, Kreiger N, et al. *Upper extremity disorders. A survey of their cost and frequency in the United States.* St Louis: CV Mosby, 1980.
61. Bamberger HB, Stern PJ, Kiefhaber TR, et al. Trapeziometacarpal joint arthrodesis: A functional evaluation. *J Hand Surg [Am]* 1992;17:605–611.
62. Carroll RE. Arthrodesis of the carpometacarpal joint of the thumb. *Clin Orthop* 1987;220:106–110.
63. Carroll RE, Hill NA. Arthrodesis of the carpometacarpal joint of the thumb. *J Bone Joint Surg Am* 1973;55:292–294.
64. Leach RE, Bolton PE. Arthritis of the carpometacarpal joint of the thumb: results of arthrodesis. *J Bone Joint Surg Am* 1968;50:1171–1177.
65. Muller GM. Arthrodesis of the trapeziometacarpal joint for osteoarthritis. *J Bone Joint Surg Br* 1949;31:540–542.
66. Badger FB. Arthrodesis of the carpometacarpal joint of the thumb. *J Bone Joint Surg Br* 1964;46:162–164.
67. Eaton RG, Lane LB, Littler JW. Ligament reconstruction for the painful thumb carpometacarpal joint. A long term assessment. *J Hand Surg [Am]* 1984;9:692–699.
68. Kleinman WB, Eckenrode JF. Tendon suspension sling arthro-

plasty for thumb trapeziometacarpal arthritis. *J Hand Surg [Am]* 1991;16:983–991.
69. Kessler I. Silicone arthroplasty of the trapeziometacarpal joint. *J Bone Joint Surg Br* 1973;55:285–291.
70. Swanson AB. Disabling arthritis of the base of the thumb: treatment by resection of the trapezium and flexible (silicone) implant arthroplasty. *J Bone Joint Surg Am* 1972;54:456–471.
71. Carroll RE. Fascial arthroplasty for carpometacarpal joint of the thumb. *Orthop Trans* 1977;1:15–19.
72. Dell PC, Brushart TM, Smith RJ. Treatment of trapeziometacarpal arthritis: results of resection arthroplasty. *J Hand Surg [Am]* 1978;3:243–249.
73. Eaton RG. Replacement of the trapezium for arthritis of the basal articulations. A new technique with stabilization by tenodesis. *J Bone Joint Surg Am* 1979;61:76–82.
74. Eaton RG, Glickel SZ, Littler JW. Tendon interposition arthroplasty for degenerative arthritis of the trapeziometacarpal joint of the thumb. *J Hand Surg [Am]* 1985;10:645–654.
75. Burton RI. Basal joint arthrosis of the thumb. *Orthop Clin North Am* 1973;4:347–348.
76. Burton RI, Pellegrini VD. Surgical management of basal joint arthritis of the thumb. Part II. Ligament reconstruction with tendon interposition arthroplasty. *J Hand Surg [Am]* 1986;11:324–332.
77. Amadio PC, Millender LH, Smith RJ. Silicone spacer or tendon spacer for trapezium resection arthroplasty—comparison of results. *J Hand Surg [Am]* 1982;7:237–244.
78. Menon J. Arthroscopic management of trapeziometacarpal joint arthritis of the thumb. *Arthroscopy* 1996;12:581–587.
79. Braun RM. Total joint arthroplasty at the carpometacarpal joint of the thumb. *Clin Orthop* 1985;195:161–167.
80. Millender LH, Nalebuff EA, Amadio P, et al. Interpositional arthroplasty for rheumatoid carpometacarpal joint disease. *J Hand Surg [Am]* 1978;3:533–541.
81. Toledano B, Terrono AL, Millender LH. Reconstruction of the rheumatoid thumb. *Hand Clin* 1992;8:121–129.

36

CRYSTALLINE ARTHROPATHIES OF THE WRIST

DAVID B. FULTON
PETER J. STERN

The crystalline arthropathies are frequently viewed as nuisance diseases without life-threatening consequences, but they can be associated with considerable morbidity. Even in asymptomatic patients, the presence of crystal deposits in the wrist can lead to degenerative changes with time (1). Gout and calcium pyrophosphate dihydrate (CPPD) crystal deposition disease are the two most common crystalline arthropathies affecting the wrist. These diseases are relatively common and can mimic processes such as infection and other arthritides (2–5). Their presentation may be acute and dramatic. Making the correct diagnosis is critical in providing appropriate patient care, as the treatment of gout and CPPD disease differs considerably from the treatment of some of the disease processes that they can mimic (6).

GOUT

Historically gout was regarded as a disease of the wealthy that was associated with rich food and wine. Leeuwenhoek in the 1600s was the first to definitively recognize gout when he identified monosodium urate crystals with his newly invented microscope. Shortly after the discovery of x-rays, in 1895, Huber gave the first radiologic description of gout (7).

Gout is the most common inflammatory arthropathy in men over 40 years of age. Women are rarely affected before menopause. Estrogen may have a protective effect on the renal clearance of uric acid. Despite the infrequent incidence in women, gout should be considered in the differential diagnosis of an older woman with an acutely swollen, warm, painful wrist if the woman is taking a thiazide diuretic, a known cause of hyperuricemia (8).

The prevalence of gout in the United States is estimated at 13.6/1,000 men and 6.4/1,000 women. An elevated level of urate in the blood (>7.0 mg/dl) is termed hyperuricemia and carries an increased risk of gout. The annual incidence rate of gout is 4.9% for urate levels greater than 9 mg/dl, but only 0.1% for urate levels less than 7.0 mg/dl.

Approximately 5% of Americans will develop hyperuricemia, but only one in five with hyperuricemia will actually develop deposits of monosodium urate crystals, or clinical gout. Approximately 10% of patients with gout are overproducers of uric acid. Mechanisms of overproduction include deficiencies in purine metabolism (e.g., hypoxanthine-guanine phosphoribosyltransferase deficiency), excessive intake of purines, diseases resulting in rapid nucleic acid turnover (myeloproliferative disorders, chemotherapeutic induction of cancers), and ethanol abuse. Increased body weight is one of the most important predictors of hyperuricemia. Obesity and ethanol are associated with an increase in the production of urate and a decrease in its excretion (5,8). The potentially reversible factors that contribute to increased urate production include a high-purine diet, obesity, and regular alcohol consumption.

Approximately 90% of patients with gout have relatively impaired excretion of uric acid as opposed to overproduction. This abnormality of underexcretion is an idiopathic abnormality in the majority of patients. The serum uric acid level is normal in as many as 30% of patients experiencing an acute gout attack (9). Determining whether a patient suffers from gout because of underexcretion or overproduction of uric acid is important in determining appropriate therapy. Decreased urinary excretion of urate can be recognized on the basis of a decrease in the 24-hour urinary excretion of urate (<330 mg per day, or approximately 2 mmol per day) while the patient is on a low-purine diet or has a low renal clearance or fractional excretion of urate (8). The clearance of urate is determined in part by genetic factors, but an acquired cause is intrinsic renal disease. Hypertension can reduce the excretion of uric acid, as can certain drugs such as

---

D. B. Fulton: The Moore Orthopaedic Clinic, Columbia, South Carolina 29203.

P. J. Stern: Department of Orthopaedic Surgery, University of Cincinnati College of Medicine, Cincinnati, Ohio 45267.

thiazides, loop diuretics, low-dose salicylate, pyrazinamide, ethambutol, and niacin (8). If the excretion of uric acid is not impaired in a patient with hyperuricemia, the problem must be overproduction.

Clinical Presentation

The most common joint affected by gout is the metatarsophalangeal joint of the great toe. The wrist is relatively infrequently involved. As opposed to many diseases, which may present gradually, the onset of gouty arthritis is sudden and dramatic. Typically a patient goes to sleep asymptomatic and is awakened by pain and swelling in the wrist. The wrist may be warm, red, and tender and appear cellulitic (1,9). The pain may be severe, and even lightly touching the surface of the affected wrist may be intolerable. The swelling and inflammation can be intense enough to produce desquamation of the skin over the wrist. Gout may be mistaken for acute pyarthrosis in the wrist (10).

It is unusual to notice tophi during the initial presentation of gout, as it takes time for them to develop. After 20 years, however, unless urate-lowering drugs are appropiately used, 70% of patients will develop tophi (9). In chronic gout, uric acid may be deposited in the carpal canal and flexor tendons so as to produce median nerve compression. Surgical intervention to remove the tophaceous material may be helpful (10,11) (Fig. 36.1). Gout may also present initially in the wrist as dorsal tenosynovitis (10).

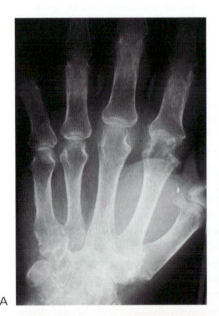
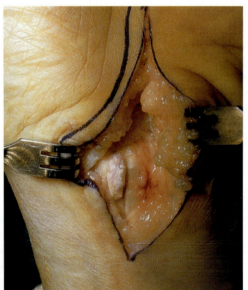
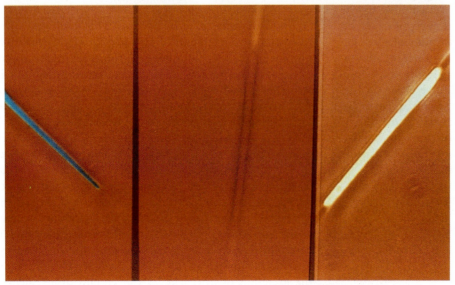

FIGURE 36.1. Carpal tunnel syndrome secondary to gout. **A:** A 57-year-old man complained of numbness and tingling in the median nerve distribution. Radiographs revealed sclerotic bone and erosions in the metacarpal heads and carpus. **B:** Tophaceous material occupying the carpal tunnel was removed in surgery, which relieved the patient's symptoms. **C:** The specimen contained negatively birefringent crystals visible under the polarized microscope (courtesy of Paul R. Fassler, M.D., Cincinnati, Ohio).

The definitive diagnosis of gout was first described by McCarty and Hollander in the 1960s (12) and consists of needle aspiration of the acutely inflamed joint or of a suspected tophus. The aspirated joint fluid should be analyzed for crystals, cell count, Gram stain, and culture. Identification of negatively birefringent needle-shaped crystals (monosodium urate) under a polarizing microscope is diagnostic of gout. Over 95% of patients who are assessed during an acute gout attack will have identifiable crystals. The diagnosis can be made only by aspirating the joint. Even if the rest of the clinical presentation is classic for gout, the diagnosis cannot be made with certainty without identification of monosodium urate crystals. If no definite exudate is aspirated, one can attempt irrigation of the joint. Laboratory values are not always helpful, as 80% of people with hyperuricemia are asymptomatic. On the contrary, the serum uric acid level may be normal in the face of an acute attack. Furthermore, a definitive diagnosis should be made before instituting treatment because many of the medications have significant side effects (8). Chronic untreated gout is a slowly destructive process punctated by acute flare-ups. Over time (average, 11.7 years), tophi will be deposited in and around joints and in soft tissue (13). As tophi become larger in size, they may calcify or ossify and impinge on adjacent structures (4,10).

Radiographic Assessment

Radiologic features are not usually seen until 6 to 12 years after the initial attack and are present in 50% of affected patients. Calcifications develop in gouty tophi of 50% of patients. Juxatarticular lobulated soft tissue masses are common. "Punched-out" bony lucencies may develop secondary to erosion from longstanding soft tissue tophi (Fig. 36.2). Erosions are usually sharply marginated and periarticular. The erosions have characteristic "overhanging edges," and pathologic fractures through gouty erosions have been reported. The erosion of joint margins resembles rheumatoid arthritis, but there is more sclerosis in gout. Erosions may be seen at the carpometacarpal, metacarpophalangeal, and interphalangeal joints. Localized osteoporosis of subchondral bone can be observed during an acute gouty attack, but extensive loss of bone density is uncharacteristic of gout and can be used to differentiate it from rheumatoid arthritis (4). Unlike rheumatoid arthritis, periarticular and articular erosions are asymmetric in distribution. Cartilage destruction does not occur until the late

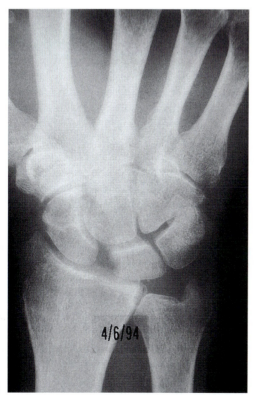
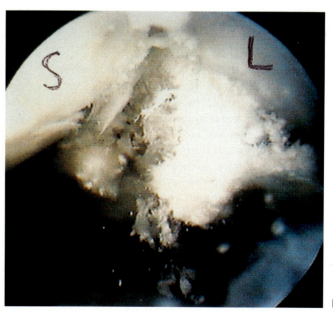

FIGURE 36.2. Gout involving the radiocarpal joint. **A:** A 63-year-old man presented with the acute onset of wrist pain. Radiographs revealed an erosive lesion in the lunate and scapholunate widening. **B:** Subsequent wrist arthroscopy revealed tophaceous deposits in the scapholunate ligament (S, scaphoid; L, lunate).

stages of disease. In fact, a normal cartilage space in articulations with extensive erosions is an important radiographic characteristic of gout. Gout may be confused with pyrophosphate arthropathy, but the presence of a soft tissue mass (tophi), an intact joint space, and asymmetric osseous erosions support the diagnosis of gout (4).

Treatment

The management of gout in the wrist is primarily medical. Operative intervention may occasionally be warranted in the chronic setting to debulk tophaceous deposits, improve tendon gliding, and decompress nerves (10). Surgical intervention is rarely necessary because medication is very effective in managing gout. Surgery may be indicated when tophi are refractory to medical management and are impairing function. This comprises fewer than 5% of patients with gout (11). Draining or infected tophi may also justify surgery.

Two classes of drugs are available: uricosuric drugs and xanthine oxidase inhibitors. Uricosuric drugs lower serum urate by increasing the urinary excretion of urate. Uricosuric drugs inhibit the tubular reabsorption of urate, thus increasing the urinary excretion of uric acid and decreasing serum urate levels. Effective uricosuria reduces the miscible urate pool, retards urate deposition, and promotes resorption of urate deposits. The most frequently used uricosuric drugs are probenecid and sulfinpyrazone. The greatest risk of therapy with uricosuric drugs is the formation of uric acid crystals in the urine and deposition of uric acid in the renal tubules, pelvis, or ureter, causing renal colic or the deterioration of renal function. These risks can be minimized by initiating therapy with a low dose (8). Uricosuric drugs are indicated in patients with low urate clearance, and a xanthine oxidase inhibitor is indicated in patients with increased urate production.

Xanthine oxidase inhibitors reduce the production of urate by blocking the final step in urate synthesis. Xanthine oxidase inhibitors result in an increase in the serum concentration of the urate precursors xanthine and hypoxanthine (8). Allopurinol is the xanthine oxidase inhibitor used to treat gout. Allopurinol is indicated for patients with gout who have urolithiasis because it has a prophylactic effect in both uric acid and calcium oxalate nephrolithiasis. Side effects occur in 3% to 5% of patients receiving allopurinol and can be severe. Hypersensitivity to allopurinol has been reported as well as life-threatening side effects including exfoliative dermatitis (<1 in 1,000 cases), vasculitis, severe rash, nephritis, and liver toxicity (8,9). Many patients have components of both low urate clearance and high dietary purine intake, and allopurinol is quite effective in most of these patients.

The medical treatment can be divided into two stages: treatment of acute inflammatory attacks and long-term uricosuric therapy to prevent the formation of destructive tophi. Acute treatment involves resting the affected joint for 48 hours and cryotherapy. Nonsteroidal antiinflammatory drugs (NSAIDs) are the preferred acute treatment in patients with no contraindications. Indomethacin, 25 to 50 mg three to four times daily for 2 to 3 days, with gradual tapering over 3 to 5 days, is usually effective. Whichever NSAID is chosen, it is important to prescribe the maximum dose as early as possible to abort the attack. Colchicine is also frequently used but has considerable side effects including nausea, vomiting, and diarrhea (8,14). The first signs of a gouty episode may be an indication to take one or two colchicine tablets (0.5–0.6 mg) in an effort to abort a full-fledged attack. Colchicine is not as effective as NSAIDs once an attack has been under way for several days and is probably not worth the side effects.

When NSAIDs are contraindicated (gastrointestinal, renal, cardiac, or hepatic diseases), corticosteroids can be effective. Intraarticular injection of depot steroid can be effective, but in about 5% of cases an injection may exacerbate inflammation by causing its own crystal-induced arthritis. A short course of systemic steroids may occasionally be helpful (8). Long-term medical management is not simple and is best supervised by an individual experienced in this area, as many agents have detrimental side effects. NSAIDs do not affect the underlying production of uric acid, nor do they prevent deposition of crystals. Long-term management decisions of hyperuricemia should not be made until the acute episode has resolved. Premature introduction of uric-acid-lowering drugs may trigger a flare-up of gouty arthritis (9).

Indications for drug therapy to lower uric acid include recurrent attacks of disabling gouty arthritis or evidence of chronic arthritis or tophi. A single gouty attack is usually not an indication because the next episode may not occur for years. The treatment goal is to reduce the serum urate concentration to about 6.0 mg/dl and preferably even lower if the patient has either clinical or radiographic evidence of tophi. Low-dose colchicine or an NSAID should be prescribed concomitantly with a urate-lowering drug to prevent breakthrough attacks. These drugs are continued for at least 3 months or until visible tophi are gone (9).

CALCIUM PYROPHOSPHATE DIHYDRATE CRYSTAL DEPOSITION DISEASE

CPPD crystal deposition disease is a general term for a disorder characterized by the presence of CPPD crystals in or around joints. This entity was originally described in 1957 by Zitnan and Sit'aj as chondrocalcinosis articularis (15). McCarty and co-workers correlated the radiologic finding of chondrocalcinosis with the clinical symptoms of "pseudogout" in 1962 (16). Pyrophosphate arthropathy is a term used to describe the distinctive pattern of structural joint damage that occurs in this disease (17). The term CPPD crystal deposition disease encompasses the clinical, radiographic, and pathologic features of this disorder. This includes the clinical presentation (pseudogout), articular and periarticular calcification, and pyrophosphate arthropathy. Patients with CPPD crystal deposition disease have CPPD crystals in the synovial fluid of the affected joint. These crystals can be distinguished from sodium urate crystals by their optical properties and by their x-ray diffraction pattern.

CPPD crystal deposition disease affects both sexes and has a predilection for middle-aged and elderly individuals. By the ninth decade, 50% of people have chondrocalcinosis on radiographs. The arthritis associated with CPPD crystal deposition disease (pyrophosphate arthropathy) has been termed "the great imitator" because it may simulate osteoarthritis, rheumatoid arthritis, ankylosing spondylitis, or an acute attack of gout, in which case it is called "pseudogout" (4,18,19).

CPPD crystal deposition disease can be familial, sporadic (most common), or associated with metabolic diseases. It occurs more often in those who have suffered previous articular trauma (9). Metabolic conditions associated with CPPD deposition include hypomagnesemia, hyperparathyroidism, hypophosphatasia, hemochromatosis, and severe hypothyroidism (18,20). The association between CPPD crystal deposition disease and hemochromatosis is particularly strong, with chondrocalcinosis being observed in 41% of patients with hemochromatosis (20). Signs and symptoms of CPPD crystal deposition disease may appear earlier in patients with metabolic diseases than in patients with idiopathic CPPD crystal deposition disease. One should consider obtaining laboratory tests including serum calcium, magnesium, phosphorus, iron, and TSH in a patient with newly diagnosed CPPD crystal deposition disease to screen for associated metabolic abnormalities.

Clinical Presentation

The wrist is commonly involved in CPPD crystal deposition disease, second in incidence only to the knee (21). The radiocarpal articulation is most frequently affected (3), and unlike rheumatoid arthritis, the distal radioulnar and trapezial–metacarpal joints are rarely affected. Acute episodes of CPPD crystal deposition disease in the wrist are characterized by acute pain and inflammation that evolve quickly and resolve without treatment over about 10 days (22). The clinical presentation may mimic septic arthritis, acute carpal tunnel syndrome (6,23,24), rheumatoid arthritis, osteoarthritis, or neurogenic arthropathy. Necrosis and collapse of the scaphoid and lunate has been reported in three cases of severe pyrophosphate arthropathy (25).

Diagnosis

Like gout, the definitive diagnosis of inflammatory arthritis caused by CPPD crystals requires the demonstration of the crystals in aspirated joint fluid. The CPPD crystals are 2 to 20 μm in length and can be in the shape of rhomboids, rods, or squares (22). Under polarized light, the crystals show a weak birefringence and positive elongation. CPPD crystals can be more difficult to see than monosodium urate crystals and as a result, a misdiagnosis of rheumatoid arthritis or osteoarthritis is common.

Radiographic Assessment

The two major radiologic manifestations of this disease are calcification and arthropathy. Articular and periarticular calcific deposits may be located in synovium, cartilage, wrist capsule, tendons, ligaments, bursae, and soft tissues (20). The calcifications are often symmetric and bilateral. Pyrophosphate arthropathy represents structural joint changes and consists primarily of joint space narrowing, subchondral cyst formation, and bone sclerosis (20,26). Calcification of the triangular fibrocartilage complex is present in 74% of cases (27) (Fig. 36.3). This appears as punctate or amorphous radiodensities extending in a horizontal fan-like fashion from the ulnar aspect of the distal radius to

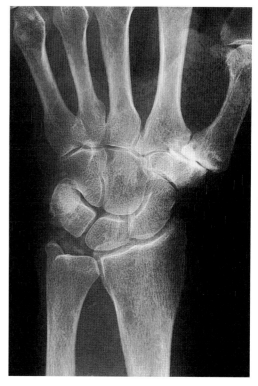

FIGURE 36.3. Calcium pyrophosphate dihydrate (CPPD) crystal deposition disease. An 80-year-old woman with CPPD crystal deposition disease presented with pain at the base of her thumb. She did not have ulnar-sided wrist pain. Radiographs revealed pantrapezial arthritis consistent with her symptoms. Calcification of the triangular fibrocartilage complex was an incidental finding.

the ulnar styloid. Hyaline cartilage calcification may occur and appears as thin, linear deposits that are parallel to, and separated from, the subjacent subchondral bone. The hyaline cartilage of the radiocarpal, midcarpal, and carpometacarpal joints is frequently affected.

Synovial calcification may be seen in the absence of cartilage involvement. The radiocarpal and distal radioulnar articulations are common sites of synovial calcification (20). Intercarpal ligament calcification occurs and is commonly seen in the scapholunate and lunotriquetral ligaments. Yang et al. reviewed the radiographs of 316 wrists in 181 patients with CPPD crystal depositon disease and found calcification in the lunotriquetral ligament in 77% of the cases (27). Disruption of the calcified scapholunate ligament may occur and lead to scapholunate dissociation and a scapholunate advanced collapse (SLAC) pattern (3,20,21). Chen et al. found SLAC wrists in 26% of cases of idiopathic CPPD crystal deposition disease (4) (Fig. 36.4). The SLAC pattern was bilateral in 63% of the cases.

The wrist arthropathy of CPPD crystal deposition disease is characteristic and has a different pattern of joint involvement than osteoarthritis or rhematoid arthritis. Pyrophosphate arthropathy in the wrist most frequently affects the radiocarpal compartment. Findings at this location include joint space narrowing, sclerosis, and discrete subchondral cysts, which can get quite large (20). Stern and Weinberg reported a pathologic fracture of the radius through a cyst caused by pyrophosphate arthropathy (26).

Narrowing of the midcarpal compartment may also be seen with particular predilection for the space between the lunate and the capitate. Distal migration of the lunate combined with proximal migration of the scaphoid may create a "stepladder" appearance suggestive of CPPD crystal depositon disease (20). The trapezioscaphoid articulation is also frequently involved and suggests the diagnosis of pyrophosphate arthropathy if the first carpometacarpal joint is normal, as this combination is uncommmon in osteoarthritis (20,21). The severity of CPPD crystal deposition disease radiographically is a very poor predictor of the clinical symptomatology (3,21). Resnick et al. found that many asymptomatic patients had calcification and arthropathy on radiographs, and many symptomatic patients had normal radiographs (21).

Treatment

Aspirating the joint to obtain crystals for diagnosis may also be somewhat therapeutic. Treatment of CPPD crystal deposition disease is largely symptomatic, using high doses of NSAIDs or intraarticular steroids to bring acute attacks of pseudogout under control. There is currently no treatment that permanently removes the CPPD crystals from the joint (18). NSAIDs or low-dose colchine may be used to reduce the incidence of recurrent attacks (8,28), but the clinical response to colchicine is not consistent. Chronic arthritis associated with this disease is treated the same as degenerative joint disease with analgesics and antiinflammatory medications.

Patients refractory to conservative management may require surgical intervention. There is a paucity of information on the surgical management of CPPD crystal deposition disease. Surgical treatment must be individualized. Limited intercarpal fusion or even total wrist arthrodesis may be necessary when medical therapy fails. The use of intraarticular injection of yttrium-90 has been useful in CPPD crystal deposition disease in the knee secondary to destruction of inflammatory synovium by local irradiation (8). The effectiveness of yttrium-90 in the wrist has not

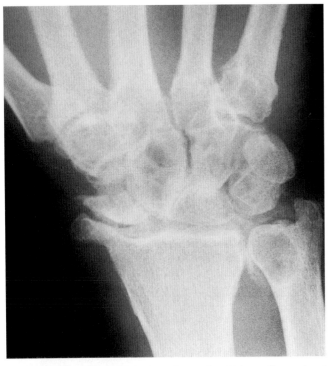

FIGURE 36.4. Pyrophosphate arthropathy. Wrist radiograph of 83-year-old patient demonstrating characteristic radiographic findings of advanced calcium pyrophosphate dihydrate (CPPD) crystal deposition disease: periarticular calcific deposits (including the triangular fibrocartilage complex), subchondral cyst formation, lunotriquetral ligament calcification, and a scapholunate advanced collapse (SLAC) pattern. **Editors' Notes:** *It should be noted that crystalline arthropathies follow a recognized degenerative pattern that is identical to SLAC wrist. The picture begins typically in the radial–scaphoid joint at the radial styloid against the articular–nonarticular junction of the scaphoid, progresses proximally between the scaphoid and radius, and, as radial support is lost with cartilage collapse, stage II SLAC occurs between the capitate and lunate and hamate and lunate. The radius–lunate joint is always preserved and is available for SLAC reconstruction. The pattern, therefore, in the human wrist is the same for rotary subluxation of the scaphoid from scapholunate dissociation, rotary subluxation from distal scaphoid instability, scaphoid fracture nonunion, Preiser's disease, and crystalline arthropathies.*

been proven. Diseases associated with CPPD disease should be identified and treated appropriately.

REFERENCES

1. Reginato AJ, Schumacher HR, Brighton CT. Experimental hydroxyapatite articular calcification. *Arthritis Rheum* 1982;25: 1239–1249.
2. Sack K. Monarthritis: differential diagnosis. *Am J Med* 1997;102: 30S–34S.
3. Resnick D. Calcium hydroxyapatite crystal deposition disease. In: Resnick D. Niwayama G, eds. *Diagnosis of bone and joint disorders.* Philadelphia: WB Saunders, 1981;1575–1597.
4. Resnick D, Niwayama G. Gouty arthritis. In: Resnick D, Niwayama G, eds. *Diagnosis of bone and joint disorders.* Philadelphia: WB Saunders, 1981;1464–1516.
5. Chiu KY, Ng WF, Wong WB, et al. Acute carpal tunnel syndrome caused by pseudogout. *J Hand Surg [Am]* 1992;17: 299–302.
6. Kann SE, Jacquemin J, Stern PJ. Simulators of hand infections. *AAOS Instr Course Lect* 1997;46:69–82.
7. Huber. Zur Verwerthung der Rontgen-Strahlen im Gebiete der inneren Medicin. *Dtsch Med Wochenschr* 1896;22.
8. Emmerson BT. The management of gout. *N Engl J Med* 1996; 334:445–451.
9. Schumacher HR Jr, Moreno Alvarez JM. Clues to common crystal-induced arthropathies. *Intern Med* 1993;14:35–47.
10. Moore JR, Weiland AJ. Gouty tenosynovitis in the hand. *J Hand Surg [Am]* 1985;10:291–295.
11. Straub LR, Smith JW, Carpenter GK Jr, et al. The surgery of gout in the upper extremity. *J Bone Joint Surg Am* 1961;43:731–751.
12. McCarty DJ Jr, Hollander JL. Identification of urate crystals in gouty synovial fluid. *Ann Intern Med* 1961;54:452–460.
13. Hench PS. The diagnosis of gout and gouty arthritis. *J Lab Clin Med* 1936;22:48–53.
14. Baker DG, Schumacher HRJ. Acute monoarthritis [see comments]. *N Engl J Med* 1993;329:1013–1020.
15. Zitnan D, Sit'aj S. Chondrocalcinosis articularis section 1. Clinical and radiological study. *Ann Rheum Dis* 1963;22:142–152.
16. McCarty DJ Jr, Kohn NN, Faires JS. The significance of calcium pyrophosphate crystals in the synovial fluid of arthritis patients: The pseudogout syndrome. *Ann Intern Med* 1962;56:711–737.
17. Resnick D, Niwayama G. *Diagnosis of bone and joint disorders with emphasis on articular abnormalities.* Philadelphia: WB Saunders, 1981.
18. Matteucci BM, Schumacher HRJ. Systemic arthritic conditions of the upper extremities—inflammatory. In: Peimer CA, ed. *Surgery of the hand and upper extremity.* New York: McGraw-Hill, 1996; 1617–1631.
19. Jones AC, Chuck AJ, Arie EA, et al. Diseases associated with calcium pyrophosphate deposition disease. *Semin Arthritis Rheum* 1992;22:188–202.
20. Resnik CS, Resnick D. Crystal deposition disease. *Semin Arthritis Rheum* 1983;12:390–403.
21. Resnik CS, Miller BW, Gelberman RH, Resnick D. Hand and wrist involvement in calcium pyrophosphate dihydrate crystal deposition disease. *J Hand Surg [Am]* 1983;8:856–863.
22. Schumacher HR. Crystal-induced arthritis: an overview. *Am J Med* 1996;100:46S–52S.
23. Beutler A, Schumacher HRJ. Gout and "pseudogout." When are arthritic symptoms caused by crystal deposition? *Postgrad Med* 1994;95:103–106.
24. McCarty DJ. Crystal identification in human synovial fluids. Methods and interpretation. *Rheum Dis Clin North Am* 1988;14: 253–267.
25. Smathers RL, Stelling CB, Keats TE. The destructive wrist arthropathy of pseudogout. *Skel Radiol* 1982;7:255–258.
26. Stern PJ, Weinberg S. Pathological fracture of the radius through a cyst caused by pyrophosphate arthropathy. Report of a case. *J Bone Joint Surg Am* 1981;63:1487–1488.
27. Yang BY, Sartoris DJ, Djukic S, et al. Distribution of calcification in the triangular fibrocartilage region in 181 patients with calcium pyrophosphate dihydrate crystal deposition disease. *Radiology* 1995;196:547–550.
28. Alvarellos A, Spilberg I. Colchicine prophylaxis in pseudogout. *J Rheumatol* 1986;13:804–805.

OVERVIEW OF ULNAR WRIST PAIN

JAMES R. SKAHEN III
ANDREW K. PALMER

The evaluation and workup of ulnar wrist pain can be a frustrating experience, even to the most seasoned hand surgeon. Over the past two decades, this frustration has resulted in an explosion of research, the results of which have forever changed our approach to the painful ulnar wrist. Through a better understanding of the anatomy, biomechanics, and pathology, we are now in a better position than ever to diagnose and treat ulnar wrist pain. Ulnar wrist pain is not a diagnosis but an invitation to investigate further.

This chapter provides an overview of the problems most commonly encountered in the differential diagnosis of ulnar wrist pain. A basic understanding of the anatomy and biomechanics, combined with history, physical examination, and appropriate diagnostic modalities, will provide solutions to a vast majority of ulnar wrist problems.

HISTORY

The evaluation of ulnar wrist pain is best approached systematically. A detailed history and physical exam can provide clues to the etiology and will help focus our diagnostic tests. Clinical examination of the wrist is a skill that can be mastered only by practice, repetition, and close attention to details.

A complete medical history and review of systems can quickly and easily be obtained by having patients complete an intake form at the initial presentation. A variety of systemic disorders including hypothyroidism, diabetes, and gout can provide important diagnostic clues. Injuries to the upper extremity and cervical spine should be noted. Past surgical history as it pertains to the cervical spine and extremity should be explored. Work history and avocations provide insight into our patient's physical demands and needs.

The mechanism of injury is very important. Biomechanics and clinical studies have taught us that various injuries follow a continuum of patterns, ranging from mild to severe (1). Understanding these mechanisms of injury can heighten our suspicion for a specific problem. Symptomatic complaints are also important. Does the patient complain of clicking, snapping, or locking, or pain in the wrist? If so, when do these symptoms occur, and what activities provoke them? Is the pain described as sharp, dull, aching, or burning in nature? Pain is a subjective complaint that is difficult to quantify and cannot be objectively confirmed. Numeric analog scales for pain, where zero represents no pain and 10 represents severe pain, can be useful in understanding our patients' interpretation of this complaint. Has the patient experienced any swelling, erythema, or ecchymosis, and, if so, where and how long did it persist? We must inquire about weakness, numbness, tingling, cold intolerance, or color changes in the hand and wrist.

Many of our patients have already been evaluated and treated by other health care professionals. Previous diagnoses, tests, treatments, and therapies are important to note because they may provide significant diagnostic clues. A complete review of the available information can greatly narrow our differential diagnoses.

A complete history provides the foundation for our examination and workup. In addition, it allows us to establish a relationship with our patient. The importance of the clinical history is expanded on later, as it is applied to a variety of clinical disorders.

PHYSICAL EXAM

The examination of upper extremity disorders is best performed with the examiner seated, facing the patient, across a hand table. A systematic exam can be done easily from this position and should be done in the same order for each patient. For example, one should examine the neurologic, vascular, and musculoskeletal systems, from proximal to distal, in each patient. This systems approach will enhance the reproducibility of one's exam and minimize the risk of missing important physical findings.

J. R. Skahen III: Department of Orthopaedic Surgery, Northeast Medical Center, and Northeast Orthopaedics, Concord, North Carolina 28025.

A. K. Palmer: Department Orthopedic Surgery, State University of New York Health Science Center at Syracuse, Syracuse, New York 13202.

Evaluation of ulnar wrist pain begins with the cervical spine. Decreased range of motion or a positive Spurling's test could indicate a cervical radiculopathy. This initial portion of the examination should include motor testing and deep tendon reflexes. Sensory examination includes two-point discrimination, Semmes-Weinstein monofilament testing, or vibration sense.

Vascular examination of the upper extremity includes Adson's and Wright's tests for thoracic outlet syndrome. In addition to the radial pulse and capillary refill, Allen's test is important to screen for ulnar artery thrombosis. Capillary refill can be assessed at the nailbeds and should be less than 1 second.

The next stage of the physical examination concentrates on the musculoskeletal system. Active and passive range of motion should be recorded for the shoulders, elbows, wrists, and digits. The contralateral extremity usually serves as a nice control. We must always keep in mind that problems at the wrist can be the result of problems elsewhere. For example, a fractured radial head can be associated with acute or chronic dysfunction of the distal radioulnar joint (DRUJ).

A variety of provocative maneuvers have been described to assist in the examination of the ulnar wrist. Although no test is pathognomonic for a specific disorder, they are very useful. Each maneuver should be done on every patient, in a specific order. We prefer to examine the scapholunate, lunotriquetral (LT), midcarpal, distal radioulnar, and pisotriquetral (PT) joints in order, followed by an examination of the triangular fibrocartilage complex (TFCC).

The *shake test* is performed by grasping the patient's forearm and gently shaking the relaxed wrist and hand. A positive shake test produces pain and protective posturing and may be consistent with inflammation or synovitis.

The LT joint can be evaluated with the *LT ballottement test* (2). The lunate is fixed with the thumb and index of one hand, and the other hand of the examiner applies a dorsal and palmar force across the LT joint. Pain, crepitus, and excessive motion are an abnormal finding. The *shuck test* is also specific to the LT joint (3). The examiner's fingers are placed in a dorsal position over the LT joint with the thumb over the pisiform. The wrist is then taken through active and passive radial and ulnar deviation. Clicking or pain may indicate LT instability.

Instability of the DRUJ can be evaluated with the *piano key* test. The radius is held in a fixed position, and the distal ulna is subjected to dorsal and palmar loading. This should be done in pronation, supination, and neutral forearm rotation. Increased translation of the ulnar head in comparison to the opposite side may indicate injury to the palmar or dorsal radioulnar ligaments of the TFCC (4). Manual compression of the DRUJ during active rotation may elicit pain or crepitus, indicating chondromalacia, impingement, or arthritis.

PT joint disorders can be assessed with provocative maneuvers (5,6). The *PT grind test* is performed by gentle compression of the pisiform onto the triquetrum with a circular motion. Pain and crepitus form a positive finding. The PT apprehension test is performed by placing an ulnar-directed force on the pisiform with the wrist in neutral position. Pain or apprehensive posturing by the patient suggests PT instability.

The *TFCC stress test* can be performed by firmly grasping the hand and the forearm. The wrist is then placed under compressive load in ulnar deviation while the carpus is flexed and extended. Pain, crepitus, or clicking is abnormal and may indicate a TFCC tear or ulnar impaction syndrome (7). Next, the extensor carpi ulnaris (ECU) tendon can be assessed for subluxation in a position of supination, ulnar deviation, and palmar flexion.

Grip strength can be easily measured in the office setting with a commercially available Jamar dynamometer. Setting I generally tests the strength of the intrinsics. Settings IV and V test the extrinsics or flexors. The settings in the midrange, II and III, test a combination of intrinsic and extrinsic strength. If strength is plotted against grip position, the normal distribution forms a bell curve. Results can obviously be altered by pain inhibition or lack of effort. The *rapid exchange grip test* is also a useful screen. In performing this test, the dynamometer is passed from one hand to another with maximal grip used each time. Normally, grip strength should decrease with each cycle, as fatigue becomes a factor. Submaximal effort will often manifest as increased grip strength with cycling or dramatically inconsistent measurements (8,9).

DIAGNOSTIC EVALUATION

A variety of diagnostic modalities are avaliable to assist us in making the correct diagnosis. These tests include radiographs, arthrograms, bone scans, computed tomography (CT) scans, magnetic resonance images (MRIs), serology, arthrocentesis, and diagnostic arthroscopy. A basic understanding of the applications and limitations of each modality will allow us to maximize our efforts.

Radiographs

Plain radiographs continue to be the mainstay of our initial workup. Simple posteroanterior (PA) and lateral radiographs of the wrist can provide much information. These films should be taken with the patient seated in neutral forearm rotation with the elbow flexed 90° and the shoulder abducted 90° (10) (Fig. 37.1). A single PA film with maximum grip may be of value if ulnar impaction is suspected. This standardized approach allows us to more accurately assess ulnar variance and carpal anatomy (11). Each radiograph should be assessed for soft tissue swelling or calcifications, arthritis and other bony pathology, carpal instability, and ulnar variance. Additional views can be added

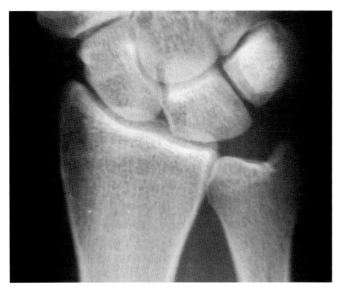

FIGURE 37.1. Single posteroanterior radiograph taken with the elbow flexed 90°, the shoulder abducted 90°, and the forearm in neutral forearm rotation. The ulnar variance is minus 1 mm.

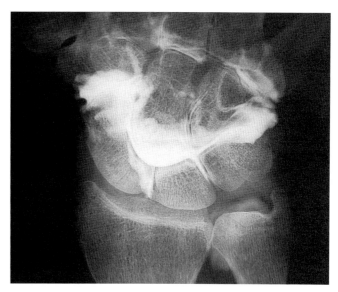

FIGURE 37.2. Normal midcarpal injection during a three-compartment arthrogram.

based on clinical suspicion. For example, a carpal tunnel view can be helpful in identifying a fracture of the hook of the hamate or PT pathology. An oblique view in 30° of supination will nicely profile the PT joint. Fluoroscopic evaluation can be helpful if ligamentous instability is suspected. It can also provide valuable information when plain radiographs are unremarkable and the physical exam is nonspecific (12).

Arthrograms

Arthrography of the wrist continues to be an important diagnostic tool (13–16). It may be used when our examination suggests abnormalities of the TFCC or the interosseous ligaments. A single radiocarpal injection of contrast and fluoroscopic examination can accurately identify many perforations in the membranous portions of the scapholunate and LT interosseous ligaments and the TFCC. However, a triple-injection arthrogram is necessary for a complete examination (Figs. 37.2 and 37.3).

The triple-injection arthrogram has two phases. The first phase begins with the injection of 1 to 3 cc of Renografin 60 and lidocaine solution into the radiocarpal joint under sterile conditions. Contrast flow is observed under fluoroscopic visualization, and appropriate spot films are taken. The wrist is then taken through dorsiflexion, palmar flexion, radial and ulnar deviation, and compression by grip to rule out small or positional leaks. The second phase of this test must be delayed for approximately 3 hours to allow for the absorption of the contrast from the radiocarpal injection. Phase 2 includes the injection of contrast and lidocaine into the DRUJ, followed by the midcarpal joint. It is important to follow the contrast fluoroscopically and to take spot films when necessary. The wrist should also be taken through a range of motion as done in phase 1. The triple-injection arthrogram enhances our ability to assess midcarpal and DRUJ pathology by identifying small, positional, or one-way communications (17). This examination should be performed by a skilled radiologist or clinician trained in the application and interpretation of this test. Digital subtraction arthrograms can more precisely determine the location of abnormal communication or perforation (18).

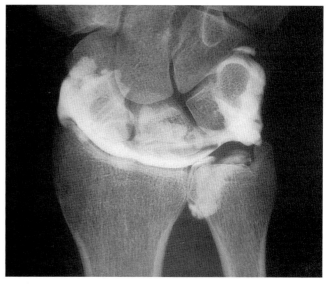

FIGURE 37.3. Triangular fibrocartilage complex perforation found during the radiocarpal injection of a three-compartment arthrogram.

Interpretation of arthrographic results must be correlated with clinical findings. It is also essential to keep in mind the age-related changes seen in the ulnar side of the wrist. Degenerative perforations of the TFCC and LT ligament do not occur before the third decade (19). This suggests that the wrist arthrogram may be more useful in the evaluation of ulnar wrist pain in those patients under age 40.

Bone Scan

Radionuclide imaging can be a useful tool in the screening of chronic ulnar wrist pain. This study typically involves the injection of ^{99}Tc-methylene diphosphate, followed by diagnostic imaging in three phases. Bone scans are highly sensitive but rather nonspecific. A recent study found that bone scans were 95% abnormal with complete intrinsic ligament tears and occult fractures (20). The bone scan is also useful in the evaluation of suspected reflex sympathetic dystrophy (RSD) (21). Typically, diffuse uptake seen in all three phases is believed to be consistent with RSD. Last, it has been suggested that the negative bone scan raises the suspicion of malingering (22).

Magnetic Resonance Imaging

MRI may become an important diagnostic tool in the evaluation of the wrist. Its unique ability to differentiate soft tissue qualities on the basis of their characteristic proton density and relaxation properties makes it ideal to evaluate the ulnar wrist. Several authors have documented the ability of MRI to identify normal and pathologic conditions of the wrist (23–29). MR imaging of the wrist can identify intrinsic and extrinsic ligament tears, TFCC injuries, tumors, occult ganglia, and avascular necrosis of the lunate (Fig. 37.4). This study requires a specially designed wrist coil, specific relaxation and echo times, and a highly skilled musculoskeletal radiologist trained in the interpretation of these images. MRI is currently overused and should not be thought of as the solution to all of our diagnostic dilemmas. It is not a substitute for physical examination, plain radiographs, and other diagnostic modalities. MRI must always be correlated with clinical findings. As our knowledge base increases, and the cost of imaging decreases, MR imaging will likely become an attractive, noninvasive diagnostic option.

Computed Tomography Scan

CT of the wrist can provide the clinician with a detailed look at the bony and articular anatomy of the wrist. Details are enhanced, and greater information can be obtained with 1- to 2-mm fine cuts with the plane of the scan appropriately directed to the suspected area of pathology (30). CT scan is useful in identifying occult fractures of the carpus (31). In particular, fractures of the hook or body of the hamate are easily identified (32). Disorders of the DRUJ such as subluxation and arthritis can be evaluated with the CT scan (33,34). Recently, three-dimensional CT of the wrist has been introduced (35). In the future, this technique may prove useful in the assessment of carpal instabilities.

Ultrasound

Diagnostic ultrasound has long been a safe and noninvasive way to evaluate soft tissue anatomy. It is commonly used in obstetrics, urology, and general surgery but rarely used in orthopedics, with the exception of evaluating developmental dislocation of the hips. Recently, it has been suggested that high-resolution ultrasound can be useful in evaluating foreign bodies, tendon ruptures or adhesions, tendinitis, or ganglion cysts (36). At this point, more research is needed to define its diagnostic applications.

Arthrocentesis

Needle aspiration of the wrist is often indicated in the workup of the painful and swollen wrist. Under sterile conditions, the radiocarpal joint is easily aspirated. It is located approximately 1 cm distal to Lister's tubercle. Gentle longitudinal traction placed across the wrist will facilitate the procedure. The fluid aspirated is then assessed for color, turbidity, and consistency. Laboratory analysis should include a complete cell count and differential, aerobic and anaerobic cultures, crystal analysis, as well as levels of glucose and protein. A properly obtained and submitted aspirate can help rule out septic arthritis, gout, calcium pyrophosphate dihydrate deposited disease (CPPD) or pseudogout, and inflammatory arthropathies.

Arthroscopy

Diagnostic arthroscopy is rapidly becoming an attractive approach in the evaluation of ulnar wrist pain. Many

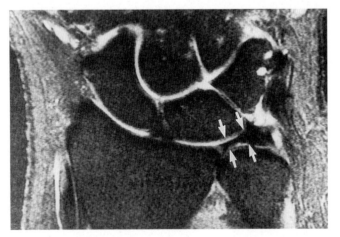

FIGURE 37.4. *White arrows* indicate an intact triangular fibrocartilage complex as seen on a T2-weighted MR image of the wrist.

authors have reported its superiority to arthrography in the diagnosis of interosseous ligament tears and TFCC tears (37–39). Studies such as the arthrogram and MRI provide us with indirect evidence of pathology. Arthroscopy, on the other hand, allows us to directly visualize the nature, location, and extent of the lesion without the need for arthrotomy (40). It also provides the opportunity for treatment. Wrist arthroscopy may be indicated in the evaluation and treatment of ulnar wrist pain if our physical examination and workup suggest an acute or chronic ligament tear, TFCC abnormality, ulnar impaction, hamate arthrosis, or loose body.

Wrist arthroscopy requires a 2.7-mm arthroscope, traction tower, and specialized instrumentation. Generally, this procedure is done under regional anesthesia, using a tourniquet. A complete evaluation of the radiocarpal joint through the 3,4 and 4,5 or 6R portals, as well as evaluation of the midcarpal joint through the midcarpal radial and ulnar portals, is required. It is also possible to evaluate the DRUJ arthroscopically. Arthroscopic findings must be clinically correlated before one proceeds with arthroscopic surgery. Diagnostic and surgical wrist arthroscopy is a learned skill that requires specialized training and a detailed understanding of the anatomy and variation of the wrist. When used in the proper setting, wrist arthroscopy can be a valuable tool in the evaluation and treatment of ulnar wrist pain.

DIFFERENTIAL DIAGNOSIS OF CHRONIC ULNAR WRIST PAIN

Triangular Fibrocartilage Complex Lesions

The TFCC is a collection of cartilaginous and ligamentous structures on the ulnar side of the wrist responsible for stabilizing the DRUJ, stabilizing the ulnar carpus, and transferring load from the ulnar carpus to the distal ulna (41,42). Anatomically, it consists of the articular disc or meniscus homolog, the dorsal and palmar radioulnar ligaments, the ulnolunate, the ulnotriquetral, and the ulnar collateral ligaments (43). These structures can be difficult to identify externally but are easily identified at the time of arthrotomy or arthroscopy (44). The peripheral 15% to 25% of the TFCC receives its blood supply from the palmar and dorsal radiocarpal branches of the ulnar artery and the dorsal and palmar branches of the anterior interosseous artery, whereas the central portion is avascular (45–47). This fact is very important when surgical repair is considered.

Lesions of the TFCC can be degenerative or traumatic. Traumatic injuries can be caused by axial loading during a fall, acute forearm rotation, or a distraction injury to the wrist (48). These injuries can occur in isolation or in conjuction with other injuries such as the fractured distal radius, the Essex-Lopresti injury, or Galeazzi fractures. Degenerative lesions may result from chronic overload of the ulnar carpus or from systemic arthropathies such as gout, CPPD, or other inflammatory arthropathies.

Patients frequently present complaining of ulnar-sided wrist pain, clicking, or snapping. Tasks that require gripping, grasping, or forearm rotation are often problematic. Physical examination will likely find tenderness and swelling around the TFCC, ulnar carpus, and DRUJ. The TFCC stress test may also be positive. The workup should initially include x-rays to assess ulnar variance and to rule out other bony or ligamentous pathology. Further studies such as the arthrogram, MRI, or wrist arthroscopy are very useful and should be employed when there is a high index of suspicion for injury to the TFCC.

Palmer has developed a classification scheme based on anatomic, biomechanical, and clinical observations, which has led to lesion-specific treatment programs (49). Class 1 abnormalities are traumatic in origin. These injuries have been further subdivided into types A through D. Class 1A lesions are traumatic tears of the articular disc, from dorsal to palmar; 1B injuries involve avulsion off the distal ulna, with or without fracture of the ulnar styloid; 1C injuries include traumatic disruption of the ulnolunate or ulnotriquetral ligaments of the TFCC; and 1D injuries include disruption of the TFCC from its attachment on the sigmoid notch of the radius. It is important to remember that class 1B through 1D injuries may be associated with significant instability of the DRUJ and ulnar carpus.

The treatment of class 1 injuries without evidence of instability should begin with a 4- to 6-week course of immobilization. Generally, a long arm cast with the forearm in neutral rotation or a short arm cast with an interosseous mold to prevent rotation is recommended. If the injury has occurred within the zone of vascularity, it has a strong chance of healing during this time. Those injuries that have failed conservative care or that present with frank instability need to be addressed surgically. Biomechanical and clinical studies have demonstrated that unstable 1B injuries, with a displaced ulnar styloid fracture, respond favorably to primary repair (50). Class 1, types A, C, and D injuries can be treated surgically (51–57).

Class 2 abnormalities are degenerative in nature and fall along a continuum from mild chondromalacia to end-stage ulnar impaction syndrome. Patients with neutral or ulnar positive variance are overrepresented in this class (58) (Fig. 37.5). It must always be remembered that many of these abnormalities can be an age-related asymptomatic phenomena (59). Therefore, findings must always be correlated with the clinical picture. In class 2A, we see mild chondromalacia of the articular disc, without evidence of perforation. Class 2B includes chondromalacia of the ulnar head and/or lunate. It is not until class 2C that the description includes a degenerative perforation of the TFCC. As we progress to 2D, the degenerative changes become more

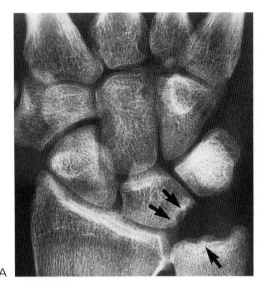 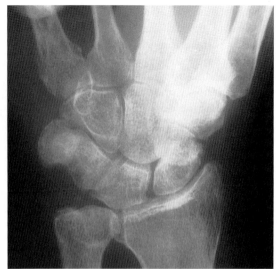

FIGURE 37.5. A: Ulnar impaction syndrome with arthritic changes in the ulnar head and cystic change in the lunate *(black arrows)*. **B:** Ulnar impaction syndrome associated with ulnar positive variance.

advanced, and the LT ligament is disrupted. Finally, 2E represents end-stage ulnar impaction with perforation of the TFCC and LT ligament and advanced arthritis of the ulnar carpus and DRUJ.

Treatment of class 2 TFCC abnormalities can also be approached conservatively. Immobilization, nonsteroidals, cortisone injections, and activity modification may prove useful. When conservative treatment has failed, a variety of surgical options have been advocated. These procedures include debridement, ulnar shortening, partial or complete excision of the ulnar head, and several techniques for interposition arthroplasty (60–65).

Ulnar Impingement Syndrome

Ulnar impingement syndrome most commonly is an iatrogenic instability problem caused by distal ulnar resection. It can also result from growth arrest of the ulnar epiphysis, or congenital abnormalities such as Madelung's deformity. The shortened distal ulna converges on the distal radius, resulting in a painful pseudarthrosis (66). This term should not be confused with ulnar impaction syndrome discussed above. Patients with ulnar impingement will demonstrate pain and crepitus in the DRUJ with pronation and supination, limited forearm rotation, tenderness over the distal ulna, weakness in grip, and possibly a positive piano key sign. Radiographs will often demonstrate scalloping of the distal radius in response to the converging and impinging distal ulna (Fig. 37.6).

Treatment involves restoring stability to the distal ulna. A variety of techniques have been developed that utilize the tenodesis effect of the ECU and/or flexor carpi ulnaris (FCU), and soft tissue interposition.

Distal Radioulnar Joint Arthritis

Arthritis in the DRUJ can be the result of trauma or systemic disorders such as rheumatoid arthritis. Patients will complain of pain, clicking, weakness of grip, and decreased range of motion. Plain radiographs may demonstrate joint narrowing, irregularities, or osteophyte formation. Perhaps the best diagnostic tool is the CT scan through the DRUJ. The opposite wrist can be used in comparison. Recently, diagnostic arthroscopy of the DRUJ was introduced (67). Although difficult to perform, it can provide direct visualization of pathology in the DRUJ.

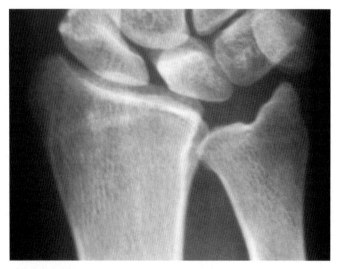

FIGURE 37.6. Ulnar impingement syndrome. Radiograph demonstrates scalloping of the sigmoid notch of the radius by the distal ulna.

Conservative care consisting of nonsteroidals, cortisone injection and activity modification may be of benefit. Immobilization will likely result in persistent disability and greater stiffness. Failure of conservative care is an indication for operative intervention. Occasionally, congruency can be restored to the DRUJ by correcting the precipitating malalignment, if the degree of degeneration is mild. For example, an osteotomy of a malunited distal radius fracture, or an ulnar shortening, may restore normal load characteristics to the DRUJ, slowing or halting degeneration. Treatment options for advanced cases include distal ulna resection, hemiresection and hemiresection with interposition. Proper patient selection, knowledge of the available procedures and experience in their application is essential to optimal outcome.

Ulnar Styloid Nonunion

Fracture of the ulnar styloid may occur in association with a distal radius fracture, or as an isolated injury. In the absence of DRUJ instability, most of these injuries respond well to a simple course of immobilization. Rarely, do these injuries result in symptomatic nonunions. Symptomatic ulnar styloid nonunions have been classified into two types, based on location and stability of the DRUJ (68) (Fig. 37.7). A stable DRUJ is found with symptomatic type 1 nonunions. These injuries may result from a direct blow, resulting in a fracture of the tip of the ulnar styloid, leaving the major attachments to the TFCC intact. Type 2 nonunions are unstable, and involve the base of the ulnar styloid. They are often the result of forced extension in a hyperpronated or hypersupinated position (69). By definition, these injuries are associated with disruption of the ulnar attachments of the TFCC, a Palmer 1B injury. Hence, the type 2 nonunion is associated with chronic instability of the DRUJ.

Clinically, these patients may complain of chronic aching ulnar wrist pain exacerbated by gripping, grasping, or twisting type activities. Physical examination will demonstrate tenderness over the ulnar styloid, and possibly clicking or grating in the DRUJ with forearm rotation. Instability should be looked for with the piano key test. Plain radiographs are useful in making the diagnosis and for screening other pathology. A CT scan of the DRUJ can be helpful in identifying subtle subluxation or instability.

Treatment of the symptomatic ulnar styloid nonunion is based on the classification scheme. Conservative treatment including immobilization, nonsteroidals, injections, and physical therapy are worth trying for 6 weeks, but it should be kept in mind that these patients have already been treated conservatively and are not likely to respond. Type 1 nonunions respond well to simple excision and early mobilization. Surgical treatment of type 2 nonunions is more complex. Large fragments are best treated by open reduction and internal fixation, using the tension band technique or screw fixation. Smaller fragments or multiple fragments are best treated with excision and reattachment of the TFCC to the distal ulna. Postoperatively, these patients are managed in a long arm cast for a minimum of 6 weeks.

Extensor Carpi Ulnaris Subluxation

The ECU tendon is located in the sixth dorsal compartment of the wrist. This fibroosseous compartment is unique in that the ECU tendon is confined to the ulnar groove by a subsheath, separate from the extensor retinaculum of the wrist (70,71). The ulnar border of the subsheath can be ruptured by forced hypersupination, palmar flexion, and ulnar deviation, resulting in subluxation or dislocation of the ECU tendon from the ulnar groove (72). Partial rupture

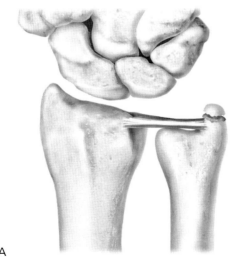
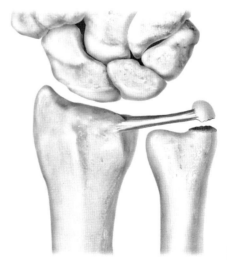

FIGURE 37.7. A: Type 1 ulnar styloid nonunion with stable distal radioulnar joint (DRUJ). **B:** Type 2 ulnar styloid nonunion with unstable DRUJ.

of the subsheath can lead to symptomatic attenuation of the ECU tendon and possibly rupture (73). Additional injuries to the TFCC must also be ruled out. This injury often goes unrecognized or is misdiagnosed as tendinitis, DRUJ instability, or TFCC injury (74).

At presentation, patients will complain of a painful snapping on the dorsal ulnar border of the wrist. Physical examination will demonstrate subluxation of the ECU tendon with supination, ulnar deviation, and palmar flexion and reduction with pronation, radial deviation, and dorsiflexion. This can also be demonstrated by grasping the ECU between the thumb and index finger and applying an ulnar directed force to the tendon, with the forearm supinated. Gross instability will be apparent. It is very important to examine the asymptomatic wrist, as mild, bilateral, asymptomatic subluxation is not uncommon. Plain radiographs will likely be normal. MRI of the DRUJ bilaterally, with the wrist supinated, extended, and ulnarly deviated, may reveal subluxation of the ECU tendon.

Theoretically, acute injuries could be treated conservatively in a long arm cast with the forearm pronated and the wrist in slight dorsiflexion and radial deviation. Unfortunately, the few acute injuries discussed in the literature have been treated surgically (75,76). It is generally agreed that chronic cases respond best to surgical reconstruction of the subsheath. A variety of techniques have been suggested and are well described is the literature cited above.

Pisotriquetral Joint Dysfunction

The pisiform is contained within the fibers of the FCU tendon and is the only sesmoid bone of the carpus. It forms a synovial articulation with the triquetrum. A variety of structures insert on the pisiform, including the FCU tendon, pisohamate ligament, pisometacarpal ligament, TFCC, transverse carpal ligament, volar carpal ligament, extensor retinaculum, abductor digiti minimi, and the PT joint capsule. The exact biomechanical function of the pisiform is not known, but it is believed to increase the flexion force of the FCU tendon by acting as a fulcrum (77). This study also found that the radial structures were the strongest, suggesting that compromise of these structures produces instability of the PT joint, with eventual degenerative arthritis (Fig. 37.8). Injury can result from a fall or blow to the hypothenar aspect of the hand and may occur in combination with other injuries of the wrist. In the acute setting, a fracture of the pisiform should be ruled out.

Patients with PT joint dysfunction complain of pain in the hypothenar region of the hand. Provocative maneuvers such as the PT grind test and the PT apprehension test will likely be positive. Up to one-third of these patients will also have an associated ulnar neuropathy (78). Because of the close proximity of the ulnar artery, an Allen's test should also be performed to rule out ulnar artery thrombosis. Radiographically, arthrosis may be identified with either a

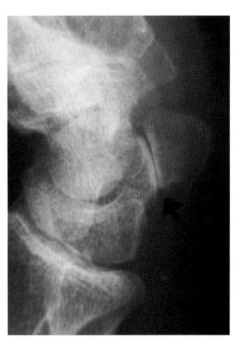

FIGURE 37.8. Pisotriquetral joint arthritis, as seen with the 30° supination view.

carpal tunnel view or a 30° supination view. On occasion, a CT scan will be helpful. Clinical suspicion can be confirmed with a local injection of lidocaine into the PT joint, producing complete, but temporary, relief.

Initial treatment of PT joint dysfunction should be conservative. Splinting, nonsteroidals, and cortisone injections may provide lasting relief. Fractures generally respond well to immobilization in a short arm cast, in slight ulnar deviation and palmar flexion, for 6 weeks. Failure of conservative care is an indication for excision of the pisiform. The pisiform can be approached through a palmar incision, splitting the fibers of the FCU. Care should be taken to protect the ulnar neurovascular bundle and ligamentous attachments. Postoperatively, patients can be managed with a soft dressing and early range of motion. Pisiformectomy can reliably relieve pain without sacrificing function (79,80). Isometric and isokinetic testing indicates that pisiformectomy decreases wrist flexion strength without functional deficit or loss of motion (81).

Hamate Fractures

The hamate is the ulnarmost bone in the distal carpal row. It forms an articulation with the bases of the ring and small finger metacarpals, capitate, triquetrum, and with type 2 lunates. The hamate is relatively fixed to the capitate, but it is subjected to motion at the carpometacarpal and triquetral hamate joints. The helical geometry of its proximal articulation with the triquetrum helps initiate flexion and extension of the proximal carpal row with wrist deviation. Dorsally, the hamate is bound by the thin dorsal triquetral ligament complex, and volarly it is bound by the pisohamate ligament and the ulnar branch of the volar arucate ligament (82). The hook of the hamate forms the ulnar wall of the carpal tunnel and serves as an attachment sight for the transverse carpal ligament. The ulnar neurovascular bundle and flexor tendons are in close proximity to the hook.

Fracture of the hamate can occur as the result of an axial blow by a clenched fist or a direct blow to the hypothenar eminence. Force directed at the hook of the hamate by a baseball bat, a golf club, or a tennis racquet can also result in fracture. These fractures not only involve the hook but can also involve the body of the hamate in coronal or sagittal planes and hence become intraarticular (83,84). Dislocations of the ring and small finger carpometacarpal joints are often associated with a fractured hamate.

Acutely, the patient will present with pain, swelling, and ecchymosis on the ulnar border of the wrist. Point tenderness over the dorsal aspect of the hamate or over the hook palmarly will be present. The carpometacarpal joints should always be checked for range of motion, stability, crepitus, and pain. The ulnar nerve, ulnar artery, and flexor tendons are at risk and should be thoroughly examined. These fractures are often missed and may present late as a nonunion with chronic ulnar wrist pain. Hamate hook fractures can also be silent and should always be excluded when a patient presents with a flexor tendon rupture to the ring or small finger (85).

Radiographic evaluation should include anteroposterior (AP), lateral, oblique, and carpal tunnel views. Fractures of the body are often not visible on standard radiographs. If an occult fracture or fracture-dislocation is suspected, an axial CT scan of the wrist is very useful (86,87) (Fig. 37.9).

Acute fractures of the hamate hook can be treated conservatively in a short arm cast. A review of the literature found that 45.9% of these fractures will unite if immobilized for 6 weeks to 4 months (88). Inclusion of the ring and small finger metacarpophalangeal joints may improve the union rate (89). For those patients who fail conservative care or cannot be immobilized for a prolonged time, surgical excision of the fragment will provide excellent results in a majority of patients (90). The hamate can be excised through the standard approach on the ulnar side of the carpal tunnel. Guyon's canal should also be released, so the ulnar neurovascular structures can be protected. The fragment can then be excised. It is recommended that the remaining hook be removed to the base, preventing a recurrent fracture and the possibility of tendon rupture in the future. Postoperatively, the wrist can be splinted for 5 to 7 days, after which range of motion can be started.

Acute fractures of the body can also be treated conservatively if they are stable and minimally displaced. Any fracture with intraarticular displacement, joint subluxation, or instability must be dealt with surgically. Reduction and fixation, with wires or mini fragment screws, can usually be accomplished through a dorsal ulnar approach. Immobilization and pins should be continued for approximately 4 to 6 weeks postoperatively.

Triquetrum Fractures

Fracture of the triquetrum can occur as an isolated injury or as part of a greater arc injury, such as a transtriquetral perilunate dislocation (91). The mechanism of injury is usually a fall on an outstretched arm with a dorsiflexed wrist. These fractures are generally believed to result from ligamentous avulsion. However, it has been suggested that the ulnar styloid can act as a chisel on the dorsum of the triquetrum during extreme dorsiflexion and ulnar deviation (92).

Patients will present with pain, swelling, tenderness, and perhaps ecchymosis over the dorsum of the triquetrum. In addition to standard radiographs, an oblique in 30° of pronation may reveal the fracture. If radiographs are negative but a high index of suspicion remains, an axial CT scan should be obtained.

Isolated triquetrum fractures respond well to 6 weeks of immobilization in a short arm cast. Those fractures associated with greater arch injuries must be surgically treated with reduction and stabilization.

Hamate Arthrosis

Arthrosis of the proximal pole of the hamate should be included in the differential diagnosis of ulnar wrist pain. A recent anatomic study found cartilage erosion at the proximal pole of the hamate in 38% of specimens (93,94). This study found a significant correlation between arthrosis and the presence of a lunate facet for the hamate, a type II lunate. Arthrosis was found in 38% of specimens with type II lunates and in only 2% with type I lunates.

Diagnosis is difficult to make clinically but should be suspected in those patients with type II lunates, where all other diagnoses have been excluded. Arthroscopically, this lesion is easily identified through the midcarpal portals. If it

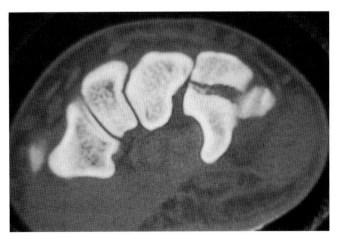

FIGURE 37.9. Coronal fracture of the body of the hamate seen only on axial computed tomography scan.

is suspected in the etiology of chronic ulnar wrist pain, arthroscopic removal of the proximal pole may provide relief by unloading its articulation with the lunate. However, this approach has not been adequately studied to be recommended as a standard of care.

Stenosing Tenosynovitis of the Extensor Carpi Ulnaris

Stenosing tenosynovitis of the sixth dorsal compartment of the wrist is an uncommon cause of chronic ulnar wrist pain but should be included in the differential diagnosis. Chronic ECU tendinitis and swelling cannot be accommodated by the relatively unyielding fibroosseous tunnel. In time, the subsheath can become thickened and stenotic, much like de Quervain's tenosynovitis, further exacerbating the problem (95).

Patients may present with pain, swelling, and tenderness along the ECU tendon. Symptoms may be exacerbated or reproduced with resisted wrist dorsiflexion and ulnar deviation, passive radial deviation, and will be relieved by injection of lidocaine into the subsheath (96). This condition can be easily confused with subluxation of the ECU tendon, and this should be ruled out.

Conservative treatments such as activity modification, nonsteroidals, cortisone injection, or casting with the wrist in slight dorsiflexion and ulnar deviation may alleviate the symptoms. Those patients who fail conservative treatments may benefit from surgical release of the sixth dorsal compartment (97). The ECU can be approached through a dorsal longitudinal incision. The extensor retinaculum is divided on the radial border of the compartment, as is the subsheath. The ulnar subsheath must not be released but, rather, is sutured to the overlying extensor retinaculum. The extensor retinaculum should also be closed. These measures will prevent subluxation of the ECU tendon from the ulnar groove. Postoperatively, the patients can be splinted or casted in slight dorsiflexion for 2 to 3 weeks, after which active range of motion can be instituted.

Lunotriquetral Ligament Tears

Disruption of the LT interosseous ligament should be included in the differential diagnosis of ulnar wrist pain. This ligament may be torn acutely by a hyperextension or twisting injury. The ligament can also be disrupted as part of the ulnar impaction syndrome.

Extrinsic ligaments stabilizing the LT joint include the dorsal radiotriquetral ligament and the volar ulnar carpal ligaments. The intrinsic LT ligament has a thickened dorsal and volar component and a thin membranous central portion. The central membranous portion is a fibrocartilaginous structure and is relatively avascular (98). Disruption of the interosseous portion of the LT ligament results in carpal instability dissociative (CID). This does not result in a volar intercalated segment instability (VISI) deformity or a carpal instability, nondissociative (CIND), which requires disruption of the LT ligament and the ulnar limb of the volar arcuate ligament (99). These injuries have been divided into three stages (100). Stage I includes partial or complete rupture of the LT interosseous ligament, without evidence for a VISI deformity. Stages II and III result in a VISI deformity.

Patients will present with ulnar wrist pain and perhaps a click or snap with wrist motion. Grip strength may be diminished. The LT ballottement test and shuck tests may be positive. Routine radiographs will likely be unremarkable, with the exception of those patients with ulnar positive variance and ulnar impaction syndrome. Wrist arthrography will demonstrate an abnormal communication between the midcarpal and radiocarpal joints through the LT interval. MRI can also demonstrate discontinuity of the LT, best represented by increased signal intensity within the LT ligament, seen on T2 images (101). Wrist arthroscopy can also be an effective tool in the investigation of LT pathology. The interpretation of these studies must always be correlated with the clinical exam. Anatomic dissections have found that LT tears are rare before age 45 but can be found in over 27% of those over age 60 (102).

Acute LT ligament sprains or tears can be initially treated in a well-molded cast for 4 to 6 weeks with good results (103). However, these same authors found that chronic LT tears responded poorly to immobilization. Patients with chronic LT tears, instability, or those who failed conservative management will likely require operative intervention such as ligament repair, reconstruction, or LT fusion.

The development of wrist arthroscopy has added greatly to the treatment of LT tears. Simple arthroscopic debridement of an isolated partial LT tear, with early mobilization, has been reported to provide relief of pain and mechanical symptoms in this select group of patients (104). Osterman believes that the midcarpal joint is the key to assessment and treatment of LT ligament problems (105). The midcarpal view allows one to assess subtle instabilities of the LT joint. He found that 80% of his patients with perforation of the LT ligament, without VISI or CIND, did well with debridement of the LT interval and arthroscopic reduction and pinning of the LT joint for 8 weeks.

EDITORS' COMMENTS

The radial side of the wrist carries the load. The ulnar side of the wrist is supportive but in general does not carry the functional responsibilities of the radial side. The DRUJ is not truly wrist but is concerned with forearm rotation. This division should probably be maintained in our clinical approach to the wrist. Abnormalities on the ulnar side of the wrist will less often shut down function than abnormalities on the load-bearing radial side of the wrist.

Clinical Examination

The clinical examination may be divided into two major components—abnormalities distal to the end of the ulna and the TFC, and abnormalities that involve these structures and those more proximal. The division is easily ascertained clinically by passively rotating the forearm from the midforearm position. Loading the rotation moment from the midforearm leaves no loads distal to the TFC and distal end of the ulna. With marked inflammation in the carpal area [i.e., severe triquetral impingement ligament tear (TILT) syndrome], one may pick up some symptoms at the extremes of supination and pronation, but usually this passive maneuver will indite or eliminate abnormalities of the TFC and DRUJ. The clinical examination remains the key feature for diagnosis on the ulnar side of the wrist. Synovium is the tissue with the greatest pain response. Following clinical examination, the x-rays are the next most important evaluation. These may rarely include CT scanning and arthroscopy. MRIs may demonstrate abnormalities that may or may not match the clinical exam and should be considered supportive, not diagnostic. Arthrograms are not indicated. No surgery should be carried out on the basis of dye passing abnormally through joints. Arthroscopy is rarely indicated. If the clinical situation dictates surgery, then open direct repair with evaluation of the associated injured structures is preferred.

Ulnar Wrist Diagnoses

The following is a breakdown based on statistical frequency of problems on the ulnar side of the wrist. It must be understood that these statistics are the result of a reconstructive hand surgery practice, where acute injuries are referred and emergency room practice is absent. There are three categories of frequency. The first category includes the most common phenomena on the ulnar side of the wrist.

Idiopathic synovitis of the DRUJ is common, frequently from an injury or an activity overload. A change in job activity will often produce a temporary synovitis of the DRUJ. These are obviously best handled with simple conservative means, followed by steroid injection if necessary.

DRUJ subluxation is fairly common. A partial ligamentous tear, which allows hypermobility of the distal end of the ulna, will produce intermittent symptoms but seldom requires surgical treatment. It is relatively common following pronation injuries.

TILT syndrome is common. Symptoms are from periostitis on the ulnar side of the triquetrum secondary to capsular pressure. It is a manifestation of ligament tear but can also be seen following removal of the distal ulna or ulnar carpal translation. Compression occurs between the ulnar aspect of the triquetrum and the ulna sling mechanism. TILT syndrome is described in more detail in Chapter 40.

DRUJ degenerative arthritis is probably the result of lifelong ligamentous tears allowing abnormal motion, which gradually destroy congruity of the DRUJ. Interestingly, the destruction always occurs proximally on the articular surface of the ulna and progresses distally. We have not infrequently been able to solve the problem with a partial arthroplasty of the DRUJ.

Degenerative arthritis at the DRUJ begins proximally and frequently produces multiple episodes of pain and limited function before total destruction of the DRUJ occurs. Limited surgery may be effective as follows.

The patient is operated on under suitable anesthesia. A longitudinal incision is made over the ulna. This can be accomplished through a transverse incision, but the potential for future matched ulnar arthroplasty makes us more comfortable with a longitudinal incision for this procedure. Dorsal blunt dissection is accomplished. The dorsal branch of the ulnar nerve is identified and retracted distally. The ulna capsule is opened from proximally until the joint can be adequately visualized. Destruction occupies the proximal half of the articular surface of the ulna. The distal half of the ulna articular surface has normal cartilage, and the matching articular surface of the sulcus joint of the radius has normal cartilage. Dental rongeurs are then used to resect the proximal half of the articular surface throughout the entire supination–pronation range. This articular surface devoid of cartilage is cut away, leaving a clean edge proximally on the remaining articular cartilage and bone.

Closure is done in standard fashion with a bulk dressing and forearm splint only, so supination and pronation are allowed immediately. The bulk dressing is reduced to a small wrist dressing in 48 hours, and full activity is allowed.

This requires that the distal half of the articular surface be adequate; it probably just delays the eventual distal ulna resection but has been symptomatically effective long term. Major degenerative arthritis of the DRUJ is best treated by matched ulnar arthroplasty.

Partial tears of the triquetrum–lunate joint seldom require limited wrist arthrodeses or other treatment. When symptomatic, they are commonly associated with ulnar impaction syndrome, and step-cut shortening of the ulna is sufficient treatment.

The second category of ulnar wrist diagnoses are less common but not rare. First in this category are symptomatic nonunions of the ulnar styloid. If the very common ulnar styloid fracture is pulled away from the distal end of the ulna, it will remain asymptomatic as a free piece (Editors' Fig. 37.1) (3 mm or more of space between the styloid and the parent ulna). If, on the other hand, the fragment is close to the ulna or touching, a picture resembling degenerative arthritis will occur between the two bones (Editors' Fig. 37.2). The bones will enlarge, osteophytes will form, and increasing symptoms will require removal of the styloid fragment (Editors' Fig. 37.3).

Pisiform degenerative arthritis falls into this middle-frequency category. Pisiformectomy, maintaining continuity of the FCU, is effective treatment (Editors' Fig. 37.4).

Nonunions of the hook of the hamate frequently follow fracture of the hamate. We have previously published work emphasizing the importance of maintaining the hook. MRI studies show a change in direction around 80° as the flexors to the ring and little fingers change direction over the hook of the hamate in full ulnar deviation power grip. Particularly in professional athletes, especially golfers, this pulley mechanism is terribly important, and the patient is best served by bone grafting; the surgery is described in Chapter 12.

ECU stenosing tenosynovitis is also a middle-frequency occurrence and is best handled by conservative means, up to, and including, steroid injection. In classic situations, a cocompartment release is the most effective

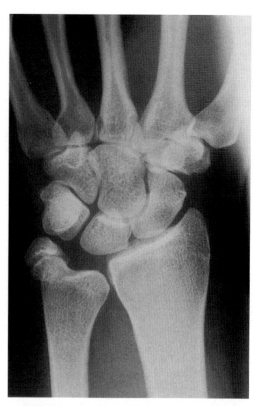

EDITORS' FIGURE 37.2. If the fragment is close to the parent bone, the fragment will enlarge with osteophyte formation and classic changes of nonunion or degenerative arthritis. This situation will usually be markedly symptomatic, requiring removal of the fragment.

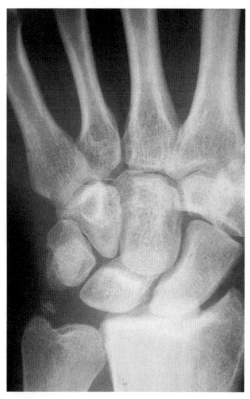

EDITORS' FIGURE 37.1. The typical ulnar styloid fracture is usually pulled far enough away from the parent bone that it remains asymptomatic and of no consequence.

treatment. This maintains the entire extensor retinaculum, requiring no secondary repair while permitting immediate mobilization. Cocompartment release is described in Chapter 76.

Localized impingement of the base of the fifth metacarpal against the hamate is relatively common. Typically, following fractures of the base of the fifth metacarpal, there is impingement of the ulnarmost aspect of the metacarpal against the ulnar aspect of the hamate requiring simple resection arthroplasty.

Ulnar impaction syndrome may be seen in young people with ulnar positive variance. *Impaction* is a term meaning an abnormal contact load between normal structures, as in positive ulnar variance. *Impingement* means abnormal contact between abnormal units such as fracture fragments, osteophytes, resected distal ulna, etc. A second category of ulnar impaction patients are those in the third and fourth decades who have had an ulnar positive variance all their lives. Some activity change or injury brings to light the destructive process slowly occurring between the distal end of the ulna and the proximal ulnar aspect of the lunate. This same group of patients will often demonstrate a partial tear of the tri-

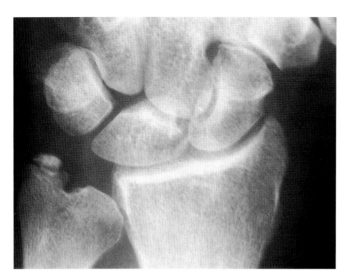

EDITORS' FIGURE 37.3. The styloid fragment is reactive to its close approximation to the ulna. Pain required removal.

quetral–lunate joint secondary to ulnar impaction. The treatment for symptomatic ulnar impaction syndrome is step-cut shortening of the ulna.

Congenital incomplete development of the triquetral–lunate joint may occur with secondary degenerative arthritis. Congenital problems with this joint are the most common congenital abnormalities of the wrist. The joint develops from distal to proximal, and the cartilage is usually normal in the distal half of the joint. The proximal portion of the joint demonstrates bone where cartilage should be. This distinguishes it from degenerative arthritis of this joint secondary to instability and classically has a fluted champagne glass appearance on x-ray. The clinical problems arise as the thin inadequate cartilage in the proximal half of the joint gradually wears out and localized degenerative arthritis occurs, producing symptoms in the third or fourth decade. Treatment is limited wrist arthrodesis of the triquetral–lunate joint.

The third and least common category of ulnar wrist diagnoses includes dislocation of the DRUJ. Complete dislocation is a traumatic event and statistically falls into the third and least common category of ulnar wrist problems. Dislocation occurs from complete rupture of either the dorsal, the volar, or both radioulnar ligaments. In an active person, this usually requires reinsertion. Fortunately, the volar and dorsal radial–ulnar ligaments usually rupture distally from the ulna, and repair is best carried out by reinserting them into the distal ulna. Tears occur between either ligament and the radius but are usually not troublesome enough to require treatment. These injuries are often picked up incidentally on exam.

Total rupture of the triquetral–lunate ligament is in this rare category. Total instability between triquetrum and lunate that is symptomatic requires limited wrist arthrodesis between these two bones.

Ulnar artery thrombosis is usually a phenomenon secondary to direct trauma, either repetitive or a single major injury. The typical picture is a worker using the hand as a hammer. Pain is often severe and out of proportion to physical findings and highly localized in the canal of Guyon. We have found that there is usually adequate collateral circulation, and removal of the artery is the simplest treatment. We have on occasion used vein grafts to maintain an ulnar artery through the canal of Guyon, believing that workers in the North might experience cold sensitivity. On an intuitive basis, this is a more appropriate approach, but we cannot find fault with the success of simple artery excision.

Nonunions of ulnar carpal bones fall into this rare category of causes of ulnar wrist pain and should be grafted.

Degenerative arthritis of the hamate–lunate joint is seldom an isolated phenomenon. In our experience, it is associated with a scapholunate advanced collapse (SLAC) wrist. There are usually some changes between the capitate and the lunate secondary to shear loading and loss of radial wrist support in one form or another. SLAC reconstruction is the usual treatment.

It is now obvious to the reader that the triangular fibrocartilage has not been mentioned in any of the three incidence categories listed above. Although we hesitate to take this position because of the preponderance of literature dealing with repairs of the TFCC, it has been our experience that tears of the ulna–triquetral and ulna–lunate ligaments and tears in the ulnar sling mechanism that do not involve destabilizing the distal ulna

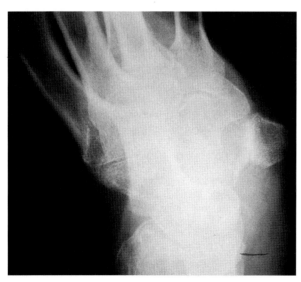

EDITORS' FIGURE 37.4. This subpisiform view demonstrates complete loss of articular cartilage between the pisiform and the triquetrum, with marked sclerosis and osteophyte formation. Pisiformectomy is the indicated procedure.

seldom require a surgical approach. Small flap tears of the triangular fibrocartilage appear to be the most commonly successful arthroscopic procedure. We have found TILT syndrome to be the most common diagnosis in patients referred to us with diagnoses of tears in the triangular fibrocartilage. One phenomenon that may play a role here includes patients with radial wrist problems that limit their load capacity. Typically they have been immobilized or been off work on total inactivity for prolonged periods of time. When first seen, these patients frequently will complain of ulnar wrist symptoms. We have found that placing these patients on 5 hours of artificial loading, usually with a Baltimore Therapeutic Equipment work simulator machine, including forceful loading in all positions, will reproduce the radial-sided symptoms and clarify the diagnosis. This is an important phenomenon in which the inactivity on the load side of the wrist allows the synovium to quiet down, the scaphoid does not displace, and the wrist becomes essentially asymptomatic. The ulnar-sided symptoms prevail. Heavily loading the wrist again makes evident a dynamic rotary subluxation (scapholunate interosseous dissociation), and the ulnar-sided symptoms by comparison diminish. Our only explanation for this phenomenon is that the repetitive injuries or injury that produced the radial-sided ligament tear produces some ulnar-sided tearing or allows some ulnar carpal translation, producing low-grade TILT syndrome, which persists even in the inactive wrist while the function-limiting radial side becomes quiescent. TILT syndrome is difficult to diagnose with an arthroscope because the involved area is under significant compression.

If the ulnar side of the wrist demonstrates a symptomatic component that interferes with the patient's quality of life or requires repair, we think the best approach is a presumptive diagnosis and open surgery with evaluation of any concomitant associated structures and definitive repair as opposed to arthroscopy.

REFERENCES

1. Mayfield JK, Johnson RP, Kilcoyne RK. Carpal dislocations: pathomechanics and progressive perilunar instability. *J Hand Surg [Am]* 1980;5:226–241.
2. Regan DS, Linscheid RL, Dobyns JH. Lunotriquetral sprains. *J Hand Surg [Am]* 1984;9:502–514.
3. Osterman AL, Seidman GD. The role of arthroscopy in the treatment of lunatotriquetral ligament injuries. *Hand Clin* 1995;11:41–50.
4. Ekenstam F. Anatomy of the distal radioulnar joint. *Clin Orthop* 1992;275:14–18.
5. Seradge H, Seradge E. Pisotriquetral pain syndrome after carpal tunnel release. *J Hand Surg [Am]* 1989;14:858–862.
6. Carroll RE, Coyle MP. Dysfunction of the pisotriquetral joint: Treatment by excision of the pisiform. *J Hand Surg [Am]* 1985;10:703–707.
7. Friedman SL, Palmer AK. The ulnar impaction syndrome. *Hand Clin* 1991;7:295–310.
8. Czitrom AA, Lister GD. Measurement of grip strength in the diagnosis of wrist pain. *J Hand Surg [Am]* 1988;13:16–20.
9. Hildreth DH, Breidenbach WC, Lister GD, et al. Detection of submaximal grip effort by use of rapid exchange grip. *J Hand Surg [Am]* 1989;14:742–745.
10. Palmer AK, Glisson RR, Werner FW. Ulnar variance determination. *J Hand Surg [Am]* 1982;7:376–379.
11. Epner RA, Bowers WH, Guilford WB. Ulnar variance—the effect of wrist positioning and roentgen filming technique. *J Hand Surg [Am]* 1982;7:298–305.
12. Hankin FM, White SJ, Braunstein EM, et al. Dynamic radiographic evaluation of obscure wrist pain in the teenage patient. *J Hand Surg [Am]* 1986;11:805–809.
13. Palmer AK, Levinsohn EM, Kuzma GR. Arthrography of the wrist. *J Hand Surg [Am]* 1983;8:15–23.
14. Mikic ZD. Arthrography of the wrist joint. An experimental study. *J Bone Joint Surg Am* 1984;66:371–378.
15. Renius WR, Hardy DC, Trotty WG, et al. Arthrographic evaluation of the carpal triangular fibrocartilage complex. *J Hand Surg [Am]* 1987;12:495–503.
16. Hardy DC, Trotty WG, Carnes KM, et al. Arthrographic surface anatomy of the carpal triangular fibrocartilage complex. *J Hand Surg [Am]* 1988;13:823–829.
17. Zinberg EM, Palmer AK, Coren AB, et al. The triple injection wrist arthrogram. *J Hand Surg [Am]* 1988;13:803–809.
18. Manaster BJ, Mann RJ, Rubenstein S. Wrist pain: Correlation of clinical and plain film findings with arthrographic results. *J Hand Surg [Am]* 1989;14:466–473.
19. Mikic ZD. Age changes in the triangular fibrocartilage of the wrist. *J Anat* 1978,126.367–384.
20. Pin PG, Semenkovich JW, Young VL, et al. Role of radionuclide imaging in the evaluation of wrist pain. *J Hand Surg [Am]* 1988;13:810–814.
21. Mackinnon SE, Holder LE. The use of three phase radionuclide bone scanning in the diagnosis of reflex sympathetic dystrophy. *J Hand Surg [Am]* 1984;9:556–563.
22. Taleisnik J. Pain on the ulnar side of the wrist. *Hand Clin* 1987;3:51–69.
23. Koenig H, Lucas D, Meissner R. The wrist: A preliminary report on high-resolution MR imaging. *Radiology* 1986;160:463–467.
24. Weiss KL, Beltran J, Shaman OM, et al. High-field MR surface coil imaging of the hand and wrist, part I. *Radiology* 1986;160:143–146.
25. Weiss KL, Beltran J, Shaman OM, et al. High-field MR surface coil imaging of the hand and wrist—part II—pathology correlations and clinical relevance. *Radiology* 1986;160:147–152.
26. Hajek PC, Baker LL, Sartoris DG, et al. MR arthrography: anatomic–pathologic investigation. *Radiology* 1987;163:141–147.
27. Skahen JR, Palmer AK, Levinsohn EM, et al. Magnetic resonance imaging of the triangular fibrocartilage complex. *J Hand Surg [Am]* 1990;15:552–557.
28. Totterman SMS, Miller RJ. Triangular fibrocartilage complex: Normal appearance on coronal three-dimensional gradient-recalled-echo MR images. *Radiology* 1995;195:521–527.
29. Smith DK, Snearly WN. Lunotriquetral interosseous ligament of the wrist: MR appearances in asymptomatic volunteers and arthrographically normal wrists. *Radiology* 1994;191:199–202.
30. Stewart NR, Gilula LA. CT of the wrist: a tailored approach. *Radiology* 1992;183:13–20.
31. Hindman BW, Kulik WJ, Lee J, et al. Occult fractures of the carpals and metacarpals: demonstrated by CT. *Am J Radiol* 1989;153:529–532.

32. Ebraheim NA, Skie MC, Savolaine ER, et al. Coronal fracture of the body of the hamate. *J Trauma* 1995;38:169–174.
33. Mino DE, Palmer AK, Levinsohn EM. The role of radiography and computed tomography in the diagnosis of subluxation and dislocation of the distal radioulnar joint. *J Hand Surg [Am]* 1983; 8:23–31.
34. Pirela-Cruz MA, Goll SR, Klug M, et al. Stress computed tomography analysis of the distal radioulnar joint: A diagnostic tool for determining translational motion. *J Hand Surg [Am]* 1991;16: 75–82.
35. Biondetti PR, Vannier MW, Gilula LA, et al. Three-dimensional surface reconstruction of the carpal bones from CT scans: transaxial vs. coronal technique. *Comp Med Imag Graph* 1988;12: 67–73.
36. Read JW, Conolly WB, Lanzetta M, et al. Diagnostic ultrasound of the hand and wrist. *J Hand Surg [Am]* 1996;21: 1004–1010.
37. Roth JH, Haddad RG. Radiocarpal arthroscopy and arthrography in the diagnosis of ulnar wrist pain. *Arthroscopy* 1986;2: 234–243.
38. Chung KC, Zimmerman NB, Travis MT. Wrist arthrography vs arthroscopy: A comparative study of 150 cases. *J Hand Surg [Am]* 1996;21:591–594.
39. Pederzini L, Luchetti R, Soragni M, et al. Evaluation of the triangular fibrocartilage tears by arthroscopy, arthrography, and magnetic resonance imaging. *Arthroscopy* 1992;8:191–197.
40. Cooney WP. Evaluation of chronic wrist pain by arthrography, arthroscopy, and arthrotomy. *J Hand Surg [Am]* 1993;18: 815–822.
41. Palmer AK, Werner FW, Glisson RR, et al. Partial excision of the triangular fibrocartilage complex: An experimental study. *J Hand Surg [Am]* 1988;13:391–394.
42. Palmer AK, Werner FW. Biomechanics of the distal radioulnar joint. *Clin Orthop* 1984;187:26–34.
43. Palmer AK, Werner FW. The triangular fibrocartilage complex of the wrist—anatomy and function. *J Hand Surg [Am]* 1981;6: 153–162.
44. Palmer AK. Triangular fibrocartilage disorders: Injury patterns and treatments. *Arthroscopy* 1990;6:125–132.
45. Thiru-Pathi RG, Ferlic DC, Clayton ML, et al. Arterial anatomy of the triangular fibrocartilage of the wrist and its surgical significance. *J Hand Surg [Am]* 1986;11:258–263.
46. Chidgey LK, Dell PC, Bittar ES, et al. Histologic anatomy of the triangular fibrocartilage. *J Hand Surg [Am]* 1991;16:1084–1100.
47. Mikic Z. The blood supply of the human distal radioulnar joint and the microvasculature of its articular disc. *Clin Orthop* 1992; 275:19–28.
48. Adams BD, Samani JE, Holley KA. Triangular fibrocartilage injury: A laboratory model. *J Hand Surg [Am]* 1996;21:189–193.
49. Palmer AK. Triangular fibrocartilage complex lesions: A classification. *J Hand Surg [Am]* 1989;14:594–606.
50. Shaw JA, Bruno A, Paul EM. Ulnar styloid fixation in the treatment of posttraumatic instability of the radioulnar joint: A biomechanical study with clinical correlation. *J Hand Surg [Am]* 1990;15:712–720.
51. Osterman AL, Terrill RG. Arthroscopic treatment of TFCC lesions. *Hand Clin* 1991;7:277–281.
52. Bednar JM, Osterman AL. The role of arthroscopy in the treatment of traumatic triangular fibrocartilage injuries. *Hand Clin* 1994;10:605–614.
53. Gan BS, Richards RS, Roth JH. Arthroscopic treatment of triangular fibrocartilage tears. *Orthop Clin North Am* 1995;26: 721–729.
54. Cooney WP, Linscheid RL, Dobyns JH. Triangular fibrocartilage tears. *J Hand Surg [Am]* 1994;19:143–154.
55. Jantea CL, Baltzer A, Ruther, W. Arthroscopic repair of radial-sided lesions of the fibrocartilage complex. *Hand Clin* 1995;11: 31–36.
56. Osterman AL. Arthroscopic debridement of triangular fibrocartilage complex tears. *Arthroscopy* 1990;6:120–124.
57. Hermansdorfer JD, Kleinman WB. Management of chronic peripheral tears of the triangular fibrocartilage complex. *J Hand Surg [Am]* 1991;16:340–346.
58. Palmer AK, Glisson RR, Werner FW. Relationship between ulnar variance and triangular fibrocartilage complex thickness. *J Hand Surg [Am]* 1984;9:681–683.
59. Viegas SF, Ballantyne G. Attritional lesions of the wrist joint. *J Hand Surg [Am]* 1987;12:1025–1029.
60. Feldon P, Terrono AL, Belsky MR. The "wafer" procedure. Partial distal ulnar resection. *Clin Orthop* 1992;275:124–129.
61. Feldon P, Terrono AL, Belsky MR. Wafer distal ulna resection for triangular fibrocartilage tears and/or ulna impaction syndrome. *J Hand Surg [Am]* 1992;17:731–737.
62. Darrach W. Partial excision of lower shaft of ulna for deformity following Colles's fracture. *Ann Surg* 1913;57:764.
63. Bowers WH. Distal radioulnar joint arthroplasty: The hemiresection–interposition technique. *J Hand Surg [Am]* 1985;10: 169–178.
64. Watson HK, Ryu J, Burgess RC. Matched distal ulnar resection. *J Hand Surg [Am]* 1986;11:812–817.
65. Darrow JC, Linscheid RL, Dobyns JH, et al. Distal ulnar recession for disorders of the distal radioulnar joint. *J Hand Surg [Am]* 1985;10:482–491.
66. Bell MJ, Hill RJ, McMurtry RY. Ulnar impingement syndrome. *J Bone Joint Surg Br* 1985;67:126–129.
67. Leibovic S, Bowers WH. Arthroscopy of the distal radioulnar joint. *Orthop Clin North Am* 1995;26:755–757.
68. Hauck RM, Skahen JR, Palmer AK. Classification and treatment of ulnar styloid nonunion. *J Hand Surg [Am]* 1996;21: 418–422.
69. Coleman HM. Injuries of the articular disc at the wrist. *J Bone Joint Surg Br* 1960;42:522–529.
70. Spinner M, Kaplan EB. Extensor carpi ulnaris: Its relationship to the stability of the distal radioulnar joint. *Clin Orthop* 1970;68: 124–129.
71. Palmer AK, Skahen JR, Werner FW, et al. The extensor retinaculum of the wrist: An anatomical and biomechanical study. *J Hand Surg [Br]* 1985;10:11–16.
72. Eckhardt WA, Palmer AK. Recurrent dislocation of extensor carpi ulnaris tendon. *J Hand Surg [Am]* 1981;6:629–631.
73. Chun S, Palmer AK. Chronic ulnar wrist pain secondary to partial rupture of the extensor carpi ulnaris tendon. *J Hand Surg [Am]* 1987;12:1032–1034.
74. Burkhart SS, Wood MB, Linscheid RL. Posttraumatic recurrent subluxation of the extensor carpi ulnaris tendon. *J Hand Surg [Am]* 1982;7:1–3.
75. Rowland SA. Acute traumatic subluxation of the extensor carpi ulnaris tendon at the wrist. *J Hand Surg [Am]* 1986;11: 809–811.
76. Paley D, McMurtry RY, Murray JF. Dorsal dislocation of the ulnar styloid and extensor carpi ulnaris tendon into the distal radioulnar joint: The empty sulcus sign. *J Hand Surg [Am]* 1987; 12:1029–1032.
77. Pevny T, Rayan GM, Egle D. Ligamentous and tendinous support of the pisiform, anatomic and biomechanical study. *J Hand Surg [Am]* 1995;20:299–304.
78. Carroll RE, Coyle MP. Dysfunction of the pisotriquetral joint: Treatment by excision of the pisiform. *J Hand Surg [Am]* 1985; 10:703–707.
79. Carroll RE, Coyle MP. Dysfunction of the pisotriquetral joint: Treatment by excision of the pisiform. *J Hand Surg [Am]* 1985; 10:703–707.

80. Paley D, McMurtry RY, Cruickshank B. Pathologic conditions of the pisiform and pisotriquetral joint. *J Hand Surg [Am]* 1987;12:110–119.
81. Arner M, Haberg L. Wrist flexion strength after excision of the pisiform bone. *Scand J Plast Reconstr Surg* 1984;18:241–245.
82. Buterbaugh GA, Palmer AK, Skahen JR. *Triquetral hamate joint instability*. Paper presented at American Society for Surgery of the Hand, 3rd Annual Residents and Fellows Conference, Las Vegas, Nevada, 1985.
83. Milch H. Fracture of the hamate bone. *J Bone Joint Surg Am* 1934;16:459.
84. Ebraheim NA, Skie MC, Savolaine ER, et al. Coronal fracture of the body of the hamate. *J Trauma* 1995;38:169–174.
85. Milek MA, Boulas HJ. Flexor tendon ruptures secondary to hamate hook fractures. *J Hand Surg [Am]* 1990;15:740–744.
86. Egawa M, Asai T. Fracture of the hook of the hamate: Report of six cases and the suitability of computed tomography. *J Hand Surg [Am]* 1983;8:393–398.
87. Uhl RL, Campbell M. Hamate fracture dislocation: A case report. *J Hand Surg [Am]* 1995;20:578–580.
88. Carroll RE, Lakin JF. Fracture of the hook of the hamate: Acute treatment. *J Trauma* 1993;34:803–805.
89. Whalen JL, Bishop AT, Linscheid RL. Nonoperative treatment of acute hamate hook fractures. *J Hand Surg [Am]* 1992;17:507–511.
90. Carroll RE, Lakin JF. Fracture of the hook of the hamate: Acute treatment. *J Trauma* 1993;34:803–805.
91. Jupiter JB. Scaphoid fractures. In: Manske PR, ed. *ASSH Hand Surgery Update*, Englewood, CO: American Society for Surgery of the Hand, 1994;1–9.
92. Garcia-Elias M. Dorsal fractures of the triquetrum—avulsion or compression fractures. *J Hand Surg [Am]* 1987;12:266–268.
93. Viegas SF, Patterson RM, Hokanson JA, et al. Wrist anatomy: Incidence, distribution, and correlation of anatomic variations, tears, and arthrosis. *J Hand Surg [Am]* 1993;18:463–475.
94. Viegas SF, Wagner K, Peterson P. Medial (hamate) facet of the lunate. *J Hand Surg [Am]* 1990;15:564–571.
95. Wood MB, Dobyns JH. Sports-related extraarticular wrist syndromes. *Clin Orthop* 1986;202:93–102.
96. Kip PC, Peimer CA. Release of the sixth dorsal compartment. *J Hand Surg [Am]* 1994;19:599–601.
97. Hajj AA, Woods MB. Stenosing tenosynovitis of the extensor capri ulnaris. *J Hand Surg [Am]* 1986;11:519–520.
98. Berger RA. General anatomy of the wrist. In: An K-N, Berger RA, Cooney SP III, eds. *Biomechanics of the wrist joint*. New York: Springer-Verlag, 1991;1–22.
99. Trumble TE, Bour CJ, Smith RJ, et al. Kinematics of the ulnar carpus related to the volar intercalated segment instability pattern. *J Hand Surg [Am]* 1990;15:384–392.
100. Viegas SF, Patterson RM, Peterson PD, et al. Ulnar-sided perilunate instability: An anatomic and biomechanical study. *J Hand Surg [Am]* 1990;15:268–278.
101. Zlatkin MB, Chao PC, Osterman AL, et al. Chronic wrist pain: Evaluation with high-resolution MR imaging. *Radiology* 1989;173:723–729.
102. Viegas SF, Patterson RM, Hokanson JA, et al. Wrist anatomy: Incidence, distribution, and correlation of anatomic variations, tears, and arthrosis. *J Hand Surg [Am]* 1993;18:463–475.
103. Regan DS, Linscheid RL, Dobyns JH. Lunotriquetral sprains. *J Hand Surg [Am]* 1984;9:502–514.
104. Ruch DS, Poeling GG. Arthroscopic management of partial scapholunate and lunotriquetral injuries of the wrist. *J Hand Surg [Am]* 1996;21:412–417.
105. Osterman AL, Seidman GD. The role of arthroscopy in the treatment of lunatotriquetral ligament injuries. *Hand Clin* 1995;11:41–50.

TRIANGULAR FIBROCARTILAGE COMPLEX INJURY AND REPAIR

SCOTT D. SAGERMAN
ANDREW K. PALMER
WALTER H. SHORT

Injuries of the triangular fibrocartilage complex (TFCC) are a well-recognized cause of ulnar wrist pain. In recent years, the anatomy and function of the TFCC have been well studied (1). Attention has now been shifted to the treatment of TFCC pathology (2).

This chapter explores the spectrum of TFCC injuries with special emphasis on the surgical treatment of traumatic lesions.

ANATOMY AND BIOMECHANICS

As its name implies, the TFCC is a complex anatomic structure (Fig. 38.1). It is comprised of the horizontal disc (TFC proper), the extrinsic ulnocarpal ligaments, ulnar collateral ligament, and the extensor carpi ulnaris (ECU) subsheath. The horizontal disc itself is divided into a central portion composed of obliquely oriented collagen, and peripheral structures composed of longitudinally oriented collagen, termed the dorsal radioulnar and palmar radioulnar ligaments. The thickness of the horizontal disc has been found to vary depending on ulnar variance (3). Vascular injection studies (4,5) have shown that the periphery of the horizontal disc contains an abundant blood supply arising from the ulnar and anterior interosseous arteries. The central portion and radial attachment are devoid of vascularity.

The primary functions of the TFCC involve transmission of load to the ulna and stabilization of the ulnocarpal and distal radioulnar joints (DRUJ). The load-bearing capability of the TFCC and its ability to resist shear and

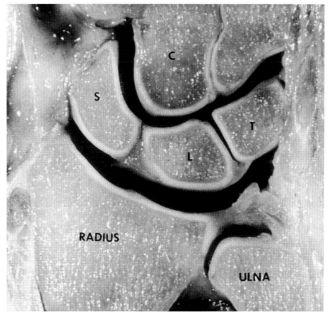

FIGURE 38.1. Cross section of cadaver wrist illustrating the triangular fibrocartilage complex and its radial and ulnar attachments. *S*, scaphoid; *C*, capitate; *L*, lunate; *T*, triquetrum.

tension forces are imparted by the characteristic arrangement of collagen fibers in the horizontal disc and radioulnar ligaments (6). Approximately 20% of axial load is transmitted across the wrist to the ulna through the TFCC. Biomechanical studies have shown that complete excision of the horizontal disc greatly alters load transmission across the wrist, although partial excision allows the TFCC to retain its load-bearing function (7,8). Sectioning of the dorsal and palmar radioulnar ligaments has also been shown to affect DRUJ stability (9,10), and avulsion of the attachment of the TFCC at the base of the ulnar styloid in association with fractures can produce clinically significant instability of the DRUJ (11,12).

S. D. Sagerman: Department of Orthopaedics, Northwestern University Medical School, Chicago, Illinois 60611; and Northwest Community Hospital, Arlington Heights, Illinois 60005.

A. K. Palmer and W. H. Short: Department of Orthopedic Surgery, State University of New York Health Science Center at Syracuse, Syracuse, New York 13202.

CLASSIFICATION

Injury to the TFCC may occur via traumatic or degenerative disruption of the horizontal disc or its peripheral attachments (13) (Table 38.1). Traumatic lesions (class 1) are thought to occur from a combination of axial loading and forearm rotation, resulting in increased compressive, tensile, and shear forces on the TFCC (14,15) (Fig. 38.2). These tears may produce acute pain and swelling localized to the ulnocarpal region. When the central avascular portion of the TFCC is involved, the healing capacity is limited, and pain may persist accompanied by clicking during forearm rotation. Peripheral tears, if incomplete or nondisplaced, have the capacity to heal without residual symptoms. However, complete avulsions may be associated with subluxation or dislocation of the DRUJ.

Degenerative lesions of the TFCC (class 2) are thought to arise from a process in which chronic loading leads to progressive wear on the horizontal disc and surrounding structures, producing a spectrum of injury termed the "ulnocarpal abutment syndrome" (16). This process is associated with positive ulnar variance, either from a congenital length discrepancy between the radius and ulna or from the dynamic changes that occur with axial loading and forearm pronation. The onset of symptoms is usually insidious, related to degenerative changes occurring at the central portion of the horizontal disc. Progressive thinning of the disc ensues until it perforates. Then, chondral changes involving the opposing articular surfaces of the ulnar head and the lunate may occur, eventually leading to lunotriquetral ligament disruption and ulnocarpal arthritis. Degenerative TFCC perforations have been shown to occur increasingly with age (17), although it does not appear that these tears necessarily result in symptoms.

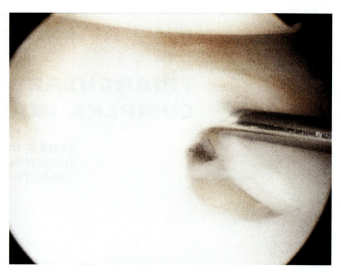

FIGURE 38.2. Arthroscopic photo of traumatic tear of the triangular fibrocartilage complex (TFCC) horizontal disc. The probe is entering the tear in the horizontal disc, and the ulnar head is visible through the defect in the TFCC.

TABLE 38.1. TRIANGULAR FIBROCARTILAGE COMPLEX ABNORMALITIES

Class 1: Traumatic
  A. Central perforation
  B. Ulnar avulsion
    with distal ulnar fracture
    without distal ulnar fracture
  C. Distal avulsion
  D. Radial avulsion
    with sigmoid notch fracture
    without sigmoid notch fracture
Class 2: Degenerative (ulnocarpal abutment syndrome)
  A. TFCC wear
  B. TFCC wear
    + lunate and/or ulnar chondromalacia
  C. TFCC perforation
    + lunate and/or ulnar chondromalacia
  D. TFCC perforation
    + lunate and/or ulnar chondromalacia
    − lunate and/or ulnar chondromalacia
  E. TFCC perforation
    + lunate and/or chondromalacia
    − LT ligament perforation
    + ulnocarpal arthritis

LT, lunotriquetral; TFCC, triangular fibrocartilage complex.

IMAGING STUDIES

Evaluation of patients presenting with ulnar wrist pain begins with a thorough history and physical examination to exclude more common conditions, such as fractures, arthritis, and tendinitis. Several diagnostic imaging studies may be useful when TFCC pathology is suspected. Plain x-rays are usually obtained first. Although the TFCC itself is not visualized, x-rays are helpful in determining ulnar variance and detecting degenerative changes of ulnocarpal abutment. If DRUJ subluxation or instability associated with TFCC disruption is suspected, a true lateral x-ray and axial CT scans in neutral, supination, and pronation are appropriate (18).

Wrist arthrography is the standard method for detection of full-thickness perforations of the TFCC (19) (Fig. 38.3). To maximize sensitivity of arthrography, the three-compartment technique is preferred (20). Passage of contrast between the radiocarpal and the DRUJ compartments is indicative of TFCC disruption, although correlation with clinical findings is warranted before one can assume that a symptomatic tear is present (21). Arthrography has been found to be extremely accurate when correlated with operative findings.

More recently, magnetic resonance imaging (MRI) has been utilized for detection of TFCC pathology (22). Although it is accurate in predicting perforations of the cen-

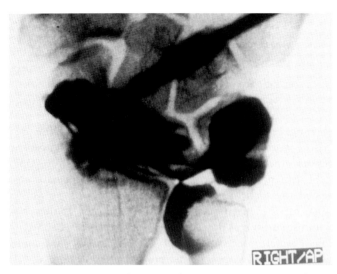

FIGURE 38.3. Wrist arthrogram demonstrating passage of contrast from the radiocarpal joint into the distal radioulnar joint through a defect in the triangular fibrocartilage complex.

tral portion of the horizontal disc, MRI is less reliable in detecting peripheral detachments of the TFCC. Although this test is noninvasive, in most centers the cost is significantly higher than that of arthrography.

Wrist arthroscopy has emerged as a valuable tool for evaluation of TFCC pathology, affording direct visualization of the articular structures (23,24). The size, location, and stability of TFCC tears can be accurately assessed. Additionally, adjacent articular structures, including cartilage surfaces, intercarpal ligaments, and the capsule can be examined. Besides aiding in diagnosis, wrist arthroscopy allows surgical intervention to proceed when TFCC tears are identified (25,26). The benefits of arthroscopic evaluation have led some authors to abandon arthrography and proceed directly to arthroscopy for patients with suspected TFCC injuries. Others prefer to document TFCC perforation via arthrography before offering an invasive surgical procedure such as arthroscopy.

TREATMENT

Treatment of TFCC tears is based on the classification scheme. This chapter will focus on traumatic (class 1) injuries, and degenerative (class 2) injuries are covered in Chapter 39.

Class 1A

Central perforations of the TFCC (class 1A) occurring the avascular region of the horizontal disc are not felt to possess the ability to heal. However, small tears may not necessarily produce significant symptoms. Therefore, in general, a trial of conservative symptomatic treatment is warranted before surgical intervention is considered. Activity modification, intermittent use of a wrist splint, and antiinflammatory medication may be helpful. A local steroid injection into the ulnocarpal joint may also be effective for diminishing local synovitis that may accompany TFCC injuries. When symptoms persist beyond a reasonable time period and interfere with performance of usual activities, surgery is indicated.

Arthroscopic debridement has emerged as the preferred surgical treatment for many traumatic central TFCC tears (2,27,28). This procedure combines the benefits of limited exposure with excellent visualization of the TFCC and neighboring structures. Arthroscopy is performed in an outpatient setting with regional or general anesthesia. Redundant or unstable flaps of the torn horizontal disc may cause mechanical irritation when interposed between the articular surfaces of the ulnocarpal joint. These tears are debrided using a variety of methods, including basket forceps, punches, arthroscopy blades, and motorized shavers. Synovectomy and debridement of intercarpal ligament tears or chondral lesions can also be done. Excision of the central portion of the TFCC has not been shown to effect its load bearing function (29). It is important, however, to preserve the peripheral rim including the dorsal and palmar radioulnar ligaments. Patients may begin early rehabilitation exercises and immobilization of the wrist is not usually necessary.

Technique

Treatment of class 1A TFCC tears basically involves removing the unstable portion of the horizontal disc while preserving the peripheral rim and ligamentous structures. The advantages of wrist arthroscopy, including illumination, magnification, and limited exposure, make this the preferred method for debridement of these tears. A thorough knowledge of arthroscopic anatomy and experience using the wrist arthroscope are essential to perform this procedure successfully and avoid complications.

Once anesthesia is administered, the arm is placed in fingertrap traction and draped sterilely. A variety of traction holding devices are now commercially available. In addition, a small joint arthroscope and a variety of arthroscopic instruments including a motorized shaver are also needed. The skin landmarks are drawn on the dorsal aspect of the wrist, the arm is exsanguinated, and a tourniquet is inflated. The standard dorsal portals are created using the recommended technique of small longitudinal incisions carried through the dermis only, subcutaneous spreading using a tentonomy scissors, and introduction of the arthroscope using a blunt trochar without injuring the articular surfaces. To begin with, the 3,4 portal between the third and fourth extensor compartments is utilized for the arthroscope, while the 4,5 and 6R portals are utilized for the arthroscopic instruments and shaver. Inflow tubing is attached to the arthroscope cannula, and outflow is not usually necessary. A systematic inspection of the radiocarpal and ulnocarpal joints is carried out using a small probe to palpate the articular structures. Once the extent of TFCC horizontal disc perforation is determined, the neighboring structures are visualized to identify accompanying pathology such as synovitis or intercarpal ligament tears. Often, it is useful to switch the arthroscope into the 4,5 or 6R portal to gain a full visualization of the ulnocarpal joint structures.

Debridement of the horizontal disc tear can be performed using a variety of instruments. For large unstable flaps, a small banana blade or hook knife is useful to trim the unstable redundant edges of the tear. This tissue can then be removed using a small grasping forceps. Smaller edges can be trimmed using a basket forceps, including straight, angled, and back-biting types. Usually, the central two-thirds of the horizontal disc is removed, preserving the dorsal and palmar radioulnar ligaments and ulnar attachment of the horizontal disc with a smooth peripheral margin. A motorized shaver with a full-radius resector can then be utilized to smooth the edges of the remaining horizontal disc as well as remove any accompanying synovitis from the ulnocarpal capsule (Fig. 38.4). It is important to be able to switch instruments and the arthroscope between the various portals in order to complete the debridement and eliminate all redundant unstable flaps of the tear. Finally, the joint should be irrigated with normal saline and any loose pieces of the TFCC removed using the motorized shaver with suction.

If general anesthesia is utilized, then the wrist may be injected with long-acting local anesthetic for postoperative analgesia. This is helpful to allow the patient to perform range-of-motion exercises in the immediate postoperative period. Usually, there is no need to immobilize the wrist following arthroscopic debridement.

Several authors have reported excellent results following arthroscopic and open debridement for isolated TFCC tears (27,28,30). Pain relief has been reliable and function of the TFCC has been preserved. Osterman reported a prospective series of patients undergoing arthroscopic debridement of TFCC tears (28). Eighty-five percent of patients experienced pain relief, and 93% noticed resolution of painful clicking. Eight-eight percent of patients considered the procedure worthwhile. Minami et al. reported 100% excellent results among 11 patients who underwent arthroscopic debridement of traumatic TFCC tears (27). Some have suggested that debridement alone in wrists showing positive ulnar variance may lead to recurrent symptoms. In these situations, additional procedures such as ulnar head shortening ("wafer procedure") (31,32) or ulnar shortening osteotomy (33) should be considered. Menon et al. reported poor results following partial TFCC excision in patients over 40 years of age with associated degenerative arthritis (30).

Peripheral tears or detachments occur in the vascularized zone of the TFCC and thus may have the ability to heal. Recent reports have suggested various repair methods for these injuries and have documented successful healing following surgical reattachment of peripheral TFCC tears (34–40).

Class 1B

Ulnar detachment (class 1B) of the TFCC from the fovea of the ulnar head, with or without an associated ulnar styloid base fracture, may result in various degrees of DRUJ instability. Incomplete or subacute tears in this region may be difficult to detect. Arthrography may not show a communication between the ulnocarpal joint and the DRUJ but may show contrast leakage into the ulnar capsule or ECU tendon sheath. Arthroscopic examination may reveal diminished tension on the horizontal disc ("trampoline effect"), suggestive of an ulnar TFCC detachment (35). Surgical reattachment of these tears is indicated when definite subluxation of the DRUJ is noted clinically or when symptoms of pain and/or instability persist despite a trial of immobilization. Both open and arthroscopic suture repair methods have been described with favorable results (35,37, 39,40). When the TFCC remains attached to a displaced fragment of the ulnar styloid, these fractures are amenable to reduction and fixation using tension-band or compression screw fixation (11,12). A period of cast immobilization is usually necessary following these procedures.

Technique

Isolated avulsions of the TFCC from its ulnar attachment, without an associated ulnar styloid fracture, are usually detected arthroscopically. The standard dorsal portals are utilized. With the arthroscope in the 3,4 portal and a small

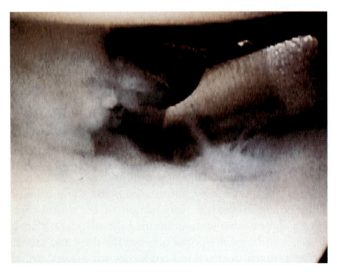

FIGURE 38.4. Class 1A. Central tear of the triangular fibrocartilage complex horizontal disc is debrided.

probe in the 6R portal, tension on the horizontal disc can be evaluated. Loss of normal tension and disruption at the ulnar attachment of the horizontal disc in the vicinity of the fovea are indicative of a class 1B tear.

The frayed edges of the tear may be debrided using a motorized shaver. This may entail switching the arthroscope from the 3,4 to the 6R viewing portal and utilizing the shaver in the 3,4 or 4,5 portal. The capsular edge should then be freshened and any synovitis removed. A variety of repair techniques have been developed allowing arthroscopically assisted suturing of these tears. The detached edge of the horizontal disc is sutured to the ulnar capsule directly opposite the site of the tear, and sutures are tied on the superficial surface of the capsule. A longitudinal incision is made on the dorsoulnar aspect of the wrist overlying the site of the tear. Typically, this involves opening the sixth extensor compartment retinaculum and retracting the ECU tendon, exposing its subsheath. Tears that occur slightly more palmarly are reattached to the ulnar capsule between the ECU and flexor carpi ulnaris (FCU). In this instance, care must be taken to identify and protect the dorsal sensory branch of the ulnar nerve. Once the capsule is exposed, sutures are then inserted using one of several techniques. For example, long straight meniscal repair needles may be utilized through an arthroscopic cannula placed in the 3,4 portal to place sutures in the edge of the TFCC; 2-0 PDS suture (Davis & Geck, Manati, PA) is typically utilized. The needles are advanced through the capsule using arthroscopic guidance and delivered through the longitudinal incision that was previously made. Depending on the size of the tear, one, two, or three sutures may be needed to reattach the torn edge of the TFCC and reestablish normal tension on the horizontal disc. The sutures are then tied over the ulnar capsule after releasing traction from the wrist with the forearm positioned in neutral rotation. Alternatively, the sutures may be inserted using a suture-passing device. Through the longitudinal incision over the capsule, sutures are placed through the capsule or ECU subsheath, depending on the location of the tear, and then into the TFCC edge. The end of the suture is then retrieved and brought back through the capsule using arthroscopic visualization. The sutures are then tied over the capsule or ECU subsheath, the retinaculum is repaired, and the skin is closed in the usual manner.

The DRUJ is immobilized using transverse K-wires between the ulna and radius proximal to the joint, and a long arm or Munster cast is then applied for 6 weeks, at which time the K-wires are removed, and the wrist is gradually mobilized.

Class 1B tears associated with ulnar styloid fractures are repaired by reduction and fixation of the ulnar styloid fragment. If nondisplaced, the ulnar styloid can be stabilized using percutaneous pin fixation under fluoroscopic guidance. Displaced fractures are best treated with open reduction utilizing a longitudinal incision over the distal ulna between the ECU and FCU tendons. Care is taken to expose and protect the dorsal ulnar sensory nerve. The fracture site is exposed subperiosteally, and the styloid fragment reduced. Fixation using tension band wire or a compression screw can be utilized. Long arm or Muenster cast immobilization with the forearm in neutral rotation for 4 to 6 weeks is necessary.

Hermansdorfer and Kleinman are reported relief of pain in 8 of 11 patients who underwent an open surgical reattachment of class 1B lesions (35). They utilized suture placement through drill holes at the base of the ulnar styloid. Cooney et al. reported good or excellent results in five patients who underwent reattachment of class 1B tears (34). Trumble et al. reported satisfactory results in nine patients who underwent an arthroscopically assisted repair of class 1B tears in nine patients (40). Sennwald et al. described a repair technique involving an osteotomy of the ulnar head with reattachment of the TFCC to the ulna styloid through drill holes with encouraging results in eight patients (39). A multicenter study reported satisfactory results in 42 of 45 patients who underwent arthroscopic repair of class 1B tears with average follow-up of 3 years (41). Shaw et al. reported satisfactory results in six patients who underwent open reduction and internal fixation of ulnar styloid avulsion fractures using K-wire fixation with no nonunions (10). Bowers suggests immobilization for nondisplaced fractures in a short arm cast in neutral rotation, whereas displaced fractures are treated with open reduction and internal fixation using intraosseous compression wiring (42).

Class 1C

Class 1C TFCC tears represent an avulsion of the horizontal disc from its distal attachments to the lunate or triquetrum in the vicinity of the ulnolunate or ulnotriquetral ligament. These injuries are seen infrequently, and there is little information concerning treatment. Repair of these lesions has been described in two recent reports (34,40). Cooney's series (34) included repair of five palmar tears of the TFCC through an open approach, which produced three good and two fair results. Three of these patients had ulnar recession performed concomitantly to assist in surgical exposure. Trumble's series (40) included two patients with class 1C tears who underwent the arthroscopic repair method used for the more common class 1B lesions. Mooney and Poehling described successful treatment of an isolated ulnolunate ligament avulsion with arthroscopic debridement (43).

Class 1D

Radial avulsions of the TFCC from the sigmoid notch of the distal radius (class 1D) have traditionally been treated with debridement. Vascular injection studies showed that no blood vessels enter the TFCC through its radial attachment, leading to the assumption that tears in this region would not heal. However, recent reports have described both open and arthroscopic repair methods that involve freshening the edge of the sigmoid notch down to bleeding bone, thereby creating the potential for vascular supply (36,38,40). It now appears that these tears can heal following surgical reattachment. Despite this, opinions differ regarding the recommended treatment for class 1D injuries. Because radial avulsions of the TFCC occur relatively infrequently, it is important to distinguish these injuries from the more common class 1A central perforations, which typically appear within a few millimeters of the sigmoid notch attachment. Repair is feasible only for those tears directly off bone, with or without an associated avulsion fracture.

Treatment for class 1D tears of the TFCC depends on the extent of detachment of the radial attachment. When the injury is confined to the central portion of the sigmoid notch preserving the dorsal and palmar peripheral attachments, these injuries can be treated similarly to class 1A lesions. Specifically, arthroscopic debridement of the redundant unstable flaps of the horizontal disc at the free edge is performed in the manner described above for class 1A injuries. When the detachment involves more than the central portion, especially when the dorsal and or palmar radioulnar ligaments are involved, then repair is indicated. Both open and arthroscopically assisted techniques have been described.

Technique

The arthroscopic method is performed using the standard 3,4, 4,5, and 6R portals. While viewing is done from the 3,4 portal, a motorized burr is used to abrade the bone edge of the sigmoid notch through the 6R portal in preparation for reattachment of the horizontal disc. Drill holes are created using small K-wires inserted through the 6R or 6U portal using an arthroscopic cannula. The holes are made from the edge of the sigmoid notch across the distal radius and the radial cortex. Using the long meniscal repair needles with 2-0 PDS suture, the edge of the TFCC is reattached to the sigmoid notch. The sutures are passed through the edge of the TFCC and then through the drill holes and tied through a skin incision against the surface of the distal radius. Usually two or three sutures are needed to perform this repair. The superficial radial nerve must be identified and protected during exposure of the suture ends on the radial aspect of the distal radius. A K-wire is inserted between the ulna and radius maintaining the forearm in neutral rotation. A long arm or Munster cast is then applied with the forearm in neutral rotation and worn for 6 weeks, at which time the K-wire is removed and range-of-motion exercise is initiated.

Cooney et al. described an open repair method of class 1D TFCC tears using transosseous sutures (34). In some cases, ulnar recession was performed to improve surgical exposure. Eighteen of 23 cases show good or excellent results with a minimum follow-up of 2 years. Trumble et al. reported excellent results in a series of patients undergoing arthroscopic reattachment of class 1D tears that comprised at least 50% of the radial attachment of the TFCC (40). Whipple described a technique of reattaching class 1D tears using small suture anchors inserted through a dorsal arthrotomy (44). An arthroscopic repair technique using a special guiding device and spinal needles was described by Jantea et al. (36).

SUMMARY

TFCC injuries are a common cause of ulnar wrist pain. Tears occur from a combination of forces secondary to axial loading and forearm rotation. A classification system has been devised distinguishing traumatic (class 1) from degenerative (class 2) injuries. Class 1 tears may occur in the central portion of the horizontal disc or as peripheral detachments distally, ulnarly, or radially. Diagnosis is accomplished by a thorough history, physical examination, and selected diagnostic studies. Central lesions possess little healing capacity, although many may become asymptomatic. Symptomatic central tears are amenable to arthroscopic debridement, preserving TFCC function. Peripheral detachments, when associated with persistent pain or DRUJ instability, are best treated with repair.

EDITORS' COMMENTS

It is unfortunate that the term "triangular fibrocartilage" exists. The term produces in the mind a complex entity that attracts the diagnostician's attention out of proportion to problems produced. Basically, there is a volar and dorsal ligament running from the radius to the rotation point of the ulna. The task of these two ligaments is the stability of the ulna. The fact that the space between these two ligaments has filled with collagen is clinically unfortunate and unimportant. Loads can be recorded across this tissue between ulna and lunate. There is no bone support within this material, and as loads increase, it collapses, and loads shift to bone. There is no responsibility for perpendicular load transfer in the TFC. The ulna may be very short where no loading occurs. Most wrists fall between these extremes, and inline loads can be demonstrated across the ulna. This occurs because it is there, but the wrist does not need loads to take this route. It is better thought of as a phylogenetic phenomenon rather than as a necessary anatomic contributor. As loads increase, the collagen compresses, bone does not, and loads shift almost entirely to the radial side of the wrist.

The capsule of the DRUJ provides the joint closure with synovial lining, but the collagen becomes tight only in maximum supination and maximum pronation, lend-ing stabilization support only in these maximum rotation positions. The two ligaments from radius to ulna serve as take-off support for the ulnotriquetral and ulnolunate ligaments. The entire ligamentous complex is a cuff-shaped apparatus whose main function is upslope support for the carpals. Dorsal fibers are transversely aligned, swing along the ulnar aspect of the carpals, and continue as volar ligament structures. We term the entire structure the *ulnar sling mechanism*. It includes the carpal ligaments, TFCC, capsular structures of the DRUJ, and the sheath of the ECU including components of the extensor retinaculum. Because the ulna is not responsible for stabilizing the carpals, the attenuation and tears that involve these ligaments seldom require repair. Tears in the ulnar sling mechanism may allow it to displace distally against the ulnar aspect of the triquetrum, producing a triquetial impaction ligament teat (TILT) syndrome.

REFERENCES

1. Palmer AK, Werner FW. The triangular fibrocartilage complex of the wrist—anatomy and function. *J Hand Surg [Am]* 1981;6:153–162.
2. Palmer AK. Triangular fibrocartilage disorders: Injury patterns and treatment. *Arthroscopy* 1990;6:125–132.
3. Palmer AK, Glisson RR, Werner FW. Relationship between ulnar nerve variance and triangular fibrocartilage thickness. *J Hand Surg [Am]* 1984;9:681–683.
4. Bednar MS, Arnoczky SP, Weiland AJ. The microvasculature of the triangular fibrocartilage complex: its clinical significance. *J Hand Surg [Am]* 1991;16:1101–1105.
5. Thiru-Pathi RG, Ferlic DC, Clayton ML, et al. Arterial anatomy of the triangular fibrocartilage of the wrist and its surgical significance. *J Hand Surg [Am]* 1986;11:258–263.
6. Chidgey LK, Dell PC, Bittar ES, et al. Histologic anatomy of the triangular fibrocartilage. *J Hand Surg [Am]* 1991;16:1084–1100.
7. Palmer AK, Werner FW. Biomechanics of the distal radioulnar joint. *Clin Orthop* 1984;187:26–35.
8. Palmer AK, Werner FW, Glisson RR, et al. Partial excision of the triangular fibrocartilage complex. *J Hand Surg [Am]* 1988;13:391–394.
9. Schuind F, An KN, Berglund L, et al. The distal radioulnar ligaments: A biomechanical study. *J Hand Surg [Am]* 1991;16:1101–1114.
10. Shaw JA, Bruno A, Paul EM. Ulnar styloid fixation in the treatment of post-traumatic instability of the radioulnar joint: A biomechanical study with clinical correlation. *J Hand Surg [Am]* 1990;15:712–720.
11. Buterbaugh GA, Palmer AK. Fractures and dislocations of the distal radioulnar joint. *Hand Clin* 1988;4:361–375.
12. Mikic ZD. Treatment of acute injuries of the triangular fibrocartilage complex associated with distal radioulnar joint instability. *J Hand Surg [Am]* 1995;20:319–323.
13. Palmer AK. Triangular fibrocartilage complex lesions: A classification. *J Hand Surg [Am]* 1989;14:594–606.
14. Adams BD, Holley KA. Strains in the articular disc of the triangular fibrocartilage complex: A biomechanical study. *J Hand Surg [Am]* 1993;18:919–925.
15. Adams BD, Samani JE, Holley KA. Triangular fibrocartilage injury: A laboratory model. *J Hand Surg [Am]* 1996;21:189–193.
16. Friedman L, Palmer AK. The ulnar impaction syndrome. *Hand Clin* 1991;7:295–310.
17. Mikic ZD. Age changes in the triangular fibrocartilage of the wrist joint. *J Anat* 1978;126:367–384.
18. Mino DE, Palmer AK, Levinsohn EM. The role of radiography and computerized tomography in the diagnosis of subluxation and dislocation of the distal radioulnar joint. *J Hand Surg [Am]* 1983;8:23–31.
19. Levinsohn EM, Palmer AK, Coren AS, et al. Wrist arthrography: the value of the three compartment injection technique. *Skel Radiol* 1987;16:539–544.
20. Zinberg EM, Palmer AK, Coren AB, et al. The triple injection wrist arthrogram. *J Hand Surg [Am]* 1988;13:803–809.
21. Cantor RM, Stern PJ, Wyrick JD, et al. The relevance of ligament tears or perforations in the diagnosis of wrist pain: an arthrographic study. *J Hand Surg [Am]* 1994;19:945–953.
22. Skahen JR, Palmer AK, Levinsohn EM, et al. Magnetic resonance imaging of the triangular fibrocartilage complex. *J Hand Surg [Am]* 1990;15:552–557.
23. Koman LA, Poehling GG, Toby EB, et al. Chronic wrist pain: Indications for wrist arthroscopy. *Arthroscopy* 1990;6:116–119.
24. Roth JH, Haddad RG. Radiocarpal arthroscopy and arthrography in the diagnosis of ulnar wrist pain. *Arthroscopy* 1986;2:234–243.
25. Pederzini L, Luchetti R, Soragni O, et al. Evaluation of the triangular fibrocartilage complex tears by arthroscopy, arthrography, and magnetic resonance imaging. *Arthroscopy* 1992;8:191–197.
26. Whipple TL, Marotta JJ, Powell JH. Techniques of wrist arthroscopy. *Arthroscopy* 1986;2:244–252.
27. Minami A, Ishikawa J, Suenaga N, et al. Clinical results of treatment of triangular fibrocartilage complex tears by arthroscopic debridement. *J Hand Surg [Am]* 1996;21:406–411.
28. Osterman AL. Arthroscopic debridement of triangular fibrocartilage complex tears. *Arthroscopy* 1990;6:120–124.
29. Adams BD. Partial excision of the triangular fibrocartilage complex articular disc. A biomechanical study. *J Hand Surg [Am]* 1993;18:334–340.
30. Menon J, Wood VE, Schoene HR, et al. Isolated tears of the triangular fibrocartilage of the wrist: Results of partial excision. *J Hand Surg [Am]* 1984;9:527–530.
31. Feldon P, Terrono AL, Belsky MR. The "wafer procedure," partial distal ulnar resection. *Clin Orthop* 1992;275:124–129.
32. Wnorowski DC, Palmer AK, Werner FW, et al. Anatomic and biomechanical analysis of the arthroscopic wafer procedure. *Arthroscopy* 1992;8:204–212.
33. Chun S, Palmer AK. The ulnar impaction syndrome: Follow-up of ulnar shortening osteotomy. *J Hand Surg [Am]* 1993;18:46–53.
34. Cooney WP, Linscheid RL, Dobyns JH. Triangular fibrocartilage tears. *J Hand Surg [Am]* 1994;19:143–154.
35. Hermansdorfer JD, Kleinman WB. Management of chronic peripheral tears of the triangular fibrocartilage complex. *J Hand Surg [Am]* 1991;16:340–346.
36. Jantea CL, Baltzer A, Ruther W. Arthroscopic repair of radial-sided lesions of the triangular fibrocartilage complex. *Hand Clin* 1995;11:31–36.
37. Melone CP, Nathan R. Traumatic disruption of the triangular fibrocartilage complex. *Clin Orthop* 1992;275:65–73.
38. Sagerman SD, Short WH. Arthroscopic repair of radial-sided triangular fibrocartilage complex tears. *Arthroscopy* 1996;12:339–342.
39. Sennwald GR, Lauterburg M, Zdravkovic V. A new technique of reattachment after traumatic avulsion of the TFCC at its ulnar insertion. *J Hand Surg [Br]* 1995;20:178–184.
40. Trumble TE, Gilbert M, Vedder N. Isolated tears of the triangular fibrocartilage: Management by early arthroscopic repair. *J Hand Surg [Am]* 1997;22:57–65.
41. Corso SJ, Savoie FH, Geissler W, et al. *Arthroscopic repair of*

peripheral avulsions of the triangular fibrocartilage complex of the wrist. Paper presented at the Arthroscopy Association of North American Annual Meeting, Orlando, FL, 1994.
42. Bowers WH. The distal radioulnar joint. In: Green DP, ed. *Operative hand surgery, 3rd ed.* Edinburgh: Churchill Livingstone, 1993;991.
43. Mooney JF, Poehling GG. Disruption of the ulnolunate ligament as a cause of chronic ulnar wrist pain. *J Hand Surg [Am]* 1991;16: 347–349.
44. Whipple TL. *Peripheral detachment of the triangular fibrocartilage complex.* Paper presented at AANA surgical skills course, "Arthroscopic surgery of the wrist," Rosemont, IL, 1996.

39

ULNAR IMPACTION SYNDROME

ANDREW K. PALMER
WALTER H. SHORT
DAVID A. TOIVONEN

Ulnar-sided wrist pain remains a difficult problem for clinicians. The list of differential diagnoses of ulnar wrist pain is extensive (Table 39.1). Diagnosis and treatment can be difficult and confusing. For many clinicians, ulnar-sided wrist pain remains the "lower back" of the upper extremity. In recent years, many new studies have contributed to our knowledge of the ulnar aspect of the wrist. These have included studies on anatomy, biomechanics, pathology, and treatment. All have advanced our understanding of this complicated condition and improved our ability to diagnose and successfully treat our patients with ulnar-sided wrist pain.

Ulnar impaction syndrome or ulnocarpal abutment syndrome is a common cause of ulnar wrist pain. Ulnar impaction syndrome is a degenerative condition related to excessive load bearing across the ulnar aspect of the wrist. It is characterized by ulnar wrist pain, swelling, and limitations in motion. Chronic impaction of the ulnar head against the triangular fibrocartilage complex (TFCC) and ulnar carpus can lead to progressive deterioration of the triangular fibrocartilage, chondromalacia of the ulnar head and lunate, and tears of the lunotriquetral ligament eventually leading to end-stage degenerative changes.

Past authors have described surgical procedures on the distal ulna for malunited Colles' fractures or dislocations in an attempt to correct the ulnar head symptoms (1–3). Darrach, in 1913, described the resection of a portion of the "low shaft of the ulna" for deformity following a Colles' fracture (2). Milch, in 1941, described impaction of the ulnar head on the carpus, resulting in pain and limitations in motion from a shortened and malunited distal radius fracture (3). He described the "cuff resection" of the distal ulna, which essentially involved resection of a portion of the ulnar diaphysis followed by fixation with a wire suture. Our recog-

A. K. Palmer and W. H. Short: Department of Orthopedic Surgery, State University of New York Health Sciences Center at Syracuse, Syracuse, New York 13202.

D. A. Toivonen: Northeast Wisconsin Center for Surgery and Rehabilitation of the Hand, Ltd., Appleton, Wisconsin 54914.

TABLE 39.1. DIFFERENTIAL DIAGNOSIS OF ULNAR-SIDED WRIST PAIN

Ulnar impaction syndrome
ECU tendinitis/subluxation
Calcific tendinitis—ECU/FCU
Ulnar head chondromalacia
Distal radioulnar joint subluxation/chondromalacia/
  degenerative joint disease
Traumatic triangular fibrocartilage tear
Midcarpal instability
Lunotriquetral instability
Ulnar styloid triquetral impaction
Ulnar impingement syndrome
Miscellaneous conditions, e.g., Kienböck's disease, tumors,
  triquetral–hamate impaction, pisotriquetral joint
  abnormalities
Inflammatory conditions, e.g., gout, rheumatoid arthritis, SLE

ECU extensor carpi ulnaris; FCU, flexor carpi ulnaris; SLE, systematic lupus erythematosis.

nition and understanding of ulnocarpal abutment syndrome was greatly enhanced by Palmer's classification system of triangular fibrocartilage lesions in 1989 (4) (Table 39.2). His classification system described the pathology we now associate with ulnar impaction syndrome, including lesions of the TFCC, lunate, ulnar head, and lunotriquetral interval.

Many terms exist in the literature for this condition. These have included ulnar impaction (5), ulnar impingement (3,5), ulnocarpal impingement (6), ulnocarpal abutment (5,7), and ulnocarpal loading (5,6). We consider *ulnar impaction syndrome* and *ulnar impingement syndrome* to be two distinctly different clinical entities (Fig. 39.1). Ulnar impingement syndrome, as described by Bell (8), results from "a short ulna impinging on the distal radius and causing a painful, disabling pseudoarthrosis." It commonly occurs with an unstable distal ulna after a previous Darrach resection. Therefore, by definition, ulnar impaction syndrome and ulnar impingement syndrome are mutually exclusive terms. The former is secondary to an excessively long ulna, whereas the latter results from an unstable short ulna.

TABLE 39.2. TRIANGULAR FIBROCARTILAGE COMPLEX CLASSIFICATION

Class 1. Traumatic
   A. Central perforation
   B. Ulnar avulsion
      With distal ulnar fracture
      Without distal ulnar fracture
   C. Distal avulsion
   D. Radial avulsion
      With sigmoid notch fracture
      Without sigmoid notch fracture
Class 2. Degenerative (ulnocarpal abutment syndrome)
   A. TFCC wear
   B. TFCC wear
      + Lunate and/or ulnar chondromalacia
   C. TFCC perforation
      + Lunate and/or ulnar chondromalacia
   D. TFCC perforation
      + Lunate and/or ulnar chondromalacia
      + LT ligament perforation
   E. TFCC perforation
      + Lunate and/or ulnar chondromalacia
      + LT ligament perforation
      + Ulnocarpal arthritis

LT, lunotriquetral; TFCC, triangular fibrocartilage complex.

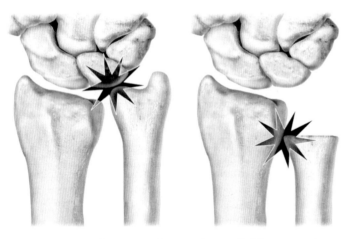

FIGURE 39.1. Ulnar impaction syndrome **(left)** versus ulnar impingement syndrome **(right)**.

ANATOMY, HISTOLOGY, AND BIOMECHANICS

The ulnar aspect of the wrist and distal radioulnar joint (DRUJ) is a complex design, both anatomically and biomechanically. Phylogenetically, it is a recent development in evolution, occurring only over the last 40 million years (9,10). The distal ulna is a fixed intraarticular structure in most animals, including lower primates. Even in monkeys, the distal ulna articulates with the triquetrum and the pisiform. The separation and proximal migration of the ulna from the carpus and formation of a separate DRUJ seen in chimpanzees, gorillas, orangutans, and humans allows for a greater degree of wrist mobility in pronation–supination and for improved functional abilities.

The distal ulna is a convex structure with articular cartilage covering 270° of its circumference (11). The articular surface height varies from approximately 5 to 8 mm surrounding the ulna at its articulation with the radius (11). The articular surface continues over the distal pole of the ulna, underlying the TFCC. Distally under the TFCC, the ulnar head is flattened. The articular surface is separated from the ulnar styloid process by the fovea, which is an area rich in vascular foramina where the TFCC inserts into the distal ulna. The distal ulna also articulates with the sigmoid notch of the distal radius. Previous articles have indicated that the articular surface of the ulnar head (the seat) and radius (sigmoid notch) at the DRUJ are angled distally and ulnarly at an angle of approximately 20° (11–13). A recent study by Sagerman and associates (14) has demonstrated a wider variation in inclination angles between the sigmoid notch and ulnar seat than previously noted. In their study, the sigmoid notch inclination averaged 7.7°, and the ulnar seat inclination averaged 21.0°. Also, the concave sigmoid notch has a greater radius of curvature than the distal ulna (4–7 mm), allowing for both rotation and translation with pronation and supination motions (11,12).

Superficially, the extensor retinaculum wraps around the distal ulna and inserts onto the palmar aspect of the carpus but has no real attachment to the ulna itself. The extensor carpi ulnaris tendon lies beneath this retinaculum and is held to the distal ulna by an extensor carpi ulnaris subsheath (11). The extensor retinaculum, in itself, provides little stability to the ulnar head.

The primary stabilizer of the DRUJ is the TFCC (4,7, 11), which is a homogeneous structure made up of dorsal and volar radial ulnar ligaments, the ulnar collateral ligament, the meniscus homolog, the sheath of the extensor carpi ulnaris, and a well-defined articular disc termed the triangular fibrocartilage proper or horizontal disc. This complex arises from the ulnar aspect of the sigmoid notch of the distal radius. It courses ulnarward to insert above the fovea at the base of the ulnar styloid. It then flows distally, joined by fibers of the ulnar collateral ligament, and becomes thickened, forming the meniscus homolog. This eventually inserts distally into the lunate, triquetrum, hamate, and base of the fifth metacarpal. Distally, there is a weak dorsal attachment to the carpus except at the dorsal lateral aspect, where the complex incorporates the floor of the sheath of the extensor carpi ulnaris. Volarly, the TFCC is strongly attached to the ulnotriquetral interosseous ligament and the triquetrum as the lunotriquetral ligament. Volarly, there is also a weaker, inconsistent attachment to the lunate known as the ulnolunate ligament. The dorsal and volar aspects of the horizontal portion of the triangular fibrocartilage are thickened on average to 4 to 5 mm and represent the dorsal and volar radial ulnar ligaments attaching the distal ulna to the radius. The horizontal triangular fibrocartilage is thickened near its strong attachment to the radius and averages approximately 2 mm in thickness. It thins out centrally in the area corresponding to the lunate–TFCC articulation and averages approximately 1 mm in thickness (15). This is a common area of perforation or degeneration. The prestyloid recess is a constant normal anatomic perforation found ulnarly and volarly in the TFCC just proximal to the thickened meniscus homolog.

The vascular anatomy of the DRUJ and TFCC has been outlined by multiple authors (16–19). Blood supply to the DRUJ is primarily derived from the palmar and dorsal branches of the anterior interosseous artery (17). The posterior interosseous artery provides some blood supply to the dorsal DRUJ capsule. The ulnar artery sends branches to the anterior ulnar capsule and the ulnar styloid area. The articular disc itself is avascular, and only its peripheral palmar, dorsal, and ulnar margins are vascularized (18,19). The extent of penetration of this vascular margin into the articular disc varies from 10% to 40%, with approximately 20% to 25% of the peripheral segment vascularized in adults (17,19). This avascular zone varies with age (17). Central and radial tears of the triangular fibrocartilage have diminished potential for repair and would be more susceptible to chronic degenerative changes.

Histologic analysis of the triangular fibrocartilage has demonstrated a variable and changing composition (20,21). The collagen fibers in the articular disc are oriented at oblique angles to one another, whereas the fibers in the radial–ulnar ligaments are oriented longitudinally along the axis of the radial origin to the ulnar insertion (19). Mikic and associates found that the articular discs of adults are primarily fibrocartilaginous tissue (20). The dorsal and palmar margins of the TFCC were more fibrous in nature, whereas the central portion was mostly chondroid in nature (20). The substance of the articular disc also changed with age. They found that the central disc in fetuses and newborns was fibrous and very cellular, but in adults it was more cartilaginous and acellular (20). In the central load-transmitting area of the TFCC, the composition is primarily cartilaginous, but in the peripheral support areas, a more fibrous ligament-like pattern is encountered.

The biomechanics of the DRUJ and ulnocarpal joint have been the subjects of multiple studies (7,11,13,21–23). Forearm rotation of up to 150° occurs through the DRUJ (22). These pronation–supination movements are accomplished by both rotation and translation. The distal ulna moves dorsally in the sigmoid notch during pronation and palmarward during supination. In addition, other studies have shown that the ulnar head moves distally in relation to the distal radius in pronation and proximally in supination, thus altering ulnar variance (23,24).

Ulnar variance is the relative lengths of the radius and ulna measured at the wrist. By convention, neutral or zero ulnar variance exists when the distal ulna cortical surface is level with the lunate fossa of the radius on a standard x-ray (23,24). An ulnar positive variant indicates that the ulna is longer than the radius, and an ulnar negative variant indicates that the ulna is shorter than the radius (Fig. 39.2).

Several methods for determining ulnar variance have been developed (23,25). The "project-a-line technique" involves a line drawn from the ulnar distal aspect of the radius articular surface toward the ulna. Variance is measured by the distance between the line and the distal cortical surface of the ulna. The "method of perpendiculars" uses a line drawn down the longitudinal axis of the radius. A second line perpendicular to the radius longitudinal axis is drawn through the distal ulnar aspect of the radius. Again, the difference between this line and the distal cortical surface of the ulna is the ulnar variance. The "method of concentric circles" involves using a template with curves of various radii (23). The template is superimposed on the radiograph, and the template curve that follows the distal radial surface is identified. The distance between the distal ulnar cortical surface and the template line that best matches the distal radial joint surface is the ulnar variance. All three of the above-described methods of ulnar variance determination have been shown to be reliable in a comparison study (25).

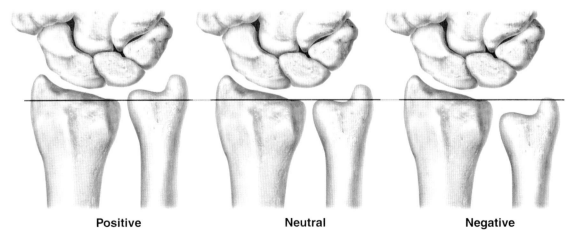

FIGURE 39.2. Ulnar variance determination.

Radiographic studies have demonstrated significant changes in ulnar variance with pronation–supination (23, 24,26) and forceful grip (27). Forearm pronation causes an increase in positive ulnar variance, whereas supination decreases ulnar variance. Epner showed that ulnar variance can change approximately 1 mm with rotation from full supination to pronation (24). Forceful grip will also increase ulnar variance. Palmer's study demonstrated that almost a 2-mm mean increase in ulnar variance can occur with maximal grip effort (28).

Compressive loads across the wrist joint have also been determined using miniature load cells in human cadaver models (7,11,22,29) (Fig. 39.3). Approximately 82% of the load applied to the wrist is borne by the distal radius, and 18% is transmitted to the ulna (11,22). Excision of the triangular fibrocartilage dramatically altered these load characteristics (11,22). With the TFCC excised, 94% of the force was transmitted to the distal radius, and 6% to the ulna. Altering ulnar variance by ulnar shortening or lengthening also had a significant affect on load transmission (11, 22). In specimens with the triangular fibrocartilage intact, surgically decreasing ulnar variance by 2.5 mm increased radius load transmission to 96% and decreased ulnar load to 4%. A surgically increased ulnar variance of 2.5 mm dropped radial load transmission to 58% and increased ulnar load transmission to 42%.

The force transmitted across the distal ulna can also be affected by dorsal tilt of the radius as in a distal radial malunion. Short and associates (30) demonstrated that an increased dorsal tilt of the distal radius leads to increased

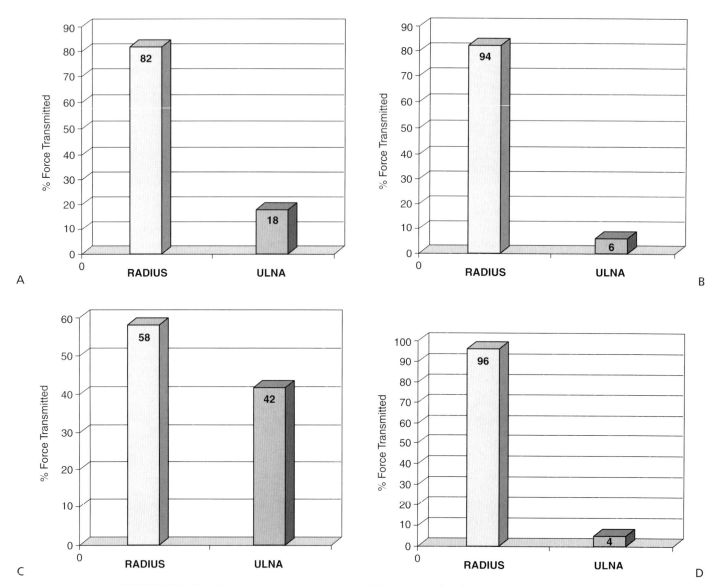

FIGURE 39.3. Graphs comparing the percentage of force transmitted through the radius to that through the ulna in an intact specimen **(A)** and specimens where the triangular fibrocartilage complex has been excised **(B)**, there is a surgically altered ulnar variance increased 2.5 mm **(C)**, and there is a surgically altered ulnar variance decreased 2.5 mm **(D)**.

force transmission across the distal ulna with axial loading of the wrist. They determined that load across the ulna increased from 21% to 67% as distal radial fragment angulation increased from 10° palmar tilt to 45° dorsal tilt.

There are no good biomechanical studies to support the hypothesis that grip or forearm position changes the relative amount of load on the radius and ulna, although previous studies demonstrated a change in variance (23,24,27). However, clinical experience has suggested that repetitive activities with a forceful grip, especially in the pronated position, contribute to ulnar impaction syndrome.

Rabinowitz and associates (21) demonstrated that both the interosseous membrane and TFCC are restraints to proximal radial migration and are involved in forearm load transmission. Birkbeck and associates (32) in 1995 confirmed this load transfer from the wrist occurring through the interosseous membrane. They found that load transmission occurred from the distal radius to the proximal ulna through the interosseous membrane. Division of the interosseous membrane eliminated this load transfer. Clearly, the interosseous membrane is a new variable that must be taken into consideration in evaluating the biomechanics of ulnar impaction syndrome. However, our concept of this relationship is just beginning, and further research in this area will be needed to clarify and improve our understanding.

PATHOLOGY

Using this biomechanical and anatomic data, we can hypothesize a mechanism for developing ulnar impaction syndrome. Repetitive activities, especially involving a forceful grip, may lead to chronic irritation among the ulnar head, TFCC, and carpus. These effects are magnified in ulnar positive variant individuals. This leads to synovitis, chondromalacia of the ulnar head, and lunate and triangular fibrocartilage perforation. Further impaction leads to lunotriquetral attenuation and disruption and, finally, to arthritis of the ulnocarpal joint and the DRUJ. A congenital ulnar positive variant would predispose these individuals to developing ulnar impaction syndrome. Other conditions that lead to an ulnar positive variant can also cause ulnar impaction syndrome. These secondary causes include a distal radius malunion, premature distal radial physeal arrest, previous radial head resection, or Essex-Lopresti injury. Prior radial shortening procedures for Kienböck's disease can also create a symptomatic ulnar positive variant.

Large cadaveric anatomic studies have looked at the incidence of degenerative lesions in human wrists (7,33,34). TFCC perforation, ulnar head and lunate chondromalacia, and lunotriquetral ligament ruptures have been found in cadaveric wrists without previous trauma history. These studies have indicated a relationship between increasing age and increasing incidence of ligamentous perforations. Mikic (33) examined 100 nontraumatized wrists and found no TFCC perforations in individuals under the age of 20. His incidence of central disc attritional lesions was 7.6% in 20- to 30-year-olds, 18.1% in 30- to 40-year-olds, and 53.1% in individuals more than 60 years of age; 100% of the individuals in their fifth decade had evidence of degenerative changes. Viegas and associates (34) reported no identifiable degenerative wrist lesions in his 100 cadaver specimens under the age of 45. He found 27.6% of his specimens 60 years of age or older had TFCC perforations. In addition, 27.6% had accompanying lunotriquetral ligament perforations. They noted that a TFCC perforation was frequently associated with a lunotriquetral tear.

Uchiyama and associates (36) studied serial radiographic changes in ulnar plus wrists over a 10-year period. Ulnar-sided degenerative changes were initially present in 17.2% of the wrists, but by final follow-up, this number had increased to 29.3%. They also noted that most of the degenerative changes in the ulnar plus wrists had progressed over the 10-year follow-up. These data, combined with biomechanical and anatomic information, suggest a causal relationship between increased force across the ulnocarpal articulation and the development and progression of degenerative changes and perforations in the ulnar wrist structures leading to ulnar impaction syndrome.

Palmer (4) in 1989 presented his classification system for TFCC lesions (Table 39.2). He divided TFCC lesions into two categories—traumatic or degenerative. Class I tears are traumatic and commonly result from falls, distraction, axial loading, or acute rotational injuries. They occur equally in ulnar positive and ulnar negative individuals. They are further divided into four categories based on location of the tears within the TFCC. A class IA tear is a traumatic perforation in the horizontal portion of the triangular fibrocartilage (Fig. 39.4), usually located 2 to 3 mm medial to the

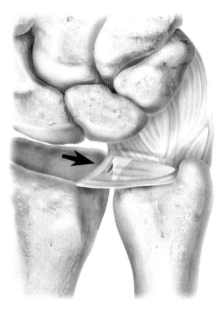

FIGURE 39.4. Palmer class IA triangular fibrocartilage complex injury.

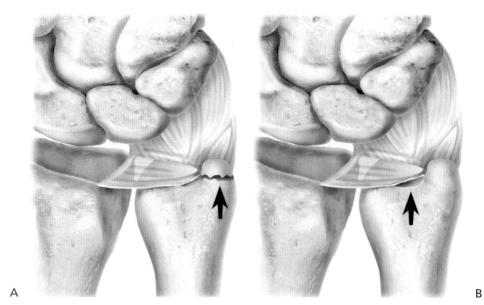

FIGURE 39.5. A: Palmer class IB triangular fibrocartilage complex (TFCC) injury (bony fracture). **B:** Palmer class IB TFCC injury (soft tissue avulsion).

radial attachment of the TFCC. This tear is usually 1 to 2 mm wide and is a slit running from the dorsal aspect of the horizontal disc in a palmarward direction. Class IB lesions represent traumatic avulsions of the triangular fibrocartilage from the distal ulna (Fig. 39.5). These may be accompanied by an ulnar styloid fracture. These lesions are usually associated with DRUJ instability. Class 1C lesions represent peripheral tears of the triangular fibrocartilage from its distal attachment (Fig. 39.6) to the lunate or the triquetrum.

Class ID tears are traumatic avulsions of the triangular fibrocartilage (Fig. 39.7) from its attachment to the radius at the sigmoid notch.

Palmer's class II tears are degenerative in nature as opposed to the traumatic origins for his class I tears. We associate class II tears with ulnar impaction syndrome. These are thought to be caused by the repetitive loading on the ulnar aspect of the wrist. Repetitive pronation and supination leads to progressive degenerative changes in the

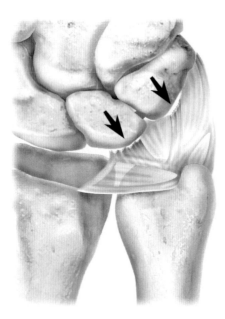

FIGURE 39.6. Palmer class IC triangular fibrocartilage complex injury.

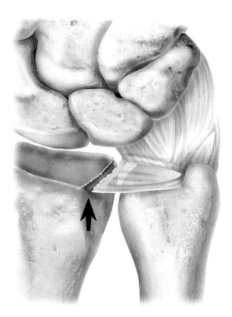

FIGURE 39.7. Palmer class ID triangular fibrocartilage complex injury.

proximal and distal aspects of the horizontal portion of the TFCC. The degenerative changes and accompanying findings are felt to increase with age and be progressive. With time and continued loading, the adjacent cartilage surfaces of the ulnar head and lunate begin to show chondromalacia changes. If the repetitive load persists, perforation of the TFCC follows. With continued loading, a significant proportion of individuals develop attenuations and ruptures of the lunotriquetral ligament. Finally, with ulnocarpal abutment and lunotriquetral instability and persistent loading on the ulnar aspect of the wrist, degenerative arthritis of the ulnocarpal, lunotriquetral, and DRUJ appears. Palmer (4) felt that the traumatic lesions were far less common than the degenerative lesions.

His degenerative lesions were broken down into five separate stages of progression, representing a continuum of pathologic changes. Class IIA (Fig. 39.8) represents wear in the horizontal portion of the TFCC without perforation. Usually, these individuals will have a neutral or positive ulnar variant, and the arthrogram will frequently be normal. Arthroscopy would best demonstrate this softening and "raggedness" in the articular disc of the TFCC.

Class IIB lesions represent continued wear in the articular disc of the TFCC (Fig. 39.9), now with chondromalacia changes present on the lunate and/or ulnar head. Arthroscopy would best demonstrate these changes, as plain radiographs and arthrograms are frequently normal other than demonstrating a positive ulnar variance and possible "raggedness" of the articular disc. Arthroscopy would demonstrate softening and fibrillations of the cartilage surface in addition to wear noted on the triangular fibrocartilage central disc.

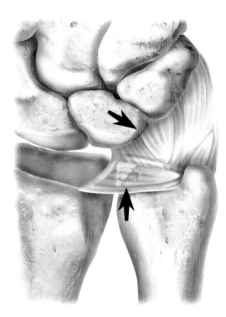

FIGURE 39.9. Palmer class IIB triangular fibrocartilage complex injury.

Class IIC lesions represent further progression and degeneration. The triangular fibrocartilage (Fig. 39.10) at this stage has a central perforation. This perforation tends to be ovoid as opposed to the slit frequently seen with traumatic central perforations. These perforations also tend to be more ulnar in location in the central disc than are found with the traumatic perforations. These degenerative lesions tend to occur in the thinner avascular portion of the central

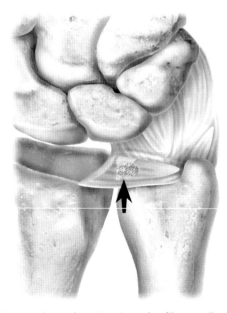

FIGURE 39.8. Palmer class IIA triangular fibrocartilage complex injury.

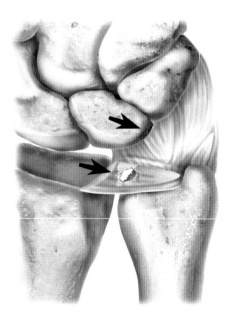

FIGURE 39.10. Palmer class IIC triangular fibrocartilage complex injury.

disc. Wrist arthrograms at this stage would demonstrate communication across the triangular fibrocartilage with either radiocarpal or DRUJ injections. There would also be continued progressive changes in the chondral surfaces on the lunate and ulnar head. At this stage, it is possible to visualize these ulnar head chondral changes on radiocarpal arthroscopy through the perforation in the central disc of the TFCC.

Class IID represents further deterioration of the process with evidence of further degenerative changes (Fig. 39.11) in the articular surface of the lunate and ulnar head associated with a large articular disc perforation. Now at this stage, lunotriquetral ligament attenuation and rupture have occurred. The arthrogram would now demonstrate the lunotriquetral perforation in addition to a large central TFCC perforation. Arthroscopy would confirm the triangular fibrocartilage horizontal disc perforation, the chondral changes on the ulnar head and accompanying lunate, and would be able to best evaluate and assess the instability at the lunotriquetral articulation. We find mid-carpal joint arthroscopy best for the assessment of lunotriquetral instability.

Class IIE represents end-stage ulnar impaction syndrome in which degenerative arthritis (Fig. 39.12) of the ulnocarpal, and occasionally the DRUJ, develops. The horizontal portion of the triangular fibrocartilage at this stage is usually completely absent, and the lunotriquetral interosseous ligament is completely disrupted.

This classification is important because it differentiates between two separate causes and types of triangular fibrocartilage pathology. Class II lesions caused by ulnar impaction syndrome demonstrate a continuum of chronic load transmission to the ulnar side of the wrist.

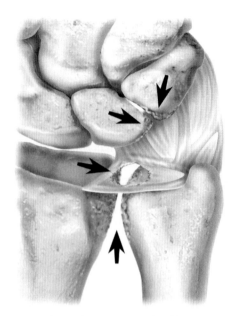

FIGURE 39.12. Palmer class IIE triangular fibrocartilage complex injury (arthritic end stage).

DIAGNOSIS

The clinical presentation of ulnar impaction syndrome is generally chronic ulnar-sided wrist pain. It is often exacerbated by activity and relieved with rest. Many patients complain of clicking and/or crepitus in the TFCC area of the wrist. Careful history and physical exam are essential in the diagnosis of ulnar impaction syndrome. See Chapter 37 for details of the history, physical exam, radiographic evaluation, and differential diagnosis of ulnar-sided wrist pain.

TREATMENT

The specific treatment of ulnar impaction syndrome must be individualized on the basis of its stage and patient symptomatology. We use Palmer's classification system as a staging guide for treatment (4). Patients with only mildly positive or neutral ulnar variance frequently will respond to nonoperative treatment. Individuals with excessive positive variance and significant structural abnormalities who are unable to abstain from aggravating activities tend to have progressive symptoms and frequently require surgical intervention. Multiple factors will influence surgical decision making. These include ulnar variance, distal radius articular surface alignment/deformity, TFCC integrity, lunotriquetral ligament status, DRUJ congruency and stability, and patient skeletal age.

Class IIA Treatment

Class IIA ulnar impaction syndrome involves TFCC wear only. At this early stage, a clinical exam in the face of an

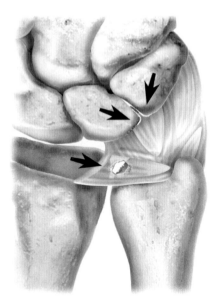

FIGURE 39.11. Palmer class IID triangular fibrocartilage complex injury.

ulnar positive variant is important in the diagnosis. Arthrography and magnetic resonance imaging (MRI) at this stage frequently are negative. Treatment should involve rest and avoidance of offending activities. Nonsteroidal antiinflammatory drugs and temporary splints may also be of benefit. Steroid injections combined with local anesthetic may be both diagnostic and therapeutic. There are no clinical studies available documenting treatment success rates in class IIA ulnar impaction syndrome.

Class IIB Treatment

Class IIB ulnar impaction syndrome involves triangular fibrocartilage wear plus ulnar head and/or lunate chondromalacia. A clinical exam of an ulnar positive variant and possibly MRI findings indicative of chondromalacia and synovitis may aid in the diagnosis at this stage. Arthrography at this stage is usually negative. However, a partial triangular fibrocartilage tear may sometimes be interpreted. Treatment at this stage begins conservatively with rest, nonsteroidal antiinflammatory drugs, splinting, and possibly injections. If symptoms persist and the condition is aggravated by work, job modifications or changes may decrease symptoms enough to avoid surgery. Frequently, class IIB ulnar impaction syndrome responds to these conservative methods. If symptoms persist, it is commonly because of progression of the disease to later stages of ulnar impaction syndrome. Arthroscopic exam with debridement of fibrillations and chondromalacia alone may alleviate some of the symptoms at this stage. Because the offending mechanical abnormality (increased load on the ulnar aspect of the wrist) has not been corrected, this treatment may provide only temporary relief. Persistent symptoms in the face of a significant ulnar positive variant at stage IIB would respond to surgical intervention to unload the ulnar carpus.

Class IIC Treatment

Class IIC ulnar impaction syndrome involves chondromalacia of the ulnar head and/or lunate and a triangular fibrocartilage horizontal disc tear. An initial trial of conservative treatment is appropriate, including nonsteroidal antiinflammatory drugs, splints, and possibly injections or vocational changes. There are numerous surgical options for class IIC ulnar impaction syndrome, and each will be examined individually.

Arthroscopic Triangular Fibrocartilage Debridement

TFCC tears have been treated by both open and arthroscopic methods (37–52). Successful results have been obtained by open debridement of the triangular fibrocartilage lesions (38–40). Open excision of a TFCC is a more invasive procedure than arthroscopic debridement. We also feel that the TFCC, ligaments, and other possible associated abnormalities in articular cartilage are better visualized through the arthroscope than in the open procedure. We feel patients have less pain and an earlier return to function, motion, and strength with the arthroscopic procedure compared to the open procedure. For these reasons, we feel that arthroscopic treatment of triangular fibrocartilage lesions is most appropriate.

The standard starting arthroscopy portal is made at the 3,4-portal region, which is located between the third and fourth extensor compartments overlying the radiocarpal joint. This is located just distal to Lister's tubercle. Our technique of portal entry is to make a small incision just through the skin with a #11 blade. Careful blunt dissection with a small mosquito hemostat is performed down to the wrist capsule. The mosquito hemostat is then used to perforate the wrist capsule to allow entry into the joint. It is important to use only blunt-tipped instruments for this. We do not routinely infiltrate the radiocarpal or midcarpal joints with saline before placement of the instrumentation. The cannula is next inserted through the capsular perforation made with the hemostat. Subsequent portals are established with needle localization techniques using a 20-gauge needle. The second portal commonly made is the 4,5-portal located between the fourth and fifth dorsal extensor compartment overlying the radiocarpal joint. We do not routinely use outflow on our arthroscopies unless there is significant bleeding or debris within the joint. The arthroscope may be exchanged between the 3,4- and the 4,5-portal to allow visualization of the entire radiocarpal joint. Other commonly used portals include the 6-ulnar (6U) and 6-radial (6R) portals based either ulnar or radial to the extensor carpi ulnaris tendon. Care must be taken to avoid injury to the ulnar nerve or the dorsal sensory branch with placement of these more ulnar portals. These portals do allow better visualization of the ulnar structures of the wrist including the lunotriquetral ligament. A 1,2-portal can also be made on the radial side of the wrist to allow better visualization of the radial structures or to allow for instrumentation. Care must be taken to avoid injury to the radial artery or superficial radial nerve along the radial aspect of the wrist.

Following diagnostic inspection and probing of the TFCC, the debridement of the triangular fibrocartilage central disc is performed. Our preferred method begins with the arthroscope in the 3,4-portal and a suction punch in the 4,5- or 6R-portal. Redundant margins at the perforation are debrided using the suction punch. Small biting arthroscopic instruments may also be used in this fashion. As the debridement progresses, it is frequently necessary to move the arthroscope from the 3,4-portal to the 4,5- or 6U-portal for complete visualization. This also allows for insertion of the arthroscopic debriding instruments into the 3,4-portal to complete the debridement. A small motorized shaver, usually in the 2.0 to 2.9 size range with a cutting blade, is next used to finally trim and complete debridement of the edges of the TFCC. On completion of the debridement, the wrist is copiously irrigated with normal saline to remove any small fragments and debris. A light sterile dressing is placed, and a small splint applied to the wrist, immobilizing it in neutral position. Progressive motion and strengthening exercises are allowed after approximately 7 to 10 days and are progressed as symptoms diminish.

With arthroscopic debridements of the triangular fibrocartilage, it is important to recognize the function of the central disc and surrounding stabilizing ligaments of the TFCC.

It is noted that multiple studies on partial excisions of the triangular fibrocartilage have not demonstrated an increase in postoperative instability (40,42,44,50). The important stabilizing function of the TFCC is maintained if no more than two-thirds (42,50) of the central disc is excised or a 2-mm-wide (50) periphery of the articular disc is preserved.

In ulnar positive variants with degenerative triangular fibrocartilage lesions, results indicate that impaction syndromes persist unless the ulnar positive variance and increased ulnar force transmission are addressed.

Osterman and associates (53) in 1996 presented a study on the natural history of untreated symptomatic TFCC tears. They found 35% of the ulnar negative to ulnar neutral patients were asymptomatic at follow-up. Symptoms in this group had not progressed, and those that diminished had done so in approximately 2 years' time. The second group of patients were ulnar positive variant individuals. This group had exhibited progression of symptoms and x-ray changes. Forty-four percent of this group had come to surgery. The study indicated that TFCC tears in ulnar negative to neutral variants did not worsen with time, and, in fact, one-third were asymptomatic at a final follow-up of approximately $9^{1}/_{2}$ years. However, TFCC tears in ulnar positive variant individuals tended to worsen both symptomatically and radiographically with time.

Wafer Procedure

The wafer procedure has been described for treatment of ulnar impaction syndrome (54–57). This involves limited resection of the distal ulnar head at its point of impaction with the ulnar carpus (Fig. 39.13). Feldon and associates (55) feel it is a viable alternative to formal ulnar shortening procedures. They do feel, however, that it is contraindicated in patients with instability of the DRUJ, DRUJ arthritis, or a positive ulnar variance of more than 4 mm. Experience with this procedure has demonstrated that approximately 6 months is needed postoperatively to reach the final satisfactory endpoint. In stage IIC and later stages of ulnar impaction syndrome, the wafer procedure can be performed arthroscopically through the large perforation in the TFCC. This has been described by Osterman (47), Buterbaugh (58),

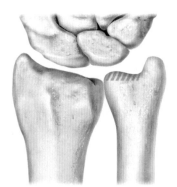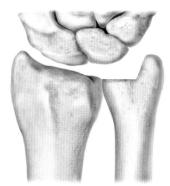

FIGURE 39.13. Ulnar impaction syndrome: wafer procedure.

Wnorowski (59), and Whipple (60). Wnorwoski and Palmar (59) demonstrated that there was significant unloading of the ulnar aspect of the wrist after excision of the central disc complex and the radial two-thirds of the ulnar head to a depth of subchondral bone. Arthroscopic wafer resections beyond 3 mm of bone do not continue to show progressive unloading of the ulnar carpus. This is critical because it is important to maintain as much of the articulation with the sigmoid notch as possible to maintain the DRUJ stability.

We cannot recommend the arthroscopic wafer procedure in stage IIB cases because of the potential for damage to adjacent structures. If the wafer procedure is to be performed in stage IIB cases, we recommend it be performed in an open fashion. The later stages of ulnar impaction syndrome with triangular fibrocartilage central disc perforation provide a portal and access point for resection of the distal head of the ulna with less risk for injury to the adjacent cartilage and ligamentous structures.

Formal Ulnar Shortening

Extraarticular ulnar shortening is very effective in the treatment of ulnar impaction syndrome and remains the "gold standard." In most cases of ulnar impaction syndrome, it has become our procedure of choice. In cases with significant DRUJ incongruity, DRUJ degenerative joint arthritis, or DRUJ deformity, other surgical alternatives should be considered. One major advantage of an ulnar shortening osteotomy is that it is an extraarticular procedure. The ulnocarpal joint and DRUJ are not directly disturbed, which theoretically lessens the risks of postoperative adhesions and stiffness. Clinical experience has shown a more rapid diminution in pain and rapid return to activity following ulnar shortening compared to wafer procedures. An additional important advantage of ulnar shortening is the possible effects on the lunotriquetral and DRUJ stability.

Linscheid, in 1987 (61), suggested that extraarticular ulnar shortening, in addition to unloading the ulnar carpus, may tighten the ulnocarpal and articular disc–carpal ligaments, thereby stabilizing the ulnar column of the wrist. Smith and associates (62) concluded that ulnar shortening plays a beneficial role in stabilizing the lunotriquetral interval, but its role may be limited.

Personal clinical experience has demonstrated that symptoms from ulnar impaction syndrome associated with mild lunotriquetral and DRUJ instability can be reliably alleviated by ulnar shortening alone.

An important consideration in an ulnar shortening osteotomy is the DRUJ congruity. A parallel alignment between the sigmoid notch and ulnar seat (ulnar articular surface at sigmoid notch) is important to prevent late ulnar head impingement and arthritic change at the DRUJ. Sagerman and associates (14), in 1995, showed that there was a wide variation in the inclination in the ulnar seat and sigmoid notch, and they suggested that ulnar shortening procedures can produce significant alterations in the DRUJ alignment and mechanics.

A potential disadvantage of the ulnar shortening osteotomy is nonunion at the osteotomy site. The risk of this can be lessened by precise rigid internal fixation, oblique osteotomies to increase bony contact area, and the use of low-speed oscillating saws with cooling irrigation. We believe that no more than 3 to 4 mm of shortening should be performed because of the risk of altering DRUJ mechanics.

Our technique for ulnar shortening osteotomy involves a longitudinal skin incision overlying the ulnar subcutaneous border of the forearm. Care must be taken to protect the dorsal sensory branch of the ulnar nerve. Subperiosteal stripping along the dorsal aspect of the ulna is performed to allow placement of a seven-hole, 3.5-mm dynamic compression plate dorsally. The plate is positioned overlying the distal ulna with the distal end of the plate a centimeter or two from the distal end of the ulna. The central hole in the plate will overlie the osteotomy site. At the proposed site of the osteotomy, the volar periosteum is stripped to afford exposure for the osteotomy. The two most distal screw holes in the plate are filled with 3.5-mm cortical screws. An oblique mark is made over the ulna at the proposed site of the osteotomy. This is made in an oblique fashion extending from the dorsal distal to proximal volar direction. This is positioned so the central hole in the plate can be filled with an interfragmentary screw perpendicular to the osteotomy, providing compression (Fig. 39.14). Next, the distal screw hole is loosened, and the other screw is removed. The plate is then swung out from the osteotomy site. The AO small distracter (63) is applied to the ulnar aspect of the distal ulna, spanning the proposed osteotomy site. The osteotomy is next completed through approximately 70% of the bone with continuous saline irrigation. A second free saw blade is then placed in the original cut, and a second cut is made parallel to the first using the free saw blade as a guide. It is important to consider the width of the saw blade in the amount of bone resected. We have in the past

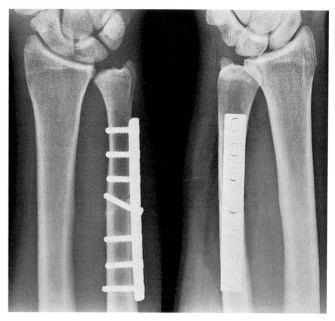

FIGURE 39.14. Radiograph demonstrating plate positioning that allows an interfragmentary screw to be set perpendicular to the osteotomy, providing compression.

stacked saw blades one upon another in an attempt to resect the width of bone desired, however, we have found that this has created excessive heat and burning of the bony edges, potentially leading to an increased incidence of nonunion. The goal of the surgery is to resect enough ulnar shaft to obtain a final ulnar variance of 0 to −1 mm. Once the cuts are completed, the resected segment of ulnar bone is removed. The AO distracter is then compressed, closing down the osteotomy site. Placement of this distracter maintains rotational alignment and simplifies fixation and stabilization of the bony ends. With the osteotomy site compressed by the AO distracter, the plate is rotated back into place overlying the dorsal aspect of the ulna. The two most distal screw holes are refilled, and the screws tightened back down. The screw hole proximal to the osteotomy site is next filled under compression. The interfragmentary screw is then placed perpendicular to the osteotomy to provide interfragmentary compression through the plate with the near cortex overdrilled. The remaining screw holes are then filled, and the distracter is removed. X-rays taken intraoperatively confirm satisfactory hardware placement and satisfactory correction of the ulnar variance. The tourniquet is let down, and hemostasis is obtained. Short arm immobilization is maintained for 3 to 4 weeks, and then a therapy program is instituted for range-of-motion and progressive strengthening.

Rayhack (64,65) has developed a precision ulnar osteotomy system for ulnar shortening procedures. It is a set of guides and clamps that aid in bone cutting and allow placement of a 3.5-mm plate. It provides a standardized "cookbook" approach to ulnar shortening osteotomies.

Rigid internal fixation of the osteotomy site is essential to prevent risk of nonunions. Generally, the best fixation can be obtained with AO principals and dynamic compression plating. The type of osteotomy utilized will also affect the healing potential. The wider the surface area of bony contact (e.g., oblique or step-cut osteotomy versus transverse), the greater the chance of union. A 45° oblique osteotomy increases the healing bone surface contact area by 40% compared to a straight transverse osteotomy (64). Rayhack (64,65) compared the healing time of transverse osteotomies to that of a 45° oblique osteotomy with the Rayhack osteotomy system. Twenty-three transverse osteotomies healed in an average of 21 weeks with one nonunion. The oblique osteotomy group healed in 11 weeks with no nonunions.

The clinical effectiveness of ulnar shortening for ulnar impaction syndrome is well documented (63–68). DRUJ arthritis or incongruity, excessive DRUJ instability, or excessive lunotriquetral instability will contribute to failure if these factors are not appreciated preoperatively. Removal of hardware after ulnar shortening osteotomies depends on patient symptoms.

Class IIC ulnar impaction syndrome is a common stage of presentation. Surgical treatment includes arthroscopic triangular fibrocartilage debridement, an open or arthroscopic wafer procedure, or a formal ulnar shortening. Our procedure of choice for class IIC ulnar impaction syndrome is the formal ulnar shortening as described above, provided there is no preexisting DRUJ incongruity.

Class IID Treatment

Class IID ulnar impaction syndrome involves progression of the disease to involve the lunotriquetral joint. Arthrography or MRI and arthroscopy will demonstrate a lunotriquetral ligament perforation. The degree of lunotriquetral instability will vary with the severity of the lunotriquetral ligament disruption and the chronicity of the ulnar impaction syndrome. Surgical treatments at this stage are similar to those for stage IIC disease. However, for cases with mild to moderate lunotriquetral instability, formal ulnar shortening is a more attractive procedure than the wafer procedure because it may tighten the ulnar ligaments, thereby stabilizing the lunotriquetral joint as previously mentioned (61,62).

The degree of lunotriquetral instability can be assessed clinically by lunotriquetral ballottement tests, etc. (69,70). The best method for assessment of lunotriquetral instability, however, is arthroscopically with mid-carpal joint inspection. Based on laboratory studies (62), severe lunotriquetral instability in late stage IID ulnar impaction syndrome will likely not be adequately stabilized by ulnar shortening alone. An approach to this problem is to perform the ulnar shortening osteotomy, rehabilitate the patient, and on subsequent reexaminations determine if there is symptomatic persistence of lunotriquetral instability. Further treatment of this lunotriquetral instability can then be performed once it has been determined that this is a significant contributing factor to the patient's symptom complex. Alternatively, at the time of formal ulnar shortening, if severe instability is noted at the lunotriquetral interval on arthroscopic examination, it may be warranted to proceed with formal treatment of the lunotriquetral instability in addition to alleviating the excessive force transmission at the distal ulna.

There are numerous reports in the literature regarding treatment options for lunotriquetral instability (69,71–77). Few of these, however, address the lunotriquetral instability specifically in cases of ulnar impaction syndrome (49,57, 71). Treatment has ranged from lunotriquetral ligament repair to reconstruction to arthroscopically assisted internal fixation to lunotriquetral fusion. Variable results have been associated with all methods (49,57,69,71–77).

Lunotriquetral repair would be an unlikely option in cases of chronic ulnar impaction syndrome as attenuation and degeneration of the ligament from chronic loading would leave inadequate substance for repair.

The most commonly described treatment for lunotriquetral instability is lunotriquetral arthrodesis. Variable results are also reported with this procedure (69,71–76). Numerous techniques for lunotriquetral arthrodesis have been described (71,73,74,76) and are outlined elsewhere in this text. Successful outcomes of lunotriquetral arthrodesis in ulnar impaction syndrome have been reported and recommended (49,57).

Formal ulnar shortening, in our opinion, is the preferred method of treatment for stage IID ulnar impaction syndrome with mild lunotriquetral instability, assuming there is no significant DRUJ arthritis or incongruity evident.

Class IIE Treatment

Class IIE ulnar impaction syndrome is the end stage for excessive ulnar column load in the wrist. It is exemplified by lunate and ulnar chondromalacia, a lunotriquetral ligament perforation, and ulnocarpal arthritis. Occasionally, this arthritis is also evident at the DRUJ. Plain-film x-rays will demonstrate the arthritic change evident at the DRUJ and ulnocarpal area, and at times, include the lunotriquetral interval. At this stage, procedures such as triangular fibrocartilage debridement, wafer procedure, or ulnar shortening that simply unload the ulnar aspect of the wrist are insufficient. End-stage arthritic joints have developed, and simply correcting the biomechanical abnormality will not alleviate the arthritic change. Treatment of the lunotriquetral joint arthritis at this stage would include a lunotriquetral arthrodesis. If other joint abnormalities are present on the radial side of the wrist, consideration for other procedures such as proximal row carpectomy or complete wrist arthrodesis may be necessary.

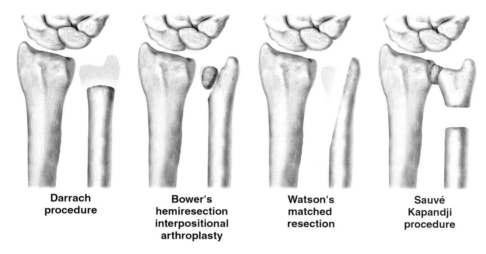

FIGURE 39.15. Ulnar impaction syndrome: distal radioulnar joint salvage procedures.

Multiple salvage procedures for treating the arthritic change have been described. The distal ulnar head resection popularized by Darrach (1,2) has been used for many years for treatment of end-stage DRUJ problems. Other modifications include Bowers' hemiresection interpositional arthroplasty or Watson's matched ulnar resection. The Sauvé-Kapandji procedure is also an option for addressing end-stage ulnar impaction syndrome associated with DRUJ arthritis. It must also be noted that frequently these procedures must be considered in earlier stages of ulnar impaction syndrome with concurrent DRUJ incongruity. A formal ulnar shortening in the face of the DRUJ incongruity would potentially worsen the DRUJ pathology and lead to progressive arthritic change and continued symptoms.

Salvage procedures for the stage IIE ulnar impaction syndrome have generally demonstrated successful results based on the literature (78–100). The choice of a Darrach resection, Bowers' hemiresection interpositional arthroplasty, Watson's matched ulnar resection, or a Sauvé-Kapandji procedure as the salvage procedure for end-stage ulnar impaction syndrome will be based on surgical preference, training, and prior experience. Each of these procedures is addressed in depth in other chapters in this text, and we refer you to those for further explanation (Fig. 39.15).

DYNAMIC ULNAR IMPACTION SYNDROME

Dynamic ulnar impaction syndrome is an uncommon condition that presents in patients with intermittent symptoms that tends to occur primarily with forceful gripping activities. Usually these patients have ulnar neutral or negative variance on their x-rays, yet their examination and history is consistent with ulnar impaction syndrome. A stress x-ray consisting of a pronated maximal grip view may be helpful in demonstrating significant dynamic positive ulnar variance. These dynamic stress x-rays and reproduction of symptoms with similar motion and activity are important in the aid and diagnosis of this condition. Arthroscopy is helpful for confirmation of the typical ulnar impaction syndrome changes on the central disc and lunate. Treatment of choice is an ulnar shortening, with generally successful results.

SECONDARY ULNAR IMPACTION SYNDROME

Ulnar impaction syndrome commonly is caused by a congenitally long ulna. This is a common finding in many individuals. There are many other causes of ulnar impaction syndrome, and these are termed secondary ulnar impaction. Other causes include a distal radius malunion, Essex-Lopresti injury, previous radial head resection, distal radial physeal injury, or previous radial shortening procedure (as in the case of Kienböck's disease). In the case of a distal radial malunion, an osteotomy of the distal radius may be most appropriate in treating the ulnar impaction syndrome.

Ulnar impaction syndrome in the case of an Essex-Lopresti injury or previous radial head resection is a much more difficult problem to treat. At this point, there are no sound solutions for this problem. Radial head replacement with implants has been described. Silastic implants have offered no long-term solutions for this because of mechanical breakdown and synovitis. Newer metallic designs have yet to be shown in long-term studies to provide satisfactory results. At times, the final solution for a persistently symptomatic Essex-Lopresti lesion is creation of a one-bone forearm.

Ulnar impaction syndrome related to previous radial growth arrests can lead to a wide variation in pathology.

The spectrum of pathology ranges from very mild ulnar positivity that can be easily treated by wafer procedures or ulnar shortening procedures to significant variance discrepancies that may require more formalized salvage procedures.

CONCLUSION

Ulnar impaction syndrome is a spectrum of clinical findings. It is secondary to impaction of the ulnar head against the TFCC and ulnar carpus, resulting in progressive deterioration of the triangular fibrocartilage, ulnocarpal joint surfaces, and lunotriquetral ligament. The disorder is characterized by an ulnar positive variance. There are multiple stages of ulnar impaction syndrome progressing to end-stage arthritis. As a general rule, surgical procedures for the treatment of ulnar impaction syndrome are successful in alleviating symptoms. Ulnar impaction syndrome without arthritic change and with a congruent DRUJ, in our opinion, is best treated by a formal ulnar shortening osteotomy. This not only unloads the excessive forces across the ulnar carpus, but also has the potential to tighten the lunotriquetral and DRUJ articulation, providing additional stability at that level. Further progression of ulnar impaction syndrome can be complicated by arthritic changes at the ulnocarpal joint and DRUJ. These will require more formalized salvage procedures including hemiresections or arthrodeses. Ulnar impaction syndrome is best treated by careful examination of the patient, determination of the stage of ulnar impaction syndrome, and application of appropriate treatment, whether conservative or surgical.

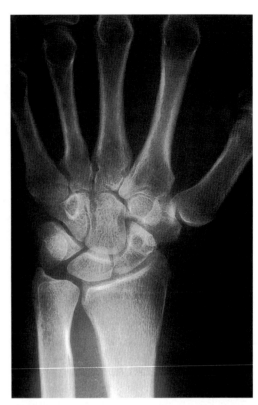

EDITORS' FIGURE 39.1. Ulnar impaction syndrome. This is a young girl demonstrating significant ulnar impaction syndrome that is totally asymptomatic. There is deformity of the lunate but adequate cartilage exists between the distal end of the ulna and the lunate. The existence of a long ulna is not in itself an indication for step-cut shortening. An intact distal radioulnar joint should be preserved if possible.

EDITORS' COMMENTS

Ulnar impaction syndrome is a single term that covers multiple clinical entities. The most common clinical entity involves a relatively normal ulnar variance with a pistoning effect of the hand and radius. Heavy loads in the hand are taken entirely by the radius and produce a proximal migration of the radius, with collapse of the cartilage at the wrist and elbow. The triquetral–lunate joint impacts on the ulna, and partial tears may be produced. Symptoms are usually low grade, temporary, and responsive to conservative treatment. Occasionally, this phenomenon will produce enough of an interference with the quality of life that surgery is indicated. Partial lunate–triquetral tearing is noted, and minimal step-cut shortening of the ulna is curative.

The second diagnosis under ulnar impaction syndrome encompasses the overly long ulnas. These can become symptomatic in teenagers, where the long ulna impacts on the carpals and symptoms are produced, or it can remain asymptomatic (Editors' Fig. 39.1). This same phenomenon is seen commonly in patients in their fourth and fifth decades, when low-grade longstanding ulna impaction has now produced a secondary degenerative arthritis between the end of the distal ulna and the proximal ulnar aspect of the lunate (Editors' Fig. 39.2). Again, if these are symptomatic enough to require some form of repair, the definitive procedure is a step-cut shortening of the ulna (Editors' Fig. 39.3). Only a few millimeters will usually suffice. The cartilage from the distal end of the ulna in a "wafer" procedure is not as satisfactory. The problem here arises because the triangular fibrocartilage must rotate through 180 degrees across the top of the ulna as the forearm supinates and pronates. Destroying the cartilage on the distal ulna produces an unsatisfactory interface between the ulna and the triangular fibrocartilage, and prolonged or permanent symptoms result.

The most common ulnar impaction syndrome is seen after a Colles' fracture. There is usually concomitant malalignment of the sulcus joint in the radius for the distal ulna, and the appropriate procedure is typically a matched ulnar arthroplasty. This is a very gratifying procedure in the less active, somewhat older patient post-Colles'. It not only takes care of their symptoms, but also

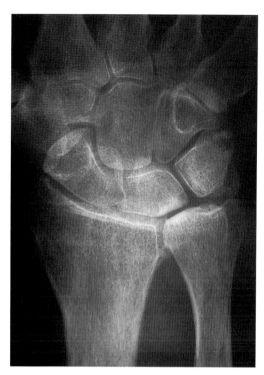

EDITORS' FIGURE 39.2. Ulnar impaction syndrome. This is an older patient with longstanding ulnar impaction syndrome, now experiencing symptoms. The cartilage is gone, and there are sclerotic changes on the opposing surfaces of the lunate and ulna.

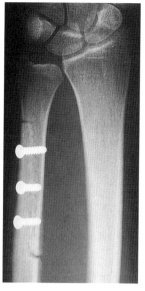 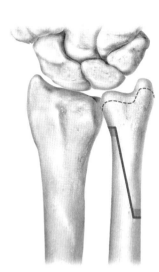

EDITORS' FIGURE 39.3. A,B: Step-cut shortening. The optimal step-cut shortening procedure will bring the distal ulna to the level of the articular surface of the radius. Screws or plates may be used for fixation. With this technique, it is most important that the base of the osteotomy for each segment be wider. Therefore, the long cut on the osteotomy is not parallel to the long axis of ulna, but slopes to prevent fracture at the stress riser areas in the two transverse portions of the osteotomy. Step-cut shortening may relieve the symptoms of triquetral impingement ligament tear (TILT) syndrome by drawing the ulnar sling mechanism proximally. In addition, it may be all that is necessary in the management of partial tears of the triquetral–lunate ligament. Matched ulnar arthroplasty is not indicated unless the distal radioulnar joint is destroyed.

increases supination–pronation and wrist flexion–extension. There are radial shortening surgeries or injuries that produce ulnar impaction syndrome. Without the Colles' fracture, there is no linear malalignment of the sulcus joint component of the DRUJ. Step-cut shortening may be carried out. The DRUJ should be maintained if it appears to be adequate. The step-cut shortening can always be converted to a matched ulnar arthroplasty if necessary.

Another category of ulnar impaction occurs in Madelung's deformity, where the etiology is the increased radioulnar slope of the radius. The carpals exceed the ability of the ligaments to maintain an upslope position, the ulna is long, and impaction on the distal ulna occurs. Most symptoms in Madelung's are secondary to ulnar impaction, although less commonly the slope of the distal radius may produce problems in itself, and osteotomy of the radius may be indicated. The treatment in Madelung's is a form of matched ulnar arthroplasty.

Ulnar impaction also occurs in rheumatoid arthritis patients, in whom ulnar carpal translation occurs secondary to panligamentous destruction. This is not an indication for a Sauvé-Kapandji procedure. The best approach is to reestablish the wrist on the distal radius with the rheumatoid arthroplasty technique described in Chapter 61 combined with a matched ulnar arthroplasty.

REFERENCES

1. Darrach W. Anterior dislocation of the head of the ulna. *Ann Surg* 1912;56:802.
2. Darrach W. Partial excision of lower shaft of ulna for deformity following Colles fracture. *Ann Surg* 1913;57:764.
3. Milch H. Cuff resection of the ulna for malunited Colles fracture. *J Bone Joint Surg* 1941;23:311–313.
4. Palmer A. Triangular fibrocartilage complex lesions: A classification. *J Hand Surg [Am]* 1989;14:594–606.
5. Friedman S, Palmer A. The ulnar impaction syndrome. *Hand Clin* 1991;7:295–310.
6. Bowers W. The distal radioulnar joint. In: Green D, ed. *Operative hand surgery, ed. 3.* New York: Churchill Livingstone, 973–1019.
7. Palmer A, Werner F. The triangular fibrocartilage complex of the wrist: Anatomy and function. *J Hand Surg [Am]* 1981;6:153–162.
8. Bell MJ, Hill RJ, McMurtry RY. Ulnar impingement syndrome. *J Bone Joint Surg Br* 1985;67:126–129.
9. Almquist EE. Evolution of the distal radioulnar joint. *Clin Orthop* 1992;275:5–13.
10. Kleinman WB, Graham TJ. Distal ulnar injury and dysfunction. In: Piemer CA, ed. *Surgery of the hand and upper extremity.* New York: McGraw-Hill, 1996;667–709.
11. Palmer AK. The distal radioulnar joint: Anatomy, biomechanics, and triangular fibrocartilage complex abnormalities. *Hand Clin* 1987;3:31–40.
12. Ekenstam F. Anatomy of the distal radioulnar joint. *Clin Orthop* 1992;275:14–18.

13. Linscheid RL. Biomechanics of the distal radioulnar joint. *Clin Orthop* 1992;275:46–55.
14. Sagerman SD, Zogby RG, Palmer AK, et al. Relative articular inclination of the distal radioulnar joint: A radiographic study. *J Hand Surg [Am]* 1995;20:597–601.
15. Mikic Z. Detailed anatomy of the articular disc of the distal radioulnar joint. *Clin Orthop* 1989;245:123–132.
16. Bednar MS, Arnoczky SP, Weiland AJ. The microvasculature of the triangular fibrocartilage complex: Its clinical significance. *J Hand Surg [Am]* 1991;16:1101–1105.
17. Mikic Z. The blood supply of the human distal radioulnar joint and the microvasculature of its articular disk. *Clin Orthop* 1992; 275:19–28.
18. Osterman AL, Hunt TR, Bednar JM, et al. *Vascularity of the triangular fibrocartilage as measured* in vivo. Paper presented at the 49th Annual ASSH Meeting, Cincinnati, OH, October 28, 1994.
19. Chidgey LK, Dell PC, Bittar ES, et al. Histologic anatomy of the triangular fibrocartilage. *J Hand Surg [Am]* 1991;16:1084–1100.
20. Mikic Z, Somer L, Somer T. Histologic structure of the articular disk of the human distal radioulnar joint. *Clin Orthop* 1992;275: 29–36.
21. Rabinowitz RS, Light TR, Havey RM, et al. The role of the interosseous membrane and triangular fibrocartilage complex in forearm stability. *J Hand Surg [Am]* 1994;19:385–393.
22. Palmer AK, Werner FW. Biomechanics of the distal radioulnar joint. *Clin Orthop* 1984;187:26–35.
23. Palmer AK, Glisson RR, Werner FW. Ulnar variance determination. *J Hand Surg [Am]* 1982;7:376–379.
24. Epner R, Bowers W, Guilford B. Ulnar variance—The effect of wrist position and roentgen filming technique. *J Hand Surg [Am]* 1982;7:298–305.
25. Steyers CM, Blair WF. Measuring ulnar variance: A comparison of techniques. *J Hand Surg [Am]* 1989;14:607–612.
26. Hardy DC, Totty WG, Reinus WR, et al. Posteroanterior wrist radiography: Importance of arm positioning. *J Hand Surg [Am]* 1987;12:504–508.
27. Friedman SL, Palmer AK, Short WH, et al. The change in ulnar variance with grip. *J Hand Surg [Am]* 1993;18:713–716.
28. Palmer AK, Glisson RR, Werner FW. Relationship between ulnar variance and triangular fibrocartilage complex thickness. *J Hand Surg [Am]* 1984;9:681–683.
29. Werner FW, Palmer AK, Fortino MD, et al. Force transmission through the distal ulna: Effect of ulnar variance, lunate fossa angulation, and radial and palmar tilt of the distal radius. *J Hand Surg [Am]* 1992;17:423–428.
30. Short WH, Palmer AK, Werner FW, et al. A biomechanical study of distal radial fractures. *J Hand Surg [Am]* 1987;12:529–534.
31. Hotchkiss RN, An KN, Sowa DT, et al. An anatomic and mechanical study of the interosseous membrane of the forearm: Pathomechanics of proximal migration of the radius. *J Hand Surg [Am]* 1989;14:256–261.
32. Birkbeck D, Failla JM, Hoshaw S, et al. *The interosseous membrane affects load distribution in the forearm.* Paper presented at the 50th Meeting of the ASSH, San Francisco, CA, September 16, 1995.
33. Mikic Z. Age changes in the triangular fibrocartilage of the wrist joint. *J Anat* 1978;126:367–384.
34. Viegas SF, Ballentyne G. Attritional lesions of the wrist joint. *J Hand Surg [Am]* 1987;12:1025–1029.
35. Shigematsu S, Abe M, Onomura T, et al. Arthrography of the normal and posttraumatic wrist. *J Hand Surg [Am]* 1989;14: 410–412.
36. Uchiyama S, Terayama K. Radiographic changes in wrists with ulnar plus variance observed over a ten-year period. *J Hand Surg [Am]* 1991;16:45–48.
37. Palmer A. Partial excision of the triangular fibrocartilage complex. In: Gelberman, RH, ed. *Master techniques in orthopedic surgery: The wrist.* New York: Raven Press, 1994;207–218.
38. Coleman H. Injuries of the articular disc at the wrist. *J Bone Joint Surg Br* 1960;42:522–529.
39. Van der Linden A. Disk lesion of the wrist joint. *J Hand Surg [Am]* 1986;11:490–497.
40. Menon J, Wood V, Schoene H, et al. Isolated tears of the triangular fibrocartilage of the wrist: Results of partial excision. *J Hand Surg [Am]* 1984;9:527–530.
41. Palmer A. Triangular fibrocartilage disorders: Injury patterns and treatment. *Arthroscopy* 1990;6:125–132.
42. Palmer A, Werner F, Glisson R, et al. Partial excision of the triangular fibrocartilage complex. *J Hand Surg [Am]* 1988;13:403–406.
43. Osterman A, Terrill R. Arthroscopic treatment of TFCC lesions. *Hand Clin* 1991;7:277–281.
44. Chidgey L. The distal radioulnar joint: Problems and solutions. *J Am Acad Orthop Surg* 1995;3:95–109.
45. Whipple T, Geissler W. Arthroscopic management of wrist triangular fibrocartilage complex injuries in the athlete. *Orthopedics* 1993;16:1061–1067.
46. Bednar J, Osterman A. The role of arthroscopy in the treatment of traumatic triangular fibrocartilage injuries. *Hand Clin* 1994; 10:605–614.
47. Osterman A. Arthroscopic debridement of triangular fibrocartilage complex tears. *Arthroscopy* 1990;6:120–124.
48. Stokes HM, Poehling GG, Trainor BC, et al. *Results of arthroscopic debridement of isolated tears of the triangular fibrocartilage complex of the wrist.* Paper presented at the ASSH 45th Annual Meeting, Toronto, Canada, September 1990.
49. Minami A, Ishikawa J, Suenaga N, et al. Clinical results of treatment of triangular fibrocartilage complex tears by arthroscopic debridement. *J Hand Surg [Am]* 1996;21:406–411.
50. Adams B. Partial excision of the triangular fibrocartilage complex articular disk: A biomechanical study. *J Hand Surg [Am]* 1993;18:334–340.
51. Hermansdorfer J, Kleinman W. Management of chronic peripheral tears of the triangular fibrocartilage complex. *J Hand Surg [Am]* 1991;16:340–346.
52. Nagle D. Arthroscopic treatment of degenerative tears of the triangular fibrocartilage. *Hand Clin* 1994;10:615–624.
53. Osterman L, Bednar J, Gambino K, et al. *The natural history of untreated symptomatic tears in the triangular fibrocartilage.* Paper presented at the ASSH 51st Annual Meeting, Nashville, TN, September 30, 1996.
54. Feldon P, Terrono A, Belsky M. The "wafer" procedure. *Clin Orthop* 1992;275:124–129.
55. Feldon P, Terrono A, Belsky M. Wafer distal ulna resection for triangular fibrocartilage tears and/or ulnar impaction syndrome. *J Hand Surg [Am]* 1992;17:731–737.
56. Feldon P. Ulnar impaction syndrome: Treatment by partial (wafer) resection of the distal ulna. *Techniques Orthop* 1992;7: 58–65.
57. Bilos J, Chamberland D. Distal ulnar head shortening for treatment of triangular fibrocartilage complex tears with ulna positive variance. *J Hand Surg [Am]* 1991;16:1115–1119.
58. Buterbaugh G. Ulnar impaction syndrome: Treatment by arthroscopic removal of the distal ulna. *Techniques Orthop* 1992; 7:66–71.
59. Wnorowski D, Palmer A, Werner F, et al. Anatomic and biomechanical analysis of the arthroscopic wafer procedure. *Arthroscopy* 1992;8:204–212.
60. Whipple T. *Arthroscopic surgery: The wrist.* Philadelphia: JB Lippincott, 1992;103–118.
61. Linscheid R. Ulnar lengthening and shortening. *Hand Clin* 1987;3:69–79.

62. Smith B, Short W, Werner F, et al. *The effect of ulnar shortening on lunotriquetral motion and instability: A biomechanical study.* Paper presented at the 12th Annual Residents and Fellows Conference in Hand Surgery—ASSH, Cincinnati, OH, October 25, 1994.
63. Wehbe M, Mawr B, Cautilli D. Ulnar shortening using the AO small distractor. *J Hand Surg [Am]* 1995;20:959–964.
64. Rayhack J. Ulnar impaction syndrome: Treatment by precision oblique ulnar shortening. *Techniques Orthop* 1992;7:49–57.
65. Rayhack J, Gasser S, Latta L, et al. Precision oblique osteotomy of shortening of the ulna. *J Hand Surg [Am]* 1993;18:908–918.
66. Darrow JC Jr, Linscheid RL, Dobyns JH, et al. Distal ulnar recession for disorders of the distal radioulnar joint. *J Hand Surg [Am]* 1985;10:482–491.
67. Boulas J, Milek M. Ulnar shortening for tears of the triangular fibrocartilaginous complex. *J Hand Surg [Am]* 1990;15:415–420.
68. Chun S, Palmer A. The ulnar impaction syndrome; follow-up of ulnar shortening osteotomy. *J Hand Surg [Am]* 1993;18:46–53.
69. Reagan DS, Linscheid RL, Dobyns JH. Lunotriquetral sprains. *J Hand Surg [Am]* 1984;9:502–514.
70. Kleinman WB. *Am Soc Surg Hand Corr Newsl* 1985;51.
71. Pin P, Young L, Gilula L, et al. Management of chronic lunotriquetral ligament tears. *J Hand Surg [Am]* 1989;14:77–83.
72. Ambrose L, Posner M. Lunate–triquetral and midcarpal joint instability. *Hand Clin* 1992;8:653–668.
73. Nelson D, Manske P, Pruitt D, et al. Lunotriquetral arthrodesis. *J Hand Surg [Am]* 1993;18:1113–1120.
74. Kirschenbaum D, Coyle M, Leddy J. Chronic lunotriquetral instability: Diagnosis and treatment. *J Hand Surg [Am]* 1993;18:1107–1112.
75. Favero KJ, Bishop AT, Linscheid RL. *Luno-triquetral ligament disruption: A comparative study of treatment methods.* Paper presented at ASSH 46th Annual Meeting, Orlando, FL, 1991.
76. Watson K, Guidera P, Zeppieri J, et al. *Luno-triquetral arthrodesis.* Paper presented at ASSH 50th Annual Meeting, San Francisco, CA, September 15, 1995.
77. Osterman A, Seidman G. The role of arthroscopy in the treatment of lunatotriquetral ligament injuries. *Hand Clin* 1995;11:41–50.
78. Ruby L. Darrach procedure. In: Gelberman, RH, ed. *Master techniques in orthopedic surgery: The wrist.* New York: Raven Press, 1994;279–285.
79. Ruby L, Ferenz C, Dell P. The pronator quadratus interposition transfer: An adjunct to resection arthroplasty of the distal radioulnar joint. *J Hand Surg [Am]* 1996;21:60–65.
80. Sotereanos D, Leit M. A modified Darrach procedure for treatment of the painful distal radioulnar joint. *Clin Orthop* 1996;325:140–147.
81. Breen T, Jupiter J. Extensor carpi ulnaris and flexor carpi ulnaris tenodesis of the unstable distal ulna. *J Hand Surg [Am]* 1989;14:612–617.
82. Tsai T, Shimizu H, Adkins P. A modified extensor carpi ulnaris tenodesis with the Darrach procedure. *J Hand Surg [Am]* 1993;18:697–702.
83. Kleinman W, Greenberg J. Salvage of the failed Darrach procedure. *J Hand Surg [Am]* 1995;20:951–958.
84. Tulipan D, Eaton R, Eberhart R. The Darrach procedure defended: Technique redefined and long-term follow-up. *J Hand Surg [Am]* 1991;16:438–444.
85. Minami A, Ogino T, Minami M. Treatment of distal radioulnar disorders. *J Hand Surg [Am]* 1987;12:189–196.
86. Nolan W, Eaton R. A Darrach procedure for distal ulnar pathology derangements. *Clin Orthop* 1992;275:85–89.
87. Bowers W. Distal radioulnar joint arthroplasty: The hemiresection–interposition technique. *J Hand Surg [Am]* 1985;10:169–178.
88. Bowers W. Distal radioulnar joint arthroplasty—Current concepts. *Clin Orthop* 1992;275:104–109.
89. Bowers W. Hemiresection interposition technique (HIT) arthroplasty of the distal radioulnar joint. In: Gelberman, RH, ed. *Master techniques in orthopedic surgery: The wrist.* New York: Raven Press, 1994;303–318.
90. Watson K, Ryu J, Burgess R. Matched distal ulnar resection. *J Hand Surg [Am]* 1986;11:812–817.
91. Watson K, Gabuzda G. Matched distal ulna resection of posttraumatic disorders of the distal radioulnar joint. *J Hand Surg [Am]* 1992;17:724–730.
92. Imbriglia J, Matthews D. The treatment of chronic traumatic subluxation of the distal ulna by hemiresection interposition arthroplasty. *Hand Clin* 1991;7:329–334.
93. Minami A, Kaneda K, Itoga H. Hemiresection–interposition arthroplasty of the distal radioulnar joint associated with repair of triangular fibrocartilage complex lesions. *J Hand Surg [Am]* 1991;16:1120–1125.
94. Bain GI, Pugh M, MacDermid J, et al. Matched hemiresection interposition arthroplasty of the distal radioulnar joint. *J Hand Surg [Am]* 1995;20:944–950.
95. Taleisnik J. The Sauvé-Kapandji procedure. *Clin Orthop* 1992;275:110–123.
96. Gordon L, Levinsohn D, Moore S, et al. The Sauvé-Kapandji procedure for the treatment of posttraumatic distal radioulnar joint problems. *Hand Clin* 1991;7:397–403.
97. Schneider L, Imbriglia J. Radioulnar joint fusion for distal radioulnar joint instability. *Hand Clin* 1991;7:391–395.
98. Sanders R, Hugh F, Hontas R. The Sauvé-Kapandji procedure: A salvage operation for the distal radioulnar joint. *J Hand Surg [Am]* 1991;16:1125–1129.
99. Johnson M, Lawrence J, Dionysian E. The Kapandji procedure for the treatment of distal radioulnar joint derangement in young patients. *Contemp Orthop* 1995;31:291–298.
100. Minami A, Suzuki K, Suenaga N, et al. The Sauvé-Kapandji procedure for osteoarthritis of the distal radioulnar joint. *J Hand Surg [Am]* 1995;20:602–608.

40

TRIQUETRAL IMPINGEMENT LIGAMENT TEAR SYNDROME

H. KIRK WATSON
JEFFREY WEINZWEIG

Ulnar wrist pain is a complex problem both diagnostically and therapeutically. Numerous etiologies, such as ulnar impaction syndrome, degenerative joint disease of the lunotriquetral (LT) joint, dislocation of the distal radioulnar joint (DRUJ), and ulnar impingement syndrome, demonstrate specific radiographic findings that indicate particular therapeutic approaches (1–5). However, distinguishing between other causes of ulnar wrist pain, such as triangular fibrocartilage complex (TFCC) tears, extensor carpi ulnaris (ECU) tendinitis, and ulnocarpal ligamentous injuries, can be challenging, especially in the absence of radiographic findings (6–10).

The symptoms of ulnar wrist pathology can vary from specific complaints of localized pain and swelling along the ulnar head or ulnar carpus to vague complaints of generalized discomfort involving that entire region of the wrist. These symptoms may or may not be the result of precedent trauma, although they are in the majority of cases. Limited wrist motion may occur along with tenderness on supination and pronation, on direct palpation of the DRUJ, at the ulnar head, over the ECU tendon or ulnar carpus, with manipulation of the TFCC, or any combination of these. Radiographic studies may demonstrate evidence of ulnar impaction syndrome, ulnar impingement syndrome, or degenerative joint disease, dislocation, or articular incongruity of the DRUJ; they may also appear normal (11–13).

The finding of very localized significant tenderness directly over the triquetrum on examination may indicate another etiology of ulnar wrist pain. When occasionally accompanied by mild to moderate swelling along the ulnar aspect of the wrist, limited wrist motion, decreased grip strength, a history of a wrist hyperflexion injury, and normal radiographs, chronic localized triquetral pain is most likely attributable to a syndrome we have termed *triquetral impingement ligament tear* (TILT) (14). This constellation of findings is usually the result of a hyperflexion pronation injury with subsequent pain on the ulnar aspect of the wrist. The mechanism of injury allows an ulnar cuff of fibrous tissue to be displaced distally from the rest of the ulnar sling and impinge against the ulnar-sloped edge of the triquetrum.

The "ulnar sling mechanism" is neither dorsal capsule nor synovium. It represents the entire ulnar cuff of ligamentous collagen ulnar to the radius. This includes the extensor retinaculum, dorsal extrinsic carpal ligaments, dorsal radioulnar ligaments, ECU sheath, volar extrinsic carpal ligaments, ulnolunate and ulnotriquetral ligaments, and triangular fibrocartilage. The short interosseous ligaments are not included. Minor ulnar translation of the carpus will produce a similar capsule–bone impingement.

This chronic impingement of a detached ulnar sling on the triquetrum causes hyperemia and articular cartilage loss with eburnation along the proximal ulnar aspect of the triquetrum and softening of the bone (Fig. 40.1).

SURGICAL TECHNIQUE FOR TILT REPAIR

The wrist is approached through an ulnar transverse incision, approximately 3 cm in length, just distal to the ulnar head. The fifth and sixth extensor compartments are retracted to reveal the underlying capsule of the carpus. The capsule is then opened, and the triquetrum inspected. The proximal ulnar region of triquetral impingement by the detached, distally displaced ulnar sling mechanism is readily apparent. The triquetrum is usually markedly

---

H. K. Watson: Connecticut Combined Hand Surgery Fellowship, Hartford Hospital, and Connecticut Children's Medical Center, Hartford, Connecticut 06106; Department of Orthopaedics, University of Connecticut School of Medicine, Farmington, Connecticut 06032; Department of Orthopedics, Rehabilitation, and Plastic Surgery, Yale University School of Medicine, New Haven, Connecticut 06520.

J. Weinzweig: Department of Plastic Surgery, Brown University School of Medicine, Rhode Island Hospital, and Hasbro Children's Hospital, Providence, Rhode Island 02905.

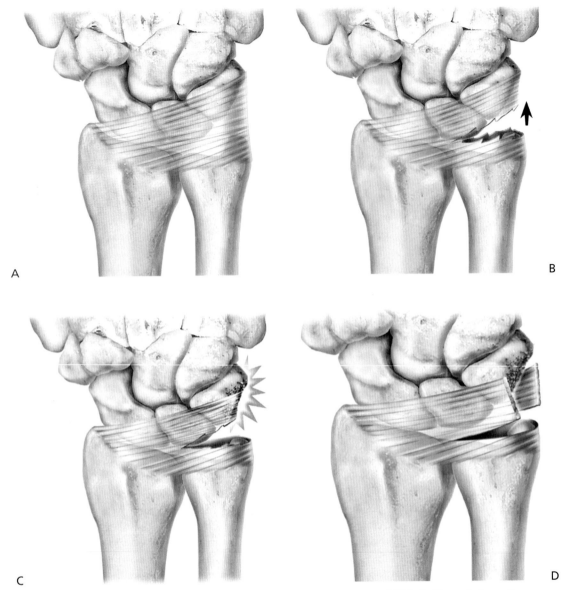

FIGURE 40.1. Mechanism of triquetral impingement ligament tear (TILT). **A:** Normal ulnar sling mechanism. **B:** Ulnar sling detached proximally and displaced distally to impinge on the triquetrum. **C:** Chronic impingement results in hyperemia and softening of the ulnar slope of the triquetrum as well as accompanying symptomatology. **D:** TILT repair is performed by excision of the impinging fibrous cuff segment.

hyperemic in this area with very soft, spongy cortex and areas of exposed subchondral bone (Fig. 40.2A,B). The fibrous cuff traversing this area is excised (Fig. 40.2C). Early in this series, the soft cortex along the ulnar aspect of the triquetrum was routinely resected (Fig. 40.2D); we no longer believe this is necessary. The LT joint, LT interosseous ligament, and TFCC are evaluated and preserved intact. The skin is then closed, and a bulky hand dressing incorporating an intrinsic plaster splint is applied. On removal of the dressing and splint 3 days postoperatively, the wrist is fully mobilized.

CLINICAL SERIES

Forty-four patients were surgically treated for TILT over a seven-year period. All patients presented with complaints of marked sensitivity and tenderness, with or without swelling along the ulnar aspect of the wrist, and decreased grip strength. Thirty-one patients also presented with complaints of postactivity ache lasting from several hours to as long as 3 weeks. Each described a precedent hyperflexion injury of the affected wrist, or blunt trauma (26 patients). Athletic injuries were another frequent cause of symptoms

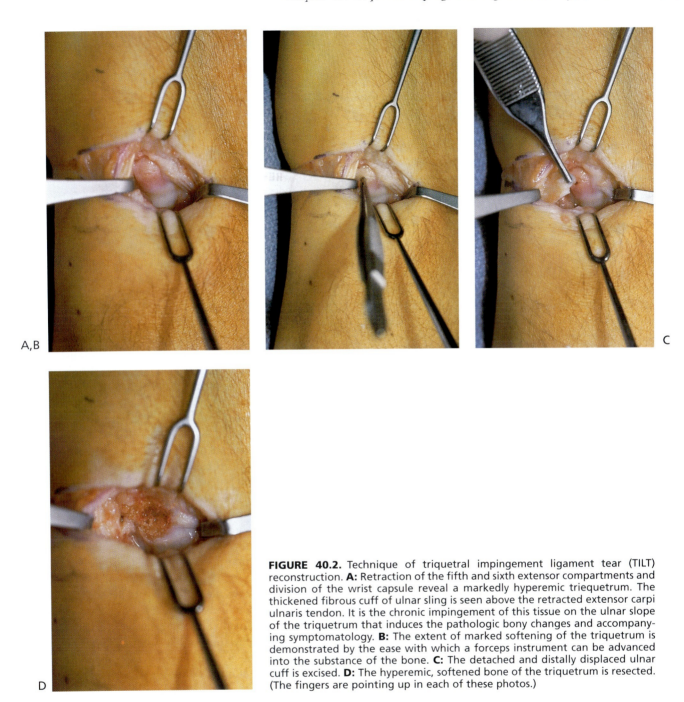

FIGURE 40.2. Technique of triquetral impingement ligament tear (TILT) reconstruction. **A:** Retraction of the fifth and sixth extensor compartments and division of the wrist capsule reveal a markedly hyperemic triequetrum. The thickened fibrous cuff of ulnar sling is seen above the retracted extensor carpi ulnaris tendon. It is the chronic impingement of this tissue on the ulnar slope of the triquetrum that induces the pathologic bony changes and accompanying symptomatology. **B:** The extent of marked softening of the triquetrum is demonstrated by the ease with which a forceps instrument can be advanced into the substance of the bone. **C:** The detached and distally displaced ulnar cuff is excised. **D:** The hyperemic, softened bone of the triquetrum is resected. (The fingers are pointing up in each of these photos.)

(seven patients), followed by falls, lifting injuries, and motor vehicle accident injuries (five, three, and three patients, respectively). Physical examination elicited the highly localized (5–7 mm area) moderate to severe pain with gentle palpation directly over the ulnar aspect of the triquetrum. There was often mild swelling along the ulnar aspect of the wrist, some degree of limited wrist motion, decreased grip strength, and mild pain with pronation and supination. These findings sufficed to make the diagnosis of TILT in each case. Except in cases where radiographic findings reflected postoperative changes following prior surgery, plain films were normal. Ulnar variance was negative in 14 cases, neutral in 24 cases, and positive in only six cases. This series of patients has been divided into two groups based on their history of prior surgical treatment related to wrist symptomatology.

Group I consisted of 26 patients, 10 female and 16 male, who had not undergone any surgical procedure related to their wrist symptoms before presentation. The mean age of patients in this group was 26.9 years (range, 15–57 years). These patients had experienced symptoms of TILT for a mean duration of 16.9 months (range, 2 months to 7 years). Seventy-three percent of these patients presented with dominant hand involvement. Preoperatively, patients demonstrated a mean loss of 13% of extension, 19% of flexion, and 1% of pronation–supination (Table 40.1).

Group II consisted of 18 patients, nine female and nine male, who had undergone a surgical procedure related to their wrist symptoms either before presentation or following evaluation. These procedures were performed before TILT repair. The mean age of patients in this group was 32.8 years (range, 23–50 years). These patients had experienced symptoms of TILT for a mean duration of 34.1 months (range, 4 months to 14 years). Seventy-eight percent of these patients presented with dominant hand involvement. Preoperatively, patients demonstrated a mean loss of 18% of extension, 28% of flexion, and 4% of pronation–supination (Table 40.1).

The 18 patients in group II had undergone a total of 22 surgical wrist procedures before presentation (Table 40.2). Ten patients underwent procedures that directly involved the ulnocarpal joint. The most common procedure performed before the development of TILT in this group of patients was matched ulnar arthroplasty; six patients underwent this operation. Two patients underwent the Darrach procedure while two others underwent an ulnar step-cut lengthening osteotomy with a concomitant matched ulnar arthroplasty. None of the procedures performed directly involved the proximal ulnar aspect of the triquetrum. The two patients in this series who underwent LT arthrodesis did not demonstrate findings consistent with TILT preoperatively or intraoperatively. They developed TILT symptomatology only following hyperflexion injury.

An impinging fibrous sling and hyperemic bone demonstrating cartilage loss and eburnation along the proximal ulnar aspect of the triquetrum, as well as synovial hyperemia, were present in every case. Histologically, the excised ulnar sling cuff appeared as dense fibrocartilaginous tissue consistent with ligament demonstrating fibrovascular proliferative changes. The resected soft cortical bone demonstrated focal periosteal atrophic changes with degeneration of the articular surface (Fig. 40.3).

In all but three cases, the TFCC and LT interosseous ligament were noted to be intact at the time of exploration. One patient demonstrated a small TFCC perforation, which was debrided at the time of TILT repair. Another patient demonstrated an insignificant LT interosseous ligament tear that required no treatment in the face of an otherwise stable LT joint. A third patient demonstrated both a TFCC tear and a complete rupture of the LT interosseous ligament with resultant instability of the LT joint that necessitated LT arthrodesis at the time of TILT repair.

Follow-up was available for 32 patients at a mean of 21.7 months postoperatively (range, 4–72 months). Group I patients maintained 92% of extension, 85% of flexion, 94% of radial deviation, 82% of ulnar deviation, 73% of grip strength, and 87% of key pinch postoperatively, compared with the normal contralateral wrist. Full pronation and supination were restored in all patients (Table 40.3). Group II patients maintained 93% of extension, 80% of flexion, 93% of radial deviation, 90% of ulnar deviation, 88% of grip strength, and 87% of key pinch postoperatively, compared with the normal contralateral wrist. Full pronation and supination were restored in all patients (Table 40.4).

Subjectively, all patients except one reported that both rest pain and activity pain along the ulnar aspect of the wrist had significantly improved following surgery. All 44 patients in the series were able to resume occupational and recreational activities within several weeks following TILT repair.

There were no complications in this series of patients.

TABLE 40.1. PREOPERATIVE WRIST RANGE OF MOTION

Motion	Mean Loss[a] (Range)
Group I	
Extension	13% (0–93%)
Flexion	19% (0–32%)
Pronation/supination	1% (0–11%)
Group II	
Extension	18% (0–92%)
Flexion	28% (0–95%)
Pronation/supination	4% (0–28%)

[a]Compared with opposite wrist.

TABLE 40.2. PRIOR SURGERY (GROUP II PATIENTS)

Matched ulnar arthroplasty	6
Darrach procedure	2
Step-cut ulna lengthening	2
DRUJ arthroplasty	2
Triscaphe arthrodesis	1
SLAC reconstruction	1
Trapezoidal osteotomy	1
TFCC repair/debridement	2
ECU release	1
Dorsal wrist syndrome	1
LT arthrodesis	2
ORIF nonunion of ulna fracture	1

DRUJ, distal radioulnar joint; ECU, extensor carpi ulnaris; LT, lunotriquetral; ORIF, open reduction with internal fixation; SLAC, scapholunate advanced collapse; TFCC, triangular fibrocartilage complex.

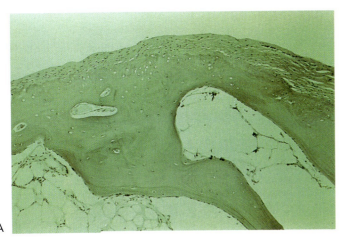 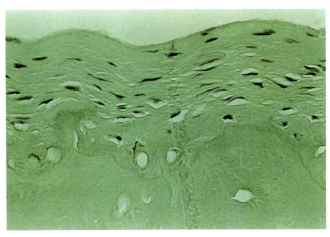

FIGURE 40.3. Histologic changes associated with triquetral impingement ligament tear syndrome. **A:** A section of the subchondral bone that has experienced chronic pressure attributable to the ulnar sling cuff demonstrates thick, reactive collagen covering the entire articular surface. There is complete absence of articular cartilage in this area (H&E, original magnification ×40). **B:** Chronic pressure has resulted in replacement of the normal articular cartilage with dense collagen overlying the bone where there would normally be hyaline cartilage (H&E, original magnification ×400).

DISCUSSION

The ulnar aspect of the carpus remains the diagnostic "Achilles heel" of the wrist. In the absence of radiographic findings consistent with bone or joint pathology, the etiology of ulnar wrist pain is often attributed to a TFCC tear (15). Interestingly, only two patients in our study (4.5%) treated for TILT were found intraoperatively to have a TFCC perforation.

TILT can be distinguished from other etiologies of ulnar wrist pain on the basis of radiographic and physical examination. The absence of radiographic findings rules out most types of bony pathology. Plain radiographic studies of each of the 26 TILT patients in group I, who had not undergone any prior surgery, did not demonstrate any evidence suggestive of ulnar impaction syndrome, ulnar impingement syndrome, or DRUJ pathology. Sixteen of the 18 patients in group II, who had undergone prior surgery, demonstrated only those radiographic changes consistent with the type of surgery they had. No additional radiographic changes were noted as possible sources for the symptomatology presented by this group of patients.

Patients with TILT experience only mild discomfort with pronation and supination, negligible reduction in the range of these motions, and no discomfort with radioulnar compression; these findings are often associated with other types of ulnar wrist pathology. Instead, they experience severe localized pain with direct palpation of the ulnar side of the triquetrum. This pain is occasionally accompanied by mild to moderate swelling along the ulnar aspect of the wrist, diminished wrist motion, decreased grip strength, and a history of a hyperflexion injury.

TABLE 40.3. POSTOPERATIVE WRIST MOTION AND STRENGTH (GROUP I)

Motion	Loss[a]
Extension	8%
Flexion	15%
Radial deviation	6%
Ulnar deviation	18%
Pronation	0%
Supination	0%
Strength	**Maintained**
Grip	73%
Key pinch	87%

[a]Compared with opposite wrist.

TABLE 40.4. POSTOPERATIVE WRIST MOTION AND STRENGTH (GROUP II)

Motion	Loss[a]
Extension	7%
Flexion	20%
Radial deviation	7%
Ulnar deviation	10%
Pronation	0%
Supination	0%
Strength	**Maintained**
Grip	88%
Key pinch	87%

[a]Compared with opposite wrist.

Intraoperatively, a thickened cuff of the ulnar sling mechanism was found impacted tightly against the triquetrum in every case. This cuff of fibrous tissue impinges unremittingly on the ulnar-sloped edge of the triquetrum, resulting in hyperemia, eburnation, and softening of the bone. The triquetral softening is often so pronounced that the tip of a forceps instrument can be easily pushed directly into the bone.

Any procedure that results in disruption of the integrity of the ulnar sling mechanism can subsequently predispose a patient to the development of TILT. Ten patients (22.7%) in the present series had previously undergone either a matched ulnar arthroplasty (six patients), a Darrach procedure (two patients), or a step-cut osteotomy for ulnar lengthening with a concomitant matched ulnar arthroplasty (two patients).

Step-cut shortening of the ulna is a relatively popular operation for the management of ulnar impaction syndrome. Interestingly, it is successful even when there is no significant ulnar impaction evident on x-ray and a neutral or even negative ulnar variance exists. It may be that these patients have TILT syndrome and the step-cut shortening of the ulna draws the ulnar sling mechanism proximally away from the triquetrum, solving the problem. If one makes the diagnosis of TILT, of course, the solution is much simpler with a straightforward TILT reconstruction and full mobilization in 48 hours.

Excision of the ulnarmost segment of the displaced fibrous cuff eliminates the offensive agent and is likely all that is actually necessary to treat this condition. Excision of the softened, hyperemic bone, early in this series thought necessary to provide a cancellous surface on which the capsule overlying the triquetrum may readily attach, is no longer performed.

REFERENCES

1. Bowers WH. Problems of the distal radioulnar joint. *Adv Orthop Surg* 1984;7:289–303.
2. Friedman SL, Palmer AK. The ulnar impaction syndrome. *Hand Clin* 1991;7:295–310.
3. Gross SC, Watson HK, Strickland JW, et al. Triquetral–lunate arthritis secondary to synostosis. *J Hand Surg [Am]* 1989;14:95–102.
4. Watson HK, Brown RE. Ulnar impingement syndrome after Darrach procedure: Treatment by advancement lengthening osteotomy of the ulna. *J Hand Surg [Am]* 1989;14:302–306.
5. Watson HK, Gabuzda GM. Matched distal ulnar resection for posttraumatic disorders of the distal radioulnar joint. *J Hand Surg [Am]* 1992;17:724–730.
6. Chun S, Palmer AK. Chronic ulnar wrist pain secondary to partial rupture of the extensor carpi ulnaris tendon. *J Hand Surg [Am]* 1987;12:1032–1035.
7. Palmer AK. Triangular fibrocartilage disorders: injury patterns and treatment. *Arthroscopy* 1990;6:125–132.
8. Palmer AK, Werner FW. The triangular fibrocartilage complex of the wrist: Anatomy and function. *J Hand Surg [Am]* 1981;6:153–172.
9. Taleisnik J. The ligaments of the wrist. *J Hand Surg [Am]* 1976;1:110–118.
10. Viegas SF, Ballantyne G. Attritional lesions of the wrist joint. *J Hand Surg [Am]* 1987;12:1025–1029.
11. Bell MJ, Hill RJ, McMurtry RY. Ulnar impingement syndrome. *J Bone Joint Surg Br* 1985;67:126–129.
12. Chun S, Palmer AK. The ulnar impaction syndrome: follow-up of ulnar shortening osteotomy. *J Hand Surg [Am]* 1993;18:46–53.
13. Stanley JK, Hodgson SP, Royle SG. An approach to the diagnosis of chronic wrist pain. *Ann Chir Main Membre Super* 1994;13:202–205.
14. Watson HK, Weinzweig J. Triquetral impingement ligament tear (TILT) syndrome. *J Hand Surg [Br]* 1999;24:350–358.
15. Taleisnik J. Clinical and technologic evaluation of ulnar wrist pain (Editorial). *J Hand Surg [Am]* 1988;13:801–802.

41

PRINCIPLES OF RHEUMATOID ARTHRITIS

H. KIRK WATSON
JEFFREY WEINZWEIG

THE RHEUMATOID FORMULA

Rheumatoid arthritis is a destructive inflammatory disease. The destruction occurs secondary to the ability of the inflamed synovium to destroy abutting tissue (1–6). In particular, placing this inflamed synovium under load enables it to destroy any tissue, including bone, fairly rapidly. A formula, therefore, can be loosely put forward to explain the deformities of rheumatoid arthritis:

$$\text{rheumatoid synovium} + \text{load} = \text{deformity}$$

Abnormal loads may be created by normal anatomy (7) such as the existence of the synovial-lined fibrous sheath pulley systems; overload may also be created by overactive muscles attempting to protect proximate joints. Anywhere there is abnormal stress on tissues combined with rheumatoid synovium, destruction of those tissues can occur. This includes ligaments, cartilage, tendon, or bone. The force may be produced by the proliferating synovium itself, as seen when total destruction and dislocation of a joint occurs secondary to massive intraarticular synovial overgrowth (3). This formula provides a general pragmatic approach to rheumatoid arthritis in that removal of either the inflamed rheumatoid synovium or the abnormal force will prevent deformity (8).

Synovium in the hand exists as a peritendinous phenomenon in the flexor fibroosseous sheaths, in the carpal tunnel, and in the six extensor retinacular tunnels. Other than this, synovium exists only in the joints. Synovial removal is more easily accomplished as a peritendinous phenomenon than as a joint treatment. The major drawback to joint synovectomy as a treatment of rheumatoid arthritis is the subsequent cartilage loss. The principal function of the synovium is to care for the cartilage, including providing nutrition, removing wastes, and providing fluid for a low-friction surface. The inadequately cared-for cartilage following synovectomy of a joint gradually deteriorates.

Treatment with the synovial-load formula in mind simplifies things in the case of tendons. The continued existence of a synovial mass in the fourth dorsal compartment dictates the need for its removal along with removal of the load component, i.e., extensor retinaculum. This assumes failure of medical treatment. One is well advised to perform a "cocompartment" release to remove the load, as some synovium remains and may regrow. Cocompartment release is simply the transecting of the septae between compartments, forming one large compartment of two. Typically, the septum between the fourth and fifth compartments is excised, producing a single large compartment that still functions with adequate retinaculum to prevent bowstringing (see Chapter 76). This removes much of the force component capable of inducing the rheumatoid synovium to erode through the tendons and rupture them (Fig. 41.1) (9). Synovectomy is the treatment of choice for carpal tunnel problems, along with opening of the tunnel, which affect both sides of the formula (10). A similar procedure is indicated for synovial overgrowth in the flexor retinaculum where the pulleys are maintained; the cruciform portions are excised, and a radical synovectomy is performed.

ULNAR DRIFT AND JOINT SUBLUXATION

Ulnar drift and volar subluxation of the metacarpophalangeal (MP) joints result primarily from the overactive pull of the intrinsic muscles (11). One of the earliest signs that a hand will deform in rheumatoid arthritis is a positive

---

H. K. Watson: Connecticut Combined Hand Surgery Fellowship, Hartford Hospital, and Connecticut Children's Medical Center, Hartford, Connecticut 06106; Department of Orthopaedics, University of Connecticut School of Medicine, Farmington, Connecticut 06032; Department of Orthopedics, Rehabilitation, and Plastic Surgery, Yale University School of Medicine, New Haven, Connecticut 06520.

J. Weinzweig: Department of Plastic Surgery, Brown University School of Medicine, Rhode Island Hospital, and Hasbro Children's Hospital, Providence, Rhode Island 02905.

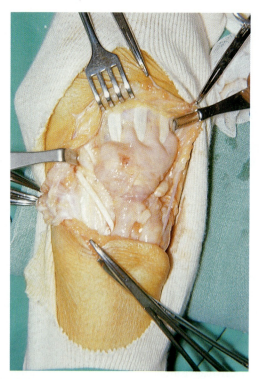

FIGURE 41.1. Peritendinous synovitis combined with the load of the extensor retinaculum invades and ruptures tendons, typically along the distal edge of the extensor retinaculum.

Bunnell test. The overpull or overactivity of the intrinsics is probably secondary to the proximity of synovially inflamed joints. The body is attempting to protect the inflamed joint with nearby muscle support similar to the back spasms that follow a facet subluxation of the spine. This protective mechanism on an ongoing basis provides the abnormal loads that cause the deformities in the digits. Because of the anatomy of the intrinsics, the major loads are placed on the dorsal radial aspect of the MP joints (12). The load in this area, following the formula of load and rheumatoid arthritis synovium, produces collagenous dissolution that results in a volar-ulnar subluxation of the MP joints. As with most deformities of rheumatoid arthritis, it is the very earliest stages of load concentration that predict the deformity. The first volar interosseous muscle to the index finger inserts on the hood. The first dorsal interosseous muscle on the radial side inserts into bone and has an effect only on radial deviation of the proximal phalanx. If both of these muscles become tight, then closing of the proximal interphalangeal (PIP) and distal interphalangeal (DIP) joints will produce an ulnar angulation at the MP joint because flexion will overtighten only the ulnar-sided first volar interosseous muscle (13). With every closing of the index finger, there is repeated load to the radial dorsal aspect of the MP joint. This initiates capsular attenuation in this area. The ulnar angulation of the proximal phalanx then increases the load on this dorsal radial aspect of the MP capsule, resulting in increased destruction and progressive drift along with volar subluxation of the proximal phalanx.

It is logical to assume that subluxation in the wrist and the ulnar approach of the extrinsic tendons to the MP joints are the etiologic factors in ulnar drift of the digits. This is not the case. The finger deformity was predicted long before these phenomena occur. The ulnar subluxation of the tendons and the increased angular approach from the ulnar side play a tertiary role in ulnar drift but not an etiologic one. Therefore, operating on the wrist is not indicated as a method of protecting the MP joints, and, indeed, a rheumatoid patient should be approached based on the anatomy that is producing that particular patient's functional deficit. There is no contraindication to operating on MP joints in the face of wrist deformity and ulnar positioning of the extensor tendons.

Once the dorsal radial capsule begins to attenuate at the MP joints, there is a progressive ulnar drift and volar subluxation of the proximal phalanx (Fig. 41.2) (14). This proximal ulnar positioning unloads the intrinsics and relieves the tight extensor hoods, thereby protecting against the development of PIP and DIP joint deformity. Early on, the tendency toward subluxation at the MP

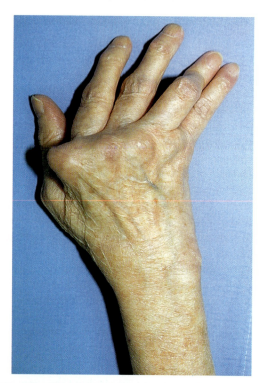

FIGURE 41.2. Rheumatoid synovium in the metacarpophalangeal (MP) joints combined with load from overactive intrinsics acts on the dorsal MP joint capsule and produces capsular and ligamentous dissolution and a volar–ulnar dislocation of the proximal phalanges. This volar–ulnar dislocation effectively lengthens the intrinsics, thereby removing the load component of the formula. As a result, the fingers remain basically protected for long periods of time.

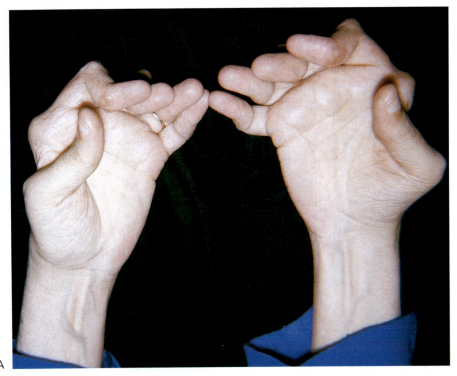
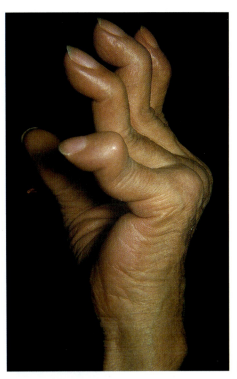

FIGURE 41.3. If the metacarpophalangeal joints do not dislocate, continued intrinsic loads on the fingers produce boutonnière **(A)** and swan-neck **(B)** deformities as well as dislocations or fusions.

joints will predict the protection of the interphalangeal (IP) joints. In contrast, if the MP joints do not have sufficient destructive synovium or the intrinsic anatomy does not tend toward a dorsal radial capsular attenuation, then the IP joints will be subjected to abnormal intrinsic loads, and the rheumatoid synovium in the joints will result in deformity. Again, load plus rheumatoid synovium equals deformity.

If the MP joints sublux, the fingers are protected. If the MP joints hold, the finger deformities will occur. The IP joint deformities are swan-necks, boutonnières, dislocations, or autofusions (Fig. 41.3) (15–17). As with the MP joint, the very earliest capsular attenuations of the IP joints will predict which of these occur. In patients with hyperextensible joints in general, the perivolar plate capsular structures may begin to attenuate. Once this begins, the forces are increasingly concentrated volarly, and a hyperextension deformity of the PIP joint results in a swan-neck deformity. If, on the other hand, the synovium in the PIP joint begins to attenuate the dorsal capsule, it will attenuate the central slip and eventually result in boutonnière deformities. The anatomy predicts the deformity defined by the synovium-load rheumatoid formula. In some patients, the capsule does not tend to attenuate. The constantly increasing pressure dissolves the cartilage, and autofusion occurs. In very late stages, synovial overgrowth within the joint will produce its own force by virtue of its growth; this force will then produce a panligamentous destruction of the proximal and distal joints, resulting in complete capsular dissolution and dislocation.

THE ZED THUMB

This entire phenomenon repeats itself in the thumb. The tight intrinsics produce the zed thumb (Fig. 41.4A). This initially manifests as dorsal capsular dissolution of the MP joint. Increased tightness of the hood produces an extension deformity of the distal phalanx (18–20). The synovial attenuation, therefore, occurs on the volar capsule of the IP joint, and the distal phalanx continues to migrate dorsally on the proximal phalanx. The end stage of this phenomenon is attenuation and rupture of the flexor pollicis longus over the volar head of the proximal phalanx at the IP joint level (21).

If the carpometacarpal (CMC) joint subluxes from synovial destruction of its capsule, the MP and IP joints are then protected, and one will not see a zed thumb or dislocations of the MP or IP joints (Fig. 41.4B). The subluxation at the CMC joint unloads the force component of the formula by effectively lengthening the intrinsics and secondarily reducing their load on the MP and IP joints. Again, the very earliest stages will predict which of the two thumb types will develop, based on the synovium-load formula.

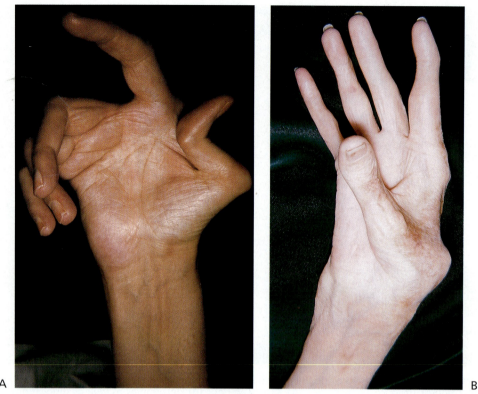

FIGURE 41.4. A: The overactivity of the intrinsics of the thumb will flex the metacarpophalangeal (MP) joint, pulling on the hood and extending the distal joint and gradually producing the classic "zed" thumb. **B:** If, on the other hand, the carpometacarpal (CMC) joint dislocates, this dislocation unloads the intrinsics by effectively shortening them and reduces their activity on the MP and interphalangeal joints, thereby preserving these joints. The CMC joint, therefore, predicts the thumb deformity.

INTRINSIC RELEASE

In the early stages of rheumatoid finger deformity, the best approach is intrinsic release (21,22). This is accomplished through a transverse dorsal incision that includes the capsular and bony insertions of the intrinsics as well as the hood insertions. The hood insertion excision will protect the IP joints, but protection of the MP joints requires removal of the muscle tendinous junction, particularly the ulnar intrinsics. If the articular cartilage in the MP joints is good, then this preservational type of surgical approach is warranted. The ulnar intrinsics are excised, the extensor tendon is recentralized if it tends toward ulnar subluxation, and a partial synovectomy of the MP joint is performed, if indicated. The radial intrinsics are unloaded by the loss of their ulnar counterpart. This procedure provides protection for the MP joints and has been effective for patients for many years.

THE DISTAL RADIOULNAR JOINT IN RHEUMATOID ARTHRITIS

The distal radioulnar joint is commonly involved. Our procedure of choice is a resection of the distal ulna. We prefer the matched ulnar arthroplasty, which does not require maintaining triangular fibrocartilage attachment, periosteum, or other soft tissue on the distal ulna, as the ulnar sling mechanism will firmly reattach to the broad cancellous surface of the ulna (see Chapter 59). Matched ulnar arthroplasty is not contraindicated in a panligamentous destruction downslope wrist, as the wrist itself must be treated at the same time.

THE ULNA IN RHEUMATOID ARTHRITIS

In the wrist, the basic problem is the panligamentous destruction and loss of upslope ligament function. Particulate silicone synovitis from silicone implants will produce a very similar panligamentous laxity and destruction, and it is this that is the major contraindication to the use of silicone scaphoids or lunates in the wrist (23,24). As the ligamentous attenuation of rheumatoid arthritis occurs, the wrist assumes its neutral anatomy position. Neutral anatomy for the wrist is a volar-ulnar subluxation, downslope on the radius, with the carpals frequently settling on the distal ulna (Fig. 41.5). The distal ulna supports the wrist under these

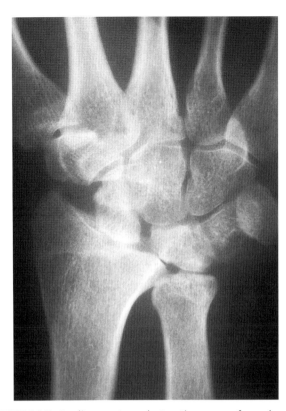

FIGURE 41.5. Panligamentous destruction occurs from rheumatoid synovium in the wrist joint. The loss of upslope ligament support allows ulnar translation, and the entire carpus often ends up sitting perched over the end of the ulna. This is not an indication for a Sauvé-Kapandji procedure. The wrist is no longer functioning as a true wrist, and these patients are best served by placing the scaphoid and lunate into a concavity on the distal radius combined with a matched ulnar arthroplasty.

rheumatoid wrist is based on limited function, be that from pain or limited motion where motion is required for that patient's quality of life (25). Even severely destroyed, displaced wrists on x-ray may function adequately for a patient if they are in keeping with the load capabilities of the rest of the tissues of that extremity and the patient's needs. If the clinical picture requires repair, the procedure of choice is "nonunion" or pseudarthrosis arthroplasty in which a cancellous concavity is formed in the distal radius and a cancellous convexity is formed from the proximal scaphoid and lunate (see Chapter 61). The wrist is then nested in the concavity with the flap of reflected wrist ligament interposed between the scaphoid and lunate and the radius cup. This is cross-pinned for 2 to 3 weeks, then mobilized (Fig. 41.6). This procedure can be carried out no matter how severe the dislocation. The wrist may lie several inches up the forearm and can still be reestablished on the distal radius (26). Frequently one or both of the carpal bones will fuse to the radius even in that short period of time, but long-term follow-up has repeatedly demonstrated that the nonunion wrists do better. This procedure is not applicable to non-rheumatoid patients but is very successful in rheumatoid arthritis. In rheumatoid arthritis, the midcarpal joint is often

conditions, but a true structural wrist no longer exists. The carpals are ulnar-subluxed. Describing this support of the wrist by the ulna as being a normal part of the ulna's responsibility is erroneous. In the normal state, the ulna needs the wrist, but the wrist does not need the ulna. The ulna may be very long or very short, but does not contribute to load transference in any significant or necessary degree. As the loads increase, they will be transmitted through bone by the scaphoid and lunate into the radius. There is, therefore, no indication for preserving the distal ulna as in a Sauvé-Kapandji procedure, and this is true even in rheumatoid arthritis with ulnar translation. The solution to the wrist is not to be sought in the ulna, which has no way of adequately articulating with the carpals or taking load. The solution lies in reestablishing load transfer from the hand through the carpals to the radius.

THE WRIST IN RHEUMATOID ARTHRITIS

It is important to recognize that it is the patient to be treated, not the x-ray. An indication for surgery on the

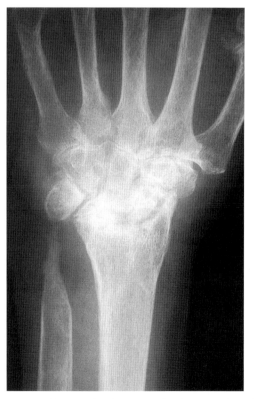

FIGURE 41.6. Following the rheumatoid wrist procedure alluded to in Fig. 41.5, it is not unusual for either the lunate or scaphoid to fuse with the radius, even with only 2 weeks of immobilization. In the present case, the lunate and radius have fused. There is motion between the radius and scaphoid and around the distal lunate.

better preserved than the radiocarpal joint, probably because it has more inherent stability, but there are occasions when the destruction is so advanced that there is almost no identifiable scaphoid or lunate, in which case the proximal carpals, be they capitate or hamate, may be placed into the concavity of the distal radius and treated in a similar fashion.

The procedure is typically combined with a matched ulnar arthroplasty. In our original description of the matched ulnar arthroplasty, it had been performed almost exclusively on patients with rheumatoid arthritis (27,28). In cases of severe progressive rheumatoid arthritis with 15-year follow-up, the nonunion wrist was often the best joint the patient had. There is little or no further deterioration. In 30 years of experience with the procedure, no patients have returned requiring revision of the wrist in late follow-up.

REFERENCES

1. Cush JJ, Lipsky PE. Cellular basis for rheumatoid inflammation. *Clin Orthop* 1991;265:9–22.
2. Ferlic DC. Management of the rheumatoid wrist. In: Clayton ML, Smythe CT, eds. *Surgery for rheumatoid arthritis.* New York: Churchill Livingstone, 1992;155–187.
3. Feldon P, Terrono AL, Nalebuff EA, et al. Rheumatoid arthritis and other connective tissue diseases. In: Green DP, Hotchkiss RN, Pederson WC, eds. *Operative hand surgery, 4th ed.* New York: Livingstone Churchill, 1998;1651–1739.
4. Taleisnik J. Rheumatoid arthritis of the wrist. *Hand Clin* 1989;5:257–278.
5. Taleisnik J. Rheumatoid synovitis of the volar compartment of the wrist joint: Its radiologic signs and its contribution to wrist and hand deformity. *J Hand Surg [Am]* 1979;4:526–535.
6. Wilson RL. Rheumatoid arthritis of the hand. *Orthop Clin North Am* 1986;17:313–343.
7. MacConaill MA. The mechanical anatomy of the carpus and its bearing on some surgical problems. *J Anat* 1941;75:166–173.
8. Shapiro JS. The wrist in rheumatoid arthritis. *Hand Clin* 1996;12:477–498.
9. Ferlic DC. Rheumatoid flexor tenosynovitis and rupture. *Hand Clin* 1996;12:561–572.
10. Millender LH, Nalebuff EA. Preventive surgery: Tenosynovectomy and synovectomy. *Orthop Clin North Am* 1975;6:765–792.
11. Flatt AE. Some pathomechanics of ulnar drift. *Plast Reconstr Surg* 1966;37:295–303.
12. Littler JW. The finger extension mechanism. *Surg Clin North Am* 1967;47:415–432.
13. Wilson RL, DeVito MC. Extensor tendon problems in rheumatoid arthritis. *Hand Clin* 1996;12:551–559.
14. Stirrat CR. Metacarpophalangeal joints in rheumatoid arthritis of the hand. *Hand Clin* 1996;12:515–530.
15. Nalebuff EA. The rheumatoid swan-neck deformity. *Hand Clin* 1989;5:203–214.
16. Rizio L, Belsky MR. Finger deformities in rheumatoid arthritis. *Hand Clin* 1996;12:531–540.
17. Shapiro JS. Wrist influence in rheumatoid swan neck deformity. *J Hand Surg* 1982;7:484–491.
18. Stein AB, Terrono AL. The rheumatoid thumb. *Hand Clin* 1996;12:541–550.
19. Terreno A, Millender LH, Nalebuff AE. Boutonniere rheumatoid thumb deformity. *J Hand Surg [Am]* 1990;15:999–1003.
20. Toledano B, Terreno A, Millender L. Reconstruction of the rheumatoid thumb. *Hand Clin* 1992;8:121–129.
21. Terreno A, Nalebuff E, Philips C. The rheumatoid thumb. In: Hunter T, ed. *Rehabilitation of the hand: Surgery and therapy.* St Louis: CV Mosby, 1995;1329–1343.
22. Littler JW. Redistribution of forces in the correction of the boutonniere deformity. *J Bone Joint Surg Am* 1967;49:1267–1274.
23. Peimer CA. Reactive synovitis after silicone arthroplasty. *J Hand Surg [Am]* 1986;11:624–638.
24. Smith RJ. Silicone synovitis of the wrist. *J Hand Surg [Am]* 1985;10:47–60.
25. Vicar AJ, Burton RI. Surgical management of the rheumatoid wrist: Fusion or arthroplasty? *J Hand Surg [Am]* 1986;11:790–797.
26. Ryu J, Watson HK, Burgess RC. Rheumatoid wrist reconstruction utilizing a fibrous nonunion and radiocarpal arthrodesis. *J Hand Surg [Am]* 1985;10:830–836.
27. Watson HK, Gabuzda GM. Matched distal ulna resection for post-traumatic disorders of the distal radioulnar joint. *J Hand Surg [Am]* 1992;17:724–730.
28. Watson HK, Ryu J, Burgess RC. Matched distal ulnar resection. *J Hand Surg [Am]* 1986;11:812–817.

42

EVALUATION AND TREATMENT OF THE RHEUMATOID WRIST

LEONARD K. RUBY
CHARLES CASSIDY

The wrist joint, comprising radiocarpal, midcarpal, and distal radioulnar articulations, is one of the most common sites of involvement in patients afflicted with rheumatoid arthritis (1). The normal wrist provides force transmission to and from the hand and positions the hand in space in conjunction with the elbow and shoulder. The wrist influences digital alignment, motion, strength, and function; therefore, it is imperative that the treating physician understand the pathology of the wrist in order to render proper treatment of the entire upper extremity.

THE PATHOMECHANICS OF RHEUMATOID ARTHRITIS OF THE WRIST

Although the natural history of rheumatoid wrist involvement for any affected individual is probably predetermined (2–8), a general pattern can be discerned and reasonably well described. Early, enzymatic degradation of the articular surfaces produces joint narrowing and functional lengthening of the stabilizing ligaments. Bone is also eroded by direct synovial invasion along nutrient foramina. This is why the waist of the scaphoid, the scapholunate area, and the ulnar styloid, all of which contain vascular channels, are such common sites for bony erosion (9) (Fig. 42.1). Simultaneous with this cartilage degradation is direct synovial invasion of the ligaments, which become even more lax from this process (10,11).

The distal radioulnar joint (DRUJ) may be the earliest and most commonly involved site in the rheumatoid wrist (12), and DRUJ pathology may have a global impact on the wrist and hand. In the region of the ulnar styloid, synovitis invades the triangular fibrocartilage complex (TFCC), the principal stabilizer of the DRUJ. Attenuation of the dorsal and volar radioulnar ligaments and functional lengthening of these structures secondary to joint surface loss produce instability of the radius–ulna relationship, and the ulnar head becomes prominent. The ulnocarpal complex is weakened as well, permitting carpal supination and possibly contributing to ulnar translocation (13).

Along the extensor carpi ulnaris (ECU) tendon, tenosynovitis stretches the restraining subsheath, allowing for volar tendon subluxation (14,15) and loss of that important dynamic distal radioulnar stabilizer.

At the radiocarpal joint, changes in the intrinsic and extrinsic ligaments, the joint surface, and altered musculotendinous forces across the wrist result in palmar and ulnar translation as well as supination with respect to the radius (11). Because the center of motion of the wrist moves palmarly and ulnarly, the moment arms of the extensor carpi radialis longus (ECRL) and brevis (ECRB) are increased while the antagonist moment arm of the flexor carpi ulnaris is decreased, creating a dynamic imbalance. This deformity, in turn, leads to radial deviation of the metacarpals, which promotes ulnar deviation of the fingers at the metacarpophalangeal (MP) joints (10,16). Further, fourth and fifth carpometacarpal joint involvement allows these joints to collapse into flexion, further exacerbating the appearance of a prominent ulnar head (17). Shapiro (10) has observed that longitudinal collapse of the wrist will alter the normal tension in the extrinsic extensors and flexors of the digits as well as the wrist motors, producing an "extrinsic minus" imbalance; this may partially explain the swan-neck deformities commonly seen in rheumatoid patients.

Eventually, the combination of articular and ligamentous damage produces one of three general patterns of deformity (18). In some instances, progressive carpal destruction is accompanied by stiffness and radiographic evidence of spontaneous ankylosis (Fig. 42.2). This type is seen most commonly in juvenile rheumatoid arthritis (JRA), although adults may develop it as well. Interestingly, a very similar process produces a very different result in the second pattern, as unyielding destruction results in complete disorganization, collapse, and a "floppy" wrist (10);

L. K. Ruby and C. Cassidy: Department of Orthopaedics, Tufts University and New England Medical Center, Boston, Massachusetts 02111.

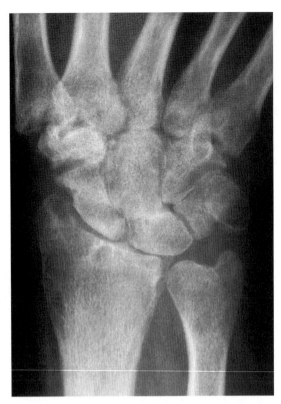

FIGURE 42.1. A wrist with moderate involvement. Note joint space narrowing, especially midcarpal, and multiple erosions in the radius at ligamentous attachments.

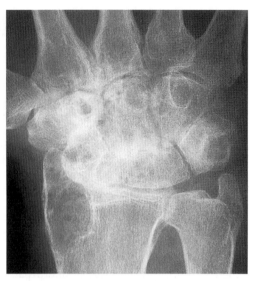

FIGURE 42.3. Note the sclerosis and joint space narrowing plus a large distal radial cyst consistent with osteoarthritis superimposed on rheumatoid arthritis.

this process is seen in the arthritis mutilans variant. In the third type, the disease may enter a quiescent phase, and the changes that were initiated by the rheumatoid synovitis lead to degenerative changes secondary to the abnormal loading of the already compromised cartilage surface (Fig. 42.3).

In JRA, the natural history is somewhat different. Premature ossification of the carpus and early closure of the radial epiphysis limit overall growth, producing a short, thin wrist. Additionally, because the ulnar physis fuses before the radial physis, the ulna is relatively short, contributing to an ulnar

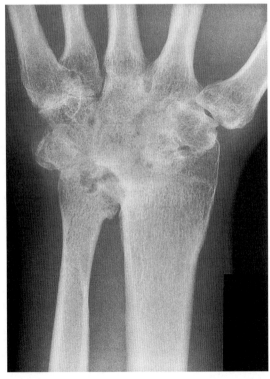

FIGURE 42.2. Spontaneous fusion of this patient's wrist in relatively good position. No treatment was necessary.

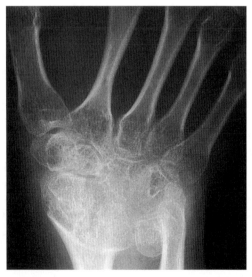

FIGURE 42.4. Spontaneous fusion of this juvenile rheumatoid arthritis wrist in typical ulnar deviation of the carpus and metacarpals.

deviation posture. Rather than becoming excessively lax, the JRA wrist fuses spontaneously in a high percentage of patients (19,20), usually in flexion and ulnar deviation (Fig. 42.4). Early intervention with wrist orthoses may promote ankylosis in a more functional position.

CLINICAL EVALUATION

Early in the disease, the patient may complain of stiffness, mild pain, swelling, and weakness (10). Often the weakness is a manifestation of the pain as well as the mechanical changes. However, because digital involvement, compressive neuropathy, and flexor tenosynovitis can also produce weakness, a thorough evaluation of the entire extremity is essential.

Wrist synovitis is often difficult to appreciate clinically because the wrist is enveloped by tendons and is covered on the palmar side by the unyielding transverse carpal ligament. A sense of fullness and limited wrist motion are the most common findings.

Significant dorsal swelling is more likely caused by extensor tenosynovitis; the classic "double hump" configuration is produced by the extensor retinaculum creating a band across the prominent extensor tenosynovium (11). Tenderness is helpful in differentiating synovitis from tenosynovitis, as the latter is usually nontender. On the volar side, tenosynovitis may be associated with findings of median nerve entrapment.

At the DRUJ, the earliest clinical findings include pain with forearm rotation and limited supination (21,22). Frequently, a prominent distal ulna is the only abnormality noted and may be caused by DRUJ instability, carpal supination, or both. Simultaneous downward-directed pressure on the ulnar head and upward pressure on the pisiform may produce the sensation of reduction of the hand and the ulna onto the radius (23).

As the disease progresses, the patient will notice increasing pain, deformity, and weakness until the disease process either burns out or continues to create a very lax, totally unstable wrist, or the wrist fuses (Fig. 42.5).

The digital extensor and flexor tendons are also commonly affected. Rupture may be the consequence of tenosynovial infiltration or attritional wear over a bony irregularity (24,25). Pain with active or resisted digital motion is a sign of impending rupture and warrants expedient tenosynovectomy. Although the classic presentation is that of an acute, sharp, painful snap associated with loss of active motion, tendon ruptures can be quite subtle and may be overlooked in the patient with severe preexisting deformity (26–28). As summarized by Nalebuff (29), several rheumatoid conditions that can mimic extensor tendon rupture must be excluded.

On the extensor side, the ulnar-sided digital tendons and the extensor pollicis longus (EPL) are the most commonly affected, whereas on the flexor side, radial-sided tendons are more likely to rupture. Arthritis of the DRUJ may predispose to attritional rupture of the extensor digiti quinti tendon (part of the so-called "caput ulnae" syndrome) (30); clinically, this is seen as a subtle loss of little finger extension. If untreated, these ruptures may progress to involve the extensor digitorum comminis to the little and ring fingers, termed the Vaughan-Jackson lesion (31–33). Surgery should include distal ulna resection in addition to tendon reconstruction.

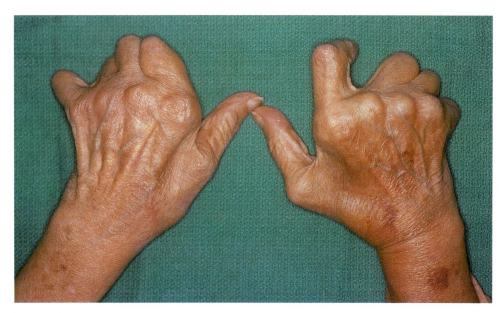

FIGURE 42.5. The right wrist in this patient demonstrates all the classic deformities of radial deviation, supination, and ulnar palmar translation with respect to the radius.

Rupture of the EPL tendon usually is the result of abrasion over an osteophyte on the dorsum of the distal radius (34). This is an isolated phenomenon and may be neglected in the patient with little functional deficit.

Less commonly, but very significantly, the patient may also suffer rupture of the flexor tendons. Loss of active thumb interphalangeal joint flexion is the most common presentation, resulting from flexor pollicis longus (FPL) tendon rupture (35). This disorder, termed the Mannerfelt lesion (35), results from attritional rupture over a bony spicule at the distal pole of the scaphoid or trapezium. If ignored, ruptures progress in a radial-to-ulnar direction, subsequently affecting the flexor digitorum profundus to the index finger.

Rupture of the sublimis tendons may be overlooked if the profundus tendons are intact. In addition, if flexor tenosynovium bridges the ruptured flexor tendons, it is difficult to diagnose tendon failure. Seldom are these isolated phenomena, and, of course, digital and wrist tendons may also rupture secondary to direct tenosynovial invasion.

RADIOGRAPHIC EVALUATION

To be of optimal value, radiographs should consist of neutral rotation, neutral deviation posteroanterior and lateral wrist views. Radiographic signs of early rheumatoid involvement include marginal erosions at the base of the ulnar styloid and the waist of the scaphoid (1). A deep erosion at the sigmoid notch of the radius, known as the "scallop sign," is worrisome, as this finding has been associated with impending extensor tendon rupture (36) (Fig. 42.6). Later findings include loss of carpal height, scapholunate dissociation, as well as the volar ulnar collapse described in the preceding section (17).

In anticipation of surgery, the physician should examine the radiographs critically in several areas. Evidence of radiocarpal instability will usually preclude soft tissue reconstructive procedures (Fig. 42.7) and would be a contraindication to an isolated distal ulna resection (37,38). Similarly, bone loss at the ulnar corner of the radius with accentuated radial inclination may predispose to ulnar translocation if the distal ulna is excised (39,40). Midcarpal joint preservation may allow for a motion-sparing partial wrist arthrodesis. Radioulnar instability may be detected on the lateral view, although this is usually more apparent clinically than radiographically. Positive ulnar variance would have an impact on the distal ulna procedure selected (see below).

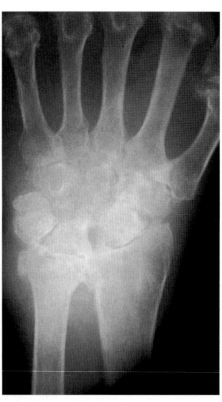

FIGURE 42.7. Although stiff and subluxed with no joint space remaining, this patient's wrist is in relatively good alignment.

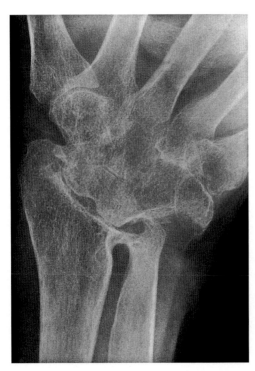

FIGURE 42.6. There is scalloping of the sigmoid notch with ulnar translation.

TREATMENT

There has been a significant advance in nonoperative treatment in the last few years, with rheumatologists using more powerful chemotherapeutic agents, such as methotrexate, as first-line drugs (41–43). Nonetheless, if nonoperative treatment, including drugs and splinting, does not arrest either tenosynovitis or synovitis within 4 to 6 months, then surgery is usually recommended (6,10,11,17). For convenience, operative procedures may be divided into either soft tissue or bony. However, in practice, it is more common than not for a combination of these to be used.

Surgical technique is discussed elsewhere in this volume, but there are some technical aspects of rheumatoid wrist surgery that warrant emphasis. Dorsal wrist exposure should be through a straight rather than a curvilinear incision, as the latter may compromise skin vascularity (10). Experience with curvilinear incisions has demonstrated a 10% slough rate (11). The length of the incision is tailored to the specific procedure. For complete exposure of the dorsal wrist joint including the DRUJ, we prefer a slightly oblique incision beginning distal-radial at the index carpometacarpal (CMC) joint and proceeding proximal-ulnar as necessary. The skin and subcutaneous tissues should be elevated as a thick flap at the level of the extensor retinaculum. Rarely is the first compartment involved with rheumatoid tenosynovitis, and so exposure of this area is not usually necessary (44). We generally try to preserve a proximal strip of retinaculum at least a centimeter in width to prevent bowstringing (Figs. 42.8 and 42.9). Following tendon repair or wrist synovectomy, the radial-based strip of retinaculum may be placed deep to the extensors to provide a gliding surface. On the palmar side, exposure is generally performed through an extended carpal tunnel incision.

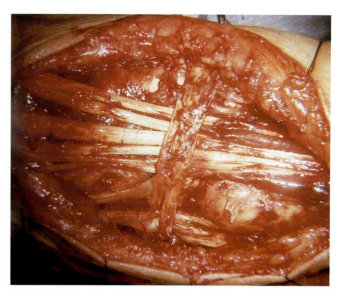

FIGURE 42.9. Intraoperative photo after complete dorsal tenosynovectomy with a proximal strip of extensor retinaculum to prevent bowstringing. If the wrist is fused or stiff, then preservation of this strip is not necessary.

Soft Tissue Procedures

Tenosynovectomy and Tendon Repairs

Rheumatoid arthritis affects the flexor and extensor tendons by both direct synovial invasion and attrition over bony prominences. Tenosynovectomy is successful in preventing rupture (44–46). The fourth extensor compartment tendons are most commonly involved, whereas first compartment tendons are usually spared (47). Of the wrist motors, the flexor carpi radialis and the ECRL and ECRB are rarely involved, but the ECU is commonly affected. The most frequent reconstruction of the wrist tendons involves redirecting the ECU to a more dorsal-radial direction and performing ECU tenosynovectomy (see below). This is almost always done in conjunction with ulnar head resection of the Darrach type. If there are ruptures of the radial wrist extensors, then soft tissue procedures are not indicated, and bony stabilization of the wrist should be performed.

Flexor tenosynovectomy is indicated for carpal tunnel syndrome, flexor tendon ruptures (48), and persistent flexor tenosynovitis (44,46). It becomes a matter of judgment on the surgeon's part of how to deal with the ruptured flexors, which may be held in functional continuity by tenosynovium. All osteophytes are trimmed, and a flap of volar capsule is used to cover bare bony surfaces. We prefer to repair the radial flap of flexor retinaculum to the ulnar aspect of the palmar fascia (49) to partially reconstruct the carpal tunnel. Digital tendon reconstruction is beyond the scope of this chapter, although end-to-side repairs for single ruptures and bridge grafts or transfers are recommended for multiple ruptures for both extensor (34,50) and flexor tendons (48).

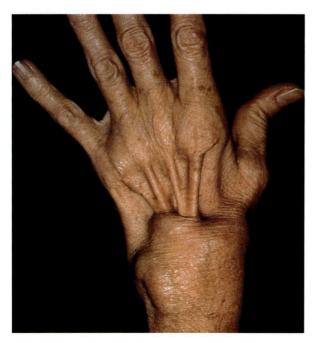

FIGURE 42.8. Typical clinical appearance of dorsal tenosynovitis.

Extensor Carpi Ulnaris Tendon Stabilization and Transfer

As discussed earlier, the ECU is an important dynamic stabilizer. Attenuation of the ECU subsheath by tenosynovitis results in volar ECU subluxation and relatively unopposed radial wrist extension (10,17). ECU stabilization is indicated in the following instances: following MP joint arthroplasty associated with correctable radial metacarpal deviation, following ECU tenosynovectomy, and following distal ulna resection. The surgical options include ECU relocation (12,37,51), ECU tenodesis as described by Rowland (52) and Leslie (53), or ECRL-to-ECU tendon transfer after the method of Clayton and Ferlic (54,55).

ECU relocation utilizes a portion of the extensor retinaculum as a pulley. If the retinaculum has been incised over the fifth or sixth compartment, then the radial flap may be looped around the ECU and sutured to itself. The ulnar flap may be utilized if the retinaculum has been incised more radially; it is divided transversely, with half placed deep to the ECU to reinforce the capsule and the other half placed dorsal to the ECU, creating a V-shaped pulley (51). The ECU relocation has the advantage of simplicity but does tend to stretch out.

ECU tenodesis is used only in the setting of distal ulna resection and is detailed fully in the chapter on the Darrach procedure (Chapter 52). The tenodesis is valuable in stabilizing the distal ulnar remnant.

Our preference in most instances is to use the ECRL-to-ECU transfer. In addition to relocating the ECU in a more dorsal position, the transfer eliminates a deforming force (the ECRL) and potentially augments ulnar deviation strength.

Synovectomy

Radiocarpal and DRUJ synovectomy have a long history. Although they may or may not prevent further progression of the disease, they do provide significant pain relief at the cost of some joint motion (56).

Larsen (57) has classified rheumatoid changes in the hand, wrist, and foot into six grades: 0 is normal; 1 is soft tissue swelling or osteoporosis or slight joint space narrowing; 2 to 5 are distinguished by increasing degrees of erosion and joint space narrowing. Stage 5 is characterized by either complete ankylosis or complete destruction ("floppy" wrist). It should be emphasized that the radiologic stage is useful, but is not the only determining factor in selecting treatment (6). In fact, a recent paper from Switzerland (18) suggests that treatment should be based on the type of destruction (spontaneous ankylosis, instability, or secondary degenerative arthritis) rather than the radiologic stage.

Most authors recommend wrist synovectomy in the early stages (Larsen stage 1–3) of disease (2,10,11,17,44–46). However, Namba (58) reviewed 36 patients who had a synovectomy on one side and no surgery on their opposite side and followed them for 8 years. Radiologically, all wrists deteriorated. Nonetheless, pain relief was 94.4% after 2 years and 80% after 8 years in the operated wrist.

Traditionally, the procedure has been performed through an open dorsal approach with its attendant morbidity including postoperative stiffness. Recently, however, arthroscopic techniques have been utilized with encouraging early results (33). Adolffson and Nylander (59) reported on arthroscopic synovectomy in 18 wrists (16 patients) with synovitis and Larsen stage 3 or better with a follow-up of 2 to 4 years. They found good pain relief, increased grip strength, and no postoperative stiffness. Although no long-term data are available, we have had good results with arthroscopic radiocarpal and midcarpal synovectomy in early cases combined with a mini-open technique for the DRUJ. It should also be mentioned that even in late cases, however, wrist synovectomy will relieve pain (58).

Synovectomy of the DRUJ poses a dilemma. Joint access is severely limited by the presence of the ulnar head. However, if the joint is mobile enough to allow for complete synovectomy, then the DRUJ is probably too unstable. It is for this reason, we believe, that no study has been published that documents the efficacy of DRUJ synovectomy with retention of the ulnar head.

We reserve mini-open DRUJ synovectomy for the patient whose primary problem is at the radiocarpal joint and whose DRUJ is stable and radiographically normal. We have no experience with arthroscopic synovectomy of the DRUJ.

Our surgical approach to the radiocarpal joint is therefore dependent on the status of the DRUJ. If the DRUJ is symptomatic and unstable or deteriorated, then we favor the standard distal ulna resection, open radiocarpal and midcarpal synovectomy, and ECU tenosynovectomy and stabilization.

Bony Procedures

For clarity, this topic is divided into separate sections addressing the management of radiocarpal and DRUJ disorder. In practice, however, rheumatoid wrist procedures usually involve the treatment of both.

Radiocarpal Joint

The two types of procedures, arthrodesis and arthroplasty, are discussed further in accompanying chapters. Arthrodesis remains the mainstay in the management of advanced rheumatoid wrist disease.

Arthrodesis

Total Wrist Arthrodesis. The indications for arthrodesis include the inability to correct the deformity of the wrist through soft tissue procedures, failure of synovectomy, infection, failure of arthroplasty, hyperlaxity, or multiple wrist tendon ruptures (11). Many techniques for total wrist arthrodesis have been described; the most popular involve use of an intramedullary rod placed either through the middle metacarpal (Fig. 42.10) or in the index–middle interspace (60–63). In addition to some technical problems with pin placement and migration (63,64), Ekerot, Jonsson, and Eiken (65) have reported carpal tunnel syndrome in 14 of 50 wrists after the Rush pin technique. We have used oblique $^3/_{32}$-in. Steinman pins placed from the radius into the carpus supplemented with local bone graft, usually from the excised ulna head (Fig. 42.11). If the bone and soft tissues are of good quality, a dorsal plate technique is acceptable (Fig. 42.12). Howard, Stanley, and Getty (66) reported on nine patients who had one-third tubular plate fusions with no failures and no complications. Most authors recommend fusing the wrist in neutral in the sagittal plane, and 5° to 10° ulnar deviation in the coronal or frontal plane to help correct ulnar deviation of the fingers at the metacarpal phalangeal joints (60–62,66,67). Vahvanen et al. (68), in a retrospective review of 62 wrist fusions, suggested that if the wrist were fused in over 5° of radial deviation, that the index finger would angulate ulnarly; if the wrist were fused in less than 5° of ulnar deviation, then the index finger would deviate radially. These authors also suggested that motion at the CMC joints is useful to the patient.

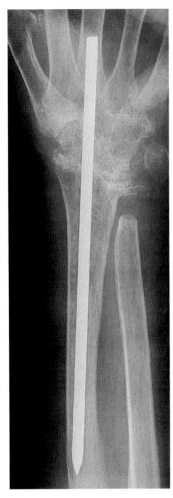

FIGURE 42.10. Total wrist arthrodesis using the intramedullary Steinman pin technique. (Courtesy of Dr. Andrew Terrono.)

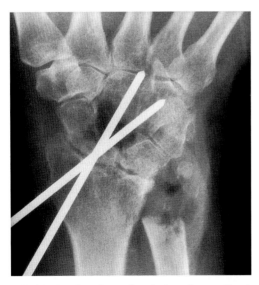

FIGURE 42.11. Total wrist arthrodesis using radius-to-carpus Steinman pin technique supplemented with bone graft from the ulna head. (Courtesy of Dr. Andrew Terrono.)

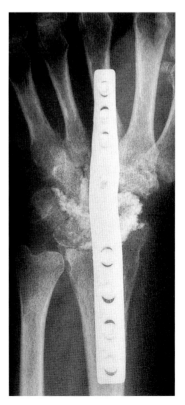

FIGURE 42.12. Total wrist arthrodesis using a dorsal plate supplemented with coralline bone substitute.

Partial Arthrodesis. Recently, several authors have described various combinations of partial fusion to gain the advantages of deformity correction and stabilization but still allow some motion (69–71). Radiolunate arthrodesis as first described by Chamay (69) has the advantage of correcting the ulnar volar translation of the carpus while allowing functional motion through the perilunate joints. The procedure is indicated when there is still relatively good preservation of the midcarpal joint, which is often the case. However, Ishikawa et al. (72) reported that after an average follow-up of 3 years, the lunate–capitate joint deteriorated in 12 of 25 wrists. Of the 25, there were 16 radiolunate and nine radioscapholunate fusions; the results were not stratified. Nevertheless, the early clinical results were good. Della Santa and Chamay (73) also found deterioration with time. In a 5-year follow-up of radiolunate arthrodesis in 26 wrists, all progressed to worse radiologic stages with time, and at the same rate as 18 unoperated contralateral wrists. The worst results were seen in the wrists with a disintegration-type pattern. Interestingly, radiolunate arthrodesis did not uniformly protect the MP joints from ulnar drift. Taleisnik (17) suggested performing radius-to-scaphoid-to-lunate arthrodesis and replacing the head of the capitate with a silicone rubber implant if the capitolunate articulation is compromised.

In our hands, radiolunate arthrodesis is performed infrequently. We reserve the procedure for the patient with preservation of the midcarpal joints and one or more of the following: painful radiocarpal arthritis with or without volar-ulnar translocation, and in conjunction with MP joint arthroplasty when uncorrectable radial wrist deviation is present. In general, we prefer total arthrodesis for bony stabilization of the wrist.

Arthroplasty

In theory, arthroplasty would be the ideal solution for the severely involved wrist, as it could correct deformity, relieve pain, and provide motion (74–78). Several types of arthroplasty have been described. Unfortunately, no technique has enjoyed predictably good results, even in this relatively low-demand population.

Fibrous stabilization or palmar shelf arthroplasty has not been shown to yield consistently good long-term results (77–81). Ryu et al. (77), in reviewing 32 patients who had undergone partial resection of the distal radius and proximal carpus (plus matched ulna resection), reported good clinical results, although 23 (72%) underwent spontaneous fusion. The results of proximal row carpectomy have been even less predictable (82). Swanson described a flexible hinge device similar to his finger joint prosthesis (83). This technique enjoyed early success (84), but late failure (85–87). Brase and Millender (87) reported on 71 Swanson silicone wrist arthroplasties and found a 25% failure rate including 14 fractured implants and four with pain and deformity. They suggested that the indications for silicone implants be narrowed to low-demand patients with good bone stock (Fig. 42.13). Vicar and Burton (88) compared their experience with fusion in 33 wrists versus arthroplasty in 37 wrists. Of these, 97% of the arthrodesis group had good or excellent results compared with 78% of the arthroplasty group. According to the authors, contraindications to arthroplasty should include the use of ambulatory aids or steroids, a prior wrist denervation procedure, severe instability with wrist dislocation, and arthritis mutilans. Arthroplasty may be indicated in the patient with bilateral disease with a fusion on the dominant side. There does seem to be some improvement in the long-term outcome if motion is limited in the early postoperative rehabilitation phase (87,88).

True total joint replacement has been described by a number of authors including Meuli (89), Volz (90), Ferlic (91), and Beckenbaugh (92). Unfortunately, they have all documented a significant incidence of complications including loosening, erosion into the carpal canal (93), infection (94), and wrist imbalance (93–97).

Ferlic et al. (97) reported on 12 metal-on-plastic total wrist arthroplasties that had failed. They noted that the salvage techniques, including replacement of the implant, resection arthroplasty, soft tissue reconstruction, or arthrodesis, were more difficult than for the silicone failures. The metal-on-plastic group required 19 operations to salvage 12 wrists. Menon (94) reported a complication rate of 44% (8 of 18) wrists treated with a modified Volz pros-

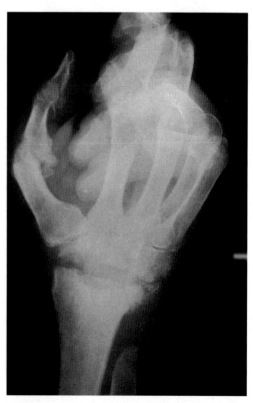

FIGURE 42.13. Patient with Swanson total wrist arthroplasty demonstrating the complication of subsidence.

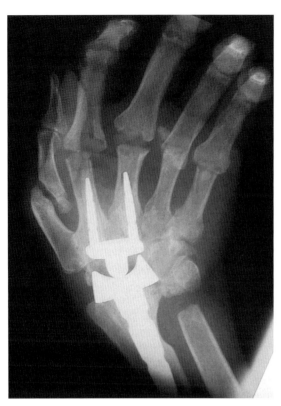

FIGURE 42.14. Patient with Volz total wrist arthroplasty showing significant imbalance.

thesis (Fig. 42.14). We have had no experience with any of the metal-on-plastic total wrist arthroplasties.

Distal Radioulnar Joint

Distal Ulna Resection

Distal ulna resection is certainly the most commonly performed procedure on the rheumatoid wrist. Fortunately, the results for any of the variety of distal ulna procedures are better in the rheumatoid than nonrheumatoid patient. Reported results include 60% to 95% pain relief and a less than 10% incidence of recurrent DRUJ synovitis or symptomatic ulnar stump instability (3,56,98–100). Rather than lose grip strength, as has been suggested in the posttraumatic population, many of the rheumatoids become stronger following distal ulna resection as the pain is eliminated (100,101).

Distal ulna resection is indicated for refractory DRUJ synovitis, especially when accompanied by radiographic change. As discussed earlier, rupture of the ulnar-sided digital extensor tendons is an indication for expedient distal ulna resection; subsequent ruptures are otherwise likely to occur (31,102). Other candidates include patients undergoing radiocarpal and/or MP joint procedures because the DRUJ is almost invariably affected as well.

Acceleration of ulnocarpal translocation has been a criticism of the distal ulna resection (103,104). However, recent data suggest that progressive ulnocarpal translocation is a consequence of the rheumatoid process itself rather than the surgery (3,105,106). Nevertheless, we do not recommend isolated distal ulna resection when in the setting of limited radiolunate contact (39,40,107), and certainly not when overt translocation is evident. In such instances, we include a limited or total wrist arthrodesis.

Many variations of the distal ulna resection have been described in an effort to minimize instability. In both Bowers' hemiresection interposition arthroplasty (108) and Watson's matched distal ulna resection (109,110), ulnar shaft–styloid continuity is retained. As stated by Bowers (108), the success of these procedures depends on integrity of the TFCC. In the majority of our rheumatoid patients, we have not been confident that the TFCC is functioning well enough to make either of these procedures worthwhile.

The modified Darrach remains our procedure of choice for distal ulna resection. The technique is discussed in detail in Chapter 52. However, several points deserve mention. We concur with many authors (12,23,100,111–114) that the best results are obtained when a minimal resection of the distal ulna is performed. The resection should be made just proximal to the ulnar articular cylinder, and the residual ulna should be beveled throughout the arc of forearm rotation to minimize radioulnar impingement and extensor tendon injury.

Meticulous soft tissue reconstruction is essential. Carpal supination is usually corrected using local tissue, either by tacking the residual TFCC to the dorsoulnar corner of the radius (115) or by suturing a distally based flap of volar capsule to the dorsal edge of the ulna (116). The distal ulna is then further stabilized, usually with an ECU tenodesis (53, 114). On occasion, we have used the pronator quadratus interposition transfer as described by Ruby et al. (117,118), especially when significant residual radioulnar impingement is evident intraoperatively. Finally, the extensor retinaculum is used to reinforce the capsular closure.

The Sauvé-Kapandji Procedure

An alternative to distal ulna resection is the Sauvé-Kapandji procedure (119). In theory, retention of the ulnar head could eliminate the complication of ulnar stump instability commonly seen following distal ulna resection. However, our experience parallels that of other authors (38,99,120), who conclude that the instability is merely transferred proximally, making salvage even more difficult. Another potential benefit, prevention of ulnocarpal translocation (40, 107), remains unsubstantiated.

The real benefit of this procedure lies in the maintenance of bone stock. Taleisnik (23,38) suggested that the Sauvé-Kapandji may be the technique of choice when a stable proximal radioulnar surface is needed for an arthroplasty or radiolunate fusion. These indications notwithstanding, we feel that the Sauvé-Kapandji procedure is unnecessarily complex for the majority of rheumatoid patients.

SUMMARY

Surgical treatment is indicated for the rheumatoid wrist when nonoperative treatment has failed to halt the disease in a reasonable time, such as 4 to 6 months. If the articular surfaces are well preserved, synovectomy of the radiocarpal and midcarpal joints, preferably through the arthroscope, combined with limited-incision synovectomy of the DRUJ is recommended. Distal ulna resection remains the standard treatment for advanced DRUJ involvement. In such instances, if the radiocarpal joint is still functional in spite of moderate x-ray changes (Larsen stage 2 or 3), we favor ulna head resection and ECU tenodesis or ECRL-to-ECU transfer with radiocarpal synovectomy through the ulnar approach. If the wrist has a fixed deformity, is totally unstable, has failed synovectomy or arthroplasty, or has had previous infection, then total wrist arthrodesis is our preference. If the midcarpal joint is preserved and motion is a priority, radiolunate or radioscapholunate arthrodesis can be considered. For the patient with a wrist fusion and contralateral disease, arthroplasty may be an attractive option. Following careful consideration of the contraindications, we may, in such instances, cautiously recommend a Swanson arthroplasty.

EDITORS' COMMENTS

The deformities of rheumatoid arthritis occur secondary to tissue destruction. Tissue destruction is synovium-related and usually ligamentous in nature. Complete destruction of joints and rupture of synovial enclosed tendons occur as severity increases. Analysis of rheumatoid arthritis deformity may be described by the equation:

$$\text{load} + \text{rheumatoid synovium} = \text{deformity}$$

Anywhere there is abnormal stress on tissue combined with rheumatoid synovium, destruction of those tissues can occur. This includes ligaments, cartilage, tendon, and bone. Removing either of the two components will prevent deformity.

Synovitis of the facet joints in the back elicits an overactivity of the back muscles in an attempt to protect the inflamed joint. This is a common physiologic response to any inflamed joint. In the hand, synovitis in the MP and interphalangeal (IP) joints produces overactivity of the local intrinsics. This constant overactivity results in fixed intrinsic tightness. The positive Bunnell test is one of the earliest objective findings in rheumatoid arthritis. These tight intrinsics are responsible for the frequent thumb deformities. As an example, the index has intrinsic insertions in the hood on the ulnar side and into the bone of the proximal phalanx on the radial side. With tightness of these intrinsics, flexing the middle and distal joints will produce a significant flexion and ulnar deviation moment at the MP joints. This produces increased pressure (load) at the dorsal radial aspect of the MP joint capsule. Rheumatoid synovium in the joint attenuates and destroys this collagen area, and the MP joint eventually subluxes volarly and ulnarly. With MP dislocation, the IP joints are protected because the tight intrinsics have been effectively released by proximal migration of their insertions. If, on the other hand, the MP joints do not sublux, the tight intrinsics will produce swan-neck deformities, boutonnière deformities, dislocations, or even fusions of the IP joints. This phenomenon of intrinsic release is repeated in the thumb, where subluxation of the CMC joint will prevent zed deformities of the thumb. All of this is independent of the angle of approach to the extensor tendons. With wrist subluxation, extensor tendons increase the ulnar subluxation force at the MP joint, but this is a terminal event and not etiologic. There is no etiologic effect of wrist position and, therefore, no reason to operate on the wrist first or in relation to finger deformity. All rheumatoid arthritis deformities should be approached as independent problems and repaired only for impaired function or to diminish pain. X-ray findings of any kind are not surgical indications.

The minor exception to these rules is the persistence of fourth dorsal compartment synovitis. The synovial mass, if not responsive to medical treatment, will invade and rupture the extensor tendons. Treatment is excision of the synovial mass, which removes the synovium portion of the formula. Combining this with a cocompartment release decreases the force component as well. The cocompartment release maintains the extensor retinaculum by cutting the septum between the fourth and fifth dorsal compartments, creating one common compartment. This significantly improves the available tendon space without interfering with the function of the extensor retinaculum.

The DRUJ is commonly involved. Our procedure of choice is a resection of the distal ulna. We prefer the matched ulnar arthroplasty, which does not require maintaining triangular fibrocartilage attachment, periosteum, or other soft tissue on the distal ulna, as the ulnar sling mechanism will firmly reattach to the broad cancellous surface of the ulna. Matched ulnar arthroplasty is not contraindicated in a panligamentous destruction downslope wrist, as the wrist itself must be treated at the same time. The procedure of choice for the rheumatoid wrist is a pseudarthrosis arthroplasty in which a cancellous concavity is formed in the distal radius along with a cancellous convexity of the scaphoid and lunate. The wrist is then nested in the concavity with the flap of reflected wrist ligament interposed between the scaphoid and lunate and the radius cup. This is cross-pinned for 2 to 3 weeks, then mobilized. The midcarpal joint is frequently better preserved than the radiocarpal joint. We find that transverse incisions in rheumatoid patients heal well, are just as exposure effective, and avoid longitudinal zigzag or curvilinear scars.

The tendon arthroplasty of the CMC joint has been a successful approach in rheumatoid as well as non-rheumatoid patients. The tendon sling mechanism of the flexor carpi radialis has excellent staying power once the radical synovectomy has been carried out at the CMC joint at the time of carpectomy.

REFERENCES

1. Hendrix RW, Urban MA, Schroeder JL, et al. Carpal predominance in rheumatoid arthritis. *Radiology* 1987;164:212–219.
2. Hanf G, Sollerman C, Elborgh R, et al. Wrist synovectomy in juvenile chronic arthritis. *Scand J Rheumatol* 1990;19:280–284.
3. Thirupathi RG, Ferlic DC, Clayton ML. Dorsal wrist synovectomy in rheumatoid arthritis—a long term study. *J Hand Surg [Am]* 1983;8:848–856.
4. Buckwalter KA, Swan JS, Braunstein EM. Evaluation of joint disease in the adult hand and wrist. *Hand Clin* 1991;7:135–151.
5. Kaye JJ, Callahan LF, Nance EP, et al. Bony ankylosis in rheumatoid arthritis—association with longer duration and greater severity of disease. *Invest Radiol* 1987;22:303–309.
6. Terrono AL, Feldon PG, Millender LH, et al. Evaluation and treatment of the rheumatoid wrist. *Inst Course Lect* 1996;45:15–26.
7. Eiken O, Haga T, Salgeback S. Assessment of surgery of the rheumatoid wrist. *Scand J Plast Reconstr Surg* 1975;9:207–215.
8. Jensen CM. Synovectomy with resection of the distal ulna in rheumatoid arthritis of the wrist. *Acta Orthop Scand* 1983;54:754–759.
9. Mannerfelt L. Surgical treatment of the rheumatoid wrist and aspects of the natural course when untreated. *Clin Rheum Dis* 1984;10:549–570.
10. Shapiro JS. The wrist in rheumatoid arthritis. *Hand Clin* 1996;12:477–498.
11. Feldon P, Millender L, Nalebuff EA. Rheumatoid arthritis in the hand and wrist. In: Green DP, ed. *Operative hand surgery, 3rd ed.* New York: Churchill Livingstone, 1993;1587–1690.
12. Flatt AE. *The care of the arthritic hand, 5th ed.* St Louis: Quality Medical Publishing, 1995.
13. Pirela-Cruz MA, Firoozbakhsh K, Moneim MS. Ulnar translocation of the carpus in rheumatoid arthritis: An analysis of five determination methods. *J Hand Surg [Am]* 1993;18:299–306.
14. Linscheid RL, Dobyns JH. Rheumatoid arthritis of the wrist. *Orthop Clin North Am* 1971;2:649–655.
15. Spinner M, Kaplan EB. Extensor carpi ulnaris. Its relationship to the stability of the distal radioulnar joint. *Clin Orthop* 1970;68:124–129.
16. Shapiro JS, Heigna W, Nasatir S. The relationship of wrist motion to ulnar phalangeal drift in the rheumatoid patient. *Hand* 1971;3:68–75.
17. Taleisnik J. Rheumatoid arthritis of the wrist. *Hand Clin* 1989;5:257–278.
18. Simmen BR, Huber H. Rheumatoid arthritis of the wrist: a new classification. *Handchir Mikrochir Plast Chir* 1994;26:182–189.
19. Evans DM, Ansen BM, Hall MA. The wrist in juvenile arthritis. *J Hand Surg [Br]* 1991;16:293–304.
20. White PH. Growth abnormalities in children with juvenile rheumatoid arthritis. *Clin Orthop* 1990;259:46–50.
21. Cracchiolo A III, Marmor L. Resection of the distal ulna in rheumatoid arthritis. *Arthritis Rheum* 1969;12:415–422.
22. Rana NA, Taylor AR. Excision of the distal end of the ulna in rheumatoid arthritis. *J Bone Joint Surg Br* 1973;55:96–105.
23. Taleisnik J. *The wrist.* New York: Churchill Livingstone, 1985;387–435.
24. Crosby EB, Linscheid RL. Rupture of the flexor profundus tendon of the ring finger secondary to ancient fracture of the hook of the hamate. Review of the literature and report of two cases. *J Bone Joint Surg Am* 1974;56:1076–1078.
25. Vaughan-Jackson OJ. Surgery of the tendons of the hands in rheumatoid arthritis. *J Bone Joint Surg Br* 1962;44:742–743.
26. Millis MB, Millender LH, Nalebuff EA. Stiffness of the proximal interphalangeal joints in rheumatoid arthritis: the role of flexor tenosynovitis. *J Bone Joint Surg Am* 1976;58:801–805.
27. Ertel AN, Millender LH, Nalebuff EA, et al. Flexor tendon ruptures in patients with rheumatoid arthritis. *J Hand Surg [Am]* 1988;13:860–866.
28. Ertel AN, Millender LH. Flexor tendon involvement in patients with rheumatoid arthritis, In: Hunter JM, Schneider LH, Mackin EJ, eds. *Tendon surgery in the hand.* St Louis: CV Mosby, 1987;370–384.
29. Nalebuff EA. The recognition and treatment of tendon ruptures in the rheumatoid hand. In: *AAOS Symposium on Tendon Surgery in the Hand.* St Louis: CV Mosby, 1975;255–269.
30. Backdahl M. The caput ulnae syndrome in rheumatoid arthritis: A study of the morphology, abnormal anatomy and clinical picture. *Acta Rheumatol Scand* 1963;Suppl 5:1–75.
31. Vaughan-Jackson OJ. Rupture of extensor tendons by attrition at the inferior radio-ulnar joint. Report of two cases. *J Bone Joint Surg Br* 1948;30:528–530.
32. Straub LR, Wilson EH. Spontaneous rupture of extensor tendons in the hand associated with rheumatoid arthritis. *J Bone Joint Surg Am* 1956;38:1208–1217.
33. Vaughan-Jackson OJ. Attrition ruptures of tendons as a factor in the production of deformities in the rheumatoid hand. *Proc R Soc Med* 1959;52:132–134.
34. Moore JR, Weiland AJ, Valdata L. Tendon ruptures in the rheumatoid hand: Analysis of treatment and functional results in fifty patients. *J Hand Surg [Am]* 1987;12:9–14.
35. Mannerfelt L, Norman O. Attrition ruptures of flexor tendons in rheumatoid arthritis caused by bony spurs in the carpal canal. A clinical and radiological study. *J Bone Joint Surg Br* 1969;51:270–277.
36. Freiberg RA, Weinstein A. The scallop sign and spontaneous rupture of finger extensor tendons in rheumatoid arthritis. *Clin Orthop* 1972;83:128–130.
37. Swanson AB. *Flexible implant resection arthroplasty in the hand and extremities.* St Louis: CV Mosby, 1973.
38. Taleisnik J. The Sauvé-Kapandji procedure. *Clin Orthop* 1992;275:110–123.
39. Black RM, Boswick JA Jr, Wiedel J. Dislocation of the wrist in rheumatoid arthritis: The relationship to distal ulna resection. *Clin Orthop* 1977;124:184–188.
40. DiBenedetto MR, Lubbers LM, Coleman CR. Long-term results of the minimal resection Darrach procedure. *J Hand Surg [Am]* 1991;16:445–450.
41. Hael L, Wagner-Weiner L, Poznanski AK, et al. Effects of methotrexate on radiologic progression in juvenile rheumatoid arthritis. *Arthritis Rheum* 1993;36:1370–1374.
42. Kasden ML, June L. Postoperative results of rheumatoid arthritis patients on methotrexate at the time of reconstructive surgery of the hand. *Orthopaedics* 1993;16:1233–1235.
43. Massarotti EM. Medical aspects of rheumatoid arthritis—diagnosis and treatment. *Hand Clin* 1996;12:463–475.

44. Millender LH, Nalebuff EA. Preventive surgery tenosynovectomy and synovectomy. *Orthop Clin North Am* 1975;6:765–792.
45. Norris SH. Surgery for the rheumatoid wrist and hand. *Ann Rheum Dis* 1990;2:863–870.
46. Stanley JK. Conservative surgery in the management of rheumatoid disease of the hand and wrist. *J Hand Surg [Br]* 1992;17:339–342.
47. Millender LH, Nalebuff EA, Albin R, et al. Dorsal tenosynovectomy and tendon transfer in the rheumatoid hand. *J Bone Joint Surg Am* 1974;56:601–610.
48. Ertel AN, Millender LH, Nalebuff EA, et al. Flexor tendon ruptures in patients with rheumatoid arthritis. *J Hand Surg [Am]* 1988;13:860–866.
49. Tanzer RC. The carpal tunnel syndrome. In: Converse JM, ed. *Reconstructive plastic surgery.* Philadelphia: WB Saunders, 1964;1787–1794.
50. Bora FW, Osterman AL, Thomas VJ, et al. The treatment of ruptures of multiple extensor tendons at wrist level by a free tendon graft in the rheumatoid patient. *J Hand Surg [Am]* 1987;12:1038–1040.
51. Cassidy C, Ruby LK. Tendon dysfunction in systemic arthritis. In: Peimer C, ed. *Surgery of the hand and upper extremity.* New York: McGraw-Hill, 1996;1645–1676.
52. Rowland SA. Stabilization of the ulnar side of the rheumatoid wrist following radiocarpal Swanson's implant arthroplasty and resection of the distal ulna. *Bull Hosp Joint Dis* 1984;44:442–448.
53. Leslie BM, Carlson G, Ruby LK. Results of extensor carpi ulnaris tenodesis in the rheumatoid wrist undergoing a distal ulnar excision. *J Hand Surg [Am]* 1990;15:547–551.
54. Clayton ML, Ferlic DC. Tendon transfer for radial rotation of the wrist in rheumatoid arthritis. *Clin Orthop* 1974;100:176–185.
55. Boyce T, Youmn Y, Sprague BL, et al. Clinical and experimental studies on the effect of extensor carpi radialis longus transfer in the rheumatoid hand. *J Hand Surg [Am]* 1978;3:390–394.
56. Brumfield R, Kuschner SH, Gellman H, et al. Results of dorsal wrist synovectomies in the rheumatoid hand. *J Hand Surg [Am]* 1990;15:733–735.
57. Larsen A, Dale K, Eek M. Radiographic evaluation of rheumatoid arthritis and related conditions by standard reference films. *Acta Radiol Diag* 1977;18:481–491.
58. Namba H. Clinical results of synovectomy for rheumatoid wrist compared with the opposite side. *J Jpn Orthop Assoc* 1981;55:527–541.
59. Adolffson L, Nylander G. Arthroscopic synovectomy of the rheumatoid wrist. *J Hand Surg [Br]* 1993;18:92–96.
60. Skak SV. Arthrodesis of the wrist by the method of Mannerfelt. A follow-up of 19 patients. *Acta Orthop Scand* 1982;53:557–559.
61. Koka R, D'Arcy JL. Stabilization of the wrist in rheumatoid disease. *J Hand Surg [Br]* 1989;14:288–290.
62. Mannerfelt L, Malmsten M. Arthrodesis of the wrist in rheumatoid arthritis. *Scand J Plast Reconstr Surg* 1971;5:124–130.
63. Millender LH, Nalebuff EA. Arthrodesis of the rheumatoid wrist. An evaluation of sixty patients and a description of a different surgical technique. *J Bone Joint Surg [Am]* 1973;55:1026–1034.
64. Turner PG, Bowker P, Noble J. Problems in rheumatoid wrist fusion. *J Hand Surg [Br]* 1985;10:256.
65. Ekerot L, Jonsson K, Eiken O. Median nerve compression complicating arthrodesis of the rheumatoid wrist. *Scand J Plast Reconstr Surg* 1983;17:257–262.
66. Howard AC, Stanley D, Getty CJM. Wrist arthrodesis in rheumatoid arthritis: A comparison of two methods of fusion. *J Hand Surg [Br]* 1993;18:371–380.
67. Kobus RJ, Turner RH. Wrist arthrodesis for treatment of rheumatoid arthritis. *J Hand Surg [Am]* 1990;15:541–546.
68. Vahvanen V, Kettunan P. Arthrodesis of the wrist in rheumatoid arthritis: A follow-up of 62 cases. *Ann Chir Gynecol* 1977;66:195–202.
69. Chamay A, Della Santa D, Vilaseca A. Radiolunate arthrodesis in rheumatoid wrist (21 cases). *Ann Hand Surg* 1991;10:197–206.
70. Nalebuff EA, Garrod KJ. Present approach to the severely involved rheumatoid wrist. *Orthop Clin North Am* 1984;15:369–381.
71. Linscheid R, Dobyns JH. Radiolunate arthrodesis. *J Hand Surg [Am]* 1985;10:821–829.
72. Ishikawa H, Hanyo T, Saito H, et al. Limited arthrodesis for the rheumatoid wrist. *J Hand Surg [Am]* 1992;17:1103–1109.
73. Della Santa D, Chamay A. Radiologic evaluation of the rheumatoid wrist after radiolunate arthrodesis. *J Hand Surg [Br]* 1995;20:146–154.
74. Beckenbaugh RD. Total joint arthroplasty: The wrist. *Mayo Clin Proc* 1979;54:513–515.
75. Liretto R, Minawl P. Biaxial total wrist arthroplasty in rheumatoid arthritis. *Can J Surg* 1995;38:51–53.
76. Robertson GA, Bailey BN. Silastic sheet arthroplasty for the painful rheumatoid wrist: A long term review. *Br J Plast Surg* 1985;38:190–196.
77. Ryu J, Watson HK, Burgess RC. Rheumatoid wrist reconstruction utilizing a fibrous nonunion and radiocarpal arthrodesis. *J Hand Surg [Am]* 1985;10:830–836.
78. Nylen S, Sollerman C, Haffajee D, et al. Swanson implant arthroplasty of the wrist in rheumatoid arthritis. *J Hand Surg [Br]* 1984;9:295–299.
79. Gellman H, Rankin G, Brumfield R, et al. Palmar shelf arthroplasty in the rheumatoid wrist. Results of long term follow-up. *J Bone Joint Surg Am* 1989;71:223–227.
80. Biyan A, Simison AJM. Fibrous stabilization of the rheumatoid wrist. *J Hand Surg [Br]* 1995;20:143–145.
81. Skoff H. Palmar shelf arthroplasty. A follow-up note. *J Bone Joint Surg Am* 1988;70:1377–1382.
82. Ferlic DC, Clayton ML, Mills MF. Proximal row carpectomy: review of rheumatoid and non-rheumatoid wrists. *J Hand Surg [Am]* 1991;16:420–424.
83. Swanson AB. Flexible implant arthroplasty for arthritic disabilities of the radiocarpal joint. *Orthop Clin North Am* 1973;4:383–394.
84. Goodman MJ, Millender LH, Nalebuff EA, et al. Arthroplasty of the rheumatoid wrist with silicone rubber: An early evaluation. *J Hand Surg [Am]* 1980;5:114–121.
85. Jolly SL, Ferlic DC, Clayton ML, et al. Swanson silicone arthroplasty of the wrist in rheumatoid arthritis: A long term follow-up. *J Hand Surg [Am]* 1992;17:142–149.
86. Fatti JF, Palmer AH, Mosher JF. The long term results of Swanson silicone rubber interpositional wrist arthroplasty. *J Hand Surg [Am]* 1986;11:166–175.
87. Brase DW, Millender LH. Failure of silicone rubber wrist arthroplasty in rheumatoid arthritis. *J Hand Surg [Am]* 1986;11:175–183.
88. Vicar AJ, Burton RI. Surgical management of the rheumatoid wrist—fusion or arthroplasty? *J Hand Surg [Am]* 1986;11:790–797.
89. Meuli HC. Arthroplastie due poignet. *Ann Chir* 1973;27:527–530.
90. Volz RG. The development of a total wrist arthroplasty. *Clin Orthop* 1976;116:209–214.
91. Ferlic DC. Management of the rheumatoid wrist. In: Clayton ML, Smythe CT, eds. *Surgery for rheumatoid arthritis.* New York: Churchill Livingstone, 1992;155–187.
92. Beckenbaugh RD. Arthroplasty of the wrist. In: Morrey BF, ed. *Joint replacement arthroplasty.* New York: Churchill Livingstone, 1991;195–215.
93. Sieminow M, Lister GD. Tendon ruptures and median nerve

damage after Hamas total wrist arthroplasty. *J Hand Surg [Am]* 1987;12:374–377.
94. Menon J. Total wrist replacement using the modified Volz prosthesis. *J Bone Joint Surg Am* 1987;69:998–1006.
95. Meuli HC, Fernandez DL. Uncemented total wrist arthroplasty. *J Hand Surg [Am]* 1995;20:115–122.
96. Bosco JA, Bynum DH, Bowers WH. Long-term outcome of Volz total wrist arthroplasties. *J Arthroplasty* 1994;9:25–31.
97. Ferlic DC, Jolly SN, Clayton ML. Salvage for failed implant arthroplasty of the wrist. *J Hand Surg [Am]* 1992;17:917–923.
98. Allieu Y, Lussiez B, Ascencio G. The long-term results of synovectomy of the rheumatoid wrist: a report of 60 cases. *Fr J Orthop Surg* 1989;3:188–194.
99. Bieber EJ, Linscheid RL, Dobyns JH, et al. Failed distal ulna resections. *J Hand Surg [Am]* 1988;13:193–200.
100. Tulipan DJ, Eaton RG, Eberhart RD. The Darrach procedure defended: Technique redefined and long-term follow-up. *J Hand Surg [Am]* 1991;16:438–444.
101. Bowers WH. The distal radioulnar joint. In: Green DP, ed. *Operative hand surgery, ed. 3.* New York: Churchill Livingstone, 1993;973–1019.
102. Vaughan-Jackson OJ. Attrition rupture of tendons in the rheumatoid hand. *J Bone Joint Surg Am* 1958;40:1431.
103. Baldwin WI. Orthopaedic surgery of injuries. In: Jones R, ed. *Pub. joint comm. of Henry Frowde, vol 1.* London: Hodder and Stoughton, 1921.
104. Goncalves D. Correction of disorders of the distal radioulnar joint by pseudarthrosis of the ulna. *J Bone Joint Surg Br* 1974;56:462–464.
105. Van Gemert AML, Spauwen PHM. Radiological evaluation of the long-term effects of resection of the distal ulna in rheumatoid arthritis. *J Hand Surg [Br]* 1994;19:330–333.
106. Nanchahal J, Sykes PJ, Williams RL. Excision of the distal ulna in rheumatoid arthritis: Is the price too high? *J Hand Surg [Br]* 1996;21:189–196.
107. Gainor BJ, Schaberg J. The rheumatoid wrist after resection of the distal ulna. *J Hand Surg [Am]* 1985;10:837–844.
108. Bowers WH. Distal radioulnar joint arthroplasty: The hemiresection–interposition technique. *J Hand Surg [Am]* 1985;10:169–178.
109. Watson HK, Gabuzda GM. Matched distal ulna resection for post-traumatic disorders of the distal radioulnar joint. *J Hand Surg [Am]* 1992;17:724–730.
110. Watson HK, Ryu J, Burgess RC. Matched distal ulna resection. *J Hand Surg [Am]* 1986;11:812–817.
111. Backhouse KM. Surgical treatment of the rheumatoid wrist. *Ann Acad Med Singapore* 1983;12:263–271.
112. Dingman PVC. Resection of the distal end of the ulna (Darrach procedure): An end-result study of 24 cases. *J Bone Joint Surg Am* 1952;34:893–900.
113. Ferlic DC, Clayton ML. Synovectomy of the hand and wrist. *Ann Chir Gynaecol* 1985;198:26–30.
114. O'Donovan TM, Ruby LK. The distal radioulnar joint in rheumatoid arthritis. *Hand Clin* 1989;5:249–256.
115. Feldon P. Rheumatoid arthritis. *Hand Surg Update* 1994;17:1–10.
116. Blatt G, Ashworth CR. Volar capsule transfer for stabilization following resection of the distal end of the ulna. *Orthop Trans* 1979;3:13.
117. Ruby LK. Darrach procedure. In: Gelberman RH, ed. *Master techniques in orthopaedic surgery, the wrist.* New York: Raven Press, 1994;279–285.
118. Ruby LK, Ferenz CC, Dell PC. The pronator quadratus interposition transfer: An adjunct to resection arthroplasty of the distal radioulnar joint. *J Hand Surg [Am]* 1996;21:60–65.
119. Sauvé L, Kapandji M. Nouvelle technique de traitement chirurgical des luxations récidivantes isolées de l'extremité inferieure du cubitus. *J Chir (Paris)* 1936;47:589–594.
120. Milroy P, Coleman S, Iver R. The Sauvé-Kapandji operation: technique and results. *J Hand Surg [Br]* 1992;17:411–414.

43

TOTAL WRIST ARTHROPLASTY

JAY MENON

HISTORICAL BACKGROUND

The first total wrist arthroplasty was performed by Themistocle Gluck, a German surgeon, over a century ago (1890) (1). The device was made of ivory and had two forks on either end to engage the radius, ulna, and the metacarpals. "A 19-year-old male whose wrist was destroyed by tuberculosis was salvaged by this operation, relieving pain and maintaining the length of the hand" (1). Despite this long history, total wrist arthroplasty has not attained widespread acceptance. In contrast, total hip and total knee replacement has become increasingly popular ever since Charnley introduced low-friction arthroplasty (2). Shoulder and elbow surgeons readily embraced this concept to manage arthritis, which resulted in a steady decline of fusion of these joints. The literature of the last 25 years is replete with information on biomaterials, implant design, implant wear, implant fixation, and implant host reaction. These scientific studies have lead to the increased durability of implants, and have contributed to the improvement of the quality of life of arthritic patients.

In spite of these advancements, when the wrist joint is involved, fusion is still the first choice of a majority of surgeons. Early failures and complications, coupled with the reigning popularity of wrist fusion, dampened the initial enthusiasm generated by total wrist arthroplasty. Lack of economic incentive and market forces discouraged manufacturers from investing money to develop new wrist designs. Wrist fusion is relatively easy to achieve, is considered very functional, and is not disabling. Widespread acceptance of this notion has hampered the development of wrist devices. Patients accepted a fixed position of the wrist—I call it "a position of compromise" because no one position is optimum for all activities—and adapted to the chores of day-to-day living. However, those who had fusion of one wrist and arthroplasty of the other preferred arthroplasty to fusion (3,4). In a report on wrist fusion by Kobus et al. (5), all the unsatisfied patients had arthroplasty on the contralateral side. A recent analysis of patients who had wrist fusion revealed that they had a great deal of difficulty in doing the activities of day-to-day living such as fastening buttons, combing hair, opening a jar, or writing (6,7). Using a fused wrist for support to sit down was also difficult. Fifty percent of the patients with wrist fusion had difficulty with perineal care. Using a cane with the wrist in a palmarflexed position was also difficult; splashing water on the face was impossible. These difficulties are compounded in patients with multiple joint involvement, as in rheumatoid arthritis. Patients in other series voiced the same concerns (8–10). Von Gemert (11) reported that only 42% of patients with wrist fusion received the expected outcome.

Swanson noted that a few degrees of wrist motion will increase the reach of the fingers in space by 5 or 6 cm (12). He pointed out that wrist motion is essential to place the hand on body surfaces. There is general agreement among hand surgeons that whenever possible, attempts must be made to preserve wrist motion if multiple joints are involved, as in rheumatoid arthritis. Flatt (13) stated that virtually all recent designs of implants for total wrist arthroplasty give good pain relief and acceptable range of motion. The lack of durability of implants is what has set wrist arthroplasty apart from other joint arthroplasties.

IMPLANTS

Fracture, loosening, and imbalance of the implants have been the most common modes of failure. A thorough knowledge of the morphology of the commonly used wrist implants is necessary to analyze the factors that lead to their early demise. The following describes the design features of some wrist implants frequently used in the United States. This information will enable readers to become familiar with implant geometry, and to make meaningful comparisons of these devices.

J. Menon (deceased): Department of Orthopaedic Surgery, Southern California Permanente Medical Group, Fontana, California 92335.

Flexible Hinge Silastic Implant

In 1967, Swanson (12) developed a double-stemmed flexible implant made of medical-grade silicone as an adjunct to resection arthroplasty of the wrist in order to maintain the joint space and alignment and, at the same time, provide some stability and motion (Fig. 43.1). The midsection is barrel shaped and flattened on the dorsal and volar surfaces. The core of the implant contains dacron reinforcement for axial stability. The implant is impregnated with barium to be visible on roentgenograms, and is available in five sizes. It acts as a stent over which the new capsuloligamentous structures develop. This phenomenon has been named an "encapsulation process." Early range-of-motion exercises orient this neocapsule along the axis of the joint, yielding functional range of motion. Since 1974, the implant has been made of high-performance silicone elastomer, and the midsection was widened. Titanium grommets were developed in 1982 to protect the midsection of the implant from shearing and frictional forces (14). Swanson deduced that an excessive arc of motion averaging 60° flexion and 60° extension with an average 28° radioulnar deviation resulted in a high incidence of fractures (14). He strongly advocated limiting the range of motion of the wrist to 30° of flexion, 30° of extension, and 10° of radioulnar deviation.

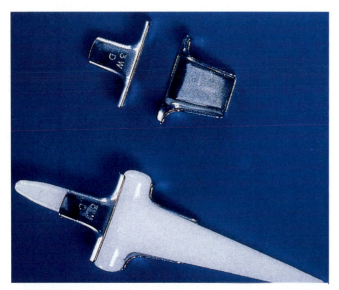

FIGURE 43.1. Swanson silastic wrist implant with titanium grommets. **Editors' Notes:** *In the normal wrist, total load is shared among multiple bones: eight carpals and five metacarpals. The underlying design deficiency of total wrist arthroplasty is the inability to incorporate all of those bones in load transference with a prosthetic implement. The designer is faced with having to choose certain small bones to take all of the loads coming through the hand. The loads on the radius are not the problem. There will probably not be a good wrist implant until a way can be found to incorporate load transference to all or most of the small bones distal to the radius.*

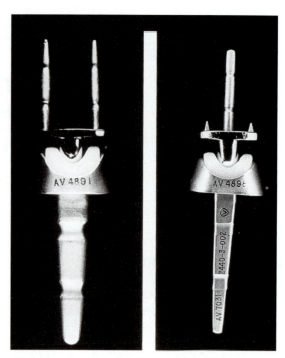

FIGURE 43.2. Volz prosthesis showing **(left)** double- and **(right)** single-prong carpal components.

The Volz Prosthesis

In 1974, Robert Volz (15) developed a unique prosthesis (Fig. 43.2). The radial component of the Volz prosthesis has a U-shaped metal-backed articular surface lined by a high-density polyethylene insert. The stem of this component is inserted into the medullary canal of the radius. The original carpal component had two prongs, and they were inserted into the medullary canals of the second and third metacarpals. The components are made of cobalt chrome. Both components are fixed using methylmethacrylate. The carpal component was later modified to a single prong in an attempt to decrease the postoperative ulnar deviation deformity caused by the increased moment arm of the ulnar deviators (15). Two sizes are available for use.

The Clayton-Volz-Ferlic Prosthesis

In 1988, a new cementless wrist prosthesis was developed to lessen the radioulnar muscle imbalance, incorporating the concept of modularity (16) (Fig. 43.3). This device was made from a titanium–aluminum–vanadium alloy. The surface of the implant was made porous by sandblasting to enhance osteointegration. The device has three modular radial sleeves and two radial stems. The radial articular surface is offset ulnarly for balancing of the wrist. The metacarpal component is made of titanium and lined with ultrahigh-density polyethylene; it has a stem that goes into the medullary canal of the third metacarpal. The components are inserted without cement.

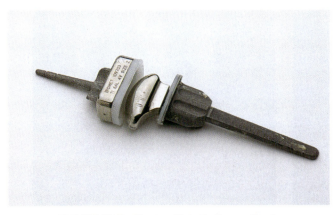

FIGURE 43.3. Clayton-Volz-Ferlic prosthesis.

The Mueli Device

The Mueli device was one of the earliest wrist implants and was first implanted in 1972 by Hans Cristoph Meuli of Berne, Switzerland (17). The prosthetic device underwent several modifications because of various problems with its performance. The current form and design (MWPIII: Meuli wrist prosthesis, third revised) was achieved in 1986 and is made of six parts titanium, seven parts aluminum, and 100 parts of the niobium wrought alloy protasul (Fig. 43.4). The surface is corundum rough-blasted. The gold-colored spherical head is coated with titanium nitride. The cup is lined by ultrahigh-molecular-weight polyethylene chirulen. It is

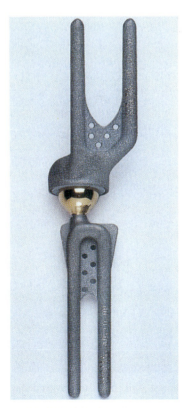

FIGURE 43.4. Mueli device.

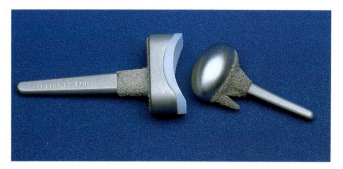

FIGURE 43.5. Biaxial wrist prosthesis.

available in two sizes and in left- and right-hand versions. The stem of the carpal component is inserted into the capitate and the second metacarpal bones without bone cement.

Biaxial Wrist Prosthesis (Mayo Clinic)

The radial component of the biaxial wrist prosthesis is a concave metal-backed polyethylene component, and the articulating surface is offset ulnarly and palmarly (18) (Fig. 43.5). The distal component is an ellipsoid metallic articulating surface with a single stem that goes into the medullary canal of the third metacarpal. The stems have a porous coating for bony ingrowth. Three sizes are available: small, medium, and large.

Trispherical Total Wrist Prosthesis

The trispherical total wrist prosthesis (19) consists of titanium alloy metacarpal and radial components with an ultrahigh-density polyethylene bearing surface (Fig. 43.6).

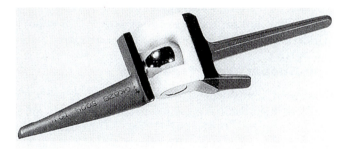

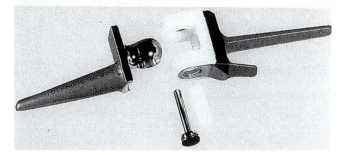

FIGURE 43.6. Trispherical wrist prosthesis. This is a constrained device. The carpal and radial components are connected by an axle.

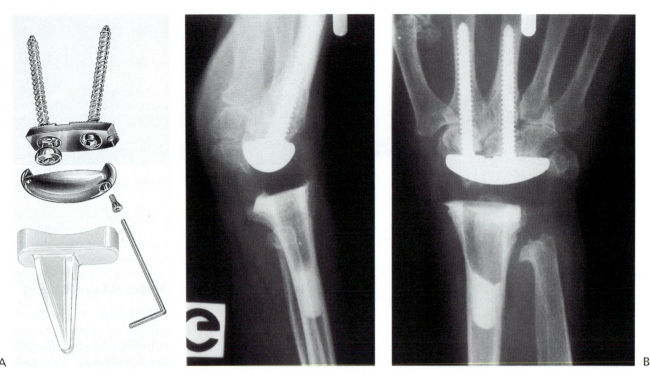

FIGURE 43.7. A: Guepar prosthesis. **B:** Radiologic appearance of a wrist with the Guepar prosthesis.

The long stem of the metacarpal component resides in the medullary canal of the third metacarpal, and the smaller stem in the second metacarpal base. The radial component has an ulnar offset to maintain the center of rotation in its normal location. The component is also tilted 12° palmarly, mimicking the palmar tilt of the articular surface of the radius. The polyethylene bearing articulates with the convex portion of the ring of the radial component. The components are then connected by an axle. This is a constrained device. The implant is designed to provide 15° of radioulnar deviation, 90° of flexion, and 85° of extension.

The Guepar Wrist Prosthesis

The radial component of the Guepar wrist prosthesis is made of high-density polyethylene with an ulnar offset articular surface (20) (Fig. 43.7). This is implanted in the radius with acrylic cement. The carpal component has two parts and is joined together by a small oblique screw. The main metal part is fixed with two screws that go into the second and third metacarpals.

The House Wrist Prosthesis

A polyethylene interface snap fits over the spherical head of the carpal component (Fig. 43.8). Radioulnar deviation occurs at this joint. Flexion–extension occurs at the junction of the polyethylene with the radial component. This prosthesis also has the potential to reconstruct the distal radioulnar joint.

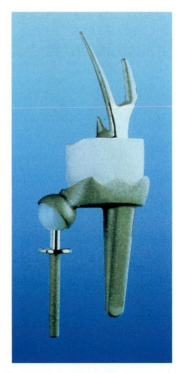

FIGURE 43.8. House wrist prosthesis with distal radioulnar joint articulation.

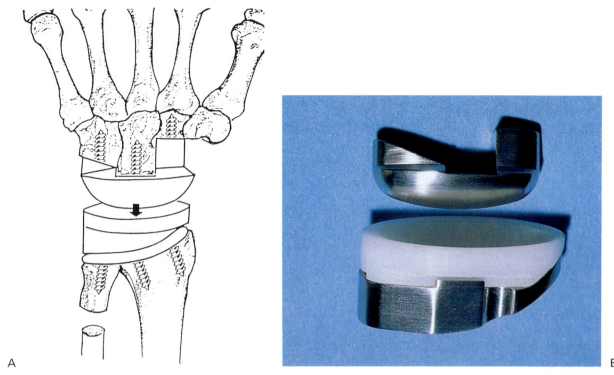

FIGURE 43.9. A: Schematic showing the method of fixation of the Giachino device. **B:** The Giachino prosthesis.

The Giachino Device

Fixation of the components of the Giachino device is achieved with screws (Fig. 43.9). Conceptually, the prosthesis has merits; clinical trials are under way in Canada.

The Universal Wrist Prosthesis

The universal wrist prosthesis (21) is a nonconstrained joint (Fig. 43.10). The carpal component is made of titanium; it is ovoid in shape and matches the cut surface of the carpal bones (Fig. 43.10B,C). The carpal plate comes in two forms, one with three screw holes (22) and the other with a central stem and two peripheral screws (Fig. 43.10E,F). The central screw and the stem are seated in the capitate. The radial peripheral screw captures the scaphoid and the trapezoid, and the screw on the ulnar side goes through the triquetrum and hamate. The stemmed version of the carpal plate is used in conjunction with bone cement (Fig. 43.10E,F). A carpal plate with three holes is fixed to the carpus by a 6.5-mm-diameter and 35-mm-long cancellous screw inserted through the central hole into the capitate (22). The peripheral screws are 4.5-mm-diameter self-tapping screws, and their length is determined in the operating room.

The articular surface of the radius is concave and is inclined 20°, similar to the articular surface of the radius (Fig. 43.10A). The concavity of the articular surface is deep enough to provide immediate stability when the components are inserted under appropriate soft tissue tension. The stem of the radial component is conical in shape and has tie mesh on either side for bony ingrowth. The component can be inserted with or without a bone carpal component. Since 1992, the tie mesh has been eliminated (Fig. 43.10F), and the radial component is inserted with bone cement only. The radial component is now made of cobalt chrome alloy to decrease polyethylene wear. A convex high-density polyethylene component slides over the pillars on the carpal plate, which functions as an interface (Fig. 43.10D). This prosthesis comes in three sizes: small, medium, and large. The polyethylene interface comes in different thicknesses to adjust soft tissue tension. Special instruments are designed to make appropriate bone cuts to obtain an optimum fit.

ANALYSIS OF WRIST ARTHROPLASTY FAILURE

Fracture of the implant has been a problem only with the Swanson silastic prosthesis. Incidence of fracture has ranged from zero to 20%, resulting in revision surgery in up to 35% of cases (23). In one series (24) followed for 5.8 years, the fracture rate was 26%. Jolly et al. (25) reported

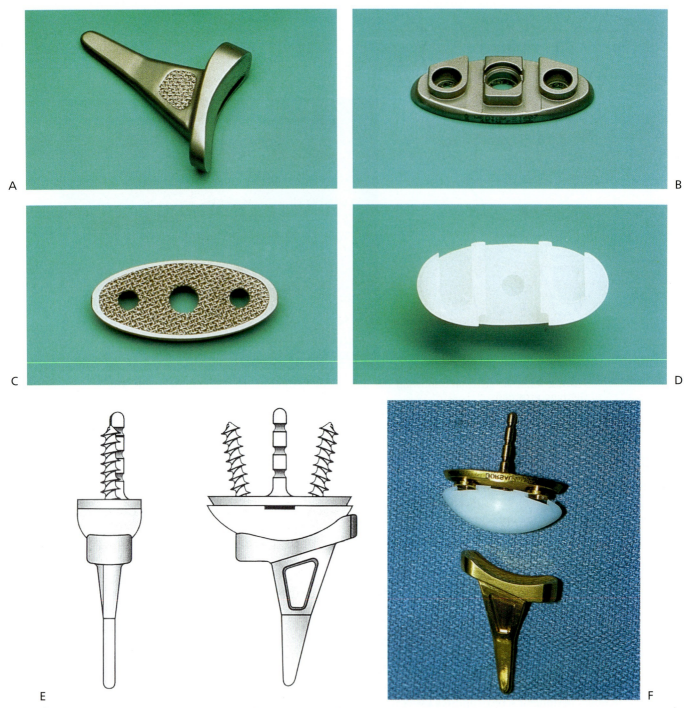

FIGURE 43.10. Universal wrist prosthesis. **A:** Radial component with tie mesh for bone ingrowth. **B:** Distal surface of the carpal plate. **C:** Proximal side of the carpal plate. Notice the three pillars over which the polyethylene insert slides. The carpal plate is fixed to the carpus by three titanium screws. **D:** Polyethylene insert. **E,F:** The carpal component with a central peg and two peripheral screws. The radial component of this version is made of cobalt chrome alloy to decrease polyethylene wear. The tie mesh has been removed. Both components are inserted with cement. The polyethylene insert comes in different thicknesses to facilitate soft tissue balance.

fracture of the implant in 52% of cases when followed for 6 years. Short-term follow-up studies reported good pain relief and satisfactory range of motion. With the passage of time, the incidence of pain relief decreased, resorption of surrounding bone occurred with settling of the prosthesis, silicone synovitis, erosion of the radius and carpal bones, and eventually failure of the implant. Hence, this implant has very limited indications and is recommended with reservation (23).

Fracture of the implant has not been a problem with any of the other implants. Two other problems that have plagued other wrist devices have been loosening and muscle imbalance. Loosening is known to occur with any prosthesis, whether in the hip or knee; unfortunately, in the case of the wrist, it happened too frequently and too soon. This was one of the major reasons why wrist arthroplasty did not become the first choice in treating arthritis of the wrist. Loosening of a prosthesis occurs from infection, mechanical failure, or asepsis. Loosening primarily occurred on the carpal side. Most of the reports on total wrist arthroplasty noted very little problem on the radial side (15,26). Mechanical failure occurs from faulty design, abnormal stresses, poor bone stock, and progressive destruction of the supporting structures from progressing disease processes.

It is important to realize the distinction between the wrist joint and other larger joints in the body when comparing implant performance and durability. The distal half of the wrist joint is composed of several small bones held together by interosseous ligaments, and the metacarpals are resting on this stack of bones held in place by carpometacarpal ligaments. In other areas of the body, a joint is essentially made up of two large bones. The carpal component of all the existing wrist devices except the universal wrist uses one or two intramedullary stems that traverse through the capitate into the medullary canal of the third metacarpal. The body of the carpal component rests on carpal bones that remain after resection. In many instances, a major portion of the carpal bones are resected. Initial stability is achieved by a press fit or by three-point fixation obtained by the slight dorsal arch of the third metacarpal. In all instances, the stem crosses the carpometacarpal joint. Some additional strength is provided by inserting methylmethacrylate into the capitate–metacarpal complex.

With time, the body of the carpal component loses support as the remaining carpal bones shift from underneath as a result of attenuation, stretching, or tearing of the extrinsic and intrinsic ligaments holding them from synovitis (Fig. 43.11). Synovitis also erodes and weakens the carpal bones. Loss of the normal geometry of these bones results in the loss of stability provided by the symmetric opposing sides of the adjacent bones. The osteoporosis that accompanies rheumatoid arthritis helps accelerate this process; further insult is added by the corticosteroids prescribed to alleviate symptoms. These markedly osteoporotic and weakened bones are subjected to the compressive forces exerted by the extrinsic tendons, resulting in disorganization and collapse of the carpus. The situation is similar to loosening of the femoral cup when inserted for avascular necrosis of the hip. The body of the carpal component is now subject to toggle as the wrist goes through its range of motion. With most of the bony support at the base having been lost, the stress now concentrates on the

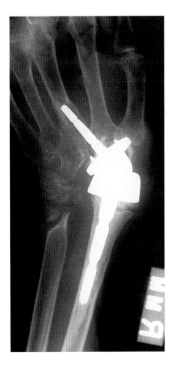
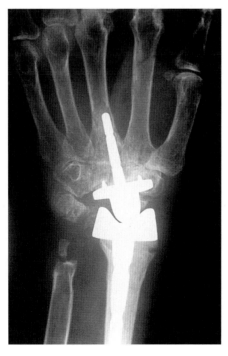

FIGURE 43.11. Loosening of the carpal component of a Volz prosthesis. Loss of bony support results in distal migration of the component and eventual loosening.

stem of the carpal implant. Motion at the carpometacarpal joint starts a line of cleavage in the cement mantle or at the bone–prosthetic interface at that joint region. This further destabilizes the carpal component and leads to clinical and radiologic loosening. The stem of the carpal component in many instances penetrates the dorsal cortex of the third metacarpal (Fig. 43.12).

The carpal component of the universal wrist prosthesis was designed with these factors taken into consideration (Fig. 43.13). Unlike other designs, the carpal plate of the universal wrist spans from the radial border of the scaphoid remnant to the ulnar border of the remaining triquetrum in the anteroposterior plane. In the lateral plane, the plate extends from the dorsal to the volar margin of the carpal bones. The carpal plate provides a solid base for the carpal bones to rest on or provides a platform for the carpal bones to be stacked on. The central screw or the stem is located primarily in the capitate and not in the medullary canal of the third metacarpal (Fig. 43.14). The peripheral screws capture the scaphoid, trapezoid, hamate, and triquetrum, and take over the function of the interosseous ligaments to prevent lateral or proximal migration of these bones. In addition, an intercarpal fusion is done (if necessary with a cancellous bone graft), which eliminates any potential source of synovitis, thereby arresting the progress of the disease. Intercarpal fusion permanently fixes the carpal bones to their anatomic position. A solid fusion converts the wrist joint into a two-bone joint similar to the larger joints in the body. Fusion could be extended to the carpometacarpal joint if longer peripheral screws are used, or if there is ligamentous laxity of these joints at the time of surgery.

Bosco et al. (26) reported their long-term experience with the Volz prosthesis. They noted progressive subsidence of the carpal component as the carpal bones deteriorated with time, and that the carpal component stabilized when it reached the metacarpal base. This finding gives credence to the concept of intercarpal fusion as recommended in the technique for the universal prosthesis.

Titanium screws are used to fix the carpal plate in the universal wrist prosthesis. Titanium is known to be osteoinductive and is widely used for dental implants (27). Titanium screws integrate with bone without any interposing connective tissue layer between the bone and the screw. Titanium implants are instantly coated with an oxide layer about 100 Å thick that facilitates osteointegration (28). Loosening of the carpal component, one of the most common modes of prosthetic failure, was not seen with the universal wrist. Lundborg et al. (29,30) have shown the clinical efficacy of threaded titanium implants in metacarpophalangeal arthroplasty and also in thumb prostheses. Cadaver studies done in our biomechanical laboratory determined that the average force required to pull out the carpal component of the universal wrist prosthesis was 825 N (unpublished data).

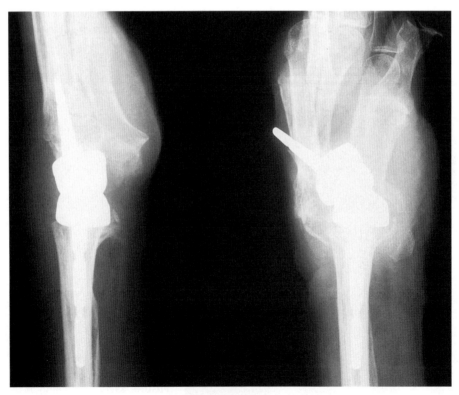

FIGURE 43.12. X-rays show gradual loss of stability of the carpal component (Volz) with eventual penetration of the stem through the dorsal cortex.

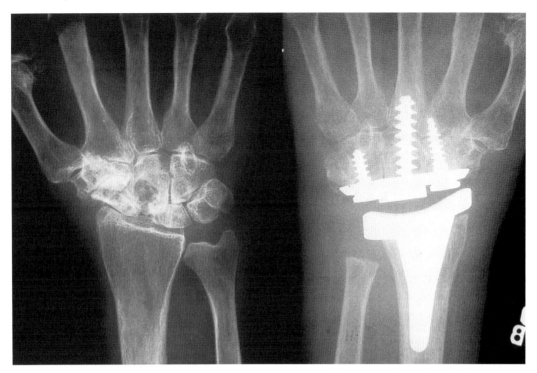

FIGURE 43.13. Pre- and 6-year postoperative appearance of the wrist with a universal wrist prosthesis. The carpal plate extends from the radial to the ulnar side. Fixation is achieved by titanium screws. Carpal bone stock is maintained by intercarpal fusion. There is no evidence of loosening.

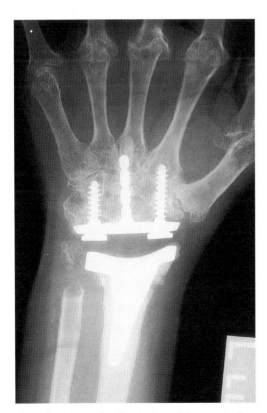

FIGURE 43.14. Universal wrist device with a central peg. Most of the capitate is retained. The peg primarily resides in the capitate. Peripheral screws may cross the carpometacarpal joints for stronger purchase.

It is now recognized that many patients on long-term medication discontinue it because of side effects or lack of response. Situnayke et al. (31) reported that only 20% of patients who are on gold, penicillamine, or sulfasalazine were still taking medication at 5 years postoperatively. Only 30% of patients on methotrexate remained on it after 5 years (32). There is no evidence that antirheumatic drugs will halt the progress of the disease (32). The original treatment protocol was often illustrated as a pyramid with a base of nonsteroidal antiinflammatory drugs, aspirin, exercise, and rest. The next step was to add disease-modifying drugs such as gold and Plaquenil. The top of the pyramid was occupied by more potent drugs such as methotrexate or azathioprine (Imuran). Physicians have now discarded this paradigm and are treating aggressively with a combination of drugs (similar to chemotherapy against cancer) to slow progression and halt irreversible damage to the bones. Stanley (33) stated that "significant mechanical problems require surgical treatment, and the surgeon is often asked to remedy these mechanical problems at a later stage in the disease when they are progressive, obvious, and medically untreatable." Hindley and Stanley (34) emphasized that the role of surgery should be viewed as prophylactic or reconstructive rather than a salvage option. An analysis of the pre- and postoperative radiographs of patients with total wrist arthroplasty published in peer-reviewed journals indeed shows this to be true. Preoperative radiographs of patients

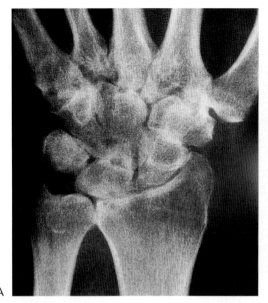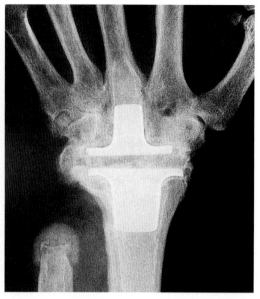

FIGURE 43.15. A: Preoperative radiograph of a rheumatoid wrist. Carpal anatomy is well preserved. **B:** Seven years postoperatively, the patient maintains an excellent pain-free functional joint. (From Swanson AB, Swanson GG. Flexible implant arthroplasty of the radiocarpal joint. *Semin Arthroplasty* 1991;2:78–84, with permission.)

with successful long-term results show very little destructive changes in the wrist (Fig. 43.15).

Loosening

Aseptic loosening of components from host reaction to polyethylene particulate debris is now a well-recognized entity (35–37). Attempts are being made to strengthen the polyethylene by gas sterilization to reduce the number of wear particles. Attribution of septic loosening to the use of cement has been found to be incorrect (35). Studies have now concluded that adding cement to the interface in rheumatoid patients enhances the bond between the implant and the bone and helps block the migration of polyethylene debris into the implant–bone interface (35, 36). Polyethylene debris has not been a problem in total wrist arthroplasty because of the low demands placed on the wrist prosthesis. However, with long-term follow-up, osteolysis (37) may become evident (Fig. 43.16), and we may see this type of loosening. The rate of wear of polyethylene is less when articulation is with a cobalt chrome surface (38). Hence, the radial articulating surface of the universal wrist prosthesis was changed from titanium to cobalt chrome.

Radial component loosening has not been a major problem with any of the devices. Third-generation cementing is recommended to achieve an optimum bond between the cement and the implant (39,40). In this technique, methylmethacrylate is mixed under a vacuum. The medullary canals are cleaned with pulsed lavage and dried.

A bone plug is utilized to restrict the cement flow and to allow introduction of the cement under pressure. Availability of a long-stem radial component will further decrease the incidence of loosening and will also help reconstruct the distal radius in cases where there is loss of bone stock.

Muscle Imbalance

In the position of rest, the wrist is dorsiflexed slightly to about 10° to 15° and deviated slightly ulnarly (41). The position of rest is assumed when the hand is resting on a horizontal plane. Dynamic support to the wrist is provided by the tendons attached to the wrist and the extrinsic tendons crossing the wrist. Twenty-four tendons participate in this balancing act. Brand (42) labeled the extensor carpi radialis longus (ECRL), the extensor carpi radialis brevis (ECRB), the flexor carpi radialis (FCR), the palmaris longus (PL), and the flexor carpi ulnaris (FCU) as dedicated wrist movers because the extrinsic muscles cannot be relied upon for wrist function, which many times conflicts with finger function. The ECRL is named as an extensor but has a large moment arm for flexion of the elbow and radial deviation of the wrist. It is most effective as a wrist extensor when radial deviation is neutralized by the ulnar deviator extensor carpi ulnaris (ECU). The ECRB is a potent wrist extensor and has a larger moment arm for wrist extension. The ECU is an important muscle that controls the balance of the wrist. By virtue of its fascial compartment, it is always held over

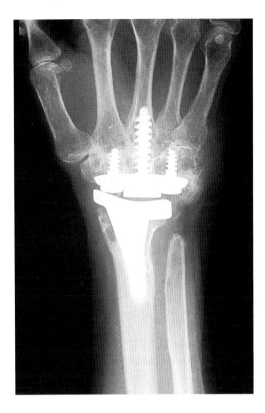
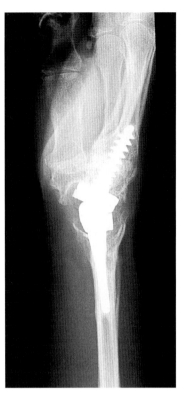

FIGURE 43.16. Radiograph seven years postoperatively, showing osteolysis around a universal wrist prosthesis. The components are not loose, and the wrist is functional. This patient will soon require bone grafting and possible revision of the components.

the distal end of the ulna. All other tendons that cross the wrist move with the radius, as the radius pronates and supinates over the fixed ulna. Because carpal bones or the wrist prosthesis moves with the radius, the ECU changes its relationship with the axes of wrist movement. It is an effective wrist extensor only in supination and may not extend the wrist when the forearm is in pronation. It is a strong ulnar deviator in pronation and supination. The FCR is as strong as the ECRB and is a wrist flexor and radial deviator. The FCU exerts the highest tension of all the muscles that cross the wrist. The insertion of this tendon into the pisiform bone, which has independent movement of its own for almost 1 cm, enhances the lever arm of the FCU.

Motor control of the carpus is achieved subconsciously even though the wrist can be moved volitionally. Concentrated efforts are generally directed to control finger activities. Analysis of muscle vector forces acting on the instant center of motion was done by Volz (43). He calculated the deforming force of each muscle by multiplying the lever arm distance from its point crossing the carpus to the instant center located in the capitate (Fig. 43.17). The mean vector force and magnitude were plotted in relationship to the planes of motion of the wrist. Volz noted that the FCU is the most powerful wrist motor tending to tilt the wrist into flexion and ulnar deviation. Brand (42) also found that the FCU has the potential to generate large force across the wrist.

Motor imbalance is defined as the inability of the patient to bring the wrist volitionally to neutral position. Imbalance

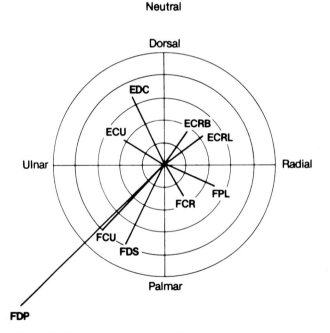

FIGURE 43.17. Vector force analysis of musculotendinous units crossing the wrist discloses that the summation of forces tends to place the wrist in a position of flexion and ulnar deviation. *ECRB,* extensor carpi radialis brevis; *ECRL,* extensor carpi radialis longus; *FPL,* flexor palmaris longus; *FCR,* flexor carpi radialis; *FDS,* flexor digitorum superficialis; *FCU,* flexor carpi ulnaris; *FDP,* flexor digitorum profundis; *ECU,* extensor carpi ulnaris; *EDC,* extensor digitorum communis. (From Volz R. Total wrist arthroplasty. In: *Review and update seminars in arthroplasty,* vol 2. Philadelphia: WB Saunders, 1991;68–77, with permission.)

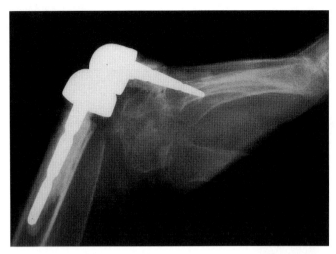

FIGURE 43.18. Radiograph showing severe flexion deformity after inserting a Volz prosthesis.

can occur in the flexion–extension (Fig. 43.18) or radioulnar plane (Fig. 43.19). Unlike muscle imbalance from paralysis of a motor nerve, the muscle imbalance in rheumatoid arthritis is caused by varying involvement of the tendons in the disease process leading to attrition or rupture. In cases where the tendon is in chronic disuse, infiltration of muscle belly with fibrous tissue robs its effective excursion, making it an ineffective wrist mobilizer and allowing the antagonist muscles and gravity to determine the resting position of the wrist. Destruction of the carpal bones and segmental collapse leads to decrease in carpal height, ulnar subluxation of the carpus resulting in ulnar soft tissue contracture, and contracture of the FCU. In advanced cases, the lines of pull and moment arms of the tendons are altered. Radial deviation of the metacarpals, seen in rheumatoid arthritis, gives undue advantage to the radial wrist movers. The best way to avoid postoperative wrist imbalance is to operate before the development of marked disorganization and deformity of the wrist.

The most common problem associated with wrist prosthesis has been a radial shift of the center of rotation, which increases the lever arm of ulnarly located wrist movers. As an example, in the original Volz wrist prosthesis, the two prongs of the carpal components were inserted into the second and the third metacarpals (15) (Fig. 43.2). This resulted in an increase of the ulnar lever arm. The design was modified, and a single-prong carpal component was developed. Designers have recognized this problem and have attempted to rectify this by shifting the radial articulating surface ulnarly. Hamas (44) emphasized the need to accurately identify the location of the center of motion, and described a method to locate the center of rotation on a preoperative radiograph using reference lines and calculations. He recognized the impracticality of this method and came up with a precentered wrist prosthesis. In this device, when the stems are centered in the medullary canal, the longitudinal axis coincides with the reference lines of the third metacarpal and the distal radius in both anteroposterior and lateral planes. He reported no imbalance in a small series of ten patients. The radial components of the trispherical Meuli, Clayton-Volz-Ferlic (CVF), and biaxial prostheses have an offset stem to position the center of rotation to a near normal position.

The distal radius is cut perpendicular to the longitudinal axis of the radius to implant the radial component of the biaxial, Meuli, trispherical, CVF, Gulpar, Volz, and house prostheses. This undoes the normal distal articular inclination and removes all of the styloid process. Making the cut parallel to the articular surface of the distal radius, as for the universal prosthesis (Fig. 43.14), preserves most of the styloid, and the architecture of the distal end is less disturbed. The radial component of the universal wrist prosthesis has 20° inclination and resurfaces the distal end of the radius to provide an articulating surface in line with the third metacarpal capitate complex. The length of the lever arms of dedicated wrist movers are only slightly affected. In addition, the large contact area of the two components is more forgiving than that of a prosthesis with smaller contact surfaces.

Despite all these built-in features to prevent it, imbalance can occur. This is where surgical judgments come into play. No amount of written detail will surpass a surgeon's knowledge of the pathophysiology of the rheumatoid wrist and the resultant vector force acting on the wrist. The surgeon must be prepared to correct preoperative contractures by capsular release and tendon lengthening. Preoperative radial deviation of the metacarpal may necessitate transfer of the ECRL to the base of the fifth metacarpal. In cases where there is fixed flexion and ulnar deviation deformity of the wrist, it is prudent to first release the contracture before the cuts are made on the bones. Always release the capsule from the radius. The extensor carpi ulnaris tendon should be brought dorsally if subluxated volarly. Balance of the wrist must be

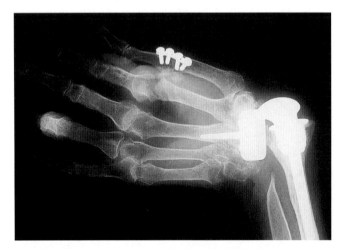

FIGURE 43.19. Severe ulnar deviation imbalance following a Clayton-Volz-Ferlic prosthesis. The components were removed, and the wrist was fused two years after the index operation.

determined at the time of trial reduction. Because the most potent deforming force is exerted by the FCU, particular care should be exerted to test the tension of this tendon by passively deviating the wrist radially and also observing the posture of the resting hand at the time of trial reduction. Ulnar deviation deformity will not correct spontaneously with time, so make all the corrections in the operating room. The general orthopedic axiom of tightening the loose structures and loosening the tight structures must be applied to achieve balance. The postoperative cast must be molded to neutralize any tendency for deformity and to facilitate the formation of a restrictive capsular scar. For example, if the wrist tends to deviate ulnarly despite adequate soft tissue release, a cast in slight radial deviation must be applied to tighten the soft tissues on the radial side. Any redundancy in the wrist extensors must be corrected by plicating the tendons to prevent late flexion deformity of the wrist.

Dislocation

A common complication with any joint replacement is dislocation of the prosthesis. Conservative bone resection, meticulous soft tissue closure, and postoperative immobilization will effectively decrease the incidence of dislocation. It is important to recognize the supination deformity of the hand in rheumatoid arthritis (45) (Fig. 43.20). To correct this, the extensor carpi ulnaris must be brought dorsally and stabilized. While the joint capsule is being closed, the components have to be held congruent. Initial postoperative immobilization must be in a long arm sugartongs splint with the forearm in as much supination as possible and the elbow flexed 90°. Supination of the forearm keeps the ECU dorsal to the ulna and positions the ulna in its anatomic position. The wrist is held in neutral or in slight radial deviation to counter the ulnar deviation force (assuming the metacarpals are in neutral position). Neutral position of the wrist allows the dorsal and volar capsules to heal with equal length. Dressing changes must not be delegated to a cast technician or someone with no knowledge of these devices.

Infection

Infection, a nightmare of total joint surgeons, is not peculiar to the wrist prosthesis. Care should be taken in handling the tissues of patients with rheumatoid arthritis. If the

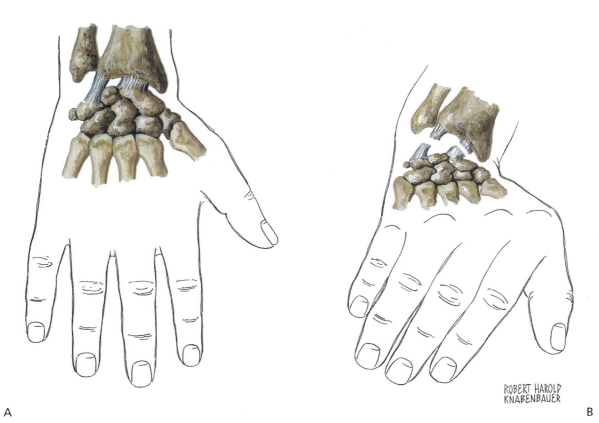

FIGURE 43.20. A: Normal wrist. **B:** Supination deformity of the hand in rheumatoid arthritis from the loss of the ulnocarpal meniscus homolog, dorsal radiotriqetral ligament, volar subluxation of the extensor carpi ulnaris, and volar flexion of the scaphoid.

(continued on next page)

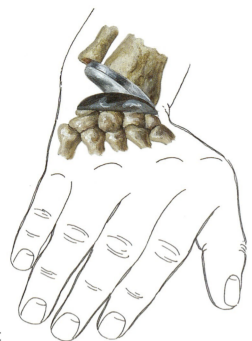

FIGURE 43.20. *(continued)* C: Incongruent reduction of the wrist prosthesis. The hand has to be pronated to get a congruent reduction with the radial component. The extensor carpi ulnaris must be brought dorsally to eliminate the deforming force.

patient is on immunosuppressive drugs, the drugs should be stopped at least two weeks before surgery. Surgery should be postponed if the patient is taking more than 10 mg of prednisone or if there is any focus of infection in the body. Prophylactic antibiotics must be administered in all cases. All traffic to and from the operating room must be restricted until after the dressings are applied.

INDICATIONS

Combined radiocarpal and midcarpal arthritis secondary to trauma, rheumatoid arthritis, osteoarthritis, and any inflammatory arthritis are candidates for total joint replacement. Surgery should not be postponed until advanced radiologic changes occur. The best results are obtained when bony architecture is preserved. *Total wrist arthroplasty should be considered a reconstructive procedure and not a salvage operation for failed medical treatment* (33).

CONTRAINDICATIONS

History of infection.
Systemic lupus erythematosus (Fig. 43.21).
Extensor tendon ruptures (multiple) (Fig. 43.22).
Manual laborer.
Nonfunctioning hand.

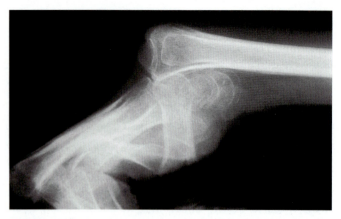

FIGURE 43.21. Radiograph of a patient with systemic lupus erythematosus. Notice the dislocation of the entire carpus. These patients have poor capsuloligamentous structures and are not candidates for nonconstrained wrist prostheses.

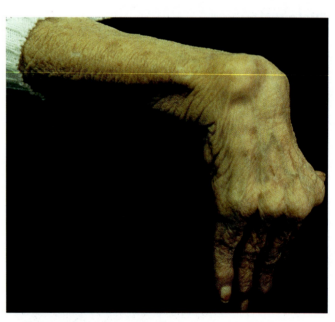

FIGURE 43.22. Flexion deformity of the wrist associated with multiple extensor tendon ruptures.

SURGICAL TECHNIQUE FOR UNIVERSAL WRIST PROSTHESIS

After adequate anesthesia, the hand is prepped and draped in the usual manner. The tourniquet is inflated to 250 mm Hg. A dorsal longitudinal incision is made along the line of the third metacarpal. The skin and the subcutaneous tissue are elevated sharply from the extensor tendons and retracted medially and laterally using 3-0 silk retraction sutures. The extensor retinaculum is then opened in a step-cut fashion and raised medially and laterally (Fig. 43.23). One-half of the retinaculum is utilized to patch any defects in the joint capsule. A synovectomy is then carried out (Fig. 43.24). The

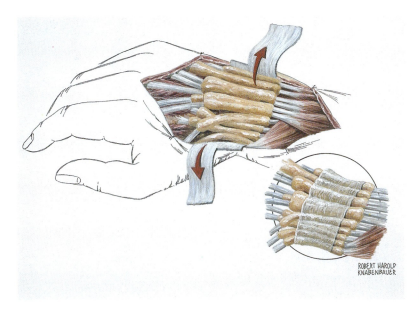

FIGURE 43.23. Extensor retinaculum is opened in a step-cut fashion. One-half is used to close any defect in the capsule.

extensor tendons are then inspected. The capsule over the distal ulna is then opened longitudinally, and the distal 1 cm of the ulna is osteotomized and removed (Fig. 43.25). A synovectomy of the ulnar compartment is then done. The radiocarpal joint is opened by detaching the capsule from the distal radius and leaving it attached distally. The extensor retinaculum is then subperiosteally elevated radially along with the brachioradialis and the tendons of first dorsal compartment muscles from the styloid process. The branch of the posterior interosseous nerve is resected, and the accompanying vessel is cauterized. The wrist is now flexed, and soft tissues are protected by Hayes retractors. The radial cutting jig is aligned along the longitudinal axis of the radius (Fig. 43.26). The dorsal lip and the articular surface are then removed using an oscillating saw. This exposes the carpal bones. In many instances the carpal bones have subluxated under the radius, and traction on the hand is necessary to expose the proximal row. The line of osteotomy of the carpal bones goes through the proximal end of the capitate (Fig. 43.26). The plan of osteotomy is perpendicular to the axis of the capitate–metacarpal complex. Osteotomy is carried out using an oscillating saw. Care is taken to positively identify the capitate before resection. Part of the scaphoid and the triquetrum remain after the resection. An intercarpal fusion is carried out by removing the articular cartilage from the capitate, scaphoid, triquetrum, and hamate using a burr or curette (Fig. 43.26). Any rents in the volar capsule are closed

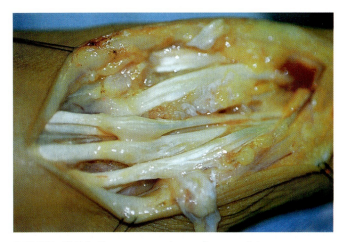

FIGURE 43.24. Extensor tendons after partial synovectomy. Integrity of the extensor carpi radialis longus and the extensor carpi radialis brevis should be checked at this time. If they are deficient, alternate treatment must be considered.

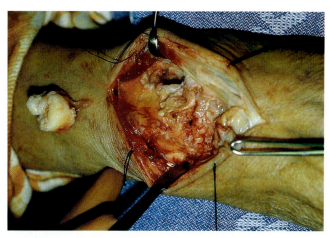

FIGURE 43.25. The distal ulna is osteotomized through a separate longitudinal incision. Synovectomy of the ulnar compartment is then done.

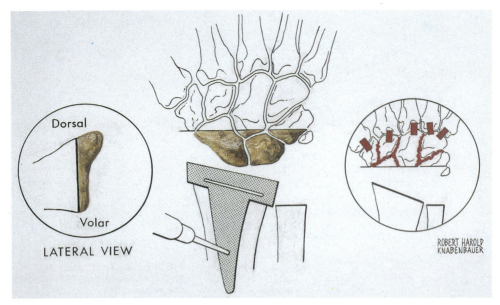

FIGURE 43.26. Radial cutting jig. The jig is aligned to the longitudinal axis of the radius. The line of osteotomy of the carpal bones goes through the proximal end of the capitate. The amount of bone removed is shown in color. An intercarpal fusion is done by removing the articular cartilage from the remaining carpal bones and packing with cancellous bone graft.

with absorbable sutures. All loose fragments of bone are removed from the joint. While the wrist is held in a flexed position, a drill hole is made in the center of the capitate–metacarpal complex with a 2.5-mm drill bit (Fig. 43.27). A probe is introduced into this hole, and the position is checked using an image intensifier in anteroposterior and lateral planes (Fig. 43.28). This is done to make sure that the tract is intraosseous. The drill has to be angled 10° dorsally to accomplish the correct alignment. Once the position is confirmed, enlarge this tract with a 3.5-mm drill bit. The surgeon now sits at the end of the hand table in order to have an end-on view of the radius. The medullary canal of the radius is then reamed with an appropriate size broach. The broach should be inserted in valgus (Fig. 43.29). Malrotation of the broach inside the medullary canal of the radius must be avoided. The second radial cutting block is aligned over the broach, and the radius is cut to match the contour of the radial component (Fig. 43.30).

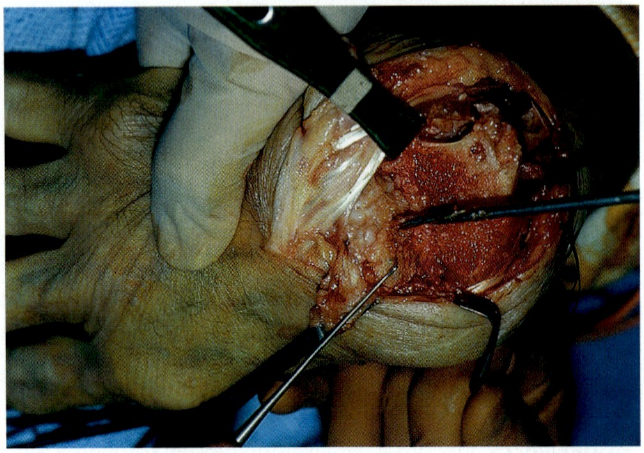

Trial Reduction

Carpal Component with Three Screws

The central screw (6.5 mm) of the carpal component is introduced into the opening in the capitate, and the carpal plate is fixed against the cut surface of the carpal bones. A drill hole is made through the radial opening of the carpal plate, into the scaphoid and the trapezoid bones, using a 2.5-mm drill (Fig. 43.31). A 20-mm-long and 4.5-mm-diameter self-tapping screw is then inserted, capturing the scaphoid and the trapezoid bones. A trial radial component is then inserted into the radius. A trial plastic carpal bearing is slid over the carpal plate, and the joint is reduced. If the joint is too tight, additional bone is removed from the radius until good flexion, extension, and radial and ulnar deviation are achieved. Release of the volar capsule and lengthening of the flexor carpi radialis or ulnaris (or both) may be required if there is fixed flexion or ulnar deviation deformity preoperatively. The trial components are then removed. The second peripheral screw (4.5 mm) is then inserted through the ulnar opening of the carpal plate. The length of screws can be determined at the time of

FIGURE 43.27. When drilling a hole in the center of the capitate, angle the drill about 10° dorsally to remain intraosseous.

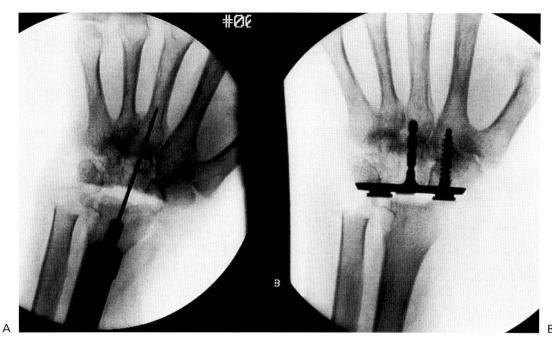

FIGURE 43.28. A: Intraoperative radiograph showing the probe inside the capitate. **B:** Trial carpal component is fixed with one screw. The length of the screws for fixing the true carpal component can be determined from this radiograph.

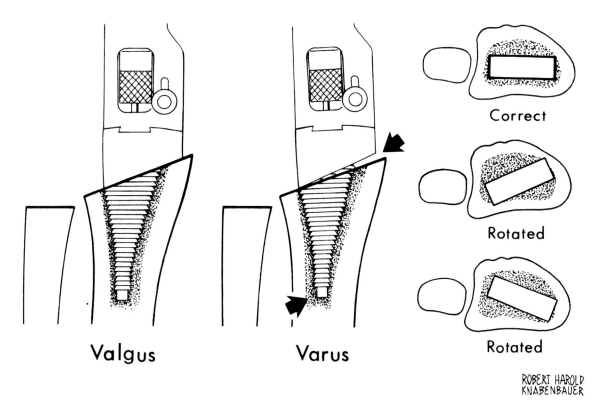

FIGURE 43.29. In order to avoid ulnar deviation deformity, the broach has to be inserted in valgus as shown. The broach should be parallel to the volar cortex of the radius and in line with the styloid process.

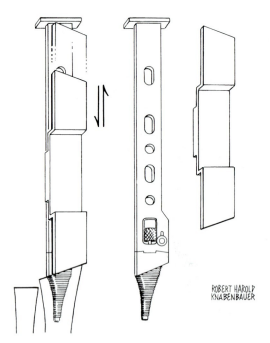

FIGURE 43.30. Second radial cutting block slides over the handle of the broach. This jig helps to make a cut that will match the obliquity of the radial component.

trial reduction using the image intensifier. Screws may cross the carpometacarpal joint in osteoporotic bones to get good purchase. The true radial component is then introduced into the radius and tapped all the way in. Care is taken to place the prosthesis in valgus. Methylmethacrylate was not used to fix either of the components in this series except in two cases on the radial side. The polyethylene interface is now slid over the carpal plate and locked in place by the locking pins. The components are then reduced, and the joint is tested for stability.

Carpal Component with Central Stem and Two Screws

The stem of the carpal component is introduced into the capitate. A drill hole is made through the radial opening, and the trial carpal component is temporarily fixed with a 20-mm-long 4.5-mm-diameter screw (Fig. 43.28). Trial radial component and plastic bearings are inserted as described earlier, and the range of motion and stability of the prosthesis are tested. Once satisfied, the trial components are removed. The wound is washed with pulsed lavage and dried. Methylmethacrylate is prepared and first introduced into the hole in the capitate. The carpal stem is then introduced into the capitate, and the component tapped all the way in. The two peripheral screws are inserted, and excess cement is removed. The medullary canal off the radius is plugged with a piece of bone to restrict the flow of the cement proximally. Bone cement is then inserted into the medullary canal of the radius. The stem of the true

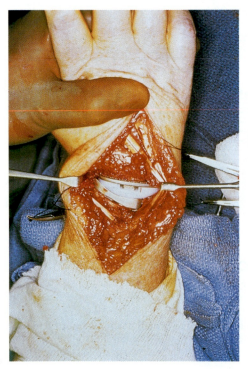
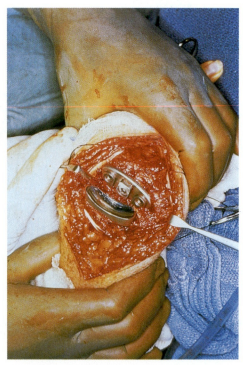

FIGURE 43.31. A: The carpal plate is fixed with three titanium screws, and the trial radial component is kept in place. **B:** Trial reduction with the polyethylene interface.

radial component is then inserted into the radius and the component is tapped in. Excess cement is removed.

The ulnar joint capsule is tightly closed, stabilizing the distal ulna. The extensor carpi ulnaris tendon is brought dorsally to stabilize the ulna and also to correct a supination deformity of the hand. The capsule of the radiocarpal joint is reattached to the radius. While closing the capsule, make sure that the components are reduced and congruent. If the capsule is deficient, one half of the retinaculum is used to cover the defects. The other half is used to reconstruct the extensor retinaculum. The skin and the subcutaneous tissue are closed in layers. A bulky hand dressing is then applied. The wrist is immobilized in neutral position, and elbow flexed 90° with the forearm in supination (see Treatment of Dislocation) in a long arm sugar-tongs splint for 3 to 4 days. After the initial dressing change, a long arm cast with the forearm in supination and wrist in neutral position is applied for a total of 4 weeks. The surgeon must supervise dressing changes to avoid inadvertent dislocation of the prosthesis.

FEATURES OF THE UNIVERSAL WRIST PROSTHESIS

1. The articular surface of the radial component is inclined 20°, similar to the distal end of the radius. This feature makes the wrist easy to balance.
2. The carpal component supports the first and the fifth rays and prevents proximal migration of these columns. Other existing designs do not support the entire carpus.
3. If the carpal bones are deficient, the carpal height can be restored by inserting a corticocancellous bone graft—a unique advantage of the universal wrist prosthesis (Fig. 43.32).
4. Oblique osteotomy removes comparatively less bone from the radius. This, coupled with the configuration of the radial component, helps to transfer the load from the carpus to the radius as *in vivo*.
5. Intercarpal fusion forms a solid bony support for the carpal component, decreases the chance of synovitis, and reduces the loosening of the carpal component by decreasing the toggle.
6. Soft tissue balancing can be achieved by choosing the appropriate size polyethylene insert.
7. Adequate bone stock is available to salvage the wrist by fusion if the prosthesis fails.

RESULTS

Universal total wrist arthroplasty was done in 63 patients. Six patients had bilateral arthroplasty, making a total of 69 cases. There were 15 men and 48 women. Their ages ranged

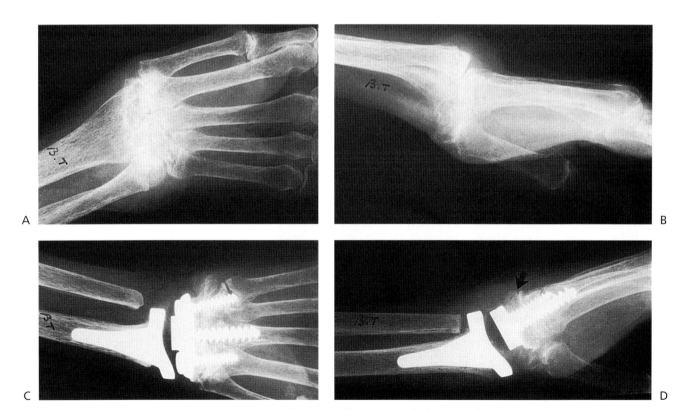

FIGURE 43.32. A,B: Preoperative radiographs of a patient with rheumatoid arthritis. Lateral view **(B)** shows the metacarpal articulating with the radius. **C,D:** Carpal height was restored with a corticocancellous iliac bone graft *(arrow)*. The wrist is functioning well eight years postoperatively.

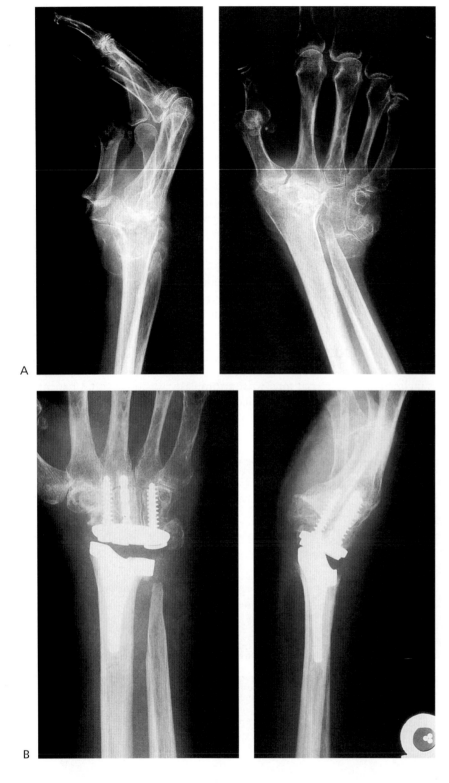

FIGURE 43.33. A: Preoperative radiograph showing marked destruction and ulnar and volar dislocation of the carpus. The styloid process is in contact with the basal joint of the thumb. **B:** Postoperative appearance of the wrist after insertion of the universal wrist prosthesis. Patient has an excellent pain-free range of motion of the wrist.

from 27 to 82 years with a mean of 58.1 years. Sixteen patients had osteoarthritis, and the remainder had rheumatoid arthritis. The universal carpal component with a central screw was used in 37 wrists. In these cases, the components were not cemented except in two cases where the radial component was cemented. In the remaining 32 cases, carpal components with a central peg and two peripheral screws were used; both components were cemented in these 32 cases. Minimum follow-up was 48 months, and the maximum was 120 months with a mean of 79.4 months (± 6.7 years) for the first 37 cases done with the carpal component with three screws. Minimum follow-up was 24 months, and the maximum was 48 months for the 32 cases done with the carpal component with a central peg. Only the carpal component with a central peg (Fig. 43.33) is approved for general use (carpal component with three screws may be obtained on a custom basis). Rettig et al. (48) and Cobb and Beckenbaugh (18) reported 15% to 17% loosening of the carpal component of the Biaxial wrist prosthesis in five years. Lirette and Kinnard (46) followed 17 biaxial wrists for 48 to 66 months without any evidence of loosening. Twenty-two percent carpal component loosening and 6% radial component loosening were noted by Bosco et al. (26) in 18 cases (Volz) followed over 8 years (103 months). Menon (47) reported symptomatic loosening of the carpal component in 19% of patients with the Volz prostheses. Sixteen percent of the Meuli (17) carpal components were loose by 4 to 5 years. In contrast, there has been no loosening of the universal carpal component fixed with three titanium screws followed for 113 months (9 years, 5 months) (22). This has been an encouraging finding to date. No loosening has occurred in the 32 cases where the cemented carpal component with a central peg was utilized. The follow-up time is shorter in this series. Carpal loosening, a nemesis of the joint replacement surgeon, can be brought under control by the concept of intercarpal fusion and screw fixation of the carpal component. Two uncemented radial components loosened, and the same radial component was reimplanted with cement. Two patients developed serious deep-seated infection of the joint. In one case, the organism grown was *Staphylococcus aureus.* Multiple drainage procedures of the wrist failed, and the prosthesis had to be removed. In the other case, the joint was infected by *Candida albicans.* This joint was saved by vigorous joint lavage and antifungal medications. Both of these patients had delayed infection and were on high doses of immunosuppressive drugs. Persistent flexion deformity with pain occurred in one patient and required removal of the implant and fusion of the joint.

Excellent pain relief was obtained in 90% of the patients: 78% to 94% relief of pain was reported by Boseo et al. (26), Meuli (17), Fourastler (20), Rettig et al. (48), and Kraay et al. (49). Postoperative range of motion was within functional range. Persistent ulnar deviation deformity (15°) developed in one patient. This patient tolerated this deformity very well. She had very good flexion and extension. A varus position of the radial component resulted in ulnar deviation deformity. Five of 18 Volz wrist arthroplasty patients developed ulnar deviation imbalance (47). Meuli (17) and Cobb (18) reported 16% and 32% incidences of abnormal wrist stance. At the time of follow-up, abnormal stance did not hinder function in all instances. Ulnar deviation can occur if the line of carpal osteotomy is oblique instead of perpendicular to the third metacarpal. If the wrist is in ulnar deviation preoperatively, the dorsally displaced ECRL may act as a wrist dorsiflexor (50,51). After surgery, the deformity was corrected, and the muscle returned to its normal position, acting as a radial deviator and leaving the wrist with no effective dorsiflexor. It is important to check the integrity of the ECRB to avoid flexion imbalance.

RESTORATION OF CARPAL HEIGHT (UNIVERSAL WRIST)

If the carpal bones are deficient, carpal height can be restored by a corticocancellous iliac bone graft (Fig. 43.32). The cancellous surface of the bone graft must face the cut surface of the carpal bones.

CONVERSION OF FUSION TO ARTHROPLASTY (UNIVERSAL WRIST)

In patients who present with spontaneous fusion in malposition secondary to rheumatoid arthritis, resection of the fusion and total wrist arthroplasty is indicated (Fig. 43.34). Technically, the procedure is easy to perform. Fusion provides excellent bone mass for fixing the carpal plate. Wrist extensors must be healthy at the time of surgery. The surgeon must be prepared to revise the fusion into a functional position if the wrist extensors are inadequate.

TREATMENT OF DISLOCATION OF THE PROSTHESIS

If dislocation is recognized early, closed reduction and immobilization in a long arm cast will be sufficient. Open reduction is recommended if closed reduction is unsuccessful or if the dislocation is detected 3 to 4 weeks after the episode. Open reduction permits atraumatic reduction of the components under direct vision. Immobilization with an external fixator guarantees maintenance of congruent reduction. The dorsoradial aspect of the distal third of the second metacarpal is exposed using a $^1\!/_2$-in. incision. A separate 1-in. incision is made over the radius to expose the middle one-third of the radius. Fixator pins are inserted under direct vision. Distal pins must be in the distal portion

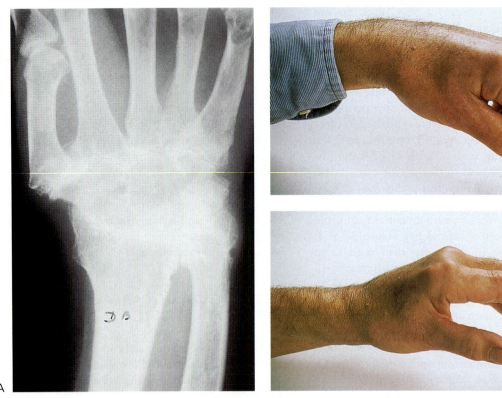

FIGURE 43.34. A: Preoperative x-ray of a 50-year-old male engineer with autofusion of the wrist in malposition. **B:** Eight years postoperatively, the patient has maintained good pain-free functional range of wrist motion. The appearance of the wrist also improved markedly.

of the metacarpal to prevent contamination of the wrist joint from pin track infection. The wrist joint is approached through a dorsal incision and the capsular flap is elevated. The components are then reduced under direct vision, and the outrigger of the external fixation device is then mounted and tightened. If there is supination deformity of the hand, the hand has to be pronated to obtain congruent reduction (Fig. 43.20). If the extensor carpi ulnaris is subluxated volarly, it should be brought up dorsally and stabilized. The external fixator is applied for 6 weeks.

SALVAGE OF FAILED ARTHROPLASTY

Revision of arthroplasty, arthrodesis, and resection with or without distraction are the options available (23). Revision of total wrist arthroplasty is desirable but is very difficult because of loss of bone from the disease process and surgical insult. It is important to assess the salvageability of a device when attempting to choose a particular wrist prosthesis. The design should have features that will make it amenable to bone grafts in case there is deficient bone stock. Rettig and Beckenbaugh (48) successfully revised 13 failed biaxial prostheses. Two and a half years after revision, eight patients remained asymptomatic, and two complained of mild to moderate pain. Their average range of motion was 36°. Two patients underwent a second revision surgery. One wrist was fused because of persistent symptoms. Ferlic (51) revised 12 metal-on-plastic implants by fusion in seven, soft tissue balancing in four, and resection arthroplasty in one. Meuli (17) was able to salvage six wrists by exchange and balancing the soft tissues, and patients in that series required a total wrist fusion. Failed silicone arthroplasties can be saved by implantation of a total wrist device or by wrist fusion. A split fibular graft is an excellent donor source for repairing defects in the radius. For adequate fusion, a corticocancellous iliac bone graft is almost always required to fill the defect left after removing the prosthesis and to maintain the carpal height (51). It is important to remove all the bone cement from the medullary canal of the radius and capitate to facilitate the healing process. Rigid fixation using an AO plate or prebend plate marketed by Synthes (Monument, CO) will increase the chances of union.

FUTURE OF WRIST ARTHROPLASTY

Wrist arthroplasty is gradually evolving. The concept of early surgery and elevating wrist arthroplasty from a salvage to a reconstructive procedure will indeed enhance the longevity of wrist arthroplasty and thus it will be more appealing to the surgeon and the patient. Newer methods of fixation, modularity, availability of components of various sizes, and varying angles and geometry will enable the surgeon to customize the needs of the patient in the operating room. Increasing demands from patients and a favorable position in the marketplace will be the driving forces behind future growth and development of wrist arthroplasty. Improvements in performance and function can be achieved only in small increments. Lessons learned from past experience should be the building blocks of the future. Total wrist arthroplasty deserves attention and should be the next frontier for the new-generation joint replacement surgeon to conquer.

EDITORS' COMMENTS

The basic problem with total wrist arthroplasty is wrist anatomy. The hand takes its loads through multiple small bones. Combined, they are sufficient to carry the needed power from the fingers to the forearm. This means, however, that total loads are shared by these multiple small bones. There is no way to attach a total wrist prosthesis to multiple small bones. Therefore, we choose the strongest components for attachment of the distal portion of the prosthesis. This has proved an inadequate approach, and in all probability there will not be an adequate total wrist prosthesis because of this fundamental problem. The digits exemplify this problem in that total joint arthroplasty of the PIP joints have very high loads for the amount of surface area between the prosthesis and the bone. Multiple phalanges and multiple digits can share these loads in the higher ranges, but all of these bones are too small for adequate prosthetic surface areas; the prosthesis loosen or cut through. The most effective interphalangeal prosthesis, therefore, have remained space-filling silicone, not hinged joints. These principles apply even more so to the small bones of the wrist. There will probably never be an adequate total wrist prosthesis of the current type; it is more likely that the solution will come in cartilage resurfacing, cadaveric transplants or stem cell cloned wrist structures.

In rheumatoid arthritis, the most effective procedure is the nonunion arthroplasty. A cancellous concavity is formed in the distal radius and a cancellous convexity formed of the remaining carpals. With or without some ligament soft tissue interposition, the convex carpals are nested in the radius concavity and cross-pinned for two weeks, after which mobilization is begun. A small degree of motion at the wrist translates into increased functional range at the tip of the fingers. Rheumatoid nonunion arthroplasty has been a highly reliable standard for 33 years. This has become basically our only procedure when major destruction, subluxation and loss of range of motion of the wrist have occurred. The patient is encouraged to get all of the mileage they can from the old wrist. Surgery is carried out when function loss and pain demand. Patients regularly request a similar approach to the opposite wrist. Patients report a lack of pain, increased power, and some functional range of motion on operated wrists.

REFERENCES

1. Ritt MJP, Stuart PR, Naggar L, et al. The early history of arthroplasty of the wrist. *J Hand Surg [Br]* 1994;19:778–782.
2. Charnley J. Total hip replacement by low friction arthroplasty. *Clin Orthop* 1970;72:7–21.
3. Vicar AJ, Burton RI. Surgical management of rheumatoid wrist—fusion or arthroplasty. *J Hand Surg [Am]* 1986;11:790–797.
4. Goodman MJ, Millender LH, Nalebuff EA, et al. Arthroplasty of rheumatoid wrist with silicone rubber. An early evaluation. *J Hand Surg [Am]* 1980;5:114–121.
5. Kobus RJ, Turner RH. Wrist arthrodesis for treatment of rheumatoid arthritis. *J Hand Surg [Am]* 1990;15:541–546.
6. Hastings H. Total wrist arthrodesis for post traumatic conditions. *Indiana Hand Ctr Newslett* 1993;1:14–15.
7. Weiss APC, Wiedeman G Jr, Owenzer D, et al. Upper extremity function after arthrodesis. *J Hand Surg [Am]* 1995;20:813–817.
8. Millender L, Nalebuff E. Arthrodesis of rheumatic wrist. *J Bone Joint Surg Am* 1973;55:1026–1034.
9. Carroll R, Dick H. Arthrodesis of the wrist in rheumatoid arthritis. *J Bone Joint Surg Am* 1971;53:1365–1369.
10. Mannerfelt L, Malmsten M. Arthrodesis of the wrist in rheumatoid arthritis. A technique without external fixation. *Scand J Plast Reconst Surg* 1971;5:124–130.
11. Van Gemert JGWN. Arthrodesis of the wrist. Clinical radiographic and ergonomic study of 66 cases. *Acta Orthop Scand [Suppl]* 1984;210:1–147.
12. Swanson AB. *Flexible implant resection arthroplasty in the hand and extremities*. St. Louis: CV Mosby, 1973;254–261.
13. Flatt AE. *The care of arthritic hand. Wrist.* St Louis: Quality Medical, 1995;175–193.
14. Swanson AB, Swanson GG. Flexible implant arthroplasty of the radiocarpal joint. *Semin Arthroplasty* 1991;2:78–84.
15. Volz R. Total wrist arthroplasty. In: *Review and update seminars in arthroplasty, vol 2*. Philadelphia: WB Saunders, 1991;68–77.
16. Ferlic DC, Clayton ML. Results of CFV total wrist arthroplasty. Review and early results. *Orthopaedics* 1995;18:1167–1171.
17. Meuli HC, Fernandez DL. Uncemented total wrist arthroplasty. *J Hand Surg [Am]* 1995;20:115–122.
18. Cobb TK, Beckenbaugh RD. Biaxial total wrist arthroplasty. *J Hand Surg [Am]* 1996;21:1011–1021.
19. Figgie MP, Ranawat CS, Inglis AE, et al. Trispherical total wrist arthroplasty in rheumatoid arthritis. *J Hand Surg [Am]* 1990;15:217–223.
20. Fourastler J, Le Breton L, Acnot J, et al. La prothè totale radiocarpienne guepar dans la chirurgie du poignet rheumatoide. *Rev Chir Orthop* 1996;82:108–115.
21. Menon J. Total wrist arthroplasty for rheumatoid arthritis. In: *Hand surgery: current practice*. London: Martin Dunitz, 1997.
22. Menon J. Universal total wrist implant. Experience with a carpal component fixed with three screws. *J Arthroplasty* 1998;13:515–523.

23. Bednar JM. Wrist joint arthroplasties. *Surg Hand Upper Extremity:* 771–794.
24. Fatti SL, Palmer AK, Greenky S, et al. Long term results of Swanson interpositional arthroplasty part II. *J Hand Surg [Am]* 1991;16:432–437.
25. Jolly SL, Ferlic DC, Clayton M, et al. Swanson silicone arthroplasty of the wrist in rheumatoid arthritis. A long term follow-up. *J Hand Surg [Am]* 1992;17:142–149.
26. Bosco JA III, Bynum DK, Bowers WH. Long term outcome of Voltz total wrist arthroplasties. *J Arthroplasty* 1996;9:25–31.
27. Branemark PI, Hansson BO, Adell R, et al. Osteointegrated implants in the treatment of edentulous jaw. Experience from a 10-year period. *Scand J Plast Reconst Surg Suppl* 1977;6:1–32.
28. Albrektson T, Branemark PI, Hansson HA, et al. Osteointegrated titanium implants: Requirements for ensuring a long lasting direct bone to implant anchorage in man. *Acta Orthop Scand* 1981;52:155–170.
29. Lundborg G, Branemark PI, Rosen T. Osteointegrated thumb prosthesis. A concept for fixation of digit prosthetic device. *J Hand Surg [Am]* 1996;21:216–221.
30. Lundborg G, Branemark PI, Carlsson I. Metacarpophalangeal joint arthroplasty based on osteointegration concept. *J Hand Surg [Br]* 1993;18:693–703.
31. Situnayake RD, Grindulis KA, McConkey B. Longterm treatment of rheumatoid arthritis with sulphasalazine, gold or pencillamine. A comparison using life table methods. *Ann Rheum Dis* 1987;46:177–183.
32. Hilliquin P, Menkes CJ. Evaluation and management of early and established rheumatoid arthritis. In: *Practical rheumatology.* St Louis: CV Mosby, 1995.
33. Stanley JK. Conservative surgery in the management of rheumatoid disease of the hand and wrist. *J Hand Surg [Br]* 1992;17:339–342.
34. Hindley CJ, Stanley JK. The rheumatoid wrist. Patterns of disease progression. *J Hand Surg [Br]* 1991;16:275–279.
35. Schmalzried TP, Jasty M, Harris WA. Periprosthetic bone loss in total hip arthroplasty, polyethylene wear and the concept of effective joint space. *J Bone Joint Surg Am* 1992;74:849–863.
36. Zicat B, Engh CA, Gokcen E. Patterns of osteolysis around total hip components inserted with and without cement. *J Bone Joint Surg Am* 1995;77:432–439.
37. Maloney W, Smith RL. Periprosthetic osteolysis in total hip arthroplasty, role of particulate debris. *J Bone Joint Surg Am* 1995;77:1448–1461.
38. Amstutz HC. Biomaterials for artificial joints. *Orthop Clin North Am* 1973;4:235–241.
39. Harris WH, Davis JP. Modern use of modern cement for total hip replacement. *Orthop Clin North Am* 1988;19:581–589.
40. Poss RP, Brick GW, Wright JR, et al. The effects of modern cementing techniques on the longevity of total hip arthroplasty. *Orthop Clin North Am* 1988;19:591–598.
41. Kaplan EB, Spinner M. *Hand as an organ.* Philadelphia: JB Lippincott, 1984.
42. Brand PW. Mechanics of individual muscles at individual joints. In: *Clinical mechanics of the hand.* St Louis: CV Mosby, 1985.
43. Volz RG. Total wrist arthroplasty. A clinical and biomechanical analysis. In: *1979 AAOS symposium on total joint replacement of the upper extremity.* St Louis: CV Mosby, 1982.
44. Hamas RS. A quantitative approach to total wrist arthroplasty: Development of a "precentered" total wrist prosthesis. *Orthopedics* 1979;2:245–253.
45. Taleisnik J. Evaluation of the wrist. In: *The wrist.* New York: Churchill Livingstone, 1985;335–356.
46. Lirette R, Kinnard P. Biaxial wrist arthroplasty in rheumatoid arthritis. *Can J Surg* 1995;38;51–53.
47. Menon J. Total wrist arthroplasty using the modified Volz prosthesis. *J Bone Joint Surg Am* 1987;69:998–1006.
48. Rettig ME, Beckenbaugh RD. Revision total wrist arthroplasty. *J Hand Surg [Am]* 1993;18:798–804.
49. Kraay MJ, Figgie MP. Wrist arthroplasty with trispherical total wrist prosthesis. *Semin Arthroplasty* 1995;6;37–43.
50. Lamberta MJ, Ferlic DC, Clayton ML. Total wrist arthroplasty in rheumatoid arthritis. *J Hand Surg [Am]* 1980;5:245–252.
51. Ferlic DC, Jolly SN, Clayton ML. Salvage for failed implant arthroplasty of the wrist. *J Hand Surg [Am]* 1992;7:917–923.

44

BENIGN TUMORS OF THE WRIST

MICHAEL J. BOTTE
HOANG N. TRAN
REID A. ABRAMS
LUKE M. VAUGHAN
RICHARD A. BROWN
MERLIN L. HAMER
CLIFFORD W. COLWELL

Soft tissue masses and benign tumors of the wrist and hand are common afflictions observed in hand and orthopedic surgery practice. Though usually not serious conditions, these tumors are a common cause of wrist pain and loss of carpal motion and can precipitate occult carpal tunnel or ulnar tunnel syndrome (1–38). These masses also produce a substantial amount of worry and stress for the patient concerned about a possible malignancy (23,39). Though malignancies of the wrist are uncommon, the possible diagnosis should still be kept in the differential, especially when there has been rapid growth, severe pain, or ulceration (23,40,41).

The following discussion on benign tumors of the wrist is divided into sections on tumors of subcutaneous tissue, tumors of vascular origin, tumors of nerves, tumors of bone, and inflammatory conditions (Table 44.1). Aspects of the tumor origin, pertinent history and physical examination findings, radiographic and laboratory assessment (when applicable), and management are discussed in each section.

M. J. Botte, H. N. Tran, and R. A. Brown: Department of Orthopaedic Surgery, University of California, San Diego, San Diego, California 92103; Department of Orthopaedic Surgery, Scripps Clinic and Research Foundation, La Jolla, California 92037.

R. A. Abrams: Department of Orthopaedics, University of California, San Diego, San Diego, California 92103.

L. M. Vaughan: Department of Orthopaedic Surgery, University of California, San Diego/Thornton Hospital, San Diego, California 92103; Department of Orthopaedics, Scripps Clinic and Research Foundation, La Jolla, California 92037.

M. L. Hamer and C. W. Colwell: Department of Orthopaedic Surgery, Scripps Clinic and Research Foundation, La Jolla, California 92037.

TABLE 44.1. BENIGN TUMORS OF THE CARPAL REGION

Tumors of subcutaneous tissue
   Ganglion cysts (dorsal, palmar)
   Epidermal inclusion cysts
   Fibroma
   Lipoma
   Fibrous xanthoma (giant cell tumor of tendon sheath)
Vascular tumors
   Aneurysms
   Hemangioma
   Arteriovenous fistula
   Lymphangioma
Tumors of nerves
   Neurofibroma
   Neurilemmoma (schwannoma)
   Lipomatous hamartoma of nerve
   Hemangioma of the median nerve
   Nerve sheath ganglion
Tumors of bone
   Enchondroma
   Multiple enchondromatosis
   Osteochondroma (multiple and solitary osteocartilaginous exostoses)
   Osteoid osteoma
   Giant cell tumor of bone
   Aneurysmal bone cyst
   Unicameral (solitary) bone cyst
Inflammatory conditions
   Rheumatoid tenosynovitis
   Rheumatoid nodules
Miscellaneous disorders
   Carpal boss
   Calcinosis

BENIGN TUMORS OF THE SUBCUTANEOUS TISSUE

Common wrist tumors of the subcutaneous tissue include the ganglion cyst (dorsal, palmar), epidermal inclusion cyst, fibroma, lipoma, and fibrous xanthoma. Though rheumatoid tenosynovitis and nodules arise in the subcutaneous tissues, these are discussed under inflammatory conditions.

Ganglion Cyst

The ganglion cyst is the most common soft tissue tumor of the wrist (2,3,42–46). It is comprised of a synovial cyst, which usually originates as an outpouching from the synovial joints of the carpus or tendon sheaths. Because it is an outpouching (and not a free, separate cyst), the cyst is connected to the associated synovial carpal joint or tendon sheath by a tube or a hollow stalk. Fluid from within the cyst originates from the joint.

Rarely, a ganglion cyst will originate from the sheath of a peripheral nerve (47,48). The usual carpal ganglion has been shown to be slightly more prevalent in women. It develops most often in the second, third, and fourth decades (2,3,42,43,45,46). Occasionally, a carpal ganglion will develop in a child (49).

The *dorsal* wrist ganglion, by far the most common type, comprises 70% of all hand and wrist ganglia (Fig. 44.1) (2,3,42,43,45,46). It usually originates from the scapholunate joint or, less commonly, from the capitohamate, scaphocapitate, or other carpal joints (2,3,43). Those originating from the scapholunate joint usually extend between the fourth and third dorsal compartments (2,3). The outpouching cyst subsequently reaches the subcutaneous tis-

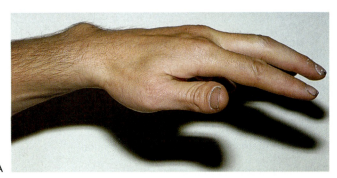
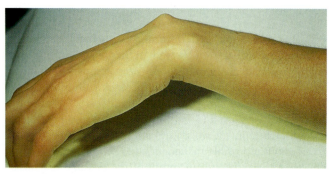

FIGURE 44.1. A,B: Typical dorsal wrist ganglion located over the middorsal area of the carpus. The ganglion usually originates from the scapholunate ligament and overlying capsule. Palmar wrist flexion accentuates the size and shape of most dorsal wrist ganglia. (From Botte MJ. Ganglion excision. In: Gelberman RH, ed. *Master techniques in orthopaedic surgery: the wrist.* New York: Raven Press, 1994;393–416, 1994, with permission.)

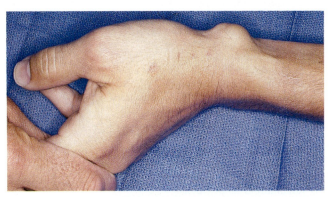
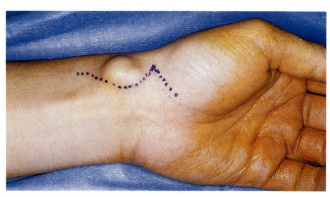

FIGURE 44.2. A,B: Palmar wrist ganglion, located on the radial side of the wrist. The palmar wrist ganglion may extend between the tendons of the flexor carpi radialis and brachioradialis, often in close proximity to the radial artery. If a palmar wrist ganglion appears to be bilobular, the "septum" may actually be the radial artery or its remnant that overlies the ganglion. Dissection of these lesions should involve identifying and protecting the radial artery before excising the mass. The origin of the palmar wrist ganglion is usually from the scaphotrapezial, trapeziometacarpal, or radiocarpal ligament and overlying capsule, but it can also originate from or extend along the tendon sheath of the flexor carpi radialis. The palmar wrist ganglion is often more subtle in physical appearance than the dorsal wrist ganglion. Dorsiflexion of the wrist can help demonstrate a small or occult palmar ganglion.

sues to form the well-known cystic mass on the middorsum of the wrist.

The *palmar* wrist ganglion is usually located on the radial aspect of the volar wrist and most often originates from the scaphotrapezial joint, trapeziometacarpal joint, or the radiocarpal joint (Fig. 44.2) (45,50,51). It can originate from the tendon sheath of the flexor carpi radialis.

History

The patient will often relate a history of the spontaneous occurrence of a painless or minimally symptomatic cystic mass on the dorsal or palmar wrist. The mass may first be noted following injury or repetitive motion. Once it has developed, the patient may relate the occurrence of spontaneous enlargement of the mass followed by regression in size. If the mass is located in the vicinity of a peripheral nerve, the patient may relate symptoms of nerve compression (43,52). A history of previous treatment including aspiration or excision is of obvious importance.

A ganglion is unique in its ability to change in size and associated symptoms. These characteristics are key history aspects in diagnosing the lesion. Ganglia often enlarge or become more symptomatic following activity and reflect an increase of fluid transfer from the joint into the cyst. The stalk of the ganglion may contain a "one-way ball valve" type of connection at the joint, and fluid may be more apt to flow into the ganglion than back into the joint. The lesions can regress in size or resolve, either spontaneously or following direct and sudden applied pressure or trauma. The regression in size represents loss of cyst fluid from either flow back into the joint or leakage into the subcutaneous tissue. Other lesions, neoplasms, or infections rarely change in size or regress as readily (43).

A history of a previous puncture wound in the presence of a wrist mass that resembles a ganglion raises the additional diagnostic considerations of an inclusion cyst, foreign body granuloma, or infectious granuloma. A history of inflammatory arthritis is significant because synovitis, tenosynovitis, rheumatoid nodules, or joint effusions can resemble a ganglion (2,3,43).

Previous trauma may be relevant if the patient has concomitant carpal instability or arthritis that may be related to the cause of the synovial fluid comprising the ganglion (2,3,38,42,45,46).

Physical Examination

The mass usually appears as a swelling on the middorsal or radiopalmar wrist. There is variable tenderness, ranging from painless to marked tenderness. It is most often cystic, but when thick-walled or loculated, it may be firm or hard and even resemble an exostosis or carpal boss. There may be an adjacent satellite lesion or loculations (Fig. 44.3). Digital

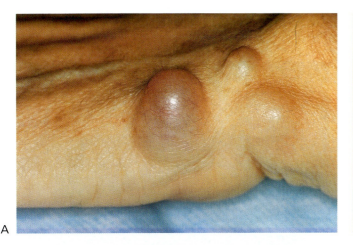

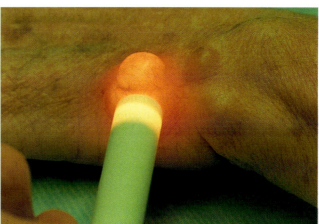

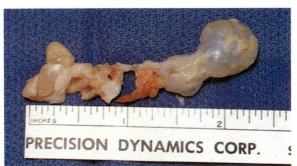

FIGURE 44.3. A: Dorsoulnar carpal ganglion, which exhibits multiple adjacent and loculated satellite lesions. **B:** Transillumination of the dorsoulnar ganglion. **C:** Excisional biopsy specimen of the ganglion with mulitple loculations and satellite lesions. (From Botte MJ. Ganglion excision. In: Gelberman R. *Master techniques in orthopaedic surgery: the wrist.* New York: Raven Press, 1994;393–416, with permission.)

compression or ballottement of the mass may help reveal the lesion's extent and the direction of the pedicle. Palmar flexion of the wrist accentuates the boundaries of the dorsal ganglion or may reveal an occult ganglion. Careful palpation may help distinguish the ganglion from extensor tenosynovitis, dorsal carpal synovitis, carpal effusion, or a carpal boss. Dorsiflexion of the wrist may accentuate the boundaries of a small or occult palmar ganglion (43).

Functional examination of the hand for a ganglion (and other benign tumors) includes active and passive motion, manual muscle testing, grip and pinch strength, and sensibility evaluation with two-point discrimination and monofilament testing. Sensibility of the dorsoradial aspect of the hand and base of the thenar eminence will reveal any possible compression of the superficial branches of the radial nerve and of the palmar cutaneous branch of the median nerve, respectively (43,52–54). Standard vascular examination includes assessment of skin color, temperature, capillary refill, turgor, palpation of pulses, and Allen's testing to demonstrate possible arterial compromise, especially with palmar ganglia located adjacent to the radial artery (51). Doppler examination may be indicated if pulses are difficult to palpate. Radial arterial palpation is performed with and without manual occlusion of the ulnar artery to eliminate retrograde pulsation. Ganglia on the ulnar side of the wrist warrant similar evaluation of the ulnar artery for occlusion. Examination for carpal instability should be undertaken with palpation for wrist clicks during active or passive motion. The scaphoid shift test is performed on both wrists for comparison to determine if scaphoid instability is present. Digital and wrist motion are assessed for mechanical block of tendon triggering, which can occur from ganglia near the extensor retinaculum or within the carpal canal. Percussion of the lesion to elicit Tinel's sign can indicate peripheral nerve encroachment.

Transillumination with a small light placed against the lesion can readily confirm the diagnosis and occasionally can establish the extent of the boundaries of the lesion (Fig. 44.3). Superficial lesions that do not transilluminate raise the suspicion of solid masses.

Radiographic Findings

Radiographs of the cystic mass may demonstrate a soft tissue shadow, which can document the size and location of the mass. Soft tissue penetration films are most likely to show the mass. Radiographs may also demonstrate carpal abnormalities possibly associated with, or related to, the development of the ganglion, including arthritis or carpal instability.

The diagnosis may be obscured in the thick-walled, deeply seated, or small lesion. Additional diagnostic tests are ultrasound and magnetic resonance imaging (MRI). Ultrasound is helpful in determining the cystic nature of the lesion. It can assess the proximity and the patency of the radial artery to a palmar carpal ganglion. Though not recommended for routine evaluation, the MRI is helpful in establishing the diagnosis in atypical, deeply seated, or occult ganglia, such as those within the carpal canal or within Guyon's canal. Though arthrograms of the wrist have demonstrated the "one-way" valve mechanism and connection of the pedicle to the main cyst, the routine use of arthrograms is not warranted (46).

Gross and Microscopic Findings

Grossly, the ganglion appears as a thin-walled translucent or transparent bluish-gray or white cyst. It may be lobulated or loculated (Figs. 44.3 and 44.4). Many fibrous septae may be present, and at times, the cyst will be thick-walled and appear more as a solid mass. The contents of the cyst consist of either viscous clear synovial-like fluid or, at times, thick gelatinous material. The fluid may be clear to yellowish. Microscopically, the lining of the cyst consists of synovium-like tissue supported by a thin fibrous connective tissue stroma.

Diagnostic Aspiration

Aspiration of the mass is useful for diagnosis (as well as treatment). If aspiration is performed for treatment as well, multiple punctures in the cyst wall are placed using digital palpation to direct the needle and compress the mass. Caution is taken during aspiration of palmar carpal ganglia to avoid injury to the radial or ulnar artery or associated

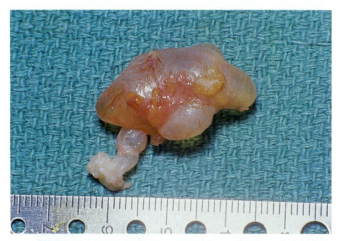

FIGURE 44.4. Example of excised dorsal carpal ganglion showing multiple loculations of the main cyst. The pedicle shows the "one-way valve" mechanism, as the fluid does not leak from the specimen. Note the portion of excised carpal joint ligament at the end of the pedicle. Excision of a portion of the ligament helps assure complete removal of the ganglion and associated synovial-type tissue, which is hoped to minimize chance of recurrence. (From Botte MJ. Ganglion excision. In: Gelberman R. *Master techniques in orthopaedic surgery: the wrist.* New York: Raven Press, 1994;393–416, with permission.)

nerves. Following aspiration, the carpus is immobilized for 3 weeks in a splint (55).

Management

If the ganglion is asymptomatic or causing minimal symptoms and the patient is reluctant to get further treatment, observation can be performed with periodic reexamination and assessment. Some patients with mild symptoms obtain reasonable relief with the use of nonsteroidal antiinflammatory medication or intermittent immobilization with a wrist splint. If, however, rapid growth, pain, or ulceration develop, excisional biopsy should be considered (43).

Aspiration, as discussed above, can also be therapeutic. Aspiration, cyst wall puncture, and injection of a steroid solution has been shown to be effective treatment (2,3,38,46,55), with 27% of dorsal carpal ganglia and 43% of palmar carpal ganglia obtaining successful resolution of symptoms. Immobilization following aspiration significantly improves results of dorsal carpal ganglion aspiration, with 40% of those immobilized for 3 weeks having no recurrence, compared to only 13% of those mobilized early having no recurrence (55). Therefore, immobilization is recommended following aspiration and cyst wall puncture for most carpal ganglia.

Operative excision of a carpal ganglion is indicated when the cystic mass is painful, interferes with function, or causes signs or symptoms consistent with nerve compression. Operative excision is also warranted when tissue for histology is desired for definitive diagnosis of a mass lesion.

Operative Excision

Dorsal Wrist Ganglion

Regional or general anesthesia is recommended for ganglion excision. The deep extension of the stalk actually necessitates placement of a small arthrotomy in the carpus for complete removal; it is difficult to obtain adequate anesthesia with local anesthesia alone. The extremity is exsanguinated gently before tourniquet inflation, with care taken to avoid ganglion rupture. If the mass is large or the diagnosis is in question (possible neoplasm or infection is suspected), exsanguination is performed with gravity, avoiding use of Esmarch compression.

A transverse incision placed along Langer's lines overlying the dorsal carpal ganglion will minimize scar contracture. The lesion is identified and mobilized from the surrounding soft tissues. The pedicle of the ganglion will often be located arising between the third and fourth dorsal compartments. The pedicle penetrates the capsule and usually originated from the scapholunate ligament and overlying capsule. The ganglion and pedicle are removed in entirety, taking a portion of connected dorsal wrist capsule and a small portion of the scapholunate (or associated ligament) to ensure thorough removal of the pedicle (Fig. 44.5). A 5 mm by 5 mm section of capsule can be removed, creating a window in the dorsal wrist capsule (43).

Because of the defect left by removal of a portion of capsule, capsular closure is neither possible or recommended (2,3,43). The wound is irrigated, tourniquet deflated, hemostasis obtained, and wound is closed, and a bulky hand dressing is applied with plaster splints. The wrist is

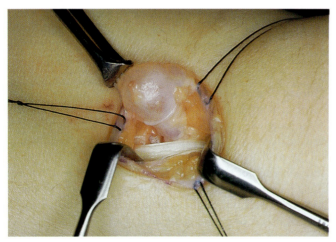
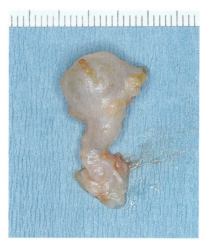
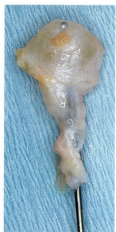

FIGURE 44.5. Excision of a dorsal wrist ganglion. **A:** A forceps gently stabilizes and helps mobilize the ganglion for excision. Note the attached synovial tube or "pedicle" of the ganglion, which originates from the dorsal carpal joints. In this patient, the ganglion originated from the dorsal capitohamate joint. **B:** Excised specimen, showing the ganglion cyst, the attached pedicle, and a small portion of the excised wrist ligaments to assure complete removal of the ganglion and associated synovial tissue. **C:** A probe has been inserted into the pedicle to demonstrate its hollow nature or tube-like structure. (From Botte MJ. Ganglion excision. In: Gelberman R. *Master techniques in orthopaedic surgery: the wrist.* New York: Raven Press, 1994;393–416, with permission.)

positioned in 30° of extension. Wrist mobilization (with the digits free) for 2 to 3 weeks allows capsular healing. Hand therapy is then performed to regain wrist motion and strength.

Palmar Wrist Ganglion

The palmar wrist ganglion is usually located radially, between the radial artery and the flexor carpi radialis tendon or the brachioradialis tendon. Although transverse incisions are preferred for most dorsal wrist ganglia, a longitudinal curved incision is optimal for the palmar ganglion because the pedicle most commonly originates from the scaphotrapezial, trapeziometacarpal, or radiocarpal joint and may tract longitudinally along the flexor carpi radialis tendon sheath to surface near or adjacent to the radial artery. The incision should not cross the wrist joint transversely, and if needed, a zigzag or curved component is added as needed to cross the wrist joint. The subcutaneous tissue is divided, the ganglion identified, and the deep fascia of the forearm divided longitudinally. The radial artery and flexor carpi radialis tendon are identified and tagged with a rubber dam. The radial artery may be found adherent to the wall of the ganglion and require careful dissection to separate it from the cyst wall (43,51).

A bilobular palmar ganglion in the vicinity of the radial artery may involve the radial artery running across the body of the cyst, thus dividing it into two lobules. The artery may not be readily apparent if adherent to the ganglion wall and may appear as a septum. Careful identification of the artery proximal to the cyst and dissection in a proximal-to-distal direction across the ganglion help avoid injury to the artery. The small superficial palmar branch of the radial artery is identified as it crosses the palmar surface of the scaphoid and preserved if possible.

The ganglion will often be found located in the interval between the flexor carpi radialis, the radial artery, and the superficial palmar branch of the median nerve. If the ganglion is located ulnar to the flexor carpi radialis tendon, the median nerve and the palmar cutaneous branch of the median nerve are identified, tagged with a rubber dam, isolated in a proximal-to-distal direction, and protected. The ganglion is freed from the surrounding soft tissues, and the pedicle is traced to its origin from the associated palmar carpal joint. Because the flexor carpi radialis tendon dives deep within a fibroosseous tunnel to reach its insertion at the base of the index and long finger metacarpals, adequate exposure of the pedicle may require opening of this tunnel and retraction of the flexor pollicis longus tendon as well. To further facilitate exposure, the base or proximal margin of the thenar muscles may be partially detached from the transverse carpal ligament, scaphoid, or trapezium. This is especially helpful if the ganglion tracks distal to the scaphotrapezial joint. The pedicle of the ganglion is traced to the carpal joint, and a small portion of capsule is removed along with the pedicle. Following excision and wound closure, the wrist is immobilized in neutral position for 2 to 3 weeks to allow for palmar capsule healing (2,3,42,43,45,46).

Ganglia from the palmar wrist are known causes of median and ulnar nerve compression. Inspection of the canal contents following open carpal tunnel release or Guyon's canal release is performed routinely to rule out an occult ganglion or other space-occupying lesion as the cause of the nerve compression syndrome (43).

Complications

Dorsal Wrist Ganglion

Complications following dorsal carpal ganglion excision include recurrence, continued pain or tenderness, wrist stiffness or weakness, neuroma formation, wound infection, and scar contracture or keloid formation (2,3,42–46). Carpal instability (including scapholunate dissociation), although possible, does not seem to be a common problem despite operative removal of a portion of capsule.

Early recurrence is usually caused by inadequate resection. This complication is best avoided by adequate resection of the pedicle and a portion of adjacent normal-appearing capsule to insure removal of all pathologic tissue. When a ganglion is excised in this manner, recurrence has been between 1% and 24% (2,3,42,46). However, when only the main cyst is excised without adequate pedicle or capsular resection, recurrence have been between 30% and 40% (2,3).

Loss of wrist palmar flexion has been reported to occur in 1% (2,3). Carpal stiffness is avoided by early active mobilization following the initial wrist postoperative immobilization period. Residual weakness of the hand and wrist are treated by hand therapy for strengthening and work hardening. Neuroma formation is avoided by identification of sensory nerves during dissection. Branches of the superficial branch of the radial nerve and of the dorsal branch of the ulnar nerve are at risk (2,3,42,52,54).

Palmar Carpal Ganglion

General complications are similar to those of the dorsal wrist ganglion, with the additional potential for injury to the radial or ulnar artery or to the palmar cutaneous branch of the median nerve. The postoperative recurrence rate is much higher for palmar ganglia, reported between 30% and 35% (compared to 1–24% for dorsal ganglia). The higher recurrence rate is thought to be related to the more variable sites of origin of palmar ganglia (2,3,45).

Epidermal Inclusion Cysts

Following the incidence of the carpal ganglion, the epidermal inclusion cyst is one of the most common masses found in the wrist and hand. This benign tumor is thought to originate from an injury that implants epithelial cells into the subcutaneous tissue. These cells survive, grow, produce keratin, slough epithelial cells into its cavity, and slowly enlarge to a significant size over months or years (56–59). The lesion is usually asymptomatic. However, when large, or in the vicinity of peripheral nerves, the tumor can cause pain or dysfunction. If the lesion is subjected to trauma, local hemorrhage and pain can follow (56–59).

History

Pertinent history includes the occurrence of a puncture wound months earlier. Some patients will relate a history of repetitive trauma to the wrist or hand or have an occupation that regularly subjects the hand and wrist to possible injury. In general, however, many patients will not recall such an injury, and frequently, an inclusion cyst will form without known etiology. The lesion will slowly increase in size; the tumor does not rapidly and intermittently enlarge and regress in size as a ganglion frequently does. The patient often complains of a painless lump or minimally symptomatic mass.

Physical Exam

An inclusion cyst usually presents as subcutaneous rubbery, firm, or hard mass that is usually mobile. Tenderness is variable. If near the surface, the lesion is usually smooth, symmetric, and without lobules. The mass does not usually adhere to tendons and thus does not move with digital or carpal motion. The inclusion cyst will not transilluminate, even when just below the surface or on the dorsum of the wrist (56–59).

Radiographic Findings

Radiographs are usually unremarkable or may show a soft tissue shadow. A soft tissue shadow can help document the size and location of the lesion. If the cyst arises in a fixed location, such as in the digit near the nail, it may rarely produce secondary bone erosion (56–59).

Gross and Microscopic Findings

The inclusion cyst appears grossly as a somewhat hollow fibrous sphere filled with thick gray or whitish "cheesy" material. The wall itself may contain a fibrous stroma, lined with epithelium. The contents of the cyst is an amorphous material, consisting of keratin, sloughed epithelial cells, and cellular debris.

Management

If the lesion is asymptomatic and not growing rapidly, expectant treatment with observation can be performed. If the lesion is symptomatic, or its tissue is desired for definitive diagnosis, excisional biopsy is performed. The lesion is carefully exposed, gently freed, isolated from soft tissues, and excised, taking care not to rupture or lacerate the lesion. If the tumor extends to bone or includes an intraosseous portion, the bone is curetted (56–59).

Fibroma and Associated Lesions

Fibromas include a large and variable of tumors, with somewhat confusing nomenclature (Fig. 44.6) (9,41,59–74). In general, these are benign tumors composed of dense fibrous connective tissue and mature fibrocytes (41). Fibrotic lesions include the nonspecific fibroma (involving soft tissue or bone), the desmoplastic fibroma, and the juvenile aponeurotic fibroma (40,41,61,62,75–78). In addition, included in this broad collection of fibrous tumors are the dermatofibroma, subdermal fibromatosis of infancy, infantile dermatofibromatosis, and palmar fibromatosis (Dupuytren's, Lederhose's, and Peyronie's) (59,60,65,67,69,72). Fibromas, in general, are more often found in the soft tissues, but also occur within bone (40,41,61).

History

The fibroma mass or masses are of variable size, shape, and lobularity. In general, fibromas can slowly enlarge and produce a wide range of symptoms, depending on size and location. Pain is associated with lesions encroaching on nerves or applying pressure to neighboring osseous structures. In some cases, especially in young patients, the clinical course is aggressive, with rapid growth. There may be a history of previous excision in childhood (62,75–78). Lesions noted at birth are among the more locally aggressive (41).

Physical Examination

The most superficial lesions are located in the subcutaneous tissues and are readily palpable. Various other locations are possible, including those adjacent to bone that cause external osseous encroachment as well as those that occur with the bone. There can be variable tenderness. With nerve encroachment, associated neuropathies can develop. Enlargement and extension may interfere with function (40,59).

Radiographic Findings

Most soft tissue fibromas are not visible on radiographs, though a soft tissue shadow may be identified if the lesion is near the surface. With the juvenile aponeurotic fibroma, stippled calcifications may be seen, which are thought to represent portions of degenerated palmar aponeuroses (79). For this reason, the term *calcifying aponeurotic fibroma* has been applied to these tumors (79).

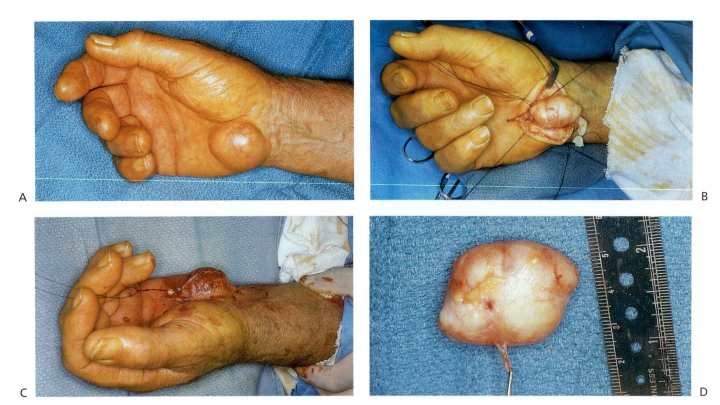

FIGURE 44.6. A: Benign fibroma overlying Guyon's canal, causing ulnar nerve compression. **B,C:** Intraoperative excision showing the encapsulated mass that was easily separated from the surrounding soft tissues. The mass was actually located superficial to Guyon's canal. **D:** Gross specimen, showing firm, whitish fibrous tissue. The histologic specimen demonstrated masses of benign fibrocytes within a thick connective stroma.

The desmoplastic fibroma of bone can resemble a simple cyst within the bone. The lesion is relatively nonspecific; it resembles other benign bone lesions on radiographs.

Gross and Microscopic Findings

Fibromas present a wide variety of sizes and shapes. Grossly, the lesion is usually smooth, firm, gray or white in color, and of variable nodularity. There is usually some component of a capsule. Microscopically, the fibroma consists of mature fibrocytes in a dense connective tissue stroma (40). The major portion of the tissue may be composed of heavy strands of mature collagen. Variable additional cells, such as inflammatory cells, can be present. Giant cells may or may not be noted. The fibrocytes can appear with varying degrees of atypia or metaplasia, and the diagnosis may not be obvious. With varying degrees of metaplasia, the determination between a malignancy may be difficult.

Management

Operative excision is the management both for symptomatic fibromas and for the asymptomatic lesion where tissue is desired for histologic examination (61). Recurrence is most common in the more aggressive, rapidly growing soft tissue fibromas in younger patients. In some cases, multiple recurrences of locally aggressive lesions have led to several operative procedures, or to amputation, to ultimately control the lesion. Histology for fibromas may be confusing and must be distinguished from aggressive fibromatosis, fibrosarcoma, fibrous histiocytoma, or other low-grade malignancies (59,79). Often, the clinical course is one of the key factors in the diagnosis (41).

Lipoma

The lipoma is a benign tumor composed of normal-appearing adipose cells and represents one of the most common solid, cellular tumors of the hand and wrist (61). The tumor may be thinly encapsulated or lobulated. Lipomas often appear much like the surrounding subcutaneous tissues in the upper limb; however, in the wrist, where large deposits of fat are unusual, identification is usually easy (20,79–81).

The lipoma is common in adults and rare in children (79). There is no relationship between the occurrence of well-localized lipomas and generalized patient obesity. The lesion is often misdiagnosed as a ganglion cyst. Larger lesions can be associated with neuropathy if local nerve compression occurs (52,54,81–84). Occult lipomas in the carpal canal or Guyon's canal are known causes of carpal tunnel syndrome and ulnar tunnel syndrome (53,84,85).

History

The history is usually of a slowly growing, painless mass. The patient may suddenly notice the mass, or palpate the lump, and subsequently notice no further growth. Functional limitations are rare but do occur as the lesion grows to a substantial size (79).

Physical Examination

The lipoma appears as a soft, subcutaneous, nontender, freely movable mass. There is a characteristic soft, spongy consistency on palpation, especially recognizable in lesions that arise in superficial tissues. Nerve dysfunction may be detectable. When large, the palmar lipoma can interfere with grasp. When it arises between the metacarpals, lateral deviation of the digits may occur (61).

Radiographic Findings

The lipoma is usually not visible on plain radiographs unless large and superficial. A soft tissue shadow may be seen; the lesion presents as fat or water density (59).

Gross and Microscopic Findings

The benign lipoma grossly and microscopically appears as normal adipose tissue. Individual cells are unremarkable. Each cell may have the typical central lipid droplet and peripherally located nucleus that form the characteristic signet-ring cell. A thin capsule may be apparent. The section of the tumor may be divided into lobules, separated by thin fibrous septae. Occasionally, the lipoma may grow to a quite large size; a fibrous capsule may surround these large lesions (59,61).

Management

Surgical excision is usually curative. Recurrences are rare (59,61,79). The lesions may be encountered unexpectedly during decompression of the carpal tunnel or Guyon's canal. Appropriate excision is then preformed as well.

Fibrous Xanthoma

The fibrous xanthoma (fibroxanthoma, giant cell tumor of tendon sheath, tendon sheath xanthoma) is among the most common solid tumors of the wrist and hand. Reported age distribution is between 8 and 80 years, and the most common locations are in the hand and wrist (61). Nomenclature and the pathologic characteristics remain an area of confusion (86–91). Although commonly found in association with tendon sheaths and joints, these tumors may have few giant cells and are often not in association with a tendon sheath (59). The origin is unknown, and various theories have been proposed. These include trauma, inflammatory causes, metabolic disturbances, and neoplasia (86,92–95).

History

The patient usually notes a slow-growing painless mass in the wrist that may be present for months or years. The lesion may reach a specific size and not change. When large, the tumor can interfere with joint motion. If local peripheral nerves are subjected to pressure, the patient may complain of associated pain, paresthesias, numbness, or weakness. In general, however, complaints are mild, and the patient is more concerned with the presence of the mass and desires diagnostic confirmation (92).

Physical Examination

The lesions are usually located in the palmar surface of the digits and thumb or on the extensor surface of the wrist or proximal palm. The mass, which may resemble a lipoma, is usually smaller than most lipomas and has a firmer, lobulated consistency. The xanthoma tends to be more firmly fixed to the deep tissues. Neurovascular compromise is unusual, but the specific location may cause local peripheral neuropathy. The benign giant cell tumor is a known cause of carpal tunnel and ulnar tunnel syndromes (53,96,97).

Radiographic Findings

Depending on the size and location of the fibrous xanthoma, a soft tissue mass may be visible. When located adjacent to a bone cortex, pressure erosion may occur and can be visualized as an indentation of the involved bone (92).

Gross and Microscopic Findings

Actual joint involvement has been reported in up to 20% of the lesions (21,95), and cartilage invasion and cystic bone destruction can occur (especially in larger joints, but rarely in the digits). The lesion is usually yellow or white, but the color may vary depending on the amount of hemosiderin pigment, number of histiocytes, and the collagen within the stroma. There may be areas of gray and orange. Its size is usually between 0.5 cm and 5 cm, and it characteristically has a firm, lumpy appearance. It may be somewhat adherent to the neighboring tendons. It may extend within a flexor tendon sheath or synovial joint. The tumor is usually not encapsulated (92).

Microscopically, the tumor has a collagenized stroma with multinucleated giant cells, characteristic polyhedral histiocytes, and hemosiderin pigment in various amounts (92,95). With time and age of the tumor, the microscopic appearance can change. Jaffe has noted this evolution of the findings; immature lesions are more cellular, whereas more advanced lesions are acellular with hyalinization of the stroma.

Management

Small asymptomatic masses in the hand may be observed if there is no functional deficit or discomfort. Symptomatic or large lesions, especially those that interfere with joint motion, warrant excision. Because these lesions are not well encapsulated, excision requires meticulous dissection to avoid incomplete excision or spillage of tumor. Recurrence is common and is probably secondary to incomplete excision (92,95,98). Even with meticulous excision, 10% recurrence has been noted (61).

BENIGN VASCULAR TUMORS

Tumors that originate from arteries or veins are relatively uncommon. When these do occur, however, the tumors are frequently located in the hands and forearm. Of 1,056 cases of blood and lymphatic tumors reviewed by Watson and McCarthy, 26% were in the extremities (99). Vascular tumors found in the region of the wrist include aneurysms, hemangiomas, arteriovenous fistulas, and lymphangiomas (100–108).

Aneurysm

Arterial aneurysms consist of 6% of all tumors of the hand and wrist (101,105,106) (Fig. 44.7). Aneurysms are not true neoplasms; most are traumatic afflictions of the arterial wall. There are two types of aneurysms found in the wrist and hand, true and false aneurysms (100–102,105, 106,108). False aneurysms account for the majority (101, 105,106).

The *true aneurysm* is a "ballooning out" of the entire arterial wall. It develops as a gradual, uniform fusiform dilation of the arterial wall components, including the endothelium, intima, and adventitia. Common sites of the true aneurysm in the wrist and hand include the hypothenar eminence involving the ulnar artery, located just distal to the pisohamate ligament (106); the base of the thenar eminence or the dorsum of the first web space, both involving

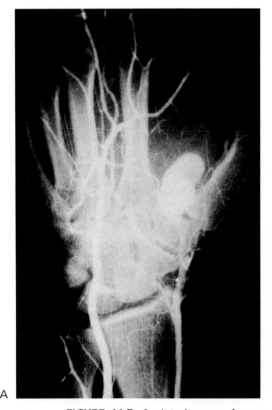
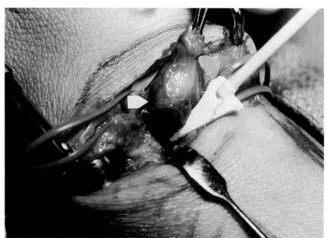

FIGURE 44.7. A: Arteriogram of an aneurysm involving the radial artery in the thumb web space. This area is a common site for both true and false aneurysms, which both can develop secondary to penetrating trauma. **B:** Operative resection of a false aneurysm *(arrow)*. The aneurysm developed from penetrating trauma that occurred previously from a smooth pin used to stabilize a scaphoid fracture.

the radial artery; and along the deep palmar arch. Besides trauma, infections (especially mycosis), atherosclerotic disease, and several other etiologies may lead to formation of a true aneurysm (Table 44.2).

The *false aneurysm,* also referred to as the *pseudoaneurysm,* is the result of partial or complete destruction of a portion of the arterial wall, with replacement by organized fibrous tissue. Penetrating trauma that damages the arterial wall is the common cause of the false aneurysm, and therefore, the false aneurysm may arise in any part of the hand or wrist subjected to injury (Table 44.2). When a penetrating injury punctures an artery, blood extravasates outside the arterial wall and forms a hematoma within the surrounding tissue (109). The arterial blood flowing into the hematoma through the arterial wall forms a cavity that eventually becomes lined with endothelium. The hematoma, which is still in continuity with the artery through the puncture site, becomes absorbed, with its wall being lined by collagen to form a scar (110). This results in a vascular "sac," which is in continuity with the artery and whose walls consists of epithelial-lined fibrous tissue (which do not contain the normal arterial constituents) (106). The turbulence of blood passing through this area can produce mural thrombi that can embolize, producing digital thrombi and associated digital ischemia. When both an artery and an adjacent vein are punctured by penetrating trauma, the resulting hematoma is more likely to form a traumatic arteriovenous fistula (106).

TABLE 44.2. ETIOLOGY OF ANEURYSMS

False aneurysms
  Penetrating
    Stab wounds
    Gunshot wounds
    Arterial punctures
    Arterial catheterization
    Surgical
    Vascular repair/reconstruction
    Regional blockade with local anesthetics
  Nonpenetrating
    Fractures
    Crush
    Hemophilic recurrent bleeding
    Mycotic infection
True aneurysms
  Arteriosclerotic
  Congenital
  Metabolic
  Disease-related
  Osteogenesis imperfecta
  Kawasaki syndrome
  Buerger's disease
  Cystic adventitial
  Hemophilic

From Koman LA, Ruch DS, Smith BP, et al. Vascular disorders. In: Green DP, Hotchkiss RN, Pederson WC, eds. *Green's operative hand surgery,* 4th ed. New York: Churchill Livingstone, 1999;2254–2302, with permission.

Though the false aneurysm usually involves some type of penetrating injury, blunt trauma can also precipitate a false aneurysm if the arterial wall is damaged and weakened to form a leak and subsequent local hematoma. This is known to occur in the hypothenar area, where the ulnar artery wall makes a sharp turn to go deep within the hand just as it passes the pisohamate ligament. The artery in this area is susceptible to trauma because of its superficial location, the sharp turn in direction, and the presence of adjacent unyielding bone (which tethers the artery and provides a solid surface on which the artery is susceptible to compression with external blunt trauma) (106). This area of the wrist is subject to blunt trauma with pneumatic tools or hammers and is, therefore, a frequent location of a false aneurysm (as well as true aneurysms) (106).

History

With either type of aneurysm, the patient may give an account of blunt or penetrating trauma (though false aneurysms are more commonly associated with a known injury incident). The occupation or hobbies may involve repetitive blunt injury to the hand or wrist. In many instances, the patient may not recall a specific injury. If the patient does recall a specific related injury, the history usually consists of the development of a tender, pulsatile mass that enlarges gradually over the following several days. The patient may note only local swelling, or, when the aneurysm is large, a visible mass may become apparent. The patients usually describe local aching pain or tenderness that is increased with local pressure or palpation. The patient may also complain of paresthesias or hypesthesias in the areas innervated by the adjacent sensory or mixed nerves. Occasionally, the patient may develop vascular compromise, resulting in painful episodes or constant blanching, pallor, or cyanotic discoloration distal to the aneurysm. These findings result either from interference with local blood flow from the aneurysm itself or from emboli thrown from the aneurysm. Emboli originate secondary to the vascular turbulence within the aneurysm. Turbulence leads to formation of mural thrombi and subsequent emboli. The emboli can cause irreversible digital ischemia and gangrene (111).

Physical Examination

A visible mass or lump may be noted in the palm (along the course of the ulnar artery or arterial arches) or in the dorsum of the first web space (along the course of the radial artery). The mass is usually tender, especially with compression, and pulsations or a systolic bruit are usually palpable or audible, respectively. The aneurysm can be distinguished from the bruit or thrill of an arteriovenous fistula, because the arteriovenous fistula usually has a continuous bruit or thrill, and the aneurysm is usually systolic (106). If the aneurysm originated from the radial or ulnar arteries at the wrist, Allen's testing may indicate poor flow or occlusion. The pulses should be evaluated proximal and distal to the aneurysm. If the ulnar artery is involved, the radial artery is manually occluded (to eliminate back flow) to evaluate pulses and patency of the involved ulnar artery. Conversely, if the radial artery is involved, the ulnar artery can be manually occluded to evaluate the pulses and patency of the radial artery. If there is encroachment of an associated major nerve, paresthesias may be elicited with percussion in the area (positive Tinel's test).

Radiographic Findings

Standard radiographs are usually normal. Contrast angiography will outline the aneurysm, showing a saccular collection of contrast material in continuity with the involved artery (Fig. 44.7A). Angiography will also help evaluate the patency and flow distal to the aneurysm. MRI can identify the lesion if the lesion is of adequate size. Additional evaluation can include pulse volume recording or radionuclide scans.

Management

Treatment of an aneurysm consists of dissecting, isolating, and resecting the lesion (Fig. 44.7B). The defect in the artery is repaired by either end-to-end arterial anastomosis, interposition vein grafting, or by a direct repair of the defect in the vessel wall (106,112). The specific type of arterial reconstruction is based on size of the vessel and the size and location of the resulting defect. Ligation of a major artery is no longer recommended, with the availability of microvascular reconstructive surgery (112).

Hemangioma

The hemangioma is a benign growth of proliferating blood vessels. In general, the hemangioma has been shown to be the fourth most common tumor of the hand (56,113). Twenty percent of 347 benign tumors of the hand were identified as a hemangioma (99,106), and the hemangioma accounts for 63% of all vascular tumors of the hand. This tumor can cause associated pain, discoloration, limb deformity, and secondary nerve compression. There are several classifications of hemangiomas described, including those based on descriptive anatomy, location, or natural history. Classifications based on descriptive anatomy include the capillary hemangioma, cavernous (venous) hemangioma, and the sclerosing hemangioma (56,106). Hemangiomas classified as to location include the superficial, subcutaneous, and intramuscular hemangiomas (105,106). Descriptive classification as to natural history includes the involuting and noninvoluting types of hemangiomas.

The *capillary hemangioma,* as the name implies, consists primarily of proliferating capillaries within the soft tissue. The tumors tend to have compact collections of endothelial cells in which there are small or no capillary lumina. These cellular proliferations tend to extend from the dermis into the subcutaneous tissue (105,106). The capillary hemangioma is among the most superficial hemangiomas, may appear red or purple, and usually has ill-defined borders. Fifty-seven percent of the subcutaneous hemangiomas are of the capillary type. It is a congenital tumor and often spontaneously regresses to complete resolution without treatment.

The *cavernous* or *venous hemangioma* consists of thin-walled sinuses with little stroma in between. The thin-walled, blood-filled spaces are widely dilated and may extend more deeply than the capillary hemangioma. The cavernous hemangioma is usually soft and compressible, and occasionally, it may cause erosion of underlying soft tissues and bone (56). Twenty-three percent of subcutaneous hemangiomas are of the cavernous type. The cavernous hemangioma develops early in childhood and usually will not regress spontaneously.

The *sclerosing hemangioma* may be a variation of the capillary hemangioma in which a perivascular thickening of histiocytes initiates a process of sclerosis. The sclerosing hemangioma tends to have more of a fibrous origin than a hematogenous origin and has also been classified as subepidermal nodular fibrosis (105,106). Ten percent of superficial hemangiomas are of the sclerosing type.

The *involuting hemangioma* tumors are usually present at birth or in infancy and go through a rapid period of growth for about 6 months. They then begin to involute and usually resolve by age 6 or 7. The involuting tumors can be either capillary, cavernous, or mixed (105,106,114). Involuting hemangiomas are usually the "strawberry nevi" of children (112).

The *noninvoluting hemangioma,* as the name implies, does not resolve with time and tends to occur later in life. The superficial, diffuse port-wine stain or nevus flammeus is a noninvoluting hemangioma (112). These flat lesions are red splotchy skin discolorations that are difficult or impossible to eradicate (105,106,114).

History

Depending on the location and type of lesion, parents will provide the history of a congenital red or purple-colored mass. In the older child, the parents may have noted growth of the lesion (involuting type). Subcutaneous hemangiomas can present with a history of throbbing pain. If in the vicinity of the median nerve at the wrist, the subcutaneous hemangioma can result in symptoms of carpal tunnel syndrome (115).

Physical Examination

A wide variety of presentations exist. Superficial lesions represent a palpable mass the can encompass a large portion of the wrist or palm. Twenty-five percent of these will have tenderness (105,106). The lesion is usually red or purple; thus, the "port-wine" description. Large lesions may be found to impair joint motion. Some appear tender, and secondary deformity of the hand or wrist can occur when there is associated bone or soft tissue deformity.

Radiographic Findings

Standard radiographs may show a soft tissue mass. Associated cortical erosion or deformity of bone has been noted in 6% (105,106). Soft tissue calcification and/or calcification of pheboliths have been noted infrequently (105,106). Preoperative arteriograms are helpful in identifying the number and location of associated "feeder" vessels to these highly vascular tumors.

Management

Treatment of hemangiomas is varied because of the diverse nature of the tumors. Those occurring early in childhood should, in general, be observed for a period because many are likely to be the involuting type and will resolve spontaneously. Surgery should be reserved only for rapidly increasing masses and for longstanding tumors in which the size of the lesion causes impaired function, pain, or deformity. Surgical excision is usually the treatment of choice for the subcutaneous hemangioma. Though a tourniquet is used, the extremity is not exsanguinated so that the entire tumor mass can be more readily identified and removed. Feeding and draining vessels are ligated or cauterized as far away from the tumor as is practical. The surgeon should be certain that the distal arterial flow will preserve the viability of the hand and fingers before attempting excision of the hemangioma. Because these tumors often bleed profusely, the tourniquet should be released before closure. Available blood for transfusion has been recommended if it should prove necessary (57).

Palmieri has noted the need for a two-stage procedure. First the tributary vessels are ligated; then, at a later date, the lesion is excised (105). If the tumor is adherent to the dermal surface and the skin is involved with the hemangioma, the skin should be excised, and the area covered with appropriate skin grafts (105,106).

The role of radiation therapy is not clear. It has been recommended specifically for control of the highly undifferentiated or infiltrating lesion (57). Radiation results in sclerosis of the hemangioma. Radiation is not felt routinely indicated (and is felt contraindicated by some authors) because it causes atrophic changes in the skin and subcutaneous tissue. Radiation therapy may also arrest skeletal growth (105,106).

The argon laser has also been recommended to treat noninvoluting superficial hemangiomas. The laser allegedly selectively damages pigmented cutaneous lesions without damaging the overlying skin, sweat gland, and hair follicles. Because hemangiomas are rich in hemoglobin pigment, which selectively absorbs the laser light, the light converts to heat, which causes coagulation of the blood vessels in the dermis to a depth of 1 mm. Scar tissue then replaces the damaged blood vessels (57,105,106). (We do not have experience with the use of the argon laser and do not specifically recommend its use.)

Sclerosing agents, such as 5% sodium morrhuate, have been advocated and will injure the tumor cells; however, the normal local tissue is also injured. Therefore, this type of treatment is not recommended (106).

Congenital Arteriovenous Fistula

The arteriovenous fistula is a communication between an artery and a vein that bypasses normal capillary circulation. The fistula may be congenital or acquired. The acquired fistulas are either traumatic or surgical in origin. The congenital arteriovenous fistula has a tendency for development in the upper limb, especially in the hand (116).

The congenital arteriovenous fistula results from a failure in the differentiation of a common embryonic vascular anlage into a true artery and vein (117). A persistent communication exists between them, and the blood is shunted through the fistula, bypassing the capillary network (118). Approximately half of the tumors appear before 2 years of age, and 60% present by the age of 10 (112).

History

The patient or parents relay a history of a slowly growing mass in the wrist or hand, often on the dorsum of the radial hand. As the tumor grows, it becomes progressively painful, partially because of ischemia. Patients often present for evaluation of a congenital arteriovenous fistula in the second decade, when symptoms or the size of the mass have become quite marked. Besides pain, symptoms and signs also consist of pulsating swelling, increased local warmth in the area of the lesion, and, conversely, cold skin, cyanosis, and pallor distal to the fistula. The patient may relate a history of persistent bleeding of a wound caused by minimal injury.

Physical Examination

A tumor mass may be visible or palpable and tender to palpation or pressure. The mass may be pulsatile from varices that arise proximal to the lesion, and a bruit may be apparent. The overlying skin is usually warm, but the skin distal to the lesion may be cooler because of vascular compromise (116). The mass may be poorly defined, fed by dilated arteries, and drained by thickened, dilated superficial veins. Edema or sweating may be present. If the fistula is active during childhood growth, there may be hypertrophy of the extremity or digits, with noticeable skeletal elongation. There may be multiple fistula sites of varying sizes. When distal circulation is markedly impaired, local signs of ischemia can occur, such as cyanosis, pallor or even ulceration (105,106,112,116).

Large congenital arteriovenous fistulas can actually produce a drop in the peripheral vascular resistance, resulting in hypotension and secondary tachycardia (106). The heart may become enlarged (116). The circulating blood volume is also secondarily increased. With large arteriovenous fistulas, proximal compression of the feeding artery of a large fistula will cause a decrease in the heart rate when the shunt is closed by the examiner's compression. The heart rate drops, and the blood pressure increases transiently (119,120). With large fistulas, the patient may develop secondary trophic changes and ischemic ulcers in the fingers secondary to shunting of large amounts of blood and the lack of oxygenated blood going distally to the digits.

Radiographic Findings

Standard radiographs will show a soft tissue mass with occasional calcification from phleboliths. Bone erosion or new bone formation is occasionally seen.

Contrast studies will help delineate the extent of the tumor and will identify the location of feeding vessels. Venous angiography or contrast arterial angiography are both helpful. Arteriograms will show a simultaneous filling of the arterial and venous systems. Pooling of the contrast material will collect in the malformation itself. The vascularity distal to the lesion may show poor filling. Multiple feeding vessels are usually noted with the congenital arteriovenous fistula.

Management

Because of the wide range of size, location, and anatomy of the congenital arteriovenous malformation, management is individualized. The lesions are difficult to treat, and operative management should be used as a last resort. Recurrence is common, and a definitive "cure" is not always possible. Koman has emphasized that the lesion is frequently more extensive than the clinical appearance suggests (121). Intervention is dependent on the symptoms, the location of the malformation, and the predominant vessels involved.

Nonoperative management includes the use of vasoactive drugs that decrease shunting and/or increase nutritional flow. Calcium channel blockers and α-adrenergic agonists may reduce symptoms (121).

Operative or interventional management consists of excision of the lesion, ligation of the arterial components feeding the lesion, or embolization techniques to obstruct the arteriovenous communication (112,116).

With a relatively small, localized lesion with only a few communicating vessels, operative excision is often feasible and successful. If the lesion is large, resection can be difficult and may require multiple procedures. An extensive lesion may be treated with subtotal resection, guided by prior arteriography to attempt to close the major arteriovenous shunts in the involved area. Subsequent staged excisions may be performed as necessary. Care must be taken to preserve circulation because distal ischemia is frequently a major complication of the lesion itself, with or without operative management. Attempted total excision and vein graft reconstruction has only limited application because of the diffuse nature of these lesions.

An alternative to excising the lesion is the use of ligation of the arterial components of the malformation. Ligation of the thin arterial branches that feed into the lesion is difficult but can be successful in the treatment, if the arteries are able to be accurately identified and obliterated (116). Ligation of the fistula itself between the arterial and venous components is, however, rarely possible because of the size or complexity of the lesion. Ligation of the proximal principal artery is also usually not successful because of a possible subsequent increase in the collateral circulation that reproduces the symptoms. In addition, ligation of the principal artery can worsen the ischemia in the distal regions of the limb.

Embolization methods are alternative techniques employed to attempt to close larger arteriovenous fistulas. An intraarterial catheter is introduced and guided by radiographs. The tip of the catheter is placed into the arteriovenous communication, and a small pellet of foreign material is left to block the communication. This procedure has fewer complication than surgery, but its efficacy in treating multiple congenital arteriovenous fistulas has not yet been adequately evaluated. The technique seems to have more application with the traumatic arteriovenous fistula (112).

For a lesion that is too extensive for resection or not amenable for ligation or embolization methods, fasciotomy has been performed as a palliative measure to decrease pain.

Additionally, large congenital arteriovenous fistulas that are considered inoperable or untreatable can be treated by limb compression garments to stabilize or minimize the dilated components.

Acquired Arteriovenous Fistula

The acquired arteriovenous fistula is traumatic (or surgical) in origin. The traumatic arteriovenous fistula usually follows a penetrating injury. The artery and adjacent vein are lacerated or pierced. The hematoma that develops causes blood to flow from the artery to the lower-pressure venous system with subsequent bypass of the capillaries. Traumatic fistulas form rapidly and have hemodynamics (and findings) similar to the congenital arteriovenous fistula. As with the congenital fistula, an arteriogram is useful in making the diagnosis, which is confirmed by noting a large single feeder vessel with rapid shunting of blood. This is in contrast to the congenital fistulas, which have multiple feeding vessels. The acquired arteriovenous fistulas should be treated early, before permanent irreversible damage occurs to the adjacent vessel walls. The fistula should be excised, and the artery and vein repaired, either by direct repair or vein graft (106).

A major associated problem of the acquired arteriovenous fistula is the distal ischemic symptoms created by the shunting of blood in the fistula from the distal limb. Cyanotic digits caused by a surgically created fistula may require takedown of the fistula or vascular bypass graft reconstruction (121). Distal finger tip necrosis can require amputation as indicated.

LYMPHANGIOMA

Lymphangiomas are rare lymph-vascular tumors that can involve the wrist and hand. The tumors have been classified into three types: simple lymphangioma, cavernous lymphangioma, and cystic lymphangioma (cystic hygromas) (122,123).

The simple lymphangioma is usually well defined and can be treated by local excision. The cavernous lymphangioma is the most common variety, appearing at birth or shortly after. The tumor consists of dilated lymphatic sinuses that present as a soft tissue mass. Congenital constriction bands are occasionally present. Treatment of the cavernous lymphangioma is by local excision and with Z-plasty of the constricting bands, as indicated. The cavernous lymphangioma can involve the entire upper extremity and can be difficult to remove (122).

BENIGN TUMORS OF NERVES

Nerve tumors represent a relatively rare but significant group of neoplasms (47,48,124–132). The most common tumors include the neurofibroma, the neurilemmoma (schawannoma), and the lipofibromatous hamartoma. Nerve sheath ganglia have also been described involving the median and ulnar nerves (47,48). Hemangioma can rarely involve the median nerve. This intraneural variation is discussed in this section because of the location within the nerve.

Neurofibroma

The neurofibroma is the most common benign nerve sheath tumor and has gained recognition because of its association with von Recklinghausen's disease (40,41,58,63, 66,127,133–140) (Fig. 44.8). The tumor is composed of a combination of proliferating nerve sheath (Schwann) cells, fibrous connective tissue, and axons. The neurofibroma may occur as a solitary lesion but is more frequently multi-

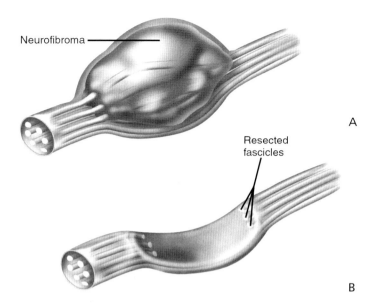

FIGURE 44.8. Schematic illustration of a neurofibroma within a major peripheral nerve. **A:** Tumor is depicted before excision. Note the fascicles entering and exiting the mass. **B:** The postexcision illustration shows the defect left by the mass along with several resected fascicles. Because the fascicles are intimately involved with the neurofibroma, excision often requires partial resection of the nerve or injury to the fascicles.

ple. It is often seen as one of the malformations of neurofibromatosis or von Recklinghausen's disease.

The neurofibroma usually originates from and eventually obliterates a small cutaneous nerve. At times, a major peripheral nerve is involved.

History

The patient usually notes a slowly enlarging, painless, soft mass. Associated complaints of pain, numbness, or paresthesias are present if the neurofibroma develops within a major peripheral nerve. Pregnancy has been noted to accelerate their growth. Despite the origin from a small cutaneous nerve, the patient does not usually complain of localized numbness or numbness in the distribution of the involved sensory nerve (unless a major nerve is involved) (129).

Physical Examination

If the solitary neurofibroma is superficial, a palpable soft or rubbery or firm mass will be noted. It is usually nontender, mobile, does not attach to neighboring tendons, and may have polypoid or nodular cutaneous characteristics. The mass does not transilluminate. Often the overlying skin will be hyperpigmented and feel soft and redundant.

The diffuse form of neurofibroma presents as a plaque-like mass that has diffusely permeated the subcutaneous tissues. The skin surface overlying the lesion develops exaggerated folds and skin creases (129).

When small, fairly localized, and involving a small cutaneous nerve, the plexiform neurofibroma may present as an ill-defined nodule. However, with time, the plexiform neurofibroma massively expands the individual nerve fascicles for long distances and cause the original nerve to twist and hang in a redundant fashion. This distorted structure may be palpable and has been likened to palpation of a "bag of worms" (63). When the tumor involves large nerves, its presentation may be similar to elephantiasis and is referred to as "elephantiasis neuromatosa" or local gigantism.

With neurofibromatosis, there may be extensive local abnormalities with erosion of adjacent bone, marked joint laxity, and large café-au-lait spots. The patients often have a family history of diffuse soft tissue and bone lesions, including congenital pseudoarthrosis of the tibia or forearm, scoliosis, and many nodular skin lesions of fibroma molluscum. There may also be gigantism of the fingers.

Radiographic Findings

Radiographic examination is usually unremarkable. If superficial in the subcutaneous tissues, and of adequate size, a soft tissue mass may be visible. If large, the mass will be identifiable with MRI and will appear as a nerve or fibrous density. If malignant degeneration of a plexiform neurofibroma is suspected, MRI may further delineate the lesion.

Gross and Microscopic Findings

On gross examination, the localized neurofibroma is usually ovoid, pale gray, and translucent (141,142). The neurofibroma contains a mixture of cells that have features of Schwann cells, perineurial cells, and fibroblasts (63,143, 144). Occasionally, myelinated and unmyelinated axonal processes are found within the lesion (63). Spindle cells are common, with elongated nuclei with pointed ends. The spindle cells are arranged in short intersecting fascicles and are accompanied by wire-like bundles of collagen (129). The proliferating cells expand the nerve and envelop the axons that course through the tumor. The stroma of the neurofibroma is frequently myxoid and contains scattered mast cells and lymphocytes.

Immunohistochemical Analysis

There are several types of immunohistochemical tests that are useful for the identification of neurofibromas. Most neurofibromas are positive for the S-100 protein and vimentin (145). Many of the lesions also stain with antibodies to Leu-7, and a minority express glial fibrillary acidic protein (145,146).

Management

Localized Cutaneous Neurofibroma

Indications for operative treatment of a suspected neurofibroma (or mass of unknown diagnosis) is pain, nerve dysfunction, and/or rapid growth. A solitary neurofibroma arising in the skin presents as a firm mass that can be managed with excisional biopsy. If, at the time of biopsy, a small cutaneous nerve is identified entering or exiting the mass, the nerve is sacrificed. Often, a nerve will not be identified in association with a solitary cutaneous neurofibroma, and the mass can be removed following dissection from the surrounding subcutaneous tissue. If the localized neurofibroma involves an identifiable branch supplying sensibility to the hand, an attempt is made to preserve the nerve. Under the dissecting microscope, the cutaneous nerve entering or exiting the mass is isolated, surgically mobilized, and followed into the mass. Because a neurofibroma is intimately intermixed with nerve fascicles, the mass is not easily separated or shelled out from the nerve (as can be done with a neurilemmoma). However, fascicles may be damaged as they are isolated from the neurofibroma (Fig. 44.8). If nerve damage does occur in the removal of a neurofibroma, and the nerve ends can be reapproximated, primary nerve repair is performed (129).

If in the exploration of a nerve tumor a large (between 2 and 6 cm), irregular, nodular lesion is encountered that is adherent to surrounding structures, one should suspect a possible malignant nerve lesion such as a malignant schwannoma (129). An incisional biopsy only is recommended when these findings are encountered.

Multiple Neurofibromas in von Recklinghausen's Disease

In the patient with classic, generalized von Recklinghausen's disease and multiple localize neurofibromas, excision of multiple asymptomatic tumors is generally not indicated (133,147). However, these patients require observation to note occurrence of new or increased symptoms, or excessive tumor growth; these are indications of possible malignant degeneration. Operative excisional biopsy is indicated in these lesions. Incisional biopsy may also be indicated for large, poorly localized lesions. Besides associated pain or increasing size of the mass, other indications for excisional biopsy include hand or wrist dysfunction caused by the mass or a subcutaneous lesion associated with infection, bleeding, or ulceration (133,147).

If an incisional biopsy histologically indicates malignant degeneration, wide *en bloc* excision is indicated (58).

Neurilemmoma (Schwannoma)

The neurilemmoma, also known as a schwannoma, is the second most common benign peripheral nerve tumor fol-

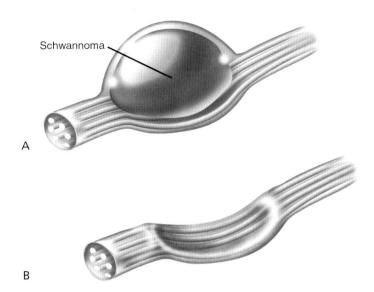

FIGURE 44.9. Schematic illustration of a schawannoma (neurilemmoma) of a major peripheral nerve. **A:** The tumor is depicted preexcision. Note the well-delineated mass, which displaces the nerve fascicles to one side. Because the fascicles are not intimately involved with the tumor, the schwannoma can be "shelled out" from the nerve trunk **(B)**, preserving the nerve fascicles.

lowing the neurofibroma in incidence (Fig. 44.9) (128–132). Eliminating the patients with multiple neurofibromas, the neurilemmoma is often considered the most common solitary peripheral nerve tumor. The tumor arises in adults along the course of the peripheral nerves. In 20% of cases, the tumor originates in the median, ulnar, or radial nerve (63,138). Involvement of the forearm, wrist, and hand is more common than in the digits (148). Most neurilemmomas are solitary, though multiple lesions have been described and may affect one or several nerves (149). Rarely, the tumor may be induced by radiation (130). The neurilemmoma is not found in the intradermal nerve ends.

Of all neurilemmomas, 20% are found in the upper extremity, 15% in the lower extremities, and the remaining found in the head or neck. Within the upper extremity, the tumor is more frequently found on the flexor than the extensor surface, and most are located near the wrist or elbow (56–58).

The neurilemmoma is usually located eccentrically within the nerve. The slow growth of these tumors is usually well accommodated by the flexible perineurium and epineurium, which dissipate the potential local compression (138). Therefore, clinical symptoms are often minimal and usually consist of only mild paresthesias, tenderness, and/or minimal nerve dysfunction (63,138,150,151).

History

Forty percent of patients complain of some local pain or tenderness. The tumor develops gradually, and therefore, the patient may relate a history of a slow-growing mass deep to the skin. Paresthesias may occur, but motor weakness is unusual.

Physical Examination

The mass may be palpable if the tumor is located within a subcutaneous nerve. The mass is soft and sometimes cystic and may be slightly tender. If superficial and well defined, the tumor may be movable from side to side, but not longitudinally. Palpation may elicit mild paresthesias, and a Tinel's sign may be present. Because of its consistency, the tumor may be confused with a lipoma or ganglion with palpation (129,148,152). Occasionally, there may be cystic degeneration within the larger neurilemmomas, and thus it may be possible to transilluminate the tumor. Transillumination may further confuse the lesion with a ganglion.

Gross and Microscopic Findings

The neurilemmoma usually appears as a round to oval, smooth, shiny and white, well-defined, encapsulated mass within the substance of the peripheral nerve. It is usually less than 5 cm in size. The mass will bulge eccentrically from the originating nerve and push aside adjacent nerve fascicles that stretch over its surface. The mass is firm to palpation and uniform in consistancy. The nerve entering and exiting the lesion will appear normal (unless multiple lesions exist within the same nerve). On cut section, the neurilemmoma is usually tan-yellow and may be partially hemorrhagic or cystic (63,129).

Histologically, the neurilemmoma contains neoplastic Schwann cells that are usually spindle-shaped and have elongated nuclei with pointed ends. The cytoplasm is eosinophilic, and the cytoplasmic borders are indistinct. The Schwann cells are characteristically arranged in alternating hypercellular and hypocellular regions, known as Antoni A and Antoni B regions, respectively (129). The blood vessels in the stroma are often dilated, have sclerotic walls, and undergo thrombosis. The resultant ischemia can result in hemorrhage, necrosis, and cystic degeneration.

A neurilemmoma can easily be confused with a sarcoma (153–156) because of the large, pleomorphic, and hyperchromatic nuclei scattered throughout the tumor (157). These cytologic changes are believed to be degenerative in nature (157). Occasionally, the tumor cells in a neurilemmoma can produce melanin and become pigmented (158). Ultrastructurally, a neurilemmoma is distinguished from other nerve tumors by the presence of only Schwann cells.

Immunohistochemical Analysis

As with the neurofibroma, several types of immunohistochemical tests are available for the identification of neurilemmomas. Most neurilemmomas are positive for vimentin, S-100, and Leu-7 (145,146,159). About one-third of neurilemmomas stain positively with antibodies recognizing glial fibrillary acidic protein and less than 10% for keratin (145).

Management

Treatment of a symptomatic neurilemmoma is operative excision. Unlike the neurofibroma (which is difficult to excise and separate from nerve fascicles), the neurilemmoma can usually be removed with little or no injury to nerve fascicles (Fig. 44.9) (80,133,138,147,152,160–162). As the tumor grows, fascicles are pushed aside and are not intimately incorporated into the tumor as usually occurs in the neurofibroma or lipofibromatous hamartoma. Therefore, a neurilemmoma is usually easily resected from the nerve; the procedure has often been likened to shelling a pea from a pod.

Results are usually favorable following excision of a neurilemmoma. There is usually relief of symptoms and recurrence is rare (80,133,138,147,152,160–162). Only occasionally have additional nerve deficits been reported following excision of this tumor (148,160,161).

Lipofibromatous Hamartoma

The lipofibromatous hamartoma of a peripheral nerve is a fibrofatty enlargement or infiltration that enlarges the involved nerve (Figs. 44.10–44.12). A hamartoma is a tumor-like aggregate of architecturally disorganized tissue composed of cell types inherent to the particular anatomical site. In lipofibromatous hamartoma, the epineurium and perineurium of the nerve are expanded and distorted by excess mature fat and fibrous tissue that infiltrates between and around nerve bundles (163,164). Since the normal nerve sheath includes fat and fibrous tissue, this process is considered a hamartoma of the nerve sheath (164–166).

The lipofibromatous hamartoma is often associated with an overgrowth or "gigantism" of the distal hand, wrist, and forearm (Fig. 44.10A). This has led to a confusing array of synonyms for the condition, which include macrodystrophia lipomatosa, macrodactyly, megalodactyly, local gigantism, infiltrating lipoma of the median nerve, perineural lipoma, and intraneural lipoma of the median nerve (82,167). The pathologic abnormalities and changes of the involved nerve are similar in cases with or without the limb overgrowth. Therefore, the current recommended terminology is lipofibromatous hamartoma with or without macrodactyly (1,4,163,168–177).

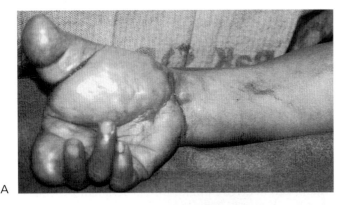

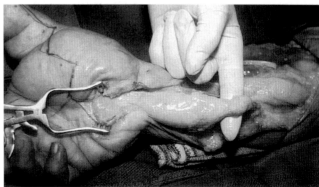

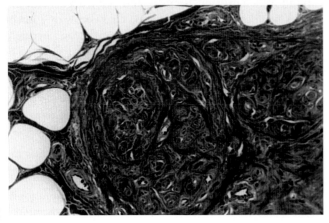

FIGURE 44.10. Upper limb containing a lipofibromatous hamartoma of the median nerve. **A:** The limb shows macrodactyly of the radial palm and hand. **B:** Median neuropathy was present, and a large lipofibromatous hamartoma of the median nerve was encountered at the time of exploration and nerve decompression. The tumor is yellowish white and appears grossly as a fusiform mass of fat. The nerve lies within the mass. **C:** Photograph of microscopic section of the lipofibromatous hamartoma. Note the fascicles and nerve fibers and the surrounding adipose tissue.

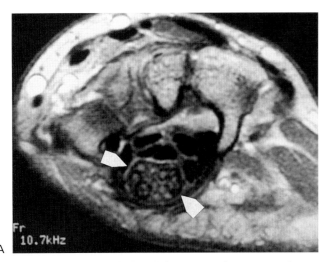 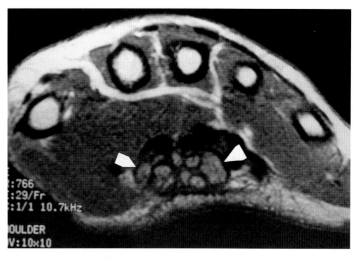

FIGURE 44.11. Magnetic resonance image of the carpal region **(A)** and the palm **(B)** of a patient with a lipofibromatous hamartoma of the median nerve *(white arrows)*. The tumor often causes signs and symptoms of median neuropathy. It is one of the more common causes of carpal tunnel syndrome in a child or adolescent.

The lipofibromatous hamartoma of nerve involves the upper extremity more often than the lower, with relatively common involvement of the wrist and palm (1,129,163, 168,170,178,179). In the upper extremity, it most commonly involves the median nerve and its digital branches. In the remaining minority of patients, the ulnar and radial nerves are involved in descending order of frequency (129,165,166,180).

History

The patient will relate a history of a long-standing mass or fullness in the forearm. Specific symptomatology is variable. Some patients may complain of minimal or no symptoms, while others will have pain, paresthesias, numbness, and motor weakness in the distribution of the involved nerve. A history similar to that of carpal tunnel syndrome or ulnar tunnel syndrome is not uncommon. When the median nerve has been involved, there may be thenar weakness with an associated history of weak grip or dropping objects. The diagnosis is suspected by history, in the child or young adult who gives an account of symptoms suggestive of carpal tunnel syndrome who has had a mass in the forearm or wrist present since birth.

Physical Examination

The lipofibromatous hamartoma may initially present as a mass or fullness in the forearm, wrist, palm, or digit (1,163,164). Depending on the nerve involved, there may be motor or sensory deficits suggestive of carpal or ulnar tunnel syndrome. Muscle atrophy of the associated muscle may be present. The patient may have mechanical dysfunction secondary to tissue overgrowth, resulting in loss of motion, pinch, or grasp (1,163,180). Tinel's sign over the involved nerve or mass may be present, with or without mild to moderate palpable tenderness. There may or may not be digital or limb gigantism in the ipsilateral limb (129).

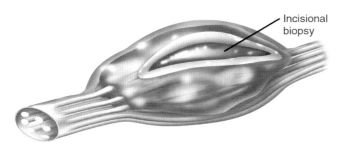

FIGURE 44.12. Schematic illustration of a lipofibromatous hamartoma of the median nerve. Note the nerve fascicles, which are intertwined within the mass. Because complete excision of the mass usually is not possible without severe injury to the nerve, aggressive tumor excision is usually not warranted for this benign process. Incisional biopsy is placed in a longitudinal fashion in line with the fascicles, with care taken to avoid injury to these structures.

Radiographic Findings

The tumor is not visible with standard radiographs. It can be deliniated with an MRI (Fig. 44.11).

Gross and Microscopic Findings

The lipofibromatous hamartoma appears grossly as a fusiform fibrofatty tissue enlargement of the associated nerve (Fig. 44.10B). The nerve may be enlarged five to six times its normal diameter, and the nerve will be slightly yellow but usually retain the glistening sheen of a normal nerve. Occasionally, the nerve may appear dull, or even appear as a fusiform mass of fat (with normal nerve entering and exiting the mass). The swelling or tumor mass shape of the nerve is usually symmetric and can extend several centimeters proximally and distally. When the median or ulnar nerve is involved at the wrist, the fatty infiltration often extends to the common or proper digital nerves as well as to the mid- or proximal forearm. The tumor may cause the nerve to bend in a redundant fashion (181). The mass may be encountered incidentally at the time of carpal tunnel release or ulnar tunnel exploration (129).

Microscopically, the nerve sheath is infiltrated and expanded by varying amounts of mature fat and fibrous tissue, which dissects between and separates individual nerve bundles. A cuff of perineural fibrosis delineates individual bundles and may extend to involve the endoneurium. The nerve fibers and axons usually appear normal (129,163). The proximal extent of nerve involvement may not be clearly delineated. Most operative explorations and biopsies are limited to the clinically affected region.

Management

Management of the lipofibromatous hamartoma of a peripheral nerve is controversial; several methods of treatment have been described (1,129,152,165,166,177, 182–185). Management has included nerve decompression and biopsy, nerve decompression and neurolysis, excision of the involved nerve, and microsurgical intraneural dissection of the tumor (1,129,147,152,165,166,177,182–185). Optimal treatment depends on specific nerve involved, the location, assocated symptoms, and the presence of macrodactyly. Because a lipofibromatous hamartoma is a benign process, less aggressive management that preserves nerve continuity is usually indicated. The tumor most commonly occurs in the median nerve in the forearm and wrist, and in these areas, the associated nerves cannot be sacrificed, as is sometimes recommended for digital nerve involvement.

Though excisional biopsy or microdissection for debulking the hamartoma has been described, nerve decompression with biopsy alone may be safer treatment in, at least, the initial treatment of these tumors. The tumor is intimately involved with nerve fascicles, and even with microdissection, further nerve injury often occurs (1,147,152). Microdissection of the nerve and aggressive neurolysis may result in disruption of vascularity, causing significant neural ischemia. Therefore, because symptoms are often relieved by decompression, aggressive tumor debulking for this benign process is probably not warranted (129,147,177,186). In addition, though the diagnosis is usually presumptively made, it cannot be confirmed without prior histologic analysis, so that if a malignancy were encountered, an excisional biopsy would cause further seeding of the tumor (147).

The recommended treatment of the lipofibromatous hamartoma involving the median or ulnar nerve in the wrist consists of nerve decompression with incisional biopsy for diagnostic confirmation. Attempts at aggressive tumor excision, even with microdissection, may result in further nerve injury and thus is not routinely warranted for most patients. Tumor excision is reserved for cases where large tumor size interferes with hand function or causes incapacitating pain (147). Although symptoms are usually initially relieved or improved after nerve decompression, the long-term prognosis is variable, and progressive loss of nerve function and pain may recur. Repeat nerve decompression, tumor excision, or opponensplasty may be required in some patients.

Guidelines for Peripheral Nerve Tumors

In dealing with all peripheral nerve tumors of the upper limb, Bogumill has presented the following useful guidelines (57,58):

1. If a well-encapsulated fusiform lesion less than 4 cm in diameter is found within the substance of the peripheral nerve and if under magnification the axons do not penetrate it, the lesion is probably a benign schwannoma (neurilemmoma) and should be enucleated, with the axons preserved.
2. A lesion 2 to 6 cm in diameter and adherent to surrounding tissues may be a malignant schwannoma. An incisional biopsy should be performed. If the diagnosis is confirmed, *en bloc* excision should be considered.
3. If a firm lesion is removed from the skin and proves to be a solitary neurofibroma, the patient should be carefully reexamined for stigmata of neurofibromatosis.
4. With neurofibromatosis, cutaneous lesions should be removed only if they are symptomatic. Skin lesions will rarely become malignant. Deeper neurofibromas should be removed if they rapidly enlarge or cause symptoms. These tumors may become malignant and should be biopsied, with radical excision if histologic examination so warrants.
5. Lipofibromas in the median nerve should be treated only by carpal tunnel release (and incisional biopsy). Intraneural dissection is indicated only if median nerve function has been severely compromised (or the mass is causing mechanical dysfunction).

Hemangioma of the Median Nerve

Hemangiomas are usually located in the subcutaneous or deeper soft tissues; however, several case reports have described intraneural hemangiomas involving nerve, approximately half of which are located within the median nerve (115,187–190). The lesion usually presents in childhood, and most reported patients have been female. This is a particularly difficult tumor to treat because of its intraneural location and common recurrence following excision.

History

The most common complaint is discomfort or pain, often associated with a palpable mass in the palmar forearm or wrist. The mass may be present for years before the patient seeks medical attention. Symptoms of carpal tunnel syndrome have been noted in some but not all patients (115,187–190).

Physical Examination

Most patients are within the first two decades of life. A tender palpable mass may be present. The mass can extend from the forearm into the palm. There may be associated nerve hyperirritability over the nerve, a positive Tinel's sign, and/or sensibility and motor deficits of carpal tunnel syndrome (115,187–190).

Radiographic Findings

Standard radiographs are usually negative. An arteriogram will often fail to show any abnormality, but may be useful to help rule out arteriovenous fistula or an aneurysm.

Gross and Microscopic Findings

Microscopically, these tumors demonstrate irregularly shaped endothelial-lined vascular cavernous spaces with the presence of scattered organizing thrombi (189).

Management

The intraneural hemangioma involving the median nerve is a difficult lesion to treat. Carpal tunnel release alone does not permanently resolve symptoms because of continued growth of the lesion and subsequent recurrence of symptoms. Partial tumor excision with microsurgical operative techniques will provide temporary relief, however, recurrences are still common. Some patients have had multiple recurrences following repeated attempts at tumor resection. Because of these recurrences, excision of the affected portion of the nerve with grafting of the defect has been recommended by some authors (188,189). The young age group affected helps provide satisfactory outcome of sensory regeneration following nerve grafting.

Nerve Sheath Ganglion

A ganglion cyst can form in the nerve sheath (Fig. 44.13). (63,129). The exact cause of this rare tumor is unknown,

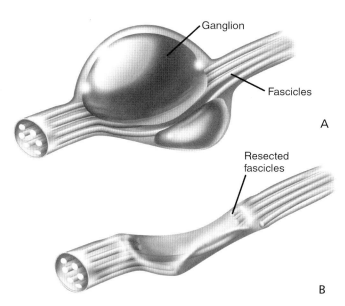

FIGURE 44.13. A: Schematic illustration of a nerve sheath ganglion, with two locules present. Nerve fascicles are depicted, showing displacement from the cystic mass. **B:** The postexcision illustration shows injury to some of the fascicles that can occur with excision.

though there is evidence that such cysts are a localized degenerative process of connective tissue secondary to a chronic mechanical irritation enzinger. The cyst can compress adjacent nerve bundles and produce motor and sensory neuropathy.

Most of these nerve ganglia arise in the peroneal nerve. However, the ulnar and median nerves are occasionally involved (63,129). The cyst pushes the nerve bundles aside so they are eccentrically located. The ganglion may be multiloculated or unilocular, and is usually filled with clear, viscous fluid similar to those found in the standard carpal ganglion. High fluid protein content has been noted (63). The ganglia lack a true cell lining and are composed of fibrous tissue with a myxoid change (129).

History and Physical Examination

The findings are similar to patients with peripheral neuropathy. A mass is usually not palpable. The tumor is usually discovered a the time of carpal tunnel or ulnar tunnel release.

Management

The diagnosis of a nerve sheath ganglion is usually obvious at the time of operative exposure, where an eccentrically located intraneural cyst mass with translucent walls is discovered. Adequate longitudinal exposure of the nerve is recommended, since the ganglion may extend several centimeters within the epineurium in between nerve fascicles. If the ganglion can be separated from the fascicles and can be easily excised without nerve injury, this is performed under magnification. Simple operative excision may be difficult if multiple locules exist along the nerve. This requires more difficult and extensive dissection for excision, with associated risks of fascicular disruption (Fig. 44.13). In these situations, incision and drainage of the ganglion may be performed instead of excision. The ganglion is incised over each accessible loculation to allow drainage (63,129).

BENIGN TUMORS OF THE BONE

Common bone tumors involving the hand and wrist include the chrondroma, osteochondroma (osteocartilaginous exostosis), giant cell tumor, osteoid osteoma, aneurysmal bone cyst (ABC), and the unicameral bone cyst.

Solitary Enchrondroma

The solitary chrondroma is a cartilage tumor that can present either as a solitary lesion located within bone (known as the enchondroma), or as a solitary lesion outside of bone, the extraosseous chrondroma (56–59,86,113,191–196). In addition, multiple enchrondramata (Ollier's Disease), a condition that rarely involves the wrist, is usually associated with deformities of the axial skeleton.

The solitary enchonroma is the most common bone tumor of the hand, and virtually always located in the phalanges and metacarpals. Involvement in the wrist is rare (56–59,86,113,191,193–196). It is thought to possibly represent a cartilage rest rather than a neoplasm (57), however, malignant degeneration to chondrosarcoma, though rare, has been reported (23). If arising from a cartilage rest, the enchondroma appears to form from misplaced islands of cartilage that are shed into the intramedullary area of bone originating from the growing epiphyseal plate (197). Reports have either shown no sex predilection or have suggested men more frequently affected than women. Most are adolescents or young adults, with the majority of patients presenting within the first four decades of life. The mean age reports varies from 22 to 40 years old, and with an age range from 10 to 70 years (56–59,86,113,191,194–197). The lesions are a generalized risk for pathological fracture, and the patient will often present only after such a fracture has occurred.

History

Many lesions are asymptomatic and are discovered only when the hand and wrist are radiographed for an unrelated injury. The patient may complain of painless swelling, or minimal tenderness. Except for pathologic fracture, most lesions will not produce pain. The patient may relate a history of minimal or substantial trauma, with acute onset of pain, swelling, and deformity indicative of pathologic fracture.

Physical Examination

In the absence of a fracture, most lesions produce few physical exam findings. Swelling and localized tenderness may be present. If the cortex is expanded in a subcutaneous location, a firm oval bulge may be palpable. With small lesions, physical examination findings are usually negative. Most lesions do not restrict motion.

When presenting with a pathological fracture, the patient will have typical findings of an acute fracture, though the mechanism or injury may be minimal. The patient will have the expected localized swelling, tenderness, motion limited by pain, and fracture deformity. Pathological fracture of the carpus will produce point tenderness and swelling; fracture deformity will be minimal (57–59).

Radiographic Findings

The enchondroma appears as a well defined, lytic bone lesion that may have calcifications or stippling. In large lesions, the entire lesion may appear to be vaguely trabeculated. The cortex is commonly expanded and thinned, and the lesion may be lined by a sclerotic margin indicative of reactive bone. The tumor does not cross the epiphyseal plate. These lesions may appear radiographically similar to the ABC or to the giant cell tumor of bone. However, the ABC usually shows more of a marked "blowout" appearance of the cortex. The giant cell tumor of bone is rarely calcified, appears near the end of the bone, and often is trabeculated (57).

Gross and Microscopic Findings

The enchondroma appears grossly as a white or bluish-white collection of friable tissue. It may extrude from the wound when the cortex is opened. Gritty islands of calcified deposits may be palpable.

On microscopic examination, there are lobules of relatively acellular cartilage with rare mitoses. If the biopsy is performed several weeks after a pathological fracture, the healing bone may be microscopically alarmingly suggestive of a malignancy. If the biopsy is made soon after the fracture, potential confusion with a malignancy is rare.

Management

For a relatively small solitary lesion that is found as an incidental radiographic finding, observation alone with periodic clinical and radiographic examination can be considered. Operative management of a solitary lesion is indicated when tissue is desired for definitive histological diagnosis, or if the lesion is large, symptomatic, or has caused deformity. Treatment is by curettage and filling the defect with autogenous bone graft (196,198–201). Even for minimally symptomatic lesions, the present authors prefer operative management, both for definitive tissue diagnosis and for the prevention of an impending pathologic fracture.

For the patient presenting with a pathological fracture, recommendations have included either (a) immobilization until the fracture has healed followed by curettage of the tumor, or (b) operative management of the lesion and fracture simultaneously. Management by immobilization until fracture healing followed by curettage of the tumor produces two periods of disability for the patient. Alternatively, the lesion can be treated at the time of acute fracture. The lesion is curetted, the bone stabilized as necessary with internal fixation, and the defect filled with an autogenous bone graft. It is advisable to obtain the graft first, or with a separate field or team, to avoid seeding the enchondroma to the bone graft donor site.

The use of implanted bone morphogenic protein may also play a potential role in the treatment and regeneration of the enchondroma defect (202).

Though rare, malignant degeneration into chondrosarcoma has been reported, arising from intraosseous enchondromas of the small bones of the hand (23). This possibility must be kept in mind during nonoperative management of these lesions, especially when new pain or swelling arises in a known lesion. Additionally, if a recurrence develops after operative management, this possibility must be kept in mind.

Multiple Enchondromatosis (Ollier's Disease)

Multiple enchondromata are far less common than solitary lesions, and rarely involve the wrist. These are mentioned only briefly to emphasize the possibility of malignant degeneration into chondrosarcoma. Multiple enchondroma lesions tend to be much larger than the solitary lesions, and are often associated with deformities of the axial skeleton (59,203). Typically, the tumors are found on only one side of the body. If bilateral, one side is usually more heavily involved than the other (57). Unlike osteochondromatosis, multiple enchondromatoses are not familial. Reports either show no significant sex predilection, or suggest a male to female ratio of 2:1 (197). Similar to the solitary enchondroma, multiple enchondromatoses are usually found in children or young adults; an average age at initial presentation is about 21 years, with a range of 9 months to 58 years (197). New lesions do not usually develop after maturity. Phalanges and metacarpals of the ulnar side of the hand are the most commonly involved area of the wrist and hand.

Multiple enchondromatosis associated with multiple hemangiomas is known as *Maffucci's syndrome*. Maffucci's syndrome is nonheritable and includes multiple enchondrally formed bones that are afflicted with proliferating masses of benign cartilage, (most of which are enchondromas), is usually found in conjunction with hemangiomatosis, and is usually located in the soft tissues (and not in bone) (197).

Management

Multiple enchondroma lesions have a considerable risk of malignant degeneration. The incidence of sarcomatous degeneration is relatively high, with 50% of patients with multiple enchondromatosis developing at least one sarcomatous lesion (57).

Indications for operative management include chronic discomfort, limb dysfunction, progressive deformity, sudden enlargement, or new onset or increase in pain (especially occurring in known, previously asymptomatic lesions) (57,59). The management of small, symptomatic lesions in the metacarpals or carpus is as described above with excision and bone grafting. With large lesions, or those with suspected malignant degeneration, incisional biopsy is indicated (59).

Osteochondroma (Solitary or Multiple)

The osteochondroma is a benign, cartilage-capped protuberance emanating from the metaphysis or diaphysis. Multiple osteochondromas, or osteochondromatosis, is a familial condition characterized by multiple lesions. Solitary or multiple osteocartilaginous exostoses may arise in the metacarpals, phalanges or both bones of the forearm (18,197,204–207). In the wrist, the distal ulna and radius are most commonly affected. Overall, in the upper extremity, the proximal humerus is the most common site (197).

Osteochondromatosis has also been referred to as multiple osteocartilaginous exostoses, hereditary multiple exostoses, diaphyseal aclasia, and hereditary deforming chondrodysplasia (57,59,204). The lesions are commonly hereditary, and appear to affect males more than females. Although an unaffected carrier male will not transmit the syndrome, the unaffected carrier female may do so.

Malignant transformation is rare in osteochondromas involving the hand or wrist. However, in general, in patients with multiple hereditary exostoses, chondrosarcomatous degeneration of the cartilage caps develops in at least one lesion in 10% to 25% of patients (57,203).

History

Because of the awareness of a strong familial history of most patients, the patient may discover a bony lump in the involved extremity. In the upper extremity, common sites are the proximal humerus and the distal forearm. Most will discover the lesions during the first decade of life. New lesions rarely develop after the patient reaches skeletal maturity. If the lesion is superficial, the patient will complain of a palpable mass, with may or may not have tenderness. When involving the distal radius or ulna, the patient will often complain of forearm deformity (ulnar deviation of the wrist) and or loss of motion (usually of forearm rotation).

Physical Examination

Involved patients are frequently of short stature, although not dwarfed (57). If the ulna is involved, the ulna is usually shorter than the radius, both bones of the forearm are frequently bowed, and there is often loss or restriction of forearm pronation/supination. The hand may be subsequently ulnarly deviated, associated with the short ulna. Deformity within the hand is usually less severe than at the forearm and wrist.

Radiographic Findings

An early osteochondroma lesion may appear or consist only of an asymmetric overgrowth of the cortex adjacent to the epiphyseal plate. As the lesion grows, there may be diffuse thickening of the involved metaphysis, with an irregular cortical outline. Subsequently, the mass matures into a bony excrescence or an elongated cortical outgrowth. Some lesions will develop in a sessile fashion, and will radiographically appear as an irregular cauliflower-shaped outline that overlies the metaphyses. There may be notable retardation of growth on the side of the tumor.

Gross and Microscopic Findings

The osteochondroma is a bony lesion comprised of a bone stalk and cartilage cap. The cartilage appears as whitish or bluish white normal cartilage covering. The bone stalk grossly appears as normal cortical bone, emanating from the metaphyseal bone. Microscopically, each lesion has a bone stalk with a central core of cancellous bone surrounded by somewhat immature cortical bone. A periosteum covers the stalk. The cartilage cap is comprised of hyaline-appearing cartilage. The cap often shows evidence of enchondral ossification and calcification.

Management

Most asymptomatic lesions without limb deformity may be treated with observation. Indications for operative management include local symptoms, (tenderness), deformity (i.e., progressive ulnar deviation of the wrist), functional disability (loss of forearm rotation or wrist motion), or the need for tissue for definitive diagnosis. Though it is usually optimal to delay operative treatment until closure of the epiphysis, this may not be indicated in those with deformity, loss of motion, or in patients with suspected malignant transformation. Malignant degeneration should be suspected in an exostosis that suddenly enlarges or becomes painful, especially after physeal closure. Small lesions are managed with excisional biopsy; large lesions, especially those that are suspected to have undergone malignant degeneration, can be treated with incisional biopsy, with definitive treatment to follow when histological analysis has been completed.

Additional causes of pain that develops in a known, previously asymptomatic osteochondroma include formation of an overlying inflamed bursa, development of an associated pseudoaneurysm, infarction of the cartilage cap or osseous portion of the osteochondroma, fracture through the stalk, mechanical irritation (to neighboring muscles, ligaments, or tendons), or nerve compression (40,41,197). Despite these other causes of pain, malignant transformation is a common cause of new symptoms, and should be treated accordingly (197).

Osteoid Osteoma

The osteoid osteoma is a small painful lesion of bone of unknown etiology (Fig. 44.14) (16,40,41,59,200,208–228). It is a distinctive, benign lesion characterized by a less than 2 cm pea-like mass of abnormal bone (the nidus) located in a shell of reactive bone. The nidus is richly innervated by nerve fibers, thereby evoking considerable pain (197).

The osteoid osteoma accounts for 2% to 3% of all excised primary bone tumors and accounts for about 11% of all benign lesions (197). The lesion frequently occurs in children and young adults, with nearly all patients less than 20 years old. The male-to-female ratio is approximately 2 to 1 (197,229). Though described as frequently occurring in the femur and tibia, these lesions also occur sporadically in the carpus (especially the capitate and scaphoid), metacarpals, and in the phalanges (215,230–242). In a recent literature review, the following distribution of the osteoid osteoma in the hand and wrist was found: 40 lesions in the phalanges, six in the metacarpals, eight in the capitate, seven in the scaphoid, and one or two in each of the other carpal bones (229).

The origin of the osteoid osteoma remains unknown. The lesion consists of a central nidus of richly vascularized mesenchymal tissue that produces irregularly arranged bars of osteoid (40,41). This central soft nidus is surrounded by shell of reactive bone and grossly has the appearance is that of a "pea within a pod" (40,41,197,243). There are usually several nerve endings within the lesion (unusual for the skeleton), which are thought to account for the common and significant amount of pain produced. In the early stages, the lesion is soft and is easily surgically removed with a curette. As the lesion ages, the osteoid material mineralizes, and the central nidus may become extremely dense. When ossification occurs in the central nidus, there remains around the periphery an area of well-vascularized mesenchymal tissue that does not calcify, so that one may find on occasion a hard central nidus lying in an envelope of fibrous connective tissue surrounded by its dense shell of reactive bone. The reactive shell surrounding an osteoid osteoma is much thicker, often two to three times as thick

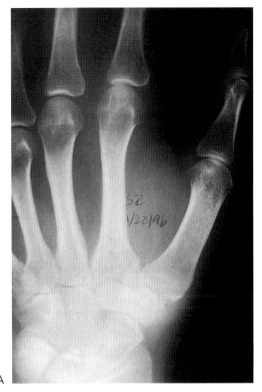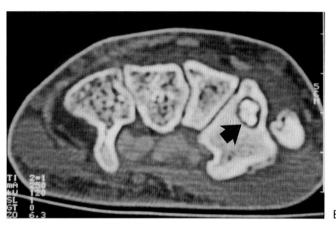

FIGURE 44.14. Radiograph **(A)** and computed tomography (CT) scan **(B)** of a wrist containing an osteoid osteoma of the trapezium. The lesion is barely visible with the standard radiographs, which demonstrate a sclerotic nidus with surrounding lucency; this, in turn, is surrounded by dense reactive bone. The lesion is clearly visible on the CT scan *(arrow)*.

as the nidus is wide, than is the reactive bone about other lesions (244). This thickened bone is among the most identifying features as seen on radiographs, computed tomography (CT) or MRI scans, or tomograms (224,245).

History

The consistent complaint is pain, often persistent, debilitating, and worse at night. Classically, the pain is markedly reduced with aspirin or other nonsteroidal antiinflammatory medications; however, wide variations occur regarding the response to these medications. There is usually no history of redness or deformity. About 12% of patients will relate the onset of symptoms to an incident of trauma, and 63% have noted swelling (229). Patients' main complaint is usually persistent pain (90% of patients), with night pain noted in 71% (229). Because of the difficulty in diagnosis, many patients will have had symptoms present for 6 to 24 months before a correct diagnosis is made. Many patients will present for a second opinion because of an initial misdiagnosis.

Physical Examination

The most consistent physical exam finding is tenderness, though the extent is dependent on the location. The tenderness may be poorly localized in deeply seated lesions. Though the cortex may be slightly expanded, the deformity is usually so slight as to not be detectable by palpation. Persistent pain may lead to loss of motion or stiffness from secondary soft tissue contracture following lack of use or self-imposed immobilization, but not from mechanical block or tumor deformity. If it is near a synovial joint, a mild sympathetic effusion may exist, but fluid analysis will be normal. In many patients, the physical examination is virtually negative, with no bone expansion, deformity, heat, redness, or loss of motion (40,41,57,243).

Radiographic Findings

On standard radiographs, the osteoid osteoma appears as an eccentric area of cortical density or sclerosis surrounding a radiolucent zone that contains a radiodense nidus (Fig. 44.14A). The entire lesion, including the surrounding sclerotic (reactive) bone, is usually less than a centimeter, and the nidus is usually 3 to 6 mm in diameter. The lesion may be difficult to demonstrate on standard radiographs, especially in the carpus. The central radiolucent area may not be visible against the irregular margins and overlapping cortices of the neighboring carpal bones. In some lesions, the entire carpal bone may appear radiodense (243).

CT scans will usually identify the lesion in detail (Fig. 44.14B). Narrow cuts in the scan will increase the number of images to identify the lesion. It is possible, though unlikely, to miss the lesion if wide cuts are obtained in the presence of a small lesion.

MRI will also identify the lesion; however, the CT scan will usually give superior detail of the osseous portions of this bone lesion (246).

Gross and Microscopic Findings

The gross appearance of the lesion is usually of a nidus of osteoid tissue within a cortical defect or a defect surrounded by sclerotic, reactive bone. The nidus of osteoid tissue appears as dark reddish-brown gritty soft tissue that is highly vascular. In the longstanding mature lesion, the nidus may have mineralized and appear as a sclerotic density within reactive bone.

Microscopically, the nidus is composed of immature trabeculae enveloped in vascular primitive mesenchymal tissue. Calcification of the trabeculae may or may not be present depending on the maturity of the lesion. The osteoid is present in waves or "bars" that are thick or plump, haphazard in arrangement. Hyperchromatic plump osteoblasts are present, which produce the osteoid. Giant cells are frequently present throughout the nidus; however, they seldom appear to be reorganizing the osteoid. If viewed out of context, the actual cellular appearance may suggest, or be confused with, osteosarcoma. However, the lesion will usually contain few mitotic cells and has no chondroid element. Within the tissue, several nerve endings may be identified. If the lesion is removed with a portion of the reactive bone, dense, thick trabecular bone will be seen, often with several osteoblasts that may be thickening the reactive trabeculae (40,41).

Management

The treatment of a carpal osteoid osteoma is complete excision or curettage (247,248). The lesion can usually be localized with intraoperative radiographs or fluoroscopy (though small lesions are not always visible and can be difficult to localize intraoperatively). Localization with radiographs will also aid in assurance of complete excision. Some authors have recommended radiographs of the excised bone and of the original tumor site to verify excision of the nidus.

The use of scintigraphy or tetracycline fluorescence has also been recommended to more precisely localize the lesion (1,249,250). In addition, percutaneous removal of an osteoid osteoma using CT control has also been described (224).

Following excision, marked relief of pain is usually obtained. Recurrence is rare, and has been attributed to incomplete removal of the nidus. Several authors have stressed the importance of complete removal of the nidus, advocating *en bloc* excision of a portion of bone and the use of radiographs to confirm complete excision. Others, however, have shown that curettage of the lesion is adequate (16,40,41,59,200,208–228).

Giant Cell Tumor of Bone

The giant cell tumor, also known as the osteoclastoma of bone, is a benign tumor that usually involves the epiphyseal region of long bones and is characterized by benign-appearing multinucleated osteoclast-like giant cells and stromal cells (56–58,86,94,97,147,251–259). The giant cell tumor represents about 5% of primary bone tumors (197). In the wrist, the distal radius and ulna are most commonly affected (Fig. 44.15). This incidence is much less than that of enchondroma, which it resembles radiographically. The mean age at presentation is 22 years (which is about 10 years younger than the reported mean age for areas other than the hand and wrist). About 12% of lesions in the hand and wrist become malignant (56–58,86,94,147,251,252,259). When the carpal bones are involved, there is a higher incidence of multicentric foci.

History

The most common symptom is pain. Patients often give a history of relatively mild trauma. Many lesions have not been diagnosed on initial presentation since the trivial nature of the reported injury and mild symptoms do not appear to warrant radiograph examination (56–58). Patients may also note a palpable tenderness, as well as a mass or swelling in the distal forearm (in distal radius or ulna lesions). Patients usually do not complain of loss of motion or dysfunction (56–58,86,94,147,251,252,259). A history of acute pain following trauma may indicate a pathological fracture through the lesion (197).

Physical Examination

Lesions that present in the distal radius and ulna are usually associated with palpable tenderness. There may also be mild

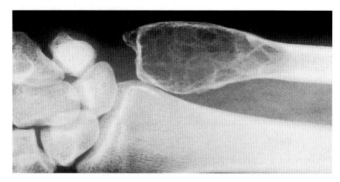

FIGURE 44.15. Radiograph of a giant cell tumor of the distal ulna, which is easily confused on radiograph with enchondroma.

swelling, and in approximately half of patients, a bony mass or expansion of the epiphyseal regions may be palpable (Bougmill). If the mass is large, wrist motion or forearm rotation may be compromised (56–58,86,94,147,251,252,259).

Radiographic Findings

Standard radiographs of the wrist usually demonstrate a radiolucent, symmetric lesion in the epiphyseal region of the distal radius or distal ulna (Fig. 44.15). Lesions in the distal radius outnumber the lesions in the distal ulna by about 10:1 (197). The lesion is usually centrally located. The cortex may be expanded, and there is often thinning and loss or destruction of both cortical and cancellous bone. The lesion may expand so that the diameter of the bone is significantly enlarged, and eventually, the cortex may be eroded or fractured. It usually does not contain stippling, calcification, or trabeculation, as is often seen in cartilaginous tumors (or in recurrent giant cell tumors previously treated with operative management) (56–58,86,94,147,251,252,259). When stippling or trabeculation is present, the lesion may resemble an enchondroma (Fig. 44.15).

Because of the high incidence of multicentric foci of giant cell tumors when the carpal bones are involved, evaluation with a bone scan or skeletal survey has been recommended when giant cell tumors are found in the carpus (56–58).

Gross and Microscopic Findings

The lesion usually has an eggshell-thin covering of periosteum or periosteal new bone formation. The end of the long bone may be visually expanded. The tumor tissue is reddish brown in color, vascular, and friable. (Its gross appearance bears no resemblance to the white glistening tissue found in enchondromas) (56–58,86,94,147,251,252, 259). Areas of hemorrhage or fibrosis may be present (197).

Microscopically, the lesion consists of many multinucleated giant cells admixed with short, round to oval, or spindle-shaped stromal cells. The stromal cells contain nuclei similar to those within giant cells. All cells that make up the tumor do not display objective anaplasia (197). The cells are suspended together loosely by a sparse intercellular matrix and vascular network (56–58,86,94,147,251,252,259).

Several bone tumors have giant cells that must be distinguished from the conventional giant cell tumor. These range from benign lesions, such as the nonossifying fibroma, to locally aggressive lesions like the ABC and high-grade sarcomas (197).

Management

If the diagnosis is in doubt, or if a possible malignancy is suspected, incisional biopsy is indicated. Once the diagnosis is made, treatment includes curettage (with or without application of concentrated phenol, alcohol, liquid nitrogen, or methyl methacrylate) or *en bloc* excision with or without reconstruction using an autologous bone graft. Partial carpectomy and arthrodesis have also been used.

Curettage, with or without bone grafting of the resulting defect, has a relative high recurrence rate. To minimize recurrence, adequate exposure and removal of tumor must be accomplished. A window is placed in the cortex that is similar in size to the lesion. This will provide wide visualization and access to the entire inner aspect of the area of bone involved. (Curettage through a small window risks recurrence because of failure to curette the overhanging edges of bone). Through the large window, the entire cavity lining is aggressively and thoroughly curetted in a systematic fashion, removing any sclerotic boundaries, which may contain microscopic extension of tumor. The cavity is irrigated, the soft tissues surrounding the lesion are protected with petrolatum gauze, and the inner surface of the tumor is treated with concentrated phenol solution or liquid nitrogen, followed by absolute alcohol, and copious saline irrigation (58). For large lesions, where potential pathologic collapse of the bone is present, methyl methacrylate may be used to fill and support the defect. The lesion can also be filled with a cancellous bone graft, with or without cortical struts for support (57,59).

Because of the high recurrence rate of the giant cell tumor following curettage, *en bloc* excision of the tumor may be more optimal as the procedure of choice after biopsy confirmation of the diagnosis, especially if the tumor is large, if there is a violation of the cortex, or if the tumor has recurred following previous treatment with curettage. Lesions of the distal ulna can be treated successfully with resection of the end of the bone. Replacement is seldom necessary for function (58). Management of lesions of the distal radius, however, is more complex, as these lesions are often extensive when initially diagnosed. When distal tumor extension from the distal radius has invaded the carpus, partial or complete carpectomy is performed followed by radiocarpal or radiometacarpal arthrodesis (56–58,86, 94,199,215,252,257,259).

Multiple giant cell tumor lesions of bone (multicentric giant cell tumor) is a rare condition, accounting for less than 1% of giant cell tumors in locations other than the hand. However, in those infrequent instances when a giant cell tumor of bone does occur in the hand or wrist, the incidence of multicentric foci is much higher than when other sites are involved. Therefore, use of a bone scan or skeletal survey should be considered in a giant cell tumor in the bones of the hand or wrist. This is particularly so when the tumor is in the carpus, for carpal bones are commonly involved in patients with multicentric giant cell tumors.

Aneurysmal Bone Cyst

The ABC is a benign lesion characterized by cyst-like walls of predominantly fibrous tissue filled with free flowing blood (197). Almost half of the cases are associated with a precursor lesion such as fibrous dysplasia, giant cell tumor, chondroblastoma, or osteosarcoma. The lesion is felt to be a vascular anomaly that is initiated by trauma or precursor tumors. The actual lesion is, therefore, neither a cyst nor a neoplasm, but rather a periosteal or intraosseous arteriovenous malformation associated with other benign or malignant afflictions. Because benign precursors are not seen in half the cases, all vestiges may be destroyed by rapid growth of the ABC (197,260–267).

Overall, unequivocal cases represent about 1% of primary bone tumors; more than 2% if small ABC components are seen and numerous other entities are included (197). The lesion is rare in the wrist and hand, representing only five cases of 492 total skeletal lesions (197). Two of these were located in the distal ulna, one in the distal radius, one in the carpus, and two in the metacarpals.

The differential diagnosis of the ABC can include fibrous dysplasia, giant cell tumor, eosinophilic granuloma, incipient lytic osteosarcoma, simple bone cyst, chondromyxoid fibroma, hyperparathyroidism, and infection. In differentiating the lesion from a giant cell tumor, the ABC usually involves a younger patient (less than 20 years old), compared to the giant cell tumor (mean age of 20–30 years old), and the ABC is usually located in the metaphysis or diaphysis, whereas the giant cell tumor is usually in the epiphysis.

Though locally aggressive, the lesion does not metastasize. The lesion is especially problematic from a diagnostic standpoint because it is easily mistaken radiographically and histologically for a malignant tumor as a result of its great rate of growth, tremendous destruction of bone, and marked cellular proliferation in its early and midphases of development (197).

History

The usual complaint is pain, usually of less than 3 months' duration. The patient may relate a history of swelling or localized mass. There is often a history of minor trauma that precipitates the symptoms.

With lesions in the long bones, 85% of patients complained of pain, and 20% presented with acute pain of a pathologic fracture (268).

Physical Examination

Visible swelling and palpable tenderness are usually present. The distal ulna and radius are the most commonly involved areas of the wrist and hand. A painful limited range of motion is possible if the lesion is located near the wrist joints. Patients with pathologic fracture will present with the expected finding of fracture pain, tenderness, swelling, and possible deformity.

Radiographic Findings

In the early phases of development, the ABC will appear radiographically as a small to large area of circumscribed or poorly demarcated lysis. There is usually little or no reactive bone or sclerotic margins. In the later or "midphase," the lesion will enlarge, and there may be marked cortical destruction. The lesion may expand the cortex, and with cortical destruction, the classical "blowout" appearance is present. In the distal portion of long bones, a Codman's triangle may be seen.

Gross and Microscopic Findings

On gross examination of the lesion *in situ*, the ABC is a blood-filled cavity with cortical expansion and destruction. The gross appearance has been likened to a bloody sponge (197).

Microscopically, the lesion consists of thin walls filled with blood cells. The walls of the lesion may resemble aberrant callus and contain exuberant spindle cells, osteoid, and woven bone slivers, with and without osteoblast rimming, osteoclast-like giant cells, and occasionally a rather peculiar characteristic lacy chondroid. The lesion pathologically can be confused with an osteosarcoma. Conversely, the telangiectatic osteosarcoma can be confused or misdiagnosed as an ABC (197).

Management

The ABC presents the difficult management challenges of eradicating vascular anomalies or cystic lesions. Described treatment has included curettage or *en bloc* bone excision. Because recurrences are common, *en bloc* excision is more often recommended (59). In the carpus, this may require secondary reconstructive procedures, similar to those described for the giant cell tumor.

Unicameral Bone Cyst

The unicameral bone cyst is a benign, simple, intraosseous cyst (197,269). It is a fluid-filled lesion lined by fibrous tissue and a single row of mesothelial-like cells. It is considered the only true cyst of primary intraosseous origin. It is relatively rare in the hands and wrist, and the distal radius is more commonly affected. The lesion is usually asymptomatic and may be an incidental finding on radiographs. Pathologic fracture may occur and account for acute pain and swelling following minimal trauma (59,197).

The unicameral bone cyst comprises about 3% of primary bone tumors. Male-to-female ratio is 2.5 to 1. The lesion is usually seen in childhood to adolescence. About 85% of patients are less than 20 years old (197).

Physical Examination

Physical examination is usually without significant findings. Some lesions will have mild tenderness. There is no deformity or swelling. If pathologic fracture occurs, expected acute localized pain, tenderness, and swelling will be present.

Radiographic Findings

The unicameral bone cyst appears as a well-defined, symmetric, purely lytic lesion usually occurring eccentrically in the metaphysis of the distal radius. The cortex may be thinned. Large lesions may have a lucent "bubbly" or multiloculated appearance (197).

Gross and Microscopic Findings

The unicameral bone cyst is usually filled with fluid. Occasionally, fibrin strands or fibroosseous tissues will be found within the cavity from prior fracture repair (197); sampling is via a #15 Craig needle with a stylet attached to a syringe plus an 18-gauge needle attached to a second syringe.

Microscopically, the lining is a thin fibrous wall lined by flat to slightly plump layers of cells of mesothelial or, less likely, endothelial origin (197).

Management

No specific treatment may be necessary for small, asymptomatic lesions discovered as incidental radiographic findings. Some lesions have undergone spontaneous healing.

For larger lesions, especially with impending pathologic fracture, corticosteroid injection treatment has been successful. The technique has been described by Scaglietti et al. (270) and Peimer et al. (59). Under fluoroscopic control, the cyst is aspirated percutaneously via large-bore needles. Cyst fluid is sent for laboratory analysis to include cell count, culture, and blood chemistry (59,270). After cyst fluid evacuation, 40 to 80 mg of methylprednisolone is injected, using up to 200 mg for large cysts. Radiographs are taken about every 6 weeks. Healing often occurs after about 8 to 12 weeks. The method may be repeated two or three times, if indicated. This treatment by intraosseous injection of methylprednisolone offers an alternative method to surgical curettage and grafting via a cortical window (59,270).

If injection fails to heal the cyst, or if the lesion is exceedingly large, operative management with curettage is recommended. Similar to the treatment of giant cell tumors, it is imperative that the cortical window be of adequate size to permit satisfactory access to the entire walls of the lesion. Sequential removal of the lining is essential to prevent recurrence. Large lesions may be grafted with cancellous graft or cortical struts as needed.

Recurrence has been noted to occur following operative management. Malignant degeneration, however, does not occur (88,194,195,271).

INFLAMMATORY DISORDERS

Inflammatory conditions commonly produce tumors or tumor-like masses in the carpal area (77,272–282). Rheumatoid arthritis can produce dorsal carpal tenosynovitis and rheumatoid nodules, two common occurrences often mistaken for tumors.

Rheumatoid Tenosynovitis

The inflammatory response associated with rheumatoid arthritis may produce tenosynovitis in the wrist and digits, resulting in a tumor-like mass. In the wrist, the dorsal carpal area is most commonly affected, associated with the extensor tendons. The tenosynovitis initially forms deep to the extensor retinaculum. It extends distally and proximally, causing swelling below the rigid ligament. When extensive, the inflammatory tissue will proliferate, forming a tumor mass on the dorsum of the wrist. The mass may be mistaken for a dorsal carpal ganglion. The inflammatory tissue may invade the extensor tendons, and tendon rupture is a well-known complication of chronic dorsal wrist tenosynovitis. Extensor tendon rupture actually results from a combination of factors: erosion caused by bone irregularity, compressive effect of the dorsal carpal retinaculum, and direct rheumatoid tenosynovitis pannus erosions into the tendons. The extensor tendons to the small and ring finger are usually the first involved, probably related to the contributing tendon erosion from the head of the ulna.

History

The tenosynovitis has variable symptoms. In some patients, it is associated with significant pain and tenderness. In others, there are minimal associated symptoms. The patient may relate a history of sudden or gradual loss of digital extensor function, indicative of an acute or gradual attenuation of the extensor tendons, respectively. The patient may relate a prior (mis)diagnosis of a dorsal carpal ganglion.

Physical Examination

The dorsal tenosynovitis is usually located in the middorsal carpal area. The inflammatory mass is soft, boggy, movable, and has variable tenderness. If inadequate digital extension is present, extensor tendon rupture must be considered. (Other causes of loss of digital extension include joint subluxation of the metacarpophalangeal joints; subluxation of the extensor tendon into the valley between the metacarpal head, causing loss of extensor efficiency; and peripheral neuropathy from posterior interosseous nerve compression following rheumatoid involvement at the elbow or in the forearm, as related to more proximal inflammatory causes.)

Radiographic Findings

Rheumatoid tenosynovitis on the dorsum of the wrist may present a soft tissue shadow. Associated carpal changes from the arthritis are usually evident.

Gross and Microscopic Findings

Rheumatoid tenosynovitis grossly appears as boggy, edematous glistening synovial tissue. It may be found adherent to the tendons and require sharp dissection to separate the tissue from the tendons. Moderate amounts of associated tendon attenuation or frank rupture may be found.

Microscopically, the tenosynovitis appears as synovial tissue, usually with abundant inflammatory cells.

Management

Initial management of rheumatoid tenosynovitis includes a regimen of conservative treatment, consisting of anti-inflammatory medication, splinting, rest, and/or physical/occupational hand therapy. Surgical excision is usually indicated if the tenosynovitis is persistent for 6 to 12 months, or if extensor rupture has occurred. Management includes resection of the tenosynovium and tendon reconstruction as necessary. The irregular ulnar head and Lister's tubercle can be resected and smoothed, and a portion of the extensor retinaculum can be transferred deep to the extensor tendons to minimize tendon contact with the carpal bones.

Rheumatoid Nodules

Firm nodules located in the subcutaneous tissues are not uncommon in rheumatoid arthritis and are occasionally seen in patients with systemic lupus erythematous (283). In the wrist, the nodules are often located on the dorsal extensor surface. Occasionally the nodules cause skin erosion and can form a draining sinus from necrosis of the central core.

History

The nodules are often painless. However, if subject to repeated trauma, the nodules can become tender and, rarely, associated with skin breakdown. Patients occasionally give a history of functional disturbance if the nodules are large.

Physical Examination

The nodules are firm, of variable tenderness. They are not attached to the underlying tendons. In the rheumatoid upper extremity, besides the dorsal wrist, common areas of nodules include the extensor surface of the forearm and the palmar aspect of the digits.

Radiographic Findings

The nodules will appear as soft tissue shadow on the standard radiograph. Associated osseous changes of rheumatoid arthritis will be noted.

Management

Symptomatic nodules can be resected (283). Homeostasis is emphasized, and the use of a drain to prevent hematoma formation suggested. These is some tendency for nodules to recur following resection, especially when associated with multiple extensive involvement (283).

ASSOCIATED DISORDERS

Carpal Boss

A carpal or carpometacarpal boss is a raised, thickened area of bone or exostosis usually located at the dorsal base of the index or long metacarpal (Fig. 44.16) (61). The origin of the mass is unknown. It is sometimes considered an osteophyte and may or may not be associated with osteoarthritis. The carpal boss may resemble a firm dorsal wrist ganglion, or vice versa (Fig. 44.16A,B).

History and Physical Examination

The mass may be painless or have varing amounts of tenderness, either from external irritation or from friction. The carpal boss can cause local encroachment of cutaneous nerves, and patients will complain of neuritic symptoms of local pain, radiation, and/or possible paresthesias. The mass may cause extensor tendon subluxation or a "snapping" phenomenon as the tendon passes over the mass. Dorsiflexion of the wrist may also precipitate symptoms, especially if there is a component of dorsal osseous impingement. Many lesions are asymptomatic; physical deformity may be the main complaint. If located deep to the overlying cutaneous nerves, tenderness and a positive Tinel's sign may be precipitated.

Radiographic Findings

The carpal boss is usually viewed on the lateral radiograph, demonstrating an exostosis on the dorsal surface of the base of the index or long metacarpal (Fig. 44.16C). A slightly

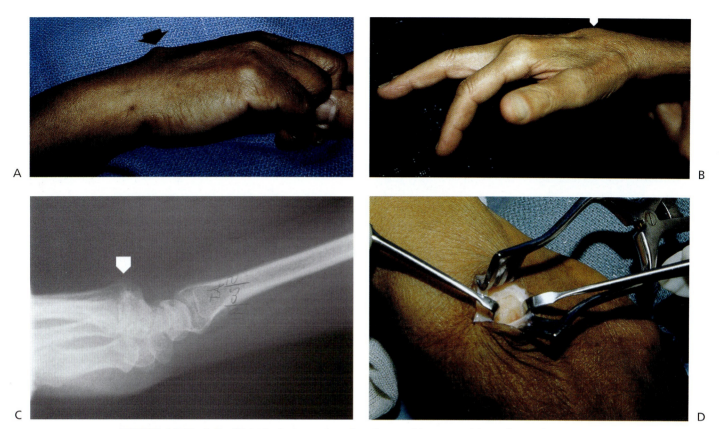

FIGURE 44.16. A,B: Clinical photographs of patients with a carpal boss *(arrows)*. Note the resemblance to a dorsal carpal ganglion or to rheumatoid tenosynovitis. The carpal boss has caused a rupture of the extensor digitorum communis *(index)* and extensor indicis proprius, resulting in loss of index finger extension **(B)**. **C:** Radiograph showing carpal boss from the base of the metacarpal *(arrow)*. **D:** Operative excision of the carpal boss.

oblique radiograph that views the mass in profile will help demonstrate the lesion.

Management

Management for asymptomatic lesions is observation and patient reassurance. Symptomatic lesions, especially those associated with painful motion, subluxing extensor tendons, or neuritic symptoms, warrant excision (Fig. 44.16D). Resection may require partial detachment (and reattachment) or the extensor carpi radialis longus or brevis or a portion of the joint capsule. Appropriate postoperative immobilization is then required.

Calcinosis

Calcinosis is a disorder of unknown etiology that involves deposition of calcium in soft tissues (Fig. 44.17). In the wrist, calcium deposition is usually in the vicinity of, or within, the insertion of tendons, such as the flexor carpi ulnaris. In the wrist and hand, the carpal area accounts for about two-thirds of cases reported (61). (Other areas include the collateral ligaments of the digits and thumb, the thumb extensor tendons, and the tendons of the intrinsic muscles). Rarely, multiple deposits are noted.

History and Physical Examination

Pain is the usually initial complaint. About one-third of patients will give a history of trauma (61). Local tenderness, pain with passive stretch or active contraction of the associated tendon is usually present.

Radiographic Findings

Radiographs obtained soon after the onset of symptoms may show a light cloudiness, suggesting a deposit (Fig. 44.17). Later, the calcium deposit will mature into a more readily outlined calcific mass. A common location is the palmar surface of the pisiform (at the insertion of the flexor carpi ulnaris), visualized radiographically on the lateral view.

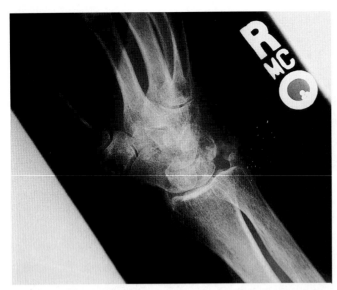

FIGURE 44.17. Radiograph showing calcium deposits distal to the ulnar head.

Management

Management is usually nonoperative, using standard methods similar to those used to treat inflammatory conditions. Heat, rest, splinting the carpus, and use of oral or local anti-inflammatory medication are initiated. Injection of local anesthetic with a steroid preparation, combined with a brief period of immobilization, is usually helpful. For large deposits, operative management may be indicated (61).

EDITORS' COMMENTS

Medicine is practiced primarily as a statistical phenomenon; that is, we look first to the more common afflictions and work our way down toward the esoteric. Under the title of masses in the hand, the five most common in order are ganglion, fibroxanthoma, epidermal inclusion cyst, foreign body granuloma, and vascular tumors, typically hemangioma. This list includes abnormal masses in the hand but excludes all skin lesions. Epidermoid inclusion tumors are included, though of skin origin.

Ganglia are by far the most common masses in the hand. They appear in three separate categories, in order of frequency: the wrist ganglion, the flexor sheath ganglion, and mucoid tumor of the distal joint.

The ganglion is a manifestation of joint overload with synovial herniation through the capsule. The communication may remain open, and the ganglion can be emptied with pressure. Frequently, the stem of the ganglion becomes constricted, allowing fluid from the joint to enter the ganglion with activity or increased intersynovial pressure from joint loading. This joint fluid will inspissate or lose some of its fluidity while stored in the ganglion and the resultant jellylike material cannot get back through the small ganglion root. This results in gradual growth of the ganglion by the accumulation of the inspissated joint fluid material, which becomes thicker and more jelly-like, and the ganglion at this point is uncollapsible. In part, it grows by virtue of this fluid hydrodynamic process. The wrist ganglia are manifestations of overload of the joints from which they arise. They can occur in young people where lax ligaments are probably a part of the etiology. These ganglia, common in young girls, can grow to a size where their cosmesis dominates a 14-year-old's life and their removal is indicated. There is seldom carpal pathology. Ganglia beyond the teens are similarly a manifestation of joint overload, but usually from some carpal pathology. The most common carpal pathology is tearing of the scapholunate interosseous system. Such tears are cumulative and increase throughout active life. Most of these ganglia arise from the dorsal scapholunate interosseous system. We have never removed a deep capsular ganglion without identifying some associated dorsal wrist syndrome components. These include bony ridging and tears of the scapholunate interosseous system. These tears begin volarly and extend around dorsally in an increasing fashion with trauma and age. There is always some ridging on the dorsum of the scaphoid and lunate. Dorsal wrist syndrome is detailed in Chapter 28.

The second most common wrist ganglion arises volarly from the radial scaphoid joint or scapholunate joint volarly and nearly equally from the scaphotrapeziotrapezoid (STT) joint. These two origins can be determined before surgery by their location. The ganglia from the STT joint will appear along the flexor carpi radialis or be wrapped around it. The ganglia from the radial scaphoid joint or volar scapholunate joint typically involve the radial artery and the space between the first dorsal compartment and the flexor carpi radialis. With scaphoradial ganglia, the capsule should be excised where the root emerges from the joint. A small excision of capsule will not interfere with the radioscaphocapitate ligament. The ganglion that traverses the tunnel of the flexor carpi radialis is more difficult to deal with. The bony ridge of the trapezium that overlies the flexor carpi radialis is removed with dental rongeurs as the root is traced to the STT joint. It is best not to create raw bone beneath the flexor carpi radialis as it traverses the carpals. Leaving a raw surface here may lead to rupture of this tendon.

Flexor sheath ganglia occur as herniations through the sheath, typically a beebee-sized lesion on the volar aspect of the fibrosseous tunnel, in the A1-A2 pulley area. There is a common association with stenosing tenosynovitis because of increased pressures in the synovial fluid space. Injecting directly into the volar surface of the fibrosseous tunnel in treating stenosing tenosynovitis can create a flexor sheath ganglion. The needle hole acts as the herniation point initiating the ganglion. It is our experience that multipuncture will eliminate the ganglion, but 90% recur in 3 to 6 weeks. At surgery, excision of a small ellipse of the sheath will prevent recurrence. The mature herniation perforation can be seen on the underside of the removed segment of sheath.

Mucoid tumors are ganglia of the distal joint. They are again a manifestation of joint overload and almost always associated with some degenerative arthritic osteophyte change in the distal joint.

Intraosseous ganglia occur from increased joint pressure and weakness of the bone wall. This weakness may be related to changes in the bone from overuse. The bone becomes edematous and hypervascular and may undergo local changes similar to Kienbock's disease. These changes may actually be Kienböck's disease in its earliest stages.

The second most common mass in the hand is the fibroxanthoma or giant cell tumor of tendon sheath. It is our experience that these arise far more commonly from joints than they do from tendon sheaths. Their growth pushes aside surrounding structures, but seldom involves them. Digital nerves, arteries, tendons, bones or joint structures may all be totally preserved at the time of excision of the fibroxanthoma. We have experienced some unusual cases involving fibroxanthoma, including one case in which recurrence occurred three times at 12-year intervals. There was no evidence of tumor in the intervening years. Fibroxanthomas are rare in the wrist.

Epidermoid inclusion tumors are manifestations of epidermal tissue being driven subdermally. They are spherical and much more painful than the other common lesions.

Foreign body granulomas demonstrate multiple presentations dependent on the foreign body and degree of inflammation.

Hemangiomas are the least common of these tumors. They are usually tender to palpation and often have bluish discoloration. There are several types. Some are congenital, whereas others appear in older age groups and may have trauma as part of their etiology. The latter occur more commonly in the hand and wrist area than in the digits. They are usually tender to palpation and often have a bluish discoloration. One patient of ours demonstrated bilateral hemangiomas associated with de Quervain's disease. Following fairly closely behind the hemangiomas in incidence are the lipomas. There are, of course, tumors that do not present as a mass in the hand. These would include the relatively common enchondroma in bone and intraosseous ganglia. Most benign tumors are treated by surgical removal. An unidentified mass in a younger person is an indication for its removal.

REFERENCES

1. Amadio PC, Reiman HH, Dobyns JH. Lipofibromatous hamartoma of nerve. *J Hand Surg [Am]* 1988;13:67–75.
2. Angelides AC, Wallace PF. The dorsal ganglion of the wrist: Its pathogenesis, gross and microscopic anatomy and surgical treatment. *J Hand Surg [Am]* 1976;1:228–235.
3. Angelides AC. Ganglions of the hand and wrist. In: Green DP, Hotchkiss RN, eds. *Operative hand surgery, 3rd ed.* New York: Churchill Livingstone, 1993;2157–2171.
4. Azouz EM, Kozlowski K, Masel J. Soft tissue tumors of the hand and wrist of children. *J Can Assoc Radiol* 1989;40:251–255.
5. Black WC. Synovioma of the hand. Report of a case. *Am J Cancer* 1936;28:481–484.
6. Botte MJ, Silver MA. Leiomyoma of a digital artery. *Clin Orthop* 1990;260:259–262.
7. Byers P, Salm R. Epidermal inclusion cysts of phalanges. *J Bone Joint Surg Br* 1966;48:544–581.
8. Carroll RE. Epidermal (epithelial) cyst of the hand skeleton. *Am J Surg* 1953;85:327.
9. Cooper PH. Fibroma of tendon sheath. *J Am Acad Dermatol* 1984;11:625–628.
10. Duhig JT, Ayer JP. Vascular leiomyoma: A study of sixty-one cases. *AMA Arch Pathol* 1959;68:424–430.
11. Duinslaeger L, Vierendeels T, Wylock P. Vascular leiomyoma in the hand. *J Hand Surg [Am]* 1987;12:624–627.
12. Fyfe IS, MacFarlane A. Pigmented villonodular synovitis of the hand. *Hand* 1980;12:179–188.
13. Gaisford JC. Tumors of the hand. *Surg Clin North Am* 1960;40:549–566.
14. Gallager RL, Helwig EM. Neurothekeoma: A benign cutaneous tumor of neural origin. *Am J Clin Pathol* 1980;74:759–764.
15. Goellner JR, Soule EH. Desmoid tumors. An ultra-structural study of eight cases. *Hum Pathol* 1980;11:43–50.
16. Herndon JH, Eaton RG, Littler JW. Carpal tunnel syndrome. An unusual presentation of osteoid osteoma with a report of 20 cases. *J Bone Joint Surg Am* 1974;56:1715.
17. Hsueh S, Cruz JS. Cartilaginous lesions of the skin and superficial soft tissue. *J Cutan Pathol* 1982;9:405–416.
18. Karr MA, Aulicino PL, DuPuy TE, et al. Osteochondromas of the hand in hereditary multiple exostosis. Report of a case presenting as a blocked proximal interphalangeal joint. *J Hand Surg [Am]* 1984;9:264–268.
19. Kawabata H, Masada K, Aoki Y, et al. Infantile digital fibromatosis after web construction in syndactyly. *J Hand Surg [Am]* 1986;11:741–743.
20. Leffert RD. Lipomas of the upper extremity. *J Bone Joint Surg Am* 1972;54:1262.
21. Moore JR, Curtis RM, Wilgis EFS. Osteocartilaginous lesions of the digits in children. An experience with 10 cases. *J Hand Surg [Am]* 1983;8:309–315.
22. Mosher JF, Peckham AC. Osteoblastoma of the metacarpal. A case report. *J Hand Surg [Am]* 1978;3:358–360.
23. Nelson DL, Abdul-Karim FW, Carter JR, et al. Chondrosarcoma of small bones of the hand arising from enchondroma. *J Hand Surg [Am]* 1990;15:655–659.
24. Nichols RW. Desmoid tumors: A report of thirty-one cases. *Arch Surg* 1923;7:227–236.
25. Poppen NK, Niebauer JJ. Recurring digital fibrous tumor of childhood. *J Hand Surg [Am]* 1977;2:253–255.
26. Posch JL. Tumors of the hand. *J Bone Joint Surg Am* 1956;38:517–527.
27. Posch JL. Tumors of the hand. In: Flynn JE, ed. *Hand surgery, 2nd ed.* Baltimore: Williams & Wilkins, 1975.

28. Ritter MA, Marshall JL, Straub LR. Extraabdominal desmoid of the hand. A case report. *J Bone Joint Surg Am* 1969;51:1641.
29. Rubenstein D, Shanker DB, Finlayson L, et al. Multiple cutaneous granular cell tumors in children. *Pediatr Dermatol* 1987;4:94–97.
30. Russell RC, Williamson DA, Sullivan JW, et al. Detection of foreign bodies in the hand. *J Hand Surg [Am]* 1991;16:2–11.
31. Schiffman KL, Harris CM, Hooper G. Hemangiopericytoma of the median nerve. *J Hand Surg [Am]* 1988;13:75–78.
32. Silva-Lopez E, Wood DK. Granular cell myoblastoma. *Curr Surg* 1983;40:202–206.
33. Smith RJ. Factitious lymphedema of the hand. *J Bone Joint Surg Am* 1975;57:89.
34. Stout AP. Tumors of soft tissue. In: *AFIP atlas of tumor pathology, fasc 1, 1st ser.* Washington, DC: Armed Forces Institute of Pathology.
35. Totty WC, Murphy WA, Lee JKT. Soft tissue tumors. *Radiology* 1986;160:135–140.
36. Upton J, Mulliken JB, Murray JE. Classification and rationale for management of vascular anomalies in the upper extremity. *J Hand Surg [Am]* 1985;10:970–974.
37. Woods JE, Murray JE, Vawter GF. Hand tumors in children. *Plast Reconstr Surg* 1970;46:130–139.
38. Zubowicz VN, Ishii CH. Management of ganglion cysts of the hand by simple aspiration. *J Hand Surg [Am]* 1987;12:618–620.
39. Bos GD, Pritchard DJ, Reiman HM, et al. Epithelioid sarcoma. An analysis of fifty-one cases. *J Bone Joint Surg Am* 1988;70:862–870.
40. Enneking WF. *Clinical musculoskeletal pathology.* Gainesville, FL: Storter, 1979.
41. Enneking WF. *Musculoskeletal tumor surgery.* New York: Churchill Livingstone, 1983.
42. Barnes WE, Larsen RD, Posch JL. Review of ganglia of the hand and wrist with analysis of surgical treatment. *Plast Reconstr Surg* 1964;34:570–577.
43. Botte MJ. Ganglion excision. In: Gelberman RH, ed. *Master techniques in orthopaedic surgery: the wrist.* New York: Raven Press, 1994;393–416.
44. Flugel M, Kessler K. Follow-up of 425 patients operated upon for ganglion cyst. *Handchir Mikrochir Plast Chir* 1986;18:47–52.
45. Greendyke SD, Wilson J, Shepler TR. Anterior wrist ganglia from the scaphotrapezial joint. *J Hand Surg [Am]* 1992;17:487–490.
46. Nelson CL, Sawmiller S, Phalen GS. Ganglions of the wrist and hand. *J Bone Joint Surg Am* 1972;54:1459–1464.
47. Gurdjian ES, Larsen RD, Linder DW. Intraneural cyst of the peroneal and ulnar nerves. *J Neurosurg* 1965;23:76–78.
48. Hartwell AS. Cystic tumor of median nerve. *Boston Med Surg J* 1901;144:582–583.
49. MacCollum MS. Dorsal wrist ganglions in children: Clinical notes. *J Hand Surg [Am]* 1977;2:325.
50. Kerrigan JJ, Bertoni JM, Jaeger SH. Ganglion cysts and carpal tunnel syndrome. *J Hand Surg [Am]* 1988;13:763–765.
51. Lister G, Smith R. Protection of the radial artery in the resection of adherent ganglions of the wrist. *Plast Reconstr Surg* 1978;61:127–129.
52. Abrams RA, Ziets RJ, Lieber RL, et al. Anatomy of the radial nerve motor branches in the forearm. *J Hand Surg [Am]* 1997;22:232–237.
53. Botte MJ, Gelberman RH. Ulnar nerve compression at the wrist. In: Szabo RM, ed. *Nerve compression syndromes: Diagnosis and treatment.* Thorofare, NJ: Slack, 1989.
54. Botte MJ, Cohen MS, Lavernia CJ, et al. The dorsal branch of the ulnar nerve: An anatomic study. *J Hand Surg [Am]* 1990;15:603–607.
55. Richman JA, Gelberman RH, Engber WD, et al. Ganglions of the wrist and digits: Results of treatment by aspiration and cyst wall puncture. *J Hand Surg [Am]* 1987;12:1041–1043.
56. Bogumill GP, Sullivan DJ, Baker GI. Tumors of the hand. *Clin Orthop* 1975;108:214–222.
57. Bogumill GP. Tumors of the hand. In: Evarts CMcC, ed. *Surgery of the musculoskeletal system, 2nd ed, vol II.* New York: Churchill Livingstone, 1990;1197–1250.
58. Bogumill GP. Tumors of the wrist. In: Lichtman DM, Alexander AH, eds. *The wrist and its disorders, 2nd ed.* Philadelphia: WB Saunders, 1997;563–581.
59. Peimer CA, Moy OJ, Dick HM. Tumors of bone and soft tissue. In: Green D, ed. *Operative hand surgery, 3rd ed.* New York: Churchill Livingstone, 1993;2225–2250.
60. Anderson WJ, Bowere WH. Chrondromyxoid fibroma of the proximal phalanx. A tumour that may be confused with chondrosarcoma. *J Hand Surg [Br]* 1986;11:144–146.
61. Calandruccio JH, Jobe MT. Tumors and tumorous conditions of the hand. In: Canle ST, ed. *Campbell's operative orthopaedics, 9th ed.* St Louis: CV Mosby, 1998;3703–3733.
62. Eisenbaum SL, Eversmann WW Jr. Juvenile aponeurotic fibroma of the hand. *J Hand Surg [Am]* 1985;10:622–625.
63. Enzinger FM, Weiss SW. *Soft tissue tumors, 2nd ed.* St Louis: CV Mosby, 1988.
64. Greene TL, Strickland JW. Fibroma of tendon sheath. *J Hand Surg [Am]* 1984;9:758–760.
65. Keasbey LE. Juvenile aponeurotic fibroma (calcifying fibroma): A distinct tumor arising in the palms and soles of young children. *Cancer* 1953;6:338–346.
66. Martuza RL, Eldridge R. Neurofibromatosis. *N Engl J Med* 1988;318:684–688.
67. Mehregan AH. Superficial fibrous tumors in childhood. *J Cutan Pathol* 1981;8:321–334.
68. Mortimer G, Gibson AAM. Recurring digital fibroma. *J Clin Pathol* 1982;35:849–854.
69. Schenkar DL, Kleinert HE. Desmoplastic fibroma of the hand. Case report. *Plast Reconstr Surg* 1977;59:128–133.
70. Seel DJ, Booher RJ, Joel R. Fibrous tumors of musculoaponeurotic origin. *Surgery* 1964;56:497–504.
71. Soule EH, Enriquez P. Atypical fibrous histiocytoma, malignant histiocytoma, and epithelioid sarcoma: A comparative study of 65 tumors. *Cancer* 1972;30:128–143.
72. Specht EE, Konkin LA. Juvenile aponeurotic fibroma. The cartilage analogue of fibromatosis. *JAMA* 1975;234:626–629.
73. Specht EE, Staheli LT. Juvenile aponeurotic fibroma. *J Hand Surg [Am]* 1977;2:256–257.
74. Stack HG. Tumors of the hand. *Br Med J* 1960;1:919.
75. Adeyemi-Doro HO, Olude O. Juvenile aponeurotic fibroma. *J Hand Surg [Br]* 1985;10:127–128.
76. Carroll RE. Juvenile aponeurotic fibroma. *Hand Clin* 1987;3:219–224.
77. Idler RS. Benign and malignant nerve tumors. *Hand Clin* 1995;11(2):203–209.
78. Iwasaki H, Kicuchi M, Eimoto T. Juvenile aponeurotic fibroma: An ultrastructural study. *Ultrastruct Pathol* 1983;4:75–83.
79. Colon R, Upton J. Pediatric hand tumors: A review of 349 cases. *Hand Clin* 1985;11(2):223–243.
80. Phalen GS, Kendrick JI, Rodriguez JM. Lipomas of the upper extremity. A series of 15 tumors of the hand and wrist and 6 tumors causing nerve compression. *Am J Surg* 1971;121:298–305.
81. Saprawi R. Acute compression ulnar neuropathy at Guyon's canal resulting from lipoma. *J Hand Surg [Am]* 1984;9:238–240.

82. Kalisman M, Dolich BH. Infiltrating lipoma of the proper digital nerves. *J Hand Surg [Am]* 1982;7:401–403.
83. Kernohan J, Dakin PK, Quain JS, et al. An unusual "giant" lipofibroma in the palm. *J Hand Surg [Br]* 1984;9:347–348.
84. Zahrawi F. Acute compression ulnar neuropathy at Guyon's canal resulting from lipoma. *J Hand Surg [Am]* 1984;9:238–240.
85. von Schroeder HP, Botte MJ. Carpal tunnel syndrome. *Hand Clin* 1996;4:643–655.
86. Jaffe HL. *Tumors and tumorous conditions of bone.* Philadelphia: Lea & Febiger, 1958.
87. Jones FE, Soule EH, Coventry MB. Fibrous xanthoma of synovium (giant-cell tumor of tendon sheath, pigmented nodular synovitis). A study of one hundred and eighteen cases. *J Bone Joint Surg Am* 1969;51:76–86.
88. Mason ML. Tumors of the hand. *Surg Gynecol Obstet* 1937;64:129–148.
89. Sapra S, Prokopetz R, Merray AH. Giant cell tumor of tendon sheath. *Int J Dermatol* 1989;28:587–590.
90. Stevenson TW. Xanthoma and giant cell tumor of the hand. *J Plast Reconstr Surg* 1950;5:75–87.
91. Vidyasagar JVS, Sharma S, Krishnakumar S, et al. Giant cell tumour of tendon sheath. *Indian J Pathol Microbiol* 1988;32:50–54.
92. Froimson AI. Benign solid tumors. *Hand Clin* 1987;3(2):213–217.
93. Jaffe HL, Lichtenstein HL, Elsutro CJ. Pigmented villonodular synovitis, bursitis, and tenosynovitis. *Arch Pathol* 1941;31:731–765.
94. Jaffe HL, Lichtenstein L, Portis R. Giant cell tumor of bone. *Arch Pathol* 1940;30:993–1031.
95. Moore JR, Weiland AJ, Curtis RM. Localized nodular tenosynovitis: Experience with 115 cases. *J Hand Surg [Am]* 1984;9:412–417.
96. Hayes JR, Mulholland RC, O'Connor BT. Compression of the deep palmar branch of the ulnar nerve. *J Bone Joint Surg Br* 1969;51:469.
97. Milberg P, Kleinert HE. Giant cell tumor compression of the deep branch of the lunar nerve. *Ann Plast Surg* 1980;4:426.
98. Phalen GS, McCormack LJ, Gazale WJ. Giant cell tumor of tendon sheath (benign synovioma) in the hand. Evaluation of 56 cases *Clin Orthop* 1959;15:140–151.
99. Watson WL, McCarthy WD. Blood and lymph vessel tumors: A report of 1956 cases. *Surg Gynecol Obstet* 1940;71:569.
100. Crawford ES, DeBakey ME, Cooley DA. Surgical considerations of peripheral arterial aneurysms: Analysis of 107 cases. *Am J Surg* 1960;100:293–302.
101. Green DP. True and false traumatic aneurysms in the hand. *J Bone Joint Surg Am* 1973;55:120.
102. Kleinert HE, Burget BC, Morgan JA, et al. Aneurysms of the hand. *Arch Surg* 1973;106:554.
103. Mulliken JB, Glowacki J. Hemangiomas and vascular malformations in infants and children. *Plast Reconstr Surg* 1982;69:412–422.
104. Niechajev IA, Karlsson S. Vascular tumors of the hand. *Scand J Plast Reconstr Surg* 1982;16:67–75.
105. Palmieri TJ. Subcutaneous hemangiomas of the hand. *J Hand Surg [Am]* 1983;8:201–204.
106. Palmieri TJ. Vascular tumors of the hand and forearm. *Hand Clin* 1987;3:225–240.
107. Stanley RJ, Cubillo E. Non-surgical treatment of arteriovenous malformations of the trunk and limb by transcatheter arterial embolization. *Radiology* 1975;115:609–612.
108. Suzuki K, Takahashi S, Nakagawa T. False aneurysm in a digital artery. *J Hand Surg [Am]* 1980;5:402–403.
109. Beck WC. Experiences with pulsating hematoma. *Am J Surg* 1947;73:580–587.
110. Baird RJ, Doran ML. The false aneurysm. *Can Med Assoc J* 1964;91:281–284.
111. Narsete EM. Traumatic aneurysm of the radial artery: A report of three cases. *Am J Surg* 1964;108:424–427.
112. Wilgis EFS. *Vascular injuries and diseases of the upper limb.* Boston: Little, Brown, 1983.
113. Pack GT. Tumors of the hands and feet. *Surgery* 1939;5:1–26.
114. Vasconez L, Morris WJ, Owsley JQ Jr. Skin tumors. In: Dunphy JE, Way LW, eds. *Current surgical diagnosis, 4th ed.* Los Altos: Lange Medical Publications, 1979;997–1000.
115. Losli EJ. Intrinsic hemangiomas of the peripheral nerves. *Arch Pathol* 1952;53:226–232.
116. Campanacci M. *Bone and soft tissue tumors.* Vienna: Springer-Verlag, 1990.
117. Sabin FR. Origin and development of the primitive vessels of the chick and of the pig. *Contrib Embryol* 1922;14:139–154.
118. Reinoff WF Jr. Congenital arteriovenous fistula: An embryological study with the report of a case. *Bull Johns Hopkins Hosp* 1924;35:271–284.
119. Branham HH. Aneurysmal varix of the femoral artery and vein following a gunshot would. *Int J Surg* 1980;3:250–251.
120. Newmeyer WL. Vascular disorders. In: Green DP, Hotchkiss RN, eds. *Operative hand surgery, 3rd ed.* New York: Churchill Livingstone, 1993;2251–2309.
121. Koman LA, Ruch DS, Smith BP, et al. Vascular disorders. In: Green DP, Hotchkiss RN, Pederson WC, eds. *Green's operative hand surgery, 4th ed.* New York: Churchill Livingstone, 1999;2254–2302.
122. Patel ME, Silver JW, Lipton DE, et al. Lipofibroma of the median nerve in the palm and digits of the hand. *J Bone Joint Surg Am* 1979;61:393–396.
123. Spitell JA Jr. Tumors of blood and lymph vessels. In: Fairburn JF, Juergens JL, Spitell JA Jr, eds. *Allen-Barker-Hines peripheral vascular disease, 4th ed.* Philadelphia: WB Saunders, 1972.
124. Angervall L, Kindblom L, Haglid K. Dermal nerve sheath myxoma. *Cancer* 1984;53:1752–1759.
125. Goldstein J, Lifshitz T. Myxoma of nerve sheath. *Am J Dermatopathol* 1985;7:423–429.
126. Holdsworth BJ. Nerve tumors in the upper limb. A clinical review. *J Hand Surg [Br]* 1985;10:236–238.
127. King DT, Barr RJ. Bizarre cutaneous neurofibroma. *J Cutan Pathol* 1980;7:21–31.
128. Kleinman GM, Sanders FJ, Gagliari JM. Plexiform schwannoma. *Clin Neuropathol* 1985;4:265–266.
129. Rosenberg AE, Dick HM, Botte MJ. Benign and malignant tumors of peripheral nerve. In: Gelberman RH, ed. *Operative nerve repair and reconstruction.* Philadelphia: JB Lippincott, 1991;1587–1625.
130. Rubenstein AB, Reichenthal E, Borohov H. Radiation-induced schwannomas. *Neurosurgery* 1989;24:929–930.
131. Silver M, Patel MR, Vigorito V. Preoperative diagnosis of a forearm peripheral schwannoma. *Orthop Rev* 1993;22:714–716.
132. White NB. Neurilemmomas of the extremities. *J Bone Joint Surg Am* 1967;49:1605.
133. Ariel IM. Current concepts in the management of peripheral nerve tumors. In: Omer GE, Spinner M, eds. *Management of peripheral nerve problems, 1st ed.* Philadelphia: WB Saunders, 1980;669–693.
134. Couturier J, Delattre O, Kujas M, et al. Assessment of chromosome 22 anomalies in neurofibromas by combined karotype and FRLP analysis. *Cancer Genet Cytogenet* 1990;45:55–62.
135. D'Agostino AN, Soule EH, Miller RH. Primary malignant neoplasms of nerves (malignant neurilemmomas) in patients without manifestations of multiple neurofibromatosis (von Recklinghausen's disease). *Cancer* 1963;16:1003–1027.
136. Krone W, Hogemann I. Cell culture studies on neurofibro-

matosis (von Recklinghausen): Monosomy 22 and other chromosomal anomalies in cultures from peripheral neurofibromatosis. *Hum Genet* 1986;74:453–455.
137. Oshman RG, Phelps RC, Kantor I. Solitary neurofibroma on the finger. *Arch Dermatol* 1988;124:1185–1186.
138. Rinaldi E. Neurilemmomas and neurofibromas of the upper limb. *J Hand Surg* 1983;8:590–593.
139. Rouleau GA, Wertelecki W, Haines JL, et al. Genetic linkage of bilateral acoustic neurofibromatosis to a DNA marker on chromosome 22. *Nature* 1987;329:246–248.
140. Williams GD, Hoffman S, Schwartz IS. Malignant transformation in a plexiform neurofibroma of the median nerve. *J Hand Surg [Am]* 1984;9:583–587.
141. Harkin JC, Reed RJ. Tumors of the peripheral nervous system. In: *Armed Forces Institues of Pathology atlas of tumor pathology, 2nd ser.* Washington DC: AFIP, 1969.
142. Harkin JC. Differential diagnosis of peripheral nerve tumors. In: Omer GE, Spinner M, eds. *Management of peripheral nerve problems.* Philadelphia: WB Saunders, 1980;657–668.
143. Dickersin GR. The electron microscopic spectrum of nerve sheath tumors. *Ultrastruct Pathol* 1987;11:103–146.
144. Erlandson RA, Woodruff JM. Peripheral nerve sheath tumors: An electron microscopic study of 43 cases. Cancer 1982;49:273–287.
145. Gray MH, Rosenberg AE, Dickersin GR, et al. Glial fibrillary acidic protein and keratin expression by benign and malignant nerve sheath tumors. *Hum Pathol* 1989;20:1089–1096.
146. Perentes E, Rubinstein LJ. Immunohistochemical recognition of human nerve sheath tumors by antileu-7 (HNK-1) monoclonal antibody. *Acta Neuropathol (Berl)* 1985;68:319–324.
147. Smith RJ, Lipke RW. Surgical treatment of peripheral nerve tumor of the upper limb. In: Omer GE, Spinner M, eds. *Management of peripheral nerve problems, 1st ed.* Philadelphia: WB Saunders, 1980;694–711.
148. Phalen GS. Neurilemmomas of the forearm and hand. *Clin Orthop* 1976;114:219.
149. Barre PS, Schaffer JW, Carter JR, et al. Multiplicity of neurilemmomas in the upper extremity. *J Hand Surg [Am]* 1987;12:307–311.
150. Louis DS, Hankin FM. Benign nerve tumors of the upper extremity. *Bull NY Acad Med* 1985;61:611–619.
151. Louis DS. Peripheral nerve tumors in the upper extremity. *Hand Clin* 1987;3:311–318.
152. Strickland JW, Steichen JB. Nerve tumors of the hand and forearm. *J Hand Surg [Am]* 1977;2:285–291.
153. Davidson SF, Das SK, Smith EE. Cellular schwannoma of the hand. *J Hand Surg [Am]* 1989;14:907–909.
154. Fletcher CDM, Chan JK-C, McKee PH. Dermal nerve sheath myxoma: A study of three cases. *Histopathology* 1986;10:135–145.
155. Fletcher CDM, Vadies SE, McKee PH. Cellular schwannoma: A distinct pseudosarcomatous entity. *Histopathology* 1987;11:21–35.
156. Woodruff JM, Godwin TA, Erlandson RA, et al. Cellular schwannoma: A variety of schwannoma sometimes mistaken for a malignant tumor. *Am J Surg Pathol* 1981;5:733–744.
157. Dahl I. Ancient neurilemmoma (schwannoma). *Acta Pathol Microbiol Scand* 1977;85:812–818.
158. Kileen RA, Davy CL, Bauserman SC. Melonocytic schwannoma. *Cancer* 1988;62:174–183.
159. Weiss SW, Langloss JM, Enzinger FM. Value of S-100 protein in the diagnosis of soft tissue tumors, with particular reference to benign and malignant Schwann cell tumors. *Lab Invest* 1983;49:299–308.
160. Barrett R, Cramer F. Tumors of the peripheral nerves and so-called "ganglia" of the peroneal nerve. *Clin Orthop* 1987;27:307–311.
161. Cooley SGE. Tumors of the hand and forearm. In: Converse JM, ed. *Reconstructive plastic surgery, 2nd ed, vol 6.* Philadelphia: WB Saunders, 1977;3449–3506.
162. Das Gupta TK, Brasfield RD, Strong EW, et al. Benign solitary schwannomas (neurilemmomas) *Cancer* 1969;24:355–366.
163. Silverman TA, Enzinger FM. Fibrolipomatous hamartoma of nerve: A clinicopathologic analysis of 26 cases. *Am J Surg Pathol* 1985;9:7–14.
164. Terzis JK, Daniel RK, Williams HB, et al. Benign fatty tumors of peripheral nerves. *Ann Plast Surg* 1978;1:193–216.
165. Paletta FX, Rybka FJ. Treatment of hamartomas of the median nerve. *Ann Surg* 1972;176:217–222.
166. Paletta FX, Senay LC Jr. Lipofibromatous hamartoma of median nerve and ulnar nerve: Surgical treatment. *Plast Reconstr Surg* 1981;68:915–921.
167. Yaghami I, McKnowne F, Alizadeh A. Macrodactylia fibrolipomatosis. *South Med J* 1976;69:1565–1568.
168. Abu Jamra FN, Rebiez JJ. Lipofibroma of the median nerve. *J Hand Surg [Am]* 1979;4:160–163.
169. Booher RJ. Lipoblastic tumors of the hands and feet. A review of the literature and a report of 33 cases. *J Bone Joint Surg Am* 1965;47:727–740.
170. Dooms GC, Hricak H, Sotlitto RA, et al. Lipomatous tumors with fatty component: MR imaging potential and comparison of MR and CT results. *Radiology* 1985;157:479–483.
171. Hajdu SE. *Pathology of soft-tissue tumors.* Philadelphia: Lea & Febiger, 1979;157–164.
172. Harrington AC, Adnot J, Chesser RS. Infiltrating lipomas of the upper extremity. *J Dermatol Surg Oncol* 1990;16(9):834–837.
173. Hoehn JG, Farber HF. Massive lipoma of the palm. *Ann Plast Surg* 1983;11:431–433.
174. Mikhail IK. Median nerve lipoma in the hand. *J Bone Joint Surg Br* 1964;46:726.
175. Pulitzer DR, Reed RJ. Nerve-sheath myxoma. *Am J Dermatopathol* 1985;7:409–421.
176. Pulvertaft RG. Unusual tumors of the median nerve. *J Bone Joint Surg Br* 1964;56:731.
177. Roland SA. Lipofibroma of the median nerve in the palm. *J Bone Joint Surg Am* 1967;49:1309.
178. Johnson RJ, Bonfiglio M. Lipofibromatous hamartoma of the median nerve. *J Bone Joint Surg Am* 1969;51:984–990.
179. Yamamoto H, Kawana T. Oral nerve sheath myxoma. *Acta Pathol Jpn* 1988;38:121–127.
180. Goldman AB, Kaye JJ. Macrodysrophia lipomatosa: Radiographic diagnosis. *Am J Roentgenol* 1977;128:101–105.
181. Dell PC. Macrodactyly. *Hand Clin* 1985;1:511–524.
182. Bergman FO, Blom SEG, Stenstrom SJ. Radical excision of a fibro-fatty proliferation of the median nerve, with no neurological loss symptoms. *Plast Reconstr Surg* 1970;46:375–380.
183. Frykman GK, Wood VE. Peripheral nerve hamartoma with macrodactyly in the hand: report of three cases and review of the literature. *J Hand Surg [Am]* 1978;3:307–312.
184. Abu Jamra FN, Rebeiz JJ. Lipofibroma of the median nerve. *J Hand Surg [Am]* 1979;4:160–163.
185. Louis DS, Hankin FM, Green TL, et al. Lipofibromas of the median nerve: Long-term follow-up of four cases. *J Hand Surg [Am]* 1985;10:403–408.
186. Rowland SA. Case report: Ten year follow-up of lipofibroma of the median nerve in the palm. *J Hand Surg [Am]* 1977;2:316–317.
187. Kojima T, Ide Y, Marumo E, et al. Haemangioma of the median nerve causing carpal tunnel syndrome. *Hand* 1976;8:62–65.

188. Kon M, Vuursteen P. An intraneural hemangioma of a digital nerve: case report. *J Hand Surg [Am]* 1981;6:357–358.
189. Patel CB, Tsai T-M, Kleinert HE. Hemangioma of the median nerve: A report of two cases. *J Hand Surg [Am]* 1986;11:76–79.
190. Peled I, Iosipovich Z, Rousso M, et al. Hemangioma of the median nerve. *J Hand Surg [Am]* 1980;5:363–365.
191. Alawneh I, Giovanini A, Willmen HR, et al. Enchondroma of the hand. *Int Surg* 1977;62:218–219.
192. Hasselgren G, Forssblad P, Tomvall A. Bone grafting, unnecessary in the treatment of enchondromas in the hand. *J Hand Surg [Am]* 1991;16:1139–1142.
193. Kuur E, Hansen SL, Lindequist S. Treatment of solitary enchondromas in fingers. *J Hand Surg [Br]* 1989;14:109–112.
194. Lucas GL. Hand tumors. A quick guide to types and treatment. *Res Staff Physician* 1979;25:76–91.
195. Mangini U. Tumors of the skeleton of the hand. *Bull Hosp Joint Dis* 1967;28:61–103.
196. McGrath MH, Watson HK. Late results with local bone graft donor sites in hand surgery. *J Hand Surg* [Am] 1981;6:234–237.
197. Mirra JM. *Bone tumors. Clinical, radiologic, and pathologic correlations.* Philadelphia: Lea & Febiger, 1989.
198. Bauer RD, Lewis MM, Posner MA. Treatment of enchondromas of the hand with allograft bone. *J Hand Surg [Am]* 1988;13:908–916.
199. Smith RJ, Brushart TM. Allograft bone for metacarpal reconstruction. *J Hand Surg [Am]* 1985;10:325–334.
200. Bednar MS, Weiland AJ, Light TR. Osteoid osteoma of the upper extremity. *Hand Clin* 1995;11:211–221.
201. Wulle C. On the treatment of enchondroma. *J Hand Surg [Br]* 1990;15:320–330.
202. Urist MR, Kovacs S, Yates KA. Regeneration of an enchondroma defect under the influence of an implant of human bone morphogenetic protein. *J Hand Surg [Am]* 1986;11:417–419.
203. Takigawa K. Chondroma of the bones of the hand. A review of 110 cases. *J Bone Joint Surg Am* 1971;53:1591–1600.
204. Fogel GR, McElfresh EC, Peterson HA, et al. Management of deformities of the forearm in multiple hereditary osteochondromas. *J Bone Joint Surg Am* 1984;66:670–680.
205. Greyson-Fleg RT, Reichmister JP, McCarthy EF, et al. Post traumatic osteochondroma. *Can Assoc Radiol J* 1987;38:195–198.
206. Shapiro F, Simon S, Glimcher MJ. Hereditary multiple exostoses: anthropometric, roentgenographic and clinical aspects. *J Bone Joint Surg Am* 1979;51:815.
207. Solomon L. Hereditary multiple exostosis. *J Bone Joint Surg Br* 1963;45:292.
208. Alaclay M, Clarac JP, Bontoux D. Double osteoid osteoma in adjacent carpal bones: A case report. *J Bone Joint Surg Am* 1982;64:779–780.
209. Allieu Y, Lussiez B, Benichou M, et al. Osteoid osteoma of the hand and wrist. *J Hand Surg [Am]* 1987;12:794–800.
210. Ambrosia JM, Wold LE, Amadio PC. Osteoid osteoma of the hand and wrist. *J Hand Surg [Am]* 1987;12:794–800.
211. Assoun J, Richardi G, Railhac JJ, et al. Osteoid osteoma: MR imaging versus CT. *Radiology* 1994;191:217–223.
212. Bauer TW, Aehr RJ, Belhobek GH, et al. Juxta-articular osteoid osteoma. *Am J Surg Pathol* 1991;15:381–387.
213. Bednar MS, McCormack RR Jr, Glasser D, et al. Osteoid osteoma of the upper extremity. *J Hand Surg [Am]* 1993;18:1019–1025.
214. Blair WR, Kube WJ. Osteoid osteoma in a distal radial epiphysis: A case report. *Clin Orthop* 1977;126:160–161.
215. Bohne WHO, Levin DB, Lyden JP. Scintimetric diagnosis of osteoid osteoma of the carpal scaphoid bone. *Clin Orthop* 1975;107:156–158.
216. Bowen CVA, Dzus AK, Hardy DA. Osteoid osteomata of the distal phalanx. *J Hand Surg [Br]* 1987;12:387–390.
217. Braun S, Chervor A, Tomeno B, et al. Phalangeal osteoid osteoma: A 13 case study. *Rev Rheum Mal Osteoart* 1979;46:225–233.
218. Carroll RE. Osteoid osteoma in the hand. *J Bone Joint Surg Am* 1953;35:888–893.
219. Cetti R, Christensen SE. Osteoid osteoma in the scaphoid bone. Case report. *Scand J Plast Reconstr Surg* 1982;16:207–209.
220. Chen SC, Caplan H. An unusual site of osteoid osteoma in the proximal phalanx of a finger. *J Hand Surg [Br]* 1989;14:341–344.
221. Cohen JD, Harrington TM, Ginsberg WW. Osteoid osteoma: 95 cases and a review of the literature. *Semin Arthritis Rheum* 1983;12:265–281.
222. DeWet IS. Osteoid osteomota: Review of the literature with a report of five cases. *S Afr J Surg* 1967;5:13.
223. Doyle LK, Ruby LK, Nalebuff EG, et al. Osteoid osteoma of the hand. *J Hand Surg [Am]* 1985;19:408–410.
224. Doyle T, King K. Percutaneous removal of osteoid osteoma using CT control. *Clin Radiol* 1989;40:514–517.
225. Dunitz NL, Lipscomb PR, Ivins JC. Osteoid osteoma of the hand and wrist. *Am J Surg* 1957;94:65–69.
226. Feldman F. Primary bone tumors of the hand and carpus. *Hand Clin* 1987;3:269–289.
227. Ghiam GF, Bora FW. Osteoid osteoma of the carpal bones. *J Hand Surg [Am]* 1978;3:280–283.
228. Jaffe HL, Mayer L. An osteoblastic osteoid tissue forming tumor of the metacarpal bone. *Arch Surg* 1932;24:550–564.
229. Alamen T, Abrams RA. Osteoid osteoma of the hand (unpublished manuscript). 1998.
230. Jensen EG. Osteoid osteoma of the capitate bone. *Hand* 1979;11:102–105.
231. Kendrick JI, Evarts CM. Osteoid osteoma: A critical analysis of 40 tumors. *Clin Orthop* 1975;54:51–59.
232. Kernohan J, Beacon JP, Dakin PK, et al. Osteoid osteoma of the pisiform. *J Hand Surg [Br]* 1985;10(3):411–414.
233. Lamb DW, Del Castillo F. Phalangeal osteoid osteoma in the hand. *Hand* 1981;13:291–295.
234. Mc Carten GM, Dixon PL, Marshall DR. Osteoid osteoma of the distal phalanx: A case report. *J Hand Surg [Br]* 1987;12:391–393.
235. McGrath BE, Bush CH, Nelson TE, et al. Evaluation of suspected osteoid osteoma. *Clin Orthop* 1996;327:247–252.
236. Meng Q, Watt I. Phalangeal osteoid osteoma. *Br J Radiol* 1989;62:321–325.
237. Muren C, Hoglund M, Engkvist O, et al. Osteoid osteomas of the hand. Report of three cases and review of the literature. *Acta Radiol* 1991;32:62–66.
238. Nakatsuchi Y, Sugimoto Y, Nakano M. Osteoid osteoma of the terminal phalanx. *J Hand Surg [Br]* 1984;9:201–203.
239. Riester J, Mosher JF. Osteoid osteoma of the capitate: A case report. *J Hand Surg [Am]* 1984;9:278–280.
240. Sullivan M. Osteoid osteoma of the fingers. *Hand* 1971;3:175–180.
241. Symeonides P, Kapetanos G. Osteoid osteoma of the capitate. *Hand* 1983;15:290–293.
242. Wiss DA, Reid BS. Painless osteoid osteoma of the fingers. *J Hand Surg [Am]* 1983;8:914–917.
243. Edeiken J, Depalma AF, Hodes PJ. Osteoid osteoma (roentgenographic emphasis). *Clin Orthop* 1966;49:201–206.
244. Simm RJ. The natural history of osteoid osteoma. *Aust NZ J Surg* 1975;45:412–415.
245. Fehring TK, Green NE. Negative radionuclide scan in osteoid osteoma: A case report. *Clin Orthop* 1984;185:245–249.

246. McConnell B III, Dell PC. Localization of an osteoid osteoma nidus in a finger by use of computed tomography: A case report. *J Hand Surg [Am]* 1984;9:139–141.
247. Marcove RC, Heelan RT, Huvos AG, et al. Osteoid osteoma. Diagnosis, localization, and treatment. *Clin Orthop* 1991;267:197–201.
248. Morrison GM, Hawes LE, Sacc JJ. Incomplete removal of osteoid-osteoma. *Am J Surg* 1950;80:476–481.
249. Gartsman GM, Ranawat CS. Treatment of osteoid osteoma of the proximal phalanx by use of cryosurgery. *J Hand Surg [Am]* 1984;9:275–277.
250. Ghelman B, Thompson FM, Arnold WD. Intraoperative radioactive localization of an osteoid-osteoma: Case report. *J Bone Joint Surg Am* 1981;63:826–827.
251. Averill RM, Smith RJ, Cambell CJ. Giant-cell tumors of the bones of the hand. *J Hand Surg [Am]* 1980;5:39–50.
252. Dahlin DC. Giant-cell bearing lesions of bone of the hands. *Hand Clin* 1987;3(2):291–297.
253. McDonald DJ, Sim FH, McLeod RA, et al. Giant-cell tumor of bone. *J Bone Joint Surg Am* 1986;68:235.
254. Peimer CA, Schiller AL, Mankin HJ, et al. Multicentric giant-cell tumor of bone. *J Bone Joint Surg Am* 1980;62:652–656.
255. Roberts A, Long J, Wickstrom J. A metacarpal giant cell tumor, a sternal osteoblastoma and a pubic osteogenic sarcoma in the same patient. *South Med J* 1976;69:660–662.
256. Shaw JA, Mosher JF. A giant-cell tumor in the hand presenting as an expansile diaphyseal lesion. Case report. *J Bone Joint Surg Am* 1983;65:692–695.
257. Smith RJ, Mankin HJ. Allograft replacement of the distal radius for giant cell tumor. *J Hand Surg [Am]* 1977;2:299–309.
258. Srivastava T, Tuli SM, Varma BP, et al. Giant cell tumor of metacarpals. *Indian J Cancer* 1975;12:164–169.
259. Szabo RM, Thorson EP, Raskind JR. Allograft replacement with distal radioulnar joint fusion and ulnar osteotomy for treatment of giant cell tumors of the distal radius. *J Hand Surg [Am]* 1990;15:929–933.
260. Barbieri CH. Aneurysmal bone cyst of the hand. An unusual situation. *J Hand Surg [Br]* 1984;9:89–92.
261. Dossing KJV. Aneurysmal bone cyst of the hand. *Scand J Plast Reconstr Hand Surg* 1990;24:173–175.
262. Frassica FJ, Amadio PC, Wold LE, et al. Aneurysmal bone cyst: Clinicopathologic features and treatment of ten cases involving the hand. *J Hand Surg [Am]* 1988;13:676–683.
263. Fuhs SE, Herndon JH. Aneurysmal bone cyst involving the hand. A review and report of two cases. *J Hand Surg [Am]* 1979;4:152–159.
264. Guy R, Langevin R, Raymond O, et al. Phalangeal aneurysmal bone cyst. *Union Med Can* 1957;86:866.
265. Harto-Garofalides G, Rigopoulos C, Fragiadakin E. Aneurysmal bone cyst of the proximal phalanx of the thumb. Successful replacement by tibial autograft. *Clin Orthop* 1967;54:125–129.
266. Johnson AD. Aneursymal bone cyst of the hand. *Hand Clin* 1987;3:299–310.
267. Mortensen NHM, Kuur E. Aneurysmal bone cyst of the proximal phalanx. *J Hand Surg [Br]* 1990;15:482–483.
268. Ruiter DJ, Van Rijssel T, Van Der Velde E. Aneurysmal bone cyst: A clinicopathologic study of 105 cases. *Cancer* 1977;39:2231.
269. Schajowicz F, Sainz MC, Slullitel JA. Juxta-articular bone cysts (intra-osseous ganglia). *J Bone Joint Surg Br* 1979;61:107.
270. Scaglietti O, Marchetti PG, Bartolozzi P. The effects of methylprednisolone acetate in the treatment of bone cysts. Results of three years follow-up. *J Bone Joint Surg Br* 1979;61:200–204.
271. Campanacci M, Capanna R, Picci P. Unicameral and aneurysmal bone cysts. *Clin Orthop* 1986;204:25–36.
272. Besser E, Roessner A, Burg E, et al. Bone tumors of the hand. A review of 300 cases documented in the Westphalian Bone Tumor Register. *Arch Orthop Trauma Surg* 1987;106:241.
273. Binkovitz LA, Berquist TH, McLeod RA. Masses of the hand and wrist: Detection and characterization with MR imaging. *AJR Am J Roentgenol* 1990;154:323–326.
274. Butler ED, Hamill JP, Seipel RS, et al. Tumors of the hand—a ten year survey and report of 437 cases. *Am J Surg* 1960;100:293–302.
275. Hoglund M, Tordai P, Engkvist O. Ultrasonography for the diagnosis of soft tissue condition in the hand. *Scand J Plast Reconstr Surg* 1991;25:225–231.
276. Lammers RL. Soft tissue foreign bodies. *Ann Emerg Med* 1988;17:1336–1337.
277. Lattes R. *Tumors of the soft tissue. Atlas of tumor pathology, 2nd ser, fasc 1, rev.* Washington, DC: Armed Forces Institute of Pathology, 1983.
278. Mankin HJ. Principles of diagnosis and management of tumors of the hand. *Hand Clin* 1987;3:185–195.
279. Pin PG, Young VL, Gilula LA, et al. Wrist pain: A systematic approach to diagnosis. *J Plast Reconstr Surg* 1990;85:42–46.
280. Saferin EH, Posch JL. Secretan's disease. Posttraumatic hard edema of the dorsum of the hand. *Plast Reconstr Surg* 1976;58:703–707.
281. Peimer CA. Long-term complications of trapeziometacarpal silicone arthroplasty. *Clin Orthop* 1987;220:86–98.
282. Peimer CA, Medige J, Eckert BS, et al. Reactive synovitis after silicone arthroplasty. *J Hand Surg [Am]* 1986;11:624–638.
283. Feldon P, Millender LH, Nalebuff EA. Rheumatoid arthritis in the hand and wrist. In: Green D, ed. *Operative hand surgery, ed 3.* New York: Churchill Livingstone, 1993;1587–1690.

BIBLIOGRAPHY

Ciccone WJ. Osteoid osteoma: A rare occurrence in the carpal navicular. *Rocky Mt Med J* 1976;73:325–327.

Dabski C, Reiman HM, Muller SA. Neurofibrosarcoma of skin and subcutaneous tissues. *Mayo Clin Proc* 1990;65:164–172.

Gelberman RH, Zakaib GS, Mubarak SJ, et al. Decompression of the forearm compartment syndromes. *Clin Orthop* 1978;134:225–229.

Geschickter CF. Tumors of peripheral nerve. *Am J Cancer* 1935;25:377–410.

Iwasaki H, Kicuchi M, Ohtsuki I, et al. Infantile digital fibromatosis. *Cancer* 1983;1:1653–1661.

Iwashita T, Enjoji M. Plexiform neurilemmoma: A clinicopathological and immunohistochemical analysis of 23 tumors from 20 patients. *Virchows Arch [A]* 1987;411:305–309.

Kaiserling E, Geerts ML. Tumor of Wagner-Meissner touch corpuscles. *Virchows Arch [A]* 1986;409:241–250.

Leroy V, Couturaud J, Lathelize H, et al. Bone scintigraphy is unreliable in studying osteoid osteoma. *Rev Rheum Mal Osteoart* 1980;47:53–56.

Lewis RC, Nannini LH, Cocke WM. Multifocal neurilemmomas of median and ulnar nerves of the same extremity—case report. *J Hand Surg [Am]* 1981;6:406–408.

Lindbom A, Lindvall N, Soderberg G, et al. Angiography in osteoid osteoma. *Acta Radiol* 1960;54:327–333.

O'Hara JP, Tegtmeyer C, Sweet DE, et al. Angiography in the diagnosis of osteoid-osteoma of the hand. *J Bone Joint Surg Am* 1975;57:163–166.

Prichard RW, Custer RP. Pacinian nuerofibroma. *Cancer* 1952;5:297–301.

Rey JA, Bello MJ, deCampos JM, et al. Cytogenetic analysis in human neurinomas. *Cancer Genet Cytogenet* 1987;28:187–188.

Shinoda M, Tsutsumi Y, Hata J, et al. Peripheral neuroepithelioma in childhood. Immunohistochemical demonstration of epithelial differentiation. *Arch Pathol Lab Med* 1988;112:1144–1158.

Taleisnik J. The palmar cutaneous branch of the median nerve and the approach to the carpal tunnel. *J Bone Joint Surg Am* 1973;55:1212–1217.

Theaker JM, Gatter KC, Puddle J. Epithelial membrane antigen expression by the perineurium of peripheral nerve and in peripheral nerve tumors. *Histopathology* 1988;13:171–179.

Tordai P, Hoglund M, Lugnegard H. Is the treatment of enchondroma in the hand by simple curettage a rewarding method? *J Hand Surg [Br]* 1990;15:331–334.

Usui M, Ishii S, Yamwaki S, et al. Malignant granular cell tumor of the radial nerve. *Cancer* 1977;19:1547–1555.

Watson-Jones R. Encapsulated lipoma of the median nerve at the wrist. *J Bone Joint Surg Br* 1964;46:736.

Yeoman PM. Fatty infiltration of the median nerve. *J Bone Joint Surg Br* 1964;46:737–739.

45

MALIGNANT TUMORS OF THE WRIST

HAROLD M. DICK
ROBERT J. STRAUCH

Malignant tumors of the wrist (from the carpometacarpal joints of the digits to the distal border of the pronator quadratus) are rare lesions. In this chapter, the principles of evaluation and biopsy of malignant tumors of the wrist are reviewed, followed by a general approach to reconstruction of these tumors and then discussion of specific tumors with case examples. The discussion is mainly confined to musculoskeletal sarcomas of the wrist.

PATIENT EVALUATION

The overwhelming majority of tumors or swellings involving the wrist will be readily diagnosable on history and physical examination. Lesions such as dorsal or volar ganglia, wrist synovitis, de Quervain's tendinitis with swelling, and other common conditions will usually be immediately recognized by the hand surgeon. Nevertheless, every painful or tumorous condition should be suspected of being a malignancy until ruled out by a careful history, physical examination, and appropriate imaging studies.

There are specific factors in the patient history that are useful in evaluating a possible malignant wrist tumor. The age of the patient will provide a clue to the type of neoplasm that may be present; for example, osteosarcoma has a bimodal age distribution with occurrence in the first two decades and then the sixth or seventh decade (1). Rhabdomyosarcoma is the most common soft tissue sarcoma found in children (2). Metastatic disease to the hand or wrist is rare under age 50 (3). The presence of pain is worrisome for malignancy when constant and present at night. Local trauma to the region does not cause a wrist malignancy but may often be the first clue to a problem when pain is produced following a pathologic fracture from a trivial injury. Local inflammation may be caused by tumor, trauma, infection, or inflammatory processes such as gout or rheumatoid arthritis, and all diagnoses should be considered and evaluated in light of the patient's history.

A detailed physical examination is useful in evaluating a possible malignant tumor. Specifically, a mass should be examined for tenderness, fixation to surrounding tissue, bruit, warmth, and regional neurovascular involvement. A solitary, freely movable mass that transilluminates will most likely be a ganglion cyst, although lipomata may also appear to transilluminate. Larger lesions (>5 cm) are more likely to be malignant. When the wrist is examined, rotation and motion of the wrist joints should be checked for mechanical blockage by tumor. Epitrochlear and axillary adenopathy should be searched for because the common soft tissue sarcomas (epithelioid and synovial cell) have a predilection for regional lymph node metastasis (4).

Laboratory or serologic evaluation should be performed in a patient with a suspected malignancy. The tests usually ordered are a complete blood count (usually normal), erythrocyte sedimentation rate (elevated in myeloma or other round-cell tumors), alkaline phosphatase (elevated in osteosarcoma), and calcium (elevated in metastatic disease) (5). If myeloma is under consideration (patient age over 40–50, multiple lytic lesions), serum and urine protein electrophoresis is obtained. Blastic bony lesions may imply prostate metastases, and a prostate-specific antigen test should be checked.

Imaging studies for evaluating suspected wrist malignancies include plain films, tomography, computed tomography (CT scan), and magnetic resonance imaging (MRI). The location of a bone lesion on plain x-rays may be useful. Giant-cell tumor (GCT) of bone and chondroblastoma are epiphyseal; round-cell tumors such as Ewing's may affect the diaphysis; metaphyseal lesions are many and include osteosarcoma, among others. Sharp delineation of a lesion from the surrounding bone with a sclerotic border is indicative of a benign lesion, whereas a "permeative" pattern and cortical destruction are seen with aggressive malignancies where the bone does not have time to mount a reactive response. Some soft tissue sarcomas may contain areas of calcification; notably synovial cell and epithelioid sarcoma (25%) (6).

H. M. Dick and R. J. Strauch: Department of Orthopaedic Surgery, Columbia University, and New York Presbyterian Hospital, New York, New York 10032.

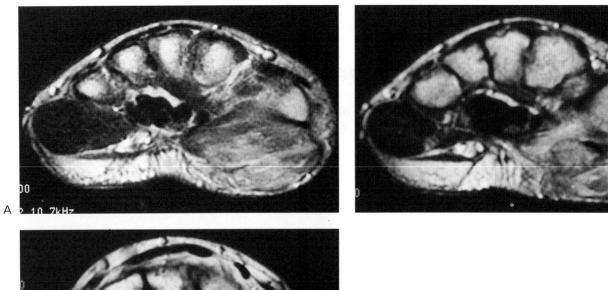

FIGURE 45.1. Magnetic resonance image of a 31-year-old man with an epithelioid sarcoma involving the right thenar area and extending deeply to the **(A)** transverse carpal ligament, **(B)** first metacarpal, and **(C)** flexor carpi radialis tendon.

CT scanning is most useful for evaluating the extent of osseous lesions but less helpful for soft tissue lesions. MRI is the technique of choice for local evaluation of soft tissue malignancies (Fig. 45.1). In combination with MRA or MRV, vascular involvement may be demonstrated without the need for angiography. It should be emphasized that although a CT scan or MRI may suggest the presence of malignancy or a benign lesion, the final diagnosis rests on histology obtained through biopsy.

If a lesion is felt to be malignant with the potential for distant metastasis, a chest x-ray and CT scan of the chest should be obtained to screen for pulmonary involvement, and a three-phase bone scan should be obtained to screen for distant bony lesions (7).

BIOPSY OF SUSPECTED MALIGNANCIES OF THE WRIST

Lesions that are suspicious for malignancy should be referred to a surgeon familiar with their treatment before biopsy. It has been shown that errors, complications, and changes in course and outcome were two to 12 times greater when the biopsy was performed in a referring institution instead of a tertiary treatment center (8). Referral to a surgeon familiar with tumor management allows coordination of the biopsy planning, pathologic interpretation, and final reconstructive plan in one center. Biopsy of a suspected malignancy can be either closed or open. Closed biopsies are obtained by percutaneous needle puncture. The advantage of a closed biopsy is that less hematoma and tumor spillage usually occurs in the surrounding tissue. The disadvantage of needle biopsy is that inadequate tumor may be removed for diagnosis (sampling error), and the needle tract may be difficult to completely excise, especially if the needle biopsy is not done by the surgeon performing the definitive procedure. Closed biopsy techniques are becoming more widespread for soft tissue malignancies and for diagnosis of metastatic lesions, recurrences, or round-cell tumors (9). Open biopsy remains the most widely used biopsy technique.

A patient who has already been operated on at another institution and referred for definitive care following "unplanned excision" of a soft tissue sarcoma is a treatment problem. This situation occasionally arises when the referring surgeon did not suspect malignancy or obtain preoperative imaging studies that would have shown the extent of the lesion, and during the course of surgery attempts to remove a malignant lesion. In this case, it has been shown that repeat excision is the best treatment course because, in one study, the margins of resection were positive 40% of the time despite negative findings on physical examination and MRI (10).

Open biopsy may be performed under tourniquet control, which we recommend, but exsanguination with an Esmarch or similar bandage should not be employed for fear of disseminating tumor hematogenously. The tourniquet may be released before skin closure to obtain hemostasis and avoid tumor seeding from a large hematoma. Drains are not usually placed because the entire drain tract would require excision at the definitive procedure; if a drain is felt essential, it should be placed in line with and close to the biopsy incision.

Transverse incisions, though widely used for their cosmetic appearance in treating dorsal carpal ganglia and other benign lesions, should not be used in planning the biopsy of a suspected malignancy. The biopsy incision should usually be longitudinal and be placed so that it can be excised *en bloc* with the final tumor resection. The radial and ulnar arteries, as well as the median and ulnar nerves, should be avoided during the biopsy if possible, because if they are exposed to tumor, they may need to be sacrificed. If the tumor involves bone but has violated the cortex, the soft tissue component alone may be biopsied because it is usually more diagnostic than the intraosseous lesion. If the lesion is entirely intracortical, a small oval cortical window may be established with fluoroscopic visualization for precise localization. The bone hole should be replaced or plugged with methylmethacrylate cement to prevent bleeding and tumor seeding (11). A representative biopsy of the tumor should always be taken, avoiding crushing of the tissue. The biopsy should endeavor to include the pseudocapsule and extend into the tumor because the central areas of the tumor are likely to be necrotic.

At the time of biopsy it is desirable to obtain a frozen section, not for definitive diagnosis, but to ensure that diagnostic tissue has been obtained before wound closure; it is disappointing to perform a repeat biopsy procedure for lack of a histologic diagnosis.

CLASSIFICATION AND STAGING

The Musculoskeletal Tumor Society employs a three-stage system for musculoskeletal sarcomas. Stage I lesions are low-grade tumors without metastases and include GCTs of bone, periosteal osteosarcoma, and other less lethal malignancies. Stage II lesions are high-grade tumors without metastatic spread; examples include synovial cell sarcoma and epithelioid sarcoma. Stage III lesions are either low- or high-grade sarcomas with regional or distant metastases. The stages I and II are further subdivided into A or B depending on whether the lesion is intra- (A) or extracompartmental (B), with a compartment being defined as a normal anatomic boundary: bone, joint capsule, or fascial compartment (12). Most malignancies involving the wrist, unless confined within a specific bone or muscle, are unfortunately extracompartmental by definition. The wrist does not lend itself readily to extraosseous compartments, and therefore, a lesion in or invading the carpal tunnel has contaminated all surrounding structures including flexor tendons, the median nerve, and likely the carpal bones as well. Only lesions that are completely intraosseous or within a well-defined muscle group (thenar, interosseous, etc.) may be classified as intracompartmental.

GENERAL PRINCIPLES OF MALIGNANT TUMOR RESECTION

Four types of wound margins have been described in the treatment of musculoskeletal malignancies: intralesional, marginal, wide, and radical (4). Each type of wound margin can be achieved by either a limb salvage or limb ablative (amputation) procedure.

The *intralesional* margin of resection implies that gross and microscopic tumor remain in the wound following the definitive surgical procedure. GCT of bone of the distal radius is commonly treated with this type of margin (curettage), although often with the addition of some adjunctive treatment such as bone cement, phenol, or liquid nitrogen. Nevertheless, recurrence rates are as high as 50%. When applied to soft tissue sarcomas, this may be termed a "debulking" procedure.

Marginal excision of a malignancy involves resection of a tumor *en bloc,* though the reactive zone between the tumor pseudocapsule and normal tissue is not entirely removed, which may leave microscopic tumor cells. A tumor that is merely "shelled out" and later is found to be malignant has likely undergone a marginal excision.

In a *wide excision,* the surgical margin passes outside of the reactive tumor zone, through normal tissue, but is still within the anatomic compartment of the tumor. Ideally, the tumor should not be visualized during the course of the procedure. In the wrist, a wide excision may be more easily achieved for sarcomas on the dorsum, where tendons may be sacrificed, flaps rotated, and tendon transfers performed for functional reconstruction. On the volar aspect of the wrist, sarcomas involving the palm and carpal tunnel area have often contaminated so many surrounding structures that a wide excision is not technically feasible.

Radical excision involves removing the tumor and the entire compartment it is contained within; removal of a small tumor within the thenar compartment would require removal of all the thenar muscles to constitute a radical resection. Similarly, a radical margin for an osteosarcoma of the distal radius would involve removal of the entire radius bone.

With respect to malignancies involving the wrist, rarely is a radical margin obtained. (Even a below-elbow amputation would not constitute a radical margin for a typical wrist malignancy.) Usually, a wide surgical margin is aimed for, but for maximal preservation of hand and wrist function, a marginal or intralesional excision may be accepted in selected cases, especially if the patient refuses a recommended amputation. The primary surgical goal, however, should always be for adequate tumor control for patient survival, with a secondary priority being to produce as little functional morbidity as possible.

How Wide Does a Wide Excision Need to Be?

Unlike more proximal lesions in the forearm, arm, thigh, or leg, where there is room for a wider resection, in the hand and wrist a 1- to 2-cm margin of normal tissue may severely compromise hand or wrist function. How much margin of normal tissue is acceptable for a "wide margin" is therefore of concern to the hand surgeon. The acceptable criteria for a wide margin of excision in the upper extremity have ranged from more than 3 cm (13) to 1 to 2 cm or less if a thick fascial barrier provides one of the margins (14). The resection is considered by some authors to have positive margins if tumor is present within 1 mm of the margin (14). For soft tissue sarcomas, it has been suggested that radiotherapy may offset the effect of positive margins (tumor at the margin of resection) by killing residual tumor cells in the surrounding tissue. The downside of leaving residual tumor behind is that local recurrence is much more likely, and it has been shown that local recurrence may lead to higher rates of metastatic disease and therefore lower survival rates (15).

A recent large study has shown that postoperative radiotherapy did not negate the effect of positive tumor margins in soft tissue sarcomas of the hand (16). In this paper, the recommendation was made that tumor-free margins must be obtained by wide local excision, or amputation if necessary, since patients with positive resection margins were much more likely to have a local recurrence despite adequate radiotherapy. Patients with a hand sarcoma with negative margins had no worse survival than patients with a sarcoma with negative margins at other anatomic sites, while the hand sarcoma group with positive margins had a significantly worse survival than patients with sarcomas with positive margins at other anatomic sites (16).

Some authors, by contrast, have found excellent results treating soft tissue sarcomas of the forearm and hand with limb salvage protocols consisting of wide or marginal excision, chemotherapy, and radiation therapy (17,18). In one of these studies, there was only an 8% recurrence rate (average follow-up less than 4 years) and a 91% survival rate, with 86% of the patients having an excellent functional result (17). Limb salvage was achieved in some cases by stripping tumor off the perineurium of the involved nerves and the peritenon from the involved tendons to allow their preservation. Surgical resections where tumor is stripped off major nerves and vessels consitute a marginal resection, by definition, and longer follow-up of these patients is mandatory.

The effect of chemotherapy has been beneficial in some series and has shown no benefit in other studies; therefore, it should not be relied on to compensate for positive margins in soft tissue sarcomas (16). Chemotherapy has been shown to improve survival in osteosarcoma (5).

Our recommendation for surgical treatment of musculoskeletal sarcomas involving the wrist and hand is that a wide margin of resection, preferably at least 1 cm, should be achieved. Postoperative radiotherapy is given following wound healing, and adjuvant chemotherapy is employed on protocol in conjunction with the oncology staff. Sarcomas treated with an amputation or wide excision where a tumor-free margin greater than 3 cm is obtained do not usually require postoperative radiotherapy.

SPECIFIC TUMORS

GCT of bone, though not generally considered a malignancy, can be extremely locally aggressive and may occasionally metastasize. GCT is therefore included in this chapter. The most common musculoskeletal soft tissue sarcomas involving the wrist include synovial cell sarcoma, epithelioid sarcoma, rhabdomyosarcoma, and malignant fibrous histiocytoma; all are discussed. One of the most common primary bone sarcomas involving the wrist is osteosarcoma, and this tumor is reviewed.

Giant-Cell Tumor of Bone

GCT of bone is an unusual lesion that, while displaying benign but locally aggressive histologic characteristics, still carries the ability to metastasize and kill the patient. In a large review of GCTs from the Istituto Rizzoli over a 70-year period, the majority of the lesions were found around the knee (63%), with the distal radius and ulna representing the second most common site (10%) (19). Fewer than 15 case reports of GCT involving the carpal bones have been found. Multicentric foci of GCT of bone may be found in up to 18% of patients with GCT involving the hand (20). Multicentric GCT of bone occurs in fewer than 1% of cases of GCT of bone overall, and it is difficult to distinguish definitively between multiple primary foci of GCT and "metatastic" GCT (21–24).

GCT of bone usually (but not always) involves the epiphyseal end of the bone following growth plate closure. It appears as an eccentric epiphyseal lytic lesion that may erode through the cortex or into the joint. Left untreated, it may grow to a huge size and destroy local structures (Fig. 45.2). The age group affected ranges from 20 to 45 years old, with tumors rarely seen before age 15 or after age 60.

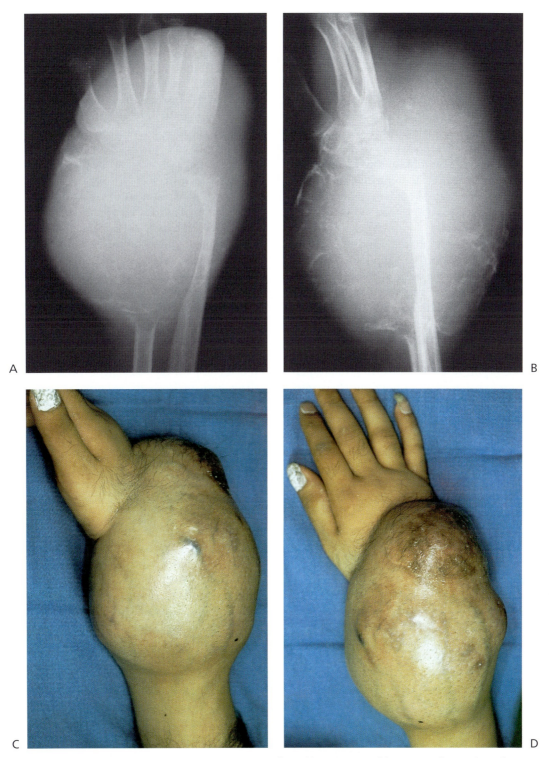

FIGURE 45.2. This rather impressive tumor was found in a 42-year-old woman who neglected a problem with her wrist for quite some time. Anteroposterior **(A)** and lateral **(B)** x-rays of a huge giant-cell tumor of bone of the distal radius. **C,D:** Clinical appearance.

There is a slight majority of women in some series (19). Most lesions have a thin covering of periosteum and appear friable and reddish-orange to brown. Histologic examination reveals a vascularized network of stromal cells and multinucleated giant cells held together by a scant intercellular matrix. The degree of histologic atypia does not correlate with its clinical behavior (Fig. 45.3).

GCT of bone involving the hand and wrist usually presents with localized pain or a tender mass. The diagnosis will usually be suggested by plain film, but MRI should be obtained to exclude extracortical or joint involvement. A chest x-ray and chest CT scan should be performed to exclude pulmonary metastases. A bone scan should be done to exclude multicentric tumors.

Treatment recommendations in the hand and carpus generally involve wide resection or amputation of the involved area. The reason for the surgical aggressiveness is the surprisingly high recurrence rate reported by Averill, Patel, and others, showing that curettage was ineffective for these hand and carpal lesions (20,25). Two patients in the series of Averill subsequently succumbed to pulmonary and visceral metastases from GCT of bone involving the metacarpals. A case report of a GCT involving the trapezium was treated by excision of the trapezium, trapezoid, partial capitate, scaphoid, first and second metacarpal excisions, removal of the thenar muscles, the distal tendons of the flexor carpi radialis (FCR), extensor carpi radialis longus (ECRL), and first dorsal compartment as well. Reconstruction was performed with iliac crest bone grafting with no recurrence reported at 30 months' follow-up (26). Another case report involving GCT of the lunate (preoperative diagnosis was Kienböck's disease) was treated with a proximal row carpectomy with limited follow-up reported (27).

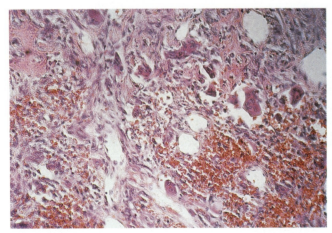

FIGURE 45.3. Photomicrograph of a giant-cell tumor of bone. Note the presence of multinucleated giant cells. Histologic appearance does not correlate with clinical behavior.

Treatment of GCT of the distal radius or ulna may involve curettage and bone graft, curettage and bone cementing (both with or without adjunctive instillation of phenol, liquid nitrogen, or another agent to maximize tumor kill), or wide resection of the involved bone followed by reconstruction with a vascularized or nonvascularized autograft or allograft. A long-term follow-up of GCT of the long bones treated with curettage, instillation of phenol, and methylmethacrylate cement revealed a recurrence rate of 50% for the distal radius, similar to rates of recurrence of 40% to 60% with curettage and bone grafting (28). Treatment of GCT of bone in the hand with radiotherapy has been condemned by some authors as producing as high as a 20% incidence of radiation sarcoma (20), though other authors have advocated radiotherapy for treatment of large, recurrent, and surgically nonresectable lesions (29,30).

En bloc resection of the distal radius requires that the radiocarpal and distal radioulnar joints be dealt with. Either the joints can be reconstructed (in an effort to preserve some wrist motion) or a radio- or ulnocarpal fusion may be performed. Options for joint reconstruction involve (a) prosthetic joint replacement, (b) free vascularized fibula or iliac crest graft, with attempted recreation of a distal graft–carpal joint, and (c) placement of a matching distal radius allograft or autograft with or without fusion of the scaphoid and lunate to the graft.

To date, prosthetic radius replacement has not enjoyed successful results in the treatment of GCT of bone of the distal radius (31,32). This is a tumor generally found in young adults who will likely wear out a prosthetic wrist replacement.

When a large resection of radius bone has been performed (>5–7 cm), a vascularized autograft may be preferred. Pho has reported five patients with a GCT of the distal radius treated by wide resection and placement of a free vascularized fibula autograft (33). In two of these patients primary wrist fusion was done. One patient had an attempted creation of a "fibula–carpal joint" and developed carpal subluxation postoperatively; this was subsequently converted to a wrist fusion. In two other patients a "fibula–carpal joint" was created, and the wrist was reported to be stable and painless with 50° to 90° of motion. It was suggested that incongruity of the articular surfaces may lead to "degenerative changes at a later stage."

Leung reported four cases of GCT of the distal radius treated by resection and reconstruction of the distal radius with a free vascularized iliac crest autograft (34). In this procedure, the iliac crest does not have an articular surface and is contoured to "look like" a distal radius articular surface. The advantages of this procedure, according to the authors, comparing the free iliac crest to the free fibula procedure with joint reconstruction, were that the operative time was shorter, less donor site morbidity was found, and the iliac crest had a higher likelihood of incorporation, being mostly corticocancellous bone, compared to the fibula cortical bone. In Leung's cases, all four patients were free of pain and had excellent motion, but "subluxation is obvious, and further follow-up study is required...." Distal radioulnar joint instability was not a reported problem in this series.

Attempting creation of a "pseudoradiocarpal joint" using either vascularized fibula or iliac crest has the inherent problem of incongruity of the articular surfaces in both procedures, combined with the difficulty of ligamentous reconstruction.

Another concept for reconstruction of the distal radius that would preserve wrist motion would be to fuse the proximal carpal row, or at least the scaphoid and lunate, to a nonvascularized (35,36) or vascularized graft (37). This would preserve midcarpal motion and should provide wrist stability as well. Such a conception using ipsilateral vascularized ulna translocation was reported by Seradge in 1982 (37). Two patients with a GCT of the distal radius were treated by resection of the tumor and translocation of the ipsilateral ulna, preserving its vascularity. The distal articular surface of the ulna was resected, and the ulna was fused to the lunate and scaphoid. Both cases achieved 85% of forearm rotation and 10° to 15° of wrist flexion–extension. No instability of the proximal ulna was reported.

Allograft replacement of the distal radius is a well-described option for reconstruction of the tumor defect. Smith has reported three cases of GCT of the distal radius treated with osteoarticular allograft replacement with reconstruction of the wrist ligaments to the allograft (38). Follow-up of under 3 years was reported without tumor recurrence, and wrist motion was between 60° and 70° without pain. One patient developed painless volar subluxation of the carpus between 1 and 2 years postoperatively.

Our recommendation for GCT of bone of the distal radius and ulna involves curettage, phenol instillation, and bone grafting if the tumor is contained within the bone. If the tumor has broken out of the bone or is growing rapidly, we favor allograft replacement of the distal radius. For distal ulnar lesions we recommend allograft replacement for large lesions, and curettage with bone graft or resection of the distal ulna for smaller lesions.

Giant-Cell Tumor
Case Studies

A 34-year-old man presented with a lytic mass of the distal radius (Fig. 45.4). An open biopsy was performed via a dorsal cortical window between the first and second compartments. Pathology revealed GCT, and he underwent curettage and iliac crest bone grafting with recurrence noted 9 months postoperatively. The decision was therefore made to perform allograft replacement of the distal radius. A dorsal approach to the wrist was utilized. The remainder of the extensor retinaculum was reflected, and the extensor tendons retracted radially and ulnarly. The distal radius was dissected out extraperiosteally in an attempt to preserve the volar and radioulnar joint ligaments (Fig. 45.4B,C). A portion of the pronator quadratus was left attached to the volar aspect of the radius. Two months postoperatively, the allograft–radius juncture was still visible on radiographs. The juncture was completely healed at 1 year postoperativly (Fig. 45.4F,G). Painless wrist range of motion of 30° flexion–extension was present.

A 26-year-old woman presented with left ulnar-sided wrist pain. X-rays revealed a lytic lesion of the distal ulna (Fig. 45.5A,B). She underwent curettage and bone graft of a GCT of bone. She developed a recurrence 6 months postoperatively, and x-ray and MRI revealed significant distal ulnar involvement (Fig. 45.5C,D). The decision was made to perform allograft replacement of the distal ulna. The ulna was exposed via a standard ulnar-border incision. It was transected proximally, leaving a 5-cm margin of uninvolved bone and levered out of the wound. Distal dissection removed all tumor and the triangular fibrocartilage complex (TFCC), and the radioulnar ligaments were cut at their ulnar border. An allograft was then inserted and held with a seven-hole plate across a step-cut osteotomy. The TFCC and radioulnar ligaments were sutured, and the distal radioulnar joint was held in neutral with a Kirschner wire (Fig. 45.5E–G). This tumor proved to be extremely aggressive, and within 1 year a local recurrence was noted involving the operative site. The allograft was removed, and a repeat excision was performed, showing recurrent GCT. Another recurrence was noted 1 year later, and at this point she underwent repeat excision and radiotherapy to the area with regression of the soft tissue lesion. Five years after the initial surgery, she presented with groin and hip pain and was found to have a large GCT involving the pelvis (Fig. 45.5H), which was resected and cemented. Shortly thereafter she developed pulmonary and rib GCT lesions and underwent resection of the left seventh rib and multiple wedge resections of the left lower and upper lobes. Subsequently she sustained a pathologic fracture (because of GCT) of T-8 and T-9 several months later and underwent T-8 and T-9 corpectomies with allograft reconstruction (Fig. 45.5I,J). Unfortunately, she developed progression of the pelvic disease (Fig. 45.5K) with severe pain requiring repeat surgery, more radiotherapy, and insertion of a pain pump for pain management. She remains alive, though functionally limited. This case demonstrates the potential aggressiveness of metastatic or multifocal GCT of bone. It is doubtful whether even a primary below-elbow amputation would have controlled her systemic disease, because it is felt that

(text continues on p. 733)

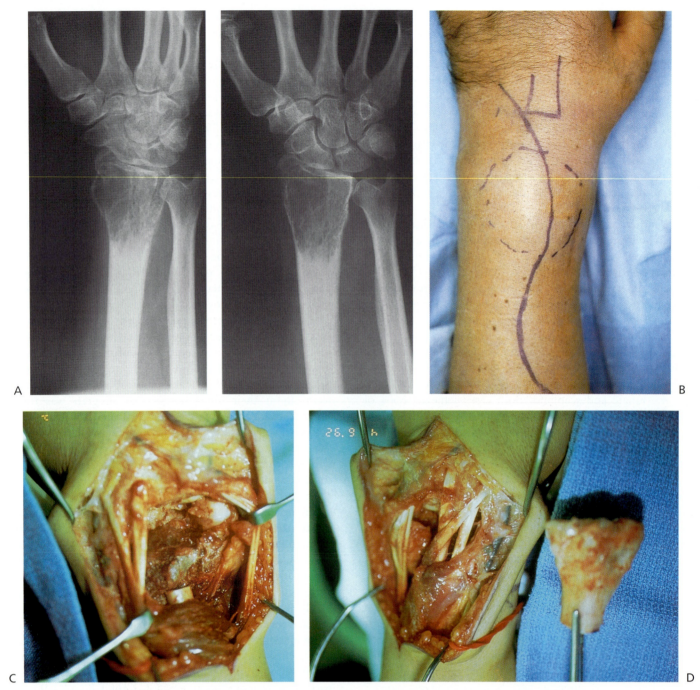

FIGURE 45.4. A 34-year-old man presented with a lytic mass of the distal radius. **A:** X-ray showing lytic lesion of distal radius. Note epiphyseal location consistent with giant-cell tumor of bone. **B:** Clinical appearance of, and surgical incision for, the dorsal exposure of the giant-cell tumor of the distal radius. **C:** The distal radius has been removed. Note the preservation of wrist, thumb, and finger extensors and margin of resection of the proximal edge of the radius. **D:** The tumor has been removed. The wrist and finger extensors have been allowed to fall back into place.

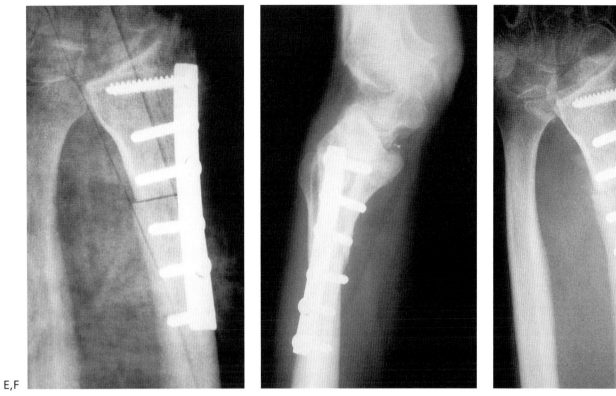

FIGURE 45.4. *(continued)* **E:** Anteroposterior x-ray 2 months postoperatively shows the allograft–radius juncture still visible. **F:** Lateral x-ray 1 year postoperatively showing that allograft–host juncture healing is complete. **G:** Anteroposterior x-ray 1 year postoperatively shows healed allograft juncture.

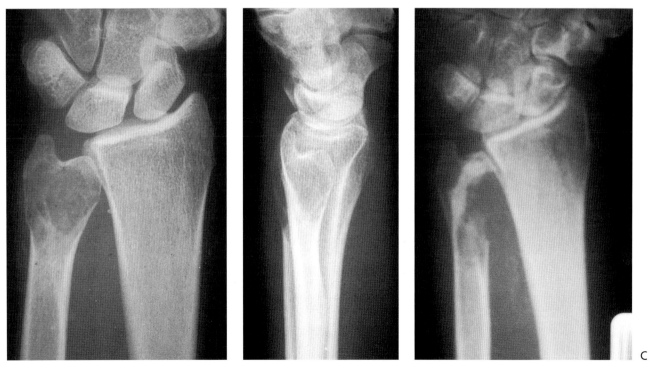

FIGURE 45.5. A 26-year-old woman presented with left ulnar-sided wrist pain. **A:** Anteroposterior x-ray showing lytic lesion of the distal ulnar epiphyseal area. The diagnosis was giant-cell tumor (GCT) of bone. **B:** Lateral x-ray of same lesion. **C:** X-ray appearance 6 months following curettage with recurrence of GCT in the bone. *(continued on next page)*

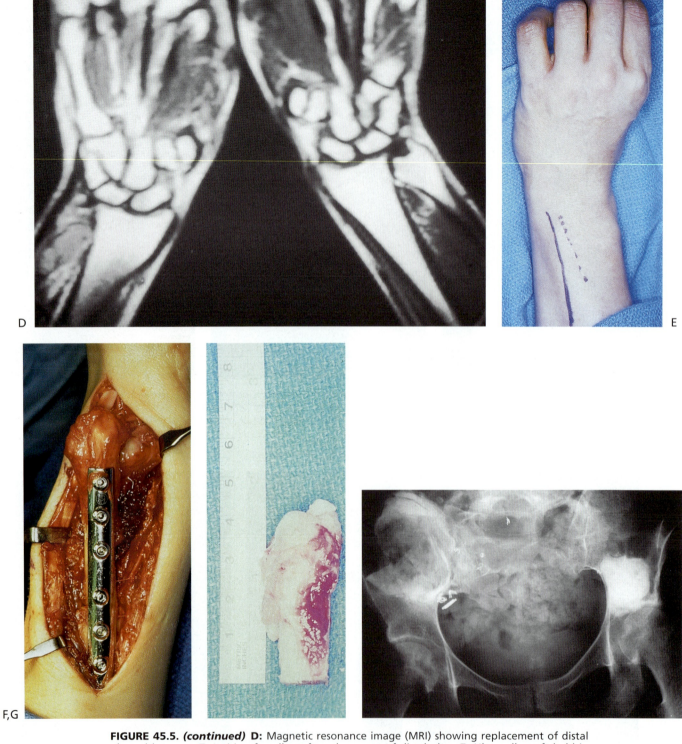

FIGURE 45.5. (continued) D: Magnetic resonance image (MRI) showing replacement of distal ulna with tumor. **E:** Incision for allograft replacement of distal ulna. **F:** Ulnar allograft held in place with plate and screw fixation. **G:** Resected segment of ulna bone. **H:** Giant-cell tumor metastasis in pelvis. X-ray of pelvis shows cement fixation of lesion following curettage.

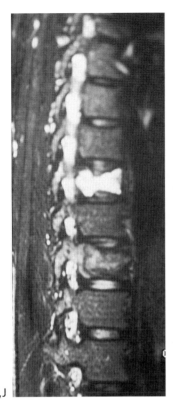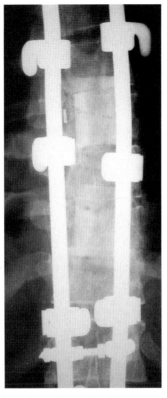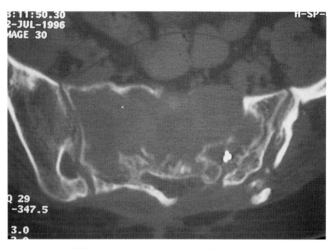

FIGURE 45.5. *(continued)* I: MRI of thoracic spine showing GCT involvement of vertebral bodies with pathologic fracture of T-8 and T-9. **J:** X-ray following T-8 and T-9 corpectomies with allograft reconstruction and spinal instrumentation. **K:** MRI showing progression of pelvic GCT disease with extensive bony destruction.

this variant of GCT may arise in separate sites. Cummins notes, in a comprehensive review of multicentric GCT, that if a second lesion at a distant location develops in a patient with GCT, there is a distinct possibility that additional lesions will develop (21). Multicentricity is particularly common with GCT involving the hands (20).

Osteosarcoma

Osteosarcoma is a rare primary bone malignancy usually occurring in the first two decades of life with a peak later in life occurring in 1% of patients with Paget's disease (secondary osteosarcoma). The metaphyseal area of long bones is the most common site of osteosarcoma, with half of tumors found around the knee; appearance in the hand and wrist is quite unusual. Usually, osteosarcoma is a lytic, destructive, intramedullary lesion (39). Advances in the past 15 years in staging, chemotherapy, and surgical management have improved survival rates from 25% to better than 60% with current adjuvant chemotherapeutic protocols (40). It has been shown that limb salvage with wide local excision produces survival rates equal to those of amputations (41). Surgical options for treatment of osteosarcoma of the distal radius parallel those for GCT of the distal radius except that curettage and bone grafting or cement is not an option; the bone must be widely resected and reconstructed.

Case Presentation: Osteosarcoma

A 29-year-old man presented with an osteosarcoma of the distal radius that had eroded the cortex (Fig. 45.6A,B). In order to obtain a wide margin of resection, both distal forearm bones as well as the proximal carpal row were resected. The entire pronator quadratus and interosseous membrane were removed with the specimen. An allograft was selected for bone reconstruction and was fused to the distal carpal row with K-wires and an intramedullary pin (Fig. 45.6C–E). The patient received postoperative chemotherapy. Unfortunately, he developed a deep postoperative wound infection beneath an area of skin necrosis and required complete removal of the allograft (Fig. 45.6F). Length was maintained with an external fixator until the wound was sterilized (Fig. 45.6G). A free vascularized osteoseptocutaneous fibula transfer (Fig. 45.6H) was performed to reconstruct the bony defect and held with an intramedullary pin. The distal juncture healed, but the proximal juncture required repeat plating to achieve union

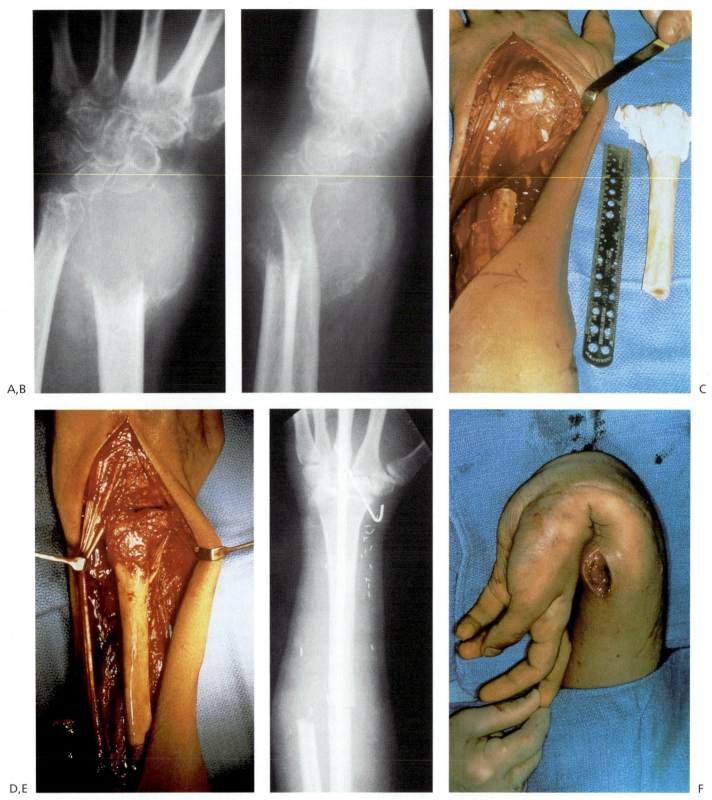

FIGURE 45.6. A 29-year-old man presented with an osteosarcoma of the distal radius that had eroded the cortex. **A:** Anteroposterior x-ray of osteosarcoma obliterating distal radius. **B:** Lateral view. **C:** Intraoperative photograph showing allograft radius replacement (right) and surgical bed following resection of radius, ulna, and proximal carpal row. **D:** Allograft secured in place. **E:** X-ray showing fixation of allograft to proximal radius with intramedullary pin and fusion to proximal row with Kirschner wire. **F:** Intraoperative photograph showing complete flaccidity of forearm following allograft removal for postoperative infection.

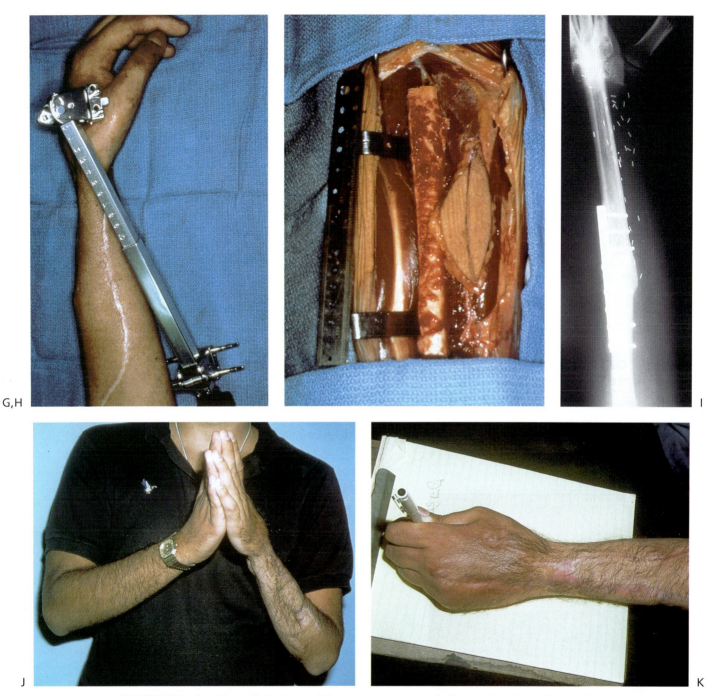

FIGURE 45.6. *(continued)* G: External fixator used to maintain forearm length until the infection cleared. **H:** Intraoperative photograph of free fibula osteoseptocutaneous transfer for bony and soft tissue reconstruction of forearm. **I:** X-ray showing fixation of free fibula transfer with compression plate and screws with healed juncture. **J:** Clinical photograph 11 years following initial tumor resection. **K:** Patient can write with reconstructed wrist, which is stable, sensate, and painless.

(Fig. 45.6I). The patient has functional use of the hand and a stable wrist and is free of disease, now 11 years following the initial surgery (Fig. 45.6J,K).

Malignant Fibrous Histiocytoma

This tumor is one of the more common soft tissue sarcomas involving the hand and wrist. It was first identified in 1964 by Brien and Stout as a biphasic tumor with fibrocytes and histiocytes. Many previous cases were likely misdiagnosed as fibrosarcoma. The most common location is the trunk, thigh, and knee area, with the upper extremity being the next most frequent site of involvement (42) (Fig. 45.7). The majority of cases occur between 50 and 70 years of age, and the tumor usually arises deep in muscular and fascial structures. It can also arise primarily within bone and extend into the soft tissues. Overall prognosis is 30% to 50% 5-year survival. Surgical therapy mandates wide local excision or amputation. Postoperative chemotherapy or radiation therapy is given on protocol.

Synovial Cell Sarcoma (Synovioma)

Synovial cell sarcoma is a "biphasic" tumor that may appear calcified 25% to 30% of the time on x-ray. It is a highly malignant tumor, but somewhat capricious in its behavior in that it may lie inactive for months or years or may metastasize aggressively and kill within months. Regional lymph node involvement may be seen and should be searched for. In some series this is the most frequent soft tissue sarcoma of the hand and wrist area (6). The average age is 26 years, and most are found under age 40, with a slight male predominance. Synovioma often is found around large joints, especially the knee. Approximately 25% of synoviomas are found in the upper extremity, with hand involvement seen in 4% to 20% of cases. Clinical symptoms include a deep palpable mass in 97% and pain in 21% to 76% (2,6). Often the mass is quite large when finally detected. Prognosis is poor overall, with many reported instances of tumor recurrence even after a 10-year disease-free survival interval. Five-year survival has been reported from 25% to 60%, but 10-year survival falls to 11% to 30%. For tumors specifically involving the hand, 9% 10-year survival is reported (43). Surgical treatment requires either adequate wide local excision or amputation. Amputation is generally associated with lower local recurrence rates but not necessarily with improved survival. We usually recommend below-elbow amputation for lesions of the carpus and wrist that are greater than 2 cm in diameter. Chemotherapy is given on protocol, and radiotherapy is given for limb-salvage cases where wide excision is performed. Regional lymph node involvement may be treated with resection or radiation.

Case Example: Synovial Cell Sarcoma

A 39-year-old man was referred following an "unplanned excision" of what was found to be a synovial cell sarcoma involving the palm. Repeat excision (Fig. 45.8) of the surgical site revealed residual tumor adjacent to the transverse carpal ligament, which was excised. Amputation was recommended for surgical control, but the patient refused. Postoperative radiotherapy was given, and the patient now remains free of disease or local recurrence 2 years following surgery.

Epithelioid Sarcoma

Epithelioid sarcoma is the most common hand sarcoma in some series. This tumor also has a predilection for regional lymph node metastasis. Epithelioid sarcoma is found in young adults, usually men, and the most common location is the upper extremity (56%) with most occurring in the hand–forearm areas. Commonly, a small superficial nodule less than 1 cm is found, but often the mass is ignored until it becomes much larger and deeper. Like synovioma, this tumor may lie dormant for years and then become aggressive. Ten-year survival has been reported between 25% and 75% (13,44,45). A recent large review of epithelioid sarcoma found that survival was significantly better at 10 years

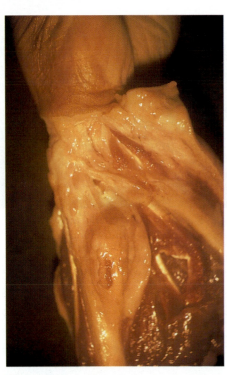

FIGURE 45.7. A 52-year-old man who developed a deeply invasive malignant fibrous histiocytoma involving the wrist and forearm. Below-elbow amputation was performed.

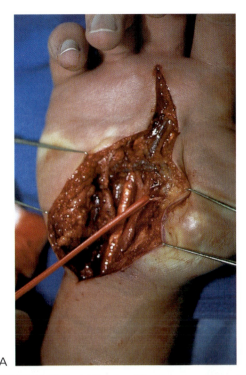 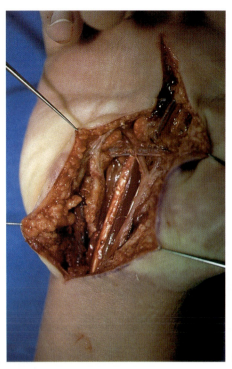

FIGURE 45.8. A 39-year-old man was referred following an "unplanned excision" of what was found to be a synovial cell sarcoma involving the palm. **A:** Intraoperative photograph showing repeat excision of a synovial cell sarcoma involving the palm. **B:** No visible tumor remains following excision of residual tumor adjacent to the transverse carpal ligament.

when a wide resection with a disease-free margin greater than 3 cm was done than when a marginal resection was performed (negative margins but through the reactive zone of the tumor). Adjuvant radiotherapy or chemotherapy did not seem to improve results following marginal resection (13).

Case Example: Epithelioid Sarcoma

A 45-year-old man presented with a soft tissue tumor involving the dorsal hand and wrist. Wide local excision of a biopsy-proven epithelioid sarcoma resulted in recurrence within 4 months. Invasion of the dorsal carpal bones and metacarpals was found, and an amputation was recommended (Fig. 45.9A). A midforearm amputation was performed with closure of the forearm muscles over the bone ends (Fig. 45.9B–D). An immediate-fit prosthesis was provided (Fig. 45.9E,F). Chemotherapy was given on protocol postoperatively, and the patient remains free of disease 2 years postoperatively.

Rhabdomyosarcoma

Rhabdomyosarcoma is the most common soft tissue sarcoma of childhood. In children, the most common type is the embryonal variety, which is seen between birth and age 15 years with an average of 8 years. Alveolar rhabdomyosarcoma is seen in an older patient group with an average age of 15 years. Typically the patient presents with a rapidly growing painless mass that spreads along lymphatic and hematogenous routes. Histologic diagnosis is often difficult. Surgical treatment involves wide local excision or marginal excision with postoperative radio- and chemotherapy. Prophylactic lymph node dissection is no longer recommended, but involved nodes should be sampled at the time of surgery. Recent advances in combined chemotherapy have improved survival rates to above 70% (6).

METASTATIC TUMORS

In general, in patients over age 40 or 50 with a suspected or known primary malignancy (usually breast, lung, or kidney), a painful radiolucent lesion involving the hand or wrist should be considered a possible metastasis. Within the hand, the distal phalanx is the most common site of metastasis, and the carpus the least likely. Overall, hand metastasis is uncommon, representing approximately 0.1% of all metastatic lesions. The prognosis of patients with hand

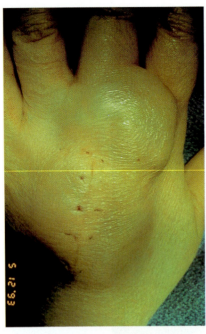
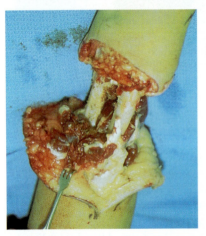
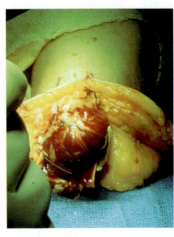
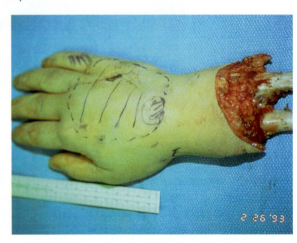
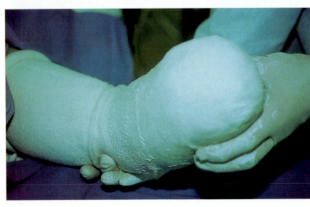
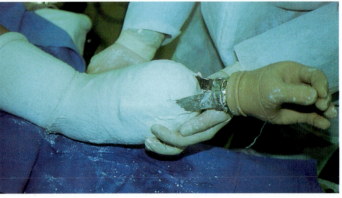

FIGURE 45.9. A 45-year-old man presented with a soft tissue tumor involving the dorsal hand and wrist. **A:** Photograph of dorsum of hand showing a recurrence of an epithelioid sarcoma 4 months following marginal excision. **B:** Intraoperative photograph showing level of resection of radius and ulna for wide excision of the tumor by below-elbow amputation. **C:** Intraoperative photograph showing "fishmouth"-type incision and closure of forearm muscles over bone ends. **D:** Tumor specimen. **E:** Construction of immediate fit plaster cast for prosthesis. **F:** Hand prosthesis in place.

metastasis is poor, with half of patients in one series expiring within 6 months (3).

CONCLUSIONS

Malignant tumors involving the wrist are quite rare, but the index of suspicion should always be high when a patient presents with an unusual or deep lesion of the wrist. Preoperative evaluation should include appropriate workup (usually involving MRI) so as to avoid the unfortunate "unplanned excision" of a soft tissue sarcoma. Biopsy should be treated with the utmost respect and preferably performed in a referral center. Surgical treatment of most malignant tumors of the wrist requires wide resection at a minimum, and for lesions of the volar aspect of the wrist or deeply invasive dorsal lesions, amputation is often required for adequate tumor control. Radiotherapy should not be relied on to "clean up" a marginal excision of most soft tissue sarcomas. Chemotherapy is useful for selected malignancies.

REFERENCES

1. Dick HM, Angelides AC. Malignant bone tumors of the hand. *Hand Clin* 1989;5:373–381.
2. Dick HM, Lee DH. Synovial sarcoma and rhabdomyosarcoma. In: Bogumill GP, Fleegler EJ, eds. *Tumors of the hand and upper limb.* New York: Churchill Livingstone, 1993;296–309.
3. Amadio PC, Lombardi RM. Metastatic tumors of the hand. *J Hand Surg [Am]* 1987;12:311–316.
4. Mankin HJ. Principles of diagnosis and management of tumors of the hand. *Hand Clin* 1987;3:185–195.
5. Dick HM, Strauch RJ. Tumors of the hand and wrist. In: Dee R, Hurst LC, Gruber MA, et al, eds. *Principles of orthopaedic practice.* New York: McGraw-Hill, 1997;1165–1171.
6. Dick HM. Synovial sarcoma of the hand. *Hand Clin* 1987;3: 241–245.
7. Simon MA, Finn HA. Diagnostic strategy for bone and soft-tissue tumors. *J Bone Joint Surg Am* 1993;75:622–631.
8. Mankin HJ, Mankin CJ, Simon MA. The hazards of the biopsy revisited. *J Bone Joint Surg Am* 1996;78:656–663.
9. Skrzynski MC, Biermann JS, Montag A, et al. Diagnostic accuracy and charge-savings of outpatient core needle biopsy compared with open biopsy of musculoskeletal tumors. *J Bone Joint Surg Am* 1996;78:644–649.
10. Noria SN, Davis A, Kandel R, et al. Residual disease following unplanned excision of a soft-tissue sarcoma of an extremity. *J Bone Joint Surg Am* 1996;78:650–655.
11. Simon MA, Biermann JS. Biopsy of bone and soft-tissue lesions. *J Bone Joint Surg Am* 1993;75:616–621.
12. Enneking WF, Spanier SS, Goodman MA. The surgical staging of musculoskeletal sarcoma. *J Bone Joint Surg Am* 1980;62: 1027–1030.
13. Steinberg BD, Gelberman RH, Mankin HJ, et al. Epithelioid sarcoma in the upper extremity. *J Bone Joint Surg Am* 1992;74: 28–35.
14. Bell RS, O'Sullivan B, Liu FF, et al. The surgical margin in soft-tissue sarcoma. *J Bone Joint Surg Am* 1989;71:370–375.
15. Creighton JJ, Peimer CA, Mindell ER, et al. Primary malignant tumors of the upper extremity: retrospective analysis of one hundred twenty-six cases. *J Hand Surg [Am]* 1985;10:805–814.
16. Brien EW, Terek RM, Geer RJ, et al. Treatment of soft-tissue sarcomas of the hand. *J Bone Joint Surg Am* 1995;77:564–571.
17. Wexler AM, Eilber FR, Miller TA. Therapeutic and functional results of limb salvage to treat sarcomas of the forearm and hand. *J Hand Surg [Am]* 1988;13:292–296.
18. Bray PW, Bell RS, Bowen CVA, et al. Limb salvage surgery and adjuvant radiotherapy for soft tissue sarcomas of the forearm and hand. *J Hand Surg [Am]* 1997;22:495–503.
19. Campanacci M, Baldini N, Boriani S, et al. Giant cell tumor of bone. *J Bone Joint Surg Am* 1987;69:106–114.
20. Averill RM, Smith RJ, Campbell CJ. Giant-cell tumors of the bones of the hand. *J Hand Surg [Am]* 1980;5:39–50.
21. Cummins CA, Scarborough MT, Enneking WF. Multicentric giant cell tumor of bone. *Clin Orthop* 1996;322:245–252.
22. Sim FH, Dahlin DC, Beabout JW. Multicentric giant-cell tumor of bone. *J Bone Joint Surg Am* 1977;57:1052–1060.
23. Peimer CA, Schiller AL, Mankin HJ, et al. Multicentric giant-cell tumor of bone. *J Bone Joint Surg Am* 1980;62:652–656.
24. Tornberg DN, Dick HM, Johnston AD. Multicentric giant-cell tumors in the long bones. *J Bone Joint Surg Am* 1975;57: 420–422.
25. Patel MR, Desai SS, Gordon SL, et al. Management of skeletal giant cell tumors of the phalanges of the hand. *J Hand Surg [Am]* 1987;12:70–77.
26. Weiner SD, Leeson MC. Giant cell tumor of the carpal trapezium. *Orthopedics* 1995;18:482–484.
27. FitzPatrick DJ, Bullough PG. Giant cell tumor of the lunate bone: A case report. *J Hand Surg [Am]* 1977;2:269–270.
28. O'Donnell RJ, Springfield DS, Motwani HK, et al. Recurrence of giant-cell tumors of the long bones after curettage and packing with cement. *J Bone Joint Surg Am* 1994;76:1827–1833.
29. Malone S, O'Sullivan B, Catton C, et al. Long-term follow-up of efficacy and safety of megavoltage radiotherapy in high-risk giant cell tumors of bone. *Int J Radiat Oncol Biol Physics* 1995;33: 689–694.
30. Bennett CJ, Marcus RB, Million RR, et al. Radiation therapy for giant cell tumor of bone. *Int J Radiat Oncol Biol Physics* 1993;26: 299–304.
31. Gold AM. Use of a prosthesis for the distal portion of the radius following resection of a recurrent giant-cell tumor. *J Bone Joint Surg Am* 1965;47:216–218.
32. Gold AM. Use of a prosthesis for the distal portion of the radius following resection of a recurrent giant-cell tumor. *J Bone Joint Surg Am* 1957;39:1374–1380.
33. Pho RWH. Malignant giant-cell tumor of the distal end of the radius treated by a free vascularized fibular transplant. *J Bone Joint Surg Am* 1981;63:877–884.
34. Leung PC, Chan KT. Giant cell tumor of the distal end of the radius treated by the resection and free vascularized iliac crest graft. *Clin Orthop* 1986;202:232–236.
35. Campbell CJ, Keokarn T. Total and subtotal arthrodesis of the wrist. *J Bone Joint Surg Am* 1964;46:1520–1533.
36. Wilson PD, Lance EM. Surgical reconstruction of the skeleton following segmental resection for bone tumors. *J Bone Joint Surg Am* 1965;47:1629–1656.
37. Seradge H. Distal ulnar translocation in the treatment of giant-cell tumors of the distal end of the radius. *J Bone Joint Surg Am* 1982;64:67–72.
38. Smith RJ, Mankin HJ. Allograft replacement of distal radius for giant cell tumor. *J Hand Surg [Am]* 1977;2:299–309.
39. Feldman F. Primary bone tumors of the hand and carpus. *Hand Clin* 1987;3:269–289.

40. Link MP, Goorin AM, Miser AW, et. al. The effect of adjuvant chemotherapy on relapse-free survival in patients with osteosarcoma of the extremity. *N Engl J Med* 1986;314:1600–1606.
41. Simon MA. Limb salvage for osteosarcoma. *J Bone Joint Surg Am* 1988;70:307–310.
42. Dick HM. Malignant fibrous histiocytoma of the hand. *Hand Clin* 1987;3:263–268.
43. Dreyfuss UY, Boome RS, Kranold DH. Synovial sarcoma of the hand—a literature study. *J Hand Surg [Br]* 1986;11:471–474.
44. Peimer CA, Smith RJ, Sirota RL, et al. Epithelioid sarcoma of the hand and wrist: patterns of extension. *J Hand Surg [Am]* 1977;2:275–282.
45. Bos GD, Pritchard DJ, Reiman HM, et al. Epithelioid sarcoma. *J Bone Joint Surg Am* 1988;70:862–870.

46

DIAGNOSIS AND MANAGEMENT OF REFLEX SYMPATHETIC DYSTROPHY (COMPLEX REGIONAL PAIN SYNDROME)

LOIS CARLSON
H. KIRK WATSON

Reflex sympathetic dystrophy (RSD) is a potential complication of any trauma to the wrist. Minor trauma combined with some unknown changes in the internal milieu can produce a devastating chain reaction that results in RSD. The injury may be as simple as catching a fingertip in a door or immobilization for any reason. There are probably patients who are predisposed to RSD, but the specific factors are yet to be defined. These are emotionally influenced and, at this point, nondefinable. The disease process begins with a breakdown in communication between the nerve and vascular systems. The nervous system helps to maintain an adequate capillary flow. At the capillary level, a lack of proper regulation results in either too little, too much, or normal blood flow to any group of cells. Both excessive and diminished flow result in sick cells. These areas of hypovascularity and color hypervascularity result in various temperature and color changes that can vary with time. Synovial tissue with its abundance of nerve endings is the predominant pain source. The process may involve only a single digit or the entire upper extremity. Some cell death occurs, resulting in scar replacement. This results in pericapsular fibrosis.

Reflex sympathetic dystrophy should be thought of as an active disease similar to infection. It should be attacked early and corrected as rapidly as possibly, as the disease process results in gradually increasing cell death and fibrosis, particularly involving joints. Clinically, symptoms include pain, edema, and vasomotor, sudomotor, and trophic changes, with decreased mobility, strength, and function. The symptoms are out of proportion to the trauma and extend beyond the site of injury.

There is continued controversy concerning appropriate nomenclature and diagnostic criteria. The actual mechanisms that initiate and maintain this abnormal constellation of symptoms are also unclear. Because of the present lack of understanding of underlying pathophysiology, the descriptive term "complex regional pain syndrome" (CRPS) (1) is now recommended by the International Association for the Study of Pain (IASP).

This chapter includes a discussion of diagnostic criteria and terminology, theoretical considerations, RSD in relation to wrist disorders, clinical assessment, and treatment options. The authors' preferred treatment approach is then highlighted.

DIAGNOSTIC CRITERIA AND TERMINOLOGY

Lankford's criteria for diagnosis of RSD have frequently been cited in the hand surgery literature (2). The cardinal signs and symptoms are pain, swelling, stiffness, and discoloration. Secondary signs include sudomotor, temperature, and trophic changes, vasomotor instability, osseous demineralization, and palmar fibromatosis. A presumptive diagnosis is made if all the cardinal and most of the secondary signs are present to a much greater degree than anticipated (2). The diagnosis is confirmed, according to Lankford, by a positive response to sympathetic block.

In 1989, the American Association for Hand Surgery (AAHS) accepted a committee report defining diagnostic criteria for RSD as diffuse pain, loss of hand function, and

---

L. Carlson: Connecticut Combined Hand Therapy, Glastonbury, Connecticut 06033, and Hartford, Connecticut 06106.

H. K. Watson: Connecticut Combined Hand Surgery Fellowship, Hartford Hospital, and Connecticut Children's Medical Center, Hartford, Connecticut 06106; Department of Orthopaedics, University of Connecticut School of Medicine, Farmington, Connecticut 06032; Department of Orthopedics, Rehabilitation, and Plastic Surgery, Yale University School of Medicine, New Haven, Connecticut 06520.

sympathetic dysfunction (3). Pain is further described as frequently being nonanatomic and out of proportion to the inciting trauma. Objective criteria for autonomic dysfunction include changes in temperature, blood flow, sweating, hair and nail growth, edema, atrophy, osteoporosis, and bone scan. This definition does not require a positive response to sympathetic block.

In a more recent classification scheme adopted by the IASP, what is commonly known as RSD is included under the term CRPS (1). Type I (RSD) and type II (causalgia) are subtypes; the terms RSD and causalgia are kept for transitional use. Sympathetically maintained pain (SMP) is not included as a separate category, but is a descriptor of a type of pain that may or may not be present (Table 46.1). Symptoms and signs of CRPS type I (RSD) include disproportionate pain (including allodynia/hyperalgesia or spontaneous pain) and evidence of edema, abnormal blood flow, or sudomotor dysfunction. Trophic changes and motor symptoms may also be present but are not necessary for diagnosis (1). A positive response to sympathetic block is also not required.

THEORETICAL CONSIDERATIONS

What Causes Reflex Sympathetic Dystrophy?

The pathophysiology of RSD is still unknown. Current theories proposed to explain RSD include peripheral and central nervous system abnormalities with and without sympathetic nervous system dysfunction. There may be different mechanisms underlying symptoms in subgroups of patients (4) or more than one mechanism in any one individual (5).

Role of the Sympathetic Nervous System

Until recently, it has generally been accepted that RSD is associated with sympathetic hyperactivity. Alternatively, decreased sympathetic activity after tissue injury may cause adaptive supersensitivity in blood vessels and nociceptive nerve endings, which then become more responsive to circulating catecholamines or norepinephrine (NE) released from sympathetic terminals (6–8). Evidence from studies of RSD patients includes lower plasma concentrations of the

TABLE 46.1. CLASSIFICATION OF COMPLEX REGIONAL PAIN SYNDROME

CRPS describes a variety of painful conditions that usually follow injury, occur regionally, have a distal predominance of abnormal findings, exceed in both magnitude and duration the expected clinical course of the inciting event, often result in significant impairment of motor function, and show variable progression over time.

CRPS Type I (RSD)
- Follows an initiating noxious event.
- Spontaneous pain or allodynia/hyperalgesia occurs beyond the territory of a single peripheral nerve, and is disproportionate to the inciting event.
- There is or has been evidence of edema, skin blood flow abnormality, or abnormal sudomotor activity in the region of the pain since the inciting event.
- This diagnosis is excluded by the existence of conditions that would otherwise account for the degree of pain and dysfunction.

CRPS Type II (Causalgia)
- This syndrome follows nerve injury. It is similar in all respects to type I.
- Is a more regionally confined presentation about a joint (e.g., ankle, knee, wrist) or area (e.g., face, eye, penis), associated with a noxious event.
- Spontaneous pain or allodynia/hyperalesia is usually limited to the area involved but may spread variably distal or proximal to the area, not in the territory of a dermatomal or peripheral nerve distribution.
- Intermitttent and variable edema, skin blood flow change, temperature change, abnormal sudomotor activity, and motor dysfunction, disproportionate to the inciting event, are present about the area involved.

Sympathetically maintained pain
- Pain that is maintained by sympathetic efferent activity or neurochemical or circulating catecholamine action, as determined by pharmacological or sympathetic nerve blockade. SMP may be a feature of several types of pain disorders, and is not an essential component of any one condition. Conditions without any response to sympathetic block are, by contrast, designated as having SIP states.

CRPS, complex regional pain syndrome; RDS, reflex sympathetic dystrophy; SIP, sympathetic independent pain; SMP, sympathetically maintained pain.
From Boas RA. Complex regional pain syndromes: symptoms, signs, and differential diagnosis. In: Janig W, Stanton-Hicks M, eds. *Reflex sympathetic dystrophy: a reappraisal*. Seattle: IASP Press, 1996:82, with permission.

sympathetic neurotransmitters NE (6,7) and neuropeptide Y (9) and increased responsiveness of venous α-adrenoceptors to local NE (8). Increased sensitivity of tissues distal to the site of trauma in response to sympathetic hypoactivity may be combined with sympathetic hyperactivity proximal to the site of trauma (10). Other theories include a failure of opioid modulation in regional sympathetic ganglia (11) or a more complex disturbance in sympathetic reflex patterns (12).

Regional Inflammatory Reaction

RSD may represent an excessive regional inflammatory reaction (13–15). The evidence to support this theory, as recently reviewed by van der Laan and Goris (14), includes increased vascular permeability for macromolecules and tissue hypoxia despite a high oxygen supply in acute RSD, evidence of oxidative stress in chronic RSD, and increased levels of bradykinin and calcitonin gene-related peptide. Results of five-phase bone scintigraphy (lateralization of regional hyperemia, increased microvascular permeability, and bone metabolism) have been reported to correlate with protein concentrations and blood cell counts that, although within normal range, suggest a subacute inflammatory process (15).

Central Sensitization

According to the classic description by Livingston, afferent impulses from a focus of irritation cause an abnormal state of activity in the internuncial pool of the spinal cord (16). This, in turn, results in abnormal sympathetic and somatic efferent output, causing vasomotor changes and muscle spasms. These peripheral abnormalities then become additional sources of abnormal afferent activity and pain (16). Roberts has proposed that SMP may be related to sympathetically induced activity in low-threshold myelinated mechanoreceptors, causing firing in wide-dynamic-range neurons in the spinal cord previously sensitized by C nociceptors (17). Variations of this theory include a need for ongoing nociceptor activity in the maintenance of central sensitization (18) and that this activity may be sympathetically dependent or independent (19) (Fig. 46.1).

Pain Component

Clinical and laboratory studies have helped identify different categories of pain and possible underlying mechanisms that may or may not involve the sympathetic nervous system (20,21). Patients with RSD may experience a variety of types of pain, including spontaneous pain, hyperalgesia (increased pain in response to stimuli that are normally painful), and allodynia (pain caused by stimuli that are not normally painful). Evoked pain may occur in response to static and dynamic mechanical stimuli as well as thermal stimuli. Pain normally occurs with injury and/or inflammation caused by activation of $A\delta$ and C nociceptors. Increased pain may occur from sensitization of these nociceptors. Central changes may cause input from $A\beta$ afferents to be interpreted as pain rather than touch.

Sympathetic–sensory coupling may occur following peripheral nerve injury and/or inflammation (22). Evidence to support such coupling includes relief of pain with sympathetic blocks and studies of RSD patients in whom application of NE increases or rekindles pain (23). Norepinephrine may have a direct effect on α-adrenoceptors of sensory afferents that are sensitized as a result of injury (24) or may trigger the release of a prostaglandin from the sympathetic postganglionic terminal, which in turn sensitizes nociceptive sensory afferents (25). Indirect coupling may also occur secondary to microvascular changes (22).

Vascular Component

Reported vascular abnormalities in RSD patients include increased, decreased, and/or variable blood flow, impaired vasomotor reflexes, and increased microvascular permeability to macromolecules (10,14,26). These vascular disturbances may reflect a combination of factors, including a localized inflammatory response, antidromic excitation of small-diameter afferents, the influence of the sympathetic nervous system, and the development of adrenergic sensitivity in microvessels.

Cooke (27) has proposed that the altered hemodynamics are caused by locally acting neuroactive and vasoactive peptides, leading to vasodilation, a low-flow state, and pain. This exaggerated response to injury may be caused by hypersensitivity to pain, inactivity, failure of inhibitors, and/or some

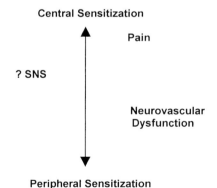

FIGURE 46.1. The pathophysiology of reflex sympathetic dystrophy (RSD) is still unknown but may involve peripheral and central sensitization of structures affecting the neurovascular and sensory systems. The role of the sympathetic nervous system (SNS) is not clear. Sympathetic activity has been proposed to be increased, decreased, or normal. Although the mechanisms underlying RSD are unclear, the clinical picture is characterized by pain and loss of normal neurovascular control.

other unknown factor. Substances released with tissue injury (such as bradykinin and prostaglandins) stimulate nociceptors and cause persistent vasodilation and inactivation of arteriovenous shunts, with loss of thermoregulatory control. The resulting tissue hypoxia initiates a sequence of events leading to continued activation of nociceptors (27).

The potential neurovascular effects of the sympathetic nervous system are complex. Sympathetic postganglionic neurons have peripheral mediator functions in addition to transmitting centrally generated impulses (22). Following tissue trauma, for example, inflammation of the joint capsule may result in part from bradykinin-stimulated production and release of a prostaglandin from sympathetic terminals, which causes increased permeability of the venules and plasma extravasation. This requires the presence of sympathetic nerve terminals but is not directly dependent on electrical activity in sympathetic neurons. Conversely, excitation of sympathetic neurons innervating the joint capsule and synovia causes vasoconstriction of the arterioles, which decreases plasma extravasation by decreasing blood flow (28).

In RSD, decreased sympathetic activity may cause an increased responsiveness of α-adrenoceptors to NE in blood vessels (8). This may explain the typical pattern of increased blood flow initially, followed by a decrease during the later stages (10). Fluctuations in vascular status may also be caused by the effects of competing influences, such as adrenergic vasoconstriction versus nociceptor-induced antidromic vasodilation (29). The relative predominance of one factor over another may vary within different vascular beds and with exposure to internal or external stressors. Trophic changes may occur secondary to neurovascular dysfunction and impaired nutritive microcirculation (30).

Psychological and Predisposing Factors

It has been proposed that psychological traits and stressful life events may predispose individuals to the development of RSD (31). Most studies comparing patients with RSD versus other types of pain, however, suggest that RSD patients do not present with a unique psychosocial disturbance (32,33). On the other hand, the pain and dysfunction accompanying RSD may cause emotional and behavioral changes that limit active use of the extremity and exacerbate the patient's level of pain (33,34).

A premorbid history of sympathetic hyperactivity or lability has also been suggested as a predisposing factor (2). This may be reflected by a previous history of migraines, cold hands and feet, fainting, blushing, and sweaty palms. Controlled, prospective studies are needed to determine the relevance of this theory. The idea that genetic factors play a role in causing certain individuals to be "at risk" for RSD also merits further study (35).

Current experimental and clinical data fail to adequately explain all aspects of RSD. Theoretically, RSD may be caused by the failure of mechanisms that normally modulate and signal the termination of the inflammatory response to injury, with peripheral and central changes that may or may not involve a sympathetically mediated process (Fig. 46.1). The pain and vascular abnormalities may both be caused by the same underlying neuroinflammatory mechanism. The evolution of trophic changes may be caused by neurovascular dysregulation compounded by a lack of use of the extremity secondary to pain.

REFLEX SYMPATHETIC DYSTROPHY AND THE WRIST

The reported incidence of RSD following wrist surgery in published studies during the past 10 years is generally 5% or less. The rate of occurrence of RSD may vary depending on the criteria used to define RSD as well as the underlying diagnosis, surgical procedure, and method of clinical management. Any source of pain may potentially increase the likelihood of the development of RSD, including tight dressings or casts, increased carpal tunnel pressure with the wrist fixed in a flexed position, compression of the superficial radial nerve, or unresolved wrist pathology. Prolonged casting may also predispose the patient to the development of this syndrome. A review of 1,077 limited wrist arthrodeses from our clinic, for example, indicates a rate of 1.9% (36) versus an overall rate of 0.5% following surgery (37).

RSD is frequently cited as a complication following distal radius fractures. Field and Atkins found an incidence of 24% in 100 patients using the criteria of finger tenderness, swelling, joint stiffness, and vasomotor instability to establish the diagnosis of RSD (38). Bickerstaff reports a similar incidence (28% in 274 patients) using the same criteria (39). A prospective study by Hove of 542 patients, however, indicated an incidence of 4% (<1% with lasting symptoms using the AAHS criteria for RSD) (40).

What are some of the factors that contribute to RSD following distal radius fractures? Field found an association between symptomless tightness of casts during the first 3 weeks after injury and development of RSD (41). Cast tightness was measured by placing an empty drip bag inside the cast, injecting air into the bag, and then taking pressure readings using a sphygmomanometer. He suggests that RSD causes the tightness, rather than the reverse (41). Method of fixation and prolonged fixation in distraction may also be related (42,43).

Bone loss has been found to be more severe and prolonged in distal radius fractures complicated by RSD, continuing for at least a year (versus a control group, in which recovery of bone occurred by 31 weeks) (44). In a long-term outcome study 10 years after a distal radius fracture in 55 patients, 26% still had features of RSD, the most common being tenderness in the fingers (45). An association was evident between continued vasomotor instability and pain, and both were associated with osteoarthritis.

CLINICAL ASSESSMENT OF REFLEX SYMPATHETIC DYSTROPHY

The evaluation should include a thorough history and examination as a baseline and guide to treatment (Table 46.2) and to rule out anatomic causes of increased pain and dysfunction, such as joint instability or peripheral nerve compression. Although most cases involve the entire hand, RSD can present in a more isolated fashion (46). Involvement of multiple limbs has also been reported (13).

Pain, Tenderness, and Sensibility

Pain may be evaluated subjectively using verbal reports, visual analog scales, and/or pain diagrams. Pain posturing and pain behaviors versus spontaneous functional use are also noted. The "volar plate test" is used to monitor joint tenderness. It is positive if there is increased pain with passive flexion of the joint, especially the proximal interphalangeal joints of the hand. This test is a quick and valuable way to monitor regional changes as the patient gets better with treatment and generally correlates with improvements in the vasomotor and trophic status.

Additional evaluation may include tests of hyperalgesia and allodynia in response to heat and cold, dynamic and static mechanical stimuli, and mechanical summation. A description of these tests has been published, including practical suggestions for testing each type of pain within a clinical setting (21). Other tests that may be of value in quantifying pain include dolorimetry (47), the McGill Pain Questionnaire (48), and the more recently developed Neuropathic Pain Scale (49).

Discriminative sensation is also assessed, including monofilament and two-point testing. Hypoesthesia or hyperesthesia may be present. Impaired discriminative ability may help identify specific patterns of nerve involvement.

Edema

Edema is measured using a volumeter and may be considered abnormal if the volume of the hand, as measured by water displacement, is greater than 5% more than that of the unaffected hand (48). Circumferential measurements may also be used to monitor changes if edema is more localized, to monitor regional improvements, or when it is not feasible to take volume measurements.

Vasomotor and Sudomotor Changes

Vasomotor and sudomotor changes are reflected clinically by alterations in color, temperature, capillary refill, and sweat pattern. Observations of color include erythema, cyanosis, mottling, and/or pallor. Temperature disturbance may be estimated by palpation or thermometry. Absolute values may not be relevant, as temperature readings vary widely with ambient temperature and stress. A difference of >1°C in comparison to the unaffected side may be significant (50). Capillary refill may be increased or decreased. Sweating may also be enhanced or diminished (hyperhidrosis or hypohidrosis). The vasomotor, sudomotor, and trophic changes tend to coincide with the pattern of pain and tenderness as described by the patient and supported by the volar plate test.

Trophic Changes

Subtle changes may be detected within weeks of the development of RSD. Trophic changes include flattening of the cuticle base (often the earliest trophic change), shiny skin, flattening of the rugae pattern, decreased pulp bulk, increased nail curvature in either plane, increased or decreased hair growth, palmar thickenings or nodules, and generalized atrophy.

Radiographic findings include "patchy" demineralization with increased juxtaarticular bone loss and swelling (51).

TABLE 46.2. CLINICAL EVALUATION

Pain, tenderness, and sensibility	Subjective description of pain
	  Verbal report
	  Visual analog scale
	  Pain diagram
	Volar plate test
	Modality-specific tests of pain
	Tests of discriminative sensibility

Edema	Volumeter Circumferential measurements

Vasomotor/sudomotor changes	Changes in color/temperature
	  Observation/palpation
	  Thermometry
	  Capillary refill test
	Sweat disturbance
	  Observation/palpation

Trophic changes	Flattening of the cuticle base Thin, shiny skin Flattening of the rugae pattern Decreased pulp bulk Increased nail curvature Hair growth abnormality Palmar thickenings or nodules Generalized atrophy Demineralization on x-ray

Mobility, strength, and function	ROM (goniometry)
	Strength (grip/pinch)
	Function
	  Observation
	  Standardized tests of function
	  Activities of daily living checklist

ROM, range-of-motion.
Clinical evaluation is critical for diagnosis, monitoring of progress, and providing objective feedback to the patient. Additional testing may be used to help substantiate the diagnosis or for research purposes. There should generally be a correlation between pain and tenderness (as measured by palpation using the volar plate test) and observable vasomotor, sudomotor, and trophic changes.

Mobility, Strength, and Function

Standard methods of evaluation are used, including goniometry, grip and pinch strength testing, and observation of function. Standardized tests of function or activity of daily living checklists may also be used to help monitor progress. Initially, motion is limited primarily by pain and edema, progressing to more fixed deformities. In addition to decreased motion and strength, movement disorders have been reported to be associated with RSD, including dystonia, spasms, and tremor (52).

Additional Testing Methods

Beyond the basic clinical evaluation, additional tests may be used to help substantiate the diagnosis of RSD, although there is no test that has been universally accepted as a "gold standard." The diagnosis of RSD can generally be made from clinical assessment; however, additional testing may be indicated in select cases and for research purposes.

A positive response to sympathetic block is no longer considered necessary for diagnosis of RSD (or CRPS type I), but a block may be used to help differentiate sympathetically maintained from sympathetically independent pain states (1). The value of diagnostic blocks without placebo control has been questioned (53).

The three-phase bone scan has been suggested as a test to help diagnose RSD. Mackinnon and Holder reported that diffuse increased periarticular uptake in the third phase (delayed image) has a sensitivity of 96% and specificity of 98% (54). From a review of published studies, Lee and Weeks suggest that this test is more accurate during the initial stage of RSD but should not be used as a major criterion in diagnosis (55).

Other tests may be used to help quantify clinical impressions of vasomotor and sudomotor changes. Methods reported to assess vasomotor status include thermography, cold stress testing, laser Doppler flowmetry, and vital capillaroscopy (26,50,56). Sudomotor function may be evaluated using resting sweat output and the quantitative sudomotor axon reflex test (57).

Differential Diagnosis

Unfortunately, the term RSD is used too frequently to diagnose any patient with unexplained pain, even in the absence of adequate objective evidence. Some of these patients in reality have an undiagnosed underlying structural problem but have been sidetracked into months of treatment for pain without adequately addressing the cause. Others may have RSD in addition to local or systemic problems (3). Factitious or conversion-type reactions may mimic RSD (58,59). Ochoa has suggested that many patients diagnosed with RSD without nerve injury have a psychogenic pseudoneuropathy (60). Objective clinical and functional testing with use of substitution maneuvers can help differentiate symptom magnifiers from true cases of RSD.

TREATMENT

Exercise plays a critical role in the management of patients with RSD. Early active motion and functional use should be encouraged to prevent the onset of RSD. If the patient is "at risk" or presents with RSD, the stress-loading program is instituted. This is the main focus of treatment within our clinic and is outlined in greater detail in the following section. Additional methods of treatment that have been reported in the literature are briefly described below.

Sympathetic interruption has traditionally been considered a primary goal of therapy. Stellate ganglion blocks have been widely used (2,61). Successful treatment with intravenous regional sympathetic blocks has been reported using a variety of agents, including guanethidine (62), reserpine (63), and bretylium (64). Other studies, however, have failed to demonstrate a significant difference in response versus placebo and have questioned the long-term effectiveness of these blocks (65). Sympathectomy is generally reserved for only the most severe cases that have had an excellent temporary response to a series of placebo-controlled sympathetic blocks. Any potential gain must be carefully weighed against the risk of serious side effects (66,67).

The wide array of drugs (oral, topical, or by injection) used in the treatment of RSD reflects the fact that there is no one "miracle drug." There are few well-controlled studies with long-term follow-up, and side effects may be significant. Adrenergic agents include clonidine (68) and phenoxybenzamine (69). The calcium channel blocker nifedipine, a vasodilator, has been reported to relieve pain (70). One study demonstrates good results using ketanserin, a serotenergic antagonist, administered intravenously (71). Antidepressants may have analgesic and modulatory effects on sympathetic hyperactivity (72). Anticonvulsants such as gabapentin (Neurontin) are recommended for the relief of lancinating pain (73). Corticosteroids have been used orally or by injection (74,75). Grundberg reported success with an intramuscular injection of methylprednisolone in conjunction with active exercise in 68% of 69 patients who were followed for at least 1 year (75). The nonsteroidal antiinflammatory ketorolac given intravenously with lidocaine resulted in partial response in 43% and complete response in 26% of 61 patients (76). Free-radical scavengers have also been used for their antiinflammatory effects (14,77). Topical administration of capsaicin has been used to decrease hypersensitivity (78). Calcitonin, more popular in Europe, is reported to have analgesic and antiosteoclastic effects (79). Bisphosphonates may also inhibit bone resorption (80). For a more in-depth review of pharmacological management, the reader is referred to recent review articles (72,81).

Although the importance of hand therapy (or physical and occupational therapy) is often alluded to in the literature, there have been few reported studies describing the efficacy of physical therapy alone or a specific treatment method. Johnson and Pannozzo reported good results in 82% of 65 patients treated with physical therapy alone using a "sensory overload" approach (82). This included exercise and exposure to a variety of stimuli, including heat and cold. Bernstein noted long-term improvement in 23 of 24 children, primarily with lower extremity RSD, using physical therapy (83). The treatment program emphasized weight-bearing activities, encouragement of activity and vigorous toweling to decrease sensitivity. Transcutaneous nerve stimulation (TENS) and electroacupuncture have been reported to be effective in the relief of pain (84–86). More recently, Grunert studied the effects of thermal biofeedback in conjunction with relaxation training and supportive psychotherapy. In a group of 20 patients, there was a significant decrease in pain (87). Current publications related to hand therapy in journals or texts are primarily descriptive and eclectic in their approach. Most warn against exacerbation of symptoms by treatment, particularly with passive mobilization. Walsh addresses treatment of pain, edema, joint stiffness, hypersensitivity, and vascular changes (88). A recent article by Hardy integrates a variety of treatment methods with theoretical considerations related to RSD and stresses "hands off" therapy. Pain is addressed first, with additional therapy aimed at resetting sensory thresholds, presenting challenges to the vasomotor system, and encouraging active motion and function (89).

Other modalities of treatment used for pain relief include local and regional somatic nerve blocks and implanted peripheral nerve stimulation. These methods may be more appropriate for treating somatic than sympathetic pain or when pain is restricted to a specific nerve distribution (90,91). Spinal cord stimulation has been recommended in cases unresponsive to other modes of treatment (85,92).

Stress-Loading (Dystrophile) Program

The most effective treatment for reflex sympathetic dystrophy is a load program (37,93). The best way to access tissue is by active demand. Stress loading employs the principle of adaptation in response to demand. It is defined as active traction and compression exercises requiring stressful use of the affected extremity, with minimal motion of painful joints. Clinically, two simple exercises are used that actively load the affected arm: scrubbing and carrying. A retrospective study using this approach was published in the *Journal of Hand Surgery* in 1987 (37). Results of long-term follow-up of 41 patients included improvement in pain in 88%, motion in 95%, and grip strength in all. The most important statistic from this study was the functional outcome. Of previously employed patients, 90% returned to work.

The program consists of two exercises as described below. Keys to the success of the program include compliance, maximum load, separation of treatment of RSD versus fibrosis, and emotional support. A home program sheet is used to increase compliance, recording each session and noting changes in weight and time. An "Activity" column is used to encourage and monitor the patient's use of the affected arm for function (Table 46.3).

1. "Scrubbing." The original version (still a viable option) simply uses a scrub brush. The patient gets down on hands and knees in a quadruped position, and scrubs a wooden board with a coarse bristled scrub brush, applying as much pressure as possible using a back and forth motion. Ideally, the patient leans forward over the affected arm, with the shoulder directly over the hand for maximum pressure and cocontraction of all muscle groups. The Dystrophile was developed to increase compliance. This is a piece of exercise equipment that simulates the scrub brush, and enables the therapist and patient to quantify the force and duration (Fig. 46.2). The timer and light on the Dystrophile are activated when the preset load is reached. Patients generally begin with 3 minutes of "scrubbing" at 4 lb pressure three times a day. The duration is increased as soon as possible up to 5 to 10 minutes. Once this level is reached, the force is then raised to tolerance. Force, not motion, is the critical factor. The patient is told to slow down if necessary to avoid tendinitis of the shoulder. A nonslip material (Scootguard or Dycem) may also be used to assist in gripping the Dystrophile.
2. "Carrying." The second part of the program involves carrying a weighted bag, briefcase, or purse in the

TABLE 46.3. STRESS LOADING (DYSTROPHILE PROGRAM) HOME PROGRAM SHEET

DYSTROPHILE PROGRAM
(Please bring this sheet with you to each therapy session.)

DYSTROPHILE: On hands and knees, push down on the handle until the light goes on. While keeping the light on, move the Dystrophile in a back and forth motion, as if scrubbing or sanding the floor. Write down the date and total minutes completed each time you "scrub."

CARRY: Carry a weighted suitcase or bag with your arm down at your side. Increase the weight as you can, and carry it whenever you are walking, even for short distances. Write down the number of pounds carried each day. Feel free to add more weight between sessions, unless your therapist had advised otherwise.

ACTIVITY LIST: Each day, write down one new activity you tried with your affected hand, or an activity that is getting easier to do.

DATE	DYSTROPHILE	CARRY	ACTIVITY
	Number/day ___	___ lb or	
	For ___ minutes	more	

affected hand, with the arm down by the side in the normal position for arm swing during ambulation (see Fig. 46.2). This is carried throughout the day whenever standing or walking. The weight should be increased to maximum tolerance (initial weight generally 1 to 5 lb). The handle can be padded or built up if needed to help hold the weight in the hand.

The typical scenario of reflex sympathetic dystrophy is an extremity so painful that it can barely be examined. To initiate the load program, the patient may be asked to use a towel to "scrub" a smooth surface for 1 to 3 minutes three times a day. They are warned to expect increased pain and swelling during the first few days, and to consider this a good sign of adequate load. A structured environment is necessary, and the patient is seen back in 24 to 48 hours. The loads are increased to 5 minutes three times a day, using a towel or, if possible, progressing to the dystrophile at its lowest setting. The patient is required to keep a daily ledger of the frequency and duration of each session. By 3 to 5 days, there is usually a decrease in pain, and the patient is better able to sleep. The involved parts of the extremity may still remain useless. The patient is progressed to 7 to 10 minutes three times a day on the dystrophile at maximum tolerable settings. By 7 to 10 days, the patient recognizes that the disease process is significantly improved and further encouragement to use the dystrophile may not necessary. The carry component is introduced when the patient is able to hold a small weight in the hand, and the weight is then gradually increased to tolerance.

All active dystrophy will respond to this load technique. Ideally, it is introduced before significant pericapsular fibrosis and the secondary changes of dystrophy have occurred. The active dystrophy can best be followed in a clinical setting by passive flexion of the proximal interphalangeal (PIP) joint. The pain of passive flexion of the PIP joint is called "the volar plate test." When there is no pain on forced passive flexion of the PIP, active dystrophy has been eradicated. The load technique is also effective in the predystrophy state (excessive pain and stiffness), as may be seen in patients after Dupuytren's surgery or Colles' fracture. Response to the dystrophile program is usually rapid and complete.

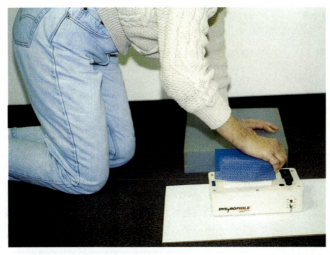
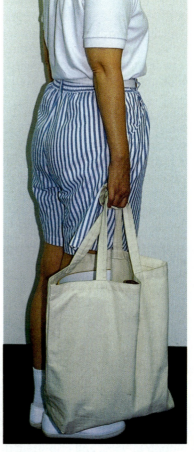

FIGURE 46.2. A: The compression technique loads the exremity with minimal joint range of motion. Basically, only the shoulder moves. All load is transferred through the tissues of the affected extremity. **B:** The carry component also loads the extremity with minimal motion but uses traction forces. The basic principle is loading of the tissues.

This concept of tissue response to active load is important not only in the treatment of the patient with RSD, but also in the rehabilitation of all patients postsurgery or injury. Full activity is allowed 48 hours postoperatively if the surgery does not require structural reattachment or bone healing, such as trigger fingers, de Quervain's, ganglia, CTS, dorsal wrist syndrome, and carpal boss repair. To emphasize this point patients are told they may "run a chainsaw." This practice limits morbidity and complications.

Although the program is quite simple, it is not always implemented in an optimum way because of failure to follow its basic principles:

1. Focus on compliance. The patient must be convinced that this approach will be successful. The patient must take an active, not passive, role in treatment and believe that progress will be made through this exercise program. The therapist and physician must be supportive, yet firm regarding the need for compliance.
2. Progress the program to maximum tolerated loads. Aggressively increase weight and duration of exercise despite temporary increases in pain and edema. Less than perfect technique or modifications may be necessary. For example, a patient in a cast may start scrubbing using a towel; the program may be modified for patients with lower extremity or back problems by scrubbing at a low table. The handle may also be modified to assist grip using thermoplastic materials (Fig. 46.3).
3. Separate treatment of RSD from treatment of fibrosis. Treat RSD first using stress loading only, both in the clinic and at home. If additional or alternative exercises are used, the principles of stress loading must be followed. For example, graded resistive pulley exercises or upper extremity "cycling" or rowing may be appropriate. Putty and other types of repetitive dynamic gripping exercises are contraindicated until the pain has subsided. Passive techniques too often cause increased synovitis and pain, aggravating the RSD, and must be avoided. Add other modalities only after the pain is significantly decreased, as measured by the volar plate test and reflected by other objective measures. Continue stress loading until the RSD is resolved and other modalities, as needed, are tolerated without relapse. Although the stress-loading program does not directly address joint motion, increased mobility usually occurs secondary to resolution of the pain and edema associated with RSD, unless the patient has progressed to fixed contractures.
4. Practice "emotional unloading." The patient is given a means to control the "disease." Give positive reinforcement, guidance, and reassurance. Demonstrate improvement at treatment sessions using measurements that are easily understood, such as volumetrics or grip strength. Encourage the patient to use the affected hand functionally and to chart improvements in daily living skills and return to normal activity for physical and emotional reasons.

Treatment of Fibrosis

Fibrosis occurs if RSD is not aggressively treated early. Treatment of fibrosis is started only after the RSD is under control. Dynamic active and resistive exercises are generally added first. Splinting is started, if needed, after the patient has successfully tolerated dynamic exercise without exacerbation of symptoms. Careful monitoring of these additions to treatment is required to avoid flaring the RSD.

If the wrist is fixed in flexion, serial static splinting may be necessary to bring the wrist into a more neutral position before final resolution of the RSD is possible. Severe wrist flexion (more than 30° flexion) puts pressure on the median nerve in the carpal canal and can significantly impair the patient's ability to grasp. This has occurred most commonly,

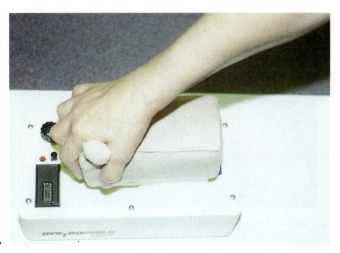
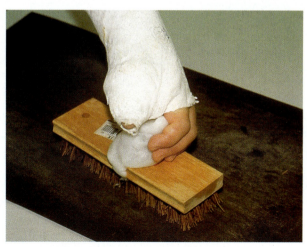

FIGURE 46.3. A,B: The Dystrophile or scrub brush can be adapted when grip is limited.

in our experience, following distal radius fractures. If this is the case, the patient is usually started on stress loading for several weeks; if wrist extension is not improving, serial plaster casting may be used to bring the wrist up to a neutral or slightly extended position. Judicious use of a circumferential thermoplastic splint as a "retaining splint" allows maintenance of gains until active wrist motion is possible. Occasionally, a hinge-type wrist splint has been used for the same purpose if this is adequate to maintain gains yet allow active wrist motion.

Anticipated Results of Treatment by Stage

Traditionally, RSD has been classified by stage, although patients do not necessarily progress through an orderly sequence within a set time frame. Both vasodilation and vasoconstriction may be present at the same time. For practical purposes, many patients may initially present with a red, hot, edematous hand (stage 1 or acute stage). Stage 2, the dystrophic stage, is characterized by fluctuations in vasomotor status and more obvious development of trophic changes and joint contractures. Stage 3, the atrophic stage, presents with fixed deformities, atrophy, severe demineralization, and often pallor.

During the acute stage, symptoms generally resolve quickly within days or weeks. Essentially full mobility and strength should be anticipated. If the patient is first seen during the dystrophic stage, the length of time required for resolution of the RSD is generally longer. Significant improvements are still noted in all parameters, including mobility, strength, and trophic changes, but additional treatment addressing fibrosis through conservative measures can be anticipated. If treatment begins in the atrophic stage, motion gains with stress loading may be minimal, although improvement in function and decrease in pain can still be achieved (Fig. 46.4). Surgical

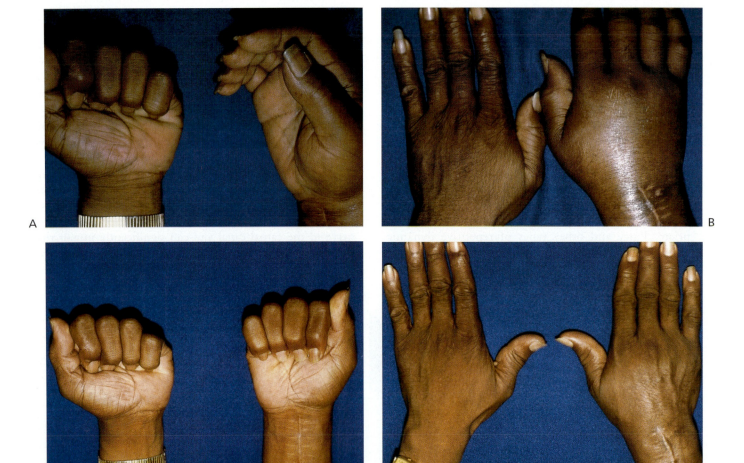

FIGURE 46.4. Stress loading can be effective at any stage of reflex sympathetic dystrophy (RSD), but residual motion deficits may occur if not treated early. **A–D:** A 42-year-old male forklift operator was referred six weeks following a distal radius fracture. Resolution of signs and symptoms of RSD was achieved using the stress-loading approach to treatment.

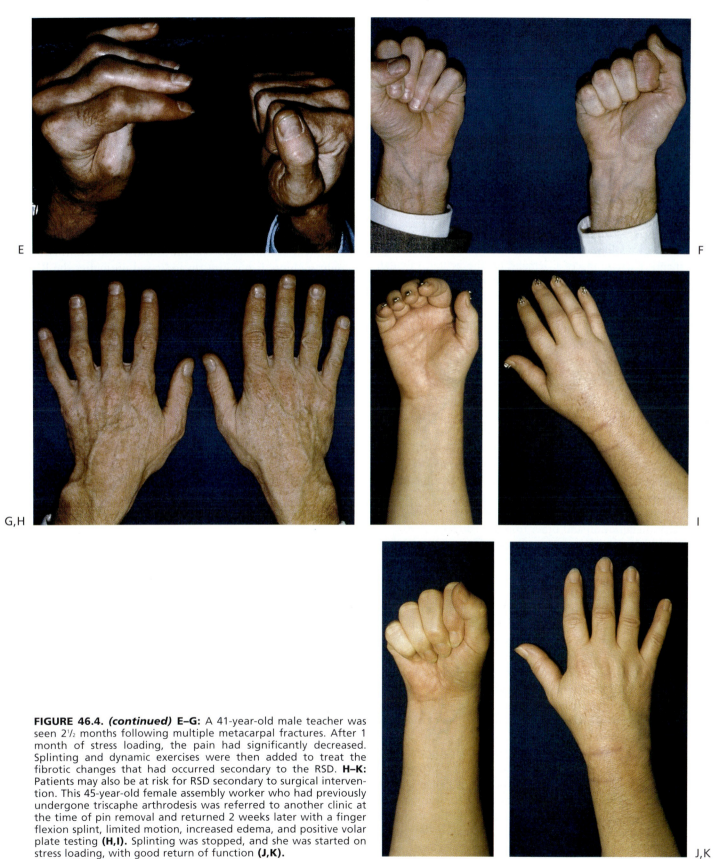

FIGURE 46.4. *(continued)* E–G: A 41-year-old male teacher was seen 2½ months following multiple metacarpal fractures. After 1 month of stress loading, the pain had significantly decreased. Splinting and dynamic exercises were then added to treat the fibrotic changes that had occurred secondary to the RSD. **H–K:** Patients may also be at risk for RSD secondary to surgical intervention. This 45-year-old female assembly worker who had previously undergone triscaphe arthrodesis was referred to another clinic at the time of pin removal and returned 2 weeks later with a finger flexion splint, limited motion, increased edema, and positive volar plate testing **(H,I)**. Splinting was stopped, and she was started on stress loading, with good return of function **(J,K)**.

intervention may include capsuloplasty of the metacarpophalangeal joints, check rein release of the proximal interphalangeal joints, and intrinsic release.

Theoretical Rationale

Theoretically, RSD may be caused by a failure to appropriately modulate and terminate the response to injury. Treatment should attempt to return the involved extremity to a state of normal homeostasis through reactivation of mechanisms that normally regulate tissue metabolism. Stressful exercise may provide such a stimulus to override what has become abnormally "normal" for the affected area.

The stress-loading program follows basic principles of exercise physiology (94). The body adapts in response to demand. Exercise places a demand on the neural, vascular, sensorimotor, and musculoskeletal systems, all of which may play a role in initiating and/or perpetuating RSD. An overload is needed to achieve a training effect. Exercise must be of sufficient intensity, duration, and frequency to achieve this training effect. Theoretically, this may be because of the effect of stress loading exercise on the following:

1. Neurovascular and inflammatory changes. Increased demand on the vascular system may stimulate reregulation of blood flow through regional and neurovascular control mechanisms. Cooke and Ward have stated that these changes in the circulation in patients with RSD may be reversible by active exercise despite an initial increase in pain (27). Normalization of nutritional blood flow to bone and other tissues may also be instrumental in the positive effects of exercise on bony demineralization and other trophic changes (95,96).
2. Central processing abnormalities. Afferent input associated with exercise may modulate or compete with the "distress" signals from other sources. Studies on normal subjects have indicated that exercise may have an inhibitory effect on cutaneous perception and pain, which may reflect inhibition of pain by muscle afferents or input from motor to sensory areas of the brain (97–99).
3. The sympathetic nervous system. One proposed theory of RSD is that decreased sympathetic activity results in "denervation supersensitivity" of sensory afferents and vascular smooth muscle. It is possible that sympathetic activation in response to exercise may result in "down-regulation" of these peripheral receptors. Another proposal by Hannington-Kiff is that RSD may be triggered by a failure of opioid modulation in regional sympathetic ganglia (11). He suggests that because increased blood concentrations of opioids occur during strenuous exercise, active use may maintain regional opioid modulation and protect the limb from RSD (11,100).

No conclusions can be drawn until more evidence is available regarding the pathophysiology of RSD and the mechanisms underlying the effectiveness of exercise in this patient population.

Stress Loading versus Other Approaches to Hand Therapy

There are three major distinctions between the stress-loading program and most other approaches as reported in the literature. First, RSD is treated only with stress loading, without interference from other modalities. Second, the stress-loading program is used despite the fact that increased pain and edema may initially occur. Most patients are able to tolerate this as long as they are convinced of the value of the program and are able to see some response to treatment within days. The third major distinction is that joint mobility is not directly addressed until after the RSD is under control. Improvement in function occurs with resolution of the underlying cause of the decreased motion, rather than treating the symptoms.

CONCLUSIONS

RSD is a potential complication of any wrist injury or surgical procedure. The clinician should be especially alert to the possibility of its development when long-term immobilization is required, with diagnoses commonly associated with RSD, or in patients with a possible predisposition for RSD.

Despite the current lack of understanding of this entity, these patients can be identified clinically and treated successfully using the stress-loading program. This exercise program can effectively resolve the constellation of signs and symptoms of RSD, including pain, edema, vasomotor, sudomotor, and trophic changes, and return these patients to an active life style. The stress-loading program should be instituted at the first sign of RSD or even on the clinician's "gut feeling" that the patient is at risk for RSD. It is a safe, successful, cost-effective treatment approach to the prevention and/or treatment of RSD. Early intervention prevents the progression of RSD. In the later stages, additional therapy must focus on correction of the fibrotic changes after the RSD is under control. Consistency in giving and receiving the message that RSD can be successfully treated is an important aspect of the therapeutic process.

REFERENCES

1. Stanton-Hicks M, Janig W, Hassenbusch S, et al. Reflex sympathetic dystrophy: changing concepts and taxonomy. *Pain* 1995;63:127–133.
2. Lankford LL. Reflex sympathetic dystrophy. In: Green DP, ed. *Operative hand surgery.* New York: Churchill Livingstone, 1993; 627–660.
3. Amadio PC, Mackinnon SE, Meritt WH, et al. Reflex sympathetic dystrophy syndrome: consensus report of an *ad hoc* com-

mittee of the American Association for Hand Surgery on the definition of reflex sympathetic dystrophy syndrome. *Plast Reconstr Surg* 1991;87:371–375.
4. Ochoa J. Human polymodal receptors in pathological conditions. *Prog Brain Res* 1996;113:185–197.
5. Moriwaki K, Yuge O, Tanaka H, et al. Neuropathic pain and prolonged regional inflammation as two distinct symptomatological components in complex regional pain syndrome with patchy osteoporosis—a pilot study. *Pain* 1997;72:277–282.
6. Drummond PD, Finch PM, Smythe GA. Reflex sympathetic dystrophy: the significance of differing plasma catecholamine concentrations in affected and unaffected limbs. *Brain* 1991; 114:2025–2036.
7. Harden RN, Duc TA, Williams TR, et al. Norepinephrine and epinephrine levels in affected versus unaffected limbs in sympathetically maintained pain. *Clin J Pain* 1994;10:324–330.
8. Arnold JM, Teasell RW, MacLeod AP, et al. Increased venous alpha-adrenoceptor responsiveness in patients with reflex sympathetic dystrophy. *Ann Intern Med* 1993;118:619–621.
9. Drummond PD, Finch PM, Edvinsson L, et al. Plasma neuropeptide Y in the symptomatic limb of patients with causalgic pain. *Clin Auton Res* 1994;4:113–116.
10. Kurvers HA, Hofstra L, Jacobs MJ, et al. Reflex sympathetic dystrophy: does sympathetic dysfunction originate from peripheral neuropathy? *Surgery* 1996;119:288–296.
11. Hannington-Kiff JG. Does failed natural opioid modulation in regional sympathetic ganglia cause reflex sympathetic dystrophy? *Lancet* 1991;338:1125–1127.
12. Baron R, Blumberg H, Janig W. Clinical characteristics of patients with complex regional pain syndrome in Germany with special emphasis on vasomotor function. In: Janig W, Stanton-Hicks M, eds. *Reflex sympathetic dystrophy: a reappraisal.* Seattle: IASP Press, 1996;25–48.
13. Veldman PH, Reynen HM, Arntz IE, et al. Signs and symptoms of reflex sympathetic dystrophy: prospective study of 829 patients. *Lancet* 1993;342:1012–1016.
14. Van der Laan L, Goris RJ. Reflex sympathetic dystrophy—an exaggerated regional inflammatory response? *Hand Clin* 1997;13: 373–385.
15. Leitha T, Korpan M, Staudenherz A, et al. Five phase bone scintigraphy supports the pathophysiological concept of a subclinical inflammatory process in reflex sympathetic dystrophy. *Q J Nucl Med* 1996;40:188–193.
16. Livingston WK. *Pain mechanisms: a physiologic interpretation of causalgia and its related states.* New York: Macmillan, 1943.
17. Roberts WJ. A hypothesis on the physiological basis for causalgia and related pains. *Pain* 1986;24:297–311.
18. Raja SN, Davis DK, Campbell JN. The adrenergic pharmacology of sympathetically maintained pain. *J Reconstr Microsurg* 1992;8:63–69.
19. Gracely RH, Lynch SA, Bennett GJ. Painful neuropathy: altered central processing maintained dynamically by peripheral input. *Pain* 1992;51:175–194.
20. Price DD, Long S, Huitt C. Sensory testing of pathophysiological mechanisms of pain in patients with reflex sympathetic dystrophy. *Pain* 1992;49:163–173.
21. Gracely RH, Price DD, Roberts WJ, et al. Quantitative sensory testing in patients with complex regional pain syndrome (CRPS) I and II. In: Janig W, Stanton-Hicks M, eds. *Reflex sympathetic dystrophy: a reappraisal.* Seattle: IASP Press, 1996;151–172.
22. Janig W, Levine JD, Michaelis M. Interactions of sympathetic and primary afferent neurons following nerve injury and tissue trauma. *Prog Brain Res* 1996;113:161–184.
23. Torebjork E, Wahren LK, Wallin G, et al. Noradrenaline-evoked pain in neuralgia. *Pain* 1995;63:11–20.
24. Rubin G, Kaspi T, Rappaport ZH, et al. Adrenosensitivity of injured afferent neurons does not require the presence of postganglionic sympathetic terminals. *Pain* 1997;72:183–191.
25. Levine JD, Taiwo YO, Collins SD, et al. Noradrenaline hyperalgesia is mediated through interaction with sympathetic postganglionic neurone terminals rather than activation of primary afferent nociceptors. *Nature* 1986;323:158–160.
26. Pollock FE, Koman LA, Smith BP, et al. Patterns of microvascular response associated with reflex sympathetic dystrophy of the hand and wrist. *J Hand Surg [Am]* 1993;18:847–852.
27. Cooke ED, Ward C. Vicious circles in reflex sympathetic dystrophy—a hypothesis. *J R Soc Med* 1990;83:96–99.
28. Miao FJ, Janig W, Levine JD. Role of sympathetic postganglionic neurons in synovial plasma extravasation induced by bradykinin. *J Neurophysiol* 1996;75:715–724.
29. Ochoa JL, Yarnitsky D, Marchettini P, et al. Interactions between sympathetic vasoconstrictor outflow and C nociceptor-induced antidromic vasodilatation. *Pain* 1993;54:191–196.
30. Kurvers HA, Jacobs MJ, Beuk RJ, et al. Reflex sympathetic dystrophy: evolution of microcirculatory disturbances in time. *Pain* 1995;60:333–340.
31. Van Houdenhove B, Vasquez G. Is there a relationship between reflex sympathetic dystrophy and helplessness? *Gen Hosp Psych* 1993;15:325–329.
32. Ciccone DS, Bandilla EB, Wu W. Psychological dysfunction in patients with reflex sympathetic dystrophy. *Pain* 1997;71: 323–333.
33. Lynch ME. Psychological aspects of reflex sympathetic dystrophy: a review of the adult and paediatric literature. *Pain* 1992; 49:337–347.
34. Covington EC. Psychological issues in reflex sympathetic dystrophy. In: Janig W, Stanton-Hicks M, eds. *Reflex sympathetic dystrophy: a reappraisal.* Seattle: IASP Press, 1996;191–215.
35. Mailis A, Wade J. Profile of Caucasian women with possible genetic predisposition to reflex sympathetic dystrophy: a pilot study. *Clin J Pain* 1994;10:210–217.
36. Watson HK, Weinzweig J, Guidera PM, et al. *One thousand intercarpal arthrodeses. J Hand Surg [Br]* 1999;24:320–330.
37. Watson HK, Carlson L. Treatment of reflex sympathetic dystrophy of the hand with an active "stress loading" program. *J Hand Surg [Am]* 1987;12:779–785.
38. Field J, Atkins RM. Algodystrophy is an early complication of Colles' fracture: What are the implications? *J Hand Surg [Br]* 1997;22:178–182.
39. Bickerstaff DR, Kanis JA. Algodystrophy: an under-recognized complication of minor trauma. *Br J Rheumatol* 1994;33: 240–248.
40. Hove LM. Nerve entrapment and reflex sympathetic dystrophy after fractures of the distal radius. *Scand J Plast Reconstr Hand Surg* 1995;29:53–58.
41. Field J, Protheroe DL, Atkins RM. Algodystrophy after Colles fractures is associated with secondary tightness of casts. *J Bone Joint Surg Br* 1994;76:901–905.
42. Lenoble E, Dumontier C, Goutallier D, et al. Fracture of the distal radius: a prospective comparison between trans-styloid and Kapandji fixations. *J Bone Joint Surg Br* 1995;77:562–567.
43. Combalia A, Suso S. Reflex sympathetic dystrophy in severe fractures of the distal radius treated with distraction devices. *J Hand Surg [Am]* 1994;19:156–157.
44. Bickerstaff DR, Charlesworth D, Kanis JA. Changes in cortical and trabecular bone in algodystrophy. *Br J Rheumatol* 1993;32: 46–51.
45. Field J, Warwick D, Bannister GC. Features of algodystrophy ten years after Colles' fracture. *J Hand Surg [Br]* 1992;17:318–320.
46. Kline SC, Beach V, Holder LE. Segmental reflex sympathetic dystrophy: clinical and scintigraphic criteria. *J Hand Surg [Am]* 1993;18:853–859.

47. Atkins RM, Kanis JA. The use of dolorimetry in the assessment of post-traumatic algodystrophy of the hand. *Br J Rheumatol* 1989;28:404–409.
48. Davidoff G, Morey K, Amann M, et al. Pain measurement in reflex sympathetic dystrophy syndrome. *Pain* 1988;32:27–34.
49. Galer BS, Jensen MP. Development and preliminary validation of a pain measure specific to neuropathic pain: the neuropathic pain scale. *Neurology* 1997;48:332–338.
50. Wilson PR, Low PA, Bedder MD, et al. Diagnostic algorithm for complex regional pain syndromes. In: Janig W, Stanton-Hicks M, eds. *Reflex sympathetic dystrophy: a reappraisal.* Seattle: IASP Press, 1996;93–105.
51. Kozin F, Genant HK, Bekerman C, et al. The reflex sympathetic dystrophy syndrome. II. Roentgenographic and scintigraphic evidence of bilaterality and of periarticular accentuation. *Am J Med* 1976;60:332–338.
52. Schwartzman RJ, Kerrigan J. The movement disorder of reflex sympathetic dystrophy. *Neurology* 1990;40:57–61.
53. Verdugo RJ, Ochoa JL. Sympathetically maintained pain. I. Phentolamine block questions the concept. *Neurology* 1994;44:1003–1010.
54. Mackinnon SE, Holder LE. The use of three-phase radionuclide bone scanning in the diagnosis of reflex sympathetic dystrophy. *J Hand Surg [Am]* 1984;9:556–563.
55. Lee GW, Weeks PM. The role of bone scintigraphy in diagnosing reflex sympathetic dystrophy. *J Hand Surg [Am]* 1995;20:458–463.
56. Koman LA, Smith BP, Smith TL. Stress testing in the evaluation of upper-extremity perfusion. *Hand Clin* 1993;9:59–83.
57. Chelimsky TC, Low PA, Naessens JM, et al. Value of autonomic testing in reflex sympathetic dystrophy. *Mayo Clin Proc* 1995;70:1029–1040.
58. Swift DW, Walker SE. The clenched fist syndrome—a psychiatric syndrome mimicking reflex sympathetic dystrophy. *Arthritis Rheum* 1995;38:57–60.
59. Chevalier X, Claudepierre P, Larget-Piet B, et al. Munchausen's syndrome simulating reflex sympathetic dystrophy. *J Rheumatol* 1996;23:1111–1112.
60. Ochoa JL, Verdugo RJ. Reflex sympathetic dystrophy—a common clinical avenue for somatoform expression. *Neurol Clin* 1995;13:351–363.
61. Linson MA, Leffert R, Todd DP. The treatment of upper extremity reflex sympathetic dystrophy with prolonged continuous stellate ganglion blockade. *J Hand Surg [Am]* 1983;8:153–159.
62. Hannington-Kiff JG. Relief of Sudeck's atrophy by regional intravenous guanethidine. *Lancet* 1977 May 28;1:1132–1133.
63. Chuinard RG, Dabezies EJ, Gould JS, et al. Intravenous reserpine for treatment of reflex sympathetic dystrophy. *South Med J* 1981;74:1481–1484.
64. Hord AH, Rooks MD, Stephens BO, et al. Intravenous regional bretylium and lidocaine for treatment of reflex sympathetic dystrophy: a randomized, double-blind study. *Anesth Analg* 1992;74:818–821.
65. Ramamurthy S, Hoffman J, Guanethidine Study Group. Intravenous regional guanethidine in the treatment of reflex sympathetic dystrophy/causalgia: a randomized, double-blind study. *Anesth Analg* 1995;81:718–723.
66. Tasker RR, Lougheed WM. Neurosurgical techniques of sympathetic interruption. In: Stanton-Hicks M, ed. *Pain and the sympathetic nervous system.* Boston: Kluwer Academic Publishers, 1990;165–190.
67. Burchiel KJ, Taha JM. Surgical intervention for reflex sympathetic dystrophy and causalgia. *Phys Med Rehabil* 1996;10:311–326.
68. Rauck RL, Eisenach JC, Jackson K, et al. Epidural clonidine treatment for refractory reflex sympathetic dystrophy. *Anesthesiology* 1993;79:1163–1169.
69. Muizelaar JP, Kleyer M, Hertogs IA, et al. Complex regional pain syndrome (reflex sympathetic dystrophy and causalgia): management with the calcium channel blocker nifedipine and/or the alpha-sympathetic blocker phenoxybenzamine in 59 patients. *Clin Neurol Neurosurg* 1997;99:26–30.
70. Prough DS, McLeskey CH, Poehling GG, et al. Efficacy of oral nifedipine in the treatment of reflex sympathetic dystrophy. *Anesthesiology* 1985;62:796–799.
71. Hanna MH, Peat SJ. Ketanserin in reflex sympathetic dystrophy. A double-blind placebo controlled cross-over trial. *Pain* 1989;38:145–150.
72. Czop C, Smith TL, Rauck R, et al. The pharmacologic approach to the painful hand. *Hand Clin* 1996;12:633–642.
73. Mellick GA, Mellick LB. Reflex sympathetic dystrophy treated with gabapentin. *Arch Phys Med Rehabil* 1997;78:98–105.
74. Kozin F, Ryan LM, Carerra GF, et al. The reflex sympathetic dystrophy syndrome. III. Scintigraphic studies, further evidence for the therapeutic efficacy of systemic corticosteroids, and proposed diagnostic criteria. *Am J Med* 1981;70:23–30.
75. Grundberg AB. Reflex sympathetic dystrophy: treatment with long-acting intramuscular corticosteroids. *J Hand Surg [Am]* 1996;21:667–670.
76. Connelly NR, Reuben S, Brull SJ. Intravenous regional anesthesia with ketorolac–lidocaine for the management of sympathetically-mediated pain. *Yale J Biol Med* 1995;68:95–99.
77. Zuurmond WW, Langendijk PN, Bezemer PD, et al. Treatment of acute reflex sympathetic dystrophy with DMSO 50% in a fatty cream. *Acta Anaesthesiol Scand* 1996;40:364–367.
78. Cheshire WP, Snyder CR. Treatment of reflex sympathetic dystrophy with topical capsaicin—case report. *Pain* 1990;42:307–311.
79. Arlet J, Mazieres B. Medical treatment of reflex sympathetic dystrophy. *Hand Clin* 1997;13:477–483.
80. Adami S, Fossaluzza V, Gatti D, et al. Bisphosphonate therapy of reflex sympathetic dystrophy syndrome. *Ann Rheum Dis* 1997;56:201–204.
81. Haddox JD, Van Alstine D. Pharmacologic therapy for reflex sympathetic dystrophy. *Phys Med Rehabil* 1996;10:297–309.
82. Johnson EW, Pannozzo AN. Management of shoulder–hand syndrome. *JAMA* 1966;195:152–154.
83. Bernstein BH, Singsen BH, Kent JT, et al. Reflex neurovascular dystrophy in childhood. *J Pediatr* 1978;93:211–215.
84. Meyer GA, Fields HL. Causalgia treated by selective large fibre stimulation of peripheral nerve. *Brain* 1972;95:163–168.
85. Robaina FJ, Rodriguez JL, de Vera JA, et al. Transcutaneous electrical nerve stimulation and spinal cord stimulation for pain relief in reflex sympathetic dystrophy. *Stereotact Funct Neurosurg* 1989;52:53–62.
86. Chan CS, Chow SP. Electroacupuncture in the treatment of post-traumatic sympathetic dystrophy (Sudeck's atrophy). *Br J Anaesth* 1981;53:899–901.
87. Grunert BK, Devine CA, Sanger JR, et al. Thermal self-regulation for pain control in reflex sympathetic dystrophy syndrome. *J Hand Surg [Am]* 1990;15:615–618.
88. Walsh MT. Therapist's management of reflex sympathetic dystrophy. In: Hunter JM, Mackin EJ, Callahan AD, eds. *Rehabilitation of the hand: surgery and therapy.* St. Louis: Mosby, 1995;817–833.
89. Hardy MA, Hardy SG. Reflex sympathetic dystrophy: the clinician's perspective. *J Hand Ther* 1997;10:137–150.
90. Cooney WP. Somatic versus sympathetic mediated chronic limb pain. *Hand Clin* 1997;13:355–361.
91. Hassenbusch SJ, Stanton-Hicks M, Schoppa D, et al. Long-term results of peripheral nerve stimulation for reflex sympathetic dystrophy. *J Neurosurg* 1996;84:415–423.

92. Kumar K, Nath RK, Toth C. Spinal cord stimulation is effective in the management of reflex sympathetic dystrophy. *Neurosurgery* 1997;40:503–509.
93. Carlson LK, Watson HK. Treatment of reflex sympathetic dystrophy using the stress-loading program. *J Hand Ther* 1988;1:149–154.
94. Astrand P, Rodahl K. *Textbook of work physiology.* New York: McGraw-Hill, 1986.
95. Maffulli N, King JB. Effects of physical activity on some components of the skeletal system. *Sports Med* 1992;13:393–407.
96. Schoutens A, Laurent E, Poortmans JR. Effects of inactivity and exercise on bone. *Sports Med* 1989;7:71–81.
97. Kosek E, Ekholm J. Modulation of pressure pain thresholds during and following isometric contraction. *Pain* 1995;61:481–486.
98. Paalasmaa P, Kemppainen P, Pertovaara A. Modulation of skin sensitivity by dynamic and isometric exercise in man. *Eur J Appl Physiol* 1991;62:279–285.
99. Pertovaara A, Kemppainen P, Leppanen H. Lowered cutaneous sensitivity to nonpainful electrical stimulation during isometric exercise in humans. *Exp Brain Res* 1992;89:447–452.
100. Thoren P, Floras JS, Hoffman P, et al. Endorphins and exercise: physiological mechanisms and clinical implications. *Med Sci Sports Exerc* 1990;22:417–428.

47

THERAPEUTIC MANAGEMENT OF THE WRIST

LOIS CARLSON
JUDY STANNARD

Rehabilitation of the wrist is guided by the need for a stable, pain-free wrist with functional mobility. Stability is needed to transmit load. Mobility is required to help position the hand for function and adjust the tension of the muscle–tendon units to the hand (1,2). Effective therapy requires an understanding of relevant anatomy, physiology, biomechanics, and pathology. To plan treatment following surgery, the therapist must also know the details of the procedure, its purpose, and the expected result.

Evaluation of the wrist and hand requires attention to detail. The hand therapist must interpret existing problems within the context of the patient's functional needs, and develop a plan of treatment that takes into account the prevention or control of complications. Lack of use or prolonged immobilization may cause unnecessary joint stiffness or symptoms of reflex sympathetic dystrophy (RSD). The outcome of treatment depends not only on the therapist's skill in developing and implementing an appropriate therapy plan, but also on the patient's ability and willingness to carry it out at home. Therapy must be an ongoing collaboration among the therapist, the surgeon, and the patient to achieve meaningful and realistic goals.

This chapter includes general evaluation and treatment parameters for patients who present with wrist dysfunction. Treatment guidelines for specific diagnostic groups are outlined, with an emphasis on postsurgical management related to the authors' clinical experience.

EVALUATION

Evaluation starts with the patient history and a basic hand examination. Upper-quarter screening may also be indicated to rule out more proximal involvement. Soft tissue testing, palpation, and provocative maneuvers help determine the causes of various limitations found during the evaluation sequence. Additional testing may be necessary to fully assess the functional implications of the physical findings.

History

The therapist should review the patient's history, including previous injuries, surgeries and medical, social, and functional status. The mechanism of injury may help identify potential areas of pathology. If the problem is not linked to a specific injury, further questioning should determine possible causes. Subjective analysis by the patient regarding symptoms, functional limitations, and goals for therapy helps focus the clinical examination. Identifying the pattern of symptoms in reference to hand use is vital. When did symptoms first occur? What activities cause pain? Does the pain continue after activity? If so, for how long? Can the pain be localized? What are the quality and severity of pain? How frequently does this occur? What makes symptoms better or worse? Are certain activities now difficult to do because of this problem? What does the patient consider the major problem requiring treatment?

Basic Hand Examination

Areas of swelling or obvious physical alterations in bony or soft tissue structures will help pinpoint the exam. General inspection includes observations related to spontaneous use, posture, deformity, skin, scar, atrophy, and vasomotor, sudomotor, and trophic status. Edema is measured using circumferential or volumetric measurements (3,4). Sensibility screening includes moving two-point and Semmes-Weinstein monofilament testing (5,6).

The reliability of goniometric measurement of the wrist has been investigated (7–9). A study by LaStayo and Wheeler (9) comparing the results of testing using ulnar, radial, or volar–dorsal alignment found the greatest reliability using the volar–dorsal alignment technique. Potential inaccuracies with the volar–dorsal technique, however, may occur with significant deformity or changes in edema (10).

L. Carlson and J. Stannard: Connecticut Combined Hand Therapy, Glastonbury, Connecticut 06033, and Hartford, Connecticut 06106.

Torque goniometry may also be used to further quantify the nature of the restriction as well as to improve the consistency of measurement (3,10–14). In addition to global active and passive range of motion, the quality of movement, end feel, and joint play are assessed. Specific provocative maneuvers have been developed to more clearly assess abnormal mobility within the wrist joint complex.

Manual muscle testing is used to test strength of specific muscles acting on the wrist (15–17). Additional methods to test muscle groups include hand-held dynamometry (18–21) or equipment commonly used in a work-conditioning program such as the Baltimore Therapeutic Equipment (BTE) Work Simulator (22). Loss of strength on functional tests of grip and pinch may reflect underlying wrist pathology. In a study by Czitrom, a significant correlation was found between decreased grip strength and wrist disorders (23).

Joint and Soft Tissue Testing

Further assessment of bony and soft tissue structures is needed to help determine the fundamental pathology causing dysfunction. The therapist should thoroughly evaluate all structures potentially causing problems in the involved area. It is not unusual to find evidence of tendon and nerve irritation in addition to joint problems. A classic example is a patient who has been treated for de Quervain's disease and carpal tunnel syndrome, who on examination exhibits rotary subluxation of the scaphoid.

Joint

Examination of the wrist joint complex requires the ability to palpate and perform specific maneuvers to identify the site and etiology of symptoms. The Cyriax evaluation assesses active, passive, and resistive motions, which may be useful in differentiating involvement of contractile and noncontractile tissues (24,25). In the Cyriax approach to evaluating the wrist complex, single-plane motions are used, making it difficult to isolate the many structures that are responsible for multiplanar motions. The present multitude of special tests widely used in the examination of the wrist supports the need for a more involved triage, with

TABLE 47.1. PROVOCATIVE TESTING: WRIST REGION

	Anatomic Unit	Test
Joint	Scaphoid-related	Finger extension test
		Articular–nonarticular junction tenderness
		Triscaphe joint synovitis
		Dorsal scapholunate synovitis
		Scaphoid shift
	Ulnar wrist	Lunotriquetral joint ballottement test (Reagan test)
		Pisotriquetral shear test
		TILT test
	DRUJ	TFCC load test
		Piano key test
		DRUJ compression
	CMC joints	Grind test (first CMC)
		Carpal boss test
Tendon	de Quervain's	Finkelstein's test
		Pain with resistance to APL/EPB
	Intersection syndrome	Pain with resistance to radial wrist extensors
		Pain, swelling, crepitus 4 cm proximal to wrist (intersection of first and second compartments)
	FCR tendinitis	Pain with resistance to radial wrist flexion
Nerve	Median, CTS	Phalen's test
		Forearm compression test
		Thenar weakness
		Sensory radial 3½ digits
		Clinical history
	Ulnar, Guyon's canal	Weakness ulnar intrinsics
		Sensory 1½ digits
		Allen's test
	Radial, superficial radial (Wartenberg's syndrome)	Stretch test

APL, abductor pollicis longus; CMC, carpometacarpal; CTS, carpal tunnel syndrome; DRUJ, distal radioulnar joint; EPB, extensor pollicis brevis; FCR, flexor carpi radialis; TFCC, triangular fibrocartilage complex; TILT, triquetral impingement ligament tear.
See Watson HK, Weinzweig J. Physical examination of the wrist. *Hand Clin* 1997;13:17–34; and Skirven T. Clinical examination of the wrist. *J Hand Ther* 1996;9:96–107 for description of testing.

each maneuver testing one of the many structures (26,27). Table 47.1 gives a summary of tests commonly used in our clinic. A discussion of specific evaluative techniques and provocative tests for the wrist is not presented here, as they are thoroughly described in Chapter 5.

Tendon

Tenosynovitis may potentially involve any of the tendons as they cross the wrist. Symptoms are elicited by applying passive stretch to the tendon or resistance to the action of the involved muscle–tendon unit. In de Quervain's disease, for example, pain may be elicited with passive stretch to the tendons of the first compartment (Finkelstein's test) or resistance to the abductor pollicus longus (APL) and extensor pollicus brevis (EPB). Other less common examples in the wrist region include intersection syndrome (28) and flexor carpi radialis tendinitis (29,30). The fourth extensor compartment is a frequent site of synovial infiltration in the patient with rheumatoid arthritis.

Restricted tendon motion may also result from scar adhesion following surgery or injury. If the wrist extensor tendons are involved, for example, active wrist extension and passive wrist flexion may be limited. Adherence of the digital extensors at or proximal to the wrist will create a seesaw effect, limiting combined flexion of the wrist and digits.

Nerve

Common nerve-related problems in the wrist region include carpal tunnel syndrome, ulnar nerve compression in Guyon's canal, and Wartenberg's syndrome (superficial radial nerve). The use of provocative tests in the evaluation of compression neuropathies is well documented (31–36). In addition, neural tissue provocation testing (NTPT) (37,38) is extremely valuable. These evaluative techniques of Elvey assess the ability of the neural tissues to comply with the physical function of the musculoskeletal system. Is there pain because the neural tissues are not able to glide through normal ranges? Or, could there simply be enough inflammation or chemical irritation of the neural tissues to create nociceptive impulses? Can this neural sensitivity cause enough reflexive muscle protection to create significant loss of musculoskeletal motion?

NTPT brings the patient through sequential active motions designed to place tension on the neural tissues. The median, radial, and ulnar nerve biases are tested separately with different patterns of movement for each. The patient with noncompliant neural tissues will use compensatory movements during active testing, resulting in a decrease in active motion and/or a lack of willingness to move through a motion. The compensatory motions serve to decrease the length of the pathway along which the sensitive nerve has to pass. Passive testing is also performed, with the therapist detecting subtle increases in muscle tone in response to neural tissue provocation. Various palpation techniques are used to assess for nerve trunk hyperalgesia and tender points that correlate with the specific peripheral nerve being tested. As part of treatment, passive oscillatory motions can be performed to gradually enhance the mobility of neural structures with the upper extremity and neck positioned in varying degrees of the testing patterns.

Vascular

Vascular problems may be suspected if there is evidence of significant color and temperature change, sensitivity to cold temperatures, or a palpable mass. Allen's test can be performed at the wrist level to test for compromise of the radial or ulnar arteries. Allen's test may be positive, for example, because of ulnar artery aneurysm or thrombosis, with tenderness in Guyon's canal, pain in the hypothenar area, and vascular symptoms in the ulnar digits (39). Pulse obliteration tests are helpful in assessing the scalene, costoclavicular, and pectoral areas when more proximal involvement is suspected.

Skin and Fascia

Skin and fascial tightness can be evaluated using skin rolling and a combination of compressive and shearing forces. Mobility should be tested in several different directions and compared to the opposite side. Although not usually a primary cause of symptoms in the wrist area, superficial tissue tightness can contribute to pain and lack of motion.

Scar

Scar mobility is most efficiently evaluated by attempting to "pinch and roll" the scar in different directions. In an area of tendon gliding, the scar can be pushed distally while the patient is asked to contract the appropriate muscle. The therapist should then watch for proximal migration of the scar during muscle contraction to see if tendon and scar are moving together rather than separately.

Functional Assessment

In general, function is assessed through patient interview, observation, and activity of daily living (ADL) checklists. Additional testing may include job simulation and functional capacity evaluation (FCE) (40,41). The FCE is especially valuable in determining work capacity when return to customary work is not feasible.

"Stress response testing" (SRT), a variation of the traditional FCE, is used in our clinic primarily for the purpose of diagnosis and clarification of symptoms, determining the functional significance of the symptoms, and establishing the consistency of the patient's performance. Patients appropriate for this type of evaluation include those with chronic complaints, unknown etiology, and/or equivocal findings. Components of the SRT include interview and medical records review, physical and functional evaluation, validity profile, and response to functional evaluation. The consistency of the patient's effort is examined using a battery of tests (42–44) as well as observation of functional task performance. Assessment of the patient's response to functional evaluation includes comparison of affected versus unaffected and pre versus post measurements of pain, strength, volume, sensibility, and motion. Of equal or greater importance is a careful reassessment of specific areas of tenderness and changes in response to provocative testing. The referring physician examines the patient immediately following the SRT for review of the therapist's findings and final evaluation of the patient. The physical effects of activity help objectify diffuse subjective complaints. Correlating these findings with specific, repeatable task components adds to the value of this diagnostic testing method.

TREATMENT

Priorities for treatment should be formulated within the context of the functional requirements of the wrist for pain-free motion and stability. Goals are based on an assessment of the underlying pathology, its impact on function, and the individual needs of the patient. Treatment methods are chosen that target the identified problems within the context of known precautions and expected outcomes.

What is a "functional range of motion" for the wrist? According to several studies, most activities of daily living are performed using less than normal motion (45–49). Frequently cited studies include those of Palmer et al. (46) (functional motion defined as 5° flexion, 30° extension, 10° radial deviation, and 15° ulnar deviation) and Ryu et al. (47) (all tasks completed using 54° flexion, 60° extension, 40° ulnar deviation, and 17° radial deviation; the majority of tasks required up to 40° each of wrist flexion/extension and 40° combined radial–ulnar deviation). A more recent study by Nelson (48) concluded that most activities studied can be completed with minimal difficulty even with all wrist motions restricted to 5° to 7° each. The effect of wrist position on grip strength has also been studied (1,50–55) According to a study by O'Driscoll et al. (53), maximum grip strength occurs with 35° extension and 7° ulnar deviation. These studies reinforce the fact that a good functional outcome is not necessarily contingent on achieving full motion.

This section reviews general treatment techniques used in rehabilitation of wrist disorders. Guidelines for treatment pertaining to specific surgical procedures follow, including discussion of possible problems, solutions, and expected outcome after surgery.

Therapeutic Exercise and Activity

Exercise can be one of the most efficient methods of accomplishing multiple goals simultaneously, including edema and pain reduction and improvement in motion, strength, and function. Early motion can enhance healing and decrease recovery time after injury or surgery (56).

Generalized joint stiffness and muscle atrophy may occur with prolonged immobilization. Active motion of uninvolved joints while still in the cast helps prevent loss of motion and promote tendon gliding. After cast removal, exercises are prescribed that emphasize combined motions of the hand and wrist as well as isolated joint exercises, in conjunction with thermal modalities and scar management techniques as needed. Achieving functional use and strength of the hand through resistive exercise and activity is emphasized (Fig. 47.1). If diffuse edema, pain, and limited motion are present during or after casting, the stress-loading approach should be considered (see Chapter 65).

The approach to exercise for the wrist depends on diagnostic and surgical variables as well as the results of the evaluation. If known degenerative change causes pain with motion, achievement of functional rather than full range is stressed; strength is increased by using isometric exercise or dynamic resistive exercises within a limited range as well as activities and exercise such as gripping that require synergistic use of the wrist musculature. If wrist instability is suspected, vigorous exercise may only exacerbate the problem. Significant carpal loading occurs with grasping (57–59) as well as with activities requiring wrist motion.

How does exercise affect the ligamentous structures of the wrist? A recent study by Crisco et al. (60) suggested that moderate exercise (gripping or push-ups) may significantly increase the laxity of the wrist. The authors suggest that an increase in joint laxity may reduce the chance of injury by reducing ligament loads within the joint. If this is so, what are the implications for patients who present with abnormal ligamentous laxity? Studies on the ligaments of the knee have demonstrated similar effects, but whether or not this is related to the ligaments themselves is not clear (61). Exercise may also have the potential to increase ligamentous strength. Significant increases in strength have been reported using exercise following periods of immobilization (61). The demonstrated effects of exercise on the strength of "normal" ligaments have not been as dramatic (62).

The ultimate goal of wrist reconstruction is functional use without pain. Therapeutic activity, work conditioning, and job simulation are all therapeutic and evaluative in nature. Activities are progressed from those requiring active wrist motion and wrist fixation during gripping and pinching to activities requiring use of the wrist under load in various positions of extension, flexion, and deviation. For example, a patient may be able to lift 50 lb from floor to waist level but be unable to lift overhead, which requires increased wrist extension. Ongoing evaluation is necessary to assess and treat the cause of limitations. Is the patient unable to perform overhead lifting because of weakness, lack of motion, or pain? If painful, what is the cause?

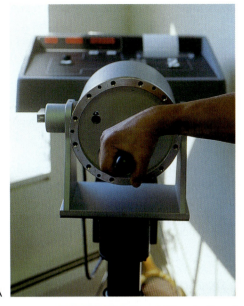
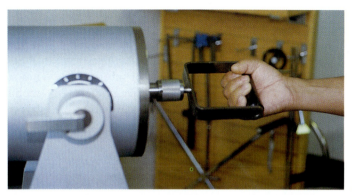

FIGURE 47.1. In addition to its primary use as a method to simulate work tasks, the Baltimore Therapeutic Equipment (BTE) work simulator can also be used for excercise programs and to objectively measure progress, for example, in both flexion **(A)** and supination **(B)**.

Splinting

Splinting is used most commonly to protect the wrist, improve functional use, or increase motion. Circumferential thermoplastic splints provide a high level of support during an intermediate stage of healing or when symptom relief is needed because of significant instability or degenerative changes (Fig. 47.2). If less rigid immobilization is required, a dorsal or volar-based thermoplastic splint or prefabricated splint may be all that is necessary.

Splinting for protection, function, or pain relief does not necessarily require static immobilization. Dynamic splints that limit motion to certain planes and ranges may be fabricated for protection after surgery or injury (63,64). Bora et al. (63) describe a wrist hinge splint used following scaphoid fracture, Colles' fracture, and intercarpal fusions. The splint may be appropriate for reliable patients after a period of casting when there is minimal tenderness and x-ray evidence of healing. Soft splinting or strapping has been reported to be effective for use with hypermobile joints (65) and to help control ulnar carpal instability (66). Wrap-around wrist supports that provide gentle compression without restricting motion may increase comfort when initially returning to work or heavy activity.

Splints worn during athletic competition must comply with regulations governing the sport in addition to providing adequate protection and function. Materials used in sport splinting include tape, padding, silicone rubber, fiberglass, and thermoplastic materials. Canelon suggests the properties of silicone rubber, including strength, durability, and relatively low rigidity, make it a good choice for stable wrist injuries (67–69). Use of such splints is also dependent on the nature of the injury and its potential for complications. A sports cast with stable middle-third scaphoid fractures, for example, has been used without complications; however, this approach may not be appropriate for fractures of the proximal third, which are prone to nonunion (70–72).

Splinting to gain motion has been used most frequently, in our experience, to increase wrist extension, which is critical for optimum grasp. According to Tubiana, contracture limiting extension occurs with involvement of the more superficial palmar ligaments and flexor carpi ulnaris; wrist flexion is limited primarily by the extensor muscles and their tendons and sheaths and only secondarily by the

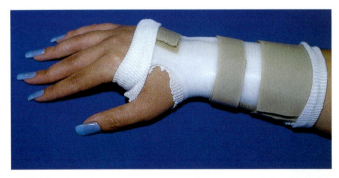

FIGURE 47.2. A circumferential splint fabricated from ¹⁄₁₆-in. Aquaplast provides total support to the wrist without unnecessary bulk.

dorsal carpal ligaments (2). Motion may also be limited in either direction by shortening or adherence of extraarticular soft tissues, including skin and fascia.

Splinting to increase motion at the wrist can be done using serial static, static progressive, or dynamic splinting (73–75). To gain joint mobility, a steady, static force is generally most effective (73). Before splinting, joint motion may be increased using heat and exercise, soft tissue techniques, and joint mobilization. Maintaining the joint in this lengthened state creates a more permanent change. Dynamic splinting, which provides an elastic force, is used to help maintain joint mobility or substitute for weak or absent muscles while allowing active motion. For example, a low-profile splint design using elastic traction and a wrist hinge made from Aquaplast tubing can be used to dynamically support the wrist in extension for function.

Serial static splints maintain the joint at the end of the available range. Changes are made by remolding or refabricating the splint as gains in motion are achieved. This method is based on the principle that tissue lengthens in response to gentle constant tension at the end of its elastic limit (76,77). Increases in joint motion have been found to be directly proportional to the length of time the joint is held at end range (78).

Serial static splinting using plaster volar and dorsal slabs is a simple, inexpensive method to achieve increased wrist mobility (Fig. 47.3). Each slab is prepared using one to two layers of cast padding and seven to eight layers of plaster. The slabs are then placed on the patient and wrapped

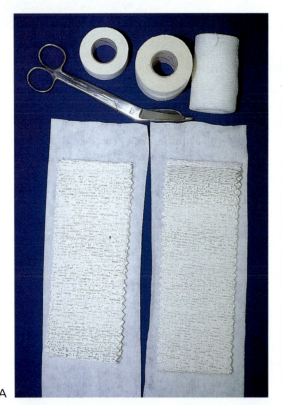
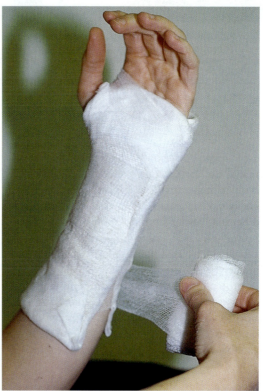
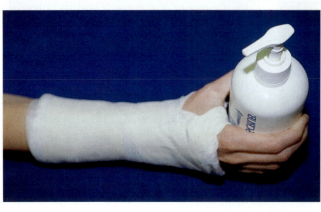

FIGURE 47.3. Plaster "pancake" splints are constructed using plaster, cast padding, gauze, and tape **(A)**. The plaster slabs are held in position with gauze while the therapist simultaneously maintains maximum range **(B)**. Once the plaster has set, the splint is secured with tape **(C)**. The splint should clear the thenar and distal palmar creases to preserve functional use.

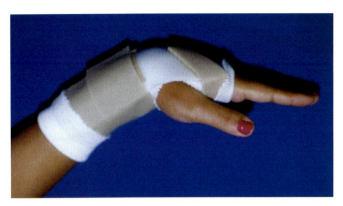

FIGURE 47.4. A serial static splint fabricated from ⅛-in. thermoplastic material can be used to increase wrist motion in less chronic cases of joint stiffness. The splint is reheated at intervals in response to gains in motion.

snugly with gauze. Steady pressure with slight traction to the wrist is applied while the plaster is hardening. The splint is then secured circumferentially with tape to maintain correction and prevent motion of the wrist within the splint. Refabrication of the splint is generally done every 2 to 3 days and continued for up to 2 weeks once gains have been achieved. The total contact and even pressure distribution with plaster also help reduce edema and increase wearing tolerance. On the negative side, this type of splinting does not allow for wrist exercise except during splint changes. This technique has been particularly effective in regaining wrist extension in patients referred late to our clinic with chronic stiffness following distal radius fractures and/or RSD. Once the targeted range is achieved, a removable thermoplastic circumferential splint may be fabricated and then gradually weaned as active range is maintained. Serial splinting may also be accomplished using QuickCast circumferential wrist splinting, which allows remolding by heating the splint while on the patient (73). Thermoplastic materials may also be effective to treat less chronic cases of joint or tendon tightness (Fig. 47.4).

Static progressive splints apply a steady, nonelastic force that can be progressed during each splinting session to accommodate improvements in motion. For the wrist, static progressive splints consist of hand and forearm components attached by a hinge, with application of a steady, inelastic force (56,73). This type of splinting has the advantage of being removable and allows reciprocal splinting into flexion and extension if required. Careful fabrication to maintain correct joint alignment is necessary.

Soft Tissue Mobilization

Scar

Scar tissue mobilization is most effectively carried out using a small piece of Theraband to help hold the tissue as it is mobilized. This prevents the skin from sliding out of the therapist's fingertips (provided the skin is free of lotion) and allows firm mobilization of the tissues. Patients should be warned that they may feel a burning stretch, and the therapist should start out somewhat gently and progress to more aggressive mobilization. Time spent on this technique should also be progressive, as some temporary soreness can be expected initially. The scar can be mobilized in circular, side-to-side, and pinch-and-roll motions. Any section that cannot be lifted or rolled should be pointed out to the patient so that greater pressure can be applied during home massage. To increase scar mobility in an area of tendon gliding, the therapist resists proximal migration of the scar during muscle contraction for approximately 10 seconds or more, as tolerated. This technique can be repeated until some release of the restriction is perceived.

Skin and Fascia

Once superficial tissue restrictions have been determined, there are several different techniques for treating this lack of gliding between tissue planes. The most basic technique is simply pushing tissue into its field of restriction. The direction of stretch should be varied and the stretch sustained until a lengthening or release of the restriction is felt by the therapist (79).

Another way to mobilize restricted tissues is to use both thumbs to push the tissue in opposing directions, thereby forming an "S" configuration with the restricted tissues (Fig. 47.5). Similarly, one can use the technique of "J-

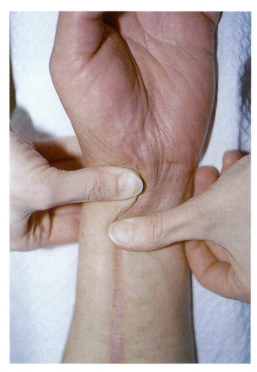

FIGURE 47.5. Both thumbs are used to stretch restricted tissues in opposing directions, forming an "S."

stroking"; this is performed using one hand to stabilize tissue while the fingertips of the other hand stroke the tissue away from the stabilizing hand using a scooping, J-shaped stroke (79).

Joint Mobilization

Reversible joint hypomobility can be effectively managed with joint mobilization (80). This controlled passive motion helps to decrease capsular tightness and thereby restore accessory joint motions. Care must be taken to thoroughly evaluate accessory motions and compare any apparent restrictions to the opposite side. This also provides information as to any hypermobility that may be present, which would be a contraindication for joint mobilization. It is imperative that the hand therapist know how to evaluate for various carpal instabilities, being cognizant of the multiplanar motion that can occur. For example, when an unstable scaphoid rotates out of position, it is not enough to passively glide this bone in an anterior–posterior direction to test its joint play (see Chapter 5).

Joint mobilization techniques described by Kaltenborn apply traction to separate joint surfaces and take up slack in the capsular structures (80). Simultaneous translational gliding and gapping (or rolling) motions are performed in low- or high-amplitude grades (80,81). Low-amplitude oscillations are indicated when the involved joint is inflamed or painful and create a vibratory stimulus for large A fibers, thus achieving pain modulation (82–85). High-grade oscillations deliver stress to the capsular tissues and, with prolonged mobilization, result in a temporary lengthening of those tissues (80,81). When wrist joint mobilization is coupled with exercise and splinting at end range, a more permanent increase in motion can be achieved.

Under the guidelines of the concave–convex rule, the direction in which a joint surface is mobilized depends on the direction of the limitation of limb movement and the nature of the joint surface. The convex joint surface is moved in the direction opposite to the limitation of motion. For example, if the limitation being treated is wrist extension (dorsally directed motion), the convex joint surface (proximal carpal row) will be mobilized in a volar direction (Fig. 47.6) (80,81). The opposite holds true for the concave joint surface. McClure and Flowers (86) point out weaknesses in the Concave-Convex rule as it applies to the glenohumeral joint, and stress the importance of aiming mobilization at those capsular tissues that are determined to be restricting a particular motion.

Adjunctive Modalities

Rehabilitation of most patients seen following wrist surgery focuses on early motion and progression of exercise and activity, with adjunctive use of other modalities as needed. The combination of heat and stretch, for example, provides more effective tissue elongation than stretch alone (87,88). Moist heat, paraffin, or fluidotherapy may be used before exercise, soft tissue mobilization, or splinting to enhance tissue elasticity (Fig. 47.7) (89). Moist heat carries the added benefit of being easily incorporated into the home program. Ultrasound can be used when selective heating of deep tissues is desired. Therapists need to determine the appropriate intensity, duration, and sound wave frequency for the tissues being targeted (90).

Another option for increasing motion is continuous passive motion (CPM) (91). CPM is useful in select cases following surgical release of severe joint restrictions or in encouraging a prescribed range of motion (see "rheumatoid wrist reconstruction" below). CPM units can be programmed to combine passive motion with prolonged stretch at end range.

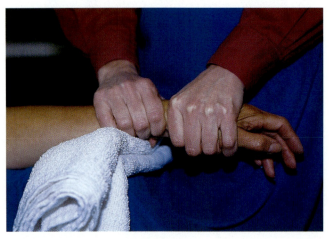

FIGURE 47.6. A ventral glide mobilization is performed at the radiocarpal joint to increase wrist extension.

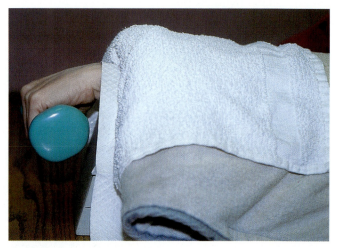

FIGURE 47.7. Application of heat to elevate tissue temperature while stretching increases tissue extensibility.

In the treatment of superficial scar, silicone gel sheeting is a useful adjunct to heat and soft tissue mobilization techniques. Although its mechanism of action is not well understood, studies do suggest that silicone gel sheeting is effective in the management of hypertrophic scar, and no significant negative effects have been reported (92).

Electrical modalities can be used to assist in decreasing acute inflammation (93,94). High-voltage galvanic electrical stimulation may be effective in decreasing nerve irritation in those patients with unresolved neural problems. Iontophoresis with dexamethasone can be helpful in treating early cases of tendinitis. Muscle reeducation and strengthening, especially after tendon transfer or nerve injury, may be improved using neuromuscular stimulation.

Returning to Work

Successful return to work requires evaluation of the job and the worker. The therapist's role begins with trying to "fit the person to the job" through patient participation in a work-conditioning program that assesses and increases abilities related to work and provides education and training in preventive and symptom-control strategies. The work conditioning program can also be used as a "lab" to try out tool modifications, supports, or other adaptations and gives the patient a chance to gain confidence in performing the job before actual return to work.

The therapist is also in a position to provide valuable information to help "fit the job to the person," which focuses on ergonomic modifications including the work station, work methods and tools, as well as organizational changes, such as rotation and job enlargement (95). Job analysis is used to identify potential risk factors, including repetitive or sustained exertions, stressful postures, forceful actions, localized mechanical stress, vibration, and cold temperatures (95,96). The literature supports the contribution of programs that focus on improving work-related function as well as ergonomic and work-style modification to increase success in returning patients with upper extremity disorders to work (97,98).

Documentation of demonstrated abilities and objective physical changes in response to work activities assists the physician in making more realistic job recommendations. Combined with an assessment of the patient's performance, recommendations for modifying the job help the patient return to work more effectively and in a timely manner with decreased potential for further injury. Return-to-work restrictions need to be defined beyond current Department of Labor physical demand categories (99), which address the issue of force without fully taking into account other factors, such as repetition and posture (100). Patient follow-up after returning to work is necessary to monitor the actual effects of work and the need for additional modification and gradual progression of work tasks. In the long run, this will help to avoid unnecessary and costly intervention.

What is known about the risk factors associated with potential wrist injury? Not surprisingly, many studies in the literature have focused on risk factors related to carpal tunnel syndrome and other cumulative trauma disorders (CTD), including force, repetition, and wrist postures deviating from neutral (101–106). Other studies suggest that velocity and acceleration parameters differentiate low- and high-risk groups, especially acceleration in the flexion–extension plane (107,108). Preliminary guidelines for maximum acceptable force in relation to repetition and wrist posture have been described (109,110). Additional research is needed to define appropriate work standards for the prevention of injury.

TREATMENT GUIDELINES FOR DIAGNOSTIC AND SURGICAL CATEGORIES

The following discussion focuses on therapy following common surgical procedures for the wrist. Rehabilitation following operative procedures developed by the senior editor (H.K.W.) are emphasized. The reader may find differences between our philosophy and time frames and those of other reports in the literature.

Limited Wrist Arthrodesis

General Comments

Therapy may be necessary before surgery to improve tissue integrity and circulation to the involved extremity. This is most critical in patients who have already been treated with casts or splints for an extended time, but may also help in general to prevent severe atrophy during the casting period (111,112). Splinting may also be required, primarily to provide pain relief while functional tasks are performed that could not otherwise be tolerated, but it should be used judiciously to avoid disuse. During preoperative visits, the therapist also reinforces information given to the patient from the surgeon regarding the surgical procedure, postoperative treatment, and anticipated outcome.

Keys to successful management following limited wrist arthrodesis include adequate immobilization, early active motion of uninvolved joints, a focus on regaining finger and thumb motion as soon as possible, and allowing the wrist to gradually adapt to its new kinematics through active exercise and use. Forceful stretching may create inflammation of ligamentous and capsular structures before the body has had a chance to "naturally" modify its anatomy in response to the altered mechanics of the wrist.

The patient is immobilized for a total of 6 weeks (long arm cast, commonly including thumb to tip with metacarpophalangeal (MP) joints of index and middle held in flexion until 3 weeks postsurgery; short arm spica for an additional 3 weeks). Patients are seen after cast application for brief evaluation and treatment as needed to increase the motion of free joints and check cast fit before and following exercise. At 6 weeks, pins are removed and active motion of all joints is initiated. Occasionally, pins cannot be removed in the office; in this case, or if healing is delayed, the patient may be fitted with a removable wrist splint for an additional 1 to 2 weeks. Resistive exercise emphasizing grip and wrist strengthening is added within the next several weeks and progresses to work conditioning and job simulation as needed. Gentle passive motion preceded by heat and scar mobilization may also be started at this time, but only if motion is not progressing to anticipated levels.

The anticipated motion varies with the surgical technique, postoperative management, and underlying pathology. Reported averages for wrist motion, from an overall review of the literature by Siegel and Ruby, are 50% for fusions of the capitate to one or more of the bones of the proximal row, 62% for fusion of the scaphoid to the trapezium and trapezoid, and 85% to 94% for fusions within the proximal row (113).

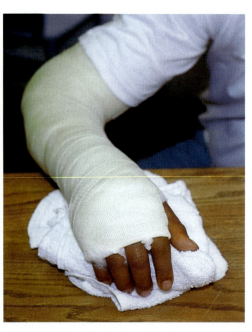

FIGURE 47.8. A "modified" stress-loading approach can be used even when the wrist is casted.

Possible Problems and Solutions

1. Motion limitations. It is usually best to concentrate on structures crossing the wrist, particularly the extensor tendons, which may limit flexion. Treatment is dependent on the cause of the limitations, e.g., tightness of the surgical scar, generalized edema, and/or joint or tendon limitations. Active, active assistive, and resistive exercise in conjunction with heat and scar mobilization techniques generally resolve these problems. Motion of the wrist is achieved primarily through exercise and normal use to achieve a pain-free functional range. Gains in motion may occur for up to a year or longer (114–116).
2. Early signs and symptoms of RSD. Prevention through early active motion and careful monitoring of casts is the ideal approach. If symptoms do occur, a modified stress-loading program can be initiated, even in the cast (Fig. 47.8; see also Chapter 65).
3. Pain. Normally, after limited wrist arthrodesis, there may be some discomfort at end range until the wrist reaches its "final range." In some cases, more isolated pain may occur from problems with the fusion itself, such as nonunion or bony impingement (113,117). Pain and edema that significantly increase over time with dynamic wrist exercise or passive stretching may be a signal to focus more on general strengthening and functional use and to reassess clinical and x-ray findings.

The two most common procedures in our experience are triscaphe arthrodesis and scapholunate advanced collapse (SLAC) wrist reconstruction. The general comments as outlined above should apply to other forms of limited arthrodesis as well.

Triscaphe Arthrodesis

Indications for triscaphe arthrodesis (fusion of the scaphoid, trapezium, and trapezoid) include rotary subluxation of the scaphoid, scaphoid nonunion, degenerative arthritis of the triscaphe joint, Kienböck's disease, and midcarpal instability (118,119). It is contraindicated if radioscaphoid degenerative change has developed. The surgical procedure now also includes a partial radial styloidectomy to avoid impingement between the scaphoid and the radial styloid (33% incidence before modification of original procedure) (120). Proper scaphoid alignment and maintenance of the external dimensions of the three bones are critical factors in preventing complications, including progressive arthritis (119,121) (see also Chapter 73). Reported nonunion rates from our clinic have been 5% or less. As a general guide, achieving a flexion–extension arc of 100° within the first month following cast removal has met with good long-term clinical results. Further study is needed to determine if there is an ideal arc of motion beyond which potential problems might emerge. In patients with Kienböck's, motion is more variable; in 32% of these patients, a second surgery has been needed to excise the lunate (122).

Expected outcomes for rotary subluxation of the scaphoid (from results in our clinic) are:

1. Range of motion approximately 80% extension–flexion and two-thirds radial–ulnar deviation. (See Table 47.2 for a breakdown by diagnosis.) (122–124). Interestingly, these correlate fairly closely to reported ranges from cadaver studies (125–127).

TABLE 47.2. TRISCAPHE ARTHRODESIS: RANGE OF MOTION (UNAFFECTED SIDE)

Diagnosis	Extension (%)	Flexion (%)	Radial deviation (%)	Ulnar deviation (%)
Rotary subluxation scaphoid	75	84	55	73
Triscaphe degenerative arthritis	82	75	59	75
Kienböck's disease	73	65	50	75

Data from Watson HK, Monacelli DM, Milford RS, et al. Treatment of Keinböck's disease with scaphotrapezio-trapezoid arthrodesis. *J Hand Surg [Am]* 1996;21:9–15; Watson HK, Ryu J, Akelman E. Limited triscaphoid intercarpal arthrodesis for rotary subluxation of the scaphoid. *J Bone Joint Surg Am* 1986;68:345–349; and Rogers WD, Watson HK. Degenerative arthritis at the triscaphe joint. *J Hand Surg [Am]* 1990;15:232–235.

2. Grip strength equal to an average of 92% of the unaffected side (123).
3. Return to work approximately 10 to 12 weeks postsurgery.

Scapholunate Advanced Collapse Pattern

SLAC wrist reconstruction (fusion of the capitate, lunate, hamate, and triquetrum, with excision of the scaphoid) (128) is indicated for the SLAC pattern of degenerative arthritis, which is the most common pattern of degenerative arthritis in the wrist (129) (see also Chapter 71). This procedure is contraindicated if there is ulnar translation or radiolunate degenerative change. The reported nonunion rate from our clinic for this procedure is 3%. Impingement may occur between the capitate and radius (13% of 100 cases reviewed), most likely because of inadequate reduction of the dorsal intercalated segment instability (DISI) position of the lunate (130).

The expected outcome (from our clinical results) is:

1. Range of motion: 53% extension–flexion and 59% radial–ulnar deviation (130).
2. Grip strength an average of 80% of the unaffected side (130).
3. Return to work approximately 10 to 12 weeks postsurgery.

Additional time may be necessary for patients returning to very heavy occupations or jobs requiring prolonged use of vibrating equipment, such as a jackhammer. Modification of job tasks or change in occupation is occasionally necessary.

Surgical Alternatives for the Treatment of Wrist Instability

Other surgical procedures that may be used for treatment of wrist instability include ligamentous repair (if seen early), dorsal capsulodesis, or soft tissue reconstruction. Immobilization periods generally range from 6 to 12 weeks. Therapy following these procedures should be gradual; passive exercise should be used with discretion to avoid overstretching the repair (131,132). Salvage procedures include proximal row carpectomy or total wrist fusion (133).

Surgical alternatives for rotary subluxation of the scaphoid include ligamentous repair and dorsal capsulodesis. After dorsal capsulodesis, Blatt begins therapy at 2 months, including active and gentle assisted exercise in conjunction with a removable splint (134). Strengthening is started at 3 months after removal of the K-wire; full activity is allowed at 6 months (134). Prosser and Herbert describe a protocol that includes early controlled active motion after scapholunate ligament repair using a range-limiting splint at 1 week following surgery (64).

Dorsal Wrist Syndrome

Dorsal wrist syndrome (DWS) (135) is defined as localized dorsal scapholunate synovitis with or without small ganglia. It is most likely caused by overstress of the ligaments from excessive activity in a normal wrist or may occur with regular use in a wrist with abnormal scaphoid motion. The patient presents with a history of activity pain, postactivity ache, and an inability to take load at the extremes of wrist extension or flexion. On examination, there is localized tenderness dorsally over the scapholunate joint with or without swelling. The finger extension test is positive.

Conservative treatment may include splinting to immobilize or restrict wrist motion and steroid injection. Surgery is generally recommended if symptoms have persisted for over 6 months and the wrist has not responded to conservative treatment. Surgical correction of this problem includes resection of abnormal ridging on the scaphoid and lunate, removal of small capsular ganglia, if present, and excision of the thickened capsule over the scapholunate joint (see also Chapter 56).

Unrestricted active motion is started in the first postoperative week, including wrist and combined wrist and finger motions. Scar management is initiated after suture removal at 2 weeks postsurgery, along with a progression of the therapy program to address strengthening and functional goals. Passive motion techniques should be used with caution if there is a tendency toward scaphoid hypermobility. If the extensor tendons of the fourth compartment become restricted at the surgical site, serial static splinting may be incorporated into the program. A dorsal thermoplastic splint is fabricated, positioning the wrist in maximum available flexion; MP flexion may also be added to put additional tension on the digital extensors, but it is generally not necessary. Active flexion of the digits is encouraged toward the end of the splinting period (1-hour sessions and/or at night, depending on the severity of the problem) for additional tendon excursion.

The expected functional outcome includes no significant limitations in range of motion (10° average loss of extension) and strength averaging 90% or better in comparison to the opposite side. Most patients are able to return to heavy work by 6 weeks or sooner following surgery. Pain that recurs following this procedure may be caused by progressive rotary subluxation of the scaphoid.

Triquetral Impingement Ligament Tear Syndrome

Triquetral impingement ligament tear (TILT) syndrome (136) is defined as chronic compression of the triquetrum by a displaced fibrous cuff from the ulnar sling mechanism, resulting in articular cartilage loss and softening of the triquetrum proximally. Clinical presentation includes localized pain over the ulnar aspect of the triquetrum, swelling of the ulnar wrist, and normal x-ray findings, often with a history of a hyperflexion injury. It is treated by surgical excision of the displaced fibrous cuff (see Chapter 40).

Active motion exercises for the wrist and forearm are started within the first week after surgery, progressing to strengthening and functional activity over the next several weeks. A soft wrist support that provides gentle compression may be used to decrease soreness and increase functional use for heavier activities during the first few weeks following surgery.

Rheumatoid Wrist

Patients with rheumatoid arthritis may be seen for conservative treatment, including exercise, joint protection, activity modification, and splinting. The most consistent positive effect of wrist splinting is relief of pain (137). Additional benefits may include increased range of motion and function and decreased swelling (138–141).

Depending on the stage of disease and surgeon's preference, surgical treatment options include synovectomy, interpositional arthroplasty, limited wrist arthrodesis, and total wrist fusion (142–144).

Rheumatoid wrist reconstruction, as described by Ryu, Watson, and Burgess (145), is the surgery of choice in our clinic for the painful rheumatoid wrist with palmar and ulnar translation. The surgical procedure produces a fibrous nonunion between the proximal carpal row and radius. Synovectomy, including extensor tendons and carpal joints, is also performed, usually combined with a matched ulna arthroplasty (see below). The wrist is pinned and immobilized for $2^{1}/_{2}$ to 3 weeks.

Active exercise of the fingers and thumb begins the first week following surgery. At $2^{1}/_{2}$ to 3 weeks, pins are removed, and the patient is started on active motion for the wrist and forearm. Although the surgical procedure is an arthrodesis-type procedure, starting motion early creates an intentional nonunion. Normally, this would be expected to be painful. The absence of pain following this procedure may reflect a combination of the lack of synovium, transection of the terminal branches of the posterior interosseous nerve during the procedure, and/or the relatively lighter activity level of many patients with rheumatoid arthritis (145).

The goal is to achieve a wrist that is functional, stable, and pain-free. Range-of-motion goals are approximately 30° to 40° of extension and flexion and at least neutral radial deviation. Attaining an adequate arc of motion and strength for wrist extension and radial deviation is an early priority of therapy. If necessary, a night splint is fabricated to maintain this position until active motion is achieved. Therapy focuses on regaining wrist motion through active range of motion, progressive resistive exercise, and gentle passive stretching as needed. CPM has also been used in select cases to achieve the targeted range.

The therapist should also be mindful of the need to promote extensor tendon gliding. During the surgical procedure, the extensor retinaculum is placed under the extensor tendons, with the exception of the extensor pollicis longus, which lessens the possibility of tendon adhesions at the surgical site. Bowstringing of extensor tendons has not been a problem, most likely because of the limited excursion of the wrist. However, adherence of tendons to overlying skin can occur, particularly in patients with delayed healing from prolonged use of corticosteroids. In most cases, this problem is adequately addressed through a standard exercise program to promote extensor tendon gliding and excursion in combination with heat and scar mobilization.

Distal Radioulnar Joint

Pain in the distal radioulnar joint (DRUJ) can occur secondary to instability, incongruity, impingement, and degenerative change (146,147). Potential causes of pain in this region include direct injury, posttraumatic malalignment after Colles' fracture, rheumatoid arthritis, osteoarthritis, and Madelung's deformity, as well as instability caused by surgery, such as a Darrach procedure.

Matched Ulna Arthroplasty

Matched ulna arthroplasty (148,149) is indicated when DRUJ congruency is lost. Surgery involves resection of a 5- to 6-cm-long area of the distal ulna in a shape that "matches" and therefore clears the contour of the radius through full pronosupination (see Chapter 59).

Following matched ulna arthroplasty, the postoperative dressing is removed approximately 3 days following the procedure. The patient is instructed in active range-of-motion exercises for the hand, wrist, and forearm and is encouraged to use the involved upper extremity as normally as possible. Active and active-assistive exercises for pronation–supination are emphasized within the first several weeks, with the patient applying overpressure at the level of the distal forearm. Active assistive pronation and supination exercises can be progressed to sustained end-range holds of 30 to 60 seconds for best results. The use of a hammer held in the patient's hand is also helpful for increasing pronosupination motion, provided the weight and torque of the hammer are tolerated (Fig. 47.9). A wrist splint may be used to prevent excessive torque at the wrist (150).

If a patient does not tolerate performing active assistive exercises independently or is slow in gaining motion, splinting can be considered. The TAP splint (Smith and Nephew), normally used as an antispasticity splint, is a neoprene wrap that provides low-level pronation or supination force (Fig. 47.10). Strengthening is started as soon as the patient has sufficient range of motion, usually 2 to 4 weeks following surgery.

From published follow-up results, the average range in comparison to the unaffected side is 98% to 99% for pronation and supination, 88% for wrist extension, and 85% for wrist flexion (149).

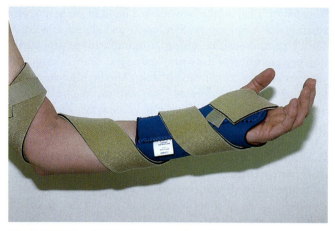

FIGURE 47.10. The spiral portion of the TAP splint can be used to increase forearm rotation in either direction. A prefabricated wrist splint assists in maintaining a steady force that is directed to the forearm rather than the wrist. If additional support is needed to prevent torque at the wrist, a custom-fabricated circumferential splint may be used.

Ulnar Osteotomy

In patients with positive ulnar variance, step-cut shortening may be required to resolve ulnar-sided wrist pain. To address ulnar impingement on the distal radius following a Darrach procedure, ulnar lengthening has been combined with matched ulna arthroplasty and reattachment of the triangular fibrocartilage complex (TFCC) and ulnar sling mechanism (151). Ulnar lengthening (or radial shortening) is also commonly used to treat Kienböck's disease during the earlier stages (152).

Ulnar osteotomy requires pinning and cast immobilization for 6 to 8 weeks. On cast removal, the patient follows a treatment regimen similar to that described for matched ulna arthroplasty, with a concentration on active assistive and strengthening exercises. Rate of exercise progression and recovery may be slower than after matched ulna arthroplasty because of immobilization and a more involved surgical procedure.

The need for splinting to increase pronation and/or supination may be greater following surgeries requiring prolonged immobilization. A custom thermoplastic static progressive splint described by Schultz-Johnson (73) is an adaptation of a design originally described by Colello-Abraham (153). The splint supports the elbow and wrist and provides static progressive traction to the forearm from laterally based outriggers. Other options include custom-fabricated serial static (73,154,155) or dynamic splints (153,156), air-bag splints (157), or commercial splints, such as the TAP splint modification described above.

Triangular Fibrocartilage Complex Repair

It is well reported that the TFCC is the main stabilizer of the DRUJ (147,158–160). Traumatic disruption is commonly

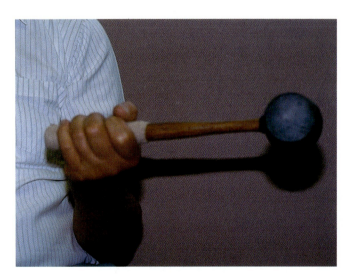

FIGURE 47.9. A hammer can be used to increase forearm rotation and strength as part of a home program.

initiated by a fall on the outstretched hand in pronation or a rotational forearm injury. Symptoms include ulnar wrist or DRUJ pain, especially during pronosupination, grip weakness or a sensation of the wrist "letting go," and clicking. Surgical techniques to correct instability of the ulna are varied and have been performed via arthroscopic and open approaches. The dorsal and volar radioulnar ligaments are the structures that must be repaired. Cast immobilization generally lasts 6 weeks in varying degrees of forearm rotation, depending on the type and location of the repair (159,161, 162). Active range of motion (ROM) is typically started after cast removal, with some surgeons avoiding radial or ulnar deviation range of motion according to which side of the TFCC was repaired (161).

Patients are progressed to active-assistive ROM and grip strengthening approximately 2 to 3 weeks after cast removal, subsequently advancing to forearm rotation strengthening. As with the previously described DRUJ surgeries, the use of heat, sustained end-range stretching, and the hammer exercise aid in gaining pronosupination. Joint mobilizations can be used, if necessary, to lengthen restricted soft tissues, provided full healing has been achieved.

Carpometacarpal Joints

Carpal Boss

Excision of a carpal boss includes removal of osteophytes, adjacent sclerotic bone, and the commonly found accessory ossicle; complete resection to a level of normal cancellous bone and articular cartilage is essential to avoid recurrence (163,164). Despite the resulting bony concavity, patients have no restrictions following removal of the postop dressing. Assisted ROM is started immediately and should include fisted wrist flexion exercises to maintain excursion of extensor tendons over the surgical area and stretch any extensor tightness that has developed as a result of muscle guarding. The patient is encouraged to use the involved hand as normally as possible; strengthening exercises and scar management are started after suture removal. Full ROM is usually attained within 2 to 4 weeks, and a full return of strength and function follows (163).

Thumb Carpometacarpal Tendon Arthroplasty

Conservative management of thumb carpometacarpal (CMC) arthritis may include steroid injection and splinting. Although the wrist must be included in the splint to effectively immobilize the CMC joint, many patients are pleased with a modified thumb–spica splint that is less bulky (Fig. 47.11). The splint is worn primarily for periods of active hand use; it can also be used during sleep to protect the joint from possible jarring motions.

After thumb CMC tendon arthroplasty, the thumb is immobilized in a plaster thumb–spica splint for 3 weeks. The patient is instructed in active ROM exercises for the fingers, elbow, and shoulder on application of the protective

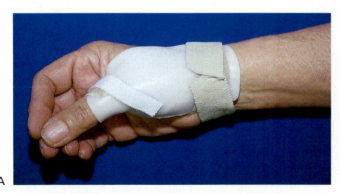
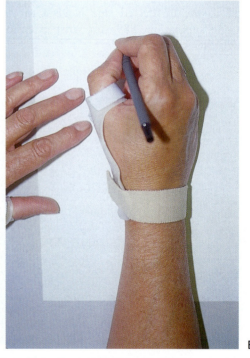

FIGURE 47.11. A modified thumb–spica splint fabricated from 1/16-in. thermoplastic material may be used for conservative treatment of carpometacarpal arthritis **(A)**. Patients have been pleased with the decrease in pain and increase in function that is possible when wearing this splint **(B)**.

splint. Patients who exhibit puffy, stiff fingers, which are possible precursors to RSD, are started on towel scrubbing, usually 3 to 5 minutes, three times a day. These patients are seen back in the office within the week to assess the need for any further preventive measures.

Patients are started on active motion exercises for the thumb and wrist on the same day that the plaster spica is removed. In addition, scar management is initiated, and any finger range of motion that is not yet full is addressed. The scar over the CMC region may become adherent, and the patient is encouraged to spend sufficient time mobilizing this scar. In 1 to 2 weeks, most patients have achieved full to nearly full thumb motion, and strengthening is started using therapy putty. A clothespin with elastics for increased resistance is a simple pinch-strengthening tool. Patients who have a tendency toward hyperextension at the MP joint of the thumb are cautioned against that motion during pinching exercises. Functional strengthening can be accomplished by having the patient perform difficult activities of daily living repetitively as exercise.

Most patients who have undergone CMC tendon arthroplasty do well with a basic home program; the occasional patient who is having difficulty attaining the last few degrees of thumb flexion is well served by the simple measure of Coban wrapping the thumb into flexion once or twice a day for 5 to 10 minutes, preferably after soaking or heating the thumb.

Therapeutic Management of Common Fractures

Distal Radius Fractures

Therapeutic guidelines for treatment of distal radius fractures have been well outlined in several recent publications (165,166). Variables affecting therapeutic management include the nature of the fracture (degree of comminution, intraarticular involvement, etc.), and the type of medical management (casting, internal and/or external fixation). The rehabilitation program is based on two major goals: prevention/control of stiffness, edema and pain in the hand and shoulder, and restoration of wrist and forearm function.

While the patient is still in a cast or external fixation device, therapy is initiated to regain active motion of the fingers and prevent shoulder stiffness, monitor cast fit and position, and instruct the patient in pin-site care, as needed. Slings should be used judiciously, if at all. Active blocking exercises are used to gain digital joint motion and stretch the intrinsic muscles. If motion is not easily achievable, blocking exercises are maintained until maximum motion is achieved (up to a 60-second practical limit). This allows the patient to overcome initial limitations caused primarily by edema. Additional exercises should address excursion and glide of extrinsic tendon systems. If all motions are painful and limited, "towel scrubbing" for 5 to 10 minutes is used prior to, or initially instead of, the active motion program until pain subsides enough to allow active motion.

Depending on healing, protective splinting may be continued for the first one to two weeks after removal of cast or external fixator with initiation of gentle active motion. Once the fracture is stable and/or clinically healed, therapy can be progressed from active motion to strengthening of the wrist and forearm. Joint mobilization and passive stretching techniques may also be useful; these techniques should be abandoned and x-rays reviewed for articular malalignment if motion is not progressing. Circumferential thermoplastic splinting to increase wrist extension may also be used, preceded occasionally by serial plaster splinting in severe cases. Splinting to increase forearm rotation may also be beneficial.

Potential complications include tendon and joint motion restrictions, nerve compression (most commonly carpal tunnel syndrome), RSD and extensor pollicus longus (EPL) rupture (167,168). Complications that are more common with external fixation devices include irritation of the superficial radial nerve, adhesions of the index and middle extensor tendons, and pin site infection (165,166). Malunion may lead to loss of articular congruency, loss of palmar tilt of the articular surface, loss of radial inclination, and radial shortening (169) (see Chapter 72).

Scaphoid Fractures

Scaphoid fractures occur most commonly in a relatively young, physically active population. Therapy following open reduction with internal fixation (ORIF) for acute fractures may include fabrication of custom wrist splints for protection during activity and exercise to increase active wrist motion. After adequate healing has been demonstrated, progressive resistive exercise and joint mobilization may be added. Joint stiffness in the hand is usually not a problem. If rigid internal fixation is used, such as the Herbert screw (170), active motion can be started as early as 10 to 14 days, with protective splinting as needed and avoidance of stress to the fracture for 6 weeks (64). Otherwise, the patient is immobilized for 6 weeks or longer, depending on healing.

Delayed healing or nonunion, a relatively frequent complication, especially in fractures of the proximal third of the scaphoid, is often managed with prolonged immobilization. This may create a picture of disuse and atrophy that must be addressed in therapy before any further surgical intervention. Therapy management following bone grafting procedures for scaphoid nonunion (171,172) is similar to the approach for acute fractures, with an increased emphasis on general strengthening and frequently a more aggressive approach to gaining wrist motion once satisfactory healing has occurred (64).

CONCLUSIONS

Therapy, especially following wrist reconstruction, has not been well documented in the literature. A review of the current literature reflects significant differences in philosophy related to the total time for immobilization and restriction of functional use as well as the rate of progression of the exercise program. In conclusion, the following general guidelines are offered:

1. Encourage early mobility of the hand through active exercise and use to prevent complications such as stiffness and RSD. The wrist is of little use without a functioning distal appendage.
2. Wrist stability must come before wrist mobility. Stability can occur without mobility, but mobility cannot be functional if pathologic movements of the carpal bones are sufficient to cause pain, impingement, and eventual progression to degenerative change.
3. Ensure adequate stability of the wrist by allowing healing of bony and soft tissue structures through appropriate immobilization, but do not immobilize longer than what can reasonably be expected to be therapeutic to avoid additional complications related to disuse. In our experience with limited wrist arthrodeses, 6 weeks of casting has been sufficient in most cases if adequate immobilization is maintained by the design of the cast. Soft tissue reconstruction may require longer periods of complete or relative immobilization. If healing of bony or soft tissues is not required for stability, such as the resection or arthroplasty-type procedures presented in this chapter, no immobilization is required beyond the initial inflammatory period.
4. Allow wrist mobility to evolve following wrist reconstruction through active exercise and use. Passive techniques may be indicated if functional motion is not progressing.
5. Once satisfactory healing has occurred, active exercise and functional activity should be progressed fairly rapidly to avoid further degeneration of tissues from immobilization and relative disuse.

REFERENCES

1. Hazelton FT, Smidt GL, Flatt AE, et al. The influence of wrist position on the force produced by the finger flexors. *J Biomech* 1975;8:301–306.
2. Tubiana R, Kuhlmann JN. Stiffness of the wrist joint. In: Tubiana R, ed. *The Hand, vol II.* Philadelphia: WB Saunders, 1985;1091–1100.
3. Brand PW. *Clinical mechanics of the hand.* St Louis: CV Mosby, 1985.
4. Waylett-Rendall J, Seibly D. A study of the accuracy of a commercially available volumeter. *J Hand Ther* 1991;4:10–13.
5. Bell-Krotoski JA. Sensibility testing: current concepts. In: Hunter JM, Mackin EJ, Callahan AD, eds. *Rehabilitation of the hand: surgery and therapy.* St Louis: CV Mosby, 1995;109–128.
6. Callahan AD. Sensibility assessment: prerequisites and techniques for nerve lesions in continuity and nerve lacerations. In: Hunter JM, Mackin EJ, Callahan AD, eds. *Rehabilitation of the hand: surgery and therapy.* St Louis: CV Mosby, 1995;129–152.
7. Horger MM. The reliability of goniometric measurements of active and passive wrist motions. *Am J Occup Ther* 1990;44:342–348.
8. Solgaard S, Carlsen A, Kramhoft M, et al. Reproducibility of goniometry of the wrist. *Scand J Rehabil Med* 1986;18:5–7.
9. LaStayo PC, Wheeler DL. Reliability of passive wrist flexion and extension goniometric measurements: a multicenter study. *Phys Ther* 1994;74:162–176.
10. Flowers KR. Invited commentary. *Phys Ther* 1994;74:174–175.
11. Breger-Lee D, Bell-Krotoski J, Brandsma JW. Torque range of motion in the hand clinic. *J Hand Ther* 1990;3:7–13.
12. Breger-Lee D, Voelker ET, Giurintano D, et al. Reliability of torque range of motion: a preliminary study. *J Hand Ther* 1993;6:29–34.
13. Flowers KR, Pheasant SD. The use of torque angle curves in the assessment of digital joint stiffness. *J Hand Ther* 1988;1:69–74.
14. Roberson L, Giurintano DJ. Objective measures of joint stiffness. *J Hand Ther* 1995;8:163–166.
15. Daniels L, Worthingham C. *Muscle testing techniques of manual examination.* Philadelphia: WB Saunders, 1986.
16. Kendall FP, McCreary EK. *Muscles: testing and function.* Baltimore: Williams & Wilkins, 1983.
17. Rancho Los Amigos Occupational Therapy Department. *Guide for muscle testing of the upper extremity.* Downey, CA: Rancho Los Amigos, 1978.
18. Andrews AW, Thomas MW, Bohannon RW. Normative values for isometric muscle force measurements obtained with hand-held dynamometers. *Phys Ther* 1996;76:248–259.
19. Bohannon RW. Test–retest reliability of hand-held dynamometry during a single session of strength assessment. *Phys Ther* 1986;66:206–209.
20. Bohannon RW, Andrews AW. Interrater reliability of hand-held dynamometry. *Phys Ther* 1987;67:931–933.
21. Rheault W, Beal JL, Kubik KR, et al. Intertester reliability of the hand-held dynamometer for wrist flexion and extension. *Arch Phys Med Rehabil* 1989;70:907–910.
22. Anderson PA, Chanoski CE, Devan DL, et al. Normative study of grip and wrist flexion strength employing a BTE work simulator. *J Hand Surg [Am]* 1990;15:420–425.
23. Czitrom AA, Lister GD. Measurement of grip strength in the diagnosis of wrist pain. *J Hand Surg [Am]* 1988;13:16–19.
24. Cyriax JH. *Textbook of orthopaedic medicine, vol 1: Diagnosis of soft tissue lesions.* London: Bailliere Tindall, 1982.
25. Ombregt L, ed. *A system of orthopaedic medicine.* London: WB Saunders, 1995.
26. Watson HK, Weinzweig J. Physical examination of the wrist. *Hand Clin* 1997;13:17–34.
27. Skirven T. Clinical examination of the wrist. *J Hand Ther* 1996;9:96–107.
28. Grundberg AB, Reagan DS. Pathologic anatomy of the forearm: intersection syndrome. *J Hand Surg [Am]* 1985;10:299–302.
29. Bishop AT, Gabel G, Carmichael SW. Flexor carpi radialis tendinitis. Part I: Operative anatomy. *J Bone Joint Surg Am* 1994;76:1009–1014.
30. Gabel G, Bishop AT, Wood MB. Flexor carpi radialis tendinitis. Part II: Results of operative treatment. *J Bone Joint Surg Am* 1994;76:1015–1018.
31. Dawson DM, Hallett M, Millender LH. *Entrapment neuropathies.* Boston: Little, Brown, 1983.
32. Eversmann WW. Entrapment and compression neuropathies. In: Green DP, ed. *Operative hand surgery.* New York: Churchill Livingstone, 1993;1341–1385.
33. Spinner M. Management of nerve compression lesions of the upper extremity. In: Omer GE, Spinner M, eds. *Management of peripheral nerve problems.* Philadelphia: WB Saunders, 1980;569–592.

34. Szabo RM. *Nerve compression syndromes—diagnosis and treatment.* New Jersey: Slack, 1989.
35. Anto C, Aradhya P. Clinical diagnosis of peripheral nerve compression in the upper extremity. *Orthop Clin North Am* 1996;27:227–236.
36. Rayan GM, ed. *Hand clinics: Nerve compression syndromes.* Philadelphia: WB Saunders, 1992.
37. Elvey RL. Physical evaluation of the peripheral nervous system in disorders of pain and dysfunction. *J Hand Ther* 1997;10:122–129.
38. Elvey RL. Treatment of arm pain associated with brachial plexus tension. *Aust J Physiother* 1986;32:225–230.
39. Newmeyer WL. Vascular disorders. In: Green DP, ed. *Operative hand surgery.* New York: Churchill Livingstone, 1993;2251–2308.
40. Schultz-Johnson K. Upper extremity functional capacity evaluation. In: Hunter JM, Mackin EJ, Callahan AD, eds. *Rehabilitation of the hand: surgery and therapy.* St Louis: CV Mosby, 1995;1739–1774.
41. Isernhagen SJ. *The comprehensive guide to work injury management.* Gaithersburg, MD: Aspen, 1995.
42. Hildreth DH, Breidenbach WC, Lister GD, et al. Detection of submaximal effort by use of the rapid exchange grip. *J Hand Surg [Am]* 1989;14:742–745.
43. King JW, Berryhill BH. Assessing maximum effort in upper-extremity functional testing. *Work* 1991;3:65–76.
44. Stokes HM. The seriously uninjured hand—weakness of grip. *J Occup Med* 1983;25:683–684.
45. Brumfield RH, Champoux JA. A biomechanical study of normal functional wrist motion. *Clin Orthop* 1984;187:23–25.
46. Palmer AK, Werner FW, Murphy D, et al. Functional wrist motion: a biomechanical study. *J Hand Surg [Am]* 1985;10:39–46.
47. Ryu JY, Cooney WP, Askew LJ, et al. Functional ranges of motion of the wrist joint. *J Hand Surg [Am]* 1991;16:409–419.
48. Nelson DL. Functional wrist motion. *Hand Clin* 1997;13:83–92.
49. Safaee-Rad R, Shwedyk E, Quanbury AO, et al. Normal functional range of motion of upper limb joints during performance of three feeding tasks. *Arch Phys Med Rehabil* 1990;71:505–509.
50. Rodgers SH. Recovery time needs for repetitive work. *Semin Occup Med* 1987;2:19–24.
51. Kraft GH, Detels PE. Position of function of the wrist. *Arch Phys Med Rehabil* 1972;53:272–275.
52. Lamoreaux L, Hoffer MM. The effect of wrist deviation on grip and pinch strength. *Clin Orthop* 1995;314:152–155.
53. O'Driscoll S, Horii E, Ness R, et al. The relationship between wrist position, grasp size, and grip strength. *J Hand Surg [Am]* 1992;17:169–177.
54. Pryce JC. The wrist position between neutral and ulnar deviation that facilitates the maximum power grip. *J Biomech* 1980;13:505–511.
55. Volz RG, Lieb M, Benjamin J. Biomechanics of the wrist. *Clin Orthop* 1980;149:112–117.
56. Thompson ST, Wehbe MA. Early motion after wrist surgery. *Hand Clin* 1996;12:87–96.
57. Friedman SL, Palmer AK, Short WH, et al. The change in ulnar variance with grip. *J Hand Surg [Am]* 1993;18:713–716.
58. Garcia-Elias M. Kinetic analysis of carpal stability during grip. *Hand Clin* 1997;13:151–158.
59. Schuind FA, Linscheid RL, An KN, et al. Changes in wrist and forearm configuration with grasp and isometric contraction of elbow flexors. *J Hand Surg [Am]* 1992;17:698–703.
60. Crisco JJ, Chelikani S, Brown RK, et al. The effects of exercise on ligamentous stiffness in the wrist. *J Hand Surg [Am]* 1997;22:44–48.
61. Maffulli N, King JB. Effects of physical activity on some components of the skeletal system. *Sports Med* 1992;13:393–407.
62. Hayashi K. Biomechanical studies of the remodeling of knee joint tendons and ligaments. *J Biomech* 1996;29:707–716.
63. Bora FW, Culp RW, Osterman AL, et al. A flexible wrist splint. *J Hand Surg [Am]* 1989;14:574–575.
64. Prosser R, Herbert T. The management of carpal fractures and dislocations. *J Hand Ther* 1996;9:139–147.
65. Colditz JC. A new wrist strap splint. *J Hand Ther* 1996;9:72–73.
66. Prosser R. Conservative management of ulnar carpal instability. *Aust J Physiother* 1995;41:41–46.
67. Canelon MF. Silicone rubber splinting for athletic hand and wrist injuries. *J Hand Ther* 1995;8:252–257.
68. Canelon MF, Karus AJ. A room temperature vulcanizing silicone rubber sport splint. *Am J Occup Ther* 1995;49:244–249.
69. Canelon MF. Material properties: A factor in the selection and application of splinting materials for athletic wrist and hand injuries. *J Orthop Sports Phys Ther* 1995;22:164–172.
70. Hunter SC, Blackburn TA. Silicone cast treatment for athletic injuries to the upper extremities. *J Med Assoc GA* 1982;71:495–497.
71. Rettig AC, Weidenbener EJ, Gloyesks R. Alternative management of midthird scaphoid fractures in the athlete. *Am J Sports Med* 1994;22:711–713.
72. Riester JN, Baker BE, Mosher JF, et al. A review of scaphoid fracture healing in competitive athletes. *Am J Sports Med* 1985;13:159–161.
73. Schultz-Johnson K. Splinting the wrist: mobilization and protection. *J Hand Ther* 1996;9:165–177.
74. Colditz J. Therapist's management of the stiff hand. In: Hunter JM, Mackin EJ, Callahan AD, eds. *Rehabilitation of the hand: surgery and therapy.* St Louis: CV Mosby, 1995;1141–1159.
75. Fess EE, Philips CA. *Hand splinting: principles and methods.* St Louis: CV Mosby, 1987.
76. Bell-Krotoski JA, Figarola JH. Biomechanics of soft-tissue growth and remodeling with plaster casting. *J Hand Ther* 1995;8:131–137.
77. Brand PW. Mechanical factors in joint stiffness and tissue growth. *J Hand Ther* 1995;8:91–96.
78. Flowers KR, LaStayo P. Effect of total end range time on improving passive range of motion. *J Hand Ther* 1994;7:150–157.
79. Sutton GS, Bartel MR. Soft-tissue mobilization techniques for the hand therapist. *J Hand Ther* 1994;7:185–192.
80. Kaltenborn FM. *Manual mobilization of the extremity joints.* Norway: Olaf Norlis Borkhandel, 1989.
81. Cookson JC, Kent BE. Orthopedic manual therapy—an overview. *Phys Ther* 1979;59:136–146.
82. Melzack R, Wall PD. Pain mechanisms: a new theory. *Science* 1965;150:971–979.
83. Basmajian JV, Nyberg RF, eds. *Rational manual therapies.* Baltimore: Williams & Wilkins, 1992.
84. Kessler RM, Hertling D. *Management of common musculoskeletal disorders.* Philadelphia: Harper & Row, 1982.
85. Paterson JK, Burn L. *An introduction to medical manipulation.* Hingham, MA: MTP Press, 1985.
86. McClure PW, Flowers KR. Treatment of limited shoulder motion: a case study based on biomechanical considerations. *Phys Ther* 1992;72:929–936.
87. Lehman JF, Masock AJ, Warren CG, et al. Effect of therapeutic temperatures on tendon extensibility. *Arch Phys Med Rehabil* 1970;51:481–487.
88. Warren CG, Lehmann JF, Koblanski JN. Heat and stretch procedures: an evaluation using rat tail tendon. *Arch Phys Med Rehabil* 1976;57:122–126.

89. Michlovitz SL. Biophysical principles of heating agents. In: Michlovitz SL, ed. *Thermal agents in rehabilitation.* Philadelphia: FA Davis, 1996;107–138.
90. Michlovitz SL. Therapeutic ultrasound. In: Michlovitz SL, ed. *Thermal agents in rehabilitation.* Philadelphia: FA Davis, 1996;168–212.
91. Salter RB. History of rest and motion and the scientific basis for early continuous passive motion. *Hand Clin* 1996;12:1–11.
92. Katz BE. Silicone gel sheeting in scar therapy. *Cutis* 1995;56:65–67.
93. Taylor Mullins PA. Use of therapeutic modalities in upper extremity rehabilitation. In: Hunter JM, Mackin EJ, Callahan AD, eds. *Rehabilitation of the hand: surgery and therapy.* St Louis: CV Mosby, 1995;1495–1519.
94. Snyder-Mackler L, Robinson AJ. *Clinical electrophysiology—electrotherapy and electrophysiologic testing.* Baltimore: Williams & Wilkins, 1989.
95. Putz-Anderson V. *Cumulative trauma disorders: a manual for musculoskeletal diseases of the upper limbs.* Bristol, PA: Taylor & Francis, 1988.
96. Sanders MJ. *Management of cumulative trauma disorders.* Boston: Butterworth-Heinemann, 1997.
97. Feuerstein M, Callan-Harris S, Hickey P, et al. Multidisciplinary rehabilitation of chronic work-related upper extremity disorders: long term effects. *J Occup Med* 1993;35:396–403.
98. Dortch HL, Trombly CA. The effects of education on hand use with industrial workers in repetitive jobs. *Am J Occup Ther* 1990;44:777–782.
99. US Department of Labor. *Dictionary of occupational titles.* Washington, DC: US Government Printing Office, 1992.
100. Carlson L, Wilson P. Cumulative trauma disorders—what does "light duty" mean? *Work* 1997;8:107–108.
101. Armstrong TJ, Fine LJ, Goldstein SA, et al. Ergonomic considerations in hand and wrist tendinitis. *J Hand Surg [Am]* 1987;12:830–837.
102. Silverstein BA, Fine LJ, Armstrong TJ. Occupational factors and carpal tunnel syndrome. *Am J Indust Med* 1987;11:343–358.
103. Masear VR, Hayes JM, Hyde AG. An industrial cause of carpal tunnel syndrome. *J Hand Surg [Am]* 1986;11:222–227.
104. Marley RJ, Fernandez JE. Psychophysical frequency and sustained exertion at varying wrist postures for a drilling task. *Ergonomics* 1995;38:303–325.
105. Malchaire JB, Cock NA, Robert AR. Prevalence of musculoskeletal disorders at the wrist as a function of angles, repetitiveness and movement velocities. *Scand J Work Environ Health* 1996;22:176–181.
106. Genaidy A, Barkawi H, Christense D. Ranking of static nonneutral postures around the joints of the upper extremity and the spine. *Ergonomics* 1995;38:1851–1858.
107. Schoenmarklin RW, Marras WS, Leurgans SE. Industrial wrist motions and incidence of hand/wrist cumulative trauma disorders. *Ergonomics* 1994;37:1449–1459.
108. Marras WS, Schoenmarklin RW. Wrist motions in industry. *Ergonomics* 1993;36:341–351.
109. Snook SH, Vaillancourt DR, Ciriello VM, et al. Psychophysical studies of repetitive wrist flexion and extension. *Ergonomics* 1995;38:1488–1507.
110. Lin ML, Radwin RG, Snook SH. A single metric for quantifying biomechanical stress in repetitive motions and exertions. *Ergonomics* 1997;40:543–558.
111. Appell HJ. Morphology of immobilized skeletal muscle and the effects of a pre- and postimmobilization training program. *Int J Sports Med* 1986;7:6–12.
112. Karpakka J, Vaananen K, Orava S, et al. The effects of preimmobilization training and immobilization on collagen synthesis in rat skeletal muscle. *Int J Sports Med* 1990;11:484–488.
113. Siegel JM, Ruby LK. A critical look at intercarpal arthrodesis: review of the literature. *J Hand Surg [Am]* 1996;21:717–723.
114. Tomaino MM. Miller RJ, Cole I, et al. Scapholunate advanced collapse wrist: proximal row carpectomy or limited wrist arthrodesis with scaphoid excision? *J Hand Surg [Am]* 1994;19:134–142.
115. Watson HK, Hempton RF. Limited wrist arthrodeses. I. The triscaphoid joint. *J Hand Surg [Am]* 1980;5:320–327.
116. Ashmead D, Watson HK. SLAC wrist reconstruction. In: Gelberman RH, ed. *Master techniques in orthopaedic surgery, the wrist.* New York: Raven Press, 1994;319–330.
117. Larsen CF, Jacoby RA, McCabe SJ. Nonunion rates of limited carpal arthrodesis: a meta-analysis of the literature. *J Hand Surg [Am]* 1997;22:66–73.
118. Watson HK, Weinzweig J. Intercarpal arthrodesis. In: Green DP, ed. *Operative hand surgery.* New York: Churchill Livingstone, 1993;108–129.
119. Watson HK, Ashmead D. Triscaphe fusion for chronic scapholunate instability. In: Gelberman RH, ed. *Master techniques in orthopaedic surgery, the wrist.* New York: Raven Press, 1994;183–192.
120. Rogers WD, Watson HK. Radial styloid impingement after triscaphe arthrodesis. *J Hand Surg [Am]* 1989;14:297–301.
121. Kleinman WB. Management of chronic rotary subluxation of the scaphoid by scapho-trapezio-trapezoid arthrodesis—rationale for the technique, postoperative changes in biomechanics, and results. *Hand Clin* 1987;3:113–133
122. Watson HK, Monacelli DM, Milford RS, et al. Treatment of Kienböck's disease with scaphotrapezio-trapezoid arthrodesis. *J Hand Surg [Am]* 1996;21:9–15.
123. Watson HK, Ryu J, Akelman E. Limited triscaphoid intercarpal arthrodesis for rotatory subluxation of the scaphoid. *J Bone Joint Surg Am* 1986;68:345–349.
124. Rogers WD, Watson HK. Degenerative arthritis at the triscaphe joint. *J Hand Surg [Am]* 1990;15:232–235.
125. Garcia-Elias M, Cooney WP, An KN, et al. Wrist kinematics after limited intercarpal arthrodesis. *J Hand Surg [Am]* 1989;14:791–799.
126. Gellman H, Kauffman D, Lenihan M, et al. An *in vitro* analysis of wrist motion: the effect of limited intercarpal arthrodesis and the contributions of the radiocarpal and midcarpal joints. *J Hand Surg [Am]* 1988;13:390–395.
127. Meyerdierks EM, Mosher JF, Werner FW. Limited wrist arthrodesis: a laboratory study. *J Hand Surg [Am]* 1987;12:526–529.
128. Watson HK, Goodman ML, Johnson TR. Limited wrist arthrodesis. Part II: Intercarpal and radiocarpal combinations. *J Hand Surg [Am]* 1981;6:223–233.
129. Watson HK, Ryu J. Evolution of arthritis of the wrist. *Clin Orthop* 1986;202:57–67.
130. Ashmead D, Watson HK, Damon C, et al. Scapholunate advanced collapse wrist salvage. *J Hand Surg [Am]* 1994;19:741–750.
131. Levine WR. Rehabilitation techniques for ligament injuries of the wrist. *Hand Clin* 1992;8:669–681.
132. Wright TW, Michlovitz SL. Management of carpal instabilities. *J Hand Ther* 1996;9:148–156.
133. Green DP. Carpal dislocations and instabilities. In: Green DP, ed. *Operative hand surgery.* New York: Churchill Livingstone, 1993;861–928.
134. Blatt G. Dorsal capsulodesis for rotary subluxation of the scaphoid. In: Gelberman RH, ed. *Master techniques in orthopaedic surgery, the wrist.* New York: Raven Press, 1994;147–165.

135. Watson HK, Weinzweig J, Zeppieri J. The natural progression of scaphoid instability. *Hand Clin* 1997;13:39–49.
136. Watson HK, Weinzweig J. Triquetral impingement ligament tear (TILT). *J Hand Surg [Br]* 1999;24:321–324.
137. Spoorenberg A, Boers M, van der Linden S. Wrist splints in rheumatoid arthritis: what do we know about efficacy and compliance? *Arthritis Care Res* 1994;7:55–57.
138. Anderson K, Maas F. Immediate effect of working splints on grip strength of arthritis patients. *Aust Occup Ther J* 1987;34:26–31.
139. Kjeken I, Moller G, Kvien TK. Use of commercially produced elastic wrist orthoses in chronic arthritis: a controlled study. *Arthritis Care Res* 1995;8:108–113.
140. Nordenskiold U. Elastic wrist orthoses—reduction of pain and increase in grip force for women with rheumatoid arthritis. *Arthritis Care Res* 1990;3:158–162.
141. Stern EB, Ytterberg SR, Krug HE, et al. Immediate and short-term effects of three commercial wrist extensor orthoses on grip strength and function in patients with rheumatoid arthritis. *Arthritis Care Res* 1996;9:42–50.
142. Brumfield R, Kuschner SH, Gellman H, et al. Results of dorsal wrist synovectomies in the rheumatoid hand. *J Hand Surg [Am]* 1990:15:733–735.
143. Dell PC, Dell RB. Management of rheumatoid arthritis of the wrist. *J Hand Ther* 1996;9:157–164.
144. Shapiro JS. The wrist in rheumatoid arthritis. *Hand Clin* 1996;12:477–498.
145. Ryu J, Watson HK, Burgess RC. Rheumatoid wrist reconstruction utilizing a fibrous nonunion and radiocarpal arthrodesis. *J Hand Surg [Am]* 1985;10:830–836.
146. Nathan R, Schneider LH. Classification of distal radioulnar joint disorders. *Hand Clin* 1991;7:239–247.
147. Bowers WH. The distal radio-ulnar joint. In: Green DP, ed. *Operative hand surgery.* New York: Churchill Livingstone, 1988; 939–985.
148. Watson HK, Ryu J, Burgess RC. Matched distal ulnar resection. *J Hand Surg [Am]* 1986;11:812–817.
149. Watson HK, Gabuzda GM. Matched distal ulna resection for posttraumatic disorders of the distal radioulnar joint. *J Hand Surg [Am]* 1992;17:724–730.
150. Jaffe R, Chidgey LK, LaStayo PC. The distal radioulnar joint: anatomy and management of disorders. *J Hand Ther* 1996;9: 129–138.
151. Watson HK, Brown RE. Ulnar impingement syndrome after Darrach procedure: Treatment by advancement lengthening osteotomy of the ulna. *J Hand Surg [Am]* 1989;14:302–306.
152. Lichtman DM, Degnan GG. Staging and its use in the determination of treatment modalities for Kienbock's disease. *Hand Clin* 1993;9:409–416.
153. Colello-Abraham K. A forearm rotation splint. In: Hunter JM, Schneider LH, Mackin EJ, et al, eds. *Rehabilitation of the hand: surgery and therapy.* St Louis: CV Mosby, 1990;1134–1139.
154. Berger-Feldscher S. Adaptation of the Murphy supination splint. *J Hand Ther* 1995;8:270–272.
155. Murphy MS. Brief or new—an adjustable splint for forearm supination. *Am J Occup Ther* 1990;44:936–939.
156. Chesher S. New spring loaded supination and pronation traction: concepts and rationale. *J Hand Ther* 1995;8:53–54
157. Barr K. The use of air bag splints to increased supination and pronation in the arm. *Am J Occup Ther* 1994;48:746–749.
158. Palmer AK, Werner FW. The triangular fibrocartilage complex of the wrist—anatomy and function. *J Hand Surg [Am]* 1981;6: 153–162.
159. Scheker LR, Belliappa PP, Acosta R, et al. Reconstruction of the dorsal ligament of the triangular fibrocartilage complex. *J Hand Surg [Br]* 1994;19:310–318.
160. Sennwald GR, Lauterburg M, Zdravkovic V. A new technique of reattachment after traumatic avulsion of the TFCC at its ulnar insertion. *J Hand Surg [Br]* 1995;20:178–184.
161. Trumble TE, Gilbert M, Vedder N. Isolated tears of the triangular fibrocartilage: management by early arthroscopic repair. *J Hand Surg [Am]* 1997;22:57–65.
162. Acosta R, Hnat W, Scheker LR. Distal radio-ulnar ligament motion during supination and pronation. *J Hand Surg [Br]* 1993;8:502–505.
163. Fusi S, Watson HK, Cuono CB. The carpal boss. A twenty-year review of operative management. *J Hand Surg [Br]* 1995;20: 405–408.
164. Cuono CB, Watson HK. The carpal boss: surgical treatment and etiological considerations. *Plast Reconstr Surg* 1979;63: 88–93.
165. Laseter GF, Carter PR. Management of distal radius fractures. *J Hand Ther* 1996;9:114–128.
166. Reiss B. Therapist's management of distal radial fractures. In: Hunter JM, Mackin EJ, Callahan AD, eds. *Rehabilitation of the hand: surgery and therapy.* St Louis: CV Mosby, 1995;337–351.
167. Palmer AK. Fractures of the distal radius. In: Green DP, ed. *Operative hand surgery.* New York: Churchill Livingstone, 1993; 929–971.
168. Frykman GK, Kropp WE. Fractures and traumatic conditions of the wrist. In: Hunter JM, Mackin EJ, Callahan AD, eds. *Rehabilitation of the hand: surgery and therapy.* St Louis: CV Mosby, 1995;315–336.
169. Watson HK, Castle TH. Trapezoidal osteotomy of the distal radius for unacceptable articular angulation after Colles fracture. *J Hand Surg [Am]* 1988;13:837–843.
170. Filan SL, Herbert TJ. Herbert screw fixation of scaphoid fractures. *J Bone Joint Surg Br* 1996;78:519–529.
171. Russe O. Fracture of the carpal navicular: diagnosis, nonoperative treatment and operative treatment. *J Bone Joint Surg Am* 1960;42:759–768.
172. Watson HK, Pitts EC, Ashmead D, et al. Dorsal approach to scaphoid nonunion. *J Hand Surg [Am]* 1993;18:359–365.

48

CASTING FOR LIMITED WRIST ARTHRODESIS

EMMANUELLA JOSEPH
RICHARD J. DEROSA, JR.
LOIS CARLSON

One of the most important outcome variables for the patient undergoing limited wrist arthrodesis is the postoperative management. Rehabilitation following wrist surgery can be complex and requires a team approach of surgeons, therapists, and cast technicians. Careful attention to detail in the postoperative dressing and casting is critical. The function of a cast is to prevent motion at the arthrodesis site while maintaining the upper extremity in a position of safety to minimize joint contractures. Casting may also serve to reduce postoperative pain. Specific types of materials for casting application, techniques, and postoperative timing vary among surgeons. This chapter emphasizes a postoperative regimen that has been effective following limited wrist arthrodesis.

AUTHOR'S PREFERRED METHOD: THEORETICAL RATIONALE

Limited wrist arthrodeses are treated with 3 weeks of long arm casting followed by 3 weeks of short arm casting or until complete radiographic union is confirmed. Smokers have a higher rate of nonunion in our experience. They are routinely casted for an additional week (a 7-week period). The proximal bones are easily held by casting the forearm and arm, but it is difficult to hold the metacarpals and distal carpal row. Maximum initial immobilization is mandatory for these small bones to fuse. Small capillaries grow rapidly into cancellous bone. The osteocytes in the cancellous graft survive, and a vascular system followed by early osteoid formation is fairly rapidly accomplished if protected by maximum immobilization. A bulky surgical dressing held with bias-cut stockinette is incorporated into a long arm plaster splint immediately postoperatively. The plaster splint is replaced with a fiberglass or plaster cast 2 to 6 days after surgery.

The "Groucho Marx" cast is a long arm cast that holds the elbow at 90°, the forearm in neutral supination–pronation, and the wrist in neutral or slight dorsiflexion. This long arm cast is reminiscent of Groucho Marx's classic pose holding a cigar (Fig. 48.1). The cast immobilizes the meta-

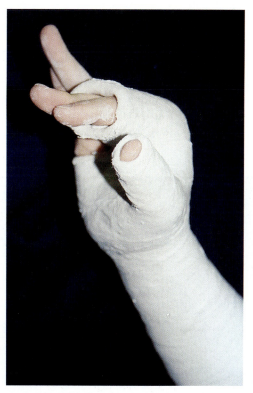

FIGURE 48.1. The "Groucho Marx" cast is a long arm cast and is applied two days after surgery. The thumb is immobilized to the tip, and the metacarpophalangeal joints of the index and middle fingers are held in full flexion. The final cast position resembles the classic pose of Groucho Marx holding a cigar.

E. Joseph: Department of Surgery, Medical College of Ohio, Toledo, Ohio 43615.

R.J. DeRosa, Jr.: Casting Section, Orthopaedic Associates of Hartford, Hartford, Connecticut 06106.

L. Carlson: Connecticut Combined Hand Therapy, Glastonbury, Connecticut 06033, and Hartford, Connecticut 06106.

carpophalangeal (MP) joints of the index and middle fingers in flexion. The index and middle metacarpals are mortised into the carpals, and their immobilization tends to hold the distal row in place. Another option is to include all of the MP joints in flexion. The cast also extends to the tip of the thumb.

At 3 weeks from the day of surgery, the long arm cast is removed. The subcuticular wire sutures are removed from the skin, and a short arm thumb–spica cast is applied from two-thirds up the forearm to the distal palmar crease. Thus, the wrist and thumb continue to be immobilized for three more weeks.

At 6 weeks postsurgery, the thumb–spica cast is removed, and x-rays are obtained to reassess the status of healing. If radiographic evidence of union is seen, the pins are removed with a few drops of lidocaine and a puncture wound over the head of each pin.

Patients are then referred to hand therapy for a progressive program of active and resistive exercise and activity.

TECHNIQUE FOR POSTOPERATIVE DRESSING AND SPLINT

Immediately after the operative procedure, a bulky compressive dressing made of fluffed gauze and simple bias or stockinette is applied (Fig. 48.2). Caution should be used when applying any elastic materials, such as Coban or Ace wraps, to avoid constriction. Fluffed gauze is used to pad the palm and support the wrist. Gauze is carefully placed between the fingers (Fig. 48.3). This separates the finger webs to prevent maceration. The gauze is packed between the fingers lightly, so that excessive pressure is not applied on the neurovascular bundles. A split dorsal long-arm plaster splint made of 10 strips of plaster is incorporated into the dressing, with one split to the thumb and a second to

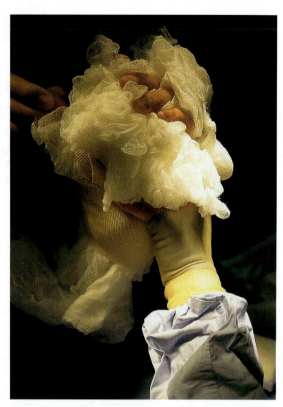

FIGURE 48.3. Fluffed gauze is used to pad the palm, support the wrist, and separate the finger web spaces.

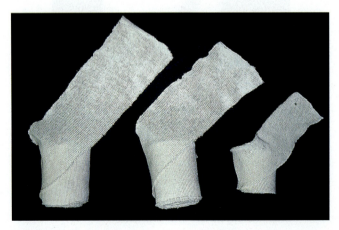

FIGURE 48.2. Stockinette is cut on a bias and used for all postoperative dressings. Use of bias provides predictable uniform compression compared to the constrictive properties of Coban or Ace wraps.

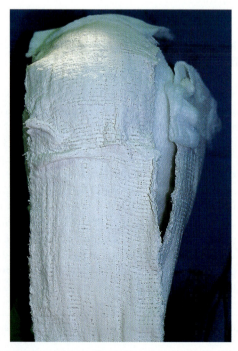

FIGURE 48.4. A plaster splint is incorporated into the dressing by splitting a section of plaster to the thumb and another to the dorsum up to the finger tips.

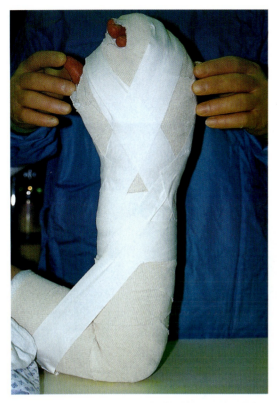

FIGURE 48.5. The postoperative bulky dressing with long arm splint.

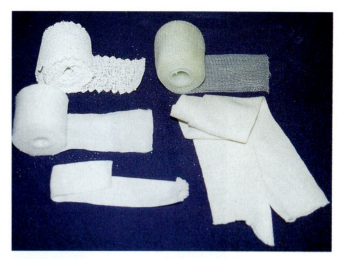

FIGURE 48.6. Supplies needed for casting: 1-in. and 3-in. stockinette, 2-in. webril, 2-in. and 3-in. rolled plaster or fiberglass.

thumb. A smaller 1-in. stockinette is placed on the thumb (Fig. 48.8).

Two-inch cast padding three layers thick is rolled from the thumb and fingertips to the upper arm (Fig. 48.9). The extremity is wrapped in cotton cast padding by partially tearing the padding after each turn to avoid wrinkles. Care

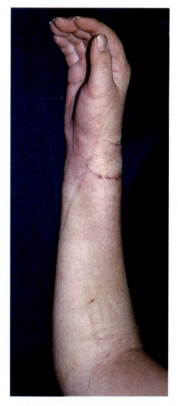

FIGURE 48.7. Positioning of the upper extremity for cast application. The thumb is positioned midway between radial and palmar abduction, the metacarpophalangeal joints are flexed, and the elbow is at 90°.

the dorsum up to the tips of the fingers (Fig. 48.4). This dressing is designed to immobilize the wrist, thumb, and fingers in addition to providing compression to minimize edema (Fig. 48.5).

TECHNIQUE FOR LONG ARM AND SHORT ARM CASTS

The long arm cast restricts pronation and supination of the forearm and prevents additional movement at the wrist. Figure 48.6 shows the supplies needed for casting of the wrist. The patient should be seated comfortably with the hand held vertically on a table. The thumb is positioned midway between radial and palmar abduction (Fig. 48.7). The MP joints of the index and middle fingers are immobilized in flexion ("Groucho Marx"), or all the MP joints are flexed. The distal edge of the cast should extend to the tip of the thumb and just proximal to the proximal interphalangeal (PIP) joints of the digits. The proximal edge of the long arm cast should reach one-half to two-thirds up the upper arm. Three- to four-inch stockinette is cut to extend beyond the proximal and distal edges of the cast so that it may be folded back and provide a soft edge after the initial layer is laid down. A hole is cut in the stockinette for the

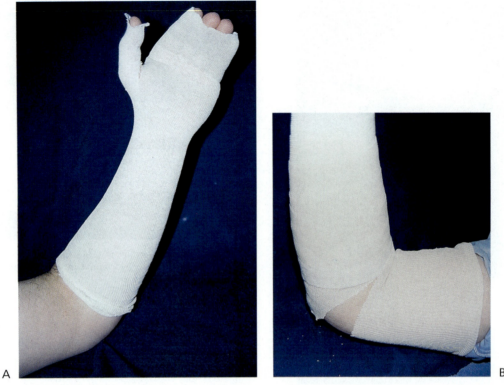

FIGURE 48.8. A: The stockinette layer. Care is taken to ensure that the stockinette remains wrinkle-free to avoid undue pressure. **B:** The stockinette is split at the elbow for long arm cast application.

is taken to add extra padding to pressure-sensitive areas or bony prominences such as the elbow joint, the MP joints, and the ulnar styloid (Fig. 48.10). The wrap should be placed from distal to proximal. The cotton cast padding should also be placed between the fingers to be included in the cast (Fig. 48.11) and should extend beyond the plaster or fiberglass to allow for proximal and distal cuffs.

Generally, 2-in. rolled plaster or fiberglass casting is used for the thumb and wrist, and 3- to 4-in. rolls for the elbow and upper arm in a long arm cast. The roll is dipped in tap water, and the excess water is *gently* squeezed out. Both the plaster and fiberglass set by an exothermic reaction. Fiberglass can release more heat than plaster during

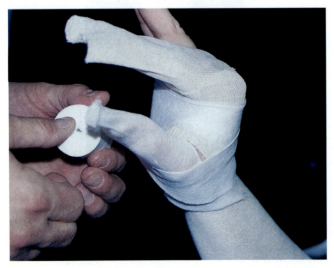

FIGURE 48.9. The application of cast padding.

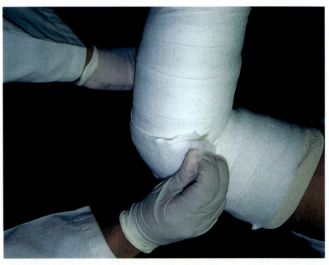

FIGURE 48.10. Padding pressure-sensitive areas and bony prominences.

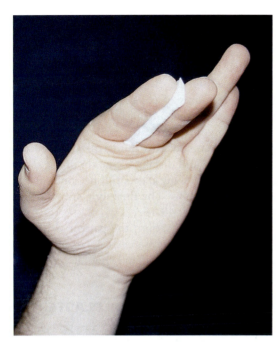

FIGURE 48.11. Cast padding placed between the fingers will prevent maceration.

this reaction. Therefore, cooler water should always be used with fiberglass. Lukewarm water is used for plaster. Using hot water will speed up the hardening time and make it difficult to apply a uniform layer for long arm casting. Caution must be taken to unroll the casting material gently while applying the cast. The "stretch–relax" technique should be used with fiberglass (Fig. 48.12A). This requires stretching the fiberglass while unwinding the roll off the extremity. The fiberglass is placed on the extremity with no tension on the roll ("relaxed"). Pulling hard on the roll will lead to a very tight and uncomfortable cast, which may lead to serious complications. Two to three layers of fiberglass are sufficient for strength, whereas at least seven layers are needed for plaster.

The proper technique for rolling plaster is shown in Fig. 48.12B. The application of the cast should begin with one rotation around the wrist, after which the roll is brought distally around the thumb. Plaster can conform easily and lay flat around the thumb web space. However, small cuts must be made in fiberglass when it is wrapped around the thumb to avoid thumb web space creases (Fig. 48.13). The cast is then wrapped distally around the palm and fingers, and proximally up the forearm. The long arm cast extends to the middle upper arm proximally with the elbow flexed at 90°, the forearm in neutral position with respect to pronation and supination, and the wrist in neutral or slight dorsiflexion. Small cuts are again made in the fiberglass when it is wrapped around the elbow to avoid volar elbow creases.

Care is taken not to go beyond the edge of the cast padding and to fold the stockinette back at both ends (Fig. 48.14). Once the cast has been rolled, any irregular or loose edges can be softened and flattened by rubbing water over the cast (Fig. 48.15). It is very important to rub the cast down whether it is

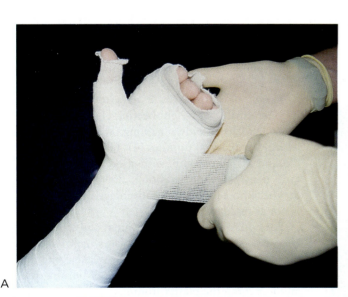
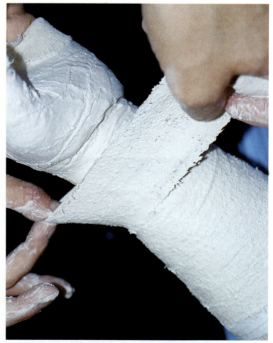

FIGURE 48.12. A: The "stretch–relax" technique for fiberglass cast application entails stretching the roll on tension when it is off the arm and relaxing on the roll before it is laid down onto the arm. **B:** When the plaster cast is rolled, the plaster should be spread off the arm and laid down without tension.

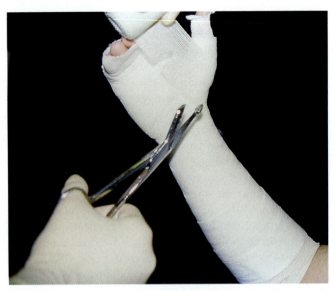

FIGURE 48.13. Small cuts are made in the fiberglass as it is wrapped around the thumb and elbow.

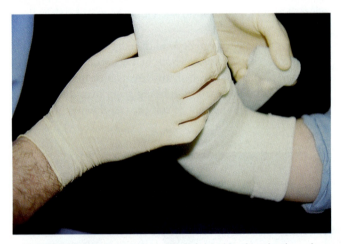

FIGURE 48.14. The stockinette is folded back at both ends.

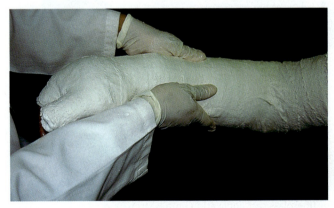

FIGURE 48.15. Polishing the final cast by rubbing it down with water.

plaster or fiberglass. Plaster may be polished by rubbing until the edges of the rolls are not visible and the cast is shiny. With plaster the expression is "rub it like you love it." Fiberglass casts need to be rubbed to ensure good lamination and smooth finish. After the cast has set, the patient should be checked for symptoms of pain, cast fit, capillary refill, and ability to move areas that are not immobilized.

The technique for short arm casting is similar, but the cast extends proximally two-thirds the distance from the wrist to the elbow and distally to the tip of the thumb and distal palmar crease. This allows full flexion and extension of the fingers and elbow. The final long arm and short arm casts are shown in Fig. 48.16.

After each cast application, the patient is instructed to keep the cast dry, and is given exercises to maintain and/or increase mobility of the hand and shoulder.

MATERIAL PROPERTIES OF PLASTER VERSUS FIBERGLASS

The two most commonly used cast materials are a bandage impregnated with plaster of Paris and a polyurethane-resin-impregnated fiberglass bandage. Knowledge of the mechanical properties and characteristics of these casting materials can improve their performance and help determine the proper setting for their use.

Plaster of Paris has been used as a casting material for hundreds of years, and its mechanics have been studied extensively. The first plaster bandages were used by Andonius Mathijen, a Flemish surgeon, in 1852 (1). Plaster is used worldwide because of its low cost and excellent molding properties. However, its application can be messy, and the cast very heavy and cumbersome. The plaster in the gauze is derived from gypsum, and starch is added as an adhesive. Plaster of Paris is made by heating and pulverizing the gypsum, which dehydrates it and produces anhydrous calcium sulfate. When water is added to plaster, crystallization is initiated, reverting the plaster back into gypsum in an exothermic reaction (1).

Plaster of Paris takes 2 days to completely dry and become capable of weight bearing (1–3). In contrast, fiberglass hardens rapidly, gaining weight-bearing strength within less than 30 minutes (4). Fiberglass is easier to handle and is lightweight, with a greater strength-to-weight ratio than plaster. In addition, fiberglass offers respiration for the skin. The major disadvantage of fiberglass is that it is not as moldable as plaster.

For both materials, water content and setting time influence cast strength. For plaster casts, cold water provides more time for cast application but weakens the final product. Hot water increases the chance of burning the patient and loosening the plaster from its fabric. The ideal temperature for crystal quality and cast strength is 30° to 40°C for plaster and 20° to 30°C for fiberglass (1).

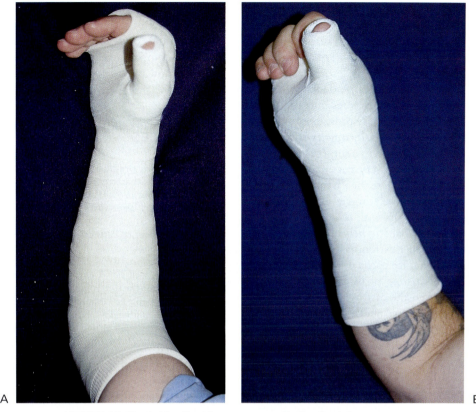

FIGURE 48.16. A: The final long arm cast. **B:** The final short arm cast.

Bone-healing rates have not been proven to be influenced by the choice of casting materials (1,2,5). It is motion within the cast that has been shown to have the most detrimental effect on union rate (2,5). In our review of 483 consecutive triscaphe limited wrist arthrodeses, in which nonunion rates of patients immobilized with plaster casts were compared to those immobilized with fiberglass casts, there was no significant difference in the nonunion rate ($p = 0.71$) (6). Prevention of nonunion in limited wrist arthrodeses is dependent on adequate immobilization, especially during the first three postoperative weeks. It is at this stage that small vascular connections are making their way through the trabecular bone graft between the bones. The slightest motion between these trabecular fragments ruptures the small capillaries, and the process must begin again. Once the initial vascular connections have been established, osteocytes will form, and new bone will be laid down among the graft trabeculae and between the graft and arthrodesing carpals. At 3 weeks, there is reasonable continuity between bones, and the arthrodesis need only be protected from any significant stress or motion (7). It is at this stage that the fingers can be freed from the cast. The cast can then be cut below the elbow to a spica splint. This cast includes the thumb and extends from the distal palmar crease to two thirds the distance between the wrist and elbow. Supination or pronation may be allowed as long as no pins have crossed into the ulna.

SPECIAL PROBLEMS

Compartment syndrome and pressure sores are significant complications of tight or unevenly distributed pressure with casting. Excessive swelling with a well-fitted cast can also lead to a compartment syndrome. Normal function of nerves and muscles is compromised, and tissue necrosis may ensue. Volkmann's ischemic contracture may occur as the residual limb deformity if the acute compartment syndrome goes untreated. Treatment is accomplished by fasciectomy to reduce the pressure caused by the swollen muscles. The most important sign of an acute compartment syndrome is pain out of proportion to what is expected and pain on passive motion of the digits. There is usually a sensory deficit, but pulses are intact with normal capillary refill. Direct measurement of an elevated pressure is the only objective finding. If impending compartment syndrome is suspected, the cast should be removed immediately.

Pressure sores may occur over bony prominences, at the edges of the cast, or over flexion surfaces. Care must be taken to add extra padding to these areas. This complication may also be avoided by uniform cast application and avoiding excess plaster or fiberglass over flexor surfaces of the joints. It is also important not to cause dents with the fingers during cast application. Pressure sores may result in total loss of soft tissue coverage over bony prominences with full bony exposure and loss of tendons, ligaments or nerves. This may require extensive reconstructive surgery with permanent major long-term deficits. Every patient complaining of pain or discomfort should have the cast immediately removed and reapplied more loosely and evenly. Pressure sores are most common in patients with sensory loss, such as peripheral nerve injuries or diabetic neuropathy.

Simple elevation of the upper extremity above the heart decreases postoperative edema. Ice packs or cooling systems are unnecessary during the casting phase because they are cumbersome and may weaken the cast by keeping it moist (2,8,9). Elevation of the extremity above the heart should be stressed throughout the entire postoperative period. It is also critical to emphasize the importance of fully moving the shoulder and digits.

Nerve injuries caused by direct compression of a nerve from the cast may occur in the ulnar nerve at the elbow, the radial nerve in the forearm, and the median nerve at the wrist. Any neurologic complaints demand immediate attention to remove or adjust the cast.

Burns may occur during casting because the materials harden in an exothermic reaction. This occurs if there is no way for the heat to dissipate. It is also more common in those patients with impaired sensation. The cast should not be set down on any impenetrable surfaces as it is hardening because the heat may not dissipate and cause a burn. Freshly set casts should not be covered if possible. The cast should not be applied more than ¼ in. thick per layer at one time. It is better to wait after the first ¼-in. layer has set before adding the next layer. Contact dermatitis is a rare complication of casting. Stockinette material is more likely to cause contact dermatitis than plaster or fiberglass.

SUMMARY

Immobilization in a properly fitted cast is essential to a successful outcome after limited wrist arthrodesis. Inadequate immobilization may lead to malpositioning, nonunion, and prolonged disability. Every effort should be made to apply the cast in the correct position. Many serious complications such as compartment syndrome, pressure sores, neuropathies and burns may be avoided by perfecting casting methods.

REFERENCES

1. Mihalko WM, Beaudoin AJ, Krause WR. Mechanical properties and material characteristics of orthopaedic casting material. *J Orthop Trauma* 1989;3:57–63.
2. Wehbe MA. Plaster uses and misuses. *Clin Orthop* 1982;167:242–249.
3. Luck JV. Plaster of Paris cast. *JAMA* 1944;124:23–29.
4. Schenck T, Somerset JH, Porter RE. Stresses in orthopeadic walking cast. *J Biomech* 1969;2:227–239.
5. Bowker P, Powell ES. A clinical evaluation of plaster-of-Paris and eight synthetic fracture splinting materials. *Injury* 1992;23:13–20.
6. Manzo R, Joseph E, Lionelli GT, et al. Comparison of non-union rates between fiberglass and plaster in limited wrist arthrodesis [abstract]. Presented at the 30th annual meeting of the American Association for Hand Surgery.
7. Watson HK, Vender MI. Wrist and intercarpal arthrodesis. In: Chapman MW, Madison M, eds. *Operative orthopaedics, 2nd ed.* Philadelphia: JB Lippincott, 1993;1363–1378.
8. Calahan, DJ, Carney DJ, Daddario N, et al. The effect of hydration water temperature on orthopedic plaster cast strength. *Orthopedics* 1986;9:683–685.
9. Weresh MJ, Bennett GL, Njus G. Analysis of cryotherapy penetration: a comparison of the plaster cast, synthetic cast, Ace wrap dressing, and Robert-Jones Dressing. *Foot Ankle Int* 1996;17:37–40.

BIBLIOGRAPHY

Davids JR, Frick SL, Skewes E, et al. Skin surface pressure beneath an above-the-knee cast: plaster cast compared with fiberglass casts. *J Bone Joint Surg Am* 1997;79:565–569.

Kaplan SS. Burns following application of plaster splint dressings. Report of two cases. *J Bone Joint Surg Am* 1981;63:670–672.

Jordan JT, Howell JM, Lauerman WC, et al. A radiographic comparison of short arm cast and plaster and fiberglass wrist splints. *Am J Emerg Med* 1993;11:590–591.13.

Patrick JH, Levack B. A study of pressures beneath forearm plasters. *Injury* 1981;13:37–41.

Richard JR. Office orthopedics: thumb spica casting for scaphoid fractures. *Am Fam Physician* 1995;52:1113–1120.

Ritchie IK, Wytch R, Wardlaw D. Flammability of modern synthetic bandages. *Injury* 1988;19:31–32.

49

CAPITATE SHORTENING WITH CAPITATE–HAMATE FUSION

EDWARD E. ALMQUIST

Capitate shortening with capitate–hamate fusion is an operative procedure in which a section of the waist or midportion of the capitate is removed. The defect created by this bone removal is closed by shortening the proximal segment onto the body of the capitate. The two segments are then stabilized by being fused to the adjacent hamate (Fig. 49.1).

For many years joint-leveling procedures were used in Scandinavia for the treatment of Kienböck's disease. I introduced radial shortening into the English literature in 1982, and more recently it became an accepted treatment for Kienböck's disease (1). The theory underlying the treatment with joint leveling developed from the observation of an increased occurrence of ulnar minus variance with Kienböck's disease. The rationale was that reestablishing a proportionate length of ulna to radius would transfer more force, acting through the carpus, towards the ulnar side and diminish pressure across the lunate (2). In its avascular softened state, rather than becoming comminuted or markedly fragmented, the unloaded lunate would have a chance for revascularization. This theory was substantiated clinically in radial shortening as well as ulnar lengthening procedures (3–8), and biomechanical cadaveric studies have also demonstrated a shift of stress from the lunate to the ulnar and radial sides of the wrist, thus unloading the lunate (9,10).

A moderate percentage of patients who develop Kienböck's disease do not have ulnar minus variance; in fact, some even have ulnar positive variance. Radial shortening without ulnar minus variance results in relative ulnar elongation, and ulnar impaction syndrome with significant clinical symptomatology can result. Even when the lunate has revascularized and become relatively asymptomatic, ulnar-sided pain and tenderness persist, associated with erosive changes of the triquetrum. Capitate–hamate fusion was introduced by Chuinard (11) and was initially viewed by this author as a substitute for radial shortening in Kienböck's patients with no ulnar minus variance. This was not substantiated in anatomic and clinical evaluations in my experience, however, and a further mechanical change was attempted through shortening the capitate by removing a segment of the waist to diminish pressure across the lunate. The anatomic feasibility was evaluated with cadaveric studies, and in these, the blood supply to the head of the capitate was observed to course through the palmar capsule and penetrate the head of the capitate through numerous small vessels. A shortening osteotomy performed from the dorsum of the capitate, not violating the palmar blood supply, would thus not cause avascular necrosis of the proximal

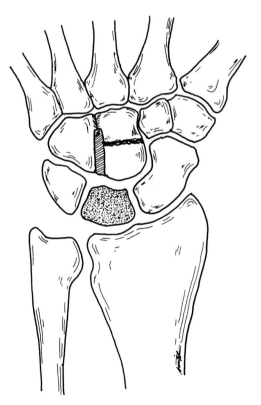

FIGURE 49.1. Diagram of capitate shortening with a capitate–hamate fusion.

E. E. Almquist: Department of Orthopaedics, University of Washington School of Medicine, Seattle, Washington 98122.

pole of the capitate. I believe that the shortening osteotomy of the capitate should be stabilized by fusing each segment to the hamate; this procedure may also further shift weight toward the ulnar side of the wrist through the fused hamate.

BIOMECHANICAL STUDIES

Several biomechanical studies have substantiated that shortening the capitate is an effective lunate-unloading procedure, diminishing the strain between the lunate and the lunate fossa of the radius. The first of these was a small cadaveric study using a strain gauge and Fuji film, showing a shift in pressure away from the lunate fossa of the radius toward the ulna through the triangular fibrocartilage complex and the head of the ulna. It also showed some increase in pressure in the scaphoid fossa of the radius through the scaphoid (12). Using a mathematical strain gauge analysis to study various procedures to unload the lunate, Horii also reported that capitate shortening diminished the load through the lunate fossa by 65% (10). Viola (13) performed a cadaveric study in which pressure-sensitive Fuji film was used on mounted specimens. He reported a decrease in pressure of 35% across the lunate fossa with capitate shortening.

INDICATIONS

The clinical indications for capitate shortening and capitate–hamate fusion are similar to those for other unloading procedures such as radial shortening or ulnar lengthening. The patient should be symptomatic, yet the condition of the lunate should not be so advanced as to preclude anatomic reconstitution of the lunate. This means that the lunate is not markedly deformed, there are no widely separated fragments or free-floating fragments, and there is a reasonable degree of congruity to the articular surfaces of the proximal and distal lunate (Fig. 49.2). In my experience, the goal of any joint-unloading procedure is to reestablish blood supply and continuity to the avascular lunate, and the procedure therefore should be limited to Kienböck's disease stages I, II, and IIIA in the Lichtman classification. In Lichtman stage IIIB with a vertical position of the scaphoid, the lunate generally is markedly flattened and fragmented so as to have lost rotational stability across the scapholunate joint. In this situation, it is unlikely for any joint-leveling procedure to be effective. If, however, the scaphoid is vertical, yet the lunate is in a reasonable degree of anatomic continuity, a decompressing procedure is feasible, and without an ulnar minus variance, capitate shortening and capitate–hamate fusion would be indicated. There appears to be better revascularization potential in younger patients, and specifically in young or teenage patients, unloading procedures are warranted even with lunate fragmentation. In patients with continuing epiphyseal growth, rather remarkable defects and gaps have been closed, and revascularization has occurred. Capitate shortening with capitate–hamate fusion may be indicated in the young adolescent population, even with quite fragmented lunates.

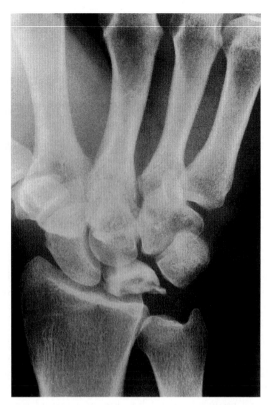

FIGURE 49.2. Posteroanterior x-ray showing lunate proximal pole collapse. This advanced stage is not amenable to decompressing procedures.

SURGICAL TECHNIQUE

The surgical technique for capitate shortening and capitate–hamate fusion is not difficult. A small segment of the waist of the capitate is removed, the capitate head is compressed against the more distal body and fixed with wires, and the capitate is then fixed to the hamate. This is accomplished by a dorsal incision made in the midportion of the wrist under tourniquet control. The wrist capsule is approached through the fourth canal, the retinaculum is incised and elevated on the ulnar border of the fourth canal for later repair, and the dorsal interosseous nerve is removed. The initial capsular incision is over the midcarpal joint, exposing the capitate, and then a very small incision is continued over the lunate, exposing the lunate fossa of the radius. This is best done along the radial border of the lunate, and it should be done in such a manner as to avoid dissecting the capsule away from the dorsal surface of the lunate. Most of the dorsal blood vessels of the lunate approach from the ulnar side, and the capsular attachment can be accessed for later revascularization. The lunate is inspected for its integrity, and it helps to have an assistant distract the carpus manually at this point. If on direct visualization the lunate is seen to be markedly fragmented and the articular surfaces very flabby and structurally destroyed to the point where revascularization and reconstitution of the lunate seem impossible, an alternative procedure such as lunate excision and capitate–scaphoid fusion should be performed. The capitate-shortening approach, in other words, allows for verification of the roentgenologic staging of the disease. It has been my experience that occasionally the roentgenologic appearance is incorrect; that is, there is so much fragmentation, separation, and destruction of the lunate noted on direct inspection that a reclassification is done, and an alternative procedure is performed. The patient should be notified of this possibility in preoperative discussion.

If the lunate appears amenable to an unloading procedure, the capsule is dissected more thoroughly away from the distal capitate to expose the capitate–hamate joint, much of the surface of the hamate, and the waist of the capitate. This permits easy visualization of the capitate–scaphoid articulation. The site for the osteotomy is selected by noting the dorsal curvature of the surface of the capitate as it moves from the proximal articular surface distally across the waist and then angles almost at 90° dorsally. This position is invariably parallel with the distal articular surface of the scaphoid. The capitate–hamate joint is exposed bluntly with a small probe, and the scaphoid–capitate joint is likewise defined. Dissection to any degree is not needed, but the boundaries of the waist of the capitate are assessed at this level. The osteotomy is performed with a thin sharp osteotome (Fig. 49.3), and is done segmentally, using a light mallet and no power tools. A segment of capitate is removed (usually 2 or 3 mm). The parallel osteotomies are done in stages, with care taken to complete the more proximal osteotomy in the mobile segment before the more distal cut is made. The osteotome should just penetrate the palmar cortex of the capitate and not pass into the capsule; the blood supply to the capitate head passes through this capsule and of course, if severed, would produce aseptic necrosis of the capitate head. The segment of resected capitate can usually be removed in one piece, and is saved for later use as a graft. After removal, a careful check of the volar surface of the margins of the capitate osteotomy is made to be sure there is no small lip of cortex to limit compression between the two fragments. The proximal capitate head is very mobile and easily manually compressed to the distal osteotomy site. A small curved blunt instrument is employed, with care taken to avoid compression clamps or any extreme pressure that could damage the articular car-

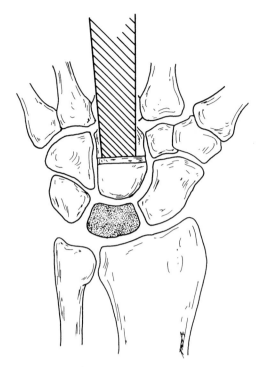

FIGURE 49.3. Surgical procedure. An osteotomy is performed with a thin osteotome, avoiding penetration of the volar capsular blood supply. A 2- to 4-mm section of the waist of the capitate is removed.

tilage. Kirschner wires are then placed across the osteotomy, passing from the dorsal distal surface of the capitate across the osteotomy and into the capitate head, just to the subchondral plate. Cross wires are used, and compression and coaptation of the osteotomy sites during this fixation are easily maintained (Fig. 49.4). Screw fixation with elaborate compressing screws requiring more complex fixation of the proximal segment could damage the articular surface, and I do not consider screw fixation to be necessary.

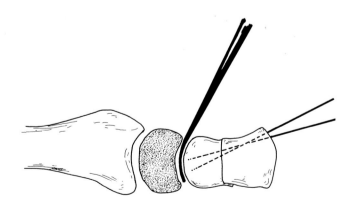

FIGURE 49.4. Surgical procedure. A blunt curved instrument compresses the head of the capitate against the body while K-wires are passed across the osteotomy.

Capitate–hamate fusion is then accomplished by decorticating the adjacent subchondral surfaces. A small curette and an osteotome are used, but this is a somewhat curved joint and has to be followed carefully to the distal edge (Fig. 49.5). The capitate–hamate joint is compressed with a clamp and fixed with Kirschner wires between the hamate and the body of the capitate, and between the hamate and the head of the capitate. Screw fixation could be used, but I believe this is not necessary. If there are any openings or areas of incomplete approximation between the capitate and hamate, the section of the waist of the capitate that was removed is used as a graft. It is packed and tamped in the crevices (Fig. 49.6).

When wire fixation is used between the hamate and capitate, care must be taken to avoid damage to the dorsal branch of the ulnar nerve, and this should be visualized in the ulnar dissection beneath the skin flaps. Care should also be taken to visualize the compressed capitate head, confirming that it is in contact throughout the entire surface of the osteotomy and not rotated with only dorsal portions in close contact. The usual reason for this rotational position is the small lip of cortex remaining on the palmar surface at the osteotomy site. The four Kirschner wires produce stable fixation and are cut off subcutaneously in a way that will avoid the tendons and the dorsal branch of the ulnar nerve. The capsule is closed, the retinaculum over the fourth canal is sewn back, and a short arm splint is applied.

Occasionally the proximal surfaces of the hamate articulates with the lunate and capitate shortening would result in

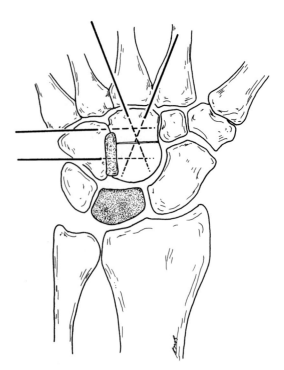

FIGURE 49.6. Surgical procedure. Transverse K-wires fix the hamate to each portion of the capitate. A bone graft is placed in the crevices as needed.

protrusion of this portion of the hamate into the lunate. In these situations the hamate may be slid distally using a compression clamp and fused to the hamate in this position. It would then be on the same plane as the proximal surface of the shortened capitate.

POSTOPERATIVE MANAGEMENT

The splint is removed at about a week, and a cast is applied when the swelling has diminished. The cast can be short arm, with cast immobilization continuing for 8 weeks. At that time, x-rays invariably reveal healing of the osteotomy site and fusion site, and the patient is usually placed in a removable splint to start some early movement. That movement should be without resistance, without lifting weights or heavy objects. The pins are removed within the next few weeks, when moderate movement has been accomplished. Avoidance of heavy strain in the wrist is recommended until revascularization occurs, and this usually entails wearing a splint during moderate activities, with avoidance of strenuous wrist use. Range of motion is commenced when the cast is off, but light resistive exercises are not begun until the pins are removed. It frequently takes up to a year to note revascularization on x-rays, and protection of the wrist should continue until that time. No electrical stimulation has been used on these patients.

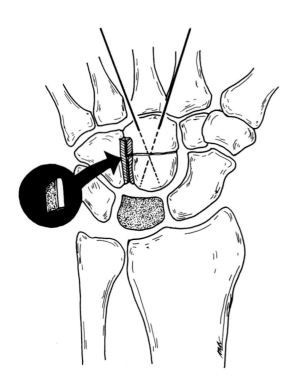

FIGURE 49.5. Surgical procedure. The adjacent surfaces of the capitate and hamate are decorticated.

CLINICAL RESULTS

The primary goal of surgical treatment of Kienböck's disease should be revascularization of the lunate; without revascularization, ultimate clinical failure will occur. It may take 5 to 10 years, but without a stable healed lunate, what initially appeared to be a good clinical response will ultimately deteriorate.

The second goal should be a return to normal or near-normal functional activities. This has been accomplished in our experience and should be expected in appropriately selected patients treated by capitate shortening (Fig. 49.7). Grip strength averaged 85% of the opposite side on long-term follow-up evaluation, and 90% returned to work or normal activity. This may include heavy manual labor, professional sports, and other vigorous activities, although, as previously noted, this should not be permitted until revascularization is accomplished.

Range of motion does not improve significantly and generally equals the average range of motion preoperatively. This is also true with radial shortening. Some patients have an acute inflammatory response during various periods of the aseptic process and temporarily become very stiff; therefore, range of motion preoperatively can vary considerably between clinic visits. After healing occurs and joint inflammation subsides, wrist range of motion becomes more constant between visits.

Pain relief in decompressing procedures is typically dramatic and is not necessarily accompanied by radiographic improvement of the lunate. This has been noted repeatedly in radial shortening procedures, is also true in capitate shortening with capitate–hamate fusion, and presumably results from a subsiding inflammatory reaction around the lunate secondary to its unloading. Diminished pain may also be related to resection of the dorsal interosseous nerve, although the same phenomenon is noted on volar

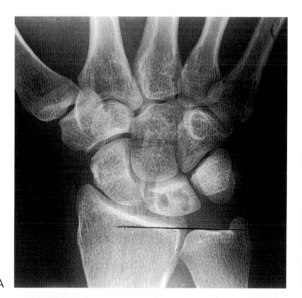

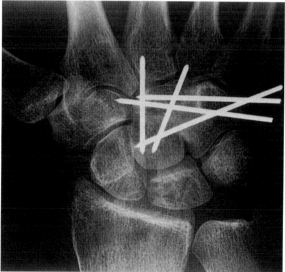

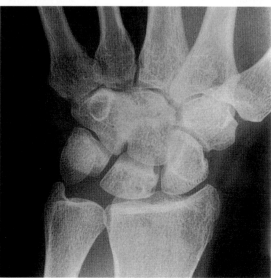

FIGURE 49.7. A: A 36-year-old woman with cystic Kienböck's disease with no architectural changes to the lunate and no ulnar minus variance. **B:** Postoperative x-ray showing capitate shortening with capitate–hamate fusion. **C:** X-ray taken 13 months postoperatively with revascularization, near-normal range of motion, and good pain relief.

approaches to radial shortening where there has been no nerve resection. Relief of pain can be expected to be lasting, and in most cases, patients experience discomfort only with heavy manual labor or stressful wrist activities.

COMPLICATIONS

The most significant complication in the surgical treatment of Kienböck's disease is failure of the lunate to revascularize. This is not a true complication but a consequence of the disease, and these patients will ultimately do poorly. Careful preoperative evaluation and selection of patients greatly reduce this possibility. In nearly 20 years of doing this procedure, I have not seen avascular necrosis of the capitate head and, in discussions with many physicians doing this procedure, have not learned of others who have observed it. I believe this is a result of careful dissection at the osteotomy site and avoidance of power tools. Pin track irritation of the extensor tendons has been noted, after which the tendons can rupture from irritation by a pin. Because of the rather prolonged use of the pins, extracutaneous placement is probably not advised. I believe care in the placement of the pins, perhaps bending the pins, cutting them close to the bone to avoid tendon irritation, and capping them appropriately, is the way to avoid this. The pins that affix the capitate to the hamate pass near the dorsal branch of the ulnar nerve, and careful avoidance of damage to that nerve during placement reduces this potential complication.

DISCUSSION

Capitate shortening is a proven procedure with validated biomechanical support for its ability to diminish stress across the lunate. If, indeed, this promotes revascularization of the lunate, the procedure has credibility, and the clinical studies and many years of experience appear to validate that conclusion. The advantages are its simplicity both in technique and in use of instrumentation: exotic and expensive equipment and implants are not needed and indeed seem contraindicated. The procedure also allows visualization of the lunate and direct classification.

When there is a hypermobile scaphoid, that is, a scaphoid that can move into vertical position quite easily, and compressing the carpus at the time of surgery allows the scaphoid to ride dorsally out of the confines of the scaphoid fossa of the radius, ligamentous stabilization of that joint seems reasonable. I have accomplished this by using a flap from the distal half of the extensor retinaculum over the fourth and fifth canals. The extensor retinaculum is mobilized from these two canals and rotated toward the radial side of the wrist while remaining attached to Lister's tubercle between the third and fourth canals. A small trough is made on the scaphoid just proximal to the distal articular surface, and this firm, thick retinacular flap is sewn through drill holes into the scaphoid, pulling the distal portion of the scaphoid dorsally, stabilizing it from vertical subluxation. This technique has also been my treatment for stage I scapholunate separation and is essentially similar to the Blatt capsulodesis technique except that the retinaculum is used rather than a capsular advancement. The rationale for performing this procedure in loose-jointed Kienböck's patients who are undergoing capitate shortening and capitate–hamate fusion is to stabilize the scaphoid to accept the greater force that will be transferred to the radial side of the wrist. It has the same rationale as a triscaphe fusion for Kienböck's disease. In my experience, however, this has rarely been necessary, as most patients with Kienböck's disease have had synovitis, an inflammation in the wrist, for a considerable period of time and already have moderate stiffness. A mobile scaphoid is usually not present unless there is marked collapse of the lunate or fragmentation of the lunate, in which case, capitate shortening is not recommended.

Radial wedge osteotomies have been advocated for Kienböck's disease without ulnar minus variance or with ulnar positive variance. Closing and opening radial- and ulnar-sided radial osteotomies have each been advocated, and biomechanical studies suggesting their effects have been presented (14–16). Although I have had no experience with these procedures, it is curious that seemingly opposite mechanical changes—either closing or opening of the radius—appear to have similar effects in unloading the lunate. I consider the straightforward and simple capitate shortening, its efficacy substantiated by several biomechanical studies, to be a more direct means of unloading the pressures across the lunate.

EDITORS' COMMENTS

The principle of circumventing load through the lunate is currently the best approach to Kienböck's disease. The lunate cannot be adequately unloaded with ulnar lengthening or radial shortening procedures, no matter their angular change. Shortening of the capitate, which is the main impresser and load transfer agent to the lunate, can unload the lunate. We would disagree with the part of the operation that transfers the load to the hamate. The hamate–triquetral joint is not optimal for in-line loading of the hand and wrist. The slopes of the ulnar intercarpal joints are not perpendicular to the loads. The ligament support between the hamate and triquetrum is lax. If loads are transferred to the triquetrum, there is no way to adequately move them onto the radius. Unloading the lunate is better done on the radial side of the wrist, and the scaphoid is the agent of transfer. The scaphoid can transfer loads around the lunate to the radius without shortening the capitate. We feel, therefore, that there is no indication for capitate shortening and capitate–hamate fusion.

REFERENCES

1. Almquist EE, Burns JF. Radial shortening for the treatment of Kienböck's disease. *J Hand Surg [Am]* 1982;7:348–352.
2. Rossak K. Druckverhaltnisse am handgelenk unter besonderer berucksichtigung von fraktur-mechanismen. *Z Orthop* 1967;103 (suppl.):269.
3. Axelsson R. Niveauoperationen bei mondbeinnekrose. *Handchirurgie* 1973;5:187.
4. Calandriello B, Palandri C. Die behandlung der lunatum malazie durch speichenverkurzung. *Z Orthop* 1966;101:531–534.
5. Eiken O, Niechajev I. Radius shortening in malacia of the lunate. *Scand J Reconstr Surg* 1980;14:191–196.
6. Kleven H. The treatment of lunatomalacia. *Tijdskr Norske Laegeforen* 1971;19:1944–1946.
7. Rosemeyer B, Artmann M, Viernstein K. Lunatum-malacie nachuntersuchungsergebnisse und therapeutische erwagungne. *Arch Orthop Unfallchir* 1976;85:119–127.
8. Viernstein K, Weigert M. Die radiusverkurzungosteotomie bei der lunatummalizie. *Munch Med Wochenschr* 1967;109:1992.
9. Trumble T, Glisson R, Seaber A, et al. A biomechanical comparison of the methods for treating Kienböck's disease. *J Hand Surg [Am]* 1986;11:88–93.
10. Horii E, Garcia-Elias M, An KN, et al. Effect on force transmission across the carpus in procedures used to treat Kienböck's disease. *J Hand Surg [Am]* 1990;15:393–400.
11. Chuinard RG, Zeman SC. Kienböck's disease: An analysis and rationale for treatment by capitate–hamate fusion. *J Hand Surg [Am]* 1980;5:290.
12. Necking L, Almquist EE. *Capitate shortening for Kienböck's disease—a biomechanical study.* Paper presented at the Proceedings of the Wrist Investigator's Workshop, Newport Beach, CA, May 15, 1990.
13. Viola RW, Kiser PK, Bach AW, et al. Biomechanical analysis of capitate shortening with capitate hamate fusion in the treatment of Kienböck's disease. *J Hand Surg [Am]* 1998;23:395–401.
14. Fu F, Simmons EH. Kienböck's disease. *Orthop Consult* 1981;2:1–7.
15. Nakamura R, Tsuge S, Watanabe K, et al. Radial wedge osteotomy for Kienböck's disease. *J Bone Joint Surg Am* 1991;73:1391–1396.
16. Werner FW, Palmer AK. Biomechanical evaluations of operative procedures to treat Kienböck's disease. *Hand Clin* 1993;9:431–443.

50

CARPAL BOSS REPAIR

JEFFREY WEINZWEIG
H. KIRK WATSON

INDICATIONS

The carpal boss is a relatively common lesion that presents as a bony protuberance on the dorsum of the wrist. Foille, in 1931, coined the term "carpe bossu" to refer to this lesion, which he described as an exostosis at the bases of the second and third metacarpals (1). The first, third, and fifth metacarpal bases are naturally prominent in the human hand. The carpal boss represents a partial or complete coalition or synchondrosis of the second (trapeziometacarpal) and third (capitometacarpal) carpometacarpal (CMC) joints as well as the trapeziocapitate joint and the 2,3-intermetacarpal joint space—collectively the "quadrangular joint." The etiology of this anomaly is abnormal bony architecture involving the dorsal aspect of the index metacarpal, trapezoid, capitate, and middle metacarpal. This abnormal architecture usually represents a congenital os that can take several forms. The os can be freestanding or fused to one or more of the four bones involved. The abnormal loading that occurs in this area produces localized degenerative arthritis on the dorsal aspect of this four-bone complex. It can become symptomatic in young people, producing local tenderness, not uncommonly ganglion formation, and eventually a marked bony prominence. This clinical entity, often mildly asymptomatic, can be very painful (2,3).

The diagnosis of carpal boss is made on physical exam by loading the "quadrangular joints." The joints are malaligned by holding the head of the index and middle metacarpals in each hand. Volarly flexing (depressing) one metacarpal head while extending the other—the "metacarpal stress test"—will reproduce the patient's symptoms. A similar provocative maneuver described by Fusi (4) has the index and middle proximal phalanges fully flexed, locking the phalanges to the metacarpal head and then rotating the metacarpals in opposite directions. This will overload the carpal boss area and reproduce symptoms. Diagnosis is confirmed radiographically by a modified lateral x-ray of the wrist, the "carpal boss view" (5), which readily demonstrates an accessory ossicle, the os styloideum (Fig. 50.1), in 50% of cases (4,6,7).

With osteophytic prominence of this area, radial and ulnar deviation of the wrist can cause a snapping of the index extensor tendons over the prominence. This is not the cause of the symptoms associated with carpal boss. Fusion of the four-bone complex is contraindicated. Resection of the abnormal congenital bone and the abnormal secondary osteoarthritis will cure the problem.

CONTRAINDICATIONS

Because the only indication for carpal boss repair is associated symptomatology, an asymptomatic boss does not require surgical intervention.

SURGICAL TECHNIQUE

The operative procedure is that described by Cuono and Watson in 1979 (2). The carpal boss is approached through a 3- to 4-cm transverse dorsal incision centered at the base of the middle finger (third) metacarpal (4). This places the incision at the summit of the carpal boss. Tendons of the fourth dorsal compartment are retracted ulnarward, and the carpal boss is approached on both sides of the extensor carpi radialis brevis tendon. A dental rongeur is used to remove the accessory ossicle along with the surrounding sclerotic bony prominence. Excavation is continued to the level of normal joint cartilage and normal cancellous bone on both

---

J. Weinzweig: Department of Plastic Surgery, Brown University School of Medicine, Rhode Island Hospital, and Hasbro Children's Hospital, Providence, Rhode Island 02905.

H. K. Watson: Connecticut Combined Hand Surgery Fellowship, Hartford Hospital, and Connecticut Children's Medical Center, Hartford, Connecticut 06106; Department of Orthopaedics, University of Connecticut School of Medicine, Farmington, Connecticut 06032; Department of Orthopedics, Rehabilitation, and Plastic Surgery, Yale University School of Medicine, New Haven, Connecticut 06520.

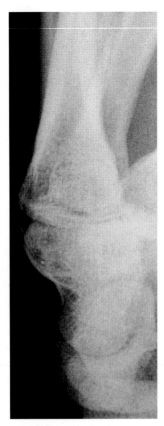

FIGURE 50.1. The lateral carpal boss view demonstrates the accessory os styloideum.

sides of all four joints. The cancellous bone should be cut away behind the joint cartilage, thus forming a slight cancellous concavity (Fig. 50.2). Aggressive resection is necessary until one can visualize normal cartilage entirely across the articular surface of each of the four bones. The involved areas of the CMC joints include only the most dorsal aspect. The great majority of each CMC joint is not involved, which predicts normal postoperative function. Any preserved dorsal wrist capsular structures are returned to their anatomic position, and the skin is closed. A bulky dressing incorporating a plaster splint is used, maintaining the wrist in moderate dorsiflexion.

POSTOPERATIVE MANAGEMENT

The dressing is maintained for 5 to 7 days, followed by early progressive mobilization.

CLINICAL SERIES

One hundred sixteen patients with a symptomatic carpal boss were surgically treated over a 20-year period (4). The mean age of this group of patients was 32 years (range, 11–75 years) and included 61 male and 55 female patients. The average duration of symptoms before presentation was 19 months. Twenty-eight patients (24%) presented following blunt trauma to the dorsum of the hand or wrist, at which time the patient became aware of the dorsal wrist prominence. The mean follow-up for this series was 42 months (range, 3 months to 16 years).

Seventy-four patients (63%) intraoperatively demonstrated an identifiable bony anomaly in the region of the quadrangular joint at the base of the index and middle metacarpals, where they articulate with the trapezoid and capitate. These anomalies were most frequently either a separate ossicle (the os styloideum) or one that was fused completely or in part to the metacarpal or carpal bones. Fused ossicles occasionally bridged the respective metacarpal and carpal bones. All patients in this series returned to full activity, usually within 2 to 3 months following surgery. None were symptomatic with stressed wrist activity, and none experienced diminished grip strength or range of motion following surgery.

COMPLICATIONS

Recurrence or persistence of carpal boss symptoms occurred in seven patients (6%) within 24 months following surgery. The development of symptoms within a matter of months suggests that the extent of the initial excision was insufficient, and degenerate joint surfaces left intact predisposed to rapid redevelopment of symptoms. Six of the seven patients underwent a secondary procedure to excise the remaining degenerative arthritic exostosis and were subsequently asymptomatic at final follow-up.

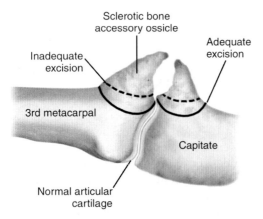

FIGURE 50.2. Resection must include the entire arthritic process dorsally. Normal cartilage must be seen on the opposing surface of all four bones at the close of the procedure. Resecting in a slightly concave fashion behind the articular cartilage will prevent bony bridging.

DISCUSSION

The carpal boss is a localized bony exostosis involving the quadrangular CMC joints of the trapezoid, capitate, and bases of the second and third metacarpals that becomes symptomatic with degenerative arthritic change. The etiology of the symptomatic carpal boss is related to maldevelopment at the quadrangular capitate–trapezoid–metacarpal joint as a result of the persistence of an accessory ossification component. The abnormal configuration of the joint complex predisposes it to the development of a highly localized and dorsal degenerative arthritic process. This area is more susceptible to the effects of repetitive trauma. Complete symptomatic relief is easily achieved but is dependent on adequate excision of the involved areas of joint.

REFERENCES

1. Fiolle J. Le "carpe bossu." *Bull Mem Soc Nat Chir* 1931;57:1687–1690.
2. Cuono CB, Watson HK. The carpal boss: Surgical treatment and etiological considerations. *Plast Reconstr Surg* 1979;63:88–93.
3. Carter R. Carpal boss: a commonly overlooked deformity of the carpus. *J Bone Joint Surg* 1941;23:935–939.
4. Fusi S, Watson HK, Cuono CB. The carpal boss: A 20-year review of operative management. *J Hand Surg [Br]* 1995;20:405–408.
5. Conway WF, Destouet JM, Gilula LA, et al. The carpal boss: An overview of radiographic evaluation. *Radiology* 1985;156:29–31.
6. Bassöe E, Bassöe HH. The styloid bone and carpe bossu disease. *Am J Roentgenol* 1955;74:886–891.
7. Thompson A. The condition of the os styloideum as attached to the III metacarpal, to the magnum, to the trapezoid. *J Anat* 1894;28:64.

51

CARPOMETACARPAL TENDON ARTHROPLASTY

H. KIRK WATSON
JEFFREY WEINZWEIG

INDICATIONS

First ray carpometacarpal (CMC) degenerative arthritis is one of the more common parawrist problems in any hand surgery practice. The solution to advanced destruction of this joint is arthroplasty or arthrodesis (1–5). Arthroplasty is by far the preferable choice because it preserves motion at the CMC joint. The success of the tendon arthroplasty technique has encouraged its use in younger and younger patients.

CONTRAINDICATIONS

Despite sacrifice of CMC joint motion, arthrodesis may be the preferable approach in the young laborer with extremely heavy work, for whom the need for absolute lifelong full strength may preclude a satisfactory result with tendon arthroplasty. Careful patient selection is crucial for a successful outcome in such cases.

SURGICAL TECHNIQUE

A transverse incision is made at the level of the CMC joint on the radial side of the wrist. The so-called "hockey stick" incision is to be avoided for all CMC surgery. The extensor pollicis brevis (EPB) is approximately in the center of this incision. A blunt spreading technique is utilized to preserve the branches of the superficial radial nerve, which are retracted volarly or dorsally. A longitudinal periosteal incision is then made on the metacarpal, just volar to the EPB, extending proximally between the EPB and the abductor pollicis longus (APL). The capsule of the CMC joint is then peeled back, using a scalpel or sharp dental osteotome. The scaphoid–trapezium joint is opened. One blade of the dental rongeur is placed in the scaphoid–trapezium joint, the other in the CMC joint, and the trapezium is osteotomized with a two-thirds segment of the trapezium dorsally and a one-third segment of the trapezium volarly. The dorsal segment is more easily removed; therefore, the dorsal segment is made larger. Care must be taken deep in the osteotomy not to injure the flexor carpi radialis (FCR) tendon, which runs in a groove in the trapezium on its deep aspect.

Small curved dental osteotomes are then used to cut the capsule between the trapezium and trapezoid and the deep capsule of the CMC joint. Once this fragment is loosened somewhat from its surrounding capsule, it can be grasped with the dental rongeurs and rotated. Four to six complete rotations or revolutions of this segment will free it from the rest of the ligamentous attachments on the deep surface of the bone and release it from the wrist. Sharp dissection with a #15 blade is then carried out on the smaller volar segment, again protecting the FCR, which is now easily visualized deep in the wound. Dental rongeurs assist in the removal of this smaller section.

The articular cartilage of the trapezoid is then removed to a cancellous surface over the entire exposed surface of trapezoid. The osteophytes are removed from the radial aspect of the base of the metacarpal, and depressing the metacarpophalangeal (MP) joint exposes the large "toe of the boot" osteophyte ulnar and deep in the wound. All of this osteophyte must be removed to the level of the cortex of the metacarpal (Fig. 51.1). One is now left with a section of cortex across the base of the metacarpal, typically just over $^1/_2$ cm in width and running from volar to dorsal. This

---

H. K. Watson: Connecticut Combined Hand Surgery Fellowship, Hartford Hospital, and Connecticut Children's Medical Center, Hartford, Connecticut 06106; Department of Orthopaedics, University of Connecticut School of Medicine, Farmington, Connecticut 06032; Department of Orthopedics, Rehabilitation, and Plastic Surgery, Yale University School of Medicine, New Haven, Connecticut 06520.

J. Weinzweig: Department of Plastic Surgery, Brown University School of Medicine, Rhode Island Hospital, and Hasbro Children's Hospital, Providence, Rhode Island 02905.

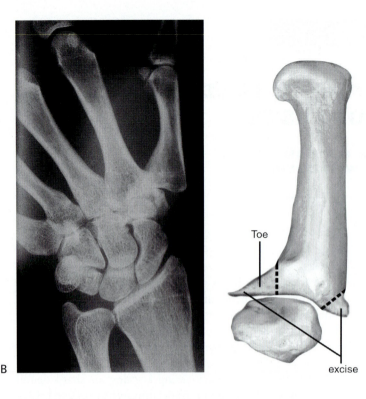

FIGURE 51.1. A,B: Carpometacarpal degenerative arthritis typically involves lateral displacement of the metacarpal shaft. The metacarpal base develops a "toe of the boot," which is the body's attempt to stabilize the metacarpal. This large osteophyte grows out ulnarward and lacks any adequate articular cartilage.

cortical bridge is maintained to prevent the collagenous anchovy from migrating into the shaft of the metacarpal (Fig. 51.2).

A small drill hole is made on the radialmost aspect of the metacarpal perpendicular to this cortical bridge and emerging in the exposed cancellous area where the "toe of the boot" osteophyte was removed. This hole is begun with a small drill, then enlarged to a drill hole that will accept approximately 50% of the FCR tendon. Attention is directed to the forearm, where a transverse incision is

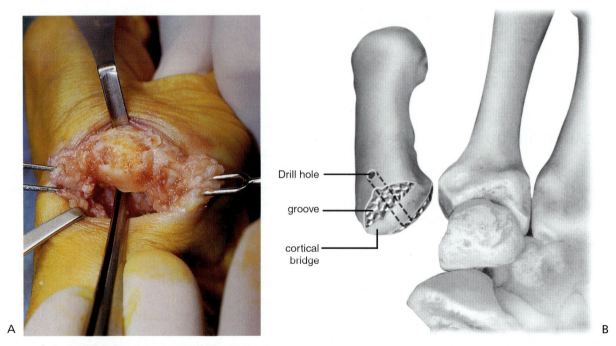

FIGURE 51.2. A cortical bridge is maintained across the base of the metacarpal to prevent the rolled-up collagenous anchovy from migrating or eroding into the metacarpal shaft.

centered over the FCR approximately 1 cm proximal to the wrist crease. Palpation of the FCR will identify the musculotendinous junction approximately 12 cm proximal to this incision. The second transverse incision is made at this level. The tendon is exposed through both wounds. Dissection is carried distally from the distal wound, elevating the communicating branch to the superficial arterial arch and cutting the fascia that overlies the FCR until one has easy access to the arthroplasty wound. The tendon fascia is incised utilizing scissors running proximally up the tendon from the distal wound and distally down the tendon from the proximal wound. The tendon is then elevated on a small retractor in the distal wound, and a suture is passed through the middle of the tendon (Fig. 51.3). Two small retractors are placed on opposite sides through the tendon. With the wrist flexed, the tendon is pulled apart into its two halves in this distal segment. A Kelly clamp is then passed from the proximal wound to the distal wound. The two ends of the suture are marked *left* and *right* by their position in the Kelly and drawn into the proximal wound. The suture is then used to saw its way through the tendon from the distal wound to the proximal wound, and the volar-ulnar half of the tendon is transected.

The ulnar half of the FCR is then delivered from the distal incision through the tunnel and into the wrist wound. The tendon is passed around the base of the metacarpal, down through the drill hole, emerging in the deep portion of the wound where the "toe of the boot" was removed. This then encircles the cortical base and is sutured with a 4-0 vicryl stitch. It is important that the proximal metacarpal be depressed toward the insertion of the FCR and that the tendon be pulled and sutured as tightly as possible. If the tendon tends to ride laterally off the metacarpal to either side, a small groove along the tendon is made to keep it centered as it crosses the base of the metacarpal and the cortical bridge. The "bitter end" of this tendon is then wrapped around the "standing part" multiple times (Fig. 51.4). This tightens the tendon suspension and provides a highly localized interposition anchovy of collagen that rests on the cortical bridge across the base of the metacarpal. The "bitter end" is then sutured to the intact FCR with a single 5-0 Dexon suture. The capsule is imbricated in an hourglass fashion and sutured with 5-0 Dexon, and the wrist and forearm wounds are closed with 4-0 subcuticular wire. A bulky standard dressing, incorporating a plaster thumb–spica splint, is applied.

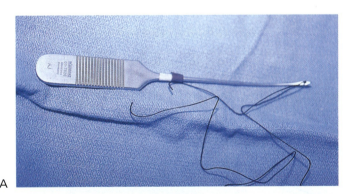

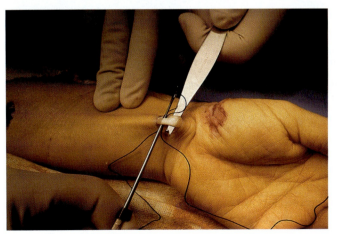

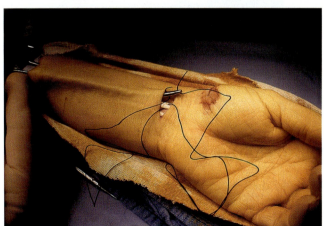

FIGURE 51.3. A,B: A sharp narrow instrument with a hole at its distal end is used to pass a suture through the flexor carpi radialis (FCR). **C:** The suture is drawn into the proximal wound and used to saw proximally, separating the two halves of the FCR. The more superficial ulnar half is transected in the forearm and drawn out to the wrist.

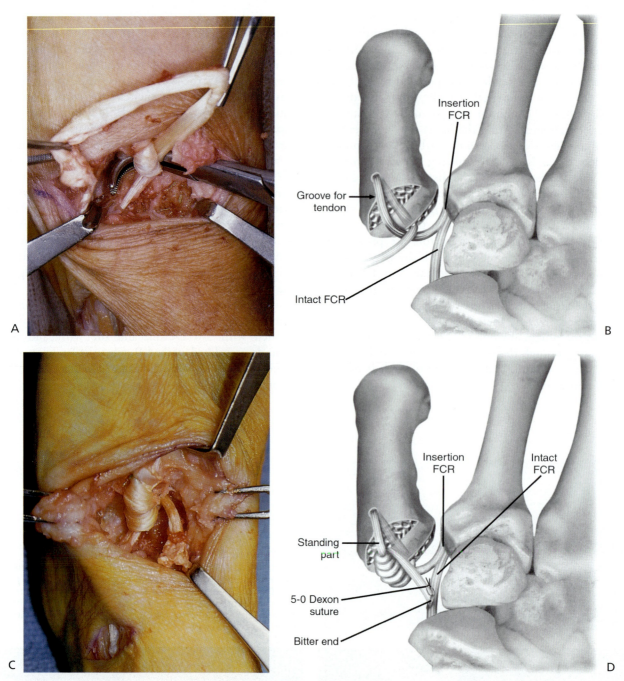

FIGURE 51.4. A,B: After the tendon has been sutured around the base of the first metacarpal through the drill hole, the "bitter end" is woven multiple times around the "standing part" using a curved snap. **C,D:** The completed suturing is shown after the excess half of the flexor carpi radialis has been completely wound around itself, producing a highly localized collagenous mass that tightens the support mechanism and serves as an interposition arthroplasty.

POSTOPERATIVE MANAGEMENT

The bulky dressing and splint are removed 2 days postoperatively, and a plaster splint, incorporating the forearm and thumb to the distal tip, is applied and maintained for 2½ to 3 weeks. The splint is then removed, and full mobilization is permitted at that time.

CLINICAL SERIES

One hundred ten patients underwent thumb CMC tendon arthroplasty over a 5-year period for treatment of pain secondary to degenerative joint disease; 11 of these patients underwent bilateral CMC tendon arthroplasty. At a mean follow-up of approximately 2 years, 61 patients were available for reevaluation. Range of motion in palmar abduction–adduction of the operative side averaged 62.6°, compared with 63.0° on the unoperated side (in unilateral cases). In thumb opposition–reposition, the operative side demonstrated a 56.1° arc compared with a 57.2° arc on the unoperated side. Key pinch averaged 11.4 lb on the operative side compared with 13.9 lb on the unoperated side (87.9%); tip pinch averaged 8.6 lb on the operative side compared with 9.9 lb on the unoperated side (93.5%). Grip strength averaged 55.3 lb on the operative side compared with 53.7 lb on the unoperated side (109%). The thumb pulp-to-palm distance was 0 cm in all unoperated thumbs as well as in 56 of 61 operated thumbs. The five patients unable to touch were short by an average of 0.5 cm (range, 0.3–0.8 cm).

Radiographic evaluation was performed on 53 thumbs, which included all thumbs except those that had had previous silicone implants, as these had undergone prior surgical shortening of the thumb metacarpal to accommodate the implant. Thumb metacarpal subluxation was present in 15 of the 53 patients. There was no erosion of the tendon into adjacent bone, and there were no cystic changes in the scaphoid or thumb metacarpal. Pain with both light use and heavy use was significantly improved in almost all patients postoperatively; only two patients reported night pain, and four patients reported occasional rest pain. Ninety-one percent of patients were satisfied with the postoperative result, and all patients who were employed before surgery returned to the same job subsequently.

COMPLICATIONS

Few complications occurred following CMC tendon arthroplasty in this series of patients. Persistent pain occurred in only six patients. One patient developed reflex sympathetic dystrophy (RSD) postoperatively, which resolved on a Dystrophile program (see Chapter 65).

We have also seen a swan-neck complication of the thumb on more than one occasion. The prerequisites for this complication are the development of a hyperextensible MP joint secondary to CMC arthritis. The destruction and lateral displacement at the base of the metacarpal produce an adduction contracture of the thumb metacarpal, resulting over time in a stretching out of the volar plate and a displacement of the sesamoid bones from their tract. Approximately 2 months following CMC tendon arthroplasty, several patients complained of pain in the A1 pulley region of the thumb with a secondary flexion deformity at the interphalangeal (IP) joint that initially appears to be the result of stenosing tenosynovitis. However, release of the A1 pulley will not release the flexion deformity of the IP joint.

Should this swan-neck phenomenon occur, we now perform check-rein capsuloplasties of the IP joint and often pin it in extension, combined with a sesamoidectomy and volar plate advancement into the metacarpal to stabilize the MP joint in flexion. On one occasion, we fused the MP joint to correct a severe hyperextension deformity.

Because the hyperextension deformity of the MP joint frequently does not require treatment, though it is commonly present with longstanding CMC joint disease, we will usually not treat MP hyperextension at the time of CMC arthroplasty. Under these circumstances, it is probably important to immobilize the IP joint in maximum extension at the time of CMC arthroplasty.

DISCUSSION

Thumb CMC osteoarthritis is a common problem resulting in pain with motion, postactivity ache, and joint instability and subluxation. The goals of surgical intervention include restoration of strength, range of motion, and painless function. Historically, approaches in the management of CMC degenerative joint disease have included arthrodesis, trapezium excision without replacement, trapezium replacement with various implants, and tendon arthroplasty with or without trapezium excision (1,6–9).

The described technique was developed to minimize the potential disadvantages of tendon arthroplasty procedures, which include postoperative weakness, decreased range of motion, proximal metacarpal migration, scaphoid impingement, and pain. This technique consists of three key components: (a) suspension of the thumb metacarpal on the FCR insertion; (b) maintenance of the cortical bridge at the base of the metacarpal; and (c) interposition of a tight collagenous (tendon) arthroplasty.

The transverse wrist incision, used to access the CMC joint, and the use of two small forearm incisions to harvest half of the FCR tendon, decrease the amount of postoperative pain and scarring. Preservation of a bridge of articular cortex at the base of the thumb metacarpal prevents erosion of the tightly packed collagen anchovy into the metacarpal, should the suspension mechanism allow proximal metacarpal migration. Passing the tendon around the base of the metacarpal and then up the shaft and down through the drill hole produces a pivot point of proximal thumb loading at the outermost metacarpal cortex. This creates an abduction moment on the metacarpal with loading. Harvesting only half of the FCR tendon has afforded us ample tendon to maintain the trapezial space by utilizing the tight roll technique. This technique prevents proximal migration, avoids sacrifice of tendon function, and avoids the need for rigid fixation while yielding painless, stable, functional thumbs.

REFERENCES

1. Burton RI, Pellegrini VD. Surgical management of basal joint arthritis of the thumb. Part II. Ligament reconstruction with tendon interposition arthroplasty. *J Hand Surg [Am]* 1986;11:324–332.
2. Carroll RE. Arthrodesis of the carpometacarpal joint of the thumb. *Clin Orthop* 1987;220:106–110.

3. Eaton RG, Lane LB, Littler JW, et al. Ligament reconstruction for the painful thumb carpometacarpal joint: A long-term assessment. *J Hand Surg [Am]* 1984;9:692–699.
4. Eaton RG, Glickel SZ, Littler JW. Tendon interposition arthroplasty for degenerative arthritis of the trapeziometacarpal joint of the thumb. *J Hand Surg [Am]* 1985;10:645–654.
5. Kleinman WB, Eckenrode JF. Tendon suspension sling arthroplasty for thumb trapeziometacarpal arthritis. *J Hand Surg [Am]* 1991;16:983–991.
6. Creighton JJ, Steichen JB, Strickland JW. Long-term evaluation of silastic trapezial arthroplasty in patients with osteoarthritis. *J Hand Surg [Am]* 1991;16:510–519.
7. Pellegrini VD, Burton RI. Surgical management of basal joint arthritis of the thumb. Part I. Long-term results of silicone implant arthroplasy. *J Hand Surg [Am]* 1986;11:309–324.
8. Swanson AB, deGroot Swanson G. Implant arthroplasty for the thumb basal joint. *Semin Arthroplasty* 1991;2:91–98.
9. Tomaino M, Pellegrini VD, Burton RI. Arthroplasty of the basal joint of the thumb. *J Bone Joint Surg Am* 1995;77:346–355.

52

THE DARRACH PROCEDURE

CHARLES CASSIDY
LEONARD K. RUBY

INDICATIONS

The distal radioulnar joint (DRUJ) may be affected by inflammatory (e.g., rheumatoid), osteoarthritic, and traumatic disorders. Because the indications and contraindications, technical concerns, and expected results following the "Darrach" may differ depending on the underlying diagnosis, rheumatoid and nonrheumatoid patients are considered separately.

The Rheumatoid Wrist

The Darrach is the procedure of choice for the management of most rheumatoid DRUJ problems (1). Therefore, any patient with symptoms referable to the DRUJ who has failed a 3- to 6-month trial of adequate nonoperative management (medications and splinting) may be considered a candidate for distal ulna resection. Preoperative complaints usually include pain, weakness, and loss of forearm rotation (primarily supination). Another important indication for distal ulna resection is rupture of the ulnar-sided digital extensor tendons—the Vaughan-Jackson lesion (2); invariably, the arthritic ulnar head has eroded through the DRUJ capsule, producing attritional tendon rupture (Fig. 52.1). Finally, distal ulna resection is often performed at the time of radiocarpal surgery (e.g., arthrodesis or arthroplasty) because the distal radioulnar disease is usually at least as severe as involvement in the remainder of the wrist.

The Posttraumatic Osteoarthritic Wrist

When the Darrach procedure is considered in the nonrheumatoid setting, patient factors are extremely important. Low-demand, older patients generally fare better than young laborers (<45 years) or those with ligamentous laxity (3). Our most frequent indication is the older woman with persistent ulnar-sided wrist pain and limited forearm rotation following a distal radius fracture. Distal ulna resection simultaneously addresses the ulnar impaction, DRUJ incongruity, and capsular contracture (Fig. 52.2).

CONTRAINDICATIONS

The Rheumatoid Wrist

Careful scrutiny of the preoperative wrist radiographs is imperative. Preexisting ulnocarpal translocation is a contraindication to isolated distal ulna resection (4,5). Similarly, bone loss at the ulnar corner of the radius or accentuated radial inclination may predispose to ulnar translocation if the radiocarpal joint is not stabilized at the time of distal ulna resection (6,7). In such instances, we prefer radiolunate or total wrist arthrodesis combined with the Darrach procedure.

At the other end of the spectrum is the rheumatoid patient with refractory wrist synovitis and normal radiographs. For this infrequent problem, we have performed an arthroscopic radiocarpal and midcarpal synovectomy combined with a mini-open DRUJ synovectomy with preservation of the ulnar head. Early results with this alternative technique are encouraging.

The Posttraumatic Osteoarthritic Wrist

As mentioned previously, failures tend to occur in younger, high-demand patients. However, the results of any distal ulna procedure are less satisfactory in this population. Consequently, whenever feasible, we prefer corrective radial osteotomy or ulnar shortening rather than the Darrach for the younger patient. In the malunited distal radius, factors

---

C. Cassidy and L. K. Ruby: Department of Orthopaedics, Tufts University School of Medicine and New England Medical Center, Boston, Massachusetts 02111.

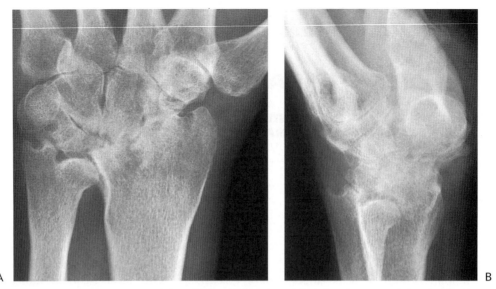

FIGURE 52.1. Posteroanterior (**A**) and lateral (**B**) radiographs of a rheumatoid distal radioulnar joint. The ulnar head is misshapen and prominent dorsally. Erosions present at the ulnar styloid and sigmoid fossa (the "scallop sign") (4) are worrisome for impending extensor tendon rupture. Advanced radiocarpal arthritis is present as well.

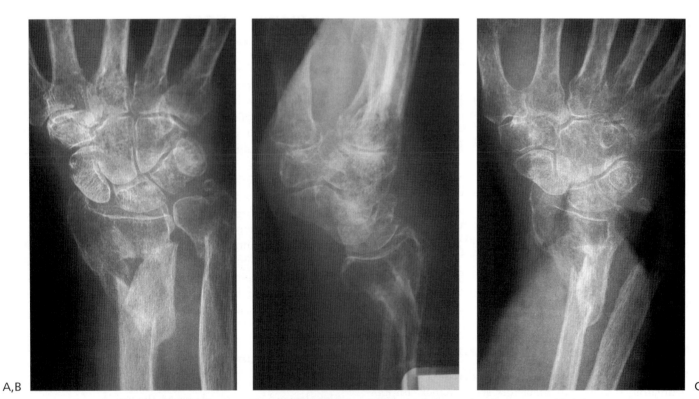

FIGURE 52.2. Posteroanterior (PA) (**A**) and lateral (**B**) wrist radiographs of a 72-year-old right-handed woman who had sustained a severely comminuted extraarticular distal radius fracture 4 months earlier. She complained of ulnar-sided wrist pain and limited forearm rotation (pronation 70°; supination –20°). Given her age, the complex deformity, and her primary complaints, Darrach resection was selected as a simple solution to a difficult problem. **C:** Intraoperative PA radiograph following distal ulna resection. Note the ulna resection level at the proximal margin of the sigmoid fossa and the contoured edge of the ulnar remnant.

in addition to the radius–ulna relationship must be considered. Significant dorsal tilt or radiocarpal articular incongruity requires radial osteotomy. In these instances, the decision whether to perform a Darrach would be based on an intraoperative assessment of the DRUJ following correction of the radius.

Distal radioulnar instability is a contraindication to distal ulna resection; such patients will be no happier with an unstable ulnar stump. Similarly, the surgeon must exercise caution in treating the ligamentously lax patient (3). Finally, although postoperative ulnar translocation is uncommon in the nonrheumatoid patient, DiBenedetto et al. (7) reported a 22% incidence of this complication. In each of the four cases, the radial inclination was more than 23°. We have yet to see this problem in our nonrheumatoid patients.

SURGICAL CONSIDERATIONS AND PITFALLS

Over 200 years of experience with distal ulna resection have led to the following conclusions: poor outcomes are almost invariably related to either improper patient selection (too young or lax), improper resection (too much), or inadequate soft tissue stabilization (too little). Ulnar stump instability resulting from excessive ulna resection is notoriously difficult to treat. We agree with Dingman (8) and others (9–12) that the best results are obtained when a minimal resection of the distal ulna is performed; the osteotomy should be made at the metaphyseal flare. To minimize radioulnar impingement and abrasion of the extensor tendons, the stump should be contoured throughout the full arc of forearm rotation.

Soft tissue reconstruction must address three issues: carpal supination, distal ulnar shaft stabilization, and extensor carpi ulnaris (ECU) stabilization (12). These considerations are especially relavent in the management of the rheumatoid wrist. Some thought to stabilization is essential before the incision is made. An incision directly through the fifth extensor compartment may not provide adequate retinaculum to reinforce the capsule.

TECHNIQUE

The Skin Incision

In many instances, especially in the rheumatoid patient, concomitant procedures will dictate the specific skin incision selected. If surgery is limited to the DRUJ, we use a longitudinal incision over the subcutaneous border of the ulna. When performing simultaneous radiocarpal and DRUJ procedures, we prefer a straight dorsal incision extending obliquely from the base of the index carpometacarpal joint to the DRUJ, modified as necessary. The skin and subcutaneous tissues are elevated as full-thickness flaps at the level of the extensor retinaculum to minimize the possibility of skin slough. Longitudinally oriented veins are preserved when possible.

The Retinacular and Capsular Incision

Several options are available for incising the retinaculum. Keep in mind that the retinaculum may be used to stabilize the ulnar stump, the ECU, or both. For the posttraumatic, stiff DRUJ, a medial-based flap of extensor retinaculum will often suffice to reinforce the capsule. Consequently, in such instances, we fashion rectangular proximal-ulnar and distal-radial retinacular flaps extending from the midfourth to the midsixth compartments.

When extensor tenolysis and/or radiocarpal surgery is necesssary in the rheumatoid patient, the fourth compartment is entered, either through a longitudinal midline incision or through extended rectangular flaps (Fig. 52.3). The medial-based flap is then elevated, dividing the septa between the fourth–fifth and fifth–sixth compartments.

A longitudinal DRUJ capsulotomy is made through the floor of the fifth compartment, stopping proximal to the triangular fibrocartilage complex (TFCC) in order to preserve the important dorsal radioulnar ligament. The floor of the retinaculum and DRUJ capsule are elevated as a single layer. Subperiosteal dissection is carried around the distal ulna for 2 to 3 cm, and Bennett retractors are placed (Fig. 52.4). In the rheumatoid patient, a separate transverse capsulotomy is made distal to the TFCC to permit access to the radiocarpal joint for synovectomy.

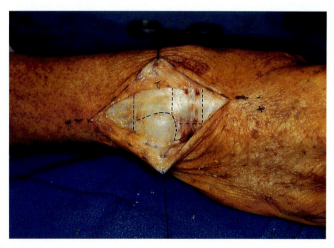

FIGURE 52.3. Proposed retinacular flaps. The ulnar-based proximal flap will be used to reinforce the capsular closure following distal ulna excision. The distal limb may be left intact to prevent bowstringing if extensor tendon surgery is not planned.

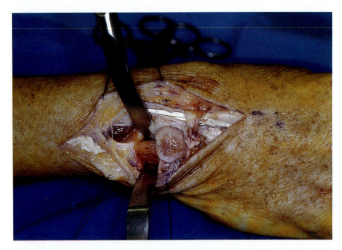

FIGURE 52.4. Subperiosteal dissection is carried proximally along the ulna for 2 to 3 cm. Care is taken to preserve the extensor carpi ulnaris sheath. Bennett retractors are placed on either side of the ulna in preparation for ostectomy.

Ulnar Head Resection

This step is the same for both rheumatoid and nonrheumatoid patients. An oscillating saw is used to perform an oblique osteotomy at the metaphyseal level of the distal ulna, with the bevel of the osteotomy oriented radially and dorsally. The ulnar head is grasped with a towel clip and is excised subperiosteally. Rather than preserve the ulnar styloid, we prefer to release the TFCC from its ulnar attachment. Care is taken to preserve the ECU subsheath and TFCC remnants (Fig. 52.5).

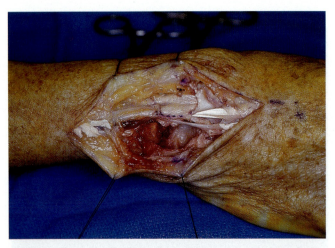

FIGURE 52.5. The ulnar head has been removed at the metaphyseal flare. The ulnar stump is then beveled along its dorsal, radial, and volar margins to eliminate any irregularities. The radius–ulna relationship is then inspected throughout the full arc of forearm rotation, and further beveling is performed as necessary.

Once the ulnar head has been removed, the ulnar stump is evaluated throughout the full arc of forearm rotation. A rongeur is used to fashion a conical shape along the radial, volar, and dorsal margins of the distal ulna. This maneuver minimizes radioulnar impingement during full pronation and supination.

Soft Tissue Reconstruction

A variety of static and dynamic slings and tethers have been described. The primary goals of these procedures are to eliminate radioulnar impingement and dorsal ulnar stump subluxation. However, in the rheumatoid patient, carpal supination and ECU subluxation must also be addressed to minimize the likelihood of progressive radiocarpal deformity. The underlying disease, the preoperative examination, and intraoperative findings will dictate which method(s) are selected. The essential factors—correction of carpal supination and stabilization of the distal ulnar shaft and ECU tendon—are discussed separately; in reality, however, they are addressed simultaneously at the time of surgery. In general, the simpler forms of stabilization are reserved for the posttraumatic group.

Carpal Supination

Several options are available to correct carpal supination. When the TFCC is present, simply suturing it tightly to the dorsoulnar corner of the radius may suffice (13). If carpal supination is extreme, we prefer the method of Blatt and Ashworth (14), suturing a distally based flap of volar capsule to the dorsal ulnar stump through drill holes.

Distal Ulnar Shaft Stabilization

For the posttraumatic patient, tight closure of the capsule with plication of the ulnar limb of retinaculum is usually sufficient. We prefer to drape the retinaculum over the ulnar stump and suture it to the volar capsule; this provides a radioulnar cushion. The radial edge of capsule is then secured to the base of the ulnar limb of the retinaculum. The radial flap of retinaculum is either approximated anatomically or looped around the ECU (see below). The radioulnar relationship is then assessed. If significant crepitation is noted, the repair is taken down, and the ulnar stump and sigmoid fossa are inspected for surface irregularities. If crepitation persists, another form of ulnar stump stabilization is selected.

A similar method of stabilizing the ulnar shaft may be used in the rheumatoid patient (Figs. 52.6 and 52.7). However, in these patients, simple plication is often inadequate. We have had experience with two other forms of stabilization: ECU tenodesis (15,16) and pronator quadratus (PQ) interposition transfer (17). Both appear to provide excellent short-term stability. Concerns regarding the durability of ECU tenodesis in nonrheumatoid patients had led one of us

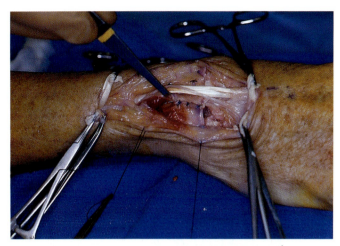

FIGURE 52.6. Following closure of the deep retinaculum and capsule, the proximal retinaculum is placed under the extensor tendons to reinforce the capsular closure. The extensor carpi ulnaris tendon is relocated.

(L.K.R.) to develop the PQ transfer. However, ECU tenodesis remains the most popular form of ulnar shaft stabilization and is our preference in most situations.

As described by O'Donovan and Ruby (15) and Leslie et al. (16), one half of the ECU tendon, harvested as a distally based slip, is passed through a drill hole in the dorsal cortex of the ulna. The tendon is then brought out through the medullary canal and is woven to itself under tension with the forearm held in supination and ulnar deviation.

The PQ interposition transfer offers the advantage of providing a muscle cushion between the radius and ulna. Undoubtedly, this muscle does atrophy with time. The PQ is harvested by elevating it along with adjacent periosteum from its ulnar attachment (Fig. 52.8). The muscle flap is then rerouted through the interosseous space and is sutured to the dorsoradial aspect of the ECU tendon sheath. The ulnar stump is manually depressed while the sutures are tied.

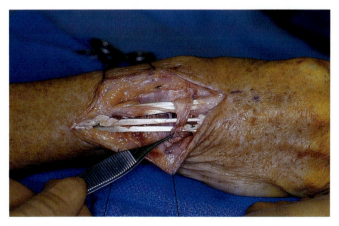

FIGURE 52.7. After completion of the extensor tendon reconstruction, the distal limb of extensor retinaculum is reapproximated anatomically to prevent bowstringing.

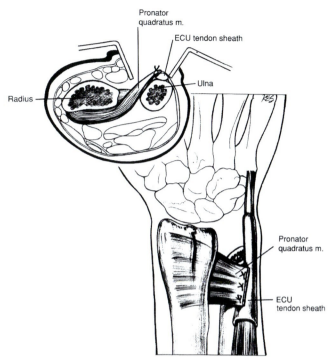

FIGURE 52.8. Pronator quadratus (PQ) interposition transfer, as viewed from the dorsum of the wrist. A tendon–periosteal flap is fashioned, and the PQ is passed through the interosseous space. The extensor carpi ulnaris tendon and sheath are mobilized dorsally, and the rerouted PQ is sutured to the dorsoradial edge of the extensor carpi ulnaris sheath while the ulnar stump is maintained in a reduced postion. (From Ruby LK, Ferenz CC, Dell PC. The PQ interposition transfer: an adjunct to resection arthroplasty of the distal radioulnar joint. *J Hand Surg [Am]* 1996;21:60–65, with permission.)

Extensor Carpi Ulnaris Stabilization

For the posttraumatic wrist, ECU subluxation may not be an issue. In such instances, anatomic retinacular closure may be adequate. However, if dorsal ulnar subluxation is evident preoperatively, we recommend some form of ECU stabilization. This may simply entail fabrication of a pulley. The radial-based distal retinacular flap may be looped around the ECU and sutured to itself. Our preference is to split the ulnar-based limb of retinaculum transversely to the edge of the fifth compartment (12) (Fig. 52.9); at the conclusion of the procedure, the distal flap is passed deep to the ECU to reinforce the capsule and provide a gliding surface. The intact ulnar edge of retinaculum acts as a pulley, maintaining the ECU in a dorsal position.

For the rheumatoid patient with correctable radial wrist deviation and an acceptable wrist joint, we prefer extensor carpi radialis longus (ECRL) transfer to the ECU (18). This transfer serves two purposes: it augments ECU function in the corrected position, and eliminates a deforming force (the ECRL). The reader is referred to the paper by Clayton and Ferlic (18) for details of the procedure.

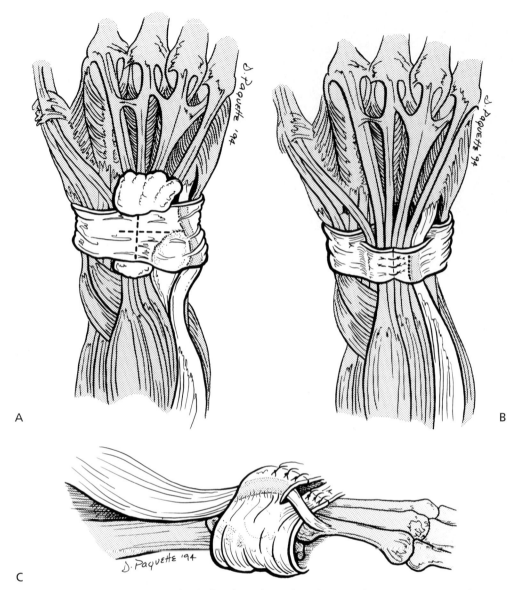

FIGURE 52.9. Extensor carpi ulnaris (ECU) tendon relocation. **A:** The extensor retinaculum is opened over the fourth compartment, and the medial flap is split transversely to the septum between the fifth and sixth compartments (*dotted lines*). **B:** Following distal ulna resection, the distal half of the retinaculum is sutured deep to the extensor tendons to augment the capsular repair and provide a smooth tendon gliding surface. **C:** The intact medial edge of the retinaculum acts as a pulley, maintaining the ECU in a dorsal position. (From Cassidy C, Ruby LK. Tendon dysfunction in systemic arthritis. In: Peimer C, ed. *Surgery of the hand and upper extremity.* New York: McGraw-Hill, 1996;1645–1676, with permission.)

POSTOPERATIVE MANAGEMENT

Following routine closure, a plaster sugar-tongs splint is applied with the forearm in 45° of supination and the wrist in neutral position. If tendon surgery has been performed, a thermoplast sugar-tongs splint with appropriate outriggers is fabricated several days postoperatively. The sutures are removed on postoperative day 10 to 12. Full-time splint wear is continued for a total of 3 weeks postoperatively; if the PQ transfer has been included, immobilization is continued for an additional week. Supervised therapy is then initiated, concentrating on forearm rotation and wrist motion. A wrist splint is worn when out of doors for an additional 2 weeks. Unlimited activity is encouraged at 6 weeks following surgery.

COMPLICATIONS

As emphasized earlier, appropriate indications and technique will minimize the likelihood of complications.

Ulnar Stump Instability

During their rehabilitation, many patients will note an intermittent clicking sensation with forearm rotation. This disturbing phenomenon is usually self-limited and disappears within several months (13).

Persistent complaints of instability are usually related to excessive resection. The tendency to shorten the ulna further must be resisted. In these difficult cases, we recommend exhausting nonoperative measures before reoperating. Our surgical preference is to bevel the existing ulnar stump and to perform a PQ transfer, possibly augmented by ECU tenodesis. One bone forearm can be considered in recalcitrant cases.

Extensor Tendon Rupture

This uncommon complication may be prevented by ensuring that the ulna resection is contoured along its dorsal aspect throughout the arc of forearm rotation. In the management of tendon ruptures, a segment of the tendon harvested for grafting may be used to reinforce the dorsal capsule.

Ulnar Translocation

As noted earlier in this chapter, radiographic signs of preexisting or impending ulnar translocation are contraindications to isolated distal ulna resection. However, longitudinal studies of post-Darrach rheumatoid patients demonstrate an incidence of ulnar translocation even if none was evident preoperatively. This problem appears to be related more to the natural history of the rheumatoid process than to the procedure itself. We find it difficult to explain how ulnar translocation could result from distal ulna resection in the nonrheumatoid patient in the absence of significant ligamentous injury. In any event, if translocation is evident preoperatively, the radiocarpal joint should be stabilized by limited or total wrist arthrodesis at the time of the Darrach procedure. Similarly, these salvage procedures are the only recourse when symptomatic translocation is evident postoperatively.

Loss of Grip Strength

We agree with Bowers (19) that reports of weakness following the Darrach procedure appear to be unsubstantiated. Our patients generally have an improvement in grip strength postoperatively that parallels their pain relief.

SUMMARY

Despite its many modifications, the Darrach procedure remains a valuable technique in the management of many difficult DRUJ disorders. An appropriate understanding of the patient, the underlying disease, and the technique will ensure that the vast majority of patients (and surgeons) are satisfied with the results.

EDITORS' COMMENTS

One must deal with two problems in considering resection of the distal ulna. The first is impingement against the radius; the second is winging or hypermobility of the distal ulna. They are obviously related. Following William Darrach's thinking through his publications, he began with a large resection, which resulted in radial impingement and winging. He then came to the conclusion that ¾ in. or less of distal ulna is the proper resection level. His last publication suggests a tepee-like closure of the periosteum with the apex of the tepee distally in hopes that some periosteum will fill in to this shape and provide connections distally. Taking this thinking a step further, the logical conclusion is to leave the bone shaped in this tepee fashion or pointed at its distal end with a shape that then parallels the radius through full supination to full pronation which tends to solve the impingement problem. The ulna length at the level of the articular surface of the radius allows attachment to the ulnar sling mechanism, preventing the winging component. Our experience with this type of distal ulnar resection dates back over 30 years. If there is any adequate cartilage in the sulcus of the radius and on the distal ulna, then a step-cut shortening of the ulna is much preferred to any resection procedure.

In degenerative arthritis of the DRUJ, the destruction is primarily on the ulnar side initially and begins proximally, progressing distally. We have successfully used a modified arthroplasty of the distal ulna, resecting the abnormal cartilageless bone on the proximal half of the ulnar head but leaving a full circumference of good cartilage distally. This often requires some resection of the proximal sulcus on the radius as well. This modified arthroplasty technique has been successful in a limited number of cases. It has not been published. One patient has returned 6 years postoperatively requesting similar surgery on early degenerative arthritis in his opposite DRUJ. No wrists with this modified arthroplasty technique of the distal ulna have, as yet, come to matched ulnar arthroplasty or another Darrach-like procedure.

Rheumatoid arthritis is not a contraindication for resection of the distal ulna when there is ulnar translation of the carpals. The answer here is the rheumatoid wrist reconstruction procedure placing the carpals back in a concavity on the distal radius and carrying out a simultaneous matched ulnar arthroplasty. The ulna head can be fused to the radius with a proximal osteotomy to restore rotation (Sauvé-Kapandji). This wrist will have symptoms with impingement of the proximal ulna shaft against the radius and symptomatic winging and is, in our view, contraindicated.

REFERENCES

1. Darrach W. Anterior dislocation of the ulna. *Ann Surg* 1912;56: 802–803.
2. Vaughan-Jackson OJ. Rupture of extensor tendons by attrition at the inferior radioulnar joint. Report of two cases. *J Bone Joint Surg Br* 1978;30:528–530.
3. Bieber EJ, Linscheid RL, Dobyns JH, et al. Failed distal ulna resections. *J Hand Surg [Am]* 1988;13:193–200.
4. Swanson AB. *Flexible implant resection arthroplasty in the hand and extremities.* St Louis: CV Mosby, 1973.
5. Taleisnik J. The Sauvé-Kapandji procedure. *Clin Orthop* 1992; 275:110–123.
6. Black RM, Boswick JA Jr, Wiedel J. Dislocation of the wrist in rheumatoid arthritis: the relationship to distal ulnar resection. *Clin Orthop* 1977;124:184–188.
7. DiBenedetto MR, Lubbers LM, Coleman CR. Long-term results of the minimal resection Darrach procedure. *J Hand Surg [Am]* 1991;16:445–450.
8. Dingman PVC. Resection of the distal end of the ulna (Darrach operation): An end-result study of 24 cases. *J Bone Joint Surg Am* 1952;34:893–900.
9. Flatt AE. *The care of the arthritic hand, 5th ed.* St Louis: Quality Medical Publishing, 1995.
10. Taleisnik J. *The wrist.* New York: Churchill Livingstone, 1985; 387–435.
11. Tulipan DJ, Eaton RG, Eberhart RE. The Darrach procedure defended: Technique redefined and long-term follow-up. *J Hand Surg [Am]* 1991;16:438–444.
12. Blank JE, Cassidy C. The distal radioulnar joint in rheumatoid arthritis. *Hand Clin* 1996;12:499–513.
13. Feldon P, Millender L, Nalebuff EA. Rheumatoid arthritis in the hand and wrist In: Green DP, ed. *Operative hand surgery.* New York: Churchill Livingstone, 1993;1623–1644.
14. Blatt G, Ashworth CR. Volar capsule transfer for stabilization following resection of the distal end of the ulna. *Orthop Trans* 1979; 3:13.
15. O'Donovan TM, Ruby LK. The distal radioulnar joint in rheumatoid arthritis. *Hand Clin* 1989;5:249–256.
16. Leslie BM, Carlson G, Ruby LK. Results of extensor carpi ulnaris tenodesis in the rheumatoid wrist undergoing a distal ulnar excision. *J Hand Surg [Am]* 1990;15:547–551.
17. Ruby LK, Ferenz CC, Dell PC. The pronator quadratus interposition transfer: an adjunct to resection arthroplasty of the distal radioulnar joint. *J Hand Surg [Am]* 1996;21:60–65.
18. Clayton ML, Ferlic DC. Tendon transfer for radial rotation of the wrist in rheumatoid arthritis. *Clin Orthop* 1974;100: 176–185.
19. Bowers WH. The distal radioulnar joint. In: Green DP, ed. *Operative hand surgery, 3rd ed.* New York: Churchill Livingstone, 1993;973–1019.
20. Freiberg RA, Weinstein A. The scallop sign and spontaneous rupture of finger extensor tendons in rheumatoid arthritis. *Clin Orthop* 1972;83:128–130.

DISTAL RADIOULNAR JOINT DISLOCATION STABILIZATION

H. KIRK WATSON
JEFFREY WEINZWEIG

"The ulna needs the wrist, but the wrist does not need the ulna."
—H. K. Watson

THEORY

Phylogenetically, the ulna is one of the component bones of the upper extremity, integral to the elbow and weight bearing in more primitive forms. In man, the wrist has left the ulna behind for increased mobility and in no way requires the ulna for its component function, including load-bearing. The distal end of the ulna, on the other hand, is basically free and unneeded but must be stabilized and maintained against its partner, the radius.

Palmer and coworkers have demonstrated that the distal end of the ulna receives 20% of the in-line load (1,2). However, this is more happenstance than functional component in that there is pressure on the end of the ulna because it is physically there; in some individuals ulnar length makes it available for loading. Several clear features substantiate the fact that this load is incidental and an unnecessary component of wrist function. In full pronation, the distal end of the ulna is almost uncovered (feel it!). In-line loads applied in this position easily circumvent the small segment of the ulna that may make carpal contact. The ulna in some individuals is significantly short of any ability to take load from the carpals except very light loads as transmitted through a very thickened triangular fibrocartilage (TFC). In addition, the intercarpal joints on the ulnar side of the wrist are much too sloped to take an in-line load. In-line load bearing would require joint surfaces lying perpendicular to the load.

H. K. Watson: Connecticut Combined Hand Surgery Fellowship, Hartford Hospital, and Connecticut Children's Medical Center, Hartford, Connecticut 06106; Department of Orthopaedics, University of Connecticut School of Medicine, Farmington, Connecticut 06032; Department of Orthopedics, Rehabilitation, and Plastic Surgery, Yale University School of Medicine, New Haven, Connecticut 06520.

J. Weinzweig: Department of Plastic Surgery, Brown University School of Medicine, Rhode Island Hospital, and Hasbro Children's Hospital, Providence, Rhode Island 02905.

The hamate–triquetral joint, for example, is too sloped for any significant load transference to the ulna.

Finally, there is a load shift phenomenon: if one were to replace the lunate with a silicone lunate and load the carpals on the radius, the initial very light loads would demonstrate nearly equal pressures on the scaphoid and silicone lunate. As the loads increase, the lunate collapses, and the load percentage will shift toward the scaphoid. When maximal loads are applied, the ultimate percentage of load transfer will be 100% through the scaphoid; because the lunate is still collapsible, at that point, 0% of the load will be transferred through it. The thickness of the TFC is a manifestation of filling the available space, not a design to transfer load to the ulna.

INDICATIONS

It is well documented that the wrist maintains normal function following matched ulnar arthroplasties (3,4) or Darrach procedures (5,6) in which the distal ulna is completely removed. These considerations confirm the fact that procedures maintaining the distal end of the ulna are not indicated because the ulna does not play a significant role in the stability or load transference of the wrist. The only time the presence of the ulna demonstrates any effect is in severe rheumatoid arthritis, where the ulnar-translocating wrist will "fetch up" on the ulna. This, of course, is no longer a "wrist" but, rather, dislocating carpal bones piling up on the ulna. Even here, the procedure of choice is recentralization of the carpals on the radius, not the maintenance of the ulnar head. Fusion of the ulnar head to the radius with osteotomy of the ulna (the Sauvé-Kapandji procedure) sets free the shaft of the ulna at a very unacceptable length. Winging is always present, and impingement on the radius almost always occurs. With each succeeding paper, Darrach demonstrated the necessity for maintaining the length of the ulna in order to address the two problems of winging and radial impingement.

A dislocated distal ulna with good cartilage is best treated by repair.

SURGICAL TECHNIQUE

Triangular Fibrocartilage Repair into the Distal Ulna

A longitudinal incision is preferable, as there is a reasonable potential here for matched ulnar arthroplasty in the future, particularly if the dislocating ulna has been present for any significant period of time. With the elbow flexed and the forearm in neutral rotation, a 6- to 8-cm incision is marked out longitudinally over the distal ulna extending a centimeter or so beyond the distal ulna. This incision is not marked out with the elbow extended and the forearm in pronation on the operating table because this will produce an oblique longitudinal incision. The operation is carried out with the surgeon seated in the axilla, the arm abducted at the shoulder, the elbow extended, and the forearm pronated (Fig. 53.1).

Following incision, a blunt spreading technique is utilized to identify the dorsal branch of the ulnar nerve. Dissection is carried deep between the extensor carpi ulnaris and the extensor digiti quinti minimi. The proximal portion of the extensor retinaculum is incised between these two tendons, and dissection is carried deep into the wrist joint distal to the TFC. The two main TFC ligaments—the dorsal and volar radioulnar ligaments—are identified. Their ulnarmost aspect is prepared for reinsertion into the distal ulna. A small hole is drilled in the distal ulna at the base of the ulnar styloid in the center of the rotational axis of the ulna. This hole aligns with the center of the shaft of the distal ulna and is equally distant from the entire articular cartilage of the ulna. This then will not create a cam effect on supination–pronation. The hole is enlarged (4–5 mm) to accept the ulnarmost aspect of the two ligaments. An 0 vicryl or similar suture is placed in the ulnar aspect of the two ligaments utilizing a Bunnell single-X or double-X suture technique. Two 1- to 2-mm drill holes are placed in the ulnarmost aspect of the ulnar cortex, approximately 2 cm proximal to the distal ulnar articular surface. The drill holes should be at least ½ cm apart and at the same level. The two suture ends are passed down the shaft of the ulna and out through each of the two drill holes. The ulnar portion of the TFC is then drawn into the drill hole in the distal ulna. The suture ends are tied securely over the cortex on the ulnar aspect of the ulnar shaft. This is accomplished with the wrist in neutral position. A fairly heavy Steinman pin is then used to transfix the radius and ulna (Fig. 53.2). Based on the size of the individual, a 2- to 3-mm–diameter pin will suffice, and this will maintain distal radioulnar joint

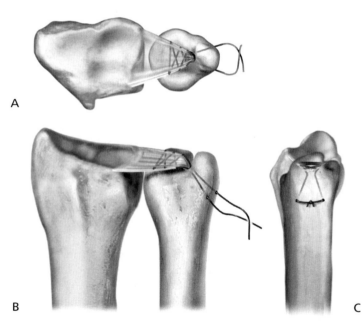

FIGURE 53.1. A–C: This distal radioulnar joint has adequate cartilage and is dislocated or significantly hypermobile, so that restabilization of the ulna to the radius is indicated. The dorsal and volar radius–ulnar ligaments typically tear out from their insertion on the ulna. A drill hole is placed in the pivot point of the distal ulna, meaning at the center of rotation when seen from distally. The Bunnell-type suture can be placed in the ulnarmost aspect of the dorsal and volar radial ulnar ligaments. A large 0 vicryl or 0 prolene suture is used to secure the ligaments into the defect in the end of the ulna. The suture ends are passed out through two small cortical holes on the ulnar aspect of the ulna and tied over that cortex. The distal radius and ulna are cross-pinned to each other for 8 weeks of immobilization. The pin may be removed in 6 weeks.

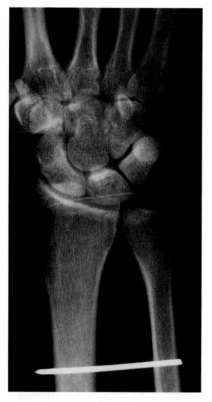

FIGURE 53.2. The suture is in place, seating the volar and dorsal radioulnar ligaments into the hole drilled in the pivot point on the end of the ulna, and tied over the ulna's lateral cortex. The radius and ulna have been cross-pinned with a large Steinmann pin left in place for 6 weeks.

DISTAL RADIUS BONE GRAFT HARVEST

JEFFREY WEINZWEIG
H. KIRK WATSON

INDICATIONS

A myriad of procedures, such as intercarpal arthrodeses, radiolunate arthrodesis, small joint arthrodesis, grafting following enchondroma curettage, and treatment of scaphoid nonunion, necessitate the use of cancellous bone graft (1–4). The distal radius is a sufficient source of cancellous graft within the same operative field.

CONTRAINDICATIONS

There are very few contraindications to harvesting cancellous bone graft from the distal radius. In the extremely elderly patient, particularly with multiple medical problems including osteoporosis, distal radius harvest may increase the risk of fracture; in such patients, fracture healing would likely also be problematic. The volume of cancellous bone harvested may be small (3 cc average), but is usually sufficient. In cases in which a moderate quantity of graft is required, reharvesting from a previously harvested distal radius can be accomplished. Nonetheless, in such cases, harvest from the contralateral distal radius is a reasonable option. Bone graft harvest in the child should be done with care to avoid injury to the epiphyseal plate. In some children, the iliac crest may be a more suitable donor site.

J. Weinzweig: Department of Plastic Surgery, Brown University School of Medicine, Rhode Island Hospital, and Hasbro Children's Hospital, Providence, Rhode Island 02905.

H. K. Watson: Connecticut Combined Hand Surgery Fellowship, Hartford Hospital, and Connecticut Children's Medical Center, Hartford, Connecticut 06106; Department of Orthopaedics, University of Connecticut School of Medicine, Farmington, Connecticut 06032; Department of Orthopedics, Rehabilitation, and Plastic Surgery, Yale University School of Medicine, New Haven, Connecticut 06520.

SURGICAL TECHNIQUE

A 3-cm transverse incision is made approximately 3 cm proximal to the radial styloid, extending from the site of Lister's tubercle dorsally to just volar to the first dorsal compartment. Spreading dissection is used to expose a flat periosteal surface between the first and second extensor compartments, which is identified by a constant periosteal artery running longitudinally in this region (5,6). Care is taken to identify and preserve the superficial branch of the radial nerve. The periosteum is incised longitudinally along this small, dispensable artery and elevated to permit removal of a teardrop-shaped cortical window approximately 2 cm long and 1.5 cm wide with a narrow, straight osteotome. The teardrop shape ensures a single stress riser aimed proximally down the long axis of the radius. The cortical window is harvested beginning distally on the radial tuberosity. Adequate cancellous bone graft is harvested with an 8-mm curette, and the cortical window is replaced. The cortical window is securely held in place by simply repositioning the overlying periosteum and extensor tendons (Fig. 54.1).

CLINICAL SERIES

Over the last 30 years, the senior author (H.K.W.) has harvested more than 1,400 bone grafts from the distal radius. This includes 906 grafts performed for triscaphe arthrodesis, 331 for scapholunate advanced collapse (SLAC) wrist reconstruction, 33 for lunotriquetral arthrodesis, and 160 for additional procedures including radiolunate arthrodesis, bony tumor excision and grafting, and management of scaphoid nonunion (Fig. 54.2).

COMPLICATIONS

Harvest of a bone graft from the distal radius has been associated with an undisplaced distal radius fracture on only

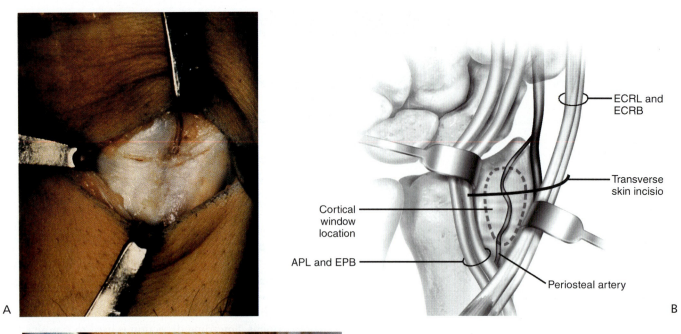
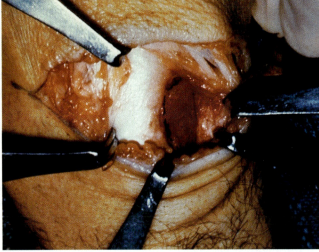

FIGURE 54.1. The first and second dorsal compartment tendons are retracted to expose the distal radius surface. A constant small periosteal artery is used as a landmark for the periosteal incision **(A,B)**. A teardrop-shaped cortical window is then removed. Cancellous bone is harvested with a curette, and the cortical window is usually replaced **(C)**.

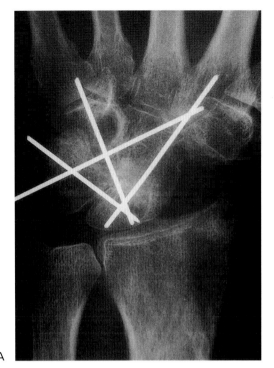 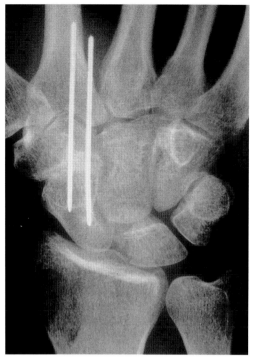

FIGURE 54.2. Limited wrist arthrodesis. The amount of bone graft needed for scapholunate advanced collapse (SLAC) wrist reconstruction **(A)**, triscaphe fusion **(B)**, or other limited wrist arthrodeses is approximately the same. There is greater grafting surface in a SLAC wrist, but some proximal migration of the capitate–hamate unit against the triquetrum–lunate unit is allowable, thus decreasing the total amount of free bone graft needed. In both examples shown, note the distal radius lucency where bone graft has been harvested.

two occasions (0.14%). In one case, this was caused by the patient falling downstairs shortly after removal of the cast. In the second case, the radius was fractured during surgery. Complications such as injury to the superficial branch of the radial nerve, infection, and hematoma have not occurred as a result of graft harvest. Twenty-four patients (1.7%) required release of the first dorsal compartment for de Quervain's disease within 5 years of bone graft surgery; this may or may not be related to the graft harvest.

DISCUSSION

The distal radius provides an ample supply of cancellous bone in the same operative field and with minimal morbidity.

REFERENCES

1. Andrews J, Miller G, Haddad R. Treatment of scaphoid nonunion by volar inlay distal radius bone graft. *J Hand Surg [Br]* 1985; 10:214–216.
2. Mirly HL, Manske PR, Szerzinski JM. Distal anterior radius bone graft in surgery of the hand and wrist. *J Hand Surg [Am]* 1995;20: 623–627.
3. Watson HK, Weinzweig J, Guidera P, et al. One thousand intercarpal arthrodeses. *J Hand Surg [Br]* 1999;24:320–330.
4. Weiss AP, Hastings H 2nd. Wrist arthrodesis for traumatic conditions: a study of plate and local bone graft application. *J Hand Surg [Am]* 1995;20:50–56.
5. McGrath MH, Watson HK. Late results with local bone graft donor sites in hand surgery. *J Hand Surg [Am]* 1981;6:234–237.
6. Watson HK, Weinzweig J. Intercarpal arthrodesis. In: Green DP, Hotchkiss RN, Pederson WC, eds. *Operative hand surgery,* 4th ed. New York: Churchill Livingstone, 1999;108–130.

55

DORSAL CAPSULODESIS FOR ROTARY SUBLUXATION OF THE SCAPHOID

GERALD BLATT

INDICATIONS

The original and primary indication for dorsal capsulodesis is a true dynamic rotary subluxation of the scaphoid (RSS) (1). RSS is a progression of the injury that created the scapholunate dissociation (2). Because radiographically evident scapholunate dissociation is a necessary and pathognomonic precursor, reduction and stabilization of the scaphoid eliminates this separation of the proximal pole from the lunate (3,4). The most obvious and presenting clinical entity is a loud click or snap emanating from the wrist on active flexion and extension. Often described as a "clunk," it may more easily be elicited by a clenched fist (carpal compression) during active range of motion. Passive or active anatomic reduction of the scaphoid remains the most important prerequisite.

Additional indications for choosing a dorsal capsulodesis to correct and control this instability are the desire and specific need to retain greater postoperative wrist range of motion than is often afforded by an intercarpal fusion (5–10). The procedure is of added benefit in the patient who demonstrates no evidence of articular injury, that is, no preoperative appearance of radioscaphoid or scaphotrapeziotrapezoid (STT) arthritis. Of particular significance is the avoidance of joint fusion in the young, growing patient with still open and active epiphyses.

CONTRAINDICATIONS

The clearest contradiction for dorsal capsulodesis is the converse of many of the presented indications. Thus, in a patient with a longstanding dissociation and a fixed RSS that does not reduce, a dynamic proximal check-rein mechanism is not beneficial. This patient has a static instability with a flexed vertical scaphoid and a dorsiflexion intercalated segment instability (DISI) deformity secondary to capsular contracture. In the absence of any articular degeneration, some have reported successful use of the dorsal capsulodesis following restoration of anatomic carpal alignment after extensive capsulotomies. I cannot offer this as a general recommendation.

An important indication would be the presence of posttraumatic or degenerative arthrosis. A procedure to restore active motion to a compromised radiocarpal or intercarpal joint may produce less than the desired clinical response.

PREOPERATIVE PLANNING

Patients present most commonly with persistent pain about the radial aspect of the wrist several weeks to months following injury. This may have been with a sudden torsional or twisting injury to the wrist or, more likely, a fall on the outstretched hand forcing the wrist into acute radial deviation. The most dramatic and significant finding is the presence of a click or snap on active motion. This disabling "clunk" is both visible and highly audible. Confirmation of probable periscaphoid ligamentous injury is obtained by the Watson test (11). The examiner's thumb is placed over the palmar tubercle of the distal pole of the scaphoid. The patient's wrist is passively brought into extension and ulnar deviation. This allows the scaphoid to assume its more vertical and longitudinal axis. With palmar pressure maintained on the distal pole of the scaphoid, the wrist is brought into flexion and radial deviation as the scaphoid fossa is compressed. Preventing the normal arc of scaphoid flexion forces the proximal pole of the scaphoid against the distal articular surface of the radius and against the lunate. Pain or a click over the middorsum of the wrist reinforces the probability of ligamentous injury.

The three standard views of the wrist—posteroanterior (PA), oblique, and lateral—may not demonstrate any pathologic changes. However, a supination anteroposterior (AP) view of the wrist, with and without carpal compression (by clenched fist), may demonstrate the gap between the scaphoid and lunate, confirming dissociation. This has been well reported as the Terry Thomas sign (Fig. 55.1).

Also noted on these views is the ring sign (12). This represents the cortical ring of the cylindrical scaphoid as seen

---

G. Blatt: Department of Orthopaedic Surgery, University of California, Los Angeles, Los Angeles, California 90024; and Department of Hand Surgery, Harbor–UCLA Medical Center, Torrance, California 90509.

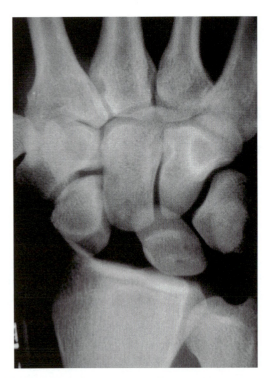

FIGURE 55.1. The classic radiograph appearance of scapholunate dissociation and rotary subluxation of the scaphoid. Note the ring and Terry Thomas signs.

in a foreshortened projection because of the flexed or vertical alignment of the scaphoid.

Dobyns et al. (13) have described the significance of the scapholunate angle. Measured from a true lateral projection, a scapholunate angle greater than 70° strongly suggests a malalignment or instability.

I have used the AP projection to measure the distance from the ring sign to the proximal cortical surface of the scaphoid. As the scaphoid rotates and becomes more flexed and vertical, this ring moves closer to the proximal pole.

The normal measurement is approximately 12 mm; in the injured or pathologic wrist, this distance is reduced by at least 4 mm.

I have found the most valuable diagnostic study to be the cineradiograph. This moving picture sequence can best demonstrate the dynamic instability of the rotary subluxation as well as the anatomic reduction.

There has also been early and interesting success with the use of a special magnetic resonance imaging (MRI) study. They have been done with a dedicated wrist coil using T2-weighted imaging and 1.0-mm Grass acquisition.

SURGICAL TECHNIQUE

The basic goal of surgery is to create a proximally based check-rein mechanism to prevent the acute flexion of the distal pole of the scaphoid and thus eliminate the rotary subluxation (Fig. 55.2). Under general anesthesia, the patient is placed supine on the operating room table, and the forearm is set in pronation on the hand table. The surgeon sits on the radial side of the wrist.

Under appropriate pneumatic tourniquet control, begin with a longitudinal dorsal incision over the wrist. As the skin flaps are elevated, the first stucture to be identified and protected is the superficial sensory branch of the radial nerve. The anatomic landmark structures to be identified include the extensor pollicis longus (EPL) and the extensor carpi radialis longus (ECRL) and brevis (ECRB). Expose the dorsal capsule of the wrist from the distal radius to the STT joint. This is accomplished by retracting the radial nerve, EPL, and ECRL radially and the ECRB ulnarward. Palpate the radiocarpal joint and the prominent proximal pole of the scaphoid. Incise the dorsal capsule along the oblique axis of the scaphoid. Progressive opening and elevation of the capsule reveals the obvious "nesting" proximal pole of the scaphoid (Fig. 55.3).

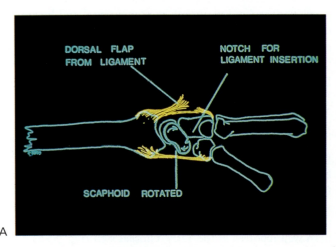
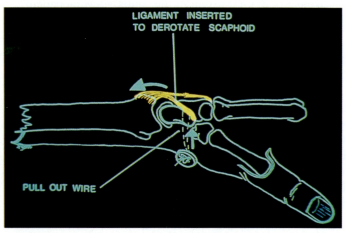

FIGURE 55.2. A,B: Graphic representation of the concept of dorsal capsulodesis to stabilize the derotated scaphoid.

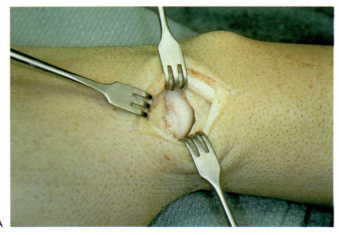 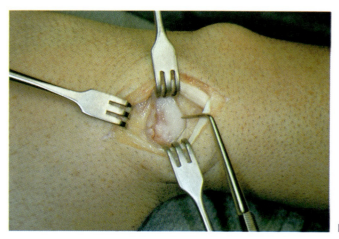

FIGURE 55.3. A: Earliest view of the proximal pole of the scaphoid. **B:** The obvious "nesting" proximal pole caused by the flexed and rotated scaphoid.

Develop the dorsal capsular flap distal to the STT joint. Develop the flap of dorsal capsule from the ulnar side of the capsule. Approximately 1.0 to 1.5 cm wide, its anatomic origin from the dorsum of the distal radius is preserved. Dissect the capsular flap as far distally to the level of the STT joint to assure adequate length of eventual insertion. Measurement of adequate length is again confirmed (Fig. 55.4). Turn the flap back proximally to further visualize and manipulate the scaphoid (Fig. 55.5).

It has been my observation that the scapholunate interosseous ligament has become atrophic and fibrotic. The joint has become filled with granulation tissue (Fig. 55.6). This is not amenable to repair and plays little role in the stability of the scaphoid. The granulation tissue is debrided with a fine rongeur, creating freshened surfaces, which are brought into apposition when the scaphoid is reduced. The long period of postoperative immobilization allows for development of an adequate scar.

Reduce the scaphoid into its anatomic alignment by applying downward and proximal pressure against the proximal pole. The scaphocapitate joint is used as an articular template to confirm reduction. While the scaphoid is being maintained in its reduced position, the distal pole of the scaphoid is internally fixed with a smooth 0.045-in. Kirschner wire (K-wire) drilled obliquely through the distal pole of the scaphoid into the capitate and base of the middle metacarpal (Fig. 55.7). Passively flex and extend the wrist to confirm stability of the scaphoid with free radiocarpal motion. With the scaphoid reduced, again measure the dorsal flap for length and adequate coverage of the proximal pole of the scaphoid.

Now create a fresh bony bed for insertion of the dorsal capsular flap, which is the next most critical step in this

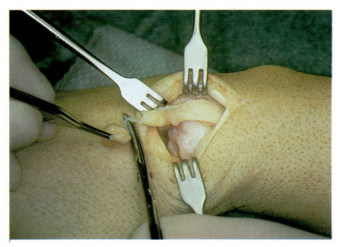

FIGURE 55.4. Completion of the flap dissection distally to approximate the longitudinal length of the scaphoid. The flap of the dorsal capsule is measured distally to ensure that adequate length has been developed for its eventual insertion.

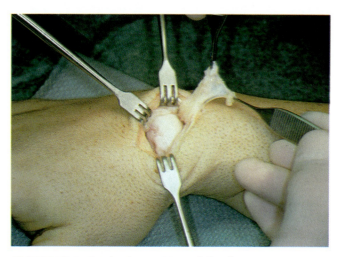

FIGURE 55.5. Proximal retraction of the flap permits greater visualization of the scaphoid.

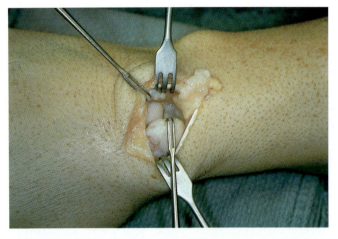

FIGURE 55.6. Note the disruption of the scapholunate (SL) joint and obvious dissociation. Fibrotic granulation of the atrophic SL ligament is seen.

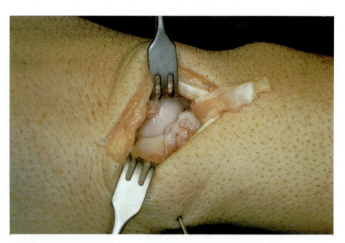

FIGURE 55.7. Internal fixation of the reduced scaphoid is achieved with a 0.045-in. smooth Kirschner wire drilled through the distal pole into the capitate and base of the middle metacarpal. The scaphocapitate joint is used as an articular template for appropriate alignment and reduction.

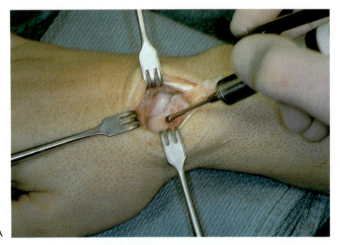

A

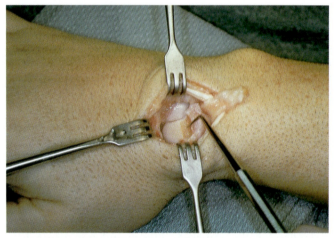

B

FIGURE 55.8. A: A site on the scaphoid proximal to the distal articular surface but distal to the midaxis of rotation is selected. A small burr in the power drill is used to denude the cortex. **B:** A trough of fresh cancellous bone is created.

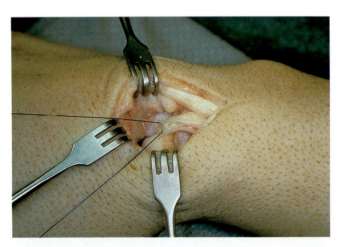

FIGURE 55.9. The dorsal capsular flap is secured with a crisscross 2-0 prolene pullout suture for its insertion into the fresh cancellous bony bed. Note the ends of the suture exiting from the distal edge of the flap.

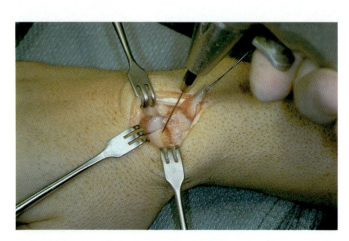

FIGURE 55.10. A length of 0.045-in. K-wire is used to create the channels in the distal pole of the scaphoid through which a straight Keith needle may be used to carry the suture ends through the scaphoid.

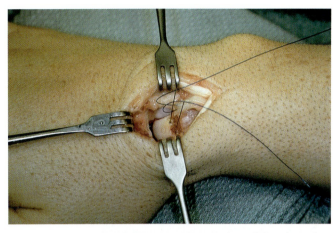 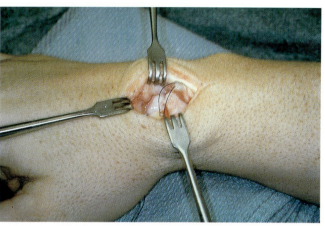

FIGURE 55.11. Construction of the ulnar channel. **A:** The ends of the prolene suture are passed through the eye of the Keith needles. **B:** The suture ends now insert into the cancellous bed and through the distal pole of the scaphoid. The suture ends may be seen exiting from the radiopalmar aspect of the wrist in the area of the scaphoid tubercle.

procedure. Using a power drill, place the small burr just proximal to the distal articular surface of the scaphoid. This insures flap insertion distal to the midaxis of the scaphoid rotation and thereby increases the mechanical leverage of the proximal check-rein effect of the capsulodesis. Denude the cortex until a fresh trough of exposed cancellous bone is achieved (Fig. 55.8). The early procedures of dorsal capsulodesis utilized a stainless steel 4-0 wire pullout suture. However, some fragmentation of this wire suture and its appearance in postoperative radiographs dictated a possible alternative technique for capsular insertion. Therefore, the recommended procedure for the dorsal capsule is to use a 2-0 prolene pullout suture (Fig. 55.9). To draw the suture through the distal pole of the scaphoid on straight Keith needles, use a 0.045-in. K-wire to drill the channels for the needles (Fig. 55.10). Pass the ends of the prolene suture through the eye of the Keith needles that have been inserted into the K-wire–created channels. Advance the needles through the scaphoid and palmar capsule, exiting at the radiopalmar aspect of the wrist, in the area of the scaphoid tubercle. This carries the suture ends down through the cancellous bed and the scaphoid (Fig. 55.11). Apply palmar and distal traction on the exiting suture ends, with the wrist in slight extension, as the dorsal capsular flap is drawn distally down into the cancellous bony trough. Securely tie the suture over a button to maintain insertion. This will eventually also be used for a pullout (Fig. 55.12).

The use of an anchor suture has become quite popular with many surgeons (14). I have occasionally used this technique. The method of insertion follows standard guidelines. However, because the suture tails rise dorsally from the distal pole of the scaphoid, I did not feel this was an

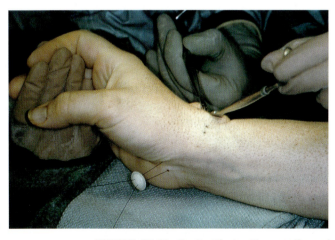 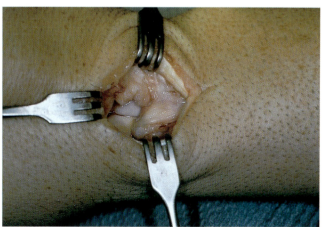

FIGURE 55.12. A: Gentle traction on the palmar-exiting suture ends, with the wrist in slight extension, advances the flap of dorsal capsule securely into the bony trough. The suture is tied over a button on the radiopalmar aspect of the wrist. **B:** Final insertion of the dorsal capsular flap with complete coverage of the scaphoid.

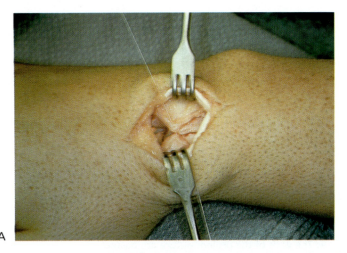 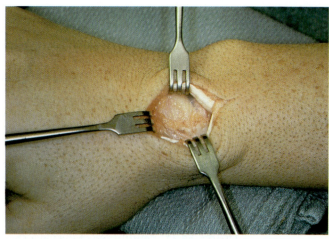

FIGURE 55.13. **A:** The radial and ulnar flaps of the dorsal wrist capsule are mobilized for direct closure, with multiple interrupted stitches of nonabsorbable suture such as 4-0 white Dacron. **B:** Completion of capsular closure easily compensating for the 1.0- to 1.5-cm gap created by construction of the flap.

efficient mechanical means of cinching the dorsal capsular flap securely into the cancellous bed.

Mobilize the radial and ulnar flaps of the dorsal capsule for direct closure. The 1.0- to 1.5-cm gap utilized to construct the dorsal capsulodesis ligament is easily compensated for. I recommend repair of this capsule with multiple interrupted 4-0 white Dacron or other nonabsorbable sutures (Fig. 55.13). The anatomic structures are allowed to resume their appropriate alignment and position, and skin closure is accomplished with multiple interrupted 5-0 nylon mattress sutures. Apply a soft compression hand dressing with additional protection provided by a palmar plaster splint.

POSTOPERATIVE MANAGEMENT

The specific postoperataive regimen has proved to be extremely important. One week to 10 days postoperative, the compressive hand dressing and splint are removed. Radiographs are obtained to assure corrective alignment of the scaphoid. Sutures are removed from the skin incision. Betadine and paper skin tapes are applied. A short arm fiberglass thumb–spica cast is now placed on the hand and wrist for a period of 2 months.

After 2 months, the cast is removed, and radiographs again obtained. The paper skin tapes are removed, leaving a fine thin incisional line. The pullout prolene suture is also removed by cutting one strand of the suture beneath the button. Gentle, steady traction on the intact strand in a palmar direction allows the suture to unravel from the now seated dorsal capsular flap, pass down through the distal pole of the scaphoid, and emerge from the area of palmar tubercle. The K-wire is not removed but left in place. The wrist is placed in a removable palmar splint (Futuro), and a therapy program is initiated.

The patient is instructed and supervised through a course of active and gentle passive-assistive range of motion. No resistive grip, twisting, or torque is permitted. This will restrict motion only to the level of the radiocarpal joint, as the presence of the K-wire will prevent midcarpal motion.

After 1 more month, now 3 months postoperative, radiographs are again obtained, and the K-wire is removed under local anesthesia in the office. The therapy program is advanced, as midcarpal and intercarpal motion may now be achieved. By this technique, the dorsal flap is subjected to a gradual and staged level of progressive stress with wrist motion. Resistive grip and an advancing program of strengthening are also now initiated as the palmar splint is discontinued. The patient is not permitted full and unrestricted activity with the wrist for an additional 3 months, that is, a total of 6 months postoperative.

It is felt that this sequential program of advancing motion and stress allows the dorsal capsular flap to adapt to the demanding arc of wrist motion in both length and tensile strength. The long-term results suggest that one might anticipate almost full recovery of wrist extension, a maximum deficit of approximately 20° of wrist flexion, and an average recovery of 80% grip strength as compared to the normal side.

COMPLICATIONS

The first potential complication to avoid is the development of a radial neuritis. Careful identification, gentle mobilization, and retraction of the superficial sensory branch of the radial nerve should provide adequate protection.

It is important to avoid making the dorsal capsular flap too narrow, which would be mechanically inadequate or subject to attrition. A good guideline is to make the flap at least as wide as the body of the scaphoid.

Incomplete reduction of the axial alignment of the scaphoid and closure of the scapholunate space is a potential complication. This may occur if there has been formation of granulation tissue or scar in the area of the old ruptured scapholunate interosseous ligament, thereby creating a mechanical block. Removal of this tissue with a fine rongeur will correct this impediment to reduction and provide fresh tissue surfaces for potential healing in the reduced position.

As alluded to earlier, the complication of a broken K-wire may be avoided by using the heavier gauge 0.045-in. wire placed through the distal pole of the scaphoid. Be sure there is stable purchase into the capitate and the base of the third metacarpal. Confirm this by passive manipulation of the wrist under direct vision.

There are no shortcuts. Strict adherence to the recommended protocol for postoperative management and restricted therapy regimen may help avoid the ultimate complication of recurrent rotary subluxation.

CLINICAL CASE

A 22-year-old college basketball player presented approximately 3 months following a severe torsion injury and fall on his right wrist. Although no acute fracture was noted on initial routine radiographs, the patient was immobilized in a splint for a short period of time. His initial complaints were of continued pain in the wrist, with an increasing snap or "clunk" on certain attempted motions.

Bilateral supination AP views confirmed a scaphoid–lunate (SL) dissociation with a shortened distance from the ring sign to the proximal pole of the scaphoid (Fig. 55.14). The dynamic instability of RSS was noted on cineradiograph. Surgical reconstruction with a dorsal capsulodesis, as described, was recommended and accomplished. The patient complied with the prescribed postoperative course and therapy regimen. He was able to return to competitive basketball by his next season.

Now 16 years postoperative, the three routine radiograph views of the wrist reveal anatomic radiocarpal and intercarpal alignment. There is no evidence of radioscaphoid or pan-scaphoid arthrosis. Supination AP views with and without carpal compression (Fig. 55.15) reveal the maintained stability of the scaphoid and closure of the SL space. For an additional perspective, an MRI study of the wrist reveals the thickened dorsal capsular flap continuing to act as a proximal check-rein mechanism on the scaphoid (Fig. 55.16). Grip strength is 10% greater in the dominant operated right hand than in the nondominant nonoperated left hand. Note the full recovery of wrist extension, with an approximate 10° deficit of full flexion. There is also excellent recovery of radial and ulnar deviation.

The patient has worked without restrictions for many years in the repair department in a major utility company and is an assistant high school basketball coach.

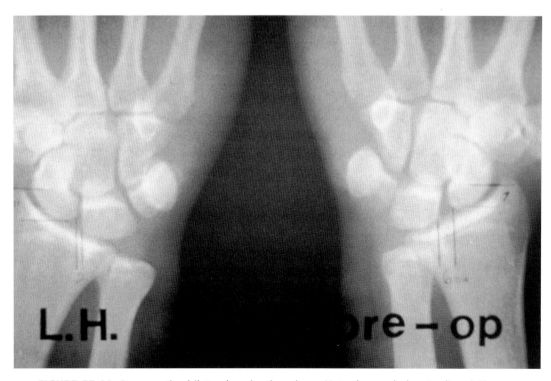

FIGURE 55.14. Preoperative bilateral supination views. Note the scapholunate dissociation on the right and the shortened distance of the ring sign to the proximal scaphoid pole.

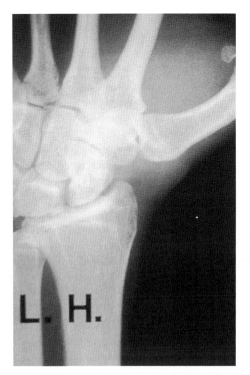
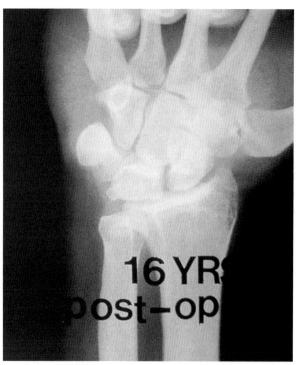

FIGURE 55.15. Same patient as in Fig. 55.14, 16 years postoperatively. Supination views of the right wrist with and without carpal compression demonstrate the stability of the scaphoid.

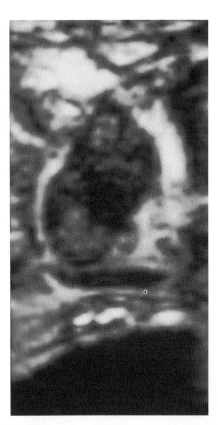

FIGURE 55.16. Magnetic resonance image of the right wrist. Orientation: proximal to the **right,** distal to the **left,** dorsal at **top,** palmar at **bottom,** carpal scaphoid in the **center.** Note the thickened flap of dorsal capsule extending from the dorsum of the distal radius to the dorsum of the distal pole of the scaphoid.

EDITORS' COMMENTS

The Blatt procedure has gradually gained acceptance both as a primary stand-alone procedure and as an adjunct to ligamentous repair for RSS. There are differences of opinion concerning its application. First, we must recognize that we are speaking of the classic RSS where the proximal pole supinates and climbs the back of the capitate with loss of scapholunate interosseous ligament support. The RSS that occurs at the STT joint with lateral displacement of the head of the scaphoid and/or hyperflexion of the scaphoid as in midcarpal instability is not amenable to the Blatt capsulodesis. We currently feel that there are patients with dynamic RSS combined with nonmaximum activity levels that can be handled by ligamentous reconstruction. These wrists can be stabilized with a modicum of range-of-motion loss, allowing the scaphoid to continue to provide adequate load transference without displacement. If the patient is a professional athlete, construction worker, avid golfer, or of similar activity level, he is better served by fusing the STT joint. If there is significant scapholunate gapping (static RSS), there is probably not an indication for a ligamentous repair of any type for this scapholunate dissociation form of rotary subluxation. This gap is indicative of total scapholunate interosseous disruption and means the scaphoid will displace under load. That displacement will lead to central destruction of the cartilage on the scaphoid and peripheral destruction of the scaphoid fossa in the radius, as in the SLAC wrist.

It is important to match the patient's needs and activity levels to the degree of scaphoid ligament disruption. Twenty-five percent of normal adults demonstrate some clinical positive scaphoid shifting, meaning for the most part some tearing of the scapholunate interosseous system. These people live and function normally and are totally asymptomatic except for perhaps certain activities and minor complaints. We are looking, therefore, at a spectrum condition where the patient's demands play as much of a role as the pathologic condition of the wrist in determining treatment. The ligamentous reconstruction for scaphoid instability must be matched to the degree of anatomic dysfunction and the patient's clinical demands.

REFERENCES

1. Blatt G. Capsulodesis in reconstructive hand surgery: dorsal capsulodesis for the unstable scaphoid and volar capsulodesis following excision of the distal ulna. *Hand Clin* 1987;3:81–102.
2. Blatt G. Scapholunate instability. In: Lichtman DM, ed. *The wrist and its disorders*. Philadelphia: WB Saunders, 1988;251–273.
3. Linscheid RL, Dobyns JH, Beabout JW, et al. Traumatic instability of the wrist. *J Bone Joint Surg Am* 1972;54:1612–1632.
4. Taleisnik J. Carpal instability: current concepts review. *J Bone Joint Surg Am* 1988;70:1262–1267.
5. Glickel SZ, Millender LH. Ligamentous reconstruction for chronic intercarpal instability. *J Hand Surg [Am]* 1984;9:514–527.
6. Goldner JL. Treatment of carpal instability without joint fusion: current assessment. *J Hand Surg [Am]* 1982;7:325–326.
7. Kleinman WB. Long-term study of chronic scapholunate instability treated by scapho-trapezium-trapezoid arthrodesis. *J Hand Surg [Am]* 1989;14:429–445.
8. Lavernia CJ, Cohen MS, Taleisnik J. Treatment of scapholunate dissociation by ligamentous repair and capsulodesis. *J Hand Surg [Am]* 1992;17:354–359.
9. Palmer AK, Dobyns JA, Linscheid RL. Management of posttraumatic instability of the wrist secondary to ligament rupture. *J Hand Surg [Am]* 1978;3:507–532.
10. Watson HK, Hempton RF. Limited wrist arthrodesis. I. The triscaphoid joint. *J Hand Surg [Am]* 1980;5:320–327.
11. Watson HK, Ashmead D, Makhlouf MV. Examination of the scaphoid bone. *J Bone Joint Surg Am* 1988;13:657–660.
12. Crittenden JJ, Jones DM, Santarelli AG. Bilateral rotational dislocation of the carpal navicular: case report. *Radiology* 1970;94:629–630.
13. Dobyns JH, Linscheid RL, Chao EYS, et al. Traumatic instability of the wrist. *Instr Course Lect* 1975;24:182–199.
14. Uhl RL, Williamson SC, Bowman MW, et al. Dorsal capsulodesis using suture anchors. *Am J Orthop* 1997;8:547–548.

56

DORSAL WRIST SYNDROME REPAIR

JEFFREY WEINZWEIG
H. KIRK WATSON

INDICATIONS

The most common manifestation of wrist pathology, which we have termed *dorsal wrist syndrome* (DWS), is the result of overload and insult to the scapholunate (SL) joint (1–3). Acute wrist trauma, in the absence of a SL interosseous ligament tear, produces SL synovitis and some degree of internal ligamentous strain in its mildest form. Repetitive minor trauma or a more substantial solitary insult to the SL region may result in DWS, which is characterized by pain on the dorsum of the wrist accompanied by significant SL synovitis with or without measurable ligamentous disruption (see Chapter 28). The surgical management of DWS is presented.

CONTRAINDICATIONS

The only relative contraindication to surgical repair of DWS is the intraoperative finding of significant (subtotal or total) SL ligamentous disruption on exploration of the SL joint. Such a finding might indicate a greater degree of carpal pathology and instability than could be satisfactorily managed without performing a triscaphe arthrodesis (4,5).

SURGICAL TECHNIQUE

Surgical management of DWS involves exploration of the SL joint with attention directed at existing soft tissue synovitis overlying the SL joint, usually including the terminal carpal branch of the posterior interosseous nerve, evaluating the integrity of the SL ligament, excision of occult ganglia, removal of the ridges on the scaphoid and lunate, and creation of cancellous surfaces for capsular adhesion.

This is accomplished through a dorsal transverse incision, approximately 3 cm in length, centered over the SL joint at the level of the radial styloid. A spreading technique is used to preserve dorsal veins and sensory nerves. The dorsal capsule is divided, and the sheath of the extensor pollicis longus is identified and traced proximally as the tendon is retracted radially. A soft tissue mass, consisting of thickened synovium and often containing ganglia (in 60% of cases) (6,7), is invariably found between the third and fourth compartments and is excised to reveal the underlying SL joint (Fig. 56.1). An occult ganglion is often identified on the dorsal SL ligamentous surface and excised. Traction of the index and middle fingers permits visualization and evaluation of the proximal portion of the SL interosseous ligament. Flexion of the distracted wrist and placement of a probe (joker) within the radiocarpal joint between the scaphoid and lunate permit evaluation of the volar portion of the SL ligament.

The partially ruptured SL ligament is often bridged by repair tissue and a synovial layer that possess negligible intrinsic strength. This layer is readily separated by the probe, and the SL joint space is entered volarly. The probe is swept proximally and then dorsally, tracing the curve of the SL joint until intact ligamentous fibers are encountered. This process permits complete evaluation of the extent of ligamentous rupture. Bony ridging on the dorsum of the scaphoid and lunate, which is present in every case, is excised using a dental rongeur (Fig. 56.2). A broad cancellous surface is thus created for capsular attachment on the dorsum of the scaphoid and lunate (Fig. 56.3). The terminal branch of the posterior interosseous nerve usually lies on the floor of the fourth dorsal compartment beneath the extensor digitorum communis tendons. Although we have not been able to demonstrate an effective difference, there are those who prefer to resect the terminal branches of the posterior interosseous nerve. This is accomplished by lifting the tendons of the fourth dorsal compartment. The nerve is

---

J. Weinzweig: Department of Plastic Surgery, Brown University School of Medicine, Rhode Island Hospital, and Hasbro Children's Hospital, Providence, Rhode Island 02905.

H. K. Watson: Connecticut Combined Hand Surgery Fellowship, Hartford Hospital, and Connecticut Children's Medical Center, Hartford, Connecticut 06106; Department of Orthopaedics, University of Connecticut School of Medicine, Farmington, Connecticut 06032; Department of Orthopedics, Rehabilitation, and Plastic Surgery, Yale University School of Medicine, New Haven, Connecticut 06520.

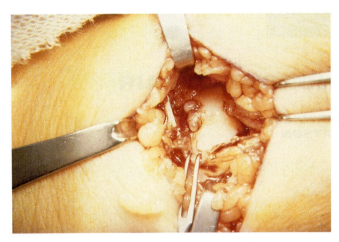

FIGURE 56.1. Two occult ganglia, identified within the scapholunate joint at the time of exploration for dorsal wrist syndrome, are excised.

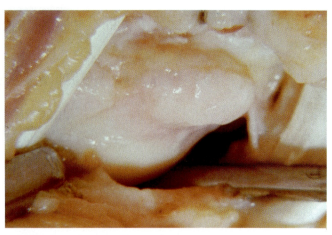

FIGURE 56.2. Marked bony ridging is seen as a large bony prominence on the dorsum of this scaphoid. This is the ridging that is excised at the time of dorsal wrist syndrome surgery. (This is the right wrist with the fingers pointing up.)

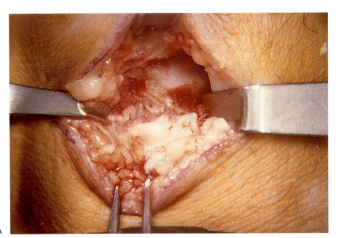
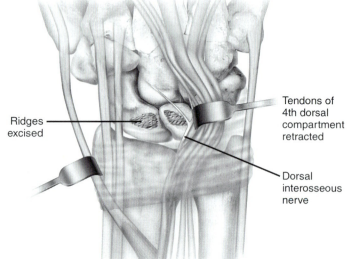

FIGURE 56.3. (A,B): Both the scaphoid and lunate had prominent bony dorsal ridges that were removed with a rongeur, leaving a broad cancellous area to which the capsule adheres, enhancing dorsal stability. (This is the right wrist with the fingers pointing up; the scaphoid is on the left, and the lunate is on the right.)

identified on the floor, deep to the tendons, and a small section is removed. The skin is then closed, and a bulky dressing incorporating a dorsal plaster splint is applied.

POSTOPERATIVE MANAGEMENT

The bulky dressing and splint are removed 3 days postoperatively, and the wrist is fully mobilized.

CLINICAL SERIES

Five hundred fifty-two patients underwent DWS surgery over an 18-year period. A subgroup of 200 consecutive patients treated for DWS over an 8-year period was reviewed (3). Wrist arthrotomies were performed on 151 of these patients (75%); the other 25% were successfully managed with conservative treatment. This group included 44 male and 107 female patients with a mean age of 30 years (range, 12–55 years). The average duration of symptoms before surgery was 24 months. Either an acute traumatic event or a history of repetitive excessive loading preceded the development of dorsal wrist pain in 64% of this group of patients (82% of male patients; 57% of female patients).

The majority of patients (75%) presented with a history of symptomatology of at least 6 months' duration. Those patients with symptoms of shorter duration were initially treated conservatively with wrist splints, steroid injection of the SL joint region, and nonsteroidal antiinflammatory medication. Indications for surgical treatment included (a) failure of a 3-month trial of conservative therapy in patients presenting with less than 6 months of symptoms or (b) more than 6 months of symptoms at the time of initial presentation.

Fifty-one patients (33%) demonstrated an intact SL ligament (type 0) with SL ridging and moderate synovitis. Sixty-three patients (42%) demonstrated a tear in the volar aspect of the SL ligament extending as far proximally as the midproximal point of the SL joint; approximately 50% of the ligament was disrupted in this group (type I). Thirty-one patients (21%) had a ligamentous tear that extended from the volar aspect of the SL ligament three-fourths the distance around the SL joint (type II). The ligamentous tear was complete in six patients (4%) (type III).

Small SL ganglia were present in 47 of these patients (31%) and excised at the time of SL exploration. Forty-four other patients (29%) had already undergone ganglion excision before their referral for continued symptoms. Fourteen patients (9.3%) required triscaphe arthrodesis following DWS treatment. Thirty-nine patients (26%) underwent carpal tunnel release before, concomitant with, or following, DWS treatment. Eighty-seven percent of all patients who had undergone surgical treatment for DWS (all but those requiring subsequent triscaphe arthrodesis) were pain-free and participating fully in both occupational and recreational activities when seen in follow-up.

COMPLICATIONS

No complications occurred following DWS repair in this series of patients. However, 14 patients required subsequent triscaphe arthrodesis because of the advanced stage of their SL ligament disruption and carpal instability.

DISCUSSION

A simple and effective technique for the surgical management of DWS, perhaps the most common manifestation of carpal pathology, is presented. This technique provides not only a therapeutic approach to the management of this condition, but also an opportunity to explore and evaluate the SL joint and interosseous ligament, thereby permitting prediction of the need for subsequent limited wrist arthrodesis (6,7).

REFERENCES

1. Watson HK, Weinzweig J, Zeppieri J. The natural progression of scaphoid instability. *Hand Clin* 1997;13(1):39–50.
2. Weinzweig J, Watson HK. Wrist sprain to SLAC wrist: a spectrum of carpal instability. In: Vastamaki M, ed. *Current trends in hand surgery.* Amsterdam: Elsevier, 1995;47–55.
3. Weinzweig J, Watson HK. Dorsal wrist syndrome: operative management of 151 patients. *Plast Surg Forum* 1998;XXI:57–60.
4. Watson HK, Hemptson RF. Limited wrist arthrodesis. Part I: The triscaphoid joint. *J Hand Surg [Am]* 1980;5:320–327.
5. Watson HK, Ottoni L, Pitts EC, et al. Rotary subluxation of the scaphoid: A spectrum of instability. *J Hand Surg [Br]* 1993;18:62–64.
6. Angelides AC, Wallace PF. The dorsal ganglion of the wrist: its pathogenesis, gross anatomy, and surgical treatment. *J Hand Surg [Am]* 1976;1:228–235.
7. Watson HK, Rodgers WD, Ashmead D. Reevaluation of the cause of the wrist ganglion. *J Hand Surg [Am]* 1989;14:812–817.

LUNOTRIQUETRAL ARTHRODESIS

H. KIRK WATSON
JEFFREY WEINZWEIG

INDICATIONS

Pathology arising from the lunotriquetral (LT) joint is a known etiology of ulnar wrist pain (1–4). Indications for limited wrist arthrodesis of this articulation include symptomatic LT joint instability, degenerative arthritis, and congenital synchondrosis or incomplete separation of the lunate and triquetrum (Fig. 57.1) (5–10).

CONTRAINDICATIONS

There are no contraindications to LT arthrodesis, a procedure specificically designed to address degenerative arthritic and instability problems associated with this joint and one with minimal morbidity. However, in cases where more extensive carpal pathology exists, such as a scapholunate advanced collapse (SLAC) wrist, a procedure that incorporates the LT fusion, such as the four-bone limited wrist arthrodesis, might be indicated.

SURGICAL TECHNIQUE

The LT joint is exposed through a transverse dorsal ulnar incision at the level of the radial styloid tip. A spreading technique is used to preserve dorsal veins and sensory nerves. The capsule is incised transversely to expose the LT joint (Fig. 57.2). The triangular fibrocartilage complex, extensor carpi ulnaris sheath, ulnar sling mechanism, and ulnar side of the triquetrum are evaluated. The adjacent articular surfaces of the lunate and triquetrum are then removed with a dental rongeur to expose cancellous bone. The opposing cortical edges are left intact to preserve the relationship of the two bones and to help maintain alignment during fixation. Removing the articular surfaces creates a biconcave cancellous space. This tends to centralize the graft and aids in preventing its displacement. Cancellous bone is harvested from the distal radius. Two 0.045-in.

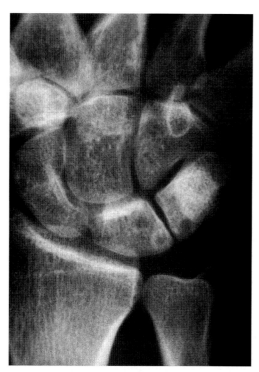

FIGURE 57.1. Congenital synchondrosis of the lunotriquetral joint. Radiographic findings in degenerative joint disease associated with congenital incomplete separation of the lunate and triquetrum include joint narrowing with bony impingement, loss of cartilaginous space, and the presence of cystic changes as seen here in both the lunate and triquetrum proximally.

H. K. Watson: Connecticut Combined Hand Surgery Fellowship, Hartford Hospital, and Connecticut Children's Medical Center, Hartford, Connecticut 06106; Department of Orthopaedics, University of Connecticut School of Medicine, Farmington, Connecticut 06032; Department of Orthopedics, Rehabilitation, and Plastic Surgery, Yale University School of Medicine, New Haven, Connecticut 06520.

J. Weinzweig: Department of Plastic Surgery, Brown University School of Medicine, Rhode Island Hospital, and Hasbro Children's Hospital, Providence, Rhode Island 02905.

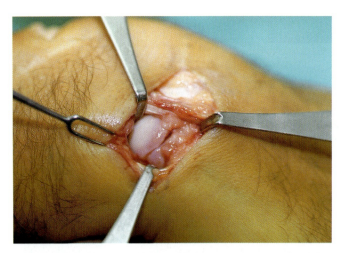

FIGURE 57.2. Exposure of the lunotriquetral joint, with fingers pointing to the right, reveals complete articular cartilage loss and destruction of the joint. Note the significant hyperemia and eburnation of the articular surfaces and subchondral bone of the lunate and triquetrum.

K-wires are preset into the triquetrum in a relatively parallel fashion. Cancellous bone graft is then densely packed into the recesses of the concave spaces. No cortical or strut graft is used. The joint is reduced with the preserved margins used as guides; the normal external dimensions of the bones are thus maintained while the K-wires are driven into the lunate but not into the scaphoid (Fig. 57.3). The remaining biconcave space is then densely packed with cancellous bone using a dental tamp. The K-wires are cut below the skin level, and the skin is closed. A bulky long arm dressing incorporating a plaster dorsal splint is applied.

POSTOPERATIVE MANAGEMENT

A short arm gauntlet cast incorporating the thumb is applied 3 to 5 days postoperatively. The rationale for incorporating the thumb is that it aids in limiting the patient's ability to use, and therefore load, the hand. At 4 weeks, the cast is changed, and sutures are removed. Six weeks postoperatively (7 weeks in smokers), the cast is removed, and radiographs of the wrist are taken. If evidence of fusion is apparent, the pins are removed in the office, and the extremity is mobilized (Fig. 57.4). Otherwise, casting is continued until healing across the fusion site has occurred.

CLINICAL SERIES

Thirty-one patients underwent 33 LT arthrodeses over a 16-year period. These patients ranged in age from 18 to 59 years; 52% were male. All patients complained of ulnar wrist pain; the majority had significant postactivity ache. Most patients could recall specific wrist trauma, including all cases in which LT instability was seen. The trauma may have been an eliciting factor and not the etiology. All patients had failed conservative treatment consisting of immobilization, steroid injection, oral antiinflammatory medications, and/or hand therapy modalities before being considered for surgery. The mean duration of symptoms before surgery was 35 months (range, 4–132 months).

Indications for LT arthrodesis included LT ligamentous injury with joint instability in 24 cases (73%). Two of these patients had already undergone unsuccessful LT arthrodesis

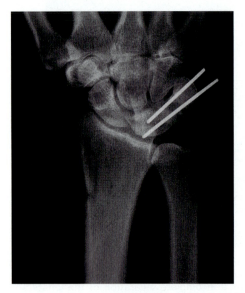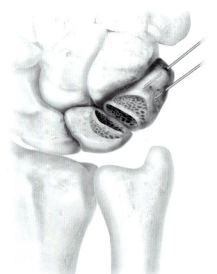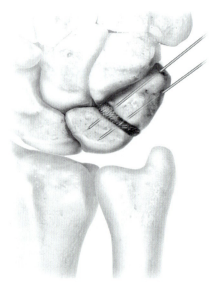

FIGURE 57.3. Following biconcave cancellous bone grafting of the lunate and triquetrum, preserving opposing cortical rims for alignment, parallel K-wires transfixing only the lunotriquetral joint stabilize the graft.

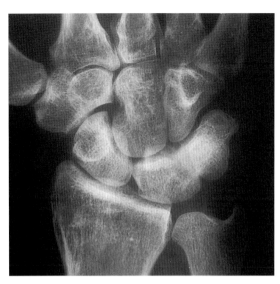

FIGURE 57.4. Twelve months after cancellous lunotriquetral (LT) arthrodesis for symptomatic degenerative joint disease, solid fusion is seen radiographically. LT limited wrist arthrodesis results in minimal mobility loss and a full-power wrist.

before referral. Nine arthrodeses were performed for degenerative arthritis (27%). Six of these nine patients had degenerative changes secondary to partial coalition of the LT joint. Additional diagnoses included triangular fibrocartilage complex injuries in four patients and ulnar impaction syndrome in three patients. Two patients underwent staged bilateral procedures. One patient underwent concomitant STT arthrodesis for dynamic rotary subluxation of the scaphoid. Another patient had concomitant step-cut ulnar shortening for ulnar impaction syndrome.

Primary union was achieved in all cases with an average period of immobilization of 48 days. The mean follow-up was 26 months following arthrodesis (range, 6–72 months). Ninety-two percent of patients reported no pain or mild pain postoperatively. Two patients reported moderate pain, and one reported severe pain postoperatively; all three had been operated on for LT instability. The average range of motion after LT arthrodesis was 68° flexion (77% of the unaffected side in patients with unilateral disease), 60° extension (80% of the unaffected side), 20° radial deviation (95%), and 33° ulnar deviation (91%), regardless of the indication for limited wrist fusion. Seventy-six percent of patients returned to their original employment after a mean period of disability of 14 weeks; an additional 12% returned to the work force after retraining. Eight percent of patients did not return to work within the follow-up period (mean, 26 months). One patient retired postoperatively.

No cases of secondary degenerative wrist disease have been seen in this series of patients.

COMPLICATIONS

Complications of 33 LT limited wrist arthrodeses performed using the cancellous biconcave technique described include reflex sympathetic dystrophy in one patient, which was successfully treated with a stress loading Dystrophile program (see Chapter 46), and pin migration necessitating early removal of the K-wires in one patient. Three patients who were operated on for LT instability demonstrated persistent pain postoperatively. There were no nonunions in this series of patients.

DISCUSSION

It is currently our impression that many of the old cases called degenerative arthritis were, in retrospect, degenerative changes secondary to incomplete joint development. The biconcave technique described for LT arthrodesis is a reliable method for addressing carpal pathology involving the LT joint without the need for permanent fixation or the use of compression screws. Strict adherence to the principles of intercarpal arthrodesis is essential. These include maintenance of the external dimensions and relationships of the carpal bones, creation of broad cancellous surfaces for grafting, utilization of a cancellous bone graft, and the use of K-wires that cross only the joints to be fused, thus allowing any loads encountered in the postoperative period to be transferred to, and diffused by, adjacent intercarpal and radiocarpal joints. This approach has resulted in 100% union with few complications, yielding functional wrists with a minimal loss of wrist motion.

REFERENCES

1. Horii E, Garcia-Elias M, An K, et al. A kinematic study of lunotriquetral dissociations. *J Hand Surg [Am]* 1991;16:355–362.
2. Kirschenbaum D, Coyle M, Leddy J. Chronic lunotriquetral instability: Diagnosis and treatment. *J Hand Surg [Am]* 1993;18: 1107–1112.
3. Lichtman DM, Noble WH, Alexander CE. Dynamic triquetrolunate instability: Case report. *J Hand Surg [Am]* 1984;9:185–188.
4. Pin P, Young V, Gilula L, et al. Management of chronic lunotriquetral ligament tears. *J Hand Surg [Am]* 1989;14:77–83.
5. Gross SC, Watson HK, Strickland JW, et al. Triquetral–lunate arthritis secondary to synostosis. *J Hand Surg [Am]* 1989;14: 95–102.
6. Nelson DL, Manske PR, Pruitt DL, et al. Lunotriquetral arthrodesis. *J Hand Surg [Am]* 1993;18:1113–1120.
7. Resnik C, Grizzard J, Simmons B, et al. Incomplete carpal coalition. *Am J Radiol* 1986;147:301–304.
8. Sennwald GR, Fischer M, Mondi P. Lunotriquetral arthrodesis. A controversial procedure. *J Hand Surg [Br]* 1995;20:755–760.
9. Watson HK, Weinzweig J. Intercarpal arthrodesis. In: Green DP, Hotchkiss RN, Pederson WC, eds. *Operative hand surgery, 4th ed.* New York: Churchill Livingstone, 1999;108–130.
10. Watson HK, Weinzweig J, Guidera P, et al. One thousand intercarpal arthrodeses. *J Hand Surg [Br]* 1999;24:320–330.

58

MATCHED HEMIRESECTION–INTERPOSITION ARTHROPLASTY

ROBERT S. RICHARDS
JAMES H. ROTH

Numerous techniques of distal radioulnar joint (DRUJ) arthroplasty have been described. The Darrach procedure was first described in 1913 and involved complete resection of the distal ulna (1). Good results have been found with this procedure in patients with rheumatoid arthritis; however, a high complication rate has been seen in nonrheumatoid patients. Complications of impingement and distal ulnar instability led to the development of multiple different procedures. The hemiresectional arthroplasty technique for DRUJ arthroplasty was first performed by Bowers in 1978 (2). The first published results of this procedure were in 1985 (3). Since then, multiple reports have been published on the results of hemiresection–interposition arthroplasty (4–10).

Watson, in 1986, reported on the results of matched resection arthroplasty (11). He noted that an advantage of matched arthroplasty of the DRUJ was a consistent distance between the radius and ulna. This was felt to minimize the risk of radioulnar impingement compared to standard hemiresectional arthroplasty procedures. Watson stated that, in his opinion, avoidance of a formal interposition arthroplasty may maximize forearm rotation. He felt that distal ulnar stability was achieved by adherence of the extensor carpi ulnaris (ECU) subsheath to the ulna.

Since 1986, one of us (J.H.R.) has performed a matched hemiresection with retinacular/capsular interposition for patients with painful disorders of the DRUJ (12). The authors feel that the matched hemiresection–interposition arthroplasty minimizes both the risk of radioulnar impingement and the risk of distal ulnar instability. During the matched hemiresection–interposition arthroplasty, the capsular retinacular interposition minimizes the risk of impingement. The stabilization of the distal ulna occurs both from the triangular fibrocartilage complex (TFCC) and stabilizing and tightening the ECU subsheath. We feel this offers the advantages of both the matched arthroplasty and the hemiresection–interposition arthroplasty.

INDICATIONS

Osteoarthritis

These patients constitute one of the best indications for a matched hemiresection–interposition arthroplasty. These are higher-demand patients than rheumatoid arthritis patients, and concern has been raised about secondary pain and instability in these patients with both the Darrach and the Sauvé-Kapandji procedures (13). The ability to preserve more of the distal ulnar stabilizers with a matched hemiresection–interposition arthroplasty may decrease the risk of secondary pain and instability.

In those patients with ulnar positive variance, secondary stylocarpal impingement has been noted after a classic hemiresection–interposition arthroplasty necessitating a concomitant ulnar shortening osteotomy. The matched hemiresection–interposition arthroplasty allows sufficient shortening of the ulnar styloid to avoid secondary stylocarpal impingement without the need for an associated ulnar shortening osteotomy or a separate anchovy in the DRUJ. The authors feel that being able to deal with various problems with one operative technique is a strength of the matched hemiresection–interposition arthroplasty.

Rheumatoid Arthritis

As a group, patients with rheumatoid arthritis do well with DRUJ arthroplasty procedures. Darrach procedures (14), the Sauvé-Kapandji procedure (15), and hemiresection–interposition arthroplasty techniques have all been reported to have good success. The advantage of both the

R.S. Richards and J.H. Roth: Department of Surgery, University of Western Ontario, and Hand and Upper Limb Centre, St. Joseph's Health Centre, London, Ontario N6A 4L6, Canada.

Sauvé-Kapandji and the hemiresection–interposition arthroplasty in preserving ulnar support for the carpus is important only in patients at an early stage of the disease. Those with late-stage disease and marked carpal subluxation have been reported to do equally well with either the Darrach or a hemiresection–interposition arthroplasty. In these patients, the ulnar head is subluxed and consequently provides little support for the ulnar side of the wrist, therefore, stabilizing the carpus with a limited wrist fusion is essential. The authors feel that their modification of the hemiresection–interposition arthroplasty with a combined capsular/retinacular flap may help stabilize the distal ulna with fewer potential problems than a Darrach procedure.

Distal Radioulnar Joint Instability and Subluxation

Before performing a matched hemiresection–interposition arthroplasty in these patients, it is critical to assess both the status of the articular surface of the DRUJ and the initial cause of the DRUJ instability. Attention should first be directed to correcting the cause of the instability before performing an arthroplasty procedure.

If the original problem is secondary to an angulated radial fracture, then correction of the radial length discrepancy is important to tension the ulnar soft tissues and stabilize the DRUJ. In patients with a primary problem of instability without a painful arthrosis, isolated matched hemiresection–interposition arthroplasty may not succeed in correcting the painful instability. Matched hemiresection–interposition arthroplasty should be reserved for patients with significant damage to the articular cartilage.

Distal Radioulnar Joint Contractures

Patients with previous DRUJ injury and loss of motion are good candidates for matched hemiresection–interposition arthroplasty. Often these are patients with a previous radioulnar dislocation and secondary contracture with arthrosis. A matched hemiresection–interposition arthroplasty deals with both the articular damage and the rotational contracture using a single dorsal incision. An excellent pain-free arc of motion is restored. In our experience, additional volar releases are not necessary after the matched hemiresection–interposition arthroplasty is performed through a dorsal approach.

SURGICAL TECHNIQUE

General or regional anesthesia is needed. An above-elbow tourniquet is used. Numerous straight and curved ulnarly based incisions have been described. Potential disadvantages of ulnarly based incisions include possible injury to the dorsal sensory branch of the ulnar nerve. Also, if further wrist surgery is required, the ulnarly based scar may make it more

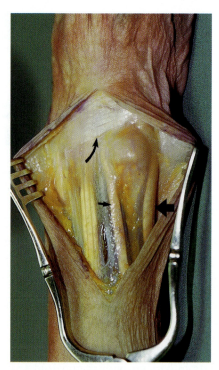

FIGURE 58.1. The skin flaps have been reflected from the dorsum of the right wrist and the extensor carpi ulnaris (ECU) tendon *(large arrow)*, the extensor digiti quinti tendon *(small arrow)*, and the extensor retinaculum *(curved arrow)* are seen. Note the position of the ECU tendon along the ulnar aspect of the head of the ulna.

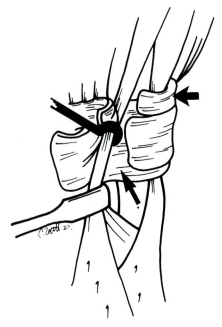

FIGURE 58.2. In this diagram, the retinaculum has been incised. The extensor digiti quinti (EDQ) tendon is retracted, and the dorsal capsule of the distal radioulnar joint *(large arrow)* is shown. The distal retinacular flap that will be repaired over the EDQ at the end of the procedure is shown *(small arrow)*.

Chapter 58: Matched Hemiresection–Interposition Arthroplasty 839

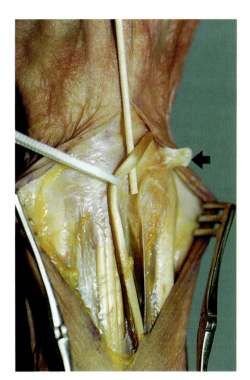

FIGURE 58.3. Here the extensor digiti quinti (EDQ) tendon has been retracted by the umbilical tape. The *pointer* shows the junction of the infratendinous portion of the retinaculum with the dorsal radioulnar joint capsule. The distal retinacular flap that will be repaired over the EDQ is seen *(arrow)*.

difficult to design skin flaps to access the radial side of the wrist. We prefer a dorsal straight midline incision as a global approach to the wrist. This incision minimizes the risk of injury to the superficial branch of the radial nerve and to the dorsal sensory branch of the ulnar nerve. Furthermore, any secondary wrist surgery from tenolysis to limited or pancarpal wrist fusions can be performed through this approach.

The skin flaps are then reflected above the level of the extensor retinaculum. At this point the extensor tendons are identified in their respective compartments (Fig. 58.1). The extensor digiti quinti (EDQ) tendon is isolated proximal to the wrist. The extensor retinaculum is then opened over the fifth compartment and the EDQ tendon is isolated on an umbilical tape (Figs. 58.2 and 58.3). At this time, the dorsal radioulnar capsular ligaments are viewed. (Figs. 58.3 and 58.4). Only very limited dissection of the infratendinous portion of the extensor retinaculum away from the dorsal radioulnar joint capsule is performed (Figs. 58.5 and 58.6). This minimizes disruption of the attachments of the ECU tendon from the TFCC (Fig. 58.6) and the distal ulna. These attachments of the ECU tendon and its subsheath to the distal ulna comprise one of the major stabilizers of the distal ulna.

The dorsal radioulnar capsule is now divided, leaving a small rim attached to the radius for later reapproximation. The ulnar head is now visualized and should be pronated and supinated to examine the joint surface (Fig. 58.6). At this time, the most proximal extent of the hemiresection is marked. Generally, the resection will extend approximately 2 cm proximal to the proximal aspect of the sigmoid notch of the radius. Fluoroscopy is useful for determining this point. A common failure in hemiresectional arthroplasty of

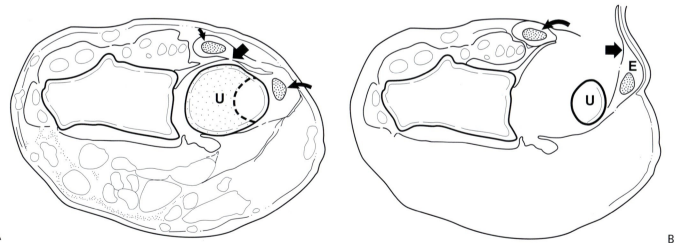

FIGURE 58.4. A: In this cross-sectional diagram, the ulnar head (U) and the junction of the infratendinous portion of the retinaculum with the dorsal radioulnar joint capsule is seen *(large arrow)*. The extensor carpi ulnaris (ECU) tendon *(curved arrow)* and the extensor digiti quinti (EDQ) tendon *(small arrow)* are also seen. **B:** The final extent of the ulnar head (U) resection is shown. The ECU tendon *(E)* and the capsular retinacular flap *(arrow)* as well as the EDQ tendon *(curved arrow)* are also seen.

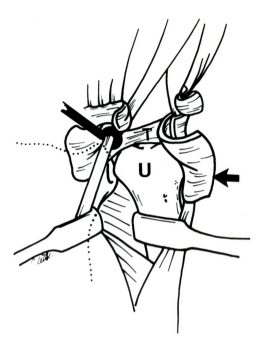

FIGURE 58.5. In this diagram, the retinaculum has been reflected in continuity with the dorsal radioulnar joint capsule *(arrow)* to expose the ulnar head *(U)* and the triangular fibrocartilage complex *(T)*.

the DRUJ is failure to extend the resection proximally enough. This makes it more difficult to accurately sculpt the ulna to avoid secondary radioulnar impingement.

With the forearm in full pronation, an oblique osteotomy extending from dorsal and ulnar to volar and radial is then created (Figs. 58.7 and 58.8). Care is taken not to disturb the ECU tendon subsheath. After the volar and radial edges are contoured to match the curve of the radius, the dorsal and ulnar aspect of the ulna is then contoured (see Fig. 58.4B). At this point, because the forearm is in full pronation, it will appear that an adequate resection has been performed. However, the forearm must now be supinated, and potential areas of impingement assessed. This is done both fluoroscopically and by direct physical examination. We have found that the simplest method of physical examination is to use the surgeon's fingertip as a guide. As the forearm is supinated, any areas that do not freely admit the tip of the index finger undergo a further bony resection. This ensures that a true matched resection with an radioulnar space that is equal in pronation and supination will be created.

The length of the ulna is now assessed. The ulna is compressed toward the radius and examined fluoroscopically. If ulnocarpal impingement is noted, then further shortening of the distal ulna is necessary. Previously, Bowers recommended a shortening osteotomy of the ulnar shaft. However, ulnocarpal impingement can be prevented in a simpler fashion by excision of the ulnar styloid. Distal ulnar instability can be avoided by leaving the ECU subsheath attached to the distal ulna and carefully performing the interposition arthroplasty.

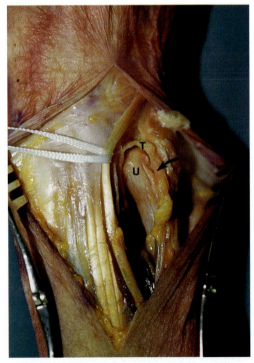

FIGURE 58.6. In this dissection, the retinaculum has been reflected in continuity with the dorsal radioulnar joint capsule *(arrow)* to expose the ulnar head *(U)* and the triangular fibrocartilage complex *(T)*.

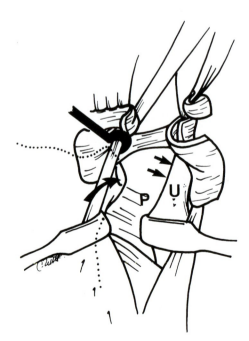

FIGURE 58.7. In this diagram, the head of the ulna *(U)* has been obliquely resected *(small arrows)*. The sigmoid notch of the radius *(curved arrow)* and the pronator quadratus muscle *(P)* are also seen. The *dotted line* outlines the distal radius.

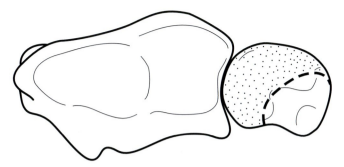

FIGURE 58.8. The extent of the ulnar head resection to obtain a matched resection of the radius is shown.

The ulnar-based retinacular and capsular flap is now mobilized to perform the interposition arthroplasty. The capsular component is mobilized and interposed between the radius and ulna (Fig. 58.9). It may be sutured to the volar aspect of the sigmoid notch. This minimizes the risk of migration. The retinacular flap is now sutured to the 1-mm stump of tissue previously left attached to the dorsal aspect of the radius (Figs. 58.9 and 58.10). This transfers the ECU tendon to the dorsal aspect of the ulna, which helps to provide distal ulna stability (Figs. 58.9 and 58.10). In addition, this tightens the ECU subsheath attachments to the distal ulna and TFCC, which also provides distal ulnar stability. The distal supratendinous portion of the retinaculum is now repaired to prevent bowstringing of the EDQ tendon. Final wound closure is performed after deflating the tourniquet and obtaining hemostasis. Drains are not required.

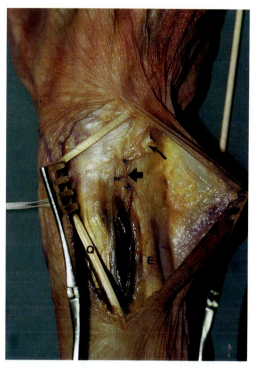

FIGURE 58.10. The repaired capsular retinacular flap is seen *(arrow)*. This completes the matched hemiresection–interposition arthroplasty. The distal retinacular flap *(curved arrow)* has not yet been sutured over the extensor digiti quinti *(Q)* tendon. The extensor carpi ulnaris *(E)* tendon has now been moved to the dorsum of the ulna in comparison to Fig. 58.1.

POSTOPERATIVE MANAGEMENT

The wrist is immobilized in a below-elbow cast for 6 weeks, at which time the patient starts a gradual return to normal activities. Hand therapy is not required for the majority of the patients. The ulnar-based interposition flap provides a secure and stable construct to stabilize the distal ulna. If concern exists about distal ulnar instability, especially in a case where the TFCC cannot be preserved, then a modified postoperative regimen has been helpful. In these occasional cases, the wrist and forearm are immobilized in a muenster cast in full supination for 6 weeks rather than being allowed immediate rotation. After the cast is removed, physiotherapy and supination splinting are then required to recover full supination, but in these patients, a pain-free DRUJ without instability has been noted.

CLINICAL CASE

A 31-year-old woman presented with a 7-year history of DRUJ pain. Physical examination, bone scans, and radiographs (Fig. 58.11) were consistent with DRUJ arthritis. Slight instability of the DRUJ was present. The patient sub-

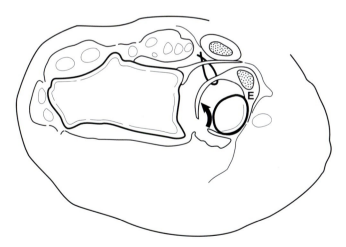

FIGURE 58.9. The interposition arthroplasty is diagrammed. The capsular flap *(curved arrow)* is interposed between the radius and the ulna. The ulnar aspect of the previously divided retinaculum is sutured to the radial remnant to stabilize the interposition. The extensor carpi ulnaris (ECU) tendon *(E)* can be seen to move to the dorsal aspect of the ulna as the ECU subsheath and the retinaculum are tightened.

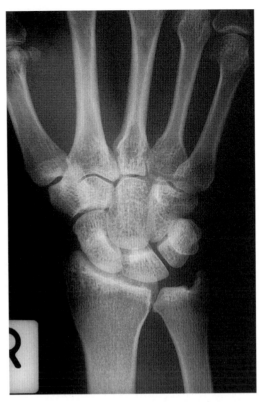

FIGURE 58.11. This posteroanterior radiograph of a 31-year-old woman shows distal radioulnar joint arthritis.

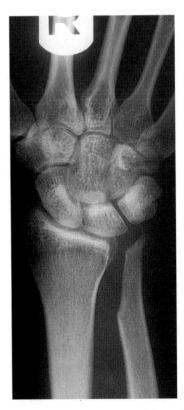

FIGURE 58.12. Postoperative posteroanterior radiograph showing the matched hemiresection–interposition arthroplasty.

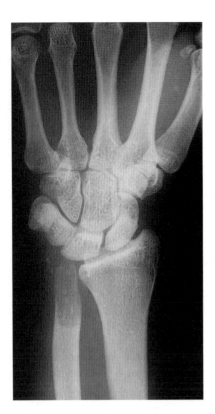

FIGURE 58.13. Postoperative posteroanterior radiograph in full supination showing the appearance of the matched hemiresection–interposition arthroplasty. No radioulnar impingement can be seen.

sequently underwent matched hemiresection–interposition arthroplasty of the DRUJ. Because of the preoperative clinical instability, she was managed with a muenster cast in full supination postoperatively. Follow-up radiographs are shown (Figs. 58.12–58.14). She is pain-free with full pronation and supination and no residual instability.

CLINICAL SERIES

A review of 49 patients at an average follow-up of 36 months (range, 12–85 months) was performed (12). Assessment consisted of objective, subjective, and functional outcomes. Thirty-five patients (72%) reported pain improvement, 10 had no change, and four were worse. Forty-one patients (84%) reported that they had a satisfactory outcome. On average, patients reported a 54% improvement in pain and a 64% satisfaction rating. Patients with rheumatoid arthritis reported an average pain improvement of 58%.

Range of motion improved postoperatively. Supination improved from 54° preoperatively to 72° postoperatively. This was 96% of the contralateral side. Pronation improved from 67° preoperatively to 72° postoperatively. This was 87% of the contralateral side.

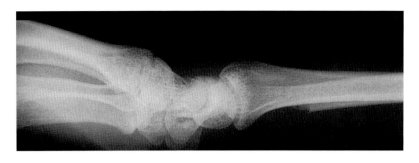

FIGURE 58.14. Although the patient had ulnar instability preoperatively, no dorsal subluxation of the ulna is present postoperatively. Clinically, the distal ulna is stable.

Functional testing was performed using the Jebsen test (16) and the Minnesota Rate of Manipulation Test (17). Patients showed difficulty in turning objects compared to published normative values. They required 86% longer to turn large objects on the Jebsen test and 53% longer to turn small objects on the Minnesota Rate of Manipulation Test.

Sixteen patients had a piano key sign with abnormal motion of the distal ulna with ballottement. In none of these patients was this symptomatic.

RADIOGRAPHIC RESULTS

Nine of the 49 patients showed x-ray film evidence of ulnocarpal impaction. Four of these patients required surgical revision, which consisted of distal ulnar shortening and a repeat matched hemiresection–interposition arthroplasty.

No patients showed radiographic signs of radioulnar impingement or scalloping.

COMPLICATIONS

One patient developed a wound infection that resolved following drainage and antibiotic therapy. One patient developed reflex sympathetic dystrophy that resolved with sympathetic blockade. One patient developed a neuroma of the dorsal sensory branch of the ulnar nerve.

Four patients required secondary surgery for ulnocarpal impaction. All patients had relief of symptoms after distal ulnar shortening. One WCB patient required secondary surgery for persistent pain. Despite removal of an ossicle from the DRUJ and further ulnar shortening, the patient continued to report pain.

There were no cases of ECU instability or subluxation. No patients required secondary surgery for distal ulnar instability. No patients required secondary surgery for radioulnar impingement.

DISCUSSION

Our technique of matched hemiresection–interposition arthroplasty differs from that described by Bowers (2,3). Separate retinacular flaps and capsular flaps are developed in Bowers' technique. The dorsal capsular flap can become thin or be button-holed during elevation. Because no attempt is made to separate the retinacular and capsular flaps, the dissection is technically simpler. In addition, the combined flap is more robust and easier to manipulate and suture. Finally, mobilizing the combined flap moves the ECU tendons to the dorsal aspect of the ulna (Figs. 58.9 and 58.10). This, combined with tightening the ECU subsheath attachments, may contribute to distal ulnar stability.

Our results are similar to both those reported by Bowers (2) as well as Watson (11). Bowers reported that 11% of patients had persistent pain, and Watson reported that 32% (11) and 25% (18) had persistent pain. Our higher incidence of persistent pain compared to Bowers' results may reflect the fact that our patients rated their own pain. Patients reported pain during heavy repetitive activities or at the extremes of rotation. Other studies have not used visual analog patient rating scales.

Ulnocarpal impaction was reported by Bowers in 5 of 38 patients (3) and by Faithfull in 2 of 155 (5). This is slightly more common than our series. We feel this results from careful fluoroscopic assessment at the time of surgery and immediate distal ulnar shortening if ulnocarpal impingement is seen. The ability to treat potential ulnocarpal impingement simply with the same surgical procedure is one of the strengths of the matched hemiresection–interposition arthroplasty.

Treatment recommendations for ulnocarpal impingement have included placement of an anchovy or ulnar shaft shortening. The authors have concerns about whether the anchovy will remain properly anchored and effective in all phases of DRUJ motion. As well, ulnar shaft shortening has the potential problem of nonunion. For this reason the authors' preferred treatment for ulnocarpal impingement is distal ulnar shortening at the time of the original procedure. If noted secondarily, distal ulnar shortening with revision of the hemiresection arthroplasty is performed. This has been successful in our patients to date.

Watson notes that one advantage of the matched resectional arthroplasty is greater forearm rotation because the interposition may hinder motion. In his published series (11,18), the postoperative forearm rotation is greater than in our patients. However, we feel that the interposition arthroplasty has an advantage in minimizing the risk of radioulnar impingement. Watson noted that 3 of 32 patients required secondary surgery for radioulnar impingement. Only one patient in our series had evidence of radioulnar impingement, with a small ossicle being present in the DRUJ. We feel that interposition arthroplasty plays a role in minimizing postoperative impingement and pain. The additional rotation of a matched ulnar arthroplasty alone may not be significant in most activities.

CONCLUSION

The primary indication for matched hemiresection–interposition arthroplasty remains pain secondary to derangements of the DRUJ. Pain relief and a high level of patient satisfaction can be expected after surgery. Although objective and functional deficits can be elicited on postoperative testing, these are not commonly associated with symptomatic problems. Ulnocarpal impingement may occur postoperatively in spite of attention to detail at the time of surgery. This can be satisfactorily treated with distal ulnar shortening and repeat matched hemiresection–interposition arthroplasty. The modified technique described here is simple to perform with a high level of patient satisfaction.

EDITORS' COMMENTS

There are many philosophies for the removal or resection of the DRUJ. The distal end of the ulna may be sacrificed without compromising wrist function. The wrist does not need the distal end of the ulna in any sense. The distal ulna will come to bear the carpals if there is panligamentous destruction as with rheumatoid arthritis or severe particulate synovitis. The wrist dislocates, downslope, over the ulna. This is not an acceptable wrist, and carpal realignment on the distal end of the radius is the best answer as described under rheumatoid wrist reconstruction.

There is no place for the Sauvé-Kapandji procedure, as under no circumstances does the wrist require the distal end of the ulna. Understanding this does not free one to resect the distal end of the ulna indiscriminately, as there are two major problems that occur following distal ulna resection: one is impingement of the ulna against the radius, and the other is winging of the free end of the remaining ulna. The best solution for a dislocated ulna or malaligned DRUJ is any procedure that will realign the DRUJ and preserve the articular cartilage on both surfaces. If there has been cartilage destruction, the solution usually requires resection. Shaping the distal end of the ulna over a prolonged sloping contour, making it parallel to the ulnar cortex of the radius, is the best solution for impingement. Leaving the ulna as long as the articular surface of the radius is the best solution for winging, as the ulnar sling mechanism will attach and stabilize the sufficiently long ulna.

The two relatively parallel surfaces between the radius and ulna are the chief defense against impingement. A sharp-cornered ulna cut off perpendicular to its long axis will impact on the radius no matter how much soft tissue is initially crammed between the two bones at surgery. It, therefore, becomes unnecessary to place any soft tissue between the two bones as long as they are relatively parallel in nature.

One need not be overly concerned with leaving periosteum or the sheath of the ECU attached to the end of the ulna. If there is a raw cancellous surface from full pronation to full supination or over the 180° surface arc of the distal ulna, the ulna sling mechanism will firmly adhere under all circumstances to the end of the ulna.

It is usually necessary to remove the ulnar styloid to achieve an ulna whose distal extent does not protrude beyond the articular surface of the radius. If one simply resects the head of the ulna, the ulna will in effect migrate radially, and the ulnar styloid will then impact on the ulnarmost carpals.

The operation is best carried out with a longitudinal incision directly over the ulna, between the ECU and the digital extensors. Resection should include 5 to 6 cm of the distal end of the remaining ulna. Immobilization is not necessary after this procedure. A bulk hand dressing with plaster splint is applied for 48 hours, and full mobilization with full activity is allowed at that time. One can not prevent adhesion of the ligamentous collagenous structures of the ulna sling mechanism to the distal end of the raw ulna. The authors mention 6 weeks of below-elbow casting, but because below-elbow immobilization limits only flexion–extension of the wrist and does not prevent full supination–pronation, these patients are effectively fully mobilized as of surgery. This may be accomplished more effectively and more comfortably without any external support. A light dressing over the wound at 48 hours will suffice.

It should be noted that the most common indication for a matched ulnar arthroplasty, with or without any capsular interposition, is following a Colles' fracture. The radius fracture shortens and usually dislocates the DRUJ. The ulna remains unfractured except, on occasion, for the styloid. The post-Colles' patient frequently is symptomatic at the DRUJ itself along with some ulnar carpal impaction component. The ulnar impaction component reduces wrist flexion–extension. These patients, often elderly, are reluctant to undergo malunion surgery to the radius. The day surgery, matched ulnar arthroplasty and 48 hours of immobilization, is minimal morbidity for a significant gain. The typical success of this procedure frequently leads the patient to more complex repair of dorsal tilt, midcarpal instability, malalignment, and other problems.

REFERENCES

1. Darrach W. Partial excision of the lower shaft of the ulna for deformity following Colles' fracture. *Ann Surg* 1913;57:764–765.
2. Bowers WH. Distal radioulnar joint arthroplasty. Current concepts. *Clin Orthop* 1992;275:104–109.
3. Bowers WH. Distal radioulnar joint arthroplasty: the hemiresection–interposition technique. *J Hand Surg [Am]* 1985;10:169–178.
4. Imbriglia JE, Matthews D. Treatment of chronic post-traumatic dorsal subluxation of the distal ulna by hemiresection–interposition arthroplasty. *J Hand Surg [Am]* 1993;18:899–907.
5. Faithfull DK, Kwa S. A review of distal ulnar hemi-resection arthroplasty. *J Hand Surg [Br]* 1992;17:408–410.
6. Minami A, Kaneda K, Itoga H. Hemiresection–interposition arthroplasty of the distal radioulnar joint associated with repair of triangular fibrocartilage complex lesions. *J Hand Surg [Am]* 1991;16:1120–1125.
7. Minami A, Suzuki K, Suenaga N, et al. Hemiresection–interposition arthroplasty for osteoarthritis of the distal radioulnar joint. *Int Orthop* 1995;19:35–39.
8. Minami A, Ogino T, Minami M. Treatment of distal radioulnar disorders. *J Hand Surg [Am]* 1987;12:189–196.
9. Imbriglia JE. Matthews D. The treatment of chronic traumatic subluxation of the distal ulna by hemiresection interposition arthroplasty. *Hand Clin* 1991;7:329–34.
10. Fernandez DL. Radial osteotomy and Bowers arthroplasty for malunited fractures of the distal end of the radius. *J Bone Joint Surg Am* 1988;70:1538–1551.
11. Watson HK, Ryu J, Burgess RC. Matched distal ulnar resection. *J Hand Surg [Am]* 1986;11:812–817.
12. Bain GI, Pugh DM, MacDermid JC, et al. Matched hemiresection interposition arthroplasty of the distal radioulnar joint. *J Hand Surg [Am]* 1995;20:944–950.
13. Bieber EJ, Linscheid RL, Dobyns JH, et al. Failed distal ulna resections. *J Hand Surg [Am]* 1988;13:193–200.
14. Kessler I, Hecht O. Present application of the Darrach procedure. *Clin Orthop* 1970;72:254–260.
15. Taleisnik J. The Sauvé-Kapandji procedure. *Clin Orthop* 1992;275:110–123.
16. Jebsen RH, Taylor N, Triesman RB, et al. An objective and standardized test of hand function. *Arch Phys Med Rehabil* 1969;50:311–319.
17. *Minnesota Rate of Manipulation Tests. Examiners Manual.* Circle Pines, MN: American Guidance Service, 1969.
18. Watson HK, Gabuzda M. Matched distal ulnar resection for posttraumatic disorders of the distal radioulnar joint. *J Hand Surg [Am]* 1992;17:724–730.

59

MATCHED ULNAR ARTHROPLASTY

JEFFREY WEINZWEIG
H. KIRK WATSON

INDICATIONS

The distal radioulnar joint (DRUJ) is a complex structure that plays a significant role in permitting normal pronosupination of the forearm and facilitating normal function of the upper extremity. A DRUJ affected by conditions such as degenerative disease, posttraumatic subluxation or dislocation, or rheumatoid arthritis will often result in pain and loss of active rotation of the forearm (1,2). DRUJ subluxation or significant ulnar positive variance may also result in ulnar impaction syndrome with substantial pain and diminished wrist function (Fig. 59.1). The matched ulnar arthroplasty addresses the problematic DRUJ articular surface or malpositioned distal ulnar head and restores painless pronosupination while preserving the triangular fibrocartilage complex (TFCC) and the ligamentous attachments of the distal ulna (Fig. 59.2) (3,4).

Preoperative evaluation of patients with carpal pathology involving the DRUJ and ulnar side of the wrist requires a focused physical examination and plain radiographic assessment. These patients usually present with complaints including generalized ulnar wrist pain, especially with attempted pronosupination, loss of strength, and considerable restriction of motion. There may or may not be a specific history of previous wrist trauma.

Physical examination usually produces pain with radioulnar compression and demonstrates significantly decreased pronation and supination. Clinical suspicion of pathology involving the DRUJ and/or distal ulna is often confirmed radiographically. Degenerative disease involving the DRUJ and pathology involving the distal ulna, such as ulnar impaction and ulnar impingement, are usually appreciated on plain radiographs without the need for additional, or more invasive, radiologic studies (Fig. 59.3).

CONTRAINDICATIONS

The success of the matched ulnar arthroplasty may be limited by concomitant carpal pathology, such as radiocarpal degenerative joint disease or carpal instability, but such pathology does not preclude the use of this technique for addressing disorders arising from the DRUJ or distal ulnar head. In addition, the matched ulnar arthroplasty is not contraindicated in the patient with ulnar impingement on the radius following a Darrach resection. Salvage is possible by combining the matched ulnar resection with a step-cut ulnar lengthening (5).

SURGICAL TECHNIQUE

The distal ulna is approached through a longitudinal incision, approximately 6 cm in length, along the lateral aspect of the ulna, beginning at the level of the ulnar head. A spreading technique is utilized to preserve superficial veins as well as the dorsal branch of the ulnar nerve, and the dissection is continued down to the ulna. The 180° arc of the ulna that is in contact with the radius from full pronation to full supination is resected in a long, sloping, convex curve averaging 5 to 6 cm in length. This convex curve matches the contour of the opposing concave radius in three dimensions, thereby ensuring that there is no impingement during full pronosupination of the forearm (Fig. 59.4). This is performed intraoperatively to verify the congruity of the opposing radial

---

J. Weinzweig: Department of Plastic Surgery, Brown University School of Medicine, Rhode Island Hospital, and Hasbro Children's Hospital, Providence, Rhode Island 02905.

H. K. Watson: Connecticut Combined Hand Surgery Fellowship, Hartford Hospital, and Connecticut Children's Medical Center, Hartford, Connecticut 06106; Department of Orthopaedics, University of Connecticut School of Medicine, Farmington, Connecticut 06032; Department of Orthopedics, Rehabilitation, and Plastic Surgery, Yale University School of Medicine, New Haven, Connecticut 06520.

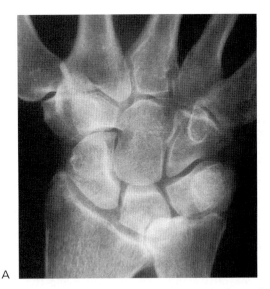 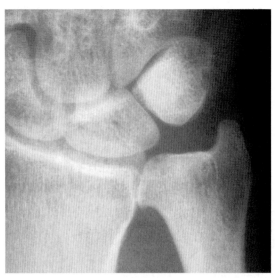

FIGURE 59.1. A,B: Complete destruction of the distal radioulnar joint is present with no remnant cartilage and no potential for preserving the distal ulna. Matched ulnar arthroplasty is indicated.

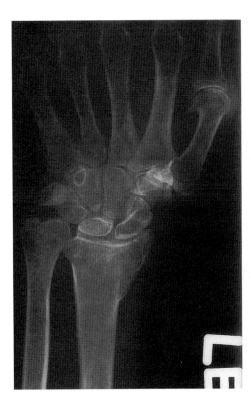 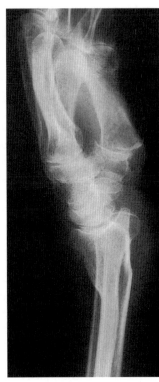

FIGURE 59.2. Dislocation or impaction and malalignment of this distal ulna is probably best managed in this age group with a matched ulnar arthroplasty. The ulna is resected from the full pronation position to the full supination position of the radius. The resection is carried out in such a manner that the shape of the ulna matches the shape of the radius. This includes resection of the dorsal flare of the radius sulcus. It is not necessary to leave soft tissue attached, as the ulnar sling mechanism will firmly reattach itself to the broad cancellous ulnar surface. The sheath of the extensor carpi ulnaris can be left on the cortical portion of the ulna, but this is not a necessary step. It is important to leave the tip of the ulna at the level of the articular surface of the radius.

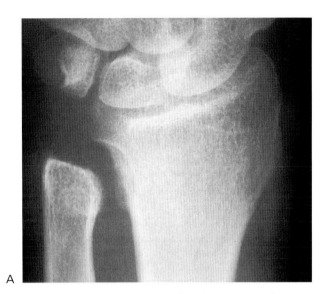
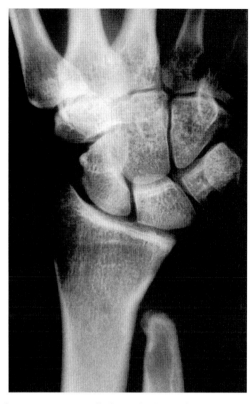

FIGURE 59.3. A,B: An ulna that is resected transversely or very proximally has a high incidence of impingement on the radius. Both views demonstrate significant symptomatic impingement of the ulna against the radius with resultant periosteal and bone reaction (see Figure 59.6).

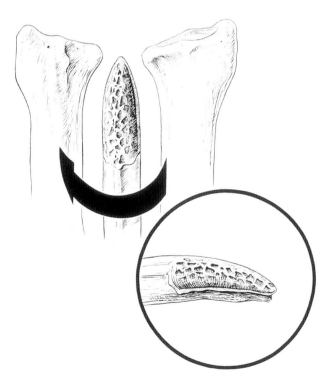

FIGURE 59.4. The alignment, position, and slope parallelism between the radius and the distal end of the ulna following matched ulnar arthroplasty are illustrated. This parallelism is maintained from full pronation to full supination.

and ulnar surfaces. Once the head of the ulna has been resected, the ulna will shift toward the radius. This usually requires ulnar styloid resection. It is important to leave the distalmost tip of the resected ulna at, or just proximal to, the level of the articular surface of the radius (Fig. 59.5).

If the ulna impinges on the carpus in ulnar deviation, only the necessary minimal amount of distal ulna is resected to permit clearance. This resection is performed without disrupting the remaining periosteum and ligamentous attachments to the distal ulna. The 180° arc of ulna cortex is maintained to the level of the articular surface of the radius. The deep fascia of the extensor carpi ulnaris sheath may remain attached to the periosteum of the ulna and contribute to stabilizing the ulna during the healing process. The large cancellous surface of the resected distal ulna will become securely adherent to the ulnar sling mechanism in any case without the need for sutures or fixation. (The ulnar sling mechanism includes the ligamentous structures that begin at the ulnarmost aspect of the distal radius and continue to the ulnar, superficial part of the extensor carpi ulnaris sheath. The TFCC and its palmar and dorsal reflections are included, as are the ulnotriquetral ligament, the ulnolunate ligament, and the DRUJ capsule.) Soft tissue interposition is not necessary. The skin incision is closed, and a bulky dressing incorporating a plaster splint to immobilize the wrist is applied.

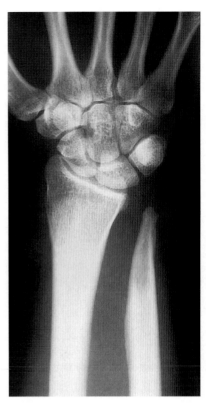

FIGURE 59.5. The ulna has been matched to the shape of the radius. The parallel surfaces cannot impinge on each other; this parallelism is preserved throughout full pronosupination. The ulna has been maintained at or near the the level of the articular surface of the distal radius, where it is long enough to be ensnared by the ulna sling mechanism, preventing winging. The preoperative radiograph for this patient is seen in Fig. 59.1B.

The radius sulcus joint presents two situations that can adversely affect the outcome of a matched ulnar arthroplasty. Occasionally, the slope of the sulcus of the radius is reversed. When seen on a posteroanterior film, the proximal portion of the radius sulcus protrudes more ulnarward than the distal portion. Thus, the slope of the radius sulcus joint in this case may be considered to be directed from proximal ulnar to distal radial. When the joint is sloped in this fashion, the proximal portion of the sulcus joint must be removed with a rongeur to prevent its impingement on the ulna. Secondly, flaring of the edges of the radius sulcus joint frequently occurs. These radial flares occur more commonly dorsally than palmarly and may be normal for a particular individual or represent secondary degenerative osteophytic formations. They can be directly palpated intraoperatively and may be significant. If they protrude ulnarward more than a few millimeters, they should be removed with a rongeur to prevent impingement of the ulna on either the palmar or dorsal flares at the extremes of supination or pronation, respectively.

POSTOPERATIVE MANAGEMENT

The bulky dressing and splint are removed 7 days postoperatively, and the wrist is fully mobilized.

CLINICAL SERIES

Eighty-eight patients (97 wrists) underwent matched ulnar arthroplasty over a 21-year period; nine patients underwent bilateral arthroplasty (6,7). The most common preoperative diagnoses were rheumatoid disease in 34 wrists (35%) and ulnar impaction syndrome in 25 wrists (26%). Additional diagnoses included degenerative disease of the DRUJ (four wrists), ulnar impingement following Darrach resection (three wrists), Colles' fractures (12 wrists), premature closure of the distal ulnar epiphysis following following fracture (one wrist), DRUJ dislocation or subluxation (three wrists), and Madelung's deformity (two wrists).

Sixty-seven patients were available for follow-up at a mean of 64 months postoperatively. Fifty-eight percent of patients were pain-free on follow-up examination, which included assessment of pronosupination and compression of the DRUJ in full pronation. An additional 32 percent of patients experienced mild pain that did not restrict use of the wrist. The remaining 10% of patients complained of moderate pain that resulted in some activity limitations; each of these patients had experienced a complicated course that included either degenerative disease of the radiocarpal joint, limited wrist arthrodesis for a scapholunate advanced collapse (SLAC) wrist or rotary subluxation of the scaphoid, comminuted intraarticular fracture of the distal radius, previous Darrach resection, bone spur formation at the site of the resected ulnar head, or previous radial osteotomy. No patient experienced severe pain that prevented the performance of work or leisure activities.

The average total arc of forearm rotation was 169°, with an average of 80.5° pronation and 88.5° supination, compared with 90° of pronation and 90° of supination on the unaffected contralateral side.

COMPLICATIONS

Few complications occurred following matched ulnar arthroplasty. A wound infection occurred in one patient; it responded well to immobilization and antibiotic therapy. Three patients experienced symptoms of radioulnar impingement secondary to periosteal bone spur formation at the site of the previous ulnar head resection. These patients responded well to excision of the spurs. One patient required reoperation for lysis of a neuroma *in situ* of the dorsal sensory branch of the ulnar nerve. Eight patients developed a triquetral impingement ligament tear (TILT) at a mean of 34 months following matched ulnar arthroplasty; two of these patients had also undergone a concomitant ulnar step-lengthening osteotomy (8). All of these patients demonstrated excellent range of motion and were pain-free following TILT repair (see Chapter 40).

MATCHED ULNAR RESECTION FOR ULNAR IMPINGEMENT

Patients who are symptomatic secondary to ulnar impingement, in whom the distal end of a shortened ulna contacts or impinges on the radius during the range of pronosupination, can be managed by performing a step-cut ulnar lengthening osteotomy along with a matched resection. This problem is not infrequently seen as a consequence of an overzealous Darrach resection in which the remaining distal ulna is left without a support mechanism. In this situation, the unstable distal ulna is free to impinge on the radius. Following appropriate lengthening and lag screw or plate fixation to restore the distal ulna to the level of the distal radius, a matched resection is performed in the manner described (Fig. 59.6).

MATCHED ULNAR ARTHROPLASTY RESECTION SALVAGE

There are times when, following even a properly done matched ulnar arthroplasty with proper length and shaping of the ulna and radius, bone overgrowth and painful impingement against the radius occur. If the ulna is simply too short, a step-cut lengthening of the ulna and matching of the newly lengthened distal segment is the best solution. If the ulna is long enough and still impacts uncomfortably on the radius, the effective salvage procedure includes the following:

1. Bony resection of the distal radius, in particular, the dorsal flare of the sulcus joint that faces the ulna, the most common area of impingement. The entire distal radius may be reshaped on its ulnar aspect to achieve

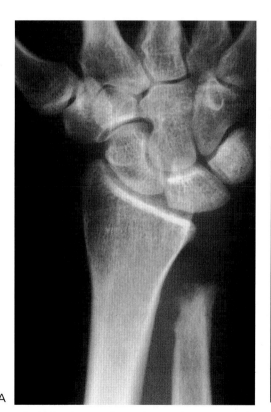 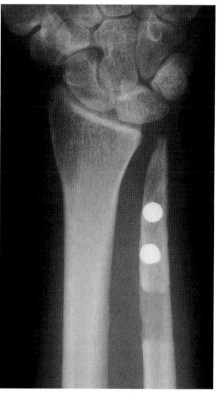

FIGURE 59.6. A: A short ulna resulting in radial impingement produces a significantly symptomatic wrist in this female patient. **B:** The only adequate solution to this problem is a step-cut lengthening of the ulna to bring it up to the ulnar sling mechanism and to reshape the distal end of the ulna at the time of osteotomy to match the shape of the radius. In essence, the result is conversion from the ulnar resection to a matched ulnar arthroplasty. It is not necessary to reattach soft tissue to the distal ulna.

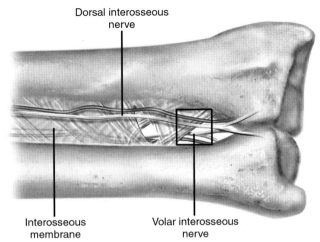

FIGURE 59.7. Interosseous neurectomy. Approximately 3 cm proximal to the distal end of the ulna, the volar and dorsal interosseous nerves lie only 1 to 2 mm apart on opposite sides of the interosseous membrane. They are readily visualized, and a 1-cm section of each is removed without disturbing the interosseous arteries lying proximate to them.

parallelism between the radius and ulna ("matched radius arthroplasty").

2. A neurectomy or transection of both the volar and dorsal interosseous nerves in the distal forearm. These are approached through the longitudinal ulnar incision by dissection across the dorsal interosseous membrane and transection of the dorsal interosseous nerve 3 to 4 in. above the wrist. A small hole in the interosseous membrane gives direct access for transection of the volar interosseous nerve, which lies immediately volar. The volar interosseous artery is protected as it lies alongside (Fig. 59.7).

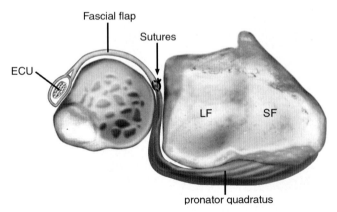

FIGURE 59.8. Pronator quadratus flap. The ulnarmost aspect of the pronator quadratus is transected from its attachments on the ulna. A flap of fascia is maintained during the approach, and the flap is sutured to the pronator quadratus, pulling viable muscle up between the radius and ulna. *ECU,* extensor carpi ulnaris.

3. The development of a dorsal flap of fascia based ulnarly on the sheath of the extensor carpi ulnaris. The ulnar attachments of the pronator quadratus are dissected free. The pronator quadratus is then brought up between the radius and ulna and attached to the fascial flap. This tends to force the ulna volarly and away from the radius (Fig. 59.8).

MODIFIED DRUJ ARTHROPLASTY FOR DEGENERATIVE ARTHRITIS

Patients who demonstrate degenerative joint disease of the DRUJ, but in whom there is adequate cartilage on the distal half of the ulnar head, may be treated with a modified DRUJ arthroplasty without the need for a formal matched ulnar arthroplasty. Thirty to fifty percent coverage of the articular surface of the distal half of the ulnar head with adequate cartilage is necessary to obtain satisfactory results with this procedure.

In these patients, a longitudinal dorsoulnar incision is used rather than a transverse incision, as a matched ulnar arthroplasty may be required in the future. A spreading technique is used to preserve the dorsal ulnar nerve and dorsal veins. The DRUJ capsule is opened proximally as the degenerative arthritic process almost always occurs proximally with subsequent distal progression.

The proximal half of the articular surface of the ulna is typically devoid of cartilage with osteophyte formation and a hyperemic, eburnated appearance consistent with periostitis. A dental rongeur is used to remove the entire proximal articular surface while preserving the healthy cartilage on the distal half of the articular head of the ulna. This is performed for the entire articular circumference from full pronation to full supination of the radius on the ulna. The skin incision is closed, and a bulky dressing is applied; 2 days following surgery, this dressing is removed, and full mobilization is begun.

This modified DRUJ arthroplasty has been employed over the past 15 years with excellent results. All patients have maintained full pronosupination and complete relief of symptoms on follow-up. None of these patients has required a subsequent matched ulnar arthroplasty.

DISCUSSION

The painful DRUJ represents a complex problem that often results in significantly diminished forearm pronosupination and wrist function. The articular surface of the ulna is a convex semicircle of 180° that opposes a concave radial sigmoid notch of 60° to 80°. Thus, at any position, 100° of ulnar articular surface is free from contact. Injury, destruction, dislocation, or subluxation of a portion of this articular surface is responsible for the clinical symptomatology seen with disorders of the DRUJ.

The earliest surgical approach to the problematic DRUJ was described by Darrach in 1912: a transverse resection of the distal ulna was performed for an unreduced dislocation of the distal ulna (9). Despite the potential for DRUJ destabilization by sacrifice of the ulnar sling mechanism, and for ulnar impingement syndrome with more proximal ulnar resections (10), the Darrach procedure remains one of the most common treatments for disorders of the DRUJ.

A number of additional procedures have been described for the management of the painful or unstable DRUJ. These include the hemiresection–interposition technique (11), stabilization of the ulna with tendon slings or capsular flaps (4,12), arthrodesis of the DRUJ with creation of a proximal pseudarthrosis by excision of a portion of the ulna (3,13,14), various ulna head resection or recession procedures (15–17), and preservation of ulnar length following distal resection with the use of silicone distal ulnar caps (18). Each of these approaches, however, is fraught with limitations. Techniques that significantly shorten the distal ulna have a greater likelihood of producing subsequent ulnar impingement syndrome (5,10). Excessive motion at the site of a pseudarthrosis will also produce impingement of the proximal ulna on the radius with resultant symptomatology. The use of silicone caps is limited by eventual loosening of the prosthesis, displacement of the cap, and sacrifice of the attachments of the ulnar sling mechanism to the ulna (18).

The matched ulnar arthroplasty technique restores painless pronosupination while preserving the full length of the ulna and structures crucial to stability of the DRUJ without the need for soft tissue interposition (6,7). The resultant range of motion is nearly full and painless, and stability of the wrist and DRUJ is maintained. Impingement between the radius and ulna does not occur because the gap between them is equal and congruous throughout the full arc of pronation and supination. The matched ulnar arthroplasty represents a reliable, predictable approach to the painful DRUJ. Patients with adequate cartilage on the distal half of the ulnar head may be treated with a modified DRUJ arthroplasty without the need for a formal matched ulnar arthroplasty.

REFERENCES

1. Bowers WH. The distal radioulnar joint. In: Green DP, Hotchkiss RN, Pederson WC, eds. *Operative hand surgery, 4th ed.* New York: Churchill Livingstone, 1999;986–1032.
2. Minami A, Ogino T, Minami M. Treatment of distal radioulnar joint disorders. *J Hand Surg [Am]* 1987;12:189–196.
3. Goncalves D. Correction of disorders of the distal radioulnar joint by articifical pseudoarthrosis of the ulna. *J Bone Joint Surg Br* 1974;56:462–464.
4. Goldner JL, Hayes MG. Stabilization of the remaining ulna using one-half of the extensor carpi ulnaris tendon after resection of the distal ulna. *Orthop Trans* 1979;3:330–331.
5. Watson HK, Brown RE. Ulnar impingement syndrome after Darrach procedure: Treatment by advancement lengthening osteotomy of the ulna. *J Hand Surg [Am]* 1989;14:302–306.
6. Watson HK, Gabuzdo GM. Matched distal ulna resection for posttraumatic disorders of the distal radioulnar joint. *J Hand Surg [Am]* 1992;17:724–730.
7. Watson HK, Ryu J, Burgess RC. Matched distal ulnar resection. *J Hand Surg [Am]* 1986;11:812–817.
8. Watson HK, Weinzweig J. Triquetral impingement ligament tear (TILT) syndrome. *J Hand Surg [Br]* 1999;24:350–358.
9. Darrach W. Anterior dislocation of the head of the ulna. *Ann Surg* 1912;56:802–803.
10. Bell MJ, Hill RJ. Ulnar impingement syndrome. *J Bone Joint Surg Br* 1985;67:126–129.
11. Bowers WH. Distal radioulnar arthroplasty: The hemiresection–interposition technique. *J Hand Surg [Am]* 1985;10:169–178.
12. Blatt G, Ashworth CR. Volar capsule transfer for stabilization following resection of the distal ulna. *Orthop Trans* 1979;3:13–14.
13. Kapandji IA. The Kapandji-Sauve procedure. *J Hand Surg [Br]* 1992;17:125–126.
14. Sauvé K. Nouvelle technique de traitement chirurgical des luxations recidivantes isolees de l'extremitie inferieure du cubitus. *J Chir* 1936;47:589–594.
15. Black RM, Boswick JA, Wiedel J. Dislocation of the wrist in rheumatoid arthritis: The relationship to distal ulna resection. *Clin Orthop* 1977;124:184–188.
16. Darrow JC, Linscheid RL, Dobyns JH, et al. Distal ulnar recession for disorders of the distal radioulnar joint. *J Hand Surg [Am]* 1985;10:482–491.
17. Jackson IT, Milward TM, Lee P, et al. Ulnar head resection in rheumatoid arthritis. *Hand* 1974;6:172–180.
18. Berg E. Indications for, and results with, the Swanson distal ulnar prosthesis. *South Med J* 1976;69:858–861.

RADIAL SHORTENING OSTEOTOMY

EDWARD A. STOKEL
THOMAS E. TRUMBLE

Avascular necrosis of the lunate, or Kienböck's disease, is thought to occur after repetitive trauma selectively loads the lunate, resulting in disruption or stasis of the intraosseous blood supply (1–3). Kienböck's disease is associated with a negative ulnar variance, and radial shortening osteotomy to level the joint surface between the radius and ulna has developed into a primary form of treatment (4,5). Clinical studies have supported the concept of shortening the radius to minimize the compressive loads across the lunate (6–15). Biomechanical studies have also confirmed that joint-leveling procedures will decompress the lunate in patients with negative ulnar variance (16–18).

INDICATIONS

Patients with a negative ulnar variance and no significant collapse or fragmentation of the lunate are ideal candidates for a radial shortening osteotomy (Lichtman class I–IIIA) (19). Some reports indicate that patients with lunate fragmentation or early degenerative changes at the radiocarpal or midcarpal joint may also benefit from the procedure (8,11,13). Once the lunate has collapsed, resulting in rotation of the scaphoid and an increase in the scapholunate angle greater than 60°, an intercarpal arthrodesis is required to maintain carpal height (8,19,20). Scaphotrapeziotrapezoid (STT) arthrodesis and scaphocapitate arthrodesis will stabilize the carpus from collapsing to a dorsal intercalated segment instability (DISI) pattern. These intercarpal arthrodeses permanently unload the lunate; therefore, revascularization is irrelevant because the lunate never bears significant load again (18). Even selected patients who are ulnar neutral may benefit from the procedure, provided there are no degenerative changes (11). A radial shortening osteotomy is not recommended for patients with an ulnar positive variance. In these rare cases, a shortening osteotomy of the capitate is recommended for patients with a positive ulnar variance and stage I to IIIA Kienböck's disease (21). In the presence of mild arthrosis, radial shortening remains the most conservative surgical choice and does not compromise later surgical options if shortening is unsuccessful. Patients with advanced degenerative changes at the radiocarpal joint are treated by wrist arthrodesis (19).

Ulnar variance determination should be performed in a standardized manner with the forearm in neutral rotation, the elbow flexed 90°, and the shoulder abducted 90° (22). Trumble et al., in a biomechanical study, concluded that 2 mm of radial shortening resulted in optimal lunate decompression (18). Greater shortening increased the risk of distal radioulnar joint disorders and ulnar impingement. This value has been corroborated by clinical studies (11,15). If ulna impingement does occur, symptoms usually resolve with ulna shortening (15,23).

SURGICAL TECHNIQUE

Shortening of the radius is performed at the distal end, through either a dorsal or volar approach. The dorsal approach avoids major neurovascular structures, involves a minimum of soft tissue dissection, and provides excellent exposure. The dorsal surface, however, is convex and irregular, and Lister's tubercle may need to be removed in order to accommodate the plate. The plate occupies a subcutaneous position and may irritate extensor tendons. Proximal dissection is somewhat limited by the extensor pollicis longus and abductor pollicis longus muscles, which cross the operative field. Postoperative scarring near the dorsal capsule may limit palmar flexion.

The volar surface of the distal radius is flat and easily accommodates a contoured plate. The overlying pronator quadratus and flexor pollicis longus muscles protect the long flexor tendons. The dissection can easily be extended proximally. The volar approach involves more dissection, and the radial artery, palmar cutaneous branches of the

---

E. A. Stokel: Private Practice, Danville, California 94526.
T. E. Trumble: Department of Orthopaedics, University of Washington, and Harborview Medical Center, Seattle, Washington 98195.

median nerve, and superficial branches of the radial nerve are at risk for injury.

We have tried both techniques and have found them equally acceptable. The advantages of one surgical approach are not clearly outweighed by the disadvantages of the other. Technically, the dorsal approach is easiest, especially if the surgeon does not have an assistant. The volar approach may cause less tendon irritation. The operation is performed under regional or general anesthesia with tourniquet control.

Volar Approach

The volar approach to the distal radius is a classic extensile approach. The patient is placed supine on the operating table with the arm in a fully supinated position on the arm board. Skin markings are made identifying the flexor carpi radialis tendon and the radial artery (Fig. 60.1). The limb is exsanguinated with an esmarch bandage, and the tourniquet is inflated. A longitudinal incision is made on the distal forearm, immediately radial and parallel to the flexor carpi radialis tendon. The incision does not need to cross the wrist crease but should extend proximally for 10 to 12 cm. The superficial veins are identified and coagulated. Superficial sensory nerve branches are identified and protected. The flexor carpi radialis and radial artery are identified, and the incision is deepened between the tendon sheath and the radial artery (Fig. 60.2). A cuff of soft tissue is preserved against the radial artery for additional protection. The pronator quadratus and the flexor pollicis longus muscles are identified on the volar surface of the distal radius. With the arm partially pronated, their insertion from the lateral aspect of the radius can be identified and the muscles mobilized by subperiosteal dissection. A cuff of

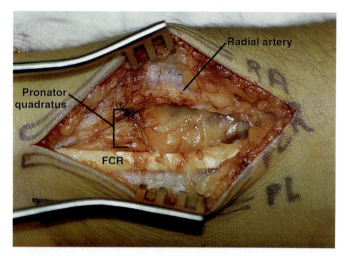

FIGURE 60.2. The flexor carpi radialis (*FCR*) and the radial artery are exposed. Note the cuff of tissue protecting the radial artery. The pronator quadratus is covered with a layer of fatty tissue.

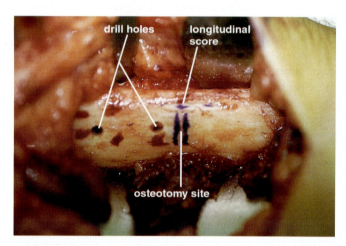

FIGURE 60.3. The volar cortex of the distal radius is exposed. Distal drill holes have already been placed. The osteotomy site is marked in pen, and longitudinal scoring is noted on the volar surface for rotational control.

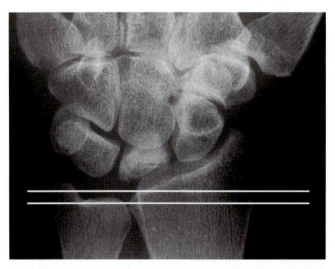

FIGURE 60.1. Avascular necrosis of the lunate with no significant arthrosis or carpal collapse. Neutral posteroanterior view demonstrates 2 mm of negative ulnar variance.

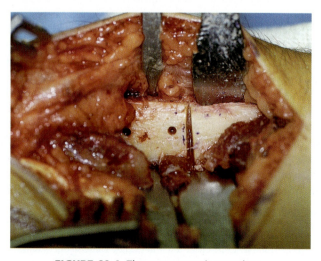

FIGURE 60.4. The osteotomy is complete.

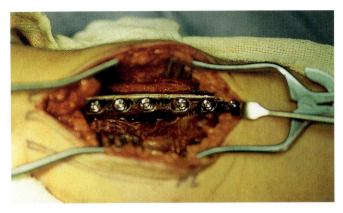

FIGURE 60.5. The six-hole DCP is applied. The three distal holes are paced in neutral fashion, and the proximal three holes are placed eccentrically away from the osteotomy site, resulting in compression across the osteotomy.

tendinous tissue at the muscles' insertion is preserved for later repair. This exposes the distal one-third of the radius.

The osteotomy site is selected at the metadiaphyseal junction and marked with a pen. The bone is scored longitudinally for correct rotational alignment. A six-hole 3.5-mm DCP or T-plate is selected, depending on the contours of the volar aspect of the radius. The plate is secured with plate-holding clamps. The distal holes are then drilled and tapped in neutral fashion to accommodate cortical screw fixation. The plate is then removed (Fig. 60.3). The osteotomy is performed with an oscillating saw. Parallel transverse cuts are made, removing 2 mm of bone, including the width of the saw blade (Fig. 60.4). Two stacked blades can also provide the necessary amount of shortening, resulting in a parallel osteotomy with a single cut. The reader is referred to the article by Labosky and Waggy for further information about the amount of bone that can be removed by the saw kerf (24). The distal cut is performed first, as it is easier to stabilize the proximal forearm when making the second cut. If necessary, the proximal cut may be slightly angled to adjust radial inclination.

The proximal and distal sections of the radius are then approximated, and the parallel contact of the osteotomized surface is verified. The plate is secured distally using the previously drilled holes. Rotation is verified using the longitudinal scoring, and the plate is clamped proximally. The proximal holes are drilled sequentially, and cortical screws are eccentrically placed away from the osteosynthesis site to provide compression (Fig. 60.5). Intraoperative anteroposterior and lateral radiographs are obtained to confirm plate placement and screw length (Fig. 60.6). Any available excess bone from the osteotomy is packed around the radius to stimulate osteosynthesis.

The pronator quadratus and flexor pollicis longus muscles are repaired to the radius using interrupted absorbable sutures (Fig. 60.7). The tourniquet can be released at this point to control hemostasis. The subcuticular structures

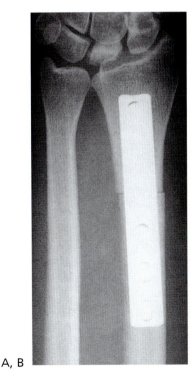 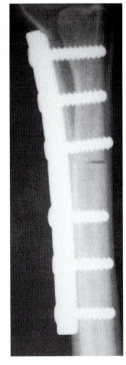 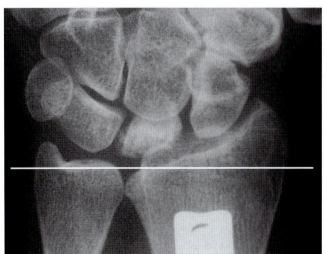

A, B   C

FIGURE 60.6. Anteroposterior **(A)** and lateral **(B)** x-rays demonstrating the osteotomy site and osteosynthesis. **C:** Postoperative neutral posteroanterior x-ray of the distal radius demonstrating the shortened radius. Compare the ulnar variance to that in Fig. 60.1.

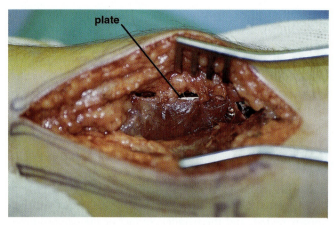

FIGURE 60.7. The pronator quadratus has been reattached to the radius with multiple sutures. A portion of the plate is visible.

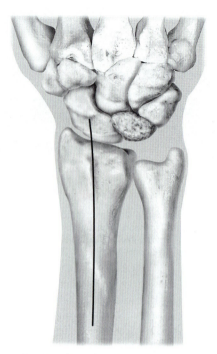

FIGURE 60.8. The dorsal approach to the distal radius extends from 2 cm distal to Lister's tubercle, proximally for 8 to 10 cm.

are closed in layers using absorbable sutures, and the skin is closed with interrupted nylon sutures. Drains are not routinely necessary. A sterile dressing is applied, followed by a plaster splint, holding the wrist in slight dorsiflexion.

Active digital motion is encouraged immediately. Sutures are removed at 14 days, and a removable wrist splint is applied. Occupational therapy to increase digital motion and begin wrist motion is started, and the splint is worn for all activities for 6 weeks. Light strengthening exercises are advanced as symptoms allow. Patients should have resumed daily activities by 6 weeks and all activities by 3 months.

Dorsal Approach

The patient is placed supine on the operating table, with the arm in a fully pronated position on the arm board. Skin markings are made identifying Lister's tubercle. The limb is exsanguinated with an esmarch bandage, and the tourniquet inflated. A longitudinal incision is made on the dorsal aspect of the distal forearm at a point 2 cm distal to Lister's tubercle and extending proximally for 8 to 10 cm (Fig. 60.8). Large superficial veins are identified and protected. Smaller veins are coagulated. Superficial sensory nerve branches are identified and retracted out of the field. The interval between the extensor pollicis longus and extensor digitorum communis is identified, and the roof of the third compartment is divided. The extensor pollicis longus tendon is retracted out of the field. The septa between the third and fourth compartments are divided proximally, and the extensor retinaculum, including the fourth compartment tendons, is subperiosteally dissected in a radial and ulnar direction (Fig. 60.9). The fourth compartment itself should be preserved to mini-

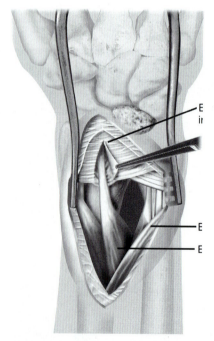

FIGURE 60.9. The third compartment has been divided, and the extensor pollicis longus tendon is retracted out of the field. The fourth compartment tendons and the proximal portion of the extensor retinaculum are subperiosteally dissected in a radial and ulnar direction, exposing the dorsum of the distal radius.

mize postoperative scarring and bowstringing of the tendons. If necessary, the entire septa between the third and fourth compartments can be divided to allow complete subperiosteal exposure of the distal radius. The interval between the extensor carpi radialis brevis and extensor digitorum communis is subperiosteally developed proximally to expose the dorsal-radial aspect of the distal radius. The extensor pollicis longus and abductor pollicis longus muscles are retracted out of the field. Two Penrose drains may be looped around opposite tendons and clamped volar to provide additional retraction.

The osteotomy site is selected at the metadiaphyseal junction, proximal to the distal radial ulnar joint (DRUJ), and marked with a pen (Fig. 60.10). The osteotomy site may be confirmed using fluoroscopy because it is important to be distal enough to take advantage of metaphyseal bone, yet proximal enough to insure that three screws can be placed in the distal fragment. The bone is also scored longitudinally for rotational alignment. A 3.5-mm T-plate is selected and contoured to the dorsal aspect of the radius. Removal of Lister's tubercle with a rongeur is usually necessary to accommodate the plate. The plate is secured with plate-holding clamps, and the distal drill holes, osteotomy, reduction, and plate fixation are identical to those described in the volar approach (Fig. 60.11). A 0.062-in. Kirschner wire may be temporarily driven through the radial styloid, across the osteotomy, and into the opposite cortex for additional stabilization. Intraoper-

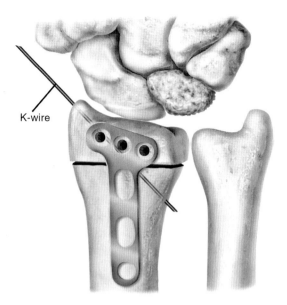

FIGURE 60.11. The T-plate is secured proximally and distally. A temporary K-wire is placed across the radial styloid for stability while the screws are placed proximally.

ative radiographs are obtained to confirm reduction and plate placement.

The extensor retinaculum is repaired using permanent sutures, allowing the extensor pollicis longus tendon to pass superficial to the extensor retinaculum. Periosteal repair is usually not possible, due to the bulk of the plate. The extensor tendons are protected by replacing the muscles over the plate. The tourniquet can be deflated at this point to control hemostasis. The subcuticular structures are closed in layers using interrupted absorbable sutures. The skin is approximated using interrupted nylon sutures and drains are not routinely necessary. A sterile dressing is applied, followed by a volar plaster splint holding the wrist is slight extension. Postoperative therapy and recovery are identical to that described previously.

COMPLICATIONS

Complications following radial shortening are rare. Persson reported three cases of nonunion and instead proposed ulna lengthening (25). Nonunion has, since then, been reported only rarely by other authors. Schattenkerk et al. (14) reported one nonunion in 20 cases, and Weiss et al. (15) reported one nonunion in 30 cases. Other authors have reported no nonunions (1,8,11,13,23). Tendinitis and irritation from retained plates are also possible. The dorsal plates should be removed approximately 12 months following complete healing to minimize tendon irritation. In general, volar plates do not need removal.

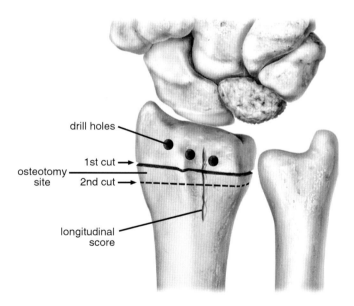

FIGURE 60.10. The osteotomy site has been selected at the metadiaphyseal junction and marked with a pen. Longitudinal scoring for correct rotational alignment is noted. The distal screw holes have already been drilled and tapped.

EDITORS' COMMENTS

Kienböck's is discussed in detail in Section IX. We have never performed a radial shortening osteotomy with or without tilting. We have never performed an ulnar lengthening or shortening osteotomy for Kienböck's disease. It is our strong assumption that the benefits from these procedures are the operative stimulus and the immobilization time that lets the lunate recover. There are many ulnas with a normal ulnar negative variance, and these patients do not develop Kienböck's disease. We would list a short ulna as one relatively small factor in the overload of the lunate and the development of fault plates within the lunate that may eventually wall off and produce areas of inadequate vascularity. Fault plates can heal with decreased load on the lunate. Lack of "intraosseous recovery time" is a major etiologic factor in Kienböck's disease. The primary treatments include prevention of the extremes of motion, prevention of load, temporary pinning of the STT joint to unload the lunate, and fusion of the STT joint to permanently unload the lunate. Almost any surgical approach with an uncollapsed early Kienböck's disease followed by weeks of immobilization for whatever procedure are probably the key factors in healing the lunate.

REFERENCES

1. Gelberman RH, Bauman TD, Menon J, et al. The vascularity of the lunate bone in Kienböck's disease. *J Hand Surg [Am]* 1980;5:272–278.
2. Jensen CH. Intraosseous pressure in Kienböck's disease. *J Hand Surg [Am]* 1993;18:355–359.
3. Schiltenwolf M, Martini AK, Mau HC, et al. Further investigation of the intraosseous pressure characteristics in necrotic lunates (Kienböck's disease). *J Hand Surg [Am]* 1996;21:754–758.
4. Gelberman RH, Salamon PB, Jurist JM, et al. Ulnar variance in Kienböck's disease. *J Bone Joint Surg Am* 1975;57:674–676.
5. Hulten O. Uber anatomische variationen der handgelenkknochen. En beitrag zur kenntnis der genese zwei verschiedener mondbein-veranderungen. *Acta Radiol* 1928;9:155–168.
6. Almquist EE, Burns JF. Radial shortening for the treatment of Kienböck's disease—a 5- to 10- year follow-up. *J Hand Surg [Am]* 1982;7:348–352.
7. Axelsson R, Moberg E. The treatment of Kienböck's disease and the role of joint levelling operations. In: *The wrist*. Edinburgh: Churchill Livingstone, 1986;194–201.
8. Condit DP, Idler RS, Fischer TJ, et al. Preoperative factors and outcome after lunate decompression for Kienböck's disease. *J Hand Surg [Am]* 1993;18:691–696.
9. Eiken O, Nicchajev I. Radius shortening in malacia of the lunate. *Scand J Plast Reconstr Surg* 1980;14:191–196.
10. Kinnard P, Tricoire JL, Basora J. Radial shortening for Kienböck's disease. *Can J Surg* 1983;26:261–262.
11. Nakamura R, Imaeda T, Miura T. Radial shortening for Kienböck's disease: Factors affecting the operative result. *J Hand Surg [Br]* 1990;15:40–45.
12. Ovesen J. Shortening of the radius in the treatment of lunatomalacia. *J Bone Joint Surg Br* 1981;63:231–232.
13. Rock MG, Roth JH, Martin L. Radial shortening osteotomy for treatment of Kienböck's disease. *J Hand Surg [Am]* 1991;16:454–458.
14. Schattenkerk ME, Nollen A, van Hussen F. The treatment of lunatomalacia. Radial shortening or ulna lengthening? *Acta Orthop Scand* 1987;58:652–654.
15. Weiss APC, Weiland AJ, Moore JR, et al. Radial shortening for Kienböck's disease. *J Bone Joint Surg Am* 1991;73:384–390.
16. Horii E, Garcia-Elias M, An KN, et al. Effect of force transmission across the carpus in procedures used to treat Kienböck's disease. *J Hand Surg [Am]* 1990;15:393–400.
17. Masear VR, Zook EG, Pichora DR, et al. Strain-gauge evaluation of lunate unloading procedures. *J Hand Surg [Am]* 1992;17:437–443.
18. Trumble T, Glisson RR, Seaber AV, et al. A biomechanical comparison of the methods for treating Kienböck's disease. *J Hand Surg [Am]* 1986;11:88–93.
19. Coe MR, Trumble TE. Biomechanical comparison of methods used to treat Kienböck's disease. *Hand Clin* 1993;9:417–429.
20. Watson HK, Monacelli DM, Milford RS, et al. Treatment of Kienböck's disease with scaphotrapezio-trapezoid arthrodesis. *J Hand Surg [Am]* 1996;21:9–15.
21. Almquist EE. Capitate shortening in the treatment of Kienböck's disease. *Hand Clin* 1993;9:505–512.
22. Palmer AK, Glisson RR, Werner FW. Ulnar variance determination. *J Hand Surg [Am]* 1982;7:376–379.
23. Almquist EE. Kienböck's disease. *Hand Clin* 1987;3:141–148.
24. Labosky DA, Waggy CA. Oblique ulnar shortening osteotomy by a single saw cut. *J Hand Surg [Am]* 1996;21:48–59.
25. Persson M. Causal treatment of lunatomalacia: further experiences of operative ulna lengthening. *Acta Chir Scand* 1950;100:531–534.

61

RADIOCARPAL ARTHRODESIS–ARTHROPLASTY FOR RHEUMATOID ARTHRITIS

H. KIRK WATSON
JEFFREY WEINZWEIG

INDICATIONS

Wrist instability and pain severely limit the function of the hand in most rheumatoid patients, 95% of whom demonstrate some degree of wrist involvement (1). Radiocarpal ligament attenuation, ulnar translocation, distal radioulnar joint dislocation, and carpal collapse are common sequelae of rheumatoid arthritis involving the wrist. Such destructive carpal processes are indications for the radiocarpal "nonunion" or pseudarthrosis arthrodesis–arthroplasty procedure (2). Matched ulnar arthroplasty and the rheumatoid wrist procedure described herein are typically performed together (Fig. 61.1). The matched ulnar arthroplasty (3,4), which restores full supination and pronation and eases positioning for the subsequent procedure, is performed first (see Chapter 59).

CONTRAINDICATIONS

A small subset of rheumatoid patients with painful wrists but with minimal destruction of bone may benefit from a simple synovectomy before the "nonunion" arthroplasty is performed. However, subsequent major cartilage loss and bony destruction are indications for performing the "nonunion" arthroplasty.

H. K. Watson: Connecticut Combined Hand Surgery Fellowship, Hartford Hospital, and Connecticut Children's Medical Center, Hartford, Connecticut 06106; Department of Orthopaedics, University of Connecticut School of Medicine, Farmington, Connecticut 06032; Department of Orthopedics, Rehabilitation, and Plastic Surgery, Yale University School of Medicine, New Haven, Connecticut 06520.
J. Weinzweig: Department of Plastic Surgery, Brown University School of Medicine, Rhode Island Hospital, and Hasbro Children's Hospital, Providence, Rhode Island 02905.

SURGICAL TECHNIQUE

The wrist procedure is begun with a dorsal transverse incision 4 to 5 mm proximal to the tip of the radial styloid. A spreading technique elevates and preserves the branches of the superficial radial nerve, dorsal ulnar nerve, and dorsal veins. The extensor retinaculum is incised on the radial border of the second dorsal compartment along the extensor carpi radialis longus tendon. The first dorsal compartment, unless significantly involved with rheumatoid synovitis, is usually not included in the procedure. The extensor retinaculum is then elevated beginning on the radial side and cutting the septa of the various intercompartment attachments, progressing from radially to ulnarward until the retinaculum is attached only ulnarly to the extensor carpi ulnaris (Fig. 61.2A). Some soft tissue is left on Lister's tubercle, as this will be used to resuture the retinaculum during closure. A #15 blade is then used to incise the dorsal extensor ligaments of the wrist. These are incised on their ulnarmost border at the triquetrum, and the entire dorsal ligamentous structure is raised as one segment and gradually cut toward the radial side until the extensor retinaculum is reflected radially but maintains its most radial attachments. A radical synovectomy is performed on all extensor compartments as the extensor retinaculum is reflected. The synovium is removed from the deep surface of this flap of extensor ligaments of the wrist. The synovium is then removed from the intercarpal and radiocarpal joints with dental rongeurs.

The wrist is flexed, and complete direct visualization of the carpals and entire distal surface of the radius is easily achieved. With a dental rongeur, the remnant of articular cartilage and cortex on the distal radius surface is removed, and a cancellous concavity is formed. On occasion, a drill is used to allow introduction of one blade of the dental rongeur. Typically, rheumatoid bone is soft enough that the

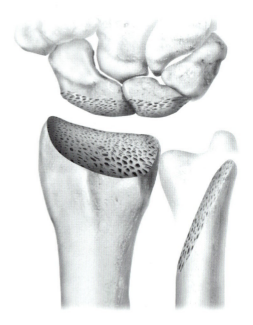

FIGURE 61.1. The "nonunion" or pseudarthrosis arthroplasty. The cancellous concavity in the distal radius and the cancellous convexity formed of the scaphoid and lunate are demonstrated. The scaphoid and lunate are nested into this concavity, cross-pinned for 2 weeks, and then fully mobilized. The procedure is combined with a matched ulnar arthroplasty.

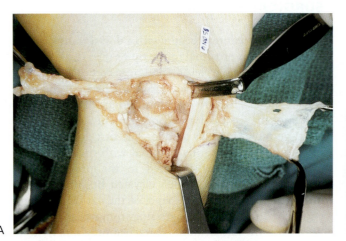
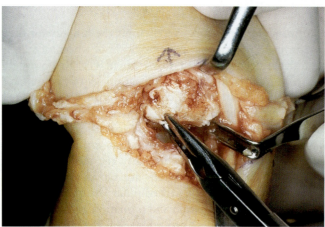
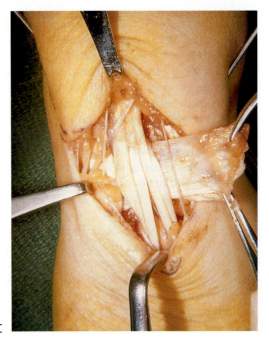

FIGURE 61.2. A: The extensor retinaculum is elevated from the extensor compartments, leaving it attached to the ulnar side of the extensor carpi ulnaris. The extensor ligaments of the wrist are cut free on the ulnar aspect and dissected free of the dorsum, leaving them attached on the radialmost aspect of the wrist. **B:** Dental rongeurs are used to remove the cartilage and subchondral bone remnants from the proximal surfaces of the scaphoid and lunate and shape these into a convexity that will fit the concavity formed in the distal radius. **C:** The ligaments of the wrist may be placed between the radius and the scaphoid and lunate or placed back across the dorsum of the wrist. The extensor retinaculum is placed deep to all tendons except the extensor pollicis longus. A stitch is placed in Lister's tubercle to hold the extensor pollicis longus in its compartment. It is the only tendon that will elevate the thumb into the plane of the fingers.

rongeur alone will easily form a cancellous concavity in the radius. The radial styloid is removed, and the dorsal ridge on the radius is also excised, particularly toward the radial side. The remnant articular cartilage and eburnated bone are then removed from the proximal surfaces of the scaphoid and lunate to form a cancellous convexity (Fig. 61.2B). The convex cancellous scaphoid and lunate are multifitted into the concavity in the radius; the triquetrum is usually partially excised to allow the lunate to sit properly in the concavity of the radius. This is necessary because the triquetrum will often impinge on the ulnarmost aspect of the radius and prevent seating of the scaphoid and lunate. When proper alignment and seating have been achieved, two 0.062-in. pins are run in retrograde crisscross fashion from the radial concavity out radially through the radius and out ulnarward, dorsal to the ulna. At this point, the scaphoid and lunate cancellous convexities are placed in the concavity of the radius. The wrist is aligned, and the pins are driven distally, often up into the metacarpals, depending on the degree of destruction in the wrist. The wrist is now maintained in place; the pins are cut off subcutaneously and left buried.

The extensor ligaments of the wrist are then laid back across the radial carpal joint. The extensor retinaculum is fed back from the ulnar side deep to the extensor carpi ulnaris, the extensor digiti quinti minimi, and the contents of the fourth dorsal compartment (Fig. 61.2C). The extensor pollicis longus, however, is placed back behind Lister's tubercle, beneath the extensor retinaculum. The extensor retinaculum is then positioned beneath the extensor carpi radialis longus and brevis on the radial side. The decreased range of motion in the wrist and the lack of significant dorsiflexion obviate the need for a retinaculum to prevent bowstringing. The extensor pollicis longus is placed beneath the retinaculum, as it is the only tendon that will raise the thumb into the plane of the fingers; unless it is maintained in its compartment, it will act simply as an abductor. The retinaculum is sutured to Lister's tubercle using 5-0 Dexon. This maintains the extensor pollicis longus in its compartment beneath the retinaculum. The radial edges of the retinaculum are sutured back to their origin on the radial aspect of the second dorsal compartment. The dorsal skin wound is closed with 4-0 subcuticular wire. A bulky dressing incorporating a dorsal plaster splint is applied in typical fashion.

On occasion, in patients with severe destruction of the midcarpal joints, in whom ligamentous structures are fairly tight, we have placed the extensor ligaments of the wrist into the concavity of the radius and set the scaphoid and lunate on this soft tissue collagenous interposition. This ensures nonunion of the scaphoid and lunate, and as long as there is an adequate concavity in the distal radius, instability has not been a problem.

Matched ulnar arthroplasty is often performed at the time of "nonunion" arthroplasty (Fig. 61.3). When it is combined with rheumatoid wrist surgery, a minor modification of the matched ulnar arthroplasty is performed. A slight degree of additional shortening of the ulna is usually necessary to prevent impaction on the carpal bones as they are settled into the concavity in the distal radius. Thus, the distal ulna may be trimmed back slightly proximal to the distal articular surface of the radius, the level to which the ulna is routinely trimmed in a nonrheumatoid matched ulnar arthroplasty.

POSTOPERATIVE MANAGEMENT

The dressing is changed in 2 days, and volar and dorsal plaster splints are applied to maintain the position of the wrist. At 2 weeks, both pins are removed, and the patient may use a volar removable splint for comfort and increased mobilization and load tolerance.

CLINICAL SERIES

Eighty-three patients with rheumatoid arthritis underwent 92 "nonunion" arthroplasty procedures over an 18-year period. Each of these patients underwent simultaneous matched ulnar arthroplasty. Additional procedures in this group included repair of ruptured extensor tendons, metacarpophalangeal (MP) joint arthrodesis of the thumb, MP arthroplasty of the thumb, and carpal tunnel release. The mean patient age at the time of surgery was 53 years (range, 14–75 years); 83% of the patients were female. All unilateral cases except three involved the dominant wrist.

Twenty-three patients (32 wrists) were evaluated at a mean follow-up period of 7.4 years following "nonunion" arthroplasty (range, 2–16 years). Nine of these patients had undergone bilateral arthroplasty. A fibrous nonunion was achieved at the radiocarpal level in 10 wrists (31.2%). These wrists were immobilized for 2 weeks with pins. Radiocarpal fusion occurred in 19 wrists (59.4%); fusion between the radius and lunate only occurred in 3 wrists (9.4%) (Fig. 61.4). None of the patients in whom a fibrous nonunion occurred experienced pain despite complaints of severe pain preoperatively. The mean arc of motion was 68° (30.5° extension, 37.5° flexion). Twelve of the 19 patients in whom a radiocarpal fusion occurred complained of mild pain that did not limit wrist loading. The mean arc of motion was 44° (18.7° extension, 25.3° flexion). One of the three patients in whom radiolunate fusion occurred complained of mild pain that did not limit activities. The mean arc of motion was 41.6° (16.6° extension, 25° of flexion). Pronation and supination were very good to excellent in most patients (mean pronation 81.7°, supination 88.9°). Subsequent carpal subluxation did not occur in any patient in this series.

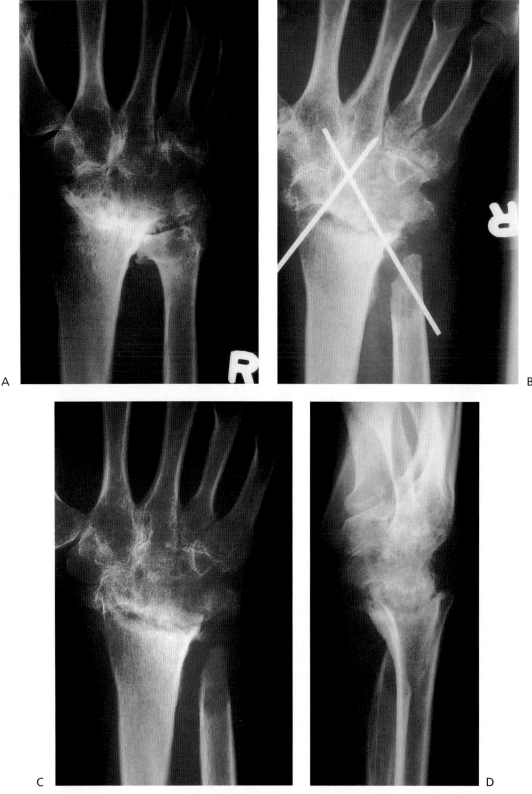

FIGURE 61.3. A: Rheumatoid destruction has obliterated the cartilage of the radial carpal joints with significant sclerosis and ulnar translation. **B:** For 2 weeks following surgery, the cross pins maintain carpal alignment and position. A matched ulnar arthroplasty has also been performed, maintaining the ulna at or near the radiocarpal joint level. **C:** Radiocarpal motion has been maintained. These motion areas are not joints and are not affected by the rheumatoid disease. They maintain their alignment, stability, and motion permanently. **D:** The plane of radiocarpal motion is demonstrated on this lateral radiograph.

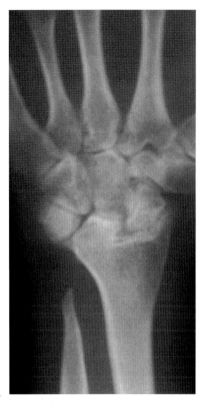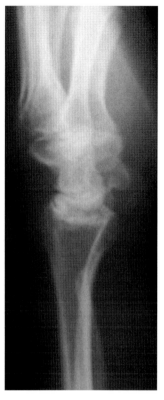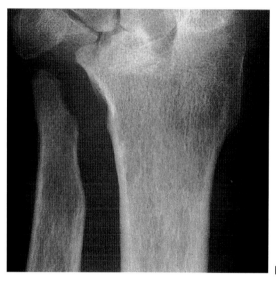

FIGURE 61.4. A: Despite early motion, a complete fusion of the radius–lunate joint has occurred. Motion is taking place in the perilunate joints following the rheumatoid wrist procedure. **B:** In this case, both the scaphoid and lunate have fused to the radius. Note the parallel surfaces between the radius and ulna following matched arthroplasty.

COMPLICATIONS

One wound infection occurred that resolved with immobilization and antibiotic therapy. No other complications occurred in this series of patients. None of the patients required a subsequent operative procedure on the wrist following the "nonunion" arthroplasty.

DISCUSSION

The painful rheumatoid wrist represents a complex problem often resulting in significantly limited hand and wrist function. A number of procedures have been described for management of the rheumatoid wrist, including complete wrist arthrodesis (5–9), limited wrist arthrodesis (10,11), soft tissue stabilization techniques (12–16), and wrist arthroplasty (17–24). Each of these is fraught with limitations. Complete wrist arthrodesis alleviates pain but also sacrifices all radiocarpal motion. This is especially debilitating in patients with MP joint involvement. Soft tissue stabilization procedures are not feasible in patients with severe deformity in which the soft tissue structures are also compromised. Silicone prostheses can result in bony impingement and pain secondary to settling of the implant into the soft bone, but use of a cemented total wrist arthroplasty remains controversial.

The "nonunion" arthroplasty is a modified form of limited wrist arthrodesis in which a radiocarpal fusion is performed; however, pin removal at 2 weeks and immediate wrist mobilization encourage formation of a radiocarpal pseudarthrosis—a "nonunion." The radiocarpal pseudarthrosis that forms permits long-term painless motion in the rheumatoid patient. Prolonged immobilization for patients undergoing combined procedures such as extensor tendon repair and thumb MP joint fusion reduces the incidence of pseudarthrosis formation. For patients in whom at least limited wrist motion is crucial, staging these procedures might more predictably yield the sought-after pseudarthrosis.

REFERENCES

1. Short CL, Bauer W, Reynolds WE. *Rheumatoid arthritis: a definition of the disease and clinical description based on a numerical study of 293 patients and controls.* Cambridge, MA: Harvard University Press, 1957.
2. Ryu J, Watson HK, Burgess RC. Rheumatoid wrist reconstruc-

tion utilizing a fibrous nonunion and radiocarpal arthrodesis. *J Hand Surg [Am]* 1985;10:830–836.
3. Watson HK, Gabuzdo GM. Matched distal ulna resection for posttraumatic disorders of the distal radioulnar joint. *J Hand Surg [Am]* 1992;17:724–730.
4. Watson HK, Ryu J, Burgess RC. Matched distal ulnar resection. *J Hand Surg [Am]* 1986;11:812–817.
5. Skak SV. Arthrodesis of the wrist by the method of Mannerfelt. A follow-up of 19 patients. *Acta Orthop Scand* 1982;53:557–559.
6. Mannerfelt L, Malmsten M. Arthrodesis of the wrist in rheumatoid arthritis. *Scand J Plast Reconstr Surg* 1971;5:124–130.
7. Millender LH, Nalebuff EA. Arthrodesis of the rheumatoid wrist. An evaluation of sixty patients and a description of a different surgical technique. *J Bone Joint Surg Am* 1973;55:1026–1034.
8. Howard AC, Stanley D, Getty CJM. Wrist arthrodesis in rheumatoid arthritis: A comparison of two methods of fusion. *J Hand Surg [Br]* 1993;18:371–380.
9. Kobus RJ, Turner RH. Wrist arthrodesis for treatment of rheumatoid arthritis. *J Hand Surg [Am]* 1990;15:541–546.
10. Ishikawa H, Hanyo T, Saito H, et al. Limited arthrodesis for the rheumatoid wrist. *J Hand Surg [Am]* 1992;17:1103–1109.
11. Chamay A, Della Santa D, Vilaseca A. Radiolunate arthrodesis in rheumatoid wrist. *Ann Hand Surg* 1991;10:197–206.
12. Leslie BM, Carlson G, Ruby LK. Results of extensor carpi ulnaris tenodesis in the rheumatoid wrist undergoing a distal ulnar excision. *J Hand Surg [Am]* 1990;15:547–551.
13. Boyce T, Youmn Y, Sprague BL, et al. Clinical and experimental studies on the effect of extensor carpi radialis longus transfer in the rheumatoid hand. *J Hand Surg [Am]* 1978;3:390–394.
14. Koka R, D'Arcy JL. Stabilization of the wrist in rheumatoid disease. *J Hand Surg [Br]* 1989;14:288–290.
15. Blatt G, Ashworth CR. Volar capsule transfer for stabilization following resection of the distal end of the ulna. *Orthop Trans* 1979;3:13.
16. Ruby LK, Ferenz CC, Dell PC. The pronator quadratus interposition transfer: An adjunct to resection arthroplasty of the distal radioulnar joint. *J Hand Surg [Am]* 1996;21:60–65.
17. Beckenbaugh RD. Total joint arthroplasty: The wrist. *Mayo Clin Proc* 1979;54:513–515.
18. Nylen S, Sollerman C, Haffajee D, et al. Swanson implant arthroplasty of the wrist in rheumatoid arthritis. *J Hand Surg [Am]* 1984;9:295–299.
19. Goodman MJ, Millender LH, Nalebuff EA, et al. Arthroplasty of the rheumatoid wrist with silicone rubber: An early evaluation. *J Hand Surg [Am]* 1980;5:114–121.
20. Jolly SL, Ferlic DC, Clayton ML, et al. Swanson silicone arthroplasty of the wrist in rheumatoid arthritis: A long term follow-up. *J Hand Surg [Am]* 1992;17:142–149.
21. Fatti JF, Palmer AH, Mosher JF. The long term results of Swanson silicone rubber interpositional wrist arthroplasty. *J Hand Surg [Am]* 1986;11:166–175.
22. Volz RG. The development of a total wrist arthroplasty. *Clin Orthop* 1976;116:209–214.
23. Beckenbaugh RD. Arthroplasty of the wrist. In: Morrey BF, ed. *Joint replacement arthroplasty.* New York: Churchill Livingstone, 1991;195–215.
24. Menon J. Total wrist replacement using the modified Volz prosthesis. *J Bone Joint Surg Am* 1987;69:998–1006.

RADIOLUNATE ARTHRODESIS

PHILIPPE SAFFAR

Radiolunate arthrodesis was first used by Chamay and Della Santa (1) to treat ulnar shift of the carpus in patients with rheumatoid arthritis but has rarely been used in posttraumatic wrists. The results have not been clearly defined in the literature because of the small number of cases (2–7).

Emergency treatment of intraarticular distal radial fractures has evolved, and reduction is performed using adapted devices, bone grafts, or arthroscopy. Knirk and Jupiter (8) demonstrated that a 2-mm residual step in the joint may result in radiocarpal osteoarthritis. Their findings have been confirmed by others (9,10). Kopylov et al. (11) and Chamay and Della Santa (1) reported good results after conservative treatment in spite of intraarticular malunion.

Few papers in the literature have dealt with the treatment of distal radius intraarticular malunions. Several types of distal radius malunions may be classified. We concentrate on malunions affecting the lunate fossa when the radioscaphoid cartilage contour is preserved. If the lunate fossa is displaced but the cartilage is preserved, osteotomy and reduction of the displaced fragment are performed. If the cartilage is destroyed, a radiolunate arthrodesis may be indicated (Fig. 62.1).

INDICATIONS

Radiolunate arthrodesis is indicated for distal radial intraarticular malunion centered on the radial lunate facet with or without dorsal subluxation of the carpus. The primary symptom is pain, but decreased motion and strength are associated complaints. Another indication for radiolunate arthrodesis is stabilization of a dorsal radiocarpal subluxation with dorsal rim impaction (Fig. 62.2). The aims are to restore carpal height and allow scaphoid realignment, to relieve pain, to restore strength and motion, and to prevent further osteoarthritis.

P. Saffar: Department of Hand Surgery, Hopitaux Boucicaut, 75730 Paris, and Institut Français de Chirurgie de la Main, 92200 Paris, France.

SURGICAL TECHNIQUE

A lazy-S dorsal wrist approach is used. It extends parallel and medial to Lister's tubercle, from 5 cm proximal to 3 cm distal to the radiocarpal joint.

The dorsal retinaculum overlying the fourth compartment is incised longitudinally. The extensor digitorum communis tendons are then retracted, and the dorsal radius periosteum is incised longitudinally in line with the dorsal wrist capsule. The periosteum is carefully elevated on each side of the incision to expose the inner part of the dorsal aspect of the radius. The status of the cartilage of the scaphoid and lunate fossae of the distal radius is assessed, as is the cartilage of the head of the capitate, proximal scaphoid, and lunate. Interosseous ligaments, particularly the scapholunate ligament, are inspected, as is the triangular fibrocartilage complex. A step-off in the articular cartilage as well as a dorsal or medial radiocarpal subluxation of the distal radius may be present.

A corticocancellous graft can be harvested from the iliac crest, the proximal end of the ulna, or from the radius as a sliding graft. When graft is taken from the radius as a sliding graft, a rectangular segment of dorsal radius cortex 4 mm thick is detached using an electric saw, 3 mm lateral to the medial border of the radius with a length of approximately 4 cm and a width of 12 mm (Fig. 62.3). A trough of the same width and depth is hollowed in the dorsomedial and distal part of the radius and in the dorsum of the lunate. The lunate is maintained in a slight dorsal intercalated segment instability (DISI) position during the excavation. Remnants of cartilage of the proximal lunate and lunate fossa are excised, and cancellous bone taken from the distal radius is packed between the two bones to restore the carpal height, which was decreased following the initial trauma (i.e., die-punch fracture, posteromedial fragment, dorsal rim fracture with subluxation). Manual distraction is applied to regain the normal carpal height and to disimpact the carpus from the radius, thus allowing the scaphoid to restore its normal alignment.

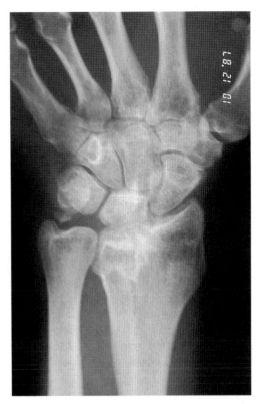

FIGURE 62.1. Intraarticular distal radius malunion localized at the lunate fossa.

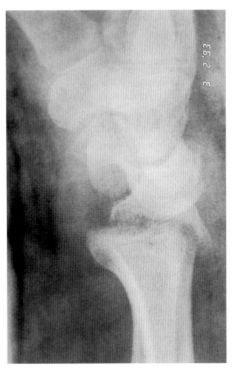

FIGURE 62.2. Dorsal radiolunate dislocation with dorsal rim impaction.

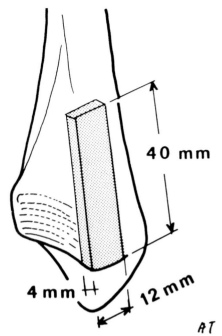

FIGURE 62.3. Graft harvested at the dorsal aspect of the distal radius.

The corticocancellous bone graft or the sliding graft is then applied in the trough (Fig. 62.4). The dorsal aspect of the graft must be at the level of the dorsal radius and thus avoid impeding the normal gliding of extensor tendons. Once the graft has been firmly secured, passive wrist motion should be assessed to rule out the possibility of impingement of the graft with the carpal bones.

Scaphoid horizontalization (Fig. 62.5) may be caused by (a) carpal impaction resulting in carpal height decrease or (b) scapholunate ligament tear. In this case, a Blatt capsulodesis procedure may be performed to restore adequate scaphoid alignment and motion. The periosteum and capsule are closed, covering the screw heads. The dorsal retinaculum and capsule are then sutured.

POSTOPERATIVE MANAGEMENT

A dressing and volar short arm splint are applied for 4 days, then replaced by a cast until union is achieved. Rehabilitation is then initiated for an average of 2 months on a daily basis to regain good range of motion.

CLINICAL SERIES

In our experience of radiolunate arthrodeses performed over a 10-year period, 15 patients (14 male, 1 female) with painful intraarticular distal radius malunions were treated. The female patient was a student. Of the 14 male patients, 12

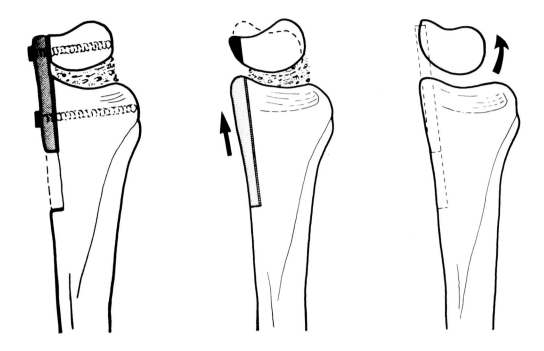

FIGURE 62.4. The graft slides dorsally and is fixed by two screws.

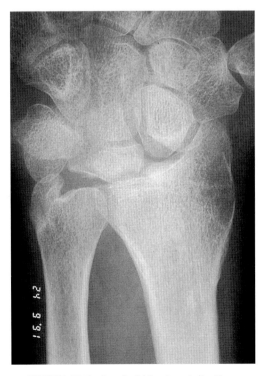

FIGURE 62.5. Scaphoid horizontalization.

were manual workers, one was a cook, and one a manager. Seven were worker's compensation cases. The average age was 33 years (range, 20–53 years). Nine of 15 involved the right hand, and 10 the dominant hand. The mechanism of injury included a fall from a height in six cases, a motorcycle injury in four, a ski accident in one, a direct blow in one, and three were unknown mechanisms. The time elapsed since injury was an average of 21.2 months (range, 2–103 months).

The initial x-rays were avalaible in 10 cases. These injuries included displaced die-punch fragments, displaced posteromedial fragments, and dorsal rim comminuted fractures often associated with dorsal subluxation. The articular step-off of the distal radius was a mean 4.4 mm (range, 3–8 mm), always with an irregular contour of the lunate fossa. In two cases, there was an irregularity of the scaphoid fossa contour. There were four cases of dorsal subluxation of the carpus.

The distance between the scaphoid and lunate, and the triquetrum and lunate, were calculated taking the proximal-lateral or proximomedial point of each bone from the corresponding point of the adjacent bone. This technique accounts for the proximal displacement of the lunate relative to the adjacent bone. The gap tended to increase on cineradiography.

Suspicion of a scapholunate interosseous ligament or a lunatotriquetral ligament tear was aroused by an increase in these gaps. The lunate presented in volar intercalated segment instability (VISI) in 11 cases and in a normal position in four cases. There was an associated dorsal tilt of the distal articular surface of the radius in three cases. Significant ulnar translation (more than 4 mm) was present in four cases. No degenerative changes were noted in the midcarpal joint, and this warrants evaluation because the residual motion will be in the perilunate and midcarpal joints. Any degenerative change of the midcarpal joint would be a contraindication to this procedure.

The distal radioulnar joint (DRUJ) was totally destroyed in four cases, and the joint surface was irregular in three cases, incongruent in five, and congruent in only three cases. There was a posterior ulnar dislocation in four cases and an anterior ulnar dislocation in one case. Four were in normal alignment.

Associated procedures are at times necessary. A distal radial osteotomy with a graft fixed with a plate and an osteotomy fixed by a screw have been performed for an associated distal radial malunion.

A carpal tunnel release was performed in two cases, one before this procedure and one at the same time. A superficial radial nerve graft was also performed in one case. A Darrach procedure was added in three cases.

A scaphoid Swanson prosthesis was inserted in two cases, one during the same procedure and one 6 months after the radiolunate procedure because of persistent radial-sided pain with an irregular radioscaphoid joint. This was at the beginning of our experience.

Combined with removal of the screws, a volar rim resection was performed for impingement of the second flexor digitorum profundus tendon against the bone.

RESULTS

Pain was present preoperatively in the majority of cases on light work. The mean preoperative range of motion was 38.6° flexion, 24.6° extension, 10° radial deviation, and 20° ulnar deviation. Grip strength measured with the Jamar dynamometer was a mean 17.7 kg (24 kg for the opposite side).

Pain decreased from continuous or present on light work to absent or climatic in all cases, stablizing after 4 months. Postoperatively, the average range of motion was 37.5° flexion, 43.3° extension, 17.9° radial deviation, and 20.8° ulnar deviation.

The average postoperative strength measured with the Jamar dynamometer was 18.5/33 kg in the opposite side compared to 17.7/24 kg preoperatively (57% of the opposite side instead of 45% preoperatively). Overuse of the noninjured side may explain the increase of strength.

The different choices of graft sources did not affect the results, and the only nonunion resulted from a fixation problem.

In 11 cases, we obtained internal fixation with two screws (Fig. 62.6), one going through the graft and the volar cortex of the radius and the second through the graft and the volar cortex of the lunate. In one case, three screws were inserted. A plate was used in one case, and staples in one case. K-wire fixation was used in one case, which resulted in the only nonunion in the series.

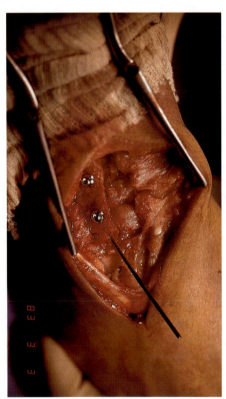 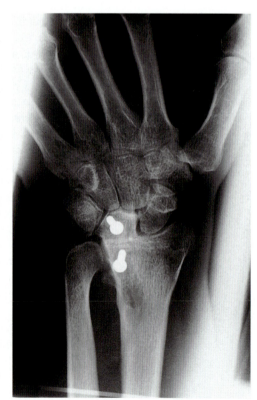 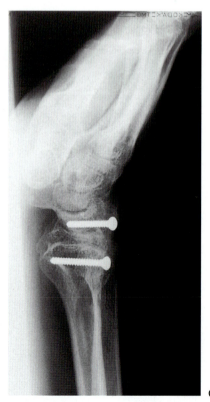

FIGURE 62.6. A: Intraoperative view of radiolunate arthrodesis. Anteroposterior **(B)** and lateral **(C)** x-rays.

POSTOPERATIVE X-RAYS

Motion of the carpus was observed on dynamic x-rays (Fig. 62.7) or cineradiographic studies and was always perilunate with occasional widening of the scapholunate space on anteroposterior views. The scaphoid did not always move normally on dynamic x-rays, which raised the question of the future evolution of the radioscaphoid joint space. On the lateral views, the motion was primarily present in the midcarpal joint.

The final position of the lunate was VISI in five cases, neutral position in four cases, and DISI in two cases. No relationship was observed between the final range of motion and the position of the lunate.

Radiographic union was achieved between 45 and 90 days in 14 of 15 cases. Extension of osteoarthritis to other joints was not observed.

One of the two scaphoid prostheses showed slight radiologic signs of "silicone synovitis" in the surrounding bones but without any clinical symptoms.

Patient satisfaction was excellent in two cases, good in five, and fair in three cases; one was unknown. Nine patients returned to their previous work, and two to lighter work; two were not recorded. The mean follow-up period was 28.5 months (range, 8–79 months).

COMPLICATIONS

There were neither infections nor cases of reflex sympathetic dystrophy. One case resulted in nonunion. It was subsequently treated by plate fixation and bone grafting with a resulting solid union.

DISCUSSION

Die-punch fractures are the result of impaction of the lunate in the lunate fossa. The pathomechanism is often a high-velocity injury with the direction of the impact in line with the forearm. The central articular fracture penetrates the subchondral bone, which is impacted and comminuted. These central fragments are difficult to reduce unless a direct approach is used. Secondary displacement and malunion are frequent. The step-off is often significant. The cartilage of the proximal lunate and of the lunate fossa is destroyed; this may be assessed by arthroscopy or CT scan after arthrography. The wrist position at the time of injury (extension, flexion, or neutral position) may result in other fracture patterns such as dorsal comminution with dorsal subluxation. This impacted fracture may be isolated or associated with other fracture lines, usually oblique, going to

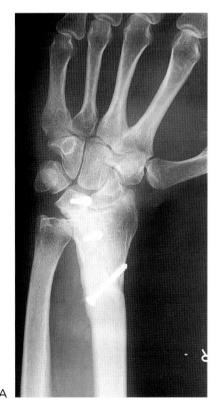 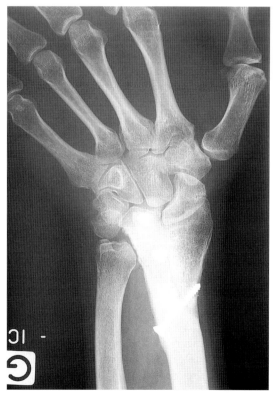

FIGURE 62.7. Postoperative dynamic x-rays. **A:** Radial deviation. **B:** Ulnar deviation.

(continued on next page)

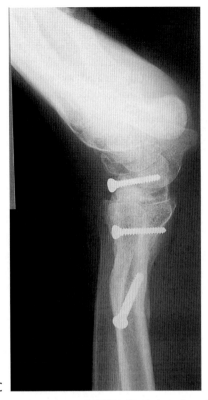 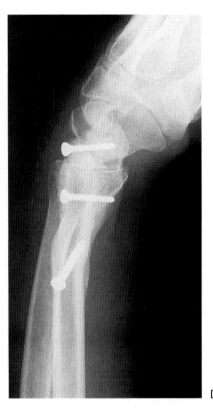

FIGURE 62.7. *(continued)* **C:** Extension. **D:** Flexion.

the radial cortex of the radius and detaching a radiostyloid fragment, which may or may not be displaced. Usually, the radioscaphoid articular space is intact. There may be an associated dorsal tilt of the distal epiphysis.

Tears of the scapholunate or triquetrolunate interosseous ligaments are commonly associated, as the lunate displaces proximally and the scaphoid and triquetrum maintain their anatomic positions. These injuries should be suspected on initial x-rays when an increased distance is seen between the proximal borders of the lunate and the adjacent bones of the first row. The horizontal position of the scaphoid can result from either scapholunate dissociation or scaphoid adaptation to a more limited space between the radius and distal carpal row. It can also be related to a distal radius malunion with a dorsal tilt. Several options are described for the surgical treatment of these malunions, including intraarticular osteotomy, limited carpal arthrodesis, proximal row carpectomy, denervation, and wrist arthroplasty. Evaluation of the cartilage status may be done preoperatively by arthroscopy or CT scan after arthrography. Such an evaluation can be of help in choosing the type of procedure to be performed.

An osteotomy of the impacted fragment can be performed if the cartilage is intact. When the cartilage of the lunate fossa is not intact, other procedures such as radioscapholunate arthrodesis or total wrist arthrodesis are indicated, but significant decrease in motion results. Proximal row carpectomy is contraindicated when the cartilage is destroyed or there is a step-off between the lunate fossa and the scaphoid fossa. Therefore, in the young manual worker, the first choice is between total and limited wrist arthrodesis.

Our experience shows that the most useful range of motion will be obtained if the lunate is fixed in a DISI position, but this has not been confirmed. Dorsal tilt of the distal articular radius should be corrected if significant.

Associated procedures may be necessary, particularly on the DRUJ, and a careful preoperative analysis should take into account the associated deformities to treat them at the same time. This makes it difficult to evaluate whether the final result is caused by radiolunate arthrodesis alone or by the combination of other procedures.

Radiolunate arthrodesis results in reduced pain while preserving a significant range of motion and could be used more frequently in the treatment of some types of distal radial intraarticular malunions.

EDITORS' COMMENTS

Radiolunate arthrodesis is a very effective procedure and an important one because it is the only good solution to destruction of the radiolunate articular surface, whether from a die-punch fracture or other articular trauma, infection, or systemic disease. The results of radiolunate

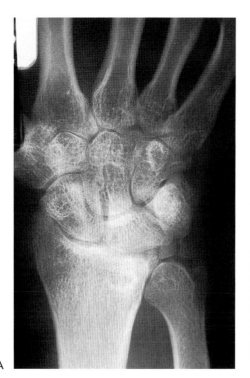 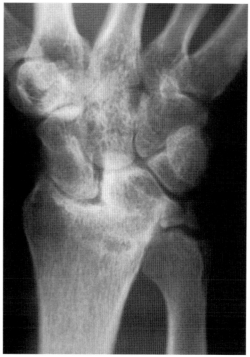

EDITORS' FIGURE 62.1. A: Three years following a die-punch fracture of the distal radius, the radiolunate joint in this patient is completely destroyed. **B:** Postoperative x-ray 3 months following radiolunate arthrodesis.

arthrodesis are highly dependent on the position of the lunate following arthrodesis. If the distal concavity of the lunate is tipped significantly in any direction, shear loading will occur between capitate and lunate and shorten the life of this main remaining motion joint in the wrist.

The second important component to the surgery is the elevation of the entire lunate away from the articular surface of the radius (Editors' Fig. 62.1). If the lunate is fused in a depressed position, the carpals on both sides will be taking excessive loads and will significantly limit range of motion. This is not as difficult as it may initially sound. The lunate can be elevated from the radius. The distal articular surface is carefully positioned, pins are driven, and the space between the cancellous radial fossa for the lunate and the cancellous lunate is then filled with a cancellous bone graft. These grafts heal well, and nonunion rates are low. An external fixator is not necessary to maintain the distally displaced lunate. For us, the procedure is carried out through a transverse incision, as are all limited wrist arthrodeses. The extensor retinaculum is maintained proximally on the radius. The capsule is incised, and the bones are approached between the third and fourth dorsal compartment contents, that is, radial to the extensor digitorum communis tendons. The edge of the scaphoid fossa on the radius is carefully delineated and marked so that the cartilage and subchondral bone are removed only from the lunate fossa. All the radius beneath the lunate is cut back to a good cancellous slightly concave surface. Dental rongeurs are then used to remove the proximal articular surface of the lunate, hyperflexing the wrist to cut away the most volar aspect to good cancellous bone. Then, 0.062-in. pins are placed, preset, retrograde, in the radius. A spacer is placed beneath the lunate. The capitate–lunate joint is directly visualized through a transverse dorsal capsular incision. The distal end of the lunate should tip neither ulnarward or radialward, and there should be no VISI or DISI positioning of the lunate. The 0.062-in. pins are run distally into the lunate but not through its distal articular surface. The crossing of these pins is sufficient to maintain the distal positioning of the lunate. The spacer can be removed, and cancellous bone packed with a dental amalgam tamped into the space between lunate and radius. Cortical bone is contraindicated, as it takes up space for cancellous bone. The graft donor site is the distal radius, approached through a transverse radial wrist incision as detailed in Chapter 54.

Bulky dressing and long arm splinting followed by a long arm Groucho Marx cast are necessary for 3 to 4

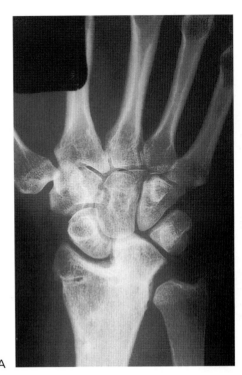
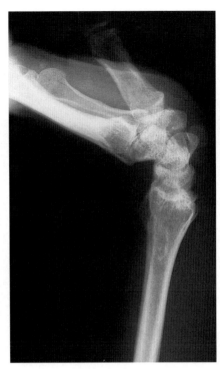
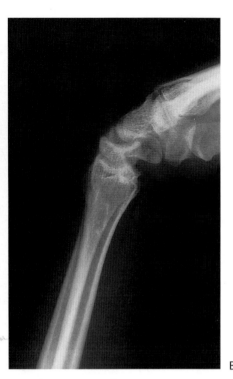

EDITORS' FIGURE 62.2. Radiolunate arthrodesis. **A:** Posteroanterior x-ray demonstrates the radiolunate arthrodesis maintaining or accentuating the normal distance between the radius and lunate. Note distal lunate positioning. **B:** Lateral x-rays of this radiolunate fusion demonstrates the significant flexion–extension arc available as a result of proper lunate positioning.

weeks; a short arm cast is then applied until 6 weeks postoperatively (Editors' Fig. 62.2).

We have not found it necessary to correct any malalignment of the distal radial articular surface as long as the lunate is elevated from the surface of the radius and aligned perpendicular to the long axis of the forearm.

REFERENCES

1. Chamay A, Della Santa D. Radiolunate arthrodesis. Factor of stability for the rheumatoid wrist. *Ann Chir Main* 1983;2:5–17.
2. Watson HK, Goodman ML, Johnson TR. Limited wrist arthrodesis. Part II: Intercarpal and radiocarpal combinations. *J Hand Surg [Am]* 1981;6:223–233.
3. Taleisnik J. Subtotal arthrodeses of the wrist joint. *Clin Orthop* 1984;187:81–88.
4. Linscheid RL, Dobyns JH. Radiolunate arthrodesis. *J Hand Surg [Am]* 1985;10:821–829.
5. Meyerdierks EM, Mosher JF, Werner FW. Limited wrist arthrodesis: a laboratory study. *J Hand Surg [Am]* 1987;12:526–529.
6. Minami A, Ogino T, Minami M. Limited wrist fusions. *J Hand Surg [Am]* 1988;13:660–667.
7. Inoue G, Tamura Y. Radiolunate and radioscapholunate arthrodeses. *Arch Orthop Trauma Surg* 1992;116:333–335.
8. Knirk JL, Jupiter JB. Intra-articular fractures of the distal end of the radius in young adults. *J Bone Joint Surg Am* 1986;68:647–659.
9. Altissimi M, Antenucci R, Fiacca C, et al. Long-term results of conservative treatment of fractures of the distal end of the radius. *Clin Orthop* 1989;206:202–210.
10. Bradway JK, Amadio PC, Cooney WP. Open reduction and internal fixation of displaced comminuted intra-articular fractures of the distal end of the radius. *J Bone Joint Surg Am* 1989;71:839–847.
11. Kopylov P, Johnell O, Redlung-Johnel I, et al. Fractures of the distal end of the radius in young adults: a 30-year follow-up. *J Hand Surg [Br]* 1993;18:45–49.

RADIOULNAR ARTHRODESIS

JOSEPH E. IMBRIGLIA
JOHN W. CLIFFORD

Rarely, severe problems of the forearm require creation of a one-bone forearm, or radioulnar synostosis. This procedure has been described in the past for salvage of traumatic forearm bone loss, paralytic problems, fixed contractures, infection, congenital problems, and tumor resection (1–8). Schneider and Imbriglia reported on its use for salvage of the unstable distal ulna following distal ulna excision (9).

Many of these problems currently are addressed by different techniques. Paralytic problems requiring forearm rotational stability rarely exist today. More complex reconstuctive procedures are used for tumor resection or traumatic bone loss. Knowledge of the radioulnar fusion technique, however, is valuable as a salvage procedure when other avenues have failed.

As Schneider and Imbriglia stated (9), this technique should be viewed as a final attempt to salvage painless forearm function at the expense of loss of forearm rotation. In the unstable distal ulna, every effort should be made to stabilize the ulna with soft tissue techniques. Failing this, fusion may be considered.

TECHNIQUE

The distal radioulnar joint (DRUJ) is approached through a dorsal incision (Fig. 63.1). The extensor retinaculum (Fig. 63.2) is entered through the fifth compartment. The retinaculum may be lengthened by extension over the fourth compartment in a step-cut fashion. The sixth compartment can be left intact and elevated off the distal ulna. The DRUJ can then be opened with a radially based U-shaped flap (Fig. 63.3).

The ulna is shortened and/or shaped to match the ulnar aspect of the radius (Fig. 63.4), depending on preexisting procedures and/or deformity at the distal ulna. The distal aspect of the ulna should be mobilized from surrounding soft tissue, and any intervening soft tissue between the radius and ulna retracted and/or removed. The radial aspect of the distal ulna should be decorticated to provide a good cancellous surface for fusion (Fig. 63.5). The ulnar aspect of the radius is then notched to accept the ulna. Cancellous bone should be exposed on the radius to provide a fusion surface (Fig. 63.6).

The radius and ulna are then coapted and held together using a bone clamp or provisional K-wires (Fig. 63.7). Fusion should be performed in 10° to 30° of pronation. Two or three screws are then placed from ulna to radius. These can be either partially threaded cancellous screws or cortical screws placed in a lag fashion across the ulna (Fig. 63.8). Bone graft is then packed around the fusion site. This can be obtained from the iliac crest, distal radius, or ulnar head. The extensor retinaculum is then repaired, and the skin is closed over a drain. Intraoperative or postoperative x-rays are taken to ensure good position and coaptation (Fig. 63.9).

AFTERCARE

The patient is placed in a well-padded sugar-tongs splint, which is converted to a long arm cast at 7 to 14 days. Above-elbow immobilization is continued until evidence of fusion is seen on x-ray, usually for 8 to 12 weeks.

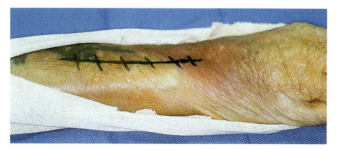

FIGURE 63.1. Dorsal incision to expose the distal radioulnar joint.

J. E. Imbriglia: Department of Orthopaedics, Western Pennsylvania Hand Center, Pittsburgh, Pennsylvania 15212.

J. W. Clifford: Department of Orthopaedics, Kaiser Santa Teresa Community Hospital, San Jose, California 95119.

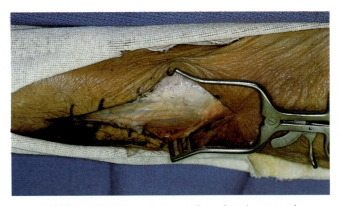

FIGURE 63.2. The extensor retinaculum is exposed.

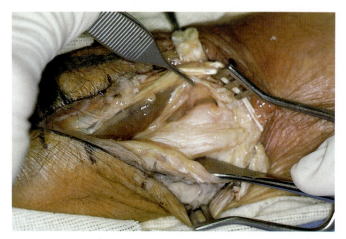

FIGURE 63.3. Exposure of the distal radioulnar joint.

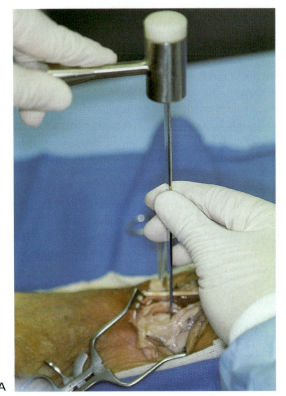

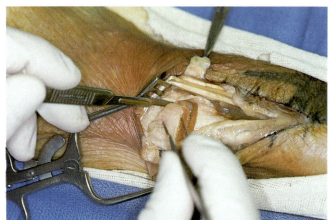

FIGURE 63.4. A,B: The ulna being contoured for arthrodesis to the radius.

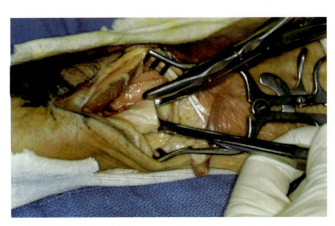

FIGURE 63.5. The radial aspect of the distal ulna is decorticated.

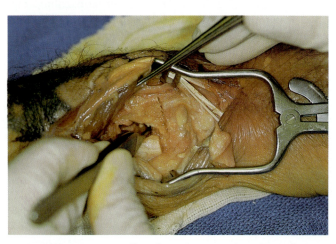

FIGURE 63.6. Cancellous bone is exposed on the radius.

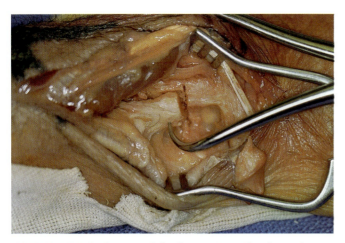

FIGURE 63.7. Reduction of the fusion site with a bone clamp.

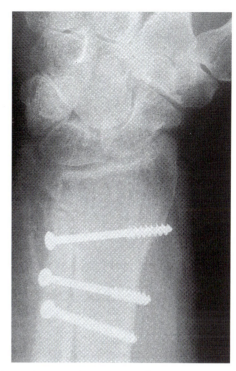

FIGURE 63.9. Fusion of the distal radioulnar joint with three lag screws.

EDITORS' COMMENTS

Fusion of the radius to the ulna creating a one-bone forearm is a salvage procedure one avoids if possible. The most reliable technical approach for us has been to create a cancellous concavity in the ulnar aspect of the shaft of the radius. The distal edge of this opening is slightly more proximal than the distal end of the ulna after the ulna has been cut back to a cancellous surface on its radial aspect. The radius is retracted, and the distal end of the ulna is placed into the cancellous end of the radius and compacted against the radius. This locks the end of the ulna into the good cancellous bone at the distal end of the radius. Pins or screws may be used from the ulna through the radial cortex of the radius. Bone graft may be added as necessary, depending on the degree of sclerosis, scarring, and other problems that are frequently associated with the need for this salvage procedure. The operation is performed through a longitudinal forearm incision.

Fixation is accomplished with either screws or heavy pins. The pins should be angled either proximally or distally as opposed to perpendicular to the long axis of the forearm. This will hold the radius in its ulnar-displaced position over the end of the ulna.

REFERENCES

1. Carroll RE, Imbriglia J. Distal radioulnar arthrodesis. *Orthop Trans* 1979;3:269.
2. Castle ME. One bone forearm. *J Bone Joint Surg Am* 1974;56:1223–1227.
3. Greenwood HH. Reconstruction of forearm after loss of radius. *Br J Surg* 1932;20:58–60.
4. Lowe HG. Radioulnar fusion for defects in the forearm bones. *J Bone Joint Surg Br* 1963;45:351–359.
5. Murray RA. The one bone forearm. *J Bone Joint Surg Am* 1955;37:366–370.
6. Reid RL, Baker GI. The single bone forearm—a reconstructive procedure. *Hand* 1973;5:214–219.
7. Vitale CC. Reconstructive surgery for defects in the shaft of the ulna in children. *J Bone Joint Surg Am* 1952;34:804–810.
8. Watson-Jones R. Reconstruction of the forearm after loss of the radius. *Br J Surg* 1934;22:23–26.
9. Schneider LH, Imbriglia JE. Radioulnar joint fusion for distal radioulnar joint instability. *Hand Clin* 1991;7:391–395.

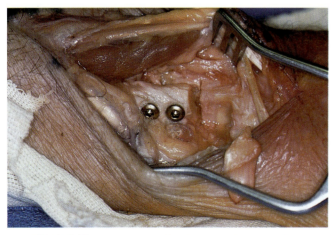

FIGURE 63.8. Lag screw placed across the fusion site.

64

ROTARY SUBLUXATION OF THE SCAPHOID

CORRECTION USING THE FLEXOR CARPI RADIALIS

GIORGIO A. BRUNELLI
GIOVANNI R. BRUNELLI

INDICATIONS

Carpal instability is still quite poorly understood and, hence, poorly treated (1–6). Wrist stability and function depend on a combination of bony, ligamentous, and muscular factors. These factors continuously interact, and the integrity of these structures is essential to the stability and function of the wrist. Many theories related to etiology remain controversial. Even the anatomy of the ligaments is variously interpreted by different authors. Consequently, the suggested treatments are quite varied, including bone fusions, capsulodesis, and ligament reconstructions.

Among the numerous types of wrist instability, the most common is scapholunate dissociation [carpal instability dissociative (CID)] (Fig. 64.1), also known as rotary subluxation of the scaphoid (RSS), which is generally accompanied by dorsal deviation of the lunate bone [dorsal intercalated segment instability (DISI)]. Almost all proposed treatments arise from the concept that the lesion responsible for the instability is rupture of the scapholunate (SL) ligaments. We believe that this idea is inaccurate, and any surgical procedure based on this assumption cannot be successful. In fact, the SL ligaments are normally loose, as they must allow the independent movements of both the scaphoid and the lunate bones, which have different degreees of movement in flexion and extension during flexion and extension and adduction and abduction of the wrist.

Rupture of the SL ligament, previously believed to be the prerequisite for dissociation, is not. Moreover (as the term "rotary subluxation" implies), the scaphoid bone in this type of carpal instability is flexed: its proximal pole tends to dislocate dorsally, and the distal pole protrudes volarly. We have demonstrated, by cutting the scapholunate ligament in fresh cadavers, that the scaphoid does not flex or subluxate.

Scapholunate ligaments are normally lax, which allows wide freedom of flexion–extension movements of the scaphoid as related to the lunate. They cannot be considered a stabilizing structure for the scaphoid. In fact, rotary subluxation of the scaphoid requires the rupture of the scaphotrapeziotrapezoid (STT) ligaments to occur. The STT ligament complex is peculiar. On the radial aspect, it consists of the continuation of the collateral radial ligament of the wrist. On the dorsal aspect, it is comprised of two fibrous branches from scaphoid to trapezium and trapezoid and by the distal band of the dorsal belt from the triquetrum to the trapezium and trapezoid.

The strongest component of the STT ligament complex, however, is located on the volar aspect and is comprised of the thick, fibrous apparatus made up of the volar STT ligaments fused with the deep layer of the sheath of the flexor carpi radialis (FCR) (Fig. 64.2). In cadaveric studies, severance of the STT ligaments, and especially of the volar component, permitted the scaphoid to rotate and flex. Therefore, we think that rupture of the (volar) STT ligament is the essential prerequisite for scaphoid rotary dislocation and that it is constant in SL dissociation.

DISI is the consequence of rotary subluxation of the scaphoid that allows proximal migration of the capitate. This, in turn, presses the lunate and brings about its gliding in order to leave the thinner dorsal bone between the radius

---

G.A. Brunelli: Foundation for Research in Spinal Cord Lesions and Department of Orthopaedics, Clinica S. Rocco, Cellatica 25060, Italy.

G.R. Brunelli: Hand Surgery Service, Institute Ortopedico Galeazzi, Milan, Italy.

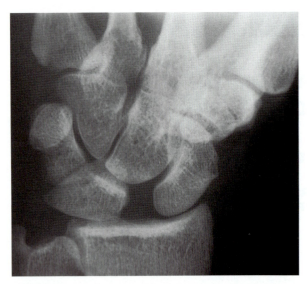

FIGURE 64.1. Scapholunate dissociation (carpal instability dissociative), also known as rotary subluxation of the scaphoid.

and capitate. The proximal movement of the capitate initiates carpal collapse, which can progress to scapholunate advanced collapse (SLAC) wrist with arthritic changes (7,8).

Many surgical procedures include various intraosseous passages of tendons in order to reconstruct the scapholu-

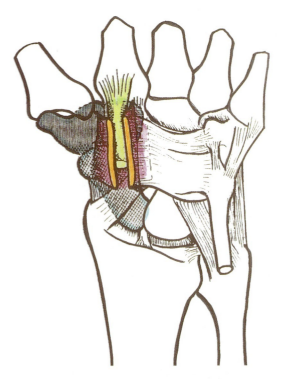

FIGURE 64.2. The strongest scaphotrapeziotrapezoid (STT) ligament is the volar one. It is comprised of the thick fibrous apparatus consisting of the volar STT ligaments fused with the deep layer of the sheath *(pink)* of the flexor carpi radialis tendons.

nate ligament. Dobyns has suggested different types of intraosseous ligaments that are modified over a period of years (1,2,7). Taleisnik takes a strip of FCR and passes it dorsally in the lunate, then throughout the scaphoid in a volar direction, and eventually in the volar edge of the radius (3,10). Other techniques aim to tie the carpal bones together or to bind the scaphoid with the lunate and the radius (9). These capsuloplasties demand perfect reduction of the position of the two bones, which is generally obtained by transfixing them by means of K-wires and by manipulation of these wires, but do not prevent the relapse of rotary subluxation because its prerequisite has not been eliminated.

Because of the inadequate results of these ligament reconstructions, many surgeons abandoned this technique in favor of partial arthrodesis in order to correct the rotary subluxation of the scaphoid. These arthrodeses, especially the STT type, however, reduce carpal mobility, modify the carpal kinetics, and aggravate the pressure against the radial glenoid with arthritic changes at short-term follow-up (11–19).

SURGICAL TECHNIQUE

We have developed a surgical technique to reduce the scaphoid to its normal position, correct the SL dissociation, reestablish the height of the carpus, and maintain the correction by reconstruction of a strong volar STT ligament. A dual approach is necessary. Through a dorsal longitudinal incision, 4 cm in length, the retinaculum of the extensor tendons is divided at the level of the dissociation. As it passes between the tendons of the extensor carpi radialis brevis and of the extensor pollicis longus, the deep fibrous layer (capsule and ligaments or their remnants) is also opened.

On the volar aspect, the skin incision follows the FCR tendon. The remains of the scar between the scaphoid and lunate are removed to allow the surgeon to see throughout the space from dorsal to volar. At this point, slight pressure exerted on the proximal pole of the scaphoid from dorsal to volar allows easy reduction of the rotary subluxation, which occurs with a slight clunk. The tendon is longitudinally split, and a 7-cm-long tendon slip is prepared that will remain attached distally (Fig. 64.3).

A tunnel with a diameter of 3 mm is created through the distal pole of the scaphoid, parallel to the distal articular surface. The tendon slip is taken with a nylon slip knot and passed through the tunnel from volar to dorsal. Pulling the tendon slip dorsally reduces the scaphoid, eliminates subluxation of the proximal pole, and corrects the SL dissociation. In fact, by going back to its articular facet of the radial glenoid, the proximal pole of the scaphoid is forced to go back to the scaphoid facet of the lunate. Also, by assuming its normal position, the scaphoid restores the normal height of the carpus, correcting its initial collapse.

The reduction is temporarily fixed by one K-wire through the scaphoid and capitate (Fig. 64.4). The K-wire will be removed after 30 days. The tendon slip is then sutured to the fibrous tissue at the dorsoulnar edge of the distal radius. If a remnant of SL ligament is identified, it will be sutured to the overlying tendon slip as it crosses the SL joint. The capsule remnants are then sutured, and the flap of the dorsal retinaculum is repaired. A plaster cast is worn for 30 days.

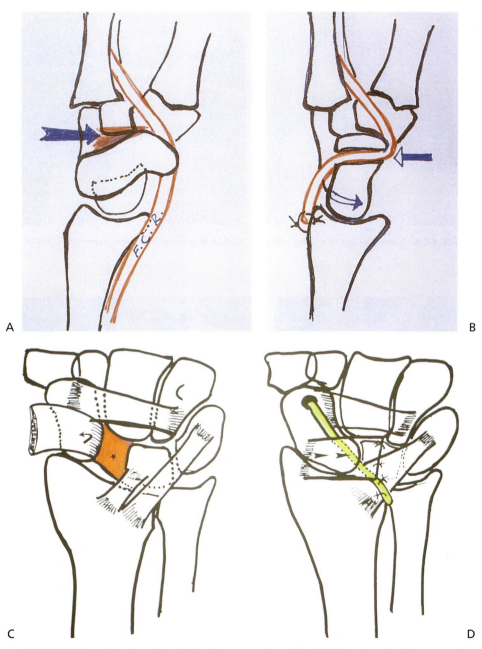

FIGURE 64.3. A,B: One slip of the flexor carpi radialis (FCR) tendon (red) is passed through a tunnel created in the distal pole of the scaphoid and pulled dorsally to reduce the subluxed scaphoid. The slip is then sutured to the dorsal edge of the distal radius near the distal radioulnar joint. **C,D:** Anteroposterior view of the procedures showing the flap over the dissociation (**C**), whereas in **D**, the slip of FCR coming out from the scaphoid and going to the dorsal edge of the distal radius is shown as well as the capsular flap put back into place.

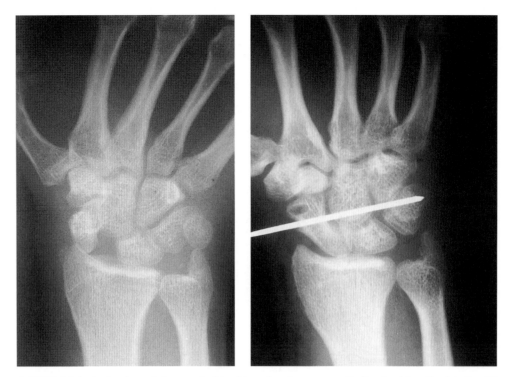

FIGURE 64.4. Reduction of the scaphoid subluxation is temporarily fixed with a K-wire (for 30 days).

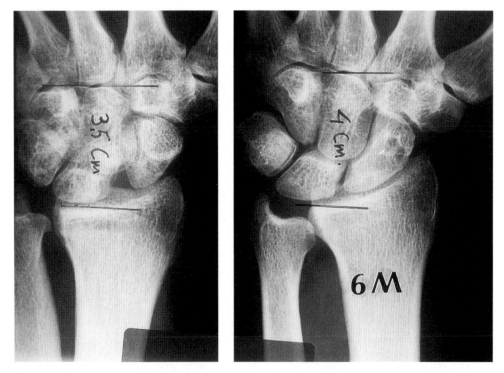

FIGURE 64.5. Carpal height is maintained after the operation (here a control is seen at 6 months).

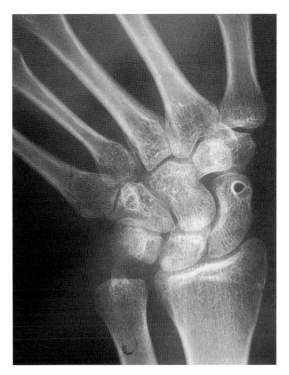 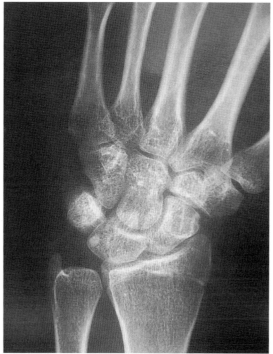

FIGURE 64.6. Following surgery, the scaphoid maintains its normal range of motion and its independence from the lunate. In this figure the scaphoid is flexed in abduction and fully extended in flexion.

CLINICAL SERIES

Our series includes 36 cases operated on over eight years with a follow-up period of 6 months to 5 years. No recurrence of rotary subluxation of the scaphoid has thus far been observed. The scaphoid has maintained its reduction in each case, and carpal height has been maintained (Fig. 64.5).

Scaphoid range of motion (ROM) was preserved with flexion during radial deviation (Fig. 64.6) of the hand and extension in ulnar deviation. The scaphoid maintains its independent movements as related to the lunate. The ROM of the wrist is on average slightly reduced in flexion (less 40–45°; maximum flexion 35–40°). This is a small price to pay to obtain a pain-free stable wrist. Extension was within normal limits in each case. Strength was reduced 35% compared to the controlateral hand, but, compared to the preoperative status, it had improved 50%. The average absence from work was 100 days. In two cases in which arthritic changes had already occurred between the distal radius and scaphoid, styloidectomy was concurrently performed. Thirty patients are completely pain-free and very satisfied. Four patients still suffer from slight pain at work. These patients had already suffered from arthritic changes before the operation, and the surgery was probably not justified. Two patients are still receiving physical therapy.

DISCUSSION

Several points warrant emphasis:

1. Rotary subluxation of the scaphoid depends mostly on the rupture of STT ligaments.
2. It is the opening of the STT joint and removal of the scar formed dorsally that allows mobilization of the scaphoid and its rather easy reduction *in situ*.
3. Scapholunate dissociation is corrected as soon as the proximal pole of the scaphoid returns to its articular facet of the radius.
4. Among the STT ligaments, the most important is the deep fibrous sheath of FCR tendon.

The technique we are suggesting is easier to perform than any other ligamentoplasty proposed to date, and our results are very encouraging.

EDITORS' COMMENTS

There are two basic types of RSS. The more common form involves release of the proximal scaphoid with rupture of the scapholunate interosseous ligament. The scaphoid flexes and supinates with the proximal pole displacing onto the dorsum of the capitate. The less common form involves the distal ligamentous scaphoid support. Scaphoid flexion occurs, often in association with a VISI deformity of the proximal row. This FCR scaphoid support operation will be more effective in the distal form of RSS.

REFERENCES

1. Dobyns JH, Linscheid RL, Chao EYS, et al. Traumatic instability of the wrist. *AAOS Instruct Course Lect* 1975;24:182–199.
2. Linscheid RL, Dobyns JH, Beabout JW, et al. Traumatic instability of the wrist. *J Bone Joint Surg Am* 1972;54:1612–1632.
3. Taleisnik J. Carpal instability: current concepts review. *J Bone Joint Surg Am* 1988;70:162–167.
4. Brunelli G, Libassi G, Stefani G. La instabilità del polso [wrist instability]. *Riv Chir Mano* 1981;18:27–46.
5. Brunelli G, Saffar P, eds. *Wrist imaging*. Paris: Springer-Verlag France, 1992.
6. Weber ER. Concepts governing the rotational shift of the intercalated segment of the carpus. *Orthop Clin North Am* 1984;15:193–207.
7. Sebald S, Dobyns JH, Linscheid RL. The natural history of collapse deformities of the wrist. *Clin Orthop* 1974;104:140–148.
8. Watson HK, Ballet FL. The SLAC wrist: scapholunate advanced collapse pattern of degenerative arthritis. *J Hand Surg [Am]* 1984;9:358–365.
9. Glickel SZ, Millendee LH. Ligamentous reconstruction for chronic intercarpal instability. *J Hand Surg [Am]* 1984;9:514–527.
10. Lavernia CJ, Cohen MS, Taleisnik J. Treatment of scapholunate dissociation by ligamentous repair and capsulodesis. *J Hand Surg [Am]* 1992;17:354–359.
11. Watson HK, Hempton RF. Limited wrist arthrodesis: the triscaphoid joint. *J Hand Surg [Am]* 1980;5:320–327.
12. Minami A, Ogino T, Minami M. Limited wrist fusions. *J Hand Surg [Am]* 1988;13:660–667.
13. Kleinman WB. Long-term study of chronic scapholunate instability treated by scaphotrapezio-trapezoid arthrodesis. *J Hand Surg [Am]* 1989;14:429–458.
14. Hom S, Ruby LK. Attempted scapholunate arthrodesis for chronic scapholunate dissociation. *J Hand Surg [Am]* 1991;16:334–339.
15. Minamikawa Y, Peimer CA, Yamaguchi T, et al. Ideal scaphoid angle for intercarpal arthrodesis. *J Hand Surg [Am]* 1992;17:370–375.
16. Augsburger S, Necking L, Horton J, et al. A comparison of scaphoid-trapezio-trapezoid fusion and four bone tendon weave for scapholunate dissociation. *J Hand Surg [Am]* 1992;17:360–369.
17. Rotman MB, Pruitt DL. Scaphocapitolunate arthrodesis. *J Hand Surg [Am]* 1993;18:26–33.
18. Fortin PT, Louis DS. Long term follow-up of scaphoid-trapezio-trapezoid arthrodesis. *J Hand Surg [Am]* 1993;18:675–681.
19. McAuliffe JA, Dell PC, Jaffe R. Complication of intercarpal arthrodesis. *J Hand Surg [Am]* 1993;18:1121–1128.

65

REFLEX SYMPATHETIC DYSTROPHY

STRESS-LOADING DYSTROPHILE PROGRAM

LOIS CARLSON
H. KIRK WATSON

INDICATIONS

Management of a patient with reflex sympathetic dystrophy (RSD) or even one "at risk" for RSD demands a specific and structured approach. First, RSD is "demystified" by giving understandable descriptions of what is happening, such as an overreaction to injury or a state in which the body acts as if the hand is still injured. Simply telling the patient that the constellation of "strange" symptoms and physical changes are all tied in and are treatable often results in a huge feeling of relief. It is emphasized that this condition can be resolved, but only if the patient is willing to comply with the home program. During the initial visit, evaluation measures are taken as a baseline for future improvements (Table 65.1). The patient is told to anticipate an initial increase in pain and probably swelling but that improvement should occur within 5 to 7 days.

DYSTROPHILE PROGRAM

The program consists of two components, "scrubbing" and "carrying," both of which require active, stressful use of the affected extremity (1–3). Force or load, not motion, is the critical factor. Keys to the success of the program include

L. Carlson: Connecticut Combined Hand Therapy, Glastonbury, Connecticut 06033 and Hartford, Connecticut 06106.

H. K. Watson: Connecticut Combined Hand Surgery Fellowship, Hartford Hospital, and Connecticut Children's Medical Center, Hartford, Connecticut 06106; Department of Orthopaedics, University of Connecticut School of Medicine, Farmington, Connecticut 06032; Department of Orthopedics, Rehabilitation, and Plastic Surgery, Yale University School of Medicine, New Haven, Connecticut 06520.

TABLE 65.1. CLINICAL EVALUATION[a]

Pain, tenderness, and sensibility	Subjective description of pain
	  Verbal report
	  Visual analog scale
	  Pain diagram
	Volar plate test
	Modality-specific tests of pain
	Tests of discriminative sensibility

Edema	Volumeter Circumferential measurements

Vasomotor/sudomotor changes	Changes in color/temperature
	  Observation/palpation
	  Thermometry
	Capillary refill test
	Sweat disturbance
	  Observation/palpation

Trophic changes	Flattening of the cuticle base Thin, shiny skin Flattening of the rugae pattern Decreased pulp bulk Increased nail curvature Hair growth abnormality Palmar thickenings or nodules Generalized atrophy Demineralization on x-ray

Mobility, strength, and function	ROM (goniometry)
	Strength (grip/pinch)
	Function
	  Observation
	  Standardized tests of function
	  Activities of daily living checklists

ROM, range of motion.
[a]Clinical evaluation is critical for diagnosis, monitoring of progress, and providing objective feedback to the patient regarding progress with treatment. There should generally be a correlation between pain and tenderness (as measured by palpation using the volar plate test) and observable vasomotor, sudomotor, and trophic changes.

TABLE 65.2. STRESS LOADING (DYSTROPHILE PROGRAM) HOME PROGRAM SHEET

DYSTROPHILE PROGRAM
(Please bring this sheet with you to each therapy session.)

DYSTROPHILE: On hands and knees, push down on the handle until the light goes on. While keeping the light on, move the Dystrophile in a back-and-forth motion, as if scrubbing or sanding the floor. Write down the date and total minutes completed each time you "scrub."

CARRY: Carry a weighted suitcase or bag with your arm down by your side. Increase the weight as you can, and carry it whenever you are walking, even for short distances. Write down the number of pounds carried each day. Feel free to add more weight between sessions, unless your therapist has advised otherwise.

ACTIVITY LIST: Each day, write down one new activity you tried with your affected hand, or an activity that is getting easier to do.

DATE	DYSTROPHILE	CARRY	ACTIVITY
	Number/day ___ For ___ minutes	___ lb or more	

compliance, maximum load, separation of treatment of RSD versus fibrosis, and emotional support. A home program sheet is used to increase compliance, recording each session and noting changes in weight and time (Table 65.2). An "Activity" column is used to encourage and monitor the patient's use of the affected arm for function.

Scrubbing

The Dystrophile device quantifies the force and duration of this exercise, which is similar to scrubbing a floor (Fig. 65.1). The timer and light on the Dystrophile are activated when the preset load is reached (Fig. 65.2). Patients generally begin with 3 minutes of "scrubbing" at 4 lb pressure three times a day.

In some cases, such as when patients are still in a cast, or when the pressure required by the Dystrophile cannot be maintained, towel scrubbing on a table may be used, again beginning at 3 minutes. This should be progressed, however, as soon as possible to the more vigorous demands of the Dystrophile technique. Towel scrubbing is also useful in many cases of patients who are "at risk" or those who simply present with increased edema following surgery that restricts general motion.

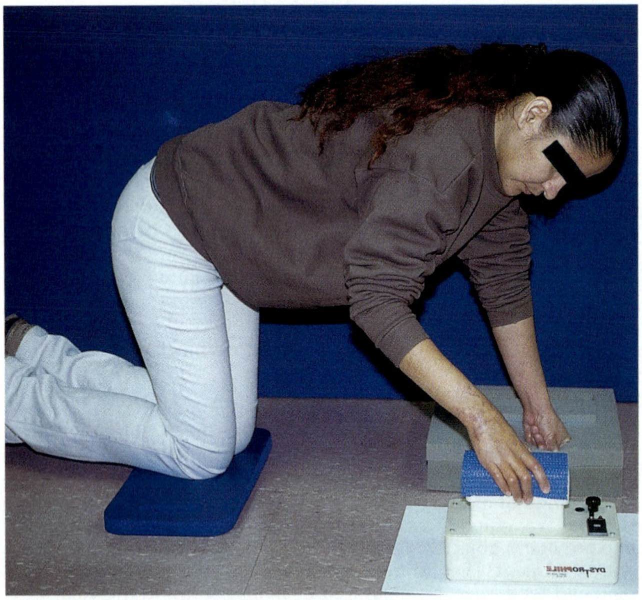

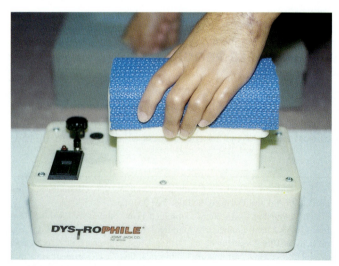

FIGURE 65.1. "Scrubbing." The patient gets down on hands and knees in a quadruped position as if scrubbing a floor and applies as much pressure as possible while moving the Dystrophile in a back-and-forth motion.

FIGURE 65.2. The Dystrophile (Joint Jack Company) was developed to increase compliance with the "scrubbing" component of the program. The timer and light are activated when the preset load is reached. Force, not motion, is the critical factor.

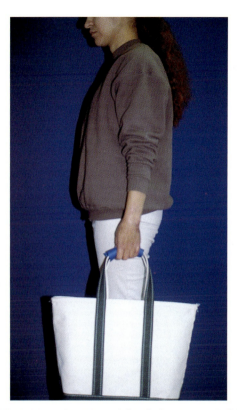

FIGURE 65.3. "Carrying." A weighted object is carried throughout the day. The weight should be increased to maximum tolerance.

Carrying

The second part of the program involves carrying a weighted bag, briefcase, or purse in the affected hand, with the arm down by the side in the normal position for arm swing during ambulation (Fig. 65.3). The patient can use simple items, such as soup cans, to increase the weight of the bag. The bag is carried throughout the day whenever standing or walking, including, for example, from the table to the refrigerator. The weight should be set at maximum tolerance (initial weight is generally 1 to 5 lb). The handle can be padded or built up if needed to facilitate holding the bag in the hand.

PROGRESSION OF THE STRESS-LOADING PROGRAM

The frequency of follow-up visits depends on the patient's need for reinforcement, supervision, support, and treatment modification. Structure and psychological support are needed to maintain compliance, including feedback regarding performance of the program and progress. In more severe cases, the patient is seen every 2 to 3 days to be given enthusiastic praise, encouragement, and objective feedback, as well as to advance and modify the program.

Ideally, patients are seen back within 48 hours of the initial visit. At that time, symptoms are often worse, and the patient needs reassurance that this is a normal response to a new exercise, but that the program must be continued. Despite possible increased pain and edema, there is often an objective indication of improvement in some component of the picture, such as a slight increase in motion or grip strength. More severe or chronic cases may take a week or more to clearly demonstrate progress, and changes may be more evident in reference to decreased pain in the joints and improved strength, rather than changes in mobility that are limited by fibrosis. The duration of scrubbing is increased up to 5 minutes, and carry load is also increased to maximum tolerance.

By 5 to 7 days, the patient will often begin to feel a difference. The scrub program is typically increased to 7 minutes three times a day, and again the carry load is increased. Load is further increased during additional visits to tolerance. For the Dystrophile, this includes increasing the force required for activation of the timer. Patients may also be started on 10 minutes two times a day as an alternative and more manageable program in terms of daily time constraints. The carry program is also advanced to maximum weight. General use of the extremity should also be encouraged and structured through written and verbal feedback from the patient and discussion with the therapist.

Throughout the course of treatment, evaluation measures are used to reinforce progress for both patient and therapist. Volumetric and grip strength measurements done before and after the program at each session will help the therapist gauge the degree to which the program can be advanced. A "good" level of stress is indicated by a slight increase in edema and decrease in strength following scrubbing. The volar plate test [pain on passive flexion of the proximal interphalangeal (PIP) joints] is an effective gauge of progress. A reduction in pain generally correlates with other objective signs of improvement, such as decreases in trophic changes and vasomotor instability. As the RSD clears, the PIP joints can be passively flexed with less and less pain. Once these joints can be forcibly passively flexed without pain (i.e., a negative volar plate test), the RSD itself is resolved. This test is also useful for noting any tendency for recurrence.

ANTICIPATED RESULTS

Resolution of problems using the stress-loading program occurs quickly in patients "at risk" for RSD, as when there is significant postoperative swelling and a tendency for the patient to be overprotective of the affected hand and limb. In acute cases of RSD, symptoms generally resolve within days or weeks. Essentially full mobility and strength should be anticipated.

If a patient is first seen during the dystrophic stage, the length of time required for resolution of the RSD is generally longer. Significant improvements are still noted in all parameters, including mobility, strength, and trophic changes, but the need for additional treatment addressing fibrosis through conservative measures can be anticipated. Other treatment techniques, such as dynamic splinting, however, should be added only after the pain and tenderness have significantly decreased, as measured by the volar plate test and reflected by other objective measures.

If treatment begins in the atrophic stage, motion gains with stress loading may be minimal, although improvement in function and a decrease in pain can still be achieved. Progress with an established home program may continue for weeks or months. Conservative management of contractures is less likely to be successful in these cases. Surgical intervention may include capsuloplasty of the metacarpophalangeal joints, check-rein release of the PIP joints, and intrinsic release.

Results of treatment using the stress-loading program in a group of 52 patients were first published in 1987 (4). Since that time, hundreds of patients have been successfully treated using this exercise program. It is a safe, cost-effective treatment approach to the prevention and treatment of RSD.

REFERENCES

1. Carlson L. The treatment of reflex sympathetic dystrophy through stress loading. *Phys Dis SIS Newslett (AOTA)* 1996;19:1–3.
2. Carlson LK, Watson HK. Treatment of reflex sympathetic dystrophy using the stress-loading program. *J Hand Ther* 1988;1:149–154.
3. Watson HK, Carlson L. Stress loading treatment for reflex sympathetic dystrophy. *Complic Orthop* 1990;5:19–28.
4. Watson HK, Carlson L. Treatment of reflex sympathetic dystrophy of the hand with an active "stress loading" program. *J Hand Surg [Am]* 1987;12:779–785.

66

SAUVÉ-KAPANDJI PROCEDURE

PETER J. MILLROY

Arthrodesis of the distal radioulnar joint with adjacent resection of the ulna neck to form a pseudarthrosis to allow pronation and supination for chronic subluxation of the ulna was first described in 1936 by Sauvé and Kapandji (1). The procedure has also been incorrectly referred to as Lauenstein's procedure. Terminology, especially in the use of eponyms, has caused confusion and errors in historical facts. In 1990, Buck-Gramcko (2) published a succinct, erudite paper correcting such errors and confusion; this is essential reading. Important historical and technical details have been supplied by Kapandji (son of the originator) in an editorial in 1992 (3).

I was taught the procedure in 1958 by my senior, Dr. Ken Watson, at the Princess Alexandra Hospital, Brisbane, as Baldwin's operation even though the distal joint was fused with a screw. I have now had extensive experience with this procedure (4).

INDICATIONS

The Sauvé-Kapandji procedure is a salvage operation and therefore is indicated when conservative treatment has failed or is obviously doomed to failure. The rates of indications for this procedure in my own series of 71 patients are presented in Table 66.1. These individuals present with significant pain, loss of function, and associated loss of pronation and supination.

In rheumatoid arthritis, where there is often a predisposition to ulnar translocation of the carpus with instability caused by ligament laxity, it is advisable to consider the Sauvé-Kapandji procedure rather than excision of the ulna head, which diminishes carpal support.

CONTRAINDICATIONS

The procedure is contraindicated when there is marked erosion, poor bone stock, or marked osteoporosis. Obviously,

P. J. Millroy: Watkins Medical Centre, Brisbane, Queensland 4000, Australia.

the procedure is not necessary at the time of simultaneous arthrodesis of the wrist. If the inferior radioulnar joint is also involved, a moderate excision of the ulna head usually suffices.

SURGICAL TECHNIQUE

Preoperative radiographs determine radius and ulna length, joint position, and bone stock. With tourniquet control, a dorsoulnar incision is made. This should not extend much beyond the tip of the ulna styloid in order to protect the dorsal branch of the ulna nerve. The sheath of the extensor carpi ulnaris is incised, and the tendon is retracted. The dorsal synovium over the ulna head is excised. The articular surface of the ulna head is exposed and removed with an osteotome and bone nibblers.

The ulna head is drilled with a 2.0-mm or 2.7-mm drill bit from the ulnar side to the center of the radial surface of the ulna head (Fig. 66.1). A 3.5-mm tap is then tapped the same distance. Note that it is technically easier because of stability to prepare the ulna head for screw insertion before performing an osteotomy of the ulna neck.

Extraperiosteal dissection exposes the ulna neck. Care must be taken on the radial side to protect the pronator quadratus attachment and also not to strip the ulna head of all soft tissue.

The next step is to create the proximal pseudarthrosis by osteotomy of the ulna neck. It is critical that this be made as far distal and close to the ulna head as possible so that the proximal stump of the ulna remains attached to the pronator quadratus. Narrow bone levers are inserted, taking care of the pronator quadratus. The lines of the osteotomies are marked (Fig. 66.2); the length of bone excised needs to be calculated from the preoperative ulna variance. The aim is to achieve a bone gap of no more than 10 mm with no ulna variance. A small power saw is used. It is more stable to cut both osteotomies not quite through and then complete the cuts with a saw or osteotome. The tubular section of ulna is then carefully excised with periosteum (Fig. 66.3). On the radial side, the pronator quadratus is detached from the

TABLE 66.1. PATIENTS FOR WHOM THE SAUVÉ KAPANDJI PROCEDURE WAS INDICATED[a]

Presentation	Number of Patients	%
Rheumatoid arthritis	31	43.7
After severe fracture of distal radius, e.g., Colles'	24	33.8
Madelung's deformity	4	5.63
Chronic instability	8	11.2
Osteoarthritis	4	5.63

[a]In a series of 71 patients.

loose bone and the distal stump. The excised ulna can be used for bone grafting the arthrodesis site if necessary, e.g., in a rheumatoid patient with bone erosion.

The ulna head is now mobile and can be controlled with a longitudinal towel clip or bone clamp. The remaining soft tissue attachments should be preserved, and any remaining cartilage can be removed. The site of the drill hole is checked. The articular facet of the radius is denuded to cancellous bone with an osteotome and bone nibbler. The ulna head at correct length can then be reduced into the radial notch to check apposition.

The radius is now drilled. The cancellous bone is often osteoporotic. Therefore, in most cases a 2-mm drill bit is used through the ulna drill hole and into the center of the radial notch under vision and hand drilled to the lateral cortex. The drill hole is not tapped; the depth is measured (usually 35 to 45 mm). A small fragment spongiosa lag screw is inserted to compress the cancellous surfaces (Fig. 66.4). If necessary, bone graft can be packed in before tightening. The screw head is coutersunk moderately to decrease irritation and the need for removal later. The rotation of the ulna head should be controlled before final compression so that the opposing ulna stumps are level. Usually, solid fixation is obtained with one screw. The position and length of the screw may be checked radiographically.

The bone gap should now be 10 mm or slightly less. Pronation and supination are tested. The gap is filled with soft tissue interposition; the pronator quadratus can usually be mobilized into the gap and attached medially. Otherwise, a subcutaneous fat and soft tissue flap (Fig. 66.5) or a slip of extensor carpi ulnaris can be used as an anchovy. Firm soft tissue closure over the proximal stump is important (Fig. 66.6). A suction drain is used. The wound is closed, and a nonadherent dressing is applied. A plaster slab is applied with the wrist in neutral.

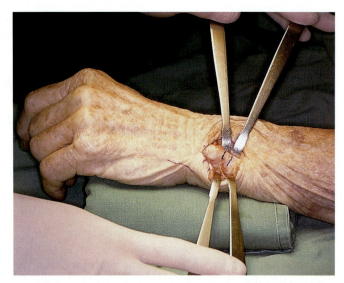

FIGURE 66.2. Ulna neck marked for osteotomies (close to the head).

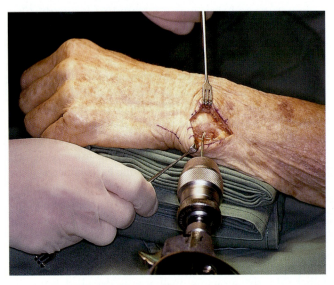

FIGURE 66.1. Drilling the ulna head.

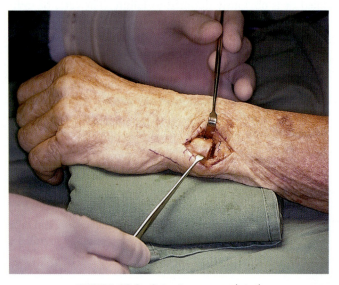

FIGURE 66.3. Osteotomy completed.

Chapter 66: Sauvé-Kapandji Procedure

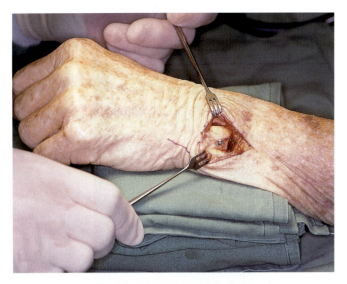

FIGURE 66.4. Lag screw being inserted.

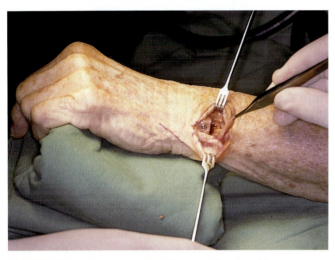

FIGURE 66.5. A fascial and flat flap mobilized to fill bone gap is sutured to the pronator.

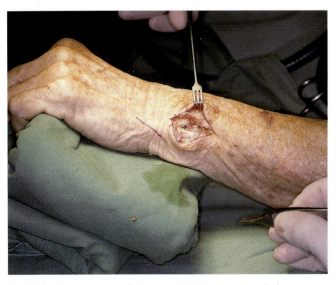

FIGURE 66.6. Strong soft tissue repair over proximal ulna stump.

POSTOPERATIVE MANAGEMENT

Elevation is maintained. Vigorous active exercises of hand, elbow, and shoulder, including pronation and supination, are encouraged immediately. The drain is removed on the first postoperative day. The plaster and sutures are removed at 10 days. An elastocrepe bandage supports the wrist for another 10 days. Hourly active mobilizing and strengthening exercises are performed. Most patients achieve full or nearly full pronation and supination without formal hand therapy.

Postoperative pain may be severe. Adequate analgesia should be prescribed so that the patient will not be apprehensive about exercise. An antiinflammatory drug such as Indocid is prescribed if it can be tolerated. It may be a factor in diminishing new bone formation.

COMPLICATIONS

Injury of the Dorsal Branch of the Ulnar Nerve

Injury of the dorsal branch of the ulnar nerve is caused by an incision made too distal because of a lack of understanding of the site of the nerve. This complication did not occur in the series presented above, and I have seen only an occasional case.

Nonunion of Arthrodesis

This complication has not occured with this technique. However, even if bone union does not occur, a reasonable fibrous union with the ulna at the correct length should not require revision.

Irritation by the Screw Head

This occurs only occasionally. Removal of the screw may be necessary.

Instability of the Proximal Ulna Stump

This occurs to varying degrees in all series. Instability with or without impingement seems to be the most serious and severe complication of this procedure. However, in most cases it results from one of two errors in technique. (a) Osteectomy was done too proximal. This is a serious error. Salvage is difficult, but prevention is simple. (b) Osteectomy was too wide. A gap greater than 10 mm will predispose to instability. The gap should be no more than 10 mm. Both complications and their prevention were stressed by Dr. A. Kapandji, son of the originator, in an informative editorial in 1992 (3).

Rothwell (5) preserves the periosteal sleeve and closes this carefully, including the sheath of extensor carpi ulnaris, to help stabilize the proximal stump. He reports no new bone formation. I have no such experience and have always carefully excised periosteum with the osteectomy, having seen new bone extend in periosteal sleeves elsewhere. Rothwell also recommends an 8-mm to 10-mm gap to improve stability.

New Bone Formation

In the series presented above, there was one such case. I have seen a few other cases. Further osteectomy was required when this occurred. Excision of periosteum, removal of bone fragments, careful irrigation, prevention of hematoma, early mobilization, and antiinflammatory drugs may be factors in prevention.

CLINICAL CASE

A 76-year-old male patient was first seen in 1994 for moderate bilateral Dupuytren's contractures. He had no symptoms in the wrist region at that time. The Dupuytren's contractures did not require operation.

He was seen again 2 years later complaining of pain on the ulnar side of the right wrist for 2 months. There was no history of injury. He noticed pain and swelling at the ulna head, aching at night, and pain with forearm rotation in the morning.

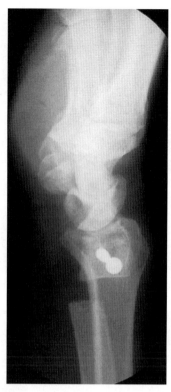

FIGURE 66.8. Lateral radiograph. Note that proximal stump is not displaced dorsally.

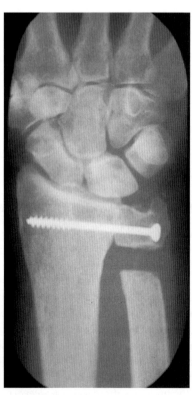

FIGURE 66.7. Radiograph taken five weeks postoperatively shows distal osteectomy and moderate bone gap.

Examination revealed a dorsally prominent right ulna head with swelling and instability on passive manipulation. A click was present on pronation and supination. Compression of the ulna head on the radius on rotation caused pain. Radiographs showed some osteoarthritis of the distal radioulnar joint and a dorsal shift of the ulna head on the lateral projection.

The symptoms did not improve with a support; a Sauvé-Kapandji procedure was then performed. The drain was removed the following day.

Postoperative care was as outlined. Ten days later the wound was well healed. The patient was encouraged to continue active exercises including pronation and supination. He had regained almost full forearm rotation 3 weeks after surgery and full rotation by 5 weeks. By 12 weeks he had good strength, no loss of function, and was using tools normally. Postoperative radiographs at five weeks show the result with the distal osteectomy and a moderate bone gap (Figs. 66.7 and 66.8).

RESULTS

I outlined the outcome of this procedure in 1992 in assessing the results of 62 operations on 53 patients (4). It was noted that any symptoms were present by 3 months after surgery.

The condition was stable by 6 months. Three patients were dissatisfied. Three others had some pain and clicking. Eight others had a tolerable click. Ninety-two percent returned to their original work. Pronation and supination were normal in 53 wrists and more than 50% in the remainder.

CONCLUSION

To obtain satisfactory results with minimal complications, it is important to resect no more than 10 mm of ulna neck distally adjacent to the ulna head.

EDITORS' COMMENTS

We include the Sauvé-Kapandji procedure for completeness; however, we feel there is no indication for this operation. The distal ulna is not necessary to the wrist or its function; it is best handled by treating dislocation or malalignment of the distal radioulnar joint (DRUJ) where adequate cartilage persists, with procedures such as ulnar lengthening and radioulnar ligament repair. When the DRUJ cannot be saved, a form of distal ulna resection is currently the best procedure. The Sauvé-Kapandji procedure has a high incidence of symptomatic distal ulna impingement against the radius. The wrist has no need for the ulna head.

REFERENCES

1. Sauvé L, Kapandji M. Une nouvelle technique de traitment chirurgical des luxations, récidivantes isolées de l'extremité cubitale inferieure. *J Chir (Paris)* 1936;47:589–594.
2. Buck-Gramcko D. On the priorities of publication of some operative procedures on the distal end of the ulna. *J Hand Surg [Br]* 1990;15:416–420.
3. Kapandji IA. Editorial: The Sauvé-Kapandji procedure. *J Hand Surg [Br]* 1992;17:125–126.
4. Millroy P, Coleman S, Ivers R. The Sauvé-Kapandji operation. *J Hand Surg [Br]* 1992;17:411–414.
5. Rothwell A, O'Neill L, Cragg K. Sauvé-Kapandji procedure for disorders of the distal radioulnar joint: A simplified technique. *J Hand Surg [Am]* 1996;21:771–777.

67

SCAPHOCAPITATE ARTHRODESIS

VILIJAM ZDRAVKOVIC
GONTRAN R. SENNWALD

INDICATIONS

Scaphocapitate arthrodesis was first described in 1946 by Sutro (1). Originally it was performed for scaphoid nonunion (1,2), but it was also used in other wrist pathologies such as scapholunate dissociation (3). Recently it has been established as an appropriate procedure for Kienböck's disease in stage IIIB (4) according to the Lichtman classification (5). It has been shown that the pattern of carpal collapse can be improved through reposition of the scaphoid, which also unloads the lunate about as well as joint-leveling procedures (6,7). It seems that the main rationale of this procedure is to prevent the progress of carpal collapse rather than to reconstruct the carpal height.

For advanced Kienböck's disease in stage IIIB, alternative procedures to scaphocapitate arthrodesis are scaphotrapeziotrapezoid (STT) arthrodesis and excision of the proximal carpal row. Leveling procedures are no longer recommended at that stage. The basic idea and biomechanical rationale for the STT and scaphocapitate arthrodeses are rather similar. However, there are several advantages in favor of the scaphocapitate arthrodesis: it is technically easier, the scaphoid can be placed more precisely, and the scapholunate ligament can be better evaluated. Further, in STT fusion, the scaphoid acts as a long lever arm in the capitate–trapezoid joint that might lead to gradual increase of scaphoid–capitate motion (8). Both limited carpal fusions lead to loss of motion in the wrist caused by bridging of the midcarpal joint. *In vitro* studies have shown that after scaphocapitate or STT fusion, flexion–extension is reduced 15%, and radioulnar deviation is decreased by 25% (9). The loss of motion *in vivo* is assumed to be a bit higher because of postoperative intraarticular and capsular fibrosis.

Compared to limited carpal fusion, excision of the proximal carpal row is more of a mutilating procedure that reduces pain but also strength because of the relative insufficiency of the flexor muscles. However, the mobility of the joint is better preserved (10). If the scapholunate ligament is ruptured, or there is arthrosis in the radioscaphoid compartment, proximal row carpectomy should be the treatment of choice, as long as the lunate notch on the radius and capitate head are intact. In young active patients, limited intercarpal fusion results in advantages, especially regarding strength.

SURGICAL TECHNIQUE

The skin incision is straight or Z-shaped and placed dorsally between the third and fourth compartments, taking into account the dorsal branch of radial nerve. Lister's tubercle is the main landmark. The extensor retinaculum is cut in U-form fashion, which allows later easier reconstruction (Fig. 67.1). We regularly resect Lister's tubercle and transfer the extensor pollicis longus tendon radially (so it will remain running over the retinaculum). The capsule should be incised longitudinally. The scaphocapitate joint can be well inspected from the dorsal approach. Scaphoid reposition is not necessary because it could produce uncontrolled constraints on the scapholunate ligament and restrict radial deviation. The goal is to preserve the acquired position of the scaphoid, which is the consequence of an irreversible remodeling process.

The dorsal capitate joint surface is cut with an oscillating saw (Fig. 67.2). The scaphoid surface is then cut parallel to the cut surface on the capitate, with the volar third maintained for better alignment. In cutting the capitate, attention must be paid not to affect the lunocapitate joint. Now the scapholunate ligament can be completely inspected and evaluated. A corticocancellous bone graft can be harvested either from the iliac crest or from the distal radius at the level of Lister's tubercle. The latter option

---

V. Zdravkovic: Kantonsspital Altstätten, CH-9450 Altstätten, Switzerland.

G. R. Sennwald: Hand Surgery Unit, Medical School of Geneva, CH1200 Geneva, Switzerland.

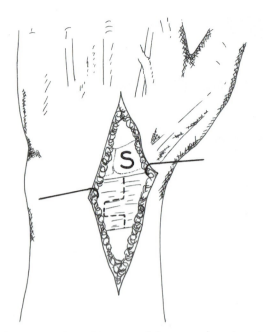

FIGURE 67.1. U-shaped incision of the extensor retinaculum. S, scaphoid.

is more convenient, and the quality of the graft is always sufficient. When the graft is harvested from the radius, the distal radius surface has to be denuded of periosteum. A vertical block is cut with the oscillating saw, taking care that cut planes be parallel and that the depth of cuts be sufficient (Fig. 67.2). The block is carefully mobilized with a chisel with great care taken to avoid breakage of the graft. To prevent bleeding, it is advantageous to fill the remaining defect on the radius with a block of artificial bone. The graft is now placed in the prepared space between the capitate and scaphoid. The fixation can be performed with two lag screws (2.0 or 2.7 mm) or with two Herbert screws (Fig. 67.3). We do not propose other fixation devices because the shear and compression forces in the midcarpal joint might be rather high. Now passive motion can be tested, especially radial deviation, which should reach at least 5°. If this is not the case, the orientation of the scaphoid (too extended) or the volume of the graft (width) should be checked. The screws should be introduced into the scaphoid at the level of its dorsal ridge between the articular surfaces for the trapezium and radius. The screw should go through the graft into the capitate. Radiologic control with an image intensifier is strongly advisable. The flexion of the scaphoid (RS angle) should not be drastically reduced compared to the preoperative situation because it could lead to contracture in ulnar deviation. The relationship among capitate, graft, and scaphoid should be tight. The dorsal capsule is closed with resorbable 3-0 stitches, and the extensor retinaculum reconstructed. After skin closure, a protective semicircular palmar cast is applied in 20° of palmar flexion to prevent a contracture of the dorsal capsule. The fingers and thumb remain free.

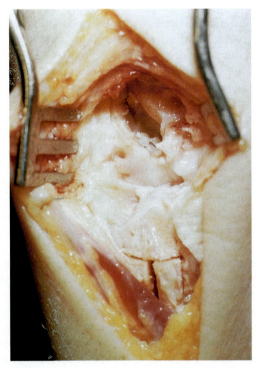

FIGURE 67.2. Intraoperative view after cutting the capitate and scaphoid surfaces. The graft on the radius has been cut but not removed.

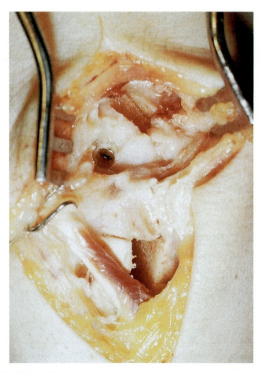

FIGURE 67.3. The graft is placed in the gap between the two bones and fixed with a screw.

POSTOPERATIVE MANAGEMENT

The wrist is immobilized for 4 to 8 weeks (depending on the quality of fixation, graft, and age of the patient) in a short arm cast without thumb fixation. The splinting position should be in neutral deviation and 20° of palmar flexion. A protective removable plastic splint should be applied for an additional 2 weeks after removal of the plaster cast. Radiographs are taken intraoperatively, at 2 weeks, and then every 2 weeks until cast removal. A CT scan might be necessary to assess bone healing. A therapy program is started after cast removal. Loading of the wrist is begun after the bony union has been radiologically ascertained.

CLINICAL SERIES

Over a 3-year period, we performed a scaphocapitate arthrodesis in 11 patients with Kienböck's disease. The mean age of the group was 30 years (range, 19–52 years). The symptoms were present for an average of 26 months (range, 5–72 months) before the first consultation at our hospital. According to Lichtman's classification (5), there were four patients with grade IIIA, six with grade IIIB, and one with grade II combined with scapholunate dissociation. The average follow-up time was 36 months (range, 13–57 months). At follow-up, radiographic and clinical examination and complete data evaluation were performed by an independent examiner.

In the early postoperative period, there were no complications that would lead to early revision or aberration from the initial therapy plan. There was no infection and no radiologic dislocation of bones or screws. Nine arthrodeses healed within 8 weeks; the remainder healed after rearthrodesis.

All patients but one were satisfied with the treatment. Pain was persistent in one patient, present only on load in three patients, and completely resolved in the remaining seven patients. Nine patients continued with their professional activities (however, two of those at a reduced level); the remaining two could no longer continue their initial profession. Detailed results are presented in Tables 67.1 and 67.2. The most significant change was loss of flexion–extension and radioulnar deviation, both reduced an average of 52%. Strength was reduced by 28%, which did not affect the working capability.

CLINICAL CASE

A young female patient presented with Kienböck's disease stage IIIA (Fig. 67.4). The dominant right hand was affected. She worked as a packaging worker and suffered wrist pain on motion for more than 2 years. The radiolunate angle was −10° (unaffected side, −14°), and the radioscaphoid angle was 56° (unaffected side, 50°). We performed the scaphocapitate arthrodesis. Follow-up examination was performed 26 months after the operation. The scaphoid and capitate were fused, and the patient had no pain. The flexion–extension arc was 40° with only 5° of radial–ulnar deviation (Fig. 67.5). This was a considerable reduction of 69% and 90% of motion of the unaffected side, respectively. Grip strength was, however, excellent, with only a 6% reduction compared to the unaffected side. The Culp wrist score was 79 points. Radiologic evaluation revealed the radiolunate angle to be −10°, and the radioscaphoid angle 32°. The patient was very satisfied with the result and resumed her original occupation.

TABLE 67.1. CLINICAL RESULTS AT FOLLOW-UP AFTER SCAPHOCAPITATE ARTHRODESIS[a]

	Average	Minimum	Maximum
Flexion/extension arc			
Affected	64°	40°	96°
Unaffected	134°	122°	150°
Loss (%)	−52		
Radial/ulnar deviation arc			
Affected	28°	5°	60°
Unaffected	59°	30°	78°
Loss (%)	−52		
Grip strength (kg)			
Affected	39	26	50
Unaffected	54	32	70
Loss (%)	−28		
Culp wrist score (points)	77	53	94

[a]n = 11.

TABLE 67.2. RADIOLOGIC RESULTS AFTER SCAPHOCAPITATE ARTHRODESIS[a]

	Average	Minimum	Maximum
Radiolunate angle			
Before	−13.6°	−22°	−4°
After	−8.7°	−22°	−2°
At followup	−9.7°	−28°	0°
Unaffected side	−11.8°	−26°	−4°
Radioscaphoid angle			
Before	56.0°	48°	62°
After	51.9°	46°	60°
At followup	50.6°	32°	74°
Unaffected side	55.0°	50°	60°

[a]n = 11.

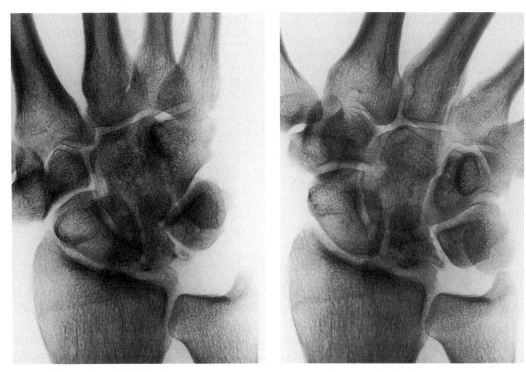

FIGURE 67.4. Preoperative x-rays in radial and ulnar deviation of the patient with Kienböck's disease.

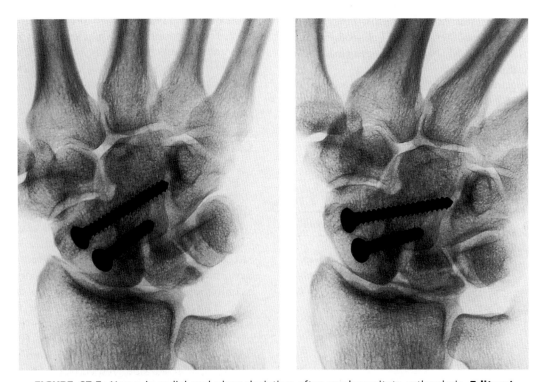

FIGURE 67.5. X-rays in radial and ulnar deviation after scaphocapitate arthrodesis. **Editors' Notes:** *It should be noted that a capitate–scaphoid fusion is much like a fused knee. The loads pass from the hand through the fusion site to the scaphoid, then to the radius. The principles behind triscaphe fusion differ significantly in that this fusion does not take the load but simply prevents the scaphoid from escaping from beneath the capitate so the loads can be taken across normal joints.*

EDITORS' COMMENTS

Scaphocapitate limited wrist arthrodesis is a procedure with limited indications. The chief indication for a scaphocapitate fusion is in salvaging a nonunion of the scaphoid that has failed several procedures and may be salvaged by fusing both the distal scaphoid to the capitate and the proximal scaphoid to the capitate. This, in effect, creates a single articular surface of the two pieces of scaphoid by virtue of their common fusion to the capitate. Scaphocapitate fusion for positioning or aligning the intact scaphoid is not indicated. A scaphocapitate fusion functions much as a knee fusion. The loads cross from the hand to the capitate to the scaphoid and then across normal cartilage into the radius. Fusing the triscaphe joint makes the loads cross from the hand to the capitate and then across a normal cartilage joint to the scaphoid and across a second normal cartilage joint to the radius. Small motion that develops at the capitate–trapezoid joint allows for a better eventual range of motion in triscaphe fusion than it does in capitate–scaphoid fusion. The principle of the triscaphe fusion is to prevent the proximal pole of the scaphoid from displacing from beneath the capitate and allow for load transference across these normal joints. Cadaver studies have shown similar ranges of motion if one simply pins the capitate–scaphoid or the triscaphe joint. This does not take into account the fact that motion develops and increases between the trapezoid and capitate following a triscaphe fusion.

REFERENCES

1. Sutro CL. Treatment of nonunion of carpal navicular. *Surgery* 1946;20:536–540.
2. Helfet AJ. A new operation for ununited fracture of the scaphoid. *J Bone Joint Surg Br* 1952;34:329.
3. Pisano SM, Peimer CA, Wheeler DR, et al. Scaphocapitate intercarpal arthrodesis. *J Hand Surg [Am]* 1991;16:328–333.
4. Sennwald GR, Ufenast H. Scaphocapitate arthrodesis for the treatment of Kienböck's disease. *J Hand Surg [Am]* 1995;20:506–510.
5. Lichtman DM, Mack FR, MacDonald RI, et al. Kienböck's disease: the role of silicone replacement arthroplasty. *J Bone Joint Surg Am* 1977;59:899–908.
6. Trumble T, Glisson RR, Seaber AV, et al. A biomechanical comparison of methods for treating Kienböck's. *J Hand Surg [Am]* 1986;11:88–93.
7. Horii E, Garcia-Elias M, Bishop AT, et al. Effect on force transmission across the carpus in procedures used to treat Kienböck's disease. *J Hand Surg [Am]* 1990;15:393–400.
8. Watson HK, Weinzweig J. Intercarpal arthrodesis. In: Green DP, Hotchkiss RN, Pederson WC, eds. *Operative hand surgery, 4th ed.* New York: Churchill-Livingstone, 1998;108–130.
9. Garcia-Elias M, Cooney WP, An KN, et al. Wrist kinematics after limited intercarpal fusion. *J Hand Surg [Am]* 1989;14:791–799.
10. Culp RW, McGuigan FX, Turner MA, et al. Proximal row carpectomy: a multicenter study. *J Hand Surg [Am]* 1993;18:19–25.

68

SCAPHOID NONUNION

BICONCAVE BONE GRAFTING

H. KIRK WATSON
JEFFREY WEINZWEIG

INDICATIONS

The appropriate management of an undisplaced, stable scaphoid fracture, including early diagnosis and sufficient immobilization, should result in union in more than 95% of cases (1). However, delayed diagnosis, inadequate treatment, and complicated fracture patterns with displacement contribute to the prevalance of scaphoid nonunion (2–4). Chronic symptomatic nonunion of the scaphoid longer than 3 to 6 months in duration requires surgical intervention to achieve bony healing (Fig. 68.1) (5–11).

CONTRAINDICATIONS

There are few contraindications to bone grafting in the management of symptomatic scaphoid nonunion. Radioscaphoid arthritis, the result of rotary subluxation of the distal pole of the scaphoid, which causes incongruity and destruction between this fragment and the corresponding articular surface of the distal radius (12), and avascular necrosis of the proximal pole (13) are contraindications to bone-grafting procedures, as they will not sufficiently address these additional underlying carpal pathologies. Such cases may require formal scapholunate advanced collapse (SLAC) wrist reconstruction (see Chapter 71).

SURGICAL TECHNIQUE

A transverse incision is made dorsally over the wrist at the level of the tip of the styloid of the radius. Blunt spreading technique is used to protect the branches of the superficial radial nerve, which are almost always retracted radially. The dorsal wrist capsule is opened over the scaphoid between the extensor carpi radialis longus and brevis. Both tendons should be free of their surrounding fascias so they may be retracted in opposite directions. The extensor pollicis longus is usually retracted ulnarward with the extensor carpi radialis brevis. The synovial and capsular attachments are cut back at the nonunion site from the dorsal ridge of the scaphoid, and the nonunion is opened (Fig. 68.2A,B).

Dental rongeurs are usually sufficient to form a cancellous concavity in each section of the scaphoid. Occasionally the use of a drill will facilitate the formation of the cavities. The drill should be a mechanical drill and rotate very slowly (a few hundred revolutions per minute), not a high-speed air drill. Cortical edges are maintained on each of the segments (Fig. 68.2C). The average depth of the cavity should be approximately 5 to 8 mm from the surface of the nonunion. If the cancellous bone appears healthy, the depth of the cavity can be less than this. If the proximal pole is small, obviously the depth will be considerably less. Attention is directed to the radius, where, through a transverse incision 2.5 to 3.0 cm proximal to the first wrist incision, bone graft is harvested from the distal radius between the first and second dorsal compartments (see Chapter 54). Only cancellous bone is taken.

A retrograde 0.045-in. Kirschner pin is run out from the concavity of the scaphoid through the distal pole of the scaphoid and out through the volar radial aspect of the wrist. A second pin is preset, running in through the skin across the dorsal surface of the radial edge of the lunate and into the proximal pole, aimed so that it will pass through the proximal pole and out through the distal scaphoid.

H. K. Watson: Connecticut Combined Hand Surgery Fellowship, Hartford Hospital, and Connecticut Children's Medical Center, Hartford, Connecticut 06106; Department of Orthopaedics, University of Connecticut School of Medicine, Farmington, Connecticut 06032; Department of Orthopedics, Rehabilitation, and Plastic Surgery, Yale University School of Medicine, New Haven, Connecticut 06520.

J. Weinzweig: Department of Plastic Surgery, Brown University School of Medicine, Rhode Island Hospital, and Hasbro Children's Hospital, Providence, Rhode Island 02905.

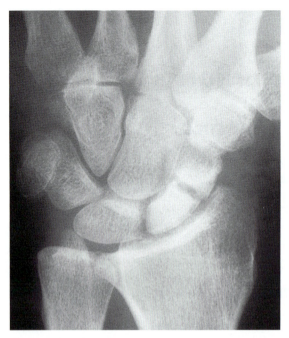

FIGURE 68.1. Longstanding scaphoid nonunion with some sclerosis of the proximal pole will require biconcave bone grafting.

With these two pins in place and drawn back, the cancellous bone graft is then packed into both concavities (Fig. 68.2D). The advantage of the dorsal approach is now evident in that the alignment of the scaphoid can be easily seen and adjusted. The capitate may be used as a template. The scaphoid is often angled, but there is also a loss of bone stock and shortening. A significant cancellous cap can be left between the two halves of the scaphoid, just as one does with a limited wrist arthrodesis (Fig. 68.3). The cancellous bone may occupy space on the articular surface between the two halves of the scaphoid without concern for the articular surface of the radius. With the scaphoid properly realigned, its typical flexion corrected, and its length corrected, the pins are driven across the nonunion site, securing both poles. The rest of the cancellous bone is then packed between the two halves, and it is not uncommon to see 1 to 2 mm of cancellous bone all the way around the nonunion site (Fig. 68.4). Pins are cut off below skin level. They pass only through the scaphoid. The capsule and other soft tissue structures are not sutured; the two dorsal skin incisions are closed with 4.0 subcuticular wires. A long arm bulky dressing incorporating plaster splints is applied.

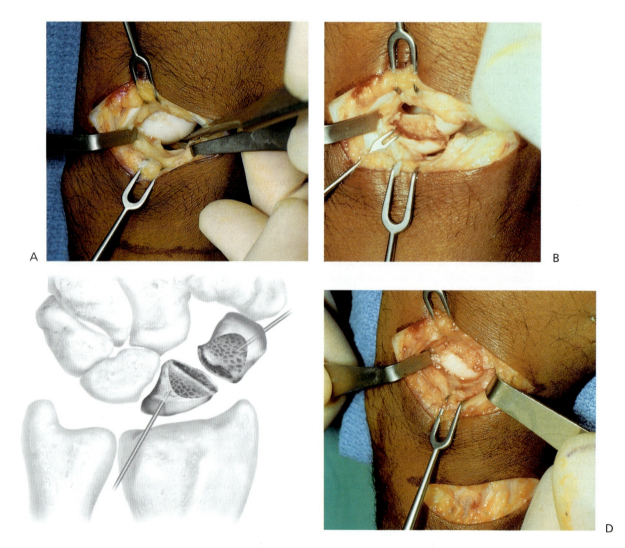

POSTOPERATIVE MANAGEMENT

The long arm splint is replaced approximately 48 hours postoperatively, and a long arm Groucho Marx cast is applied (see Chapter 48). This cast includes the proximal phalanges of the index and middle fingers, with slight flexion at the metacarpophalangeal and interphalangeal joints, and the thumb to its tip in opposition. If there is significant sclerosis and cyst formation by x-ray in a longstanding nonunion, then the long arm cast is maintained for 4 weeks. If the nonunion is relatively recent with good bone stock on both sides, then 3 weeks in the long arm cast is sufficient. A short arm gauntlet cast is then applied for an additional 3 weeks, at which time x-rays are obtained out of plaster, and a decision is made to either remove the pins and begin mobilization or continue in the short arm gauntlet for an additional week or two.

CLINICAL SERIES

The results of 36 patients who underwent biconcave bone grafting for scaphoid nonunion are reviewed (14). These patients ranged in age from 9 to 65 years (mean 28 years); 89% of the patients were male, and 56% of the cases

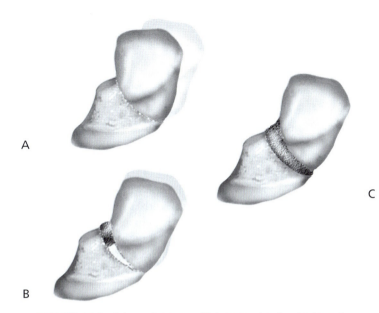

FIGURE 68.3. It is no longer sufficient to simply obtain union. **A,B:** Volar grafting will correct the angulation but not reestablish adequate scaphoid length. Longstanding nonunion usually demonstrates a collapse between the two fragments of bone. **C:** Bringing the bone out to length, correcting its angulation, and filling the defect with cancellous bone will achieve the desired result. The dorsal approach allows use of the capitate as a template.

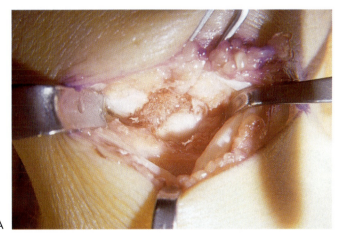
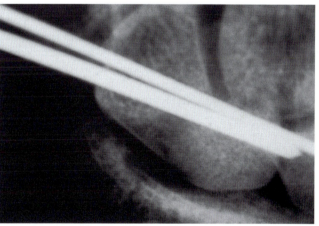

FIGURE 68.4. A: The dorsum of the right wrist with the fingers up demonstrates a scaphoid nonunion that has now been bone grafted. The cancellous bridge between the proximal and distal halves of the scaphoid is very broad but necessary in this case to realign the scaphoid. A cancellous concavity is created in which the proximal and distal segment cortices are separated, with cancellous bone filling the defect. The gap in cartilage will not produce degenerative arthritis because the loads are taken on the proximal and distal poles simultaneously. **B:** Solid scaphoid healing has occurred 6 weeks following biconcave bone grafting despite the gap seen between the cortical edges.

FIGURE 68.2. Grafting technique. **A,B:** The dorsal approach provides excellent exposure while permitting correction of the abnormal angulation of the proximal and distal poles of the scaphoid. **C:** Drilling, rongeuring, and curetting are the methods of choice for removing the bone from the proximal and distal portions of the scaphoid, forming a cancellous concavity. **D:** Note the broad cancellous surface filling the defect between the proximal and distal poles. There is no bone contact between the proximal and distal poles in this patient. Note the proximal incision utilized for distal radius bone graft harvest.

involved the dominant hand. Eleven of the 36 fractures were diagnosed at the time of injury. The mechanism of injury included extension injuries in 14 cases, direct blows to the carpus in four cases, a neutral impact (fist) injury in two cases, and a flexion injury in one case. The time interval between initial fracture and biconcave bone grafting ranged from 3 months to 20 years (mean 3 years). During this interval, 61% of the patients underwent some form of treatment. Nineteen fractures were casted; four were treated surgically, three with palmar bone grafting and one with an associated styloidectomy. Physical examination demonstrated a decreased range of motion, localized synovitis, and a change in the mobility of the scaphoid compared with the opposite wrist. Radiographic examination confirmed the clinical impression of scaphoid nonunion in each case. The distribution of fractures included 50% waist fractures, 28% proximal pole fractures, and 22% distal pole fractures. All 32 patients underwent biconcave bone grafting of the scaphoid nonunion as described.

Eighty-nine percent of the scaphoid nonunions (32 of 36 patients) healed. All proximal and all distal pole nonunions healed. Follow-up ranged from 3 months to 11 years (mean 5 years). Four failures occurred in the waist fracture group. Two of these patients demonstrated fibrous stability requiring no further treatment. The other two patients each underwent an additional procedure: a scaphocapitate fusion in one and a scaphoid replacement in the other. The patients with healed scaphoids had flexion–extension averaging 76% of the opposite wrist; grip strength averaged 88% of the opposite wrist. Twenty-five percent of patients complained of some degree of postactivity ache; 35% reported some pain with heavy use of the surgically treated wrist. Ninety-one percent of employed patients returned to their original jobs; 76% resumed all recreational sports activities.

COMPLICATIONS

Potential complications in the management of scaphoid nonunion include persistent nonunion following bone grafting, avascular necrosis, graft extrusion, pin tract infection, and progressive degenerative changes.

In the present series, four of the 32 patients demonstrated a persistent nonunion, two of whom required an additional procedure. One patient with a healed scaphoid nonunion complained of pain with light use of the surgically treated wrist. Postoperative radiographs demonstrated marked static rotary subluxation of the scaphoid, a dorsal intercalated segment instability (DISI) deformity of the lunate, and a scapholunate angle of 95° (the preoperative films could not be found to determine whether this problem was new since surgery). In this series, the scapholunate angle averaged 60° (range, 40–95°). No other complications occurred in this series of patients.

DISCUSSION

The biconcave technique described for the management of scaphoid nonunion is a reliable method for addressing problematic or longstanding nonunions without the need for permanent fixation or the use of compression screws. The principles employed in this approach to scaphoid nonunion reflect those utilized in performing intercarpal arthrodeses. These include maintenance of the external

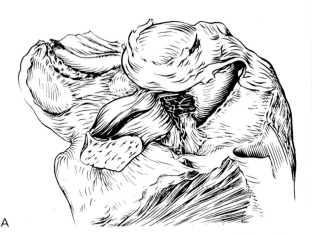
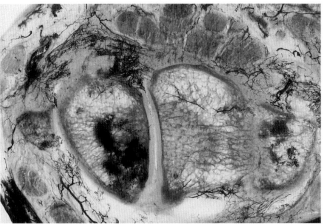

FIGURE 68.5. Diagrammatic **(A)** and dye-study **(B)** demonstrations of the vascularity to the proximal pole of the scaphoid. Despite dye studies to the contrary, Kauer (15) has demonstrated that there is ligament vascularity to the proximal pole of the scaphoid. The vessels of the volar radial scapholunate ligament are coiled like a telephone cord and capable of significant elongation. This ligament probably represents a recruitment ligament for forearm musculature as much as it does a restraining ligament for the carpals. Dye studies by Kauer have demonstrated the blood supply from this ligament to the proximal scaphoid pole.

dimensions and relationships of the carpal bones (in this case, the proximal and distal poles of the scaphoid), creation of broad cancellous surfaces for grafting (in this case, sufficient biconcave surfaces), utilization of cancellous bone graft, and the use of K-wires that cross only the joints to be fused (in this case, the nonunion site). This approach results in an excellent union rate with few complications, yielding functional wrists with minimal loss of wrist motion. In 30 years of experience, we have never created an avascular necrosis of the proximal pole of the scaphoid by approaching it for bone grafting from the dorsal aspect (Fig. 68.5).

REFERENCES

1. Cooney WP, Linscheid RL, Dobyns JH. Fractures and dislocations of the wrist. In: Rockwood CA, Green DP, eds. *Fractures in adults, vol 1*. Philadelphia: JB Lippincott, 1991;638–647.
2. Cooney WP, Dobyns JH, Linscheid RL. Nonunion of the scaphoid: analysis of the results from bone grafting. *J Hand Surg [Am]* 1980;5:343–354.
3. Cooney WP, Linscheid RL, Dobyns JH, et al. Scaphoid nonunion: role of anterior interpositional bone grafts. *J Hand Surg [Am]* 1988;13:635–650.
4. Fisk G. Carpal instability and the fractured scaphoid. *Ann R Coll Surg Engl* 1970;46:63–76.
5. Stark HH, Rickard TA, Zemel NP, et al. Treatment of ununited fractures of the scaphoid by iliac bone grafts and Kirschner wire fixation. *J Bone Joint Surg Am* 1988;70:982–991.
6. Herbert TJ, Fisher WE. Management of the fractures scaphoid using a new bone screw. *J Bone Joint Surg Br* 1984;66:114–123.
7. Schneider LH, Aulicino P. Nonunion of the carpal scaphoid: the Russe procedure. *J Trauma* 1982;22:315–319.
8. Andrews J, Miller G, Haddad R. Treatment of scaphoid nonunion by volar inlay distal radius bone graft. *J Hand Surg [Br]* 1985;10:214–216.
9. Zaidemberg C, Siebert JW, Angrigiani C. A new vascularized bone graft for scaphoid nonunion. *J Hand Surg [Am]* 1991;16:474–478.
10. Mack GR, Bosset MJ, Gelberman RH. The natural history of scaphoid nonunion. *J Bone Joint Surg Am* 1984;66:504–509.
11. Dooley BJ. Inlay bone grafting for nonunion of the scaphoid bone by the anterior approach. *J Bone Joint Surg Br* 1968;50:102–109.
12. Vender MI, Watson HK, Wiener BD, et al. Degenerative change in symptomatic scaphoid nonunion. *J Hand Surg [Am]* 1987;12:514–519.
13. Green DP. Russe technique. In: Gelberman RH, ed. *Master techniques in orthopedic surgery: The wrist*. New York: Raven Press, 1994;107–118.
14. Watson HK, Pitts EC, Ashmead D, et al. Dorsal approach to scaphoid nonunion. *J Hand Surg [Am]* 1993;18:359–365.
15. Kauer JMG. Radioscaphoid ligament (RSL). *Acta Anat* 1984;120:36–37.

SCAPHOID NONUNION

VASCULARIZED BONE GRAFTING

ALEXANDER Y. SHIN
ALLEN T. BISHOP

Approximately 90% of scaphoid fractures are successfully united by immobilization, electrical stimulation, open reduction with internal fixation, and/or conventional bone grafting (1–5). In those that do not unite, additional treatment is required to prevent arthritic degeneration. Conventional bone grafts with wedge or inlay graft techniques are successful in 70% to 90% of scaphoid nonunions (6–9). However, when conventional bone grafting fails, when avascular necrosis is present, or when the nonunion occurs in the proximal third of the scaphoid, conventional bone grafting may be less effective. Vascularized pedicled dorsal distal radius bone grafts have demonstrated a very high success rate in healing these difficult scaphoid nonunions. The surgical technique is relatively simple and requires a single incision for both graft harvest and scaphoid fixation (10–13).

INDICATIONS

Vascularized pedicled bone grafts are indicated in the treatment of scaphoid nonunions, particularly those with proximal third fractures, avascular necrosis, or failed prior grafts (13–22). Patients with acute scaphoid fractures requiring bone grafting may also benefit from vascularized bone grafts.

A.Y. Shin: Department of Orthopaedic Surgery, University of California, San Diego, San Diego, California 92103; and Division of Hand and Microvascular Surgery, Department of Orthopaedic Surgery, Naval Medical Center San Diego, San Diego, California 92134.

A. T. Bishop: Department of Orthopaedic Surgery, Mayo Medical School, and Division of Hand Surgery, Department of Orthopaedic Surgery, Mayo Clinic, Rochester, Minnesota 55905.

ANATOMY

Comprehensive knowledge of the vascular anatomy and nomenclature of the distal radius and ulna is essential for performing this vascularized bone graft. The blood supply to the distal dorsal radius is constant and robust, supplied by a series of longitudinal vessels that demonstrate consistent spatial relationships to surrounding structures.

The radial, ulnar, anterior interosseous, and posterior interosseous arteries are the four extraosseous vessels that contribute nutrient vessels to the distal radius and ulna. The anterior interosseous artery divides into anterior and posterior divisions proximal to the distal radioulnar joint. The posterior division and the radial artery form the primary sources of orthograde blood flow to the distal dorsal radius (Fig. 69.1).

The vessels directly supplying nutrient branches to the dorsal radius and ulna are best described by their relationship to the extensor compartments of the wrist and extensor retinaculum. They are considered compartmental when lying within an extensor compartment and intercompartmental when located between compartments.

Two consistent vessels are found within the fourth and fifth compartments. They lie on the surface of the radius in the floor of the fourth and fifth extensor compartments and are named the fourth and fifth extensor compartment arteries (ECA) (Fig. 69.2, Tables 69.1 and 69.2).

The fourth ECA lies directly adjacent to the posterior interosseous nerve on the radial aspect of the fourth extensor compartment. Proximally, this artery originates from the posterior division of the anterior interosseous artery or its fifth extensor compartment branch. It anastomoses distal to the radius with the dorsal intercarpal arch and the radiocarpal arch. The fourth ECA is a source of numerous nutrient arteries to the dorsal radius that penetrate deeply into cancellous bone.

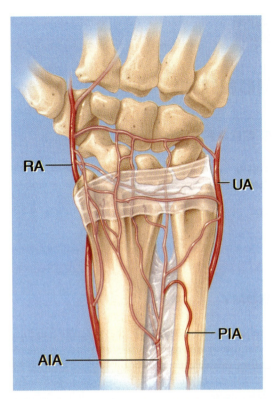

FIGURE 69.1. The sources of orthograde blood flow to the distal radius include the radial artery (RA), anterior interosseous artery (AIA), and posterior interosseous artery (PIA). The ulnar artery (UA) does not directly supply the radius. (Reproduced by permission of the Mayo Foundation.)

The fifth ECA is the largest of the four dorsal vessels. It is located in the radial floor of the fifth extensor compartment, passing at times through the 4,5 septum. This vessel is supplied by the posterior division of the anterior interosseous artery and anastomoses distally with the dorsal intercarpal arch. It may also make anastomoses to the fourth ECA, the dorsal radiocarpal arch, the 2,3 intercompartmental supraretinacular arteries (2,3-ICSRA), and/or the oblique dorsal artery of the distal ulna. Its large diameter and multiple anastomoses makes it a desirable source of retrograde blood flow. Unlike the other three dorsal vessels, however, it seldom provides direct nutrient branches to the radius.

There are two consistent intercompartmental vessels. They lie superficial to the retinaculum and are further described as supraretinacular. These two vessels, the 1,2- and 2,3-ICSRA, are located superficial to the retinaculum between their numbered compartments (Fig. 69.2). The retinaculum under these vessels is adherent to an underlying bony tubercle separating the compartments, allowing nutrient vessels to penetrate bone.

The 1,2-ICSRA originates from the radial artery approximately 5 cm proximal to the radiocarpal joint and courses beneath the brachioradialis muscle to lie on the dorsal surface of the extensor retinaculum. Distally, it enters the anatomic snuffbox to anastomose to the radial artery and/or the radiocarpal arch. It is accompanied by venae comitantes and is the smallest of the four vessels.

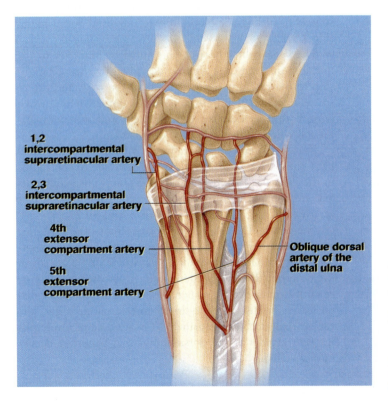

FIGURE 69.2. Four longitudinal vessels may supply the dorsal distal radius with nutrient vessels. These include two deep vessels, the fourth and fifth extensor compartment arteries. These vessels lie on the surface of the bone on the radial aspect of the fourth or fifth extensor compartment. Two superficial vessels are identified on the surface of the extensor retinaculum, the 1,2- and 2,3-intercompartmental supraretinacular arteries. Each provides nutrient vessels to the radius through a bony tubercle separating the first from the second or second from the third dorsal compartments. (From the Mayo Foundation, with permission.)

TABLE 69.1. EXTRAOSSEOUS VESSEL CHARACTERISTICS: DISTAL RADIUS VESSELS

Artery	Artery Present (%)	Internal Diameter: Mean (Range) (mm)	Provides Nutient Arteries to Bone (Y/N)
Postdivision AIA	100	0.71 (0.20–1.18)	N
1,2-ICSRA	94	0.30 (0.14–0.58)	Y
Second EC branch of 1,2 ICSRA	56	0.16 (0.14–0.19)	Y
2,3-ICSRA	100	0.35 (0.14–0.55)	Y
Fourth ECA	100	0.38 (0.28–0.72)	Y
Fifth ECA	100	0.49 (0.27–0.76)	N

AIA, anterior interosseous artery; EC, extensor compartment; ECA, extensor compartment artery; ICSRA, intercompartmental supraretinacular artery; N, no; Y, yes.
From Sheetz KK, Bishop AT, Berger RA. The arterial blood supply of the distal radius and its potential use in vascularized pedicled bone grafts. J Hand Surg [Am] 1995;20:902–914, with permission.

The distal origin is the "ascending irrigating branch" previously described by Zaidemberg et al. (14). Its superficial location makes its dissection straightforward. Although its pedicle has a short arc of rotation and its nutrient artery branches to bone are small in number and caliber (Tables 69.1 and 69.2), it is ideally located for grafts to the scaphoid.

The 2,3-ICSRA originates proximally from the anterior interosseous artery or its posterior division. It lies superficial to the extensor retinaculum directly on Lister's tubercle and anastomoses with the dorsal intercarpal arch, the dorsal radiocarpal arch, or the fourth extensor compartmental artery. Its nutrient artery branches penetrate deep into cancellous bone (Tables 69.1 and 69.2). Like the 1,2-ICSRA, the 2,3-ICSRA is easily harvested and used as a vascularized pedicled bone graft. The arc of rotation is much greater and can reach the entire proximal row.

A series of arterial arches across the dorsum of the hand and wrist provide a distal anastomotic network for the intercompartmental and compartmental arteries. These include the dorsal intercarpal arch (dICa), dorsal radiocarpal arch, and the dorsal supraretinacular arch (Fig. 69.3). The dICa is an important part of several potential grafts because of its anastomotic connections with the 1,2-ICSRA, 2,3-ICSRA, fourth ECA, fifth ECA, and the dorsal radiocarpal arch. The arch can be used as a source of retrograde arterial flow following proximal vessel ligation and graft mobilization.

TABLE 69.2. NUTRIENT ARTERY CHARACTERISTICS

Artery Supplying Nutrient Arteries	Number of Nutrient Arteries [Mean (Range)]	Nutrient Artery Internal Diameter (mm) [Mean (Range)]	Distance from Nutrient Artery Penetration to RC joint (mm) [Mean (Range)]	Percent of Nutrient Arteries That Penetrate Cancellous Bone (%)
1,2-ICSRA	3.2 (0–9)	<0.10 (<0.05–0.15)	15 (4–26)	6
Second EC branch of 1,2-ICSRA	1 (1)	0.16 (0.14–0.19)	21 (17–28)	57
2,3-ICSRA	1.8 (0–5)	0.11 (0.07–0.19)	13 (3–24)	22
Second EC branch of 2,3-ICSRA	1.4 (1–4)	0.19 (0.09–0.28)	18 (14–32)	48
Fourth ECA	3.2 (1–6)	0.16 (0.07–0.29)	11 (3–19)	45
Fourth EC br of fifth ECA	1.2 (1–2)	0.15 (0.15)	10 (6–12)	43

RC, radiocarpal; EC, extensor compartment; ECA, extensor compartment artery; ICSRA, intercompartmental supraretinacular artery.
From Sheetz KK, Bishop AT, Berger RA. The arterial blood supply of the distal radius and its potential use in vascularized pedicled bone grafts. J Hand Surg [Am] 1995;20:902–914, with permission.

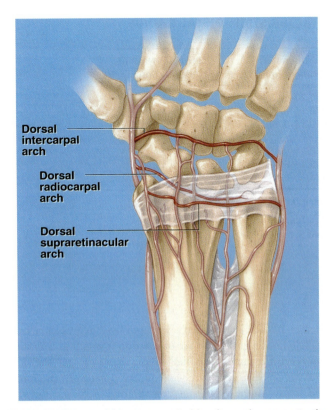

FIGURE 69.3. A rich anastomotic blood supply connects the proximal forearm arteries and dorsal radius longitudinal vessels. The distal anastomotic connections include a series of transverse arches, including the dorsal supraretinacular arch (dSRa), dorsal radiocarpal arch (dRCa), and dorsal intercarpal arch (dICa). The dICa or dRCa may be used as a source of retrograde arterial flow to vascularized grafts following proximal vessel ligation. (From the Mayo Foundation, with permission.)

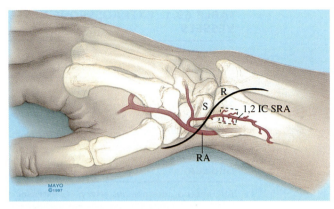

FIGURE 69.4. A gentle curvilinear dorsal radial incision is used to expose the scaphoid and graft donor site. *IC*, intercarpal; *RA*, radial artery; *SRA*, supraretinacular arch; *S*, scaphoid. (From the Mayo Foundation, with permission.)

SURGICAL TECHNIQUE

Scaphoid Nonunion

Pedicled bone grafts based on the 1,2-ICSRA are useful for most scaphoid nonunions. A dorsal approach is used for both graft harvest and exposure of the scaphoid. The extremity is elevated, and a tourniquet inflated. Exsanguination with an elastic wrap makes the vessel identification more difficult and is to be avoided. A gentle curvilinear dorsal radial incision is used to expose the scaphoid and bone graft donor site (Fig. 69.4). Branches of the superficial radial nerve are identified and protected. Subcutaneous tissues are gently retracted, and the 1,2-ICSRA and venae comitantes are visualized on the surface of the retinaculum between the first and second extensor tendon compartments. The vessels are dissected toward their distal anastomosis with the radial artery (within the anatomic snuff box). The first and second dorsal extensor compartments are opened to either side of the bone graft site, creating a cuff of retinaculum that includes the 1,2-ICSRA. The graft is centered approximately 1.5 cm proximal to the radiocarpal joint to include the nutrient vessels. Before elevation of the bone graft, a transverse dorsal-radial capsulotomy is made to expose the scaphoid nonunion site (Fig. 69.5).

In proximal pole fracture nonunions, a dorsal inlay graft is most appropriate. Fibrous tissue is removed from the nonunion site with curettes. Curettes and osteotomes are used to prepare a slot that spans the fracture site to receive the bone graft (Fig. 69.6). If the proximal pole fragment is small, the graft may instead be placed within the concavity of the proximal pole. After preparation of the nonunion site, the graft is elevated. The 1,2-ICSRA and accompanying veins are ligated proximal to the graft. The graft dimensions and location are measured to conform to the prepared scaphoid slot and centered 1.5 cm proximal to the joint line. The vessels are carefully mobilized distal to the outlined graft. An

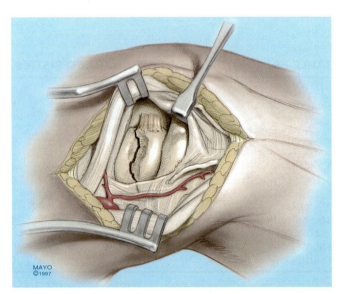

FIGURE 69.5. A dorsal radial capsulotomy is made to expose the scaphoid nonunion once the vascular pedicle is identified and protected. (From the Mayo Foundation, with permission.)

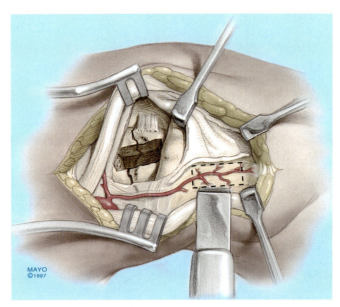

FIGURE 69.6. Dorsal inlay graft. A high-speed burr prepares a slot spanning the nonunion site when a dorsal inlay graft is used. (From the Mayo Foundation, with permission.)

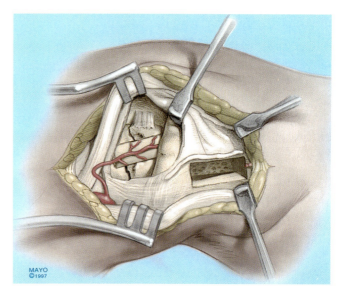

FIGURE 69.8. Dorsal inlay graft. The graft is transposed to the scaphoid and gently impacted into the prepared slot. (From the Mayo Foundation, with permission.)

osteotome is used to elevate the graft, performing the distal osteotomy in two stages, moving the pedicle radial then ulnarward to prevent injury. The graft is then gently levered out to create a distally based pedicle (Fig. 69.7).

Once the graft is harvested, the tourniquet is deflated, and the bone graft vascularity is observed. The graft is trimmed as needed using bone cutters and transposed beneath the radial wrist extensors to the scaphoid. The graft is gently press-fit into the prepared slot (Fig. 69.8). Supplemental internal fixation with K-wires or a scaphoid screw is next performed. Either may be safely placed dorsal to the graft without jeopardy to the pedicle. The wrist capsule and extensor retinaculum are closed, protecting the vascular pedicle. A bulky postoperative dressing incorporating a long arm plaster thumb–spica splint is then applied.

Interpositional Wedge Graft for Scaphoid Nonunion

When scaphoid foreshortening and angular (humpback) deformity are present, an interpositional bone graft is required. A vascularized wedge graft may be placed through a dorsoradial approach as an alternative to a conventional iliac crest graft. The incision is placed as before, and the scaphoid prepared before graft elevation. Any dorsal intercalated segment instability (DISI) carpal collapse is corrected by flexing the wrist until the lunate is in neutral flexion–extension. Its position is fixed with a radiolunate pin. Extension of the wrist then corrects the scaphoid shortening (Fig. 69.9). Fibrous tissue is removed and the dimensions of the defect are noted (Fig. 69.10). When used as a wedge, the 1,2-ICSRA pedicled graft is oriented to place the vessels and radial cortex palmarly for stability. A graft sufficiently large to fill the internal scaphoid deffect is harvested as previously described (Fig. 69.11). The graft is carefully trimmed to match the dimensions of the defect, often requiring a greater length of internal cancellous than palmar cortical bone. The graft is then inserted into the defect and secured with K-wires or by compression screw fixation (Fig. 69.12). The wound is closed, and the wrist splinted as previously described.

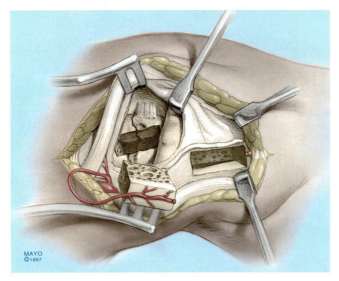

FIGURE 69.7. Dorsal inlay graft. The graft is elevated using sharp osteotomes and centered 1.5 cm proximal to the joint line. Distally, the pedicle must be carefully elevated from the radial styloid to prevent inadvertent injury. (From the Mayo Foundation, with permission.)

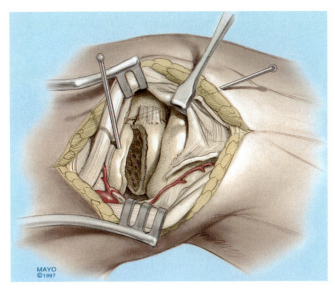

FIGURE 69.9. Wedge graft. A vascularized wedge graft may be placed from the same approach to correct a humpback deformity. Dorsal intercalated segment instability collapse is corrected by flexing the wrist under image intensification to correct lunate extension and maintained with one or two radiolunate pins. Extension of the wrist then corrects scaphoid shortening. (From the Mayo Foundation, with permission.)

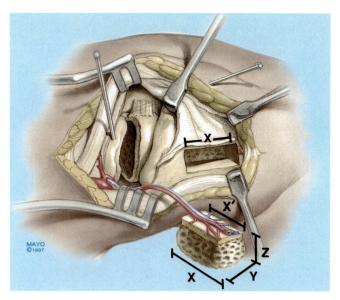

FIGURE 69.11. Wedge graft. A graft sufficiently large to correct the scaphoid shortening and fill any internal defect is planned, with the 1,2-ICSRA pedicle placed palmarly. (From the Mayo Foundation, with permission.)

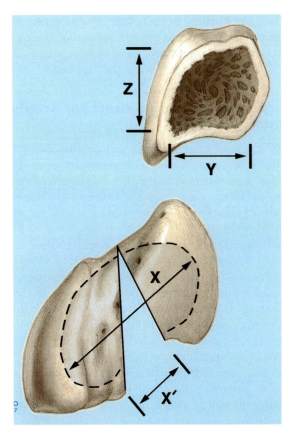

FIGURE 69.10. Wedge graft. Fibrous tissue is removed, and the dimensions of the defect are noted. (From the Mayo Foundation, with permission.)

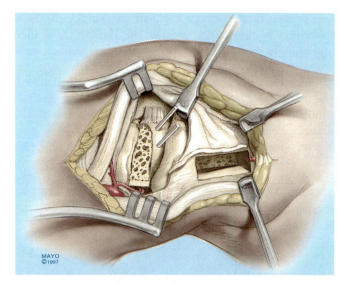

FIGURE 69.12. Wedge graft. The graft is carefully placed and secured with K-wires or a compression screw. (From the Mayo Foundation, with permission.)

POSTOPERATIVE MANAGEMENT

Active and passive range-of-motion (ROM) exercises of the digits and shoulder, as well as antiedema measures, may begin immediately. The postoperative dressing and sutures are removed 10 to 14 days later, and a long arm thumb–spica cast in neutral forearm rotation is placed for 6 weeks. Radiographs and computed tomography or trispiral tomograms are then obtained to evaluate fracture healing. A short arm thumb–spica cast is continued until evidence of healing is seen on tomograms. After the fracture has healed, wrist motion and strengthening exercises commence.

CLINICAL SERIES

Fifteen patients with established nonunions were treated with pedicled vascularized distal radius bone grafts as described previously (16). All patients were male with an average age of 27.6 years (range, 17–42 years) and had an average time interval between injury and surgery of 36.2 months (range, 3 months to 10 years). Six patients had scaphoid waist fractures, and seven demonstrated proximal-third fractures. Five patients had a previous conventional bone graft that failed. Six patients demonstrated radiographic and magnetic resonance imaging evidence of proximal pole avascular necrosis. Twelve patients had the graft placed as a dorsal inlay, and three had an interpositional wedge graft placed to correct scaphoid malalignment. Fracture fixation was with Kirschner wires or Herbert screws. All patients were casted until healing was demonstrated by trispiral tomograms.

Follow-up averaged 2.5 years (range, 1–4 years). All patients achieved fracture union, with a time to union averaging 11.1 weeks (range, 5.5–16 weeks). Patients demonstrated a flexion–extension arc averaging 90° and a radial–ulnar deviation arc of 42°. Scapholunate and capitolunate angles averaged 58.3° and 8.8°, respectively. The average carpal height index was 0.54, and the interscaphoid angulation averaged 23.6° posteroanteriorly and 24.6° laterally.

Three patients, all with preoperative degenerative changes, had additional surgery. The majority of patients were satisfied, with no or occasional pain and a functional range of motion. Radiographic measures of carpal alilgnment were within normal limits. Fair and poor results, seen in five patients, correlated with degenerative arthritis resulting from longstanding nonunions.

CLINICAL CASE

A 28-year-old man with an established proximal pole scaphoid nonunion (Fig. 69.13) underwent vascularized bone grafting utilizing the 1,2-ICSRA pedicled bone graft. A curvilinear dorsal radial incision exposing the first and second extensor compartments was made, and the 1,2-ICSRA was easily identified. The first and second extensor compartments were opened, creating a cuff of retinaculum containing the 1,2-ICSRA. Through a dorsoradial capsulotomy, the scaphoid nonunion site was exposed, and a slot was created to accept the vascularized pedicled bone graft. The bone graft was outlined 15 mm proximal to the radiocarpal joint overlying the 1,2-ICSRA. Once the graft was harvested, the tourniquet was deflated, demostrating excellent blood flow to the graft. The graft was gently impacted into the recipient slot, and a scaphoid screw placed across the graft (Fig. 69.14). The fracture healed at 6 weeks without complication (Fig. 69.15).

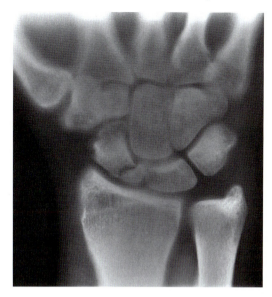

FIGURE 69.13. Anteroposterior tomogram of an established proximal pole scaphoid nonunion in a 28-year-old man. (From the Mayo Foundation, with permission.)

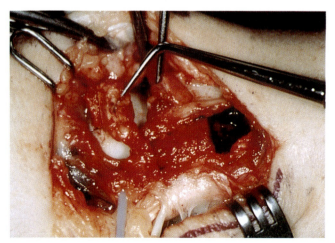

FIGURE 69.14. The graft has been placed into the slot, and a scaphoid screw advanced across the nonunion. (From the Mayo Foundation, with permission.)

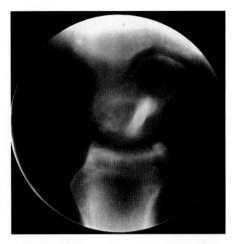

FIGURE 69.15. Tomogram taken at six weeks demonstrates fracture healing in lateral projection. (From the Mayo Foundation, with permission.)

CONCLUSIONS

Vascularized pedicled bone grafts from the dorsal distal radius are based on constant longitudinally oriented vessels with predictable distal anastomoses. For scaphoid nonunions, a reverse-flow pedicle based on the 1,2-ICSRA may be harvested and transposed to the scaphoid through a single incision. Rapid, reliable union of even difficult established scaphoid nonunions with avascular proximal poles or small proximal fragments is predictable. A good clinical outcome is dependent on the absence of degenerative changes.

REFERENCES

1. Cooney WP, Linscheid RL, Dobyns JH, et al. Scaphoid nonunion: role of anterior interpositional bone grafts. *J Hand Surg [Am]* 1988;13:635–650.
2. Stark HH, Rickard TA, Zemel NP, et al. Treatment of ununited fractures of the scaphoid by iliac bone grafts and Kirschner-wire fixation. *J Bone Joint Surg Am* 1988;70:982–991.
3. Manske PR, McCarthy JA, Strecker WB. Use of the Herbert bone screw for scaphoid nonunions. *Orthopedics* 1988;11:1653–1661.
4. Herbert TJ, Fisher WE. Management of the fractured scaphoid usiing a new bone screw. *J Bone Joint Surg Br* 1984;66:114–123.
5. Schneider LH, Aulicino P. Nonunion of the carpal scaphoid: the Russe procedure. *J Trauma* 1982;22:315–319.
6. Cooney WP, Dobyns JH, Linscheid RL. Nonunion of the scaphoid: analysis of the results from bone grafting. *J Hand Surg [Am]* 1980;5:343–354.
7. Green DP. The effect of avascular necrosis on Russe bone grafting for scaphoid nonunion. *J Hand Surg [Am]* 1985;10:597–605.
8. Andrews J, Miller G, Haddad R. Treatment of scaphoid nonunion by volar inlay distal radius bone graft. *J Hand Surg [Br]* 1985;10:214–216.
9. Mazet RJ, Hohl M. Radial styloidectomy and styloidectomy plus bone graft in the treatment of old ununited carpal scaphoid fractures. *Ann Surg* 1960;152:296–302.
10. Mazur KU, Bishop AT, Berger RA. *Vascularized bone grafting for Kienböck's disease: Method and results of retrograde-flow metaphyseal grafts and comparison with cortical graft sites (SS-03).* Paper presented at the 51st Annual Meeting of the American Society for Surgery of the Hand, Nashville, Tennessee, 1996.
11. Sheetz KK, Bishop AT, Berger RA. The arterial blood supply of the distal radius and its potential use in vascularized pedicled bone grafts. *J Hand Surg [Am]* 1995;20:902–914.
12. Bishop AT. Vascularized bone grafting. In: Green DP, Hotchkiss RN, Peaerson WC, eds. *Green's operative hand surgery*, 4th ed. New York: Churchill Livingstone, 1999; 1221–1250.
13. Bishop AT. Vascularized pedicle grafts from the dorsal distal radius: Design and application for carpal pathology. In: Saffar P, Amadio PC, Foucher G, eds. *Current practice in hand surgery*. London: Martin Dunitz, 1997;307–313.
14. Zaidemberg C, Siebert JW, Angrigiani C. A new vascularized bone graft for scaphoid nonunion. *J Hand Surg [Am]* 1991;16:474–478.
15. Roy-Camille R. Fractures et pseudarthroses du scaphoide moyen. Utilisation d'un greffo pedicule. *Act Chir Orthop R Poincare* 1965;4:197–214.
16. Steinman SP, Bishop AT, Berger RA. *Vascularized bone graft for scaphoid nonunion.* Paper presented at the 51st Annual Meeting of the American Society for Surgery of the Hand, Nashville, Tennessee, 1996.
17. Braun RM. *Pronator pedicle bone grafting in the forearm and proximal carpal row.* Paper presented at the Annual Meeting of the American Society for Surgery of the Hand, Anaheim, California, 1983.
18. Braun RM. Viable pedicle bone grafting in the wrist. In: Urbaniak JR, ed. *Microsurgery for major limb reconstruction*. St Louis: CV Mosby, 1987;220–229.
19. Chacha PB. Vascularized pedicular bone grafts. *Int Orthop* 1984;8:117–138.
20. Guimberteau JC, Panconi B. Recalcitrant non-union of the scaphoid treated with a vascularized bone graft based on the ulnar artery. *J Bone Joint Surg Am* 1990;72:88–97.
21. Kawai H, Yamamoto K. Pronator quadratus pedicled bone graft for old scaphoid fractures. *J Bone Joint Surg Br* 1988;70:829–831.
22. Kuhlmann JN, Mimoun M, Boabighi A, et al. Vascularized bone graft pedicled on the volar carpal artery for non-union of the scaphoid. *J Hand Surg [Br]* 1987;12:203–210.

70

SCAPHOLUNATE LIGAMENT RECONSTRUCTION UTILIZING A BONE–RETINACULUM–BONE AUTOGRAFT

MICHAEL T. LEGEYT
ARNOLD-PETER C. WEISS

In the evaluation of wrist pain, the hand surgeon is charged with identifying the cause of symptoms from a multitude of differential diagnoses (1). As understanding of wrist biomechanics and pathoanatomy has developed, injury to the scapholunate interosseous ligament (SLIL) has received considerable attention as an etiology of the painful wrist (2). Currently, static and dynamic dorsal intercalated segmental instability (sDISI and dDISI, respectively) are thought to be the result of injury to the SLIL.

A long-term history of untreated sDISI and dDISI leads to progressive, severe, and disabling arthrosis following a predictable course known as the scapholunate advanced collapse (SLAC) pattern (3). It is for this reason that the treatment of SLIL injuries warrants early surgical intervention. A wide range of procedures have been advocated in managing this injury, including ligament repair (4), tendon weaves (5,6), ligament reconstruction (7), capsulodesis (8), numerous types of limited intercarpal arthrodesis (9–13), and proximal row carpectomy (14,15). Although each of these procedures has its own advantages, disadvantages, and specific indications, in the patient who demonstrates a dDISI pattern of deformity without degenerative changes, we have found successful outcomes with the use of a bone–retinaculum–bone autograft.

INDICATIONS

The treating surgeon must not only identify the SLIL as the cause of symptoms, but also accurately stage the injury according to several key features. This will allow proper selection, from the various surgical procedures, of that which provides the patient with the best relief of symptoms and also provides for the best functional outcome. Determining that the deformity is dDISI, whether by provocative maneuvers on examination (e.g., the scaphoid shift maneuver), stress radiographs (e.g., clenched-fist posteroanterior view), and/or cineradiography, is crucial for success. Just as important is the determination of the presence or absence of arthrosis at the radiocarpal and intercarpal articulations. We recommend confirmation of the absence of arthrosis by both radiographic and arthroscopic examination because early degenerative changes in articular cartilage can be missed on routine radiographs and are a contraindication to SLIL reconstruction. In addition, confirmation of the SLIL tear and the extent of the tear can also be determined by arthroscopic examination, thereby determining if repair or reconstruction should be selected as the treatment option. If there remains any question of the quality of the torn ligament ends to withstand a primary repair, determination can be made at the surgical setting via direct inspection before harvesting the bone–retinaculum–bone autograft.

Once it has been determined that the patient has dDISI and that primary ligament repair cannot be performed, treatment consisting of bone–retinaculum–bone autograft reconstruction is recommended as the procedure of choice. Previous work has shown this graft to have adequate soft tissue, histologic, and biomechanical properties to make it a good choice for graft material (16). This will best restore the normal anatomic relations between the scaphoid and the lunate and provide the least loss of radiocarpal and intercarpal motion. Therefore, the main indications for this procedure are (a) dynamic instability of the scapholunate joint that is reducible intraoperatively and (b) acute scapholunate

---

M. T. LeGeyt: Department of Orthopaedic Surgery, Bristol Hospital, Bristol, Connecticut 06010.

A-P. C. Weiss: Department of Orthopaedics, Brown University School of Medicine, Providence, Rhode Island 02903.

ligament disruption (regardless of the scapholunate gap on radiographs).

CONTRAINDICATIONS

By far the most important factor determining success of treating SLIL injuries lies in the accurate evaluation and staging of the injury. Bone–retinaculum–bone autograft reconstruction is not currently recommended in the treatment of more severe injuries to the carpus (e.g., perilunate dislocations). Careful evaluation by a complete history and physical examination is key to making the diagnosis. Further evaluation utilizing routine and stress radiographs as well as advanced techniques such as cineradiography are warranted if any question remains as to the possibility of additional injuries to the carpal complex. We also recommend careful intraoperative evaluation of the scapholunate interval before harvesting the bone–retinaculum–bone autograft to give final confirmation of the diagnosis and extent of the injury.

In addition to other ligamentous injuries to the wrist, any evidence of arthrosis, whether by radiography or arthroscopy, is also a contraindication to performing bone–retinaculum–bone autograft reconstruction. Furthermore, patients with certain underlying systemic disorders such as rheumatologic diseases, concurrent infection, sarcoidosis, metabolic disorders, and crystalline arthropathies are also contraindicated for bone–retinaculum–bone autograft reconstruction. Patients with chronic scapholunate dissociation and longstanding static dissociation of the scapholunate interval are better treated by alternative methods (generally involving limited arthrodesis) because of the difficulty of obtaining and maintaining a satisfactory intraoperative reduction.

SURGICAL TECHNIQUE

The procedure can be performed with a variety of anesthetic techniques including a Bier block, axillary block, and general anesthesia. We routinely give a preoperative dose of antibiotic, usually a first-generation cephalosporin, 30 minutes before beginning the procedure. Exsanguinate the arm with an esmarch bandage and inflate the tourniquet placed above the elbow to 250 mm Hg. Proceed by mapping out a straight 5- to 6-cm dorsal incision placed just ulnar to Lister's tubercle. Carry out the dissection down through the skin and subcutaneous tissue to identify the extensor retinaculum, taking care to avoid cutaneous branches of the radial nerve and to ligate or cauterize small vessels (Fig. 70.1). Open the third dorsal compartment of the wrist and transpose the extensor pollicis longus (EPL) tendon radially. Incise the wrist capsule longitudinally and elevate from proximal to distal and from radial to ulnar,

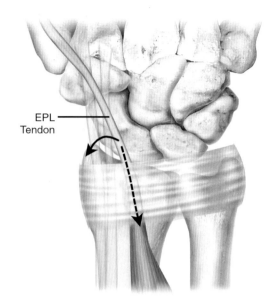

FIGURE 70.1. After careful dissection through the dorsal wrist subcutaneous tissues, the third extensor compartment is opened, continuing distally through the dorsal wrist capsule and allowing transposition radially of the extensor pollicis longus (EPL) tendon.

identifying the scaphoid and lunate. At this time, inspect the SLIL and judge whether primary repair will be successful. If not, proceed by harvesting a bony block of 20 × 8 × 8 mm (adjusted for patient size) with the overlying attached periosteum and retinaculum from Lister's tubercle using a small osteotome (Fig. 70.2). Wrap the autograft in

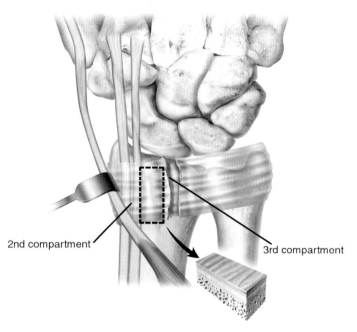

FIGURE 70.2. A 20 mm × 8 mm area over Lister's tubercle is incised with a #15 blade, and then, with a sharp osteotome, a bone block is removed with the overlying periosteum and retinaculum intact.

saline-soaked gauze until it is ready to be implanted. Next, remove any remaining ligamentous debris from the scaphoid and lunate. Kirschner wires (K-wires) are then drilled into the scaphoid and lunate to be used as joysticks. Reduce the scapholunate joint and drill two 0.045-in. K-wires across from the anatomic snuffbox to the lunate (Fig. 70.3). Confirm the reduction and the position of the K-wires with intraoperative fluoroscopy; then remove the joysticks. Using a small osteotome, fashion a trough in the proximal aspect of the scaphoid and lunate to accept the autograft (Fig. 70.4).

Using a fine ronguer, remove a narrow midportion of the cancellous and cortical bone from the autograft while taking care to leave the overlying periosteum and retinaculum intact (Fig. 70.5). Now place the autograft into the scaphoid and lunate with firm digital pressure (Fig. 70.6). Distract the wrist and extend it 30°, locking the autograft into place using the dorsal lip of the distal radius (Fig. 70.7). Once the graft is in adequate position and stable, repair the capsule with some measure of imbrication to maintain pressure on the graft. It is important to emphasize the fact that if the troughs are slightly undersized with respect to the graft, it will stay with little effort. If the graft is not stable in its bed, then consider stabilizing it with temporary K-wires or miniscrew fixation.

Confirm the position of the graft and the reduction of the scapholunate interval with fluoroscopy; then close the wound in layers leaving the EPL tendon transposed radially. Immobilize the wrist in a short arm splint with the wrist in 30° of extension.

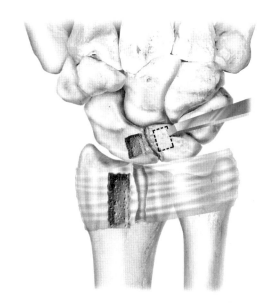

FIGURE 70.4. Troughs measuring approximately 8 mm high and 6 to 7 mm wide are fashioned using an osteotome and curette in the dorsal proximal scaphoid and dorsal radial lunate.

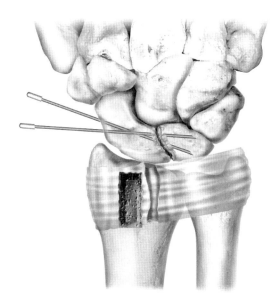

FIGURE 70.3. After appropriate reduction of the scapholunate interval, the scaphoid should be transfixed to the lunate by two crossed Kirschner wires.

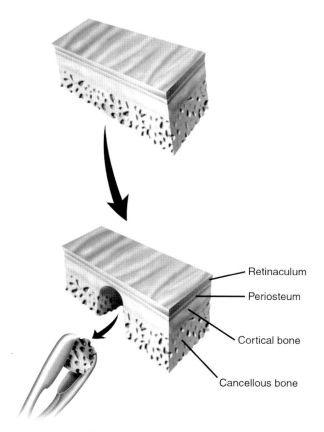

FIGURE 70.5. A fine rongeur is used to remove the midportion of cancellous and cortical bone, resulting in a bone–retinaculum–bone autograft.

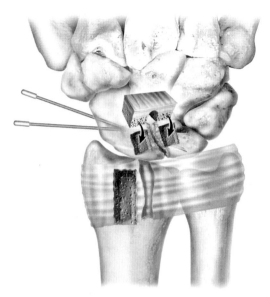

FIGURE 70.6. The autograft is then placed with firm digital pressure, matching the bony block sizes, into the troughs fashioned into the dorsal scaphoid and lunate.

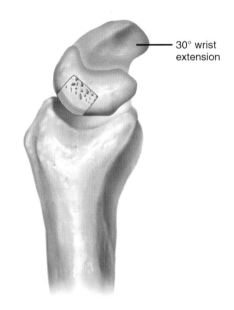

FIGURE 70.7. With slight distraction and extension to 30°, the dorsal lip of the distal radius locks the bone–retinaculum–bone autograft into place.

POSTOPERATIVE MANAGEMENT

Place the patient in a short arm cast 2 weeks after surgery when the sutures are removed. When the cast is applied at 2 weeks postoperatively, the wrist is placed in 10° of extension for an additional 6 weeks. The cast can be removed and therapy begun once the graft has incorporated, usually at 8 weeks.

The goal after soft tissue reconstruction is to provide the patient with a stable, functional, pain-free wrist. Therapy should begin while the patient is casted with edema management (elevation, retrograde massage and compression wraps for the digits), tendon gliding exercises to prevent adhesions, and active/passive range of motion (A/PROM) for the uninvolved joints as needed to prevent stiffness. After cast removal, initiate scar massage, begin PROM for the wrist, and finally commence AROM exercises with strengthening.

Slow steady gains in wrist ROM are optimal. One should not push to regain full motion too quickly in our experience, as ROM of the wrist continues to improve up to several years. Patient education on the benefits of a stable pain-free wrist rather than one with full motion that is lax and painful may be necessary. Soft tissue reconstruction generally affords greater ROM than a limited wrist arthrodesis, and in some cases full ROM may be achieved.

Some patients develop excessive capsular tightness limiting wrist flexion. PROM of the wrist may be required but should be initiated only after adequate soft-tissue healing has taken place. The use of heat and stretch in conjunction can be effective in eliciting elongation of the periarticular tissues. Function may be addressed as soon as pain and healing permit. Begin by involving the affected extremity in self-care tasks, progressing to activities of daily living (ADLs), and finally to full functional use as tolerated. This process can take several weeks. Progressive resistive exercises may be needed to regain full use. Usually, the length of therapy is approximately 3 months with significant improvement continuing for up to 6 months and, in some cases, up to several years after surgical reconstruction.

TECHNICAL ALTERNATIVES

Should the surgeon feel that after performing bone–retinaculum–bone autograft reconstruction the patient needs additional protection, a capsulodesis as described by Blatt (8) may be added to the surgical technique already described with only minor changes. In these cases we have found it useful to perform a "reverse Blatt" capsulodesis. That is to say, the distal aspect of the capsule is left attached to the scaphoid, and the proximal aspect, where it attaches to the distal radius, is imbricated.

If Lister's tubercle is unsatisfactory as a graft (generally only in patients with a history of previous dorsal wrist surgery), the surgeon has several alternatives. Possible alternative donor sites include the contralateral distal radius, the dorsal tarsometatarsal ligament, the dorsal metatarsal ligament of the fourth or fifth metatarsals, or the dorsal calcaneocuboid ligament of the foot (17). These alternative graft sites have a degree of morbidity, and we would not recommend these as a primary choice of grafts. Although allografts have been used with considerable success in other orthopedic surgeries, the risks of transmitted disease, however small, preclude them from our recommending them to patients currently.

CLINICAL SERIES

In the index study describing the bone–retinaculum–bone autograft reconstruction technique, all patients with dynamic instability had substantial relief of wrist pain (7). Although two patients had pain with heavy activity, 12 of the 14 patients were completely pain-free. There was an average decrease in the wrist flexion and extension arc after reconstruction from 69/72° to 52/67°. However, radial–ulnar deviation and supination–pronation arcs of motion were insignificantly affected. Grip strength demonstrated an improvement from 27 kg to 39 kg. Thirteen of 14 patients with dynamic instability were completely satisfied with their result at average follow-up of 3.6 years.

ACKNOWLEDGMENT

We would like to thank Nancy R. Feinberg, M.H.S., O.T.R./L., for her contribution to this chapter.

> ### EDITORS' COMMENTS
>
> The scapholunate ligament is the chief culprit in the wrist. Statistically, most wrist problems revolve around tearing of the SLIL, usually through multiple traumas over time. The tears of the scapholunate ligament system begin volarly and progress dorsally, eventually destroying the dorsal ligaments if traumatic incidents continue. An ideal ligament repair would entail some manner of reestablishing the volar scapholunate interosseous system. The bone–retinaculum–bone autograft increases the stability of the dorsalmost ligaments and might in time prove an effective procedure, particularly if used volarly.

REFERENCES

1. Weiss A-PC, Akelman E. Diagnostic imaging and arthroscopy for chronic wrist pain. *Orthop Clin North Am* 1995;26:759–767.
2. Mayfield JK. Patterns of injury to carpal ligaments. A spectrum. *Clin Orthop* 1984;187:36–42.
3. Watson HK, Ballet FL. The SLAC wrist: scapholunate advanced collapse pattern of degenerative arthritis. *J Hand Surg [Am]* 1984;9:358–365.
4. Lavernia CJ, Cohen JS, Taleisnik J. Treatment of scapholunate dissociation by ligamentous repair and capsulodesis. *J Hand Surg [Am]* 1992;17:354–359.
5. Almquist EE, Bach AW, Sack JT, et al. Four-bone ligament reconstruction for treatment of chronic complete scapholunate separation. *J Hand Surg [Am]* 1991;16:322–327.
6. Minami A, Kaneda K. Repair and/or reconstruction of scapholunate interosseous ligament in lunate and perilunate dislocations. *J Hand Surg [Am]* 1993;18:1009–1106.
7. Weiss A-PC. Scapholunate ligament reconstruction using a bone–retinaculum–bone autograft. *J Hand Surg [Am]* 1998;23:205–215.
8. Blatt G. Capsulodesis in reconstructive hand surgery: dorsal capsulodesis for the unstable scaphoid and volar capsulodesis following excision of the distal ulna. *Hand Clin* 1987;3:81–102.
9. Eckenrode JF, Louis DS, Greene TL. Schapoid–trapezium–trapezoid fusion in the treatment of chronic scapholunate instability. *J Hand Surg [Am]* 1986;11:497–502.
10. Hom S, Ruby LK. Attempted scapholunate arthrodesis for chronic scapholunate dissociation. *J Hand Surg [Am]* 1991;16:334–339.
11. Watson HK, Goodman ML, Johnson TR. Limited wrist arthrodesis. Part II: intercarpal and radiocarpal combinations. *J Hand Surg [Am]* 1981;6:223–233.
12. Watson HK, Hempton RF. Limited wrist arthrodeses. Part I: The triscaphoid joint. *J Hand Surg [Am]* 1980;5:320–327.
13. Watson HK, Ryu J, Akelman E. Limited triscaphoid intercarpal arthrodesis for rotatory subluxation of the scaphoid. *J Bone Joint Surg Am* 1986;68:345–349.
14. Tomaino MM, Delsignore J, Burton RI. Long-term results following proximal row carpectomy. *J Hand Surg [Am]* 1994;19:694–703.
15. Tomaino MM, Miller RJ, Cole I, et al. Scapholunate advanced collapse wrist: proximal row carpectomy or limited wrist arthrodesis with scaphoid excision? *J Hand Surg [Am]* 1994;19:134–142.
16. Shin SS, Moore DC, McGovern RD, et al. Scapholunate ligament reconstruction using a bone–retinaculum–bone autograft: a biomechanic and histologic study. *J Hand Surg [Am]* 1998;23:216–221.
17. Svoboda SJ, Eglseder A Jr, Belkoff SM. Autografts from the foot for reconstruction of the scapholunate interosseous ligament. *J Hand Surg [Am]* 1995;20:980–985.

71

SCAPHOLUNATE ADVANCED COLLAPSE WRIST RECONSTRUCTION

JEFFREY WEINZWEIG
H. KIRK WATSON

INDICATIONS

Scapholunate advanced collapse (SLAC) is the most common pattern of degenerative disease of the wrist (1). The most common etiology of SLAC wrist is rotary subluxation of the scaphoid (RSS) followed by scaphoid nonunion. Other conditions that will produce SLAC degeneration include Preiser's disease, midcarpal instability, intraarticular fractures involving the radioscaphoid or capitate–lunate joints, and Kienböck's disease tertiary to the secondary RSS (2–5). The key to reconstruction of the SLAC wrist lies in the radiolunate articulation. Because this is preserved at all stages of the SLAC sequence because of its spherical configuration, virtually all patients with a SLAC wrist are candidates for this type of reconstruction, regardless of the etiology of the degenerative process (6).

CONTRAINDICATIONS

SLAC wrist reconstruction involves excision of the scaphoid and arthrodesis of the capitate, lunate, hamate, and triquetrum. This procedure is also referred to as a "four-bone fusion." Successful reconstruction depends on a normal radiolunate articulation through which load transfer can occur postoperatively. Patients who present with SLAC wrist in conjunction with lunate or radiolunate pathology are not candidates for this type of reconstruction. Significant ulnar translation, which disrupts the concentric congruity of the radiolunate articulation and predictably leads to joint destruction, osteonecrosis of the lunate as in Kienböck's disease, and preexisting radiolunate degenerative change are absolute contraindications to SLAC wrist reconstruction (7,8). The salvage procedures under these conditions include radius lunate arthrodesis proximal row carpectomy and wrist arthrodesis.

SURGICAL TECHNIQUE

The surgical approach is identical to that used for triscaphe limited wrist arthrodesis (see Chapter 73). Two parallel incisions are made: one overlying the radiocarpal joint dorsally, and one proximally over the distal radial aspect of the radius for harvest of a cancellous bone graft (Fig. 71.1). After the extensor retinaculum is incised along the third compartment, a transverse incision is made through the wrist capsule at the level of the capitate–lunate joint. The scaphoid is approached in the interval between the extensor carpi radialis longus and brevis and removed in piecemeal fashion with a dental rongeur (Fig. 71.2). Care is taken to preserve the radial and palmar ligamentous structures.

Longitudinal traction on the fingers permits exposure of the radiolunate joint and confirmation that it is well preserved. With this done, articular cartilage and subchondral bone are removed from the adjacent surfaces of the capitate, lunate, hamate, and triquetrum using a dental rongeur until a broad cancellous surface is obtained (Fig. 71.3). Longitudinal traction also assists in visualizing the intercarpal joints, especially the volar aspect of the capitate–lunate joint.

Cancellous bone is then harvested from the distal radius through the proximal incision (see Chapter 54). Somewhat less bone graft is required for SLAC reconstruction than is required for triscaphe arthrodesis, as it is not necessary to maintain the original external dimensions of the capitate–lunate–hamate–triquetrum joints. Some degree of

---

J. Weinzweig: Department of Plastic Surgery, Brown University School of Medicine, Rhode Island Hospital, and Hasbro Children's Hospital, Providence, Rhode Island 02905.

H. K. Watson: Connecticut Combined Hand Surgery Fellowship, Hartford Hospital, and Connecticut Children's Medical Center, Hartford, Connecticut 06106; Department of Orthopaedics, University of Connecticut School of Medicine, Farmington, Connecticut 06032; Department of Orthopedics, Rehabilitation, and Plastic Surgery, Yale University School of Medicine, New Haven, Connecticut 06520.

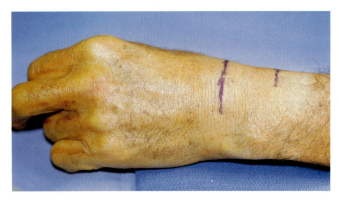

FIGURE 71.1. The distal incision is placed at the level of the radiocarpal joint; the proximal incision is placed over the distal radial aspect of the radius, 2.0 to 2.5 cm proximal to the distal incision.

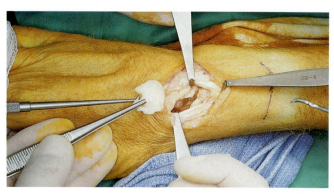

FIGURE 71.2. The scaphoid is excised in piecemeal fashion. The scaphoid is more easily removed if it is osteotomized through its central portion, the proximal pole removed first, and the distal pole removed with curved dental curettes, maintaining external ligamentous support.

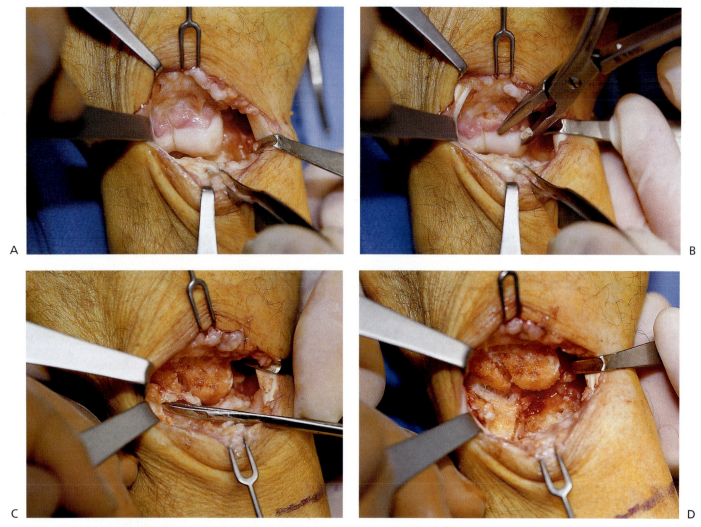

FIGURE 71.3. A: With distal traction on the middle and index fingers, the proximal articular surfaces of the capitate and hamate can be visualized between the third and fourth dorsal compartments. **B:** The cartilage and subchondral bone from the proximal joint between the capitate and hamate are removed down to cancellous bone with a dental rongeur. **C:** A small curette is useful for removal of cartilage and subchondral bone within the narrow joint spaces. **D:** The adjacent articular surfaces of the capitate, hamate, lunate, and triquetrum have been removed (in each of these images of a left wrist, the fingers are pointing up).

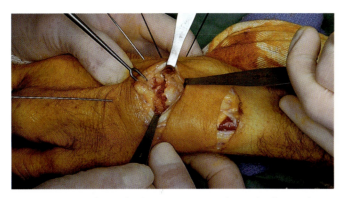

FIGURE 71.4. Three K-wires are preset through the capitate, hamate, and triquetrum up to the fusion site to be driven into the lunate. A fourth wire is preset into the triquetrum to be driven into the capitate. Part of the cancellous graft is then packed in the deep interval between the capitate and lunate. The dorsal intercalated segment instability deformity of the lunate is reduced (note a visible portion of proximal articular surface), and the K-wires are driven across to maintain carpal alignment. Note the proximal incision used to harvest distal radius bone graft.

collapse of the capitate and hamate on the lunate and triquetrum is tolerated because all load will pass directly through the single fused unit and subsequently through the preserved radiolunate joint. No other joints will be affected by this alignment change.

Three 0.045-in. Kirschner wires are passed percutaneously and preset through the capitate, hamate, and triquetrum up to the fusion site to be driven into the lunate. A fourth wire is preset into the triquetrum to be driven into the capitate. Part of the cancellous graft is then packed in the deep interval between the capitate and lunate (Fig. 71.4).

The single most important step in SLAC reconstruction is correction of the common tendency for dorsal intercalated segment instability (DISI) deformity of the lunate. The capitate must be volarly displaced on the lunate to prevent its fusion on the dorsum of the lunate with the lunate in DISI position. A buttress pin running dorsally into the lunate abutting the dorsal edge of the radius can be used to maintain the lunate in a slight volar intercalated segment instability (VISI) position. A joker placed across the distal lunate surface and used as a lever will suffice for lunate position control. It is important to bring the capitate ulnarly and align it centered on the lunate. This tightens upslope ligaments such as the radioscaphocapitate ligament and maintains radial positioning of the lunate. The preset pins are then driven into the lunate from the capitate, hamate, and triquetrum and from the triquetrum into the capitate. The intercarpal spaces are then densely packed with remaining bone graft using a dental tamp (Fig. 71.5). All pins are cut off below skin level, and a single layer intracuticular monofilament closure is used for the skin (Fig. 71.6). The hand is placed in a protected position with the wrist in slight extension and radial deviation, the forearm neutral, and the elbow at 90° (Fig, 71.7).

Since the original description of the SLAC wrist in 1984 (1), we have abandoned the use of silicone implants for replacement of the excised scaphoid during SLAC reconstruction. The incidence of particulate silicone synovitis, an unacceptable complication requiring implant removal in eight patients, and the realization that a scaphoid spacer is entirely unnecessary to prevent radial deviation of the wrist following scaphoid removal resulted in technique modification in 1988. Subsequent comparison of functional outcomes in patients with and without silicone implants supports these conclusions.

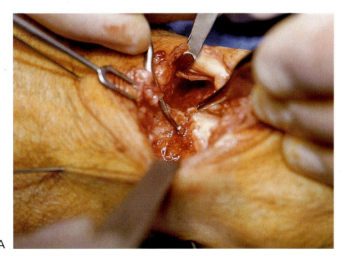 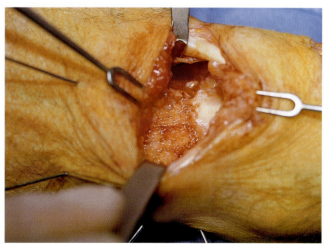

FIGURE 71.5. A,B: The intercarpal spaces are completely filled with cancellous graft using a dental tamp (in both of these images of a left wrist, the fingers are pointing to the left).

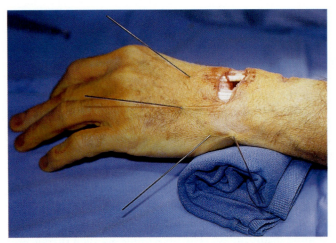

FIGURE 71.6. Appearance once the four K-wires have been driven across the fusion sites. All wires are cut off below skin level before the incisions are closed.

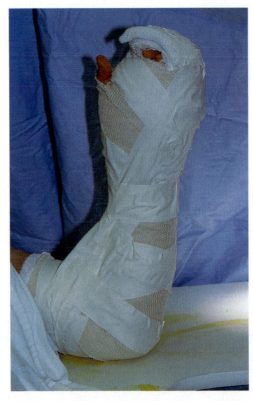

FIGURE 71.7. The intraoperative bulky dressing incorporates a long arm plaster splint that maintains the wrist in slight extension and radial deviation, the forearm neutral, and the elbow at 90°.

POSTOPERATIVE MANAGEMENT

Postoperative immobilization and management are similar to that described for triscaphe arthrodesis. Maximum initial immobilization is mandatory for these small bone fusions. Three to five days following surgery, the bulky dressing is removed, and a long arm thumb–spica cast is applied (see Chapter 48). Three weeks following limited wrist arthrodesis, the long arm cast and intracuticular sutures are removed. A short arm thumb–spica cast is applied for an additional 3 weeks. Only the thumb is included in this cast. In patients over the age of 55, 2 weeks in a long arm cast followed by 4 weeks in a short arm cast is sufficient. Six weeks postoperatively, the short arm cast is removed, and radiographs are obtained (Fig. 71.8). If radiographic evidence of union is seen, the pins are removed in the office, and the patient is referred for hand therapy for full wrist mobilization. Patients who are smokers, or those in whom there is any doubt as the status of bony healing, may occasionally be splinted for an additional week or two.

The average range of motion after SLAC reconstruction is approximately 60% of the contralateral normal wrist while average grip strength is usually greater than 90%. Long-term radiographic follow-up has demonstrated no secondary degenerative change at the radiolunate joint or other adjacent joints (2).

CLINICAL SERIES

Three hundred thirty-one patients underwent SLAC wrist reconstruction over a 22-year period. These patients were aged from 19 to 82 years and included 187 men and 65 women. The etiologies of SLAC wrist and indications for reconstruction included chronic rotary subluxation of the scaphoid, established scaphoid nonunion, advanced radioscaphoid SLAC, advanced midcarpal SLAC, distal radial fracture resulting in dislocation or disruption of the scaphoid fossa, congenital preaxial hypoplasia, fracture of the capitate, and Preiser's disease (9).

The mean duration of symptoms was 52 months (range, 1–516 months). The preoperative range of motion was limited in all cases, with a mean flexion–extension arc of 88°. Radiographic assessment revealed evidence of radioscaphoid degenerative change alone (stage I SLAC wrist) in 40% of wrists. 60% of wrists demonstrated progressive collapse with midcarpal degenerative change as well (stage II SLAC wrist). Mean follow-up was 44 months (range, 12–136 months).

Primary union occurred in 97% of cases with a mean period of immobilization of 47 days (range, 21–98 days). Ninety-one percent of patients reported that pain was better or much better following the SLAC reconstruction. Mean wrist flexion and extension was 53% of the normal opposite wrist. Mean radial and ulnar deviation was 59% of the unaffected opposite side. Mean grip strength was 80% of the opposite side.

Eighty percent returned to their original employment after a mean period of disability of 14 weeks from surgery (range, 24–98 days). Ninety-two percent of patients expressed satisfaction with the arthrodesis and stated they would undergo the procedure again if faced with the same

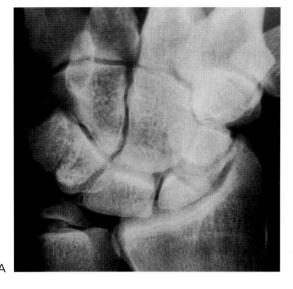
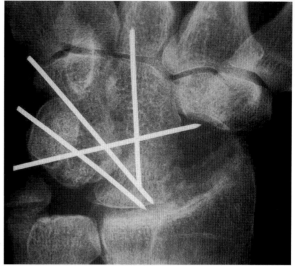
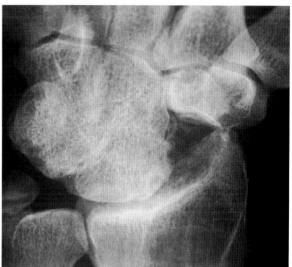

FIGURE 71.8. Scapholunate advanced collapse (SLAC) wrist reconstruction. **A:** Stage I SLAC wrist secondary to scaphoid nonunion. **B:** Postoperative radiograph 6 weeks after SLAC reconstruction with limited wrist arthrodesis and scaphoid excision demonstrates typical pin placement and adequate bony consolidation. **C:** Six months after reconstruction, the arthrodesis is radiographically solid. Note the ulnar displacement of the capitate on the lunate which tightens the radioscaphocapitate ligament and prevents ulnar translation.

situation. No secondary degenerative changes have been noted in this series on follow-up radiographs.

COMPLICATIONS

Complications after more than 300 SLAC wrist reconstructions include nonunion in 1% of cases, wound infection in 1%, and reflex sympathetic dystrophy in 1.5%. The most probable causes of nonunion in intercarpal arthrodesis are inadequate immobilization and insufficient preparation of the bones to be fused. One patient underwent total wrist arthrodesis for persistent pain in the absence of secondary degenerative changes on wrist radiographs.

Dorsal impingement among the capitate, bone graft, and radius following SLAC reconstruction required revision arthroplasty in 13% of patients. Radiographic evaluation suggested that this was technique-related. Inadequate reduction of the DISI deformity of the lunate at the time of arthrodesis not only leads to loss of carpal height but limits the available arc of radiolunate motion. Excessive graft can heal and impinge dorsally. During wrist extension, the capitate approaches the dorsal lip of the radius, where impingement may occur with associated pain. Coaxial alignment of the lunate with the capitate is essential for optimal outcome.

DISCUSSION

SLAC wrist reconstruction represents an evolution of concepts over a period of three decades. Excision of the scaphoid with arthrodesis of the capitate, lunate, hamate, and triquetrum as a "four-corner" fusion has proven to be a reliable, effective procedure for the management of SLAC wrist, the most common pattern of degenerative disease of the wrist, regardless of the etiology. The fusion block provides a stable column for load transfer through an intact radiolunate articulation, resulting in a painless wrist with preserved function.

REFERENCES

1. Watson HK, Ballet FL. The SLAC wrist: scapholunate advanced collapse pattern of degenerative arthritis. *J Hand Surg [Am]* 1984;9:358–365.
2. Watson HK, Goodman ML, Johnson TR. Limited wrist arthrodesis. Part II: Intercarpal and radiocarpal combinations. *J Hand Surg [Am]* 1981;6:223–232.
3. Watson HK, Hempton RE. Limited wrist arthrodesis. Part I: The triscaphoid joint. *J Hand Surg [Am]* 1980;5:320–327.
4. Watson HK, Weinzweig J, Guidera P, et al. One thousand intercarpal arthrodeses. *J Hand Surg [Br]* 1999;24:307–315.
5. Watson HK, Weinzweig J, Zeppieri J. The natural progression of scaphoid instability. *Hand Clin* 1997;13:39–50.
6. Watson HK, Weinzweig J. Intercarpal arthrodesis. In: Green DP, Hotchkiss RN, Pederson WC, eds. *Operative hand surgery*, 4th ed. New York: Churchill Livingstone, 1998;108–130.
7. Ashmead D, Watson HK, Damon C, et al. Scapholunate advanced collapse wrist salvage. *J Hand Surg [Am]* 1994;19:741–750.
8. Ashmead D, Watson HK. SLAC wrist reconstruction. In: Gelberman R, ed. *Mater techniques in orthopaedic surgery: The wrist.* New York: Raven Press, 1994;319–330.
9. Weinzweig J, Watson HK. Wrist sprain to SLAC wrist: a spectrum of carpal instability. In: Vastamaki M, ed. *Current trends in hand surgery.* Amsterdam: Elsevier, 1995;47–55.

72

TRAPEZOIDAL OSTEOTOMY OF THE DISTAL RADIUS

JEFFREY WEINZWEIG
H. KIRK WATSON

INDICATIONS

Malunion following a Colles' fracture is usually accompanied by loss of the normal palmar tilt of the articular surface of the distal radius, loss of the normal radial inclination, and shortening and supination of the distal fragment. As a result of these deformities, proper function of the distal radioulnar, radiocarpal, and midcarpal joints is impaired (1–5) (see Chapter 21). Indications for trapezoidal osteotomy of the distal radius include functional compromise of the wrist with significant loss of pronosupination, radiocarpal pain or instability, and persistent weakness secondary to abnormal carpal biomechanics resulting from reversal of the normal palmar tilt of the distal radial articular surface (6–9).

CONTRAINDICATIONS

The only relative contraindication to performing a trapezoidal osteotomy of the distal radius is previous harvest of sufficient cortical bone graft from this region as to preclude safely reharvesting additional graft. In such rare circumstances, the contralateral wrist could serve as the bone graft donor site.

SURGICAL TECHNIQUE

A dorsal transverse incision approximately 4 cm in length is made along the radial aspect of the wrist 3 cm proximal to the radial styloid. The transverse incision lies halfway between the level of the radiocarpal joint and the proximal edge of the trapezoidal bone graft. This allows access to all components of the surgery. Spreading technique is used to preserve superficial veins and nerves, including the superficial branch of the radial nerve. At the proximal edge of the extensor retinaculum, the periosteum of the distal radius is elevated, and two K-wires can be placed in the dorsal cortex on either side of the proposed osteotomy site. The proximal pin is placed perpendicular to the cortex of the radius. The distal pin is placed parallel to the malpositioned articular surface on direct visualization. These will guide the degree of correction later in the procedure.

The dorsal transverse osteotomy, which is performed within 1.0 cm of the radiocarpal joint, should be perpendicular to the long axis of the radius in the posteroanterior (PA) plane but sloped to match the articular surface of the radius, dorsal to volar. The palmar periosteum should be left undisturbed. The osteotomy is opened dorsally until the K-wires subtend an angle equal to the palmar tilt desired (Fig. 72.1). Ten degrees of palmar tilt of the articular surface is ideal. This position can be confirmed by intraoperative radiographs, if desired. To reestablish radial inclination, the osteotomy must open more on the radial side. The extra length required on the radial side can be measured directly on the preoperative anteroposterior (AP) radiograph, or it can be determined radiographically intraoperatively.

The osteotomy site is now seen as a trapezoid and must be filled with a bone graft of similar dimensions. The shape and dimensions of the trapezoid are transposed to the dorsal surface of the proximal radial fragment, where the osteotomy is outlined with multiple holes using a K-wire or drill bit (Fig. 72.2A). The donor site abuts the transverse osteotomy such that the longer radial margin of the trapezoidal graft comes from the distal edge of the graft. The corticocancellous graft is removed from the radial metaphysis using a $^3/_{16}$-in. osteotome.

J. Weinzweig: Department of Plastic Surgery, Brown University School of Medicine, Rhode Island Hospital, and Hasbro Children's Hospital, Providence, Rhode Island 02905.

H. K. Watson: Connecticut Combined Hand Surgery Fellowship, Hartford Hospital and Connecticut Children's Medical Center, Hartford, Connecticut 06106; Department of Orthopaedics, University of Connecticut School of Medicine, Farmington, Connecticut 06032; Department of Orthopedics, Rehabilitation, and Plastic Surgery, Yale University School of Medicine, New Haven, Connecticut 06520.

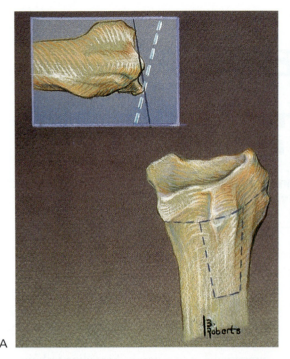
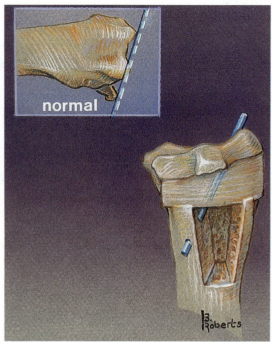
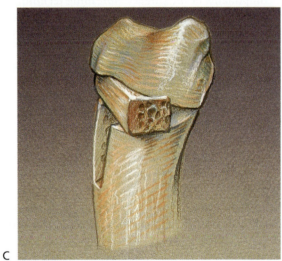

FIGURE 72.1. Trapezoidal osteotomy technique. **A:** The volar articular tilt of the radius is restored with an opening wedge osteotomy. Surgery is accomplished through a transverse incision midway between the articular surface of the radius and the most proximal aspect of the trapezoidal-shaped graft. **B:** If radial lengthening is indicated, the slightly wider aspect of the trapezoidal graft is placed radially as the opening wedge osteotomy is accomplished. The graft will lock against the cortices proximally and against the broad cancellous surface of the distal segment. A 0.045-in. Kirschner wire can be used to "cage" the graft. The graft may be rectangular if no radial lengthening is indicated. **C:** The degree of volar angulation can be controlled and modified by moving the graft volarly or dorsally.

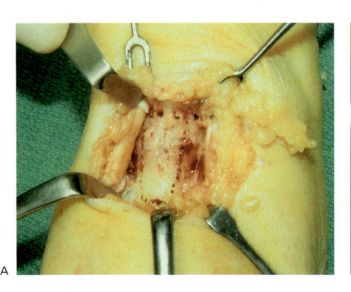
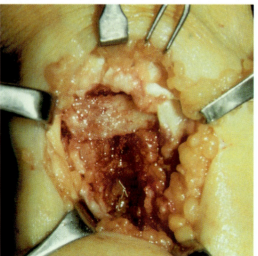

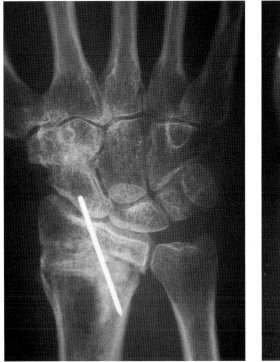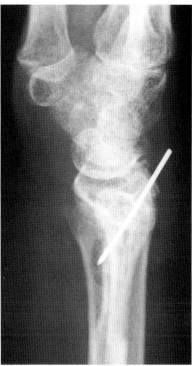

FIGURE 72.3. Posteroanterior **(A)** and lateral **(B)** radiographs 6 weeks following trapezoidal osteotomy. The volar slope of the distal radius has been restored, and healing is solid. The caging pin is removed in the office at this time.

With the transverse osteotomy site again held open by two small osteotomes, the trapezoidal graft is turned 90° and placed into position (Fig. 72.2B). A very stable construct is thus created by a combination of soft tissue tension and slight impaction of the graft, placing the trapezoidal cortex deep to the dorsal radial cortex. Sufficient fixation is obtained when the graft is "caged" using one or two K-wires through Lister's tubercle, through the cortex of the graft, and out through the ulnar aspect of the radius shaft (Fig. 72.3). After the pins are placed, gentle passive supination and pronation are effected to assess the distal radioulnar joint. In the case of significant limitation of motion, a matched ulnar arthroplasty is performed (see Chapter 59). The pins are then cut off below skin level, and the skin incision is closed. The extremity is immobilized in a bulky long arm dressing incorporating a dorsal plaster splint in 90° of elbow flexion, neutral rotation, and slight wrist extension.

POSTOPERATIVE MANAGEMENT

The bulky dressing and splint are removed 3 to 5 days postoperatively, and a long arm cast is applied including the thumb, index, and long fingers to their tips in the intrinsic plus position ("Groucho Marx" cast; see Chapter 48). At 4 weeks, a short arm cast is substituted for an additional 2 weeks. The "cage" pins are removed in the office at 6 weeks, following radiographic confirmation of bony healing, and range-of-motion excercises are begun.

CLINICAL SERIES

A dorsal opening corrective trapezoidal osteotomy of the radius was performed on 41 patients for treatment of malunion of Colles' fractures. In each case, a closed extraarticular fracture, usually the result of a fall, had initially been

FIGURE 72.2. Trapezoidal osteotomy technique. **A:** The osteotomy is best performed with multiple drill holes connected by a fine osteotome rather than with any high-speed instruments, which would produce bone necrosis. **B:** The graft is turned 90°, and cancellous bone graft is then pushed from the radius proximally up under the trapezoidal graft distally. No other grafting is necessary. Postoperatively, there is volar angulation and restoration of radial length. The graft is healed at 6 weeks.

treated with closed reduction and plaster fixation before referral. Patients presented with complaints of pain, deformity, and significant limitations in range of motion and power, and demonstrated reversal of the normal palmar tilt of the distal radial articular surface. These patients had an average dorsal tilt of −18.8° (range, −5° to −35°), compared with the normal palmar tilt of 11°. Seventy-five percent of cases involved the dominant wrist; the average age at operation was 43 years (range, 15–78 years) (9).

Trapezoidal osteotomy resulted in an excellent correction of distal radial deformity. The average plamar tilt of the distal radial articular surface averaged 12.4° following trapezoidal osteotomy (range, 4–30°), which compared favorably with the normal average palmar tilt. Radial length was similarly maintained in all patients except one who developed a nonunion. Radial inclination was increased to an average of 17.8° (normal, 22°) following trapezoidal osteotomy.

COMPLICATIONS

Few complications occurred following trapezoidal osteotomy. One patient developed a nonunion requiring plate and screw fixation and iliac crest bone graft. Another patient developed reflex sympathetic dystrophy that was treated with a Dystrophile program (see Chapter 65).

DISCUSSION

Loss of the normal palmar tilt of the distal radius, which often accompanies a malunion of a Colles' fracture, has a profound effect on wrist function and dynamics (1,4,5,10). The distal radial surface normally directs loads across the carpus onto the strong palmar ligaments. With reversal of this tilt following malunion of a Colles' fracture, loads are directed dorsally. However, the radiocarpal and intercarpal joints are not adapted for dorsal loading, which will result in significant symptoms in the active patient and, ultimately, carpal instability (1,5).

Two types of wrist instability may develop, depending on maintenance of the integrity of the carpal ligaments. With intact intercarpal ligaments, dorsal carpal translocation may occur in which a collinear lunate and capitate are translocated dorsal to the axis of the radius. With intercarpal ligamentous compromise, a midcarpal dorsal intercalated segment instability (DISI) pattern will develop. The lunate is blocked from translating palmarly by the malunion. In this case, the radius, lunate, and capitate will not be collinear. Correction of these conditions, which are often accompanied by a profound cosmetic deformity of the distal radius and carpus, requires an osteotomy of the distal radius. Fernandez states that symptoms will develop if angular deformity exceeds 25° to 30° in the sagittal plane or if radial shortening exceeds 6 mm (11). We believe the development of symptoms is much more difficult to categorize because the activity level of the patient is the main predictor. Many osteotomies have been described for the correction of malunited distal radius fractures (6,8,11–16). Each of these, however, has been fraught with compromise or complication. The technique described herein of trapezoidal osteotomy of the distal radius provides excellent results using a local corticocancellous bone graft and simple pin fixation (16).

REFERENCES

1. Bickerstaff DR, Bell MJ. Carpal malalignments in Colles' fractures. *J Hand Surg [Br]* 1989;14:155–160.
2. Cooney WD, Dobyns JH, Linscheid RL. Complications of Colles' fracture. *J Bone Joint Surg Am* 1980;62:613–619.
3. Jenkins NH, Mintowt-Czyz WJ. Malunion and dysfunction in Colles' fractures. *J Hand Surg [Br]* 1988;13:291–293.
4. Pogue DJ, Viegas SF, Patterson RM, et al. Effects of distal radius fracture malunion on wrist joint mechanics. *J Hand Surg [Am]* 1990;15:721–727.
5. Taleisnik J, Watson HK. Midcarpal instability caused by malunited fractures of the distal radius. *J Hand Surg [Am]* 1984;9:350–357.
6. Brown JN, Bell MJ. Distal radial osteotomy for malunion of wrist fractures in young patients. *J Hand Surg [Br]* 1994;19:589–593.
7. Milch H. Treatment of instabilities following fractures of the lower end of the radius. *Clin Orthop* 1963;29:157–163.
8. Posner MA, Ambrose L. Malunited Colles' fractures: correction with a biplanar closed wedge osteotomy. *J Hand Surg [Am]* 1991;16:1017–1026.
9. Watson HK, Castle TH. Trapezoidal osteotomy of the distal radius for unacceptable articular angulation after Colles' fracture. *J Hand Surg [Am]* 1988;13:837–843.
10. Jupiter JB, Masem M. Reconstruction of post-traumatic deformity of the distal radius and ulna. *Hand Clin* 1988;4:377–390.
11. Fernandez DL. Correction of post-traumatic wrist deformity in adults by osteotomy, bone grafting and internal fixation. *J Bone Joint Surg Am* 1982;64:1164—1178.
12. Af Ekenstam F, Hagert CG, Engkuist O. Corrective osteotomy of malunited fractures of the distal end of the radius. *Scand J Plast Reconstr Surg Hand Surg* 1985;19:175–187.
13. Campbell WC. Malunited Colles' fractures. *JAMA* 1937;109:1105–1108.
14. Darrach W. Partial excision of the lower shaft of the ulna for deformity following Colles' fracture. *Ann Surg* 1913;57:764–765.
15. McMurtry RY, Axelrod T, Paley D. Distal radial osteotomy. *Orthopedics* 1989;12:149–155.
16. Mudgal CS, Jones WA. Scapholunate diastasis: A component of fractures of the distal radius. *J Hand Surg [Br]* 1990;15:503–505.

73

TRISCAPHE ARTHRODESIS

H. KIRK WATSON
JEFFREY WEINZWEIG

INDICATIONS

Indications for triscaphe arthrodesis include dynamic or static rotary subluxation of the scaphoid (RSS), persistent symptomatic predynamic RSS with instability, degenerative disease of the triscaphe joint, nonunion of the scaphoid, Kienböck's disease, scapholunate (SL) dissociation, traumatic dislocations, midcarpal instability, and congenital synchondrosis of the triscaphe joint (1–11).

CONTRAINDICATIONS

Triscaphe arthrodesis is contraindicated if significant degenerative change is found at the radioscaphoid joint (12,13).

SURGICAL TECHNIQUE

The triscaphe joint is approached through a 4.0-cm transverse dorsal wrist incision just distal to the radial styloid (Fig. 73.1). Spreading technique is used to preserve dorsal veins and branches of the superficial branch of the radial nerve. The radial styloid is exposed through an incision in the capsule overlying the radial styloid–scaphoid junction, and the distal 5 mm of the styloid is removed with a rongeur, sloping volarly from distal to proximal (Fig. 73.2). A transverse incision in the dorsal capsule is then made, and the radioscaphoid joint is inspected (Fig. 73.3). If significant degenerative disease is found here, despite the absence of radiographic evidence preoperatively, our procedure of choice is scapholunate advanced collapse (SLAC) reconstruction (see Chapter 71) rather than triscaphe arthrodesis. The distal aspect of the extensor retinaculum is then opened along the extensor pollicis longus, and the triscaphe joint is approached through a transverse capsular incision between the extensor carpi radialis longus and brevis tendons (Fig. 73.4).

The entire articular surfaces of the scaphoid, trapezium, and trapezoid are then removed with a rongeur, with care taken to remove only the proximal half of the trapezium–trapezoid articulation. This is best done with a small angled curette. It is mandatory that the subchondral hard cancellous bone also be removed and the softer cancellous surfaces exposed. The cortex dorsal to the articular cartilage on the trapezium and trapezoid is also removed to broaden the surface area for grafting (Figs. 73.5 and 73.6). The volar lip of the scaphoid is rongeured by inserting a dental rongeur deep in the joint and levering the handle distally. Cancellous bone graft is then harvested from the distal radius (see Chapter 54).

Two 0.045-in. K-wires are then driven percutaneously in preset fashion from the distal aspect of the dorsal trapezoid proximally. The first, radially positioned, K-wire is passed to the point of just touching the surface of the scaphoid. The second, ulnarly positioned, K-wire is passed proximally to the point of entering the scaphotrapezoid space. In large individuals, one or both of these K-wires may be a 0.062-in. wire. A 5-mm spacer, usually the handle of a small hook, is placed into the scaphotrapezoid space to maintain the original external dimensions of the triscaphe joint. The wrist is then placed in full radial deviation and 45° of dorsiflexion while the scaphoid tuberosity is reduced by the surgeon's thumb to prevent scaphoid overcorrection (Fig. 73.7). The radial K-wire is driven into the scaphoid, avoiding placement into the radioscaphoid joint. The spacer is now removed, and the ulnar K-wire is similarly driven into the scaphoid. Care must be taken when the pins are driven proximally into the scaphoid to avoid placement of the K-wires into the radioscaphoid joint space or the radius itself (Fig. 73.8). After pinning, the scaphoid should lie at approximately 55° to 60° of palmar flexion relative to the long axis of the radius when seen from the lateral view. This

---

H. K. Watson: Connecticut Combined Hand Surgery Fellowship, Hartford Hospital, and Connecticut Children's Medical Center, Hartford, Connecticut 06106; Department of Orthopaedics, University of Connecticut School of Medicine, Farmington, Connecticut 06032; Department of Orthopedics, Rehabilitation, and Plastic Surgery, Yale University School of Medicine, New Haven, Connecticut 06520.

J. Weinzweig: Department of Plastic Surgery, Brown University School of Medicine, Rhode Island Hospital, and Hasbro Children's Hospital, Providence, Rhode Island 02905.

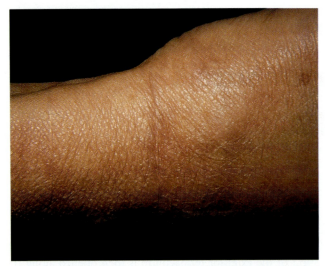

FIGURE 73.1. Wrist surgery with few exceptions is best carried out through transverse incisions. These are the recently healed transverse incisions utilized for a triscaphe limited wrist arthrodesis. Proximally on the radius one sees the transverse incision for the bone graft donor site. The bone graft can be obtained through the distal wrist incision used to perform the arthrodesis; however, the degree of traction necessary to harvest bone graft through this incision usually means a greater cosmetic defect in the transverse wrist incision than that resulting from two transverse incisions properly handled to produce minimal cosmetic deficit.

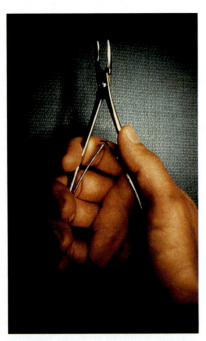

FIGURE 73.2. An essential instrument for performing a limited wrist arthrodesis is the dental rongeur. Placing the instrument deep along the distal articular surface of the scaphoid and levering the handle distally allows excision of the cartilage and subchondral bone from even the volar aspect of the distal articular surface of the scaphoid.

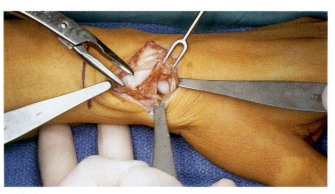

FIGURE 73.3. A limited radial styloidectomy has been performed with the dental rongeur. This provides broader access to the radioscaphoid joint and prevents postoperative radial styloid impingement. The smooth proximal pole of the scaphoid can be easily visualized. (Fingers are pointing to the right.)

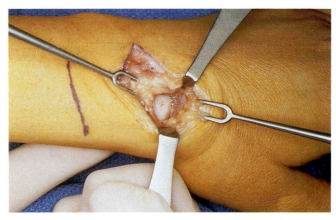

FIGURE 73.4. The triscaphe joint is best visualized between the two radial wrist extensors. The distal pole of the scaphoid and proximal articular surfaces of the trapezium and trapezoid are shown. (Fingers are pointing to the right.)

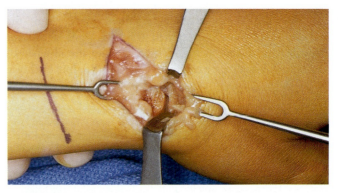

FIGURE 73.5. Bony resection commences with rongeur excision of the dorsal nonarticular surface of the distal scaphoid, which provides a broader cancellous surface for fusion. (Fingers are pointing to the right.)

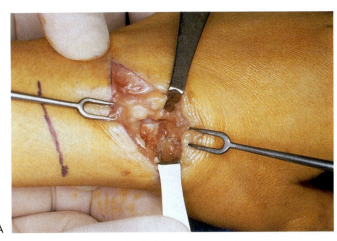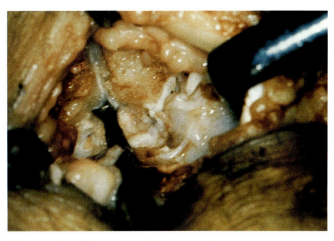

FIGURE 73.6. A: The scaphotrapeziotrapezoid joint as well as the trapezoid–trapezium interspace have been excavated using both a rongeur and curette to create a broad space for cancellous grafting. The preset K-wires are then driven from trapezoid to scaphoid, and the open space is densely packed with cancellous bone graft. (Fingers are pointing to the right.) **B:** A curette is utilized to remove the proximal half of the articular cartilage and subchondral bone between the trapezium and trapezoid.

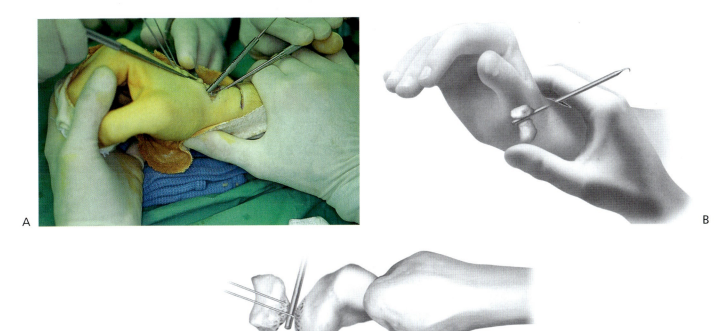

FIGURE 73.7. A,B: The key to triscaphe limited wrist arthrodesis is scaphoid position. This is easily controlled with an automated technique by placing a 5-mm spacer between the scaphoid and trapezoid. The wrist is then fully radially deviated and dorsiflexed 45°. The surgeon's thumb maintains the scaphoid within these constraints. **C:** The assistant or scrub nurse can run the preset pins, which are aligned to cross into the scaphoid. The scaphoid should lie more flexed than in a normal wrist at 55° to 60° to the long axis of the forearm.

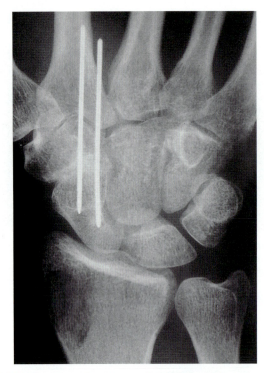

FIGURE 73.8. The relatively parallel pins from the trapezoid to the scaphoid allow muscular tone to maintain compression on the bone grafts until healing is complete at 6 weeks. The pins are removed in the office at that time.

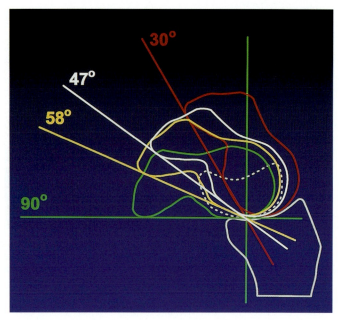

FIGURE 73.9. The normal scaphoid lies at an approximate angle of 47° to the long axis of the forearm. With rotary subluxation of the scaphoid, that angle can reach 90° or greater. There is a temptation to overcorrect the scaphoid during the triscaphe limited wrist procedure, bringing it up into a position less than 47° *(white)*, such as the 30° *(red)*. This is unacceptable and will result in highly limited motion and early degenerative change on the apex of that scaphoid against the radius. Ideally, the scaphoid should be fused between 55° and 60° of flexion *(yellow)*. This is more flexion than normal and is necessary because of the change in wrist mechanics.

ensures optimal radioscaphoid congruity and maximizes postoperative range of motion. It is not necessary to correct any abnormal rotation of the lunate. The scaphoid should not be overcorrected by placing its long axis in line with the forearm and, thus, markedly decreasing the SL angle. This will limit the motion obtained after surgery and run the risk of cartilage destruction on the proximal pole of the scaphoid.

The major concern in triscaphe arthrodesis is overcorrection; this cannot be overemphasized. The neutral scaphoid normally lies 47° to the long axis of the radius. Following triscaphe arthrodesis, the mechanics of load transfer have changed. The radial styloid must be removed, and the scaphoid must lie significantly more flexed than normal (i.e., 55–60°) in relation to the long axis of the radius (Fig. 73.9).

Cancellous bone, harvested from the distal radius, is then densely packed into the spaces between the scaphoid, trapezium, and trapezoid using a dental amalgam tamp. Maintenance of the original external dimensions of the triscaphe joint usually translates to a 4- to 8-mm gap among the three bones, which is filled with the cancellous bone graft. The pins are cut beneath the skin level, and the skin incisions are closed with a single-layer subcuticular monofilament suture (stainless steel or prolene). The wrist capsule and extensor retinaculum are simply realigned without suturing.

The postoperative dressing consists of a bulky noncompressive wrap incorporating a long arm plaster splint. The hand is placed in a protected position with the wrist in slight extension and radial deviation, the forearm neutral, and the elbow at 90°.

POSTOPERATIVE MANAGEMENT

Our postoperative management is similar for most intercarpal arthrodeses. Maximum initial immobilization is mandatory for these small bone fusions. Three to five days following surgery, the bulky dressing is removed, and a long arm thumb–spica cast is applied.

The proximal carpal row is easily immobilized by casting the forearm and arm, but it is difficult to adequately maintain the position of the distal carpal row. Therefore, the metacarpophalangeal (MP) joints of the index and middle fingers are flexed to 80° to 90° and included in the long arm cast while the interphalangeal joints are left free. The index and middle metacarpals are mortised into the carpals as the "fixed unit" of the hand. Thus, their immobilization tends to maintain the position of the distal carpal row. Because there is relatively free motion at the base of the ring and little

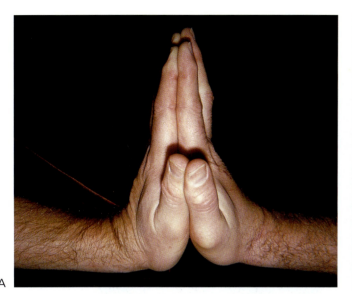 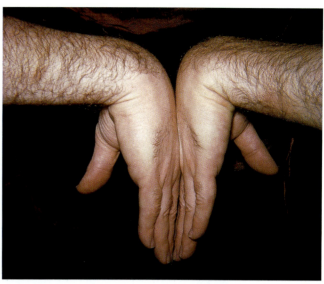

FIGURE 73.10. Over 25 years of experience with more than 900 triscaphe limited wrist arthrodeses demonstrates average dorsiflexion **(A)** and palmar flexion **(B)** arcs of just under 80% those of the normal unoperated wrist.

metacarpals, they are not included in the cast. As with any thumb–spica cast, the thumb is immobilized to the tip. We refer to this type of immobilization as a "Groucho Marx" cast, as it is reminiscent of the comedian's classic pose holding a cigar.

Three weeks following limited wrist arthrodesis, the long arm cast and intracuticular sutures are removed. A short arm thumb–spica cast is applied for an additional 3 weeks. Only the thumb is included in this cast.

Six weeks postoperatively, the short arm cast is removed, and radiographs are obtained. If radiographic evidence of union is seen, the pins are removed in the office, and the patient is referred for hand therapy for full wrist mobilization. Patients may occasionally be splinted for an additional week or two if there is any doubt as to the status of bony healing. This applies especially to large individuals who smoke.

In our experience, triscaphe limited wrist arthrodesis has yielded excellent functional results and pain-free, stable wrists. After 4 to 6 weeks of hand therapy, the average range of motion is usually 50% to 70% of the contralateral normal wrist, increasing to an average of 80% by 1 year following surgery (Fig. 73.10). Grip strength has averaged 90% of that of the unaffected wrist.

CLINICAL SERIES

Nine hundred six patients underwent triscaphe arthrodesis over a 25-year period. They ranged in age from 17 to 74; 54% were male. All patients presented with pain, swelling, and usually decreased range of motion of the wrist. The mean duration of symptoms before arthrodesis was 24.6 months (range, 1–204 months), and mean follow-up was 52 months (range, 12–197 months).

Triscaphe arthrodesis was performed for symptomatic RSS in 68% of the patients who underwent this procedure (Fig. 73.11). Other indications included Kienböck's disease in 10%, triscaphe degenerative disease in 8%, and scaphoid nonunion in 2%. Additional indications included midcarpal instability, avascular necrosis of the scaphoid, and symptomatic congenital synchondrosis of the triscaphe joint. The mean postoperative immobilization, used as a measure of time to bony fusion, was 48 days (range, 30–294 days).

Primary union was achieved in 96% of the cases. Eighty-six percent of patients rated the postoperative wrist function as better or much better than it had been preoperatively. Eighty-eight percent returned to their original employment with a mean period of disability of 14.7 weeks (range 1–56 weeks). The mean range of wrist flexion and extension, and ulnar deviation, was 75% of the opposite unaffected side. Mean power and key and tip pinch grips were more than 80% of the unaffected side. Radial styloidectomy was added to the procedure in 1987 to alleviate frequent symptomatic styloid impingement (12).

A careful review of patients and radiographs by us and by independent investigators demonstrated no secondary degenerative disease of the radioscaphoid joint or other joints of the wrist.

Eighty-one percent of the 90 patients who underwent triscaphe arthrodesis for Kienböck's disease reported no pain or mild pain at rest. Seventy-one percent had no pain with normal activity levels. Eighty-six percent returned to

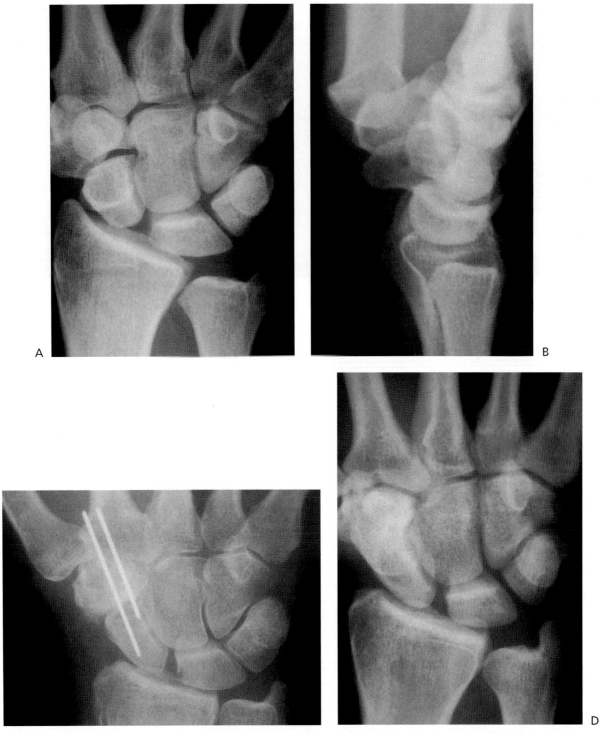

FIGURE 73.11. Triscaphe arthrodesis. Rotary subluxation of the scaphoid secondary to rupture of the scapholunate interosseous ligament is evidenced by a widened scapholunate interval, foreshortening of the scaphoid, a positive ring sign on posteroanterior view **(A)**, and a scapholunate angle of approximately 90° on lateral view **(B)**. Triscaphe limited wrist arthrodesis was performed with typical pin placement from trapezoid to scaphoid with concomitant radial styloidectomy. Following triscaphe arthrodesis, the mechanics of the wrist are such that the long elliptical scaphoid fossa of the radius interferes with function and creates radial styloid impingement. Radial styloidectomy is, therefore, a standard part of the triscaphe arthrodesis technique **(C)**. Six weeks postoperatively, solid bony fusion is demonstrated following pin removal **(D)**.

their original employment with a mean period of disability of 14.8 weeks. The postoperative range of motion in this series was slightly less than that for all triscaphe arthrodesis patients. Mean wrist flexion was 57%, and extension was 73% of the opposite unaffected side. Mean grip strength was 92% of the unaffected side.

COMPLICATIONS

Triscaphe arthrodesis has been an extremely reliable procedure and complications relatively few with more than 900 having been performed. In early cases there had been a significant incidence of radial styloid impaction. The stabilized scaphoid is unable to flex and avoid abutting the styloid in radial deviation. Among these early cases, approximately 20% required a subsequent styloidectomy, which achieved an improvement in radial deviation and relief of impaction symptoms. Since 1987, radial styloidectomy has been routinely performed as part of the triscaphe arthrodesis procedure to avoid this problem (12).

Nonunion has been extremely uncommon, with a rate of 1% to 3%, depending on the indication for limited wrist arthrodesis. We believe this rate of nonunion is kept low by the broad cancellous surface created at the time of articular resection and the large volume of cancellous graft used in performing the fusion. Infection, hematoma, and transient neurapraxias have been exceedingly rare in our experience and should be completely avoidable. One patient required drainage and antibiotics for a postoperative wound infection. Fifteen patients (2%) were treated for postoperative reflex sympathetic dystrophy with a stress-loading regimen consisting of compression (scrubbing tasks) and traction (carrying weights) modalities referred to as a "Dystrophile" program (14) (see Chapter 65).

Although degenerative change at the radioscaphoid joint, consistent with SLAC wrist, occurred in 1.5% following triscaphe arthrodesis and thus necessitated subsequent SLAC reconstruction, radiolunate degenerative change was not observed in any cases. One and a half percent of triscaphe arthrodeses thus required conversion to SLAC reconstruction. This entailed osteotomy through the triscaphe fusion, carpectomy of the scaphoid, and arthrodesis of the capitate, lunate, hamate, and triquetrum. Pain was the usual indication, but radioscaphoid degenerative joint disease (DJD) occurred in patients who had some DJD at the time of the original surgery.

There were several cases in which patients were willing to accept expected future degenerative arthritis in exchange for shorter term, full-power, asymptomatic function with increased range of motion. This allowed them to finish out careers during their exceptional remuneration years. Several professional athletes and one world-class wrestler demonstrated eburnated bone with complete cartilage loss involving the proximal scaphoid pole (Fig. 73.12). This approach

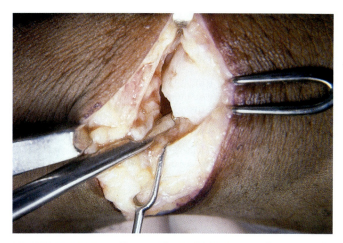

FIGURE 73.12. A professional basketball player with rotary subluxation of the scaphoid demonstrates a central area of destruction in the proximal pole articular surface, actually placing this in the realm of a scapholunate advanced collapse (SLAC) wrist. The triscaphe arthrodesis places this destroyed area of the scaphoid in the normal cartilage in the center of the radial fossa and provides a functionally asymptomatic wrist for many years. This may be converted to a SLAC reconstruction following an osteotomy of the triscaphe fusion at a later date. Profesional athletes with high, but relatively short-term, earning capacities warrant this approach.

is successful because the central portion of the scaphoid pole is destroyed while the periphery of the scaphoid fossa of the radius is destroyed. Triscaphe arthrodesis places the damaged proximal pole back in the center of the preserved cartilage of the scaphoid fossa.

DISCUSSION

Triscaphe arthrodesis addresses a diverse spectrum of carpal pathology, including scapholunate dissociation, midcarpal instability, and Kienböck's disease. It provides a stable radial column for load transfer across the wrist to the radius and permits the unloading of carpal units no longer capable of bearing load, such as the lunate in Kienböck's disese. In addition, it provides stability and strength to a wrist affected by the pathomechanics of RSS or midcarpal instability, resulting in a painless, functional wrist.

Although other procedures, such as scapholunate ligamentous reconstruction, joint-leveling procedures, and scaphocapitate arthrodesis, have been advocated for the management of the diverse group of carpal disorders for which we advocate triscaphe arthrodesis, we believe that this limited wrist arthrodesis provides the most reliable and enduring means of stabilizing the scaphoid and permitting efficient load transfer across the wrist.

Long-term radiographic follow-up has revealed only rare instances of progressive radioscaphoid or intercarpal degenerative change, and only in those patients who had some evidence of disease in these joints at the time of original surgery (5,15–17).

REFERENCES

1. Vender MI, Watson HK, Wiener BD, et al. Degenerative change in symptomatic scaphoid non-union. *J Hand Surg [Am]* 1987;12:514–519.
2. Viegas SF, Patterson RM, Peterson PD, et al. Evaluation of the biomechanical efficacy of limited intercarpal fusions for the treatment of scapho-lunate dissociation. *J Hand Surg [Am]* 1990;15:120–128.
3. Watson HK, Ashmead D. Triscaphe fusion for chronic scapholunate instability. In: Gelberman R, ed. *Master techniques in orthopaedic surgery: The wrist.* New York: Raven Press, 1994;183–194.
4. Watson HK, Fink JA, Monacelli DM. Use of triscaphe fusion in the treatment of Kienböck's disease. *Hand Clin* 1993;9:493–499.
5. Watson HK, Hempton RE. Limited wrist arthrodesis. Part I: The triscaphoid joint. *J Hand Surg [Am]* 1980;5:320–327.
6. Watson HK, Ryu J, DiBella A. An approach to Kienböck's disease: Triscaphe arthrodesis. *J Hand Surg [Am]* 1985;10:179–187.
7. Watson HK, Ryu J, Akelman E. Limited triscaphoid intercarpal arthrodesis for rotary subluxation of the scaphoid. *J Bone Joint Surg Am* 1986;68:345–349.
8. Watson HK, Weinzweig J. Intercarpal arthrodesis. In: Green DP, Hotchkiss RN, Pederson WC, eds. *Operative hand surgery, 4th ed.* New York: Churchill Livingstone, 1998;108–130.
9. Watson HK, Weinzweig J, Zeppieri J. The natural progression of scaphoid instability. *Hand Clin* 1997;13:39–50.
10. Watson HK, Weinzweig J. Treatment of Kienböck's disease with triscaphe arthrodesis. In: Vastamaki M, Vilkki S, Goransson H, et al, eds. *Proceedings of the 6th Congress of the International Federation of Societies for Surgery of the Hand.* Bologna: Monduzzi Editore, 1995;347–349.
11. Weinzweig J, Watson HK, Herbert TJ, et al. Congenital synchondrosis of the scaphotrapezio-trapezoid joint. *J Hand Surg [Am]* 1997;22:74–77.
12. Rogers WD, Watson HK. Radial styloid impingement after triscaphe arthrodesis. *J Hand Surg [Am]* 1989;14:297–301.
13. Trumble T, Bour C, Smith R, et al. Intercarpal arthrodesis for static and dynamic volar intercalated segment instability. *J Hand Surg [Am]* 1988;13:396–402.
14. Watson HK, Carlson L. Treatment of reflex sympathetic dystrophy of the hand with an active "stress loading" program. *J Hand Surg [Am]* 1987;12:779–785.
15. Watson HK, Goodman ML, Johnson TR. Limited wrist arthrodesis. Part II: Intercarpal and radiocarpal combinations. *J Hand Surg [Am]* 1981;6:223–232.
16. Watson HK, Ottoni L, Pitts EC, et al. Rotary subluxation of the scaphoid: A spectrum of instability. *J Hand Surg [Br]* 1993;18:62–64.
17. Watson HK, Weinzweig J, Guidera P, et al. One thousand intercarpal arthrodeses. *J Hand Surg [Br]* 1999;24:320–330.

ULNAR LENGTHENING

HERMANN KRIMMER
ULRICH LANZ

Joint-leveling procedures are commonly performed to change the distribution of loads across the wrist joint. The idea for lengthening the ulna for treatment of Kienböck's disease is based on the association of this disorder with ulnar minus variance. Hulten (1) coined this term to describe a wrist in which the distal articular surface of the radius extends beyond that of the ulna. In his 1928 report, Hulten analyzed 400 normal wrist radiographs and found an ulnar minus variance in only 23%, in contrast to an incidence of 74% in wrists with necrosis of the lunate. No patient with Kienböck's disease had ulnar positive variance; however, 16% of the normal group demonstrated this pattern.

Because the lunate articulates with the radius and the ulnocarpal complex, he concluded that ulnar minus increases the load on the radial aspect of the lunate favoring shear stress and impairment of blood flow. These abnormal forces lead to small repetitive compression fractures, especially at the rim of the radius. His theory correlates well with the description of Kienböck (2), who had demonstrated that the radial aspect of the lunate proximal articular surface characteristically is damaged, whereas the ulnar aspect and the distal articular surface remained well preserved.

In 1945, Persson (3) proposed ulnar lengthening for removing the concentration of stress produced at the radiolunate articulation. He proposed that the majority of the load transmission is through the firm articular surface of the radius and that the relatively shorter ulna offers only the softer triangular fibrocartilage complex. He theorized that shifting some pressure from the radiolunate to the ulnolunate side would change this unfavorable mechanical relationship to allow healing and reconstitution of the lunate. In cases in which carpal height had been lost (stage IIIB), leveling operations could prevent further carpal collapse by reducing the load from the radiolunate joint to allow remodeling.

INDICATIONS

For patients with Kienböck's disease and ulnar minus or neutral variance without carpal collapse or pancarpal arthrosis, ulnar lengthening should be considered as a treatment alternative for procedures that involve the carpus. Preoperative radiographs should include a posteroanterior (PA) view in neutral forearm rotation, anteroposterior (AP) grip, and lateral views. Magnetic resonance imaging (MRI) with gadolinium can assist in staging the severity of lunate involvement.

In Lichtman stage IIIB wrists demonstrating slight carpal collapse, ulnar lengthening should be considered as the initial treatment, as it leaves open the possibility for salvage procedures such as intercarpal arthrodesis or proximal row carpectomy. In selected cases, ulnar lengthening can be combined with vascularized bone grafting. Patients presenting with radioscaphoid degenerative disease or Lichtman stage IV disease should be excluded.

SURGICAL TECHNIQUE

Persson (3) originally described a method in which the ulna was osteotomized obliquely and the fragments distracted by oblique sliding and then wired in the new position. The technique required long immobilization times because of the high risk of nonunion, and several authors have recommended a transverse ulnar osteotomy with interposition of a bicortical bone graft (4,5). This technique requires plate fixation for more control and better stabilization of the lengthened ulna.

We favor a combination of these methods consisting of oblique sliding with fixation by dynamic AO compression

---

H. Krimmer and U. Lanz: University of Würzburg, and Klinik fur Handchirurgie, Rhön-Klinikum, 97616 Bad Neustadt, Germany.

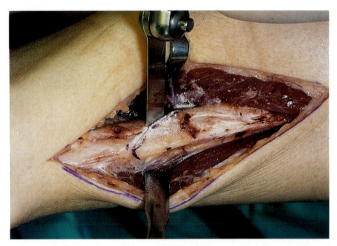

FIGURE 74.1. An oblique osteotomy at an angle less than 45° to the long axis of the ulna is performed.

extensor carpi ulnaris. A seven-hole dynamic compression AO plate is applied palmarly and first fixed distally through the first and third holes. After removal of the plate, an oblique osteotomy is performed at the level of the central hole rectangular to the plate. The osteotomy should lie in an angle of less than 45° to the long axis of the ulna (Fig. 74.1).

The plate is replaced and fixed distally by screws. With a bone-bending instrument, the oblique surfaces of the ulna are pressed together until the desired length increase of 2 to 4 mm is achieved under x-ray control (Fig. 74.2). The plate is fixed proximally, and an interfragmentary compression screw is inserted (Fig. 74.3). The wound is closed over a suction drain, and postoperative immobilization in an upper arm cast for 3 weeks is recommended.

CLINICAL SERIES

In their first report based on 20 patients followed at Mayo Clinic for 37 months, Armistead et al. (4) found complete pain relief in seven, minor symptoms under stress in 11, and incomplete relief in two patients. Preoperatively, 11 were classified as Lichtman stage IIIA, and nine as Licht-

plate, avoiding the need of bone graft from the iliac crest. The procedure is performed under axillary block with a pneumatic tourniquet applied to the patient's arm. The forearm is supinated, and the incision is made along the distal palmar border of the ulna. The distal third of the ulna is exposed between the flexor carpi ulnaris and the

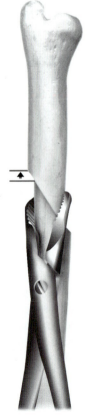
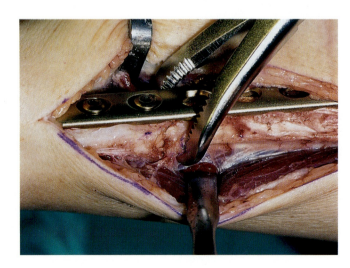

A,B

FIGURE 74.2. A: Illustration of the oblique sliding technique. **B:** The AO dynamic compression plate is fixed distally, and the oblique surfaces of the ulna are pressed together until the desired length increase is achieved.

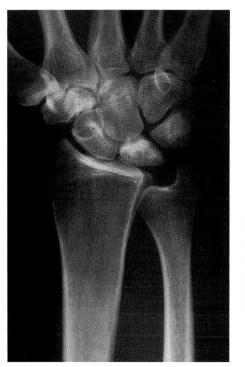 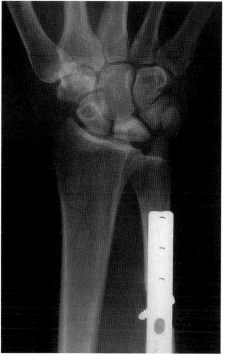

FIGURE 74.3. A: Preoperative x-ray demonstrating ulnar minus variance in Kienböck's disease. **B:** Intraoperative x-ray after ulnar lengthening of 2.5 mm. Note the interfragmentary compression screw.

man stage IIIB. The authors used a transverse osteotomy and plate fixation augmented by bone graft, and nonunion complicated treatment in three cases. All but one patient demonstrated neutral or ulna plus variance of 1 to 2 mm. Increased carpal collapse occurred in only one patient. It is noteworthy that nine patients showed a slight increase in carpal height. In 1993, Quenzer and Linscheid (6) presented a second series of 59 patients at the Mayo Clinic reexamined with a questionnaire at an average follow-up of 94 months. Overall satisfaction was high in 90%, and grip strength had improved to 70% of the opposite side. Range of motion was unchanged and did not decrease with time. Delayed union or nonunion occurred in nine patients (16%), and seven (12%) patients needed further surgery. No patients progressed to the next stage.

Our own results of 14 patients using the oblique sliding technique with plate fixation were comparable with an overall satisfaction of 85%. Grip strength measured 73% of the opposite side. There were no nonunions. The amount of lengthening ranged from 2 to 4 mm with an average of 3.2 mm (Fig. 74.4).

DISCUSSION

Recent biomechanical studies have confirmed the rationale for correcting the ulnar minus variance for treatment of Kienböck's disease. Palmer and Werner (7) demonstrated in a human cadaver model that 82% of the compressive load is transmitted through the radiocarpal articulation and 18% through the ulnocarpal articulation. A 2.5-mm increase in ulnar length increased the ulnar load to 42%, and a 2.5-mm decrease lowered the ulnar load to 43%. Using a two-dimensional rigid body spring model (RBSM) technique, Iwasaki et al. (8) showed 55% of force transmission at the radioscaphoid joint, 28% at the radiolunate, 13% at the ulnolunate, and 4% at the ulnotriquetral joint. These findings are constant through stages I, II, and IIIA of Kienböck's disease. In stage IIIB, however, a 41% increase of load occurred at the radiolunate joint as a result of flexion of the scaphoid. In their study, normal and ulnar minus wrists were not differentiated. It can be concluded from these findings that ulnar lengthening to neutral or to 1 mm ulnar positive variance significantly changes load transfer at the radiocarpal and ulnocarpal joint. This likely occurs by lowering the pressure at the the radial portion of the lunate and by enhancing the pressure area at the ulnolunate side with increased support through the triangular fibrocartilage complex. This may allow healing or at least partial remodeling of the lunate to prevent further collapse.

Lengthening of the ulna by 2 to 4 mm in our series did not create problems at the distal radioulnar joint. The oblique sliding technique with fixation by an AO compres-

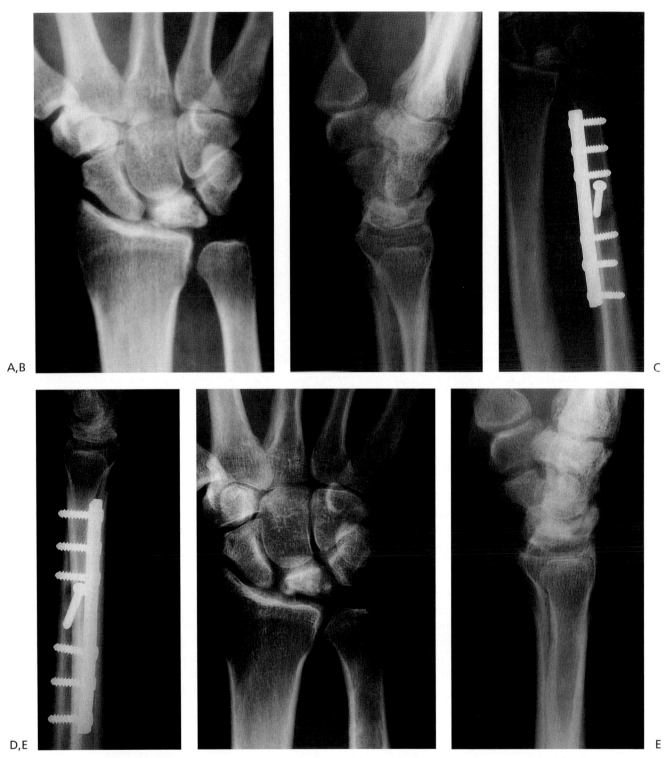

FIGURE 74.4. A,B: Preoperative x-ray of a 23-year-old man with ulnar minus variance in Kienböck's disease stage IIIA. **C,D:** Six-month follow-up. The osteotomy has healed with an ulnar lengthening of 2.3 mm. **E,F:** Seven-year follow-up. The plate has been removed. There is no increase in carpal collapse, and the patient remains free of symptoms.

sion plate provides sufficient lengthening without the need of additional bone graft from the iliac crest. The risk of nonunion is decreased with this technique by the creation of a single healing site and by the use of a compression screw across the osteotomy. Overall satisfaction with longer follow-up to 8 years remained constant at 85%.

Regarding alternative joint-leveling procedures, the clinical results for radial shortening proved to be roughly equivalent (9). Radial shortening provides a relative lengthening of the extrinsic musculotendinous units traversing the carpus and a resultant decrease in the force transmission across the carpus. One disadvantage of this technique may be that dissection of the radius involves more soft tissue structures and that the scar is more obvious at the radial side of the distal forearm than on the ulnar aspect, where it is often hardly visible. Both procedures leave the wrist uninvolved, which allows other treatment options in case of failure.

For patients with ulnar positive variance, shortening the radius or lengthening the ulna would create an impaction syndrome of the ulna head against the carpus. For this group, capitate shortening is another type of decompressive procedure that should be considered to enhance lunate revascularization and healing. Overall satisfaction is comparable at about 80%. This procedure is recommended in early stages of Kienböck's disease, when no carpal collapse and no ulnar minus variance is present (10).

Operative treatment of Kienböck's disease is not entirely predictable. Comparing 21 cases of Kienböck's disease treated with various techniques with 22 other cases treated conservatively, Delaere et al. (11) found no superiority of operative over conservative treatment at a mean follow-up time of 65 months. Moreover, surgery resulted in loss of 24% of range of motion, leading to a change in social activities in roughly a quarter of the patients. These findings outline our belief that joint-leveling procedures should be regarded as the first choice for treatment of symptomatic Kienböck's disease in case of ulnar minus variance. We have found ulnar lengthening by the described oblique sliding technique to be a very satisfactory alternative to other current procedures.

ACKNOWLEDGMENT

We thank Scott Wolfe for revising the manuscript.

EDITORS' COMMENTS

Our chief application of ulnar lengthening has been in the salvaging of previously performed Darrach procedures. The transverse excision of the distal ulna, particularly if a significant amount of bone has been removed, results in an ulnar impingement syndrome. The ulna impacts against the radius, usually producing marked symptoms.

Our solution has been a lengthening osteotomy of the ulna, usually with the use of a plate and screws combined with a matched ulna arthroplasty. This has effectively salvaged failed Darrachs. Insofar as Kienböck's disease is concerned, we have never done, nor feel there is any indication for, an ulnar lengthening procedure (see Editors' Comments in Chapter 60).

REFERENCES

1. Hulten O. Über anatomische Variationen der Handgelenkknochen. *Acta Radiol* 1928;9:155–168.
2. Kienböck R. Über die traumatische Malazie des Mondbeins und ihre Folgezustände: Entartungsformen und Kompressionsfrakturen. *Fortschr Röntgenstr* 1910;16:77–103.
3. Persson M. Pathogenese der Kienböckschen Lunatummalazie: Die Frakturtheorie im Lichte der Erfolge operativer Radiusverkürzung (Hulten) und einer neuen Operationsmethode Ulnaverlängerung. *Acta Chir Scand* 1945;92(Suppl 98):80–106.
4. Armistead RB, Linscheid RL, Dobyns JH, et al. Ulnar lengthening in the treatment of Kienböck's disease. *J Bone Joint Surg Am* 1982;64:170–178.
5. Rettig E, Linscheid RL. Ulnar lengthening osteotomy. In: Blair WF, ed. *Techniques in hand surgery.* Baltimore: Williams & Wilkins, 1996;1075–1079.
6. Quenzer DE, Linscheid RL. Ulnar lengthening procedures. *Hand Clin* 1993;9:467–474.
7. Palmer AK, Werner FW. Biomechanics of the distal radioulnar joint. *Clin Orthop* 1984;187:26–35.
8. Iwasaki N, Eiichi G, Minami A, et al. Force transmission through the wrist joint in Kienböck's disaease: A two-dimensional theoretical study. *J Hand Surg [Am]* 1998;23:415–424.
9. Weiss APC. Radial shortening. *Hand Clin* 1993;9:475–482.
10. Almquist EE. Capitate shortening in the treatment of Kienböck's disease. *Hand Clin* 1993;9:505–512.
11. Delaere O, Dury M. Molderez A, et al. Conservative versus operative treatment for Kienböck's disease. *J Hand Surg [Br]* 1998;23:33–36.

75

WRIST DENERVATION

GUY FOUCHER
ALLEN T. BISHOP

A painful wrist can be difficult to treat, especially when arthrosis is present. A proximal row carpectomy or limited radiocarpal or intercarpal arthrodesis may at times relieve pain and stop the progressive degeneration (1). Such procedures frequently allow return to full activity after a substantial initial recovery period. In the elderly, low demands make other options desirable. An ideal treatment should relieve pain while maintaining useful motion with a minimal recovery period. In such cases, wrist denervation is an appealing alternative.

The idea of reducing joint pain by division of articular branches of sensory nerves was first introduced for the hip joint by Camitz in 1933 (2) and refined in 1942 by Tavernier and Truchet (3). In 1966, Wilhelm described the innervation of the wrist joint and published the first clinical series of wrist denervation in 21 patients (4). Since then, the majority of the articles devoted to the topic have come from Germany (4–7). We have used this procedure since 1977, initially as a "partial" denervation in all dorsal approaches to the wrist.

INDICATIONS

The main indication for wrist denervation is wrist pain not amenable to other treatment modalities. An ideal candidate for wrist denervation would be a 50-year-old active patient with moderate posttraumatic arthritis following a scaphoid nonunion, causing considerable functional impairment in a wrist with a useful range of movement. After total wrist denervation, he could expect a short off-work period (average 19 days) and gradual improvement in his pain over a 16-month period.

G. Foucher: Clinique de la Faculté de Strasbourg, Strasbourg 67000, France.
A. T. Bishop: Department of Orthopedic Surgery, Mayo Medical School and Mayo Clinic, Rochester, Minnesota 55905.

CONTRAINDICATIONS

No true contraindications to the procedure have been reported. Poorer results may be expected in displaced intraarticular radius fractures or carpal instability (8) because progression of the disease is expected. Similarly, pain from advanced arthrosis is less reliably relieved, perhaps because it consists of bone- rather than joint-capsule-mediated pain.

ANATOMY

If the innervation of the wrist capsule were precise and constant, complete surgical denervation would result in complete joint anesthesia and, ultimately, a Charcot joint. In fact, neither of these occurs. This may be explained not only by inconstant anatomy but also by incomplete division of some fibers as a result of difficult access or visualization.

As Wyke described (9), joints are likely to have both primary and accessory innervation. Primary nerves innervate the capsule directly, whereas accessory nerves arise from primarily motor or cutaneous sensory branches. The posterior interosseous nerve is the only primary articular nerve for the wrist; all other contibuting nerves have an accessory role. Since the first work by Wilhelm, anatomic studies have reported variable contributions from the palmar cutaneous branch of the median nerve, the deep branch of the ulnar nerve, the anterior interosseous nerve, and others. Ferreres (10) has demonstrated a large discrepancy between microdissection and histologic studies. He demonstrated potential contributions from the median, radial, and ulnar as well as the lateral, medial, and posterior antebrachial cutaneous nerves.

The median nerve contributes joint intervation via the anterior interosseous nerve and the palmar cutaneous branch. The anterior interosseous nerve (nervi interosseus antebrachii anterior) courses through the deep substance of the pronator quadratus and emerges from its distal border as first drawn by Leonardo da Vinci. It is adherent successively to the interosseous membrane proximally and the lip of the radius distally, as described by Dellon (11). It contributes variably to the radioulnar and radiocarpal joint innervation (11–13). Articular branches were found in only 2 of 500 dissections by Cozzi (12). Fukumota found some anterior interosseous contribution to the radiocarpal joint in 59% and the distal radioulnar joint in 17% (13). The role of the palmar cutaneous branch of the median nerve (ramus palmaris nervi mediani) has been a matter of controversy. Although Fukumoto found a constant articular branch at the radial styloid (13), no or infrequent branches were seen by others (4,10,14). The palmar cutaneous branch of the median nerve usually originates from the radial aspect of the main trunk at a mean 4.1 cm (range, 2–7 cm) proximal to the distal wrist crease (15), but occasionally as high as 11 cm (16). No direct articular branch from the median nerve has been described.

The radial contribution comes from the posterior interosseous nerve and the superficial cutaneous branch. The posterior interosseous nerve (nervi interosseus antebrachii posterior), after giving off its last motor branch to the extensor indicis, lies proximally on the interosseous membrane adjacent to the posterior division of the anterior interosseous artery. Distally, it is found within the fourth extensor compartment, close to Lister's tubercle. It gives off an articular branch (41% of 57 cadavers) for the radioulnar joint 2.7 cm proximal to the radiocarpal joint (range, 1.5–3.3 cm) (17). This branch, constant for Fukumoto (13), was found in only 6%, and 5 cm proximal to the joint line, by McCarthy et al. (18).

The cutaneous branch of the radial nerve emerges into the subcutaneous space approximately 9 cm proximal to the radial styloid and divides into terminal branches 5.1 cm proximal to the same landmark (19). A mean of six branches (range, 3–10) were found at the styloid level (20). They provide occasional branches to the capsule—in only 10% in one study (13). Finally, the first dorsal digital branch or the dorsal radial branch to the index finger gives a recurrent branch (nervi articularis spatii interossei) at the first interosseous space level as described first by Winckler in 1953 (21). It has a close relationship with the venous network and needs careful dissection. Its contributes only to the first and second carpometacarpal joints (13).

The ulnar nerve innervates the wrist through branches from the main trunk, the dorsal cutaneous branch, and the deep or muscular (rather than "motor") branch, which contains 40% sensory fibers (22). The dorsal cutaneous branch pierces the antebrachial fascia at the dorsomedial border of the flexor carpi ulnaris, 5 cm proximal to the pisiform. It provides one or multiple branches to the joint (13,23,24). Fukumoto (13) found one unique branch in 70% of specimens, located 1.8 cm proximal to the styloid. Similarly, Lourie et al. found a consistent (82%) transverse branch, participating in skin and distal radioulnar joint innervation (24).

The contribution of the muscular branch to the joint is less certain. Wilhelm (4) described branches transversing the proximal interosseous spaces with a recurrent course to the dorsal capsule. Cozzi (12), Dubert (14), and Ferreres (10) have been unable to find such branches. Some volar contributions of this nerve likely exist. Finally, a branch to the pisotriquetral joint may arise from the main ulnar nerve trunk (55%) (13).

The lateral antebrachial cutaneous nerve has a variable course in the distal forearm, but its overlapping with the radial nerve is well established. It contributes a direct branch to the wrist, the rami articularis nervi cutaneous antebrachii radialis first described by Cruveilhier in 1852 (25). It may be identified running alongside the radial nerve beginning 3.1 cm proximal to the styloid (13).

The medial and posterior antebrachial cutaneous nerves may also contribute to ulnodorsal wrist innervation. The medial cutaneous nerve occasionally gives a branch 1.6 cm proximal to the ulna styloid in 10%, and the posterior cutaneous nerve a contribution in only 5% of 20 cadaver dissections (13).

There is general agreement that some branches are identifiable and resectable by microdissection (posterior interosseous nerve, recurrent branch of the first dorsal digital nerve, and branches from the lateral antebrachial cutaneous nerve). Others are difficult to identify surgically, requiring blunt dissection between the nerves and capsule to divide articular branches. Finally, some known branches do not allow efficient or safe surgical approach, such as the contributions from the deep branch to the ulnar nerve. Even though the contribution of some nerves is inconstant, it seems logical to find a technique that cuts most potential contributors to the wrist joint capsule without jeopardizing cutaneous sensibility or motor function of the forearm and hand.

SURGICAL TECHNIQUE

Since 1982, we no longer carry out preoperative diagnostic nerve blocks, as suggested by Wilhelm, because we have found no correlation between surgical and preoperative block results (5). In addition, we found the block, by diffusion to other structures, often provided the patient with additional anaesthesia and unrealistic expectations of the surgical result.

The technique used differs in several respects from the original method proposed by Wilhelm (4) and popularized by Buck-Gramcko (8,26) in the English literature. The operation is carried out under axillary nerve block using loupe magnification and a tourniquet with incomplete exsanguination. We use four incisions, one anterior and three on the posterior aspect of the wrist and hand (Fig. 75.1).

The palmar incision (incision 1) is curved concave laterally, drawn on the distal quarter of the forearm (Fig. 75.1).

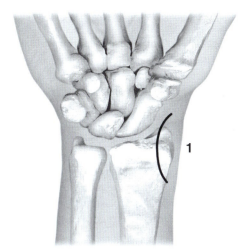
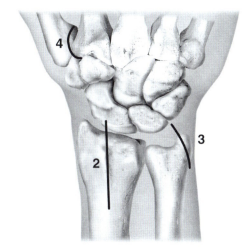

FIGURE 75.1. Skin incisions (1–4) required to carry out complete denervation of the wrist.

It is approximately 5 cm long, centered on the radial artery. The first step is to denude the radial artery over a length of approximately 2 cm and to ligate and resect the venae comitantes to ensure that branches arising from the lateral antebrachial cutaneous nerve are cut (Fig. 75.2). They must not be confused with the much larger and more superficial cutaneous branches that sometimes arise from the radial lateral antebrachial cutaneous nerves. The sheath of the flexor carpi radialis is then opened, and the palmar cutaneous branch of the median nerve is freed until it passes superficially in the subcutaneous tissue at the distal palmar wrist crease.

The skin of the lateral border of the incision is then elevated, dissecting deeply adjacent to bone and extensor retinaculum to protect and elevate the superficial branch of the radial nerve in the subcutaneous tissue of the skin flap. All of its branches that descend toward the carpus are coagulated and divided. Some of these are found regularly, including a branch from the dorsal radial nerve of the thumb to the first carpometacarpal joint, arising adjacent to the radial styloid (12). This step of the operation is completed by using the index to undermine the dorsal flap as far distally as the first interosseous space, dorsally as far as possible, and 5 cm proximally to the radial styloid process.

The next step is to sever the small, unidentifiable, inconstant branches from the anterior interosseous nerve. The flexor tendons and the median nerve are retracted ulnarly. The distal border of pronator quadratus is exposed and cauterized (Fig. 75.3). The periosteum of the the anterior surface of the radius is elevated over a distance of 1 cm to ensure that no branches remain intact. A periosteal elevator is directed to the radioulnar joint ulnarly, and toward the radial styloid radially. Developing this plane ensures that any remaining branches from the lateral cutaneous, radial, or cutaneous branch of the median nerve are divided (Fig. 75.4). The anterior incision is left open while the dorsal incisions are made.

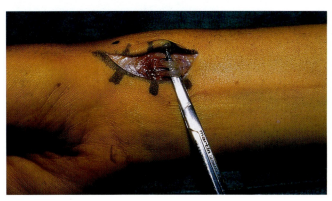

FIGURE 75.2. Through incision 1, veins are resected on both sides of the radial artery to destroy the articular branch of the lateral cutaneous nerve. (Number refers to labels in Fig. 75.1.)

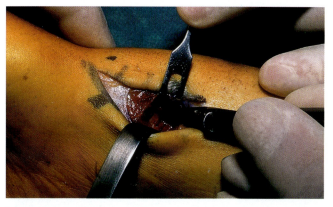

FIGURE 75.3. Through incision 1, the mass of flexor tendons is retracted to expose the distal border of the pronator quadratus muscle and destroy articular branches of the anterior interosseous nerve. (Number refers to labels in Fig. 75.1.)

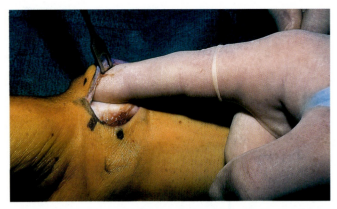

FIGURE 75.4. Through incision *1*, the skin is undermined in a dorsal direction after cutting of the articular branches arising from the radial nerve. This nerve is elevated with the skin. (Number refers to labels in Fig. 75.1.)

Rather than using the proximal short transverse dorsal incisions described by the German authors to divide the posterior interosseous nerve, we favor a 5-cm longitudinal medial incision (incision 2) centered distally on Lister's tubercle (Figs. 75.1 and 75.5). The plane of dissection is directly superficial to the dorsal retinaculum. A finger is used to undermine deep to the skin, joining the previous dissection radially and extending distally to the base of the carpometacarpal joint and ulnarly to the dorsal ulna. The posterior interosseous nerve is easily identified by entering the radial part of the fourth extensor compartment and elevating it close to Lister's tubercle. The diameter of this nerve is sometimes as large as that of a collateral digital nerve. The nerve is dissected from its accompanying vessels proximally at least 4 cm in order to visualize the ulnar branch to the distal radioulnar joint. This entire length of the posterior interosseous nerve is resected, beginning just proximal to the distal radioulnar branch.

A 3-cm incision is performed on the ulnar border of the wrist (incision 3), oblique in a dorsal and distal direction, centered on the distal ulnar head (Fig. 75.1). The sensory branch of the ulnar nerve is frequently found deeply embedded in fascia, adherent to the distal capsule (Fig. 75.6). This may explain why simply undermining the skin from incision 2 is not sufficient. Once it is elevated, all of its deep branches are divided, with care taken to avoid injuring the dorsal transverse cutaneous sensory branch, which remains with the skin. Again, skin undermining from incision 2 has to extend proximally to include any contribution from the medial and/or posterior cutaneous nerves.

An additional dorsal incision (incision 4) is needed to complete the denervation (Fig. 75.1). It is curved and centered on the apex of the first interosseous space. This allows access to the dorsal radial nerve of the index finger, which provides a deep recurrent branch to the wrist (Fig. 75.7A). This branch can be easily identified with loupe magnification. It must not be confused with the dorsal branch of the index itself. When the dorsal nerve proper is lifted, it may appear to have a deep course because of the crossing of a superficial vein (Fig. 75.8). It must be freed, and its two distal branches for the thumb and index identified. The recurrent branch can then be identified adjacent to a constant anastomotic vein between the superficial network and the venae comitantes of the radial artery (Fig. 75.7B). Once identified, it is divided.

We no longer use the two other transverse incisions recommended by Wilhelm at the base of the second and third intermetacarpal spaces (4). These incisions were to be used to divide articular branches arising from the "muscular"

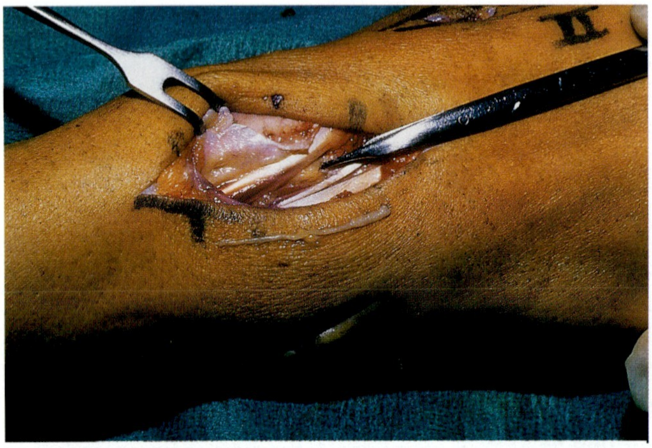

FIGURE 75.5. Incision *2* allows the opening of the fourth extensor compartment to resect the posterior interosseous nerve. (Number refers to labels in Fig. 75.1.)

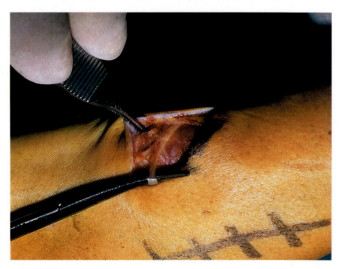

FIGURE 75.6. Through incision *3*, the cutaneous branch of the ulnar nerve is elevated to cut all branches going to the radioulnar joint. (Number refers to labels in Fig. 75.1.)

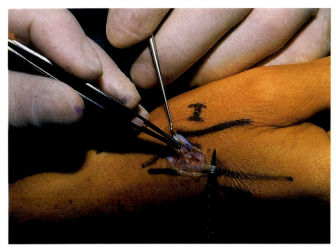 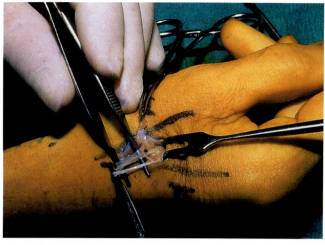

FIGURE 75.7. A,B: Through incision *4*, the first dorsal finger nerve is dissected free to look for the recurrent branch. (Number refers to labels in Fig. 75.1.)

branch of the ulanr nerve. No other authors have found these branches (10,12,14).

Finally, the incisions are closed without drainage. A light moist compression dressing is then applied, as described by Littler. No splint is used unless another surgical procedure is associated. The sutures are removed after the tenth day.

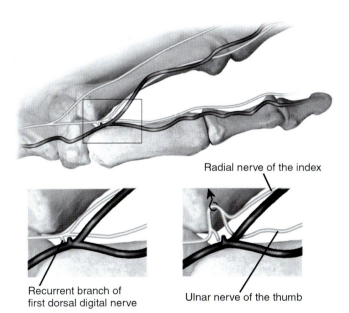

FIGURE 75.8. A pitfall in sectioning the recurrent branch of the first dorsal digital branch of the radial nerve. When the nerve is lifted, the vein shifts the course of the dorsal radial branch of the index. The radial sensory branch to the index appears to dive into the first interosseous space and may be mistaken for its recurrent branch.

CLINICAL SERIES

We performed wrist denervations in 142 patients at SOS Main Strasbourg over an 18-year period. Of these, 52 "complete" and 40 partial denervations were combined with other procedures, and 50 complete denervations were performed as isolated procedures. We have found partial denervation to be less effective than complete denervation, with frequent recurrence of the pain at 12 months (27–29). The results of isolated complete wrist denervation in 50 cases are reviewed with an average follow-up of 5 years. This operation was used when no reconstructive procedure was possible; the main indication was osteoarthritis of the wrist.

RESULTS

The assessment of patients following complete denervation is, of necessity, subjective, based on a pain-rating method, the visual analog scale (VAS) of Huskisson, and patient satisfaction. There was no significant difference between pre- and postoperative grip strength (preoperative 70/130; postoperative 90/140) or range of motion (preoperative 41/50°, postoperative 45/55°). This demonstrantes that strength and motion limitations are not caused solely by pain. That strength was preserved over time despite the the patients' advanced age demonstrates continued manual activity.

We found improvement in pain to be gradual in this group of 50 patients, with maximum benefit after a mean of 16 months. Two patients had no improvement, and one, aged 54, had a recurrence of the pain 6 months after the operation. None of the patients deteriorated. Thirty-seven patients (74%) felt significant improvement and were classified as having a good result with a score over 70 on the VAS (average, 75%). Only six patients (12%) were completely free of pain. The remaining 10 patients (the three failures being excluded) had some improvement in their pain, but this was less than 70% (average, 47%). They were classified as having a fair result.

When correlated with etiology, the lowest scores (mean, 72%) were observed in Kienböck's disease, whereas the highest scores (mean, 86%) were in posttraumatic arthritis following scaphoid nonunion or scapholunate advanced collapse (SLAC) wrist. Others, with arthrosis following intraarticular radius fractures, carpal fractures other than scaphoid, and fracture-luxations, were too small in number to allow any conclusions to be drawn. A relationship could be established between increasing age and the level of improvement of the pain. The average age was 49 years, but in the group below 40 years the average pain improvement was 58% compared with 84% for the group above 50 years ($p > 0.05$).

Our results are in accordance with the literature (5–8,26,30). Unfortunately, most of these studies have not separated the results of those patients who underwent complete and partial wrist denervation and isolated denervation versus denervation associated with reconstructive procedures. A previous comparison (27) has shown the variability of results obtained by partial denervation—a fact already underlined by Geldmacher (5)—and the frequent relapse of pain at 12 months in such cases. This fact could be explained by nerve regeneration, nerve overlapping, or anatomic variation and progression of arthritis in a wrist submitted to stress in the absence of pain. This does not mean that partial denervation is not useful as an adjunct, and we continue to perform a dorsal skin undermining and a resection of the dorsal interosseous nerve in all dorsal approaches to the wrist.

The best results were provided by Cozzi (12) and Fukumoto (13), with 90% to 95% good results in series of 130 and 20 patients, respectively. The Cozzi study does not clearly state assessment criteria or follow-up details. A multicenter German and Swiss series (8) studying 195 patients operated on by seven surgeons reported that 69% of patients experienced no or only slight pain on heavy activity and that 26% were improved. Only 5% remained unchanged in their symptoms. The best results occurred in patients with nonunion of the scaphoid (76%), as compared to those with Kienböck's disease (60%). At an average follow-up of 4.1 years, progression of arthrosis was present in 17%, a result similar to our experience (23%). Geldmacher (5) reported overall 84.4% positive results, including 62.5% excellent results in a series of 35 patients that included 26 total denervations. Seventy-five percent of Lanz's 45 patients reported improvement in pain when followed for 10.5 years (7). All of these published series reported a very low complication rate.

COMPLICATIONS

This operation has been carried out on an outpatient basis in all our cases. On the whole series of 142 operations, few complications occurred, but these are worth mentioning. One painful neuroma of the dorsal collateral nerve to the index finger, accidentally cut, was cured by a secondary intraossous transposition. Three cases of temporary radial nerve paresthesias resolved over 3 to 12 weeks. Anecdotally, the rarity of such dysesthesia despite some traction on the radial nerve might be explained by the effect of posterior interosseous nerve transection, as proposed by Lluch (31). No patient developed a Charcot joint. X-rays were available for long-term evaluation (more than 4 years postoperatively) in only 47 patients. Eleven of these patients showed a radiologic progression of osteoarthritis (23%). The 142 patients were an average age of 49 years. Of 66 individuals working before surgery, 59 (89%) resumed work after an average period of 64 days (19 days for those with an isolated denervation procedure). Among 12 patients engaged in heavy manual work, four had to shift to a lighter activity. Seven patients were unable to return to their previous employment. The average age of these patients was 56 years, and all opted for early retirement.

DISCUSSION

Denervation of the wrist is a simple technique, involves only a short period off work, has a low complication rate, and is effective in reducing pain. Seventy percent of our patients noted an improvement of pain greater than 70% on the visual analog scale. We believe that it is a useful operation in those patients in whom surgery on the underlying lesion is not possible. It remains to be seen how many years can be gained by this procedure before an arthrodesis is finally required, which still remains a technical possibility in these patients.

EDITORS' COMMENTS

The authors have no conclusive experience with denervation as a treatment option for painful wrist. We have been unable to substantiate any effective response from transecting the terminal branch of the dorsal interosseous nerve at the time of dorsal wrist syndrome repair. We will transect both the volar and dorsal interosseous nerves, 10 cm or so proximal to the wrist, when salvaging a symptomatic Darrach procedure. The effectiveness of this is not documented.

REFERENCES

1. Foucher G, Chmiel Z. Proximal row carpectomy. A study of 21 patients. *J Orthop Surg* 1992;6:367–372.
2. Camitz H. Die deformierende Hüftgelenksarthritis und speziell ihre Behandlung. *Acta Orthop Scand* 1933;4:193–213.
3. Tavernier AL, Truchet P. La section des branches articulaires du nerf obturateur dans le traitement de l'arthrite chronique de la hanche. *Rev Orthop* 1942;28:62–68.
4. Wilhelm A. Die Gelenksdenervation und ihre anatomischen Grundlagen. Em neues Behandlungsprinzip in der Handchirurgie. *Hefte Unfallheilkd* 1966;86:1–109.
5. Geldmacher J, Legal HR, Luther R. Results of denervation of the wrist and wrist joint by Wilhelm's method. *Hand* 1972;4:57–59.
6. Helbig B, Geldmacher J, Luther R. Indikation, Technik, und Ergebnisse der Handgelenksdenervation nach Wilhelm bei Knöchernen Veränderungen im Handwurzelbereich. *Orthop Praxis* 1977;13:96–98.
7. Lanz U, Lehmann L. Denervazione del polso: indicazioni e resultati. *Riv Chir Mano* 1987;13:79–84.
8. Buck-Gramcko D. Wrist denervation procedures in the treatment of Kienbock's disease. *Hand Clin* 1993;9:517–520.
9. Wyke BD. The neurology of joints: a review of general principles. *Clin Rheum Dis* 1991;7:223–239.
10. Ferreres A, Suso S, Ordi J, et al. Wrist denervation. Anatomical considerations. *J Hand Surg [Br]* 1995;20:761–768.
11. Dellon AL, MacKinnon SE, Daneshvar A. Terminal branch of anterior interosseous nerve as source of wrist pain. *J Hand Surg [Br]* 1984;9:316–322.
12. Cozzi EP. Denervation des articulations du poignet et de la main. In: Tubiana R, Masson ED, eds. *Traité de chirurgie de la main, tome IV*. Paris: Masson, 1991;781–787.
13. Fukumoto K, Kojima T, Kinoshita Y, et al. An anatomic study of the innervation of the wrist joint and Wilhelm's technique for denervation. *J Hand Surg [Am]* 1993;18:484–489.
14. Dubert T, Oberlin C, Alnot JY. Anatomie des nerfs articulaires du poignet. Application à la technique de dénervation. *Ann Chir Main Membre Sup* 1990;9:15–21.
15. Dowdy PA, Richards RS, McFarlane RM. The palmar cutaneous branch of the median nerve and the palmaris longus tendon: a cadaveric study. *J Hand Surg [Am]* 1994;19:199–202.
16. Naff N, Dellon AL, MacKinnon SE. The anatomical course of the palmar cutaneous branch of the median nerve, including a description of its own unique tunnel. *J Hand Surg [Br]* 1993;18:316–317.
17. Reissis N, Stirrat A, Manek S, et al. The terminal branch of posterior interosseous nerve: a useful donor for digital nerve grafting. *J Hand Surg [Br]* 1992;17:638–640.
18. McCarty CK, Breen TF. Arborization of the distal posterior interosseous nerve. *J Hand Surg [Am]* 1995;20:218–220.
19. Abrams RA, Brown RA, Botte MJ. The superficial branch of the radial nerve: an anatomic study with surgical implications. *J Hand Surg [Am]* 1992;17:1037–1041.
20. Auerbach DM, Collins ED, Kunkle KL, et al. The radial sensory nerve. An anatomical study. *Clin Orthop* 1994;308:241–249.
21. Winckler G. Le nerf articulaire dorsal du premier espace interosseux de la main. *Arch Anat Histol Embryol* 1953;36:61–68.
22. Dykes RW, Terzis JK. Functional anatomy of deep motor branch of ulnar nerve. *Clin Orthop* 1977;128:167–170.
23. Botte MJ, Cohen MS, Lavernia CJ, et al. Dorsal branch of the ulnar nerve: an anatomic study. *J Hand Surg [Am]* 1990;15:603–607.
24. Lourie GM, King J, Kleinman WB. The transverse radioulnar branch from the dorsal sensory ulnar nerve: its clinical and anatomical significance further defined. *J Hand Surg [Am]* 1994;19:241–245.
25. Cruveilhier J. *Traité d'anatomie descriptive, vol IV*. Paris: Paris Labé, 1852.
26. Buck-Gramcko D. Denervation of the wrist joint. *J Hand Surg [Am]* 1977;2:54–61.
27. Ferreres A, Suso S, Foucher G, et al. Wrist denervation. Surgical considerations. *J Hand Surg [Br]* 1995;20:769–772.
28. Foucher G. Technique de dénervation du poignet. *Ann Chir Main* 1989;8:84–87.
29. Foucher G, Da Silva JB, Ferreres A, et al. Total denervation of the wrist. A review of 50 cases. *J Orthop Surg* 1992;6:214–218.
30. Rostlund T, Somnier F, Axelsson R. Denervation of the wrist joint—an alternative in conditions of chronic pain. *Acta Orthop Scand* 1980;51:609–616.
31. Lluch AL, Beasley RW. Treatment of dysaesthesia of the sensory branch of the radial nerve by distal posterior interosseous neurectomy. *J Hand Surg [Am]* 1989;14:121–124.

WRIST STENOSING TENOSYNOVITIS

COCOMPARTMENT RELEASE

H. KIRK WATSON
JAMES MICHAEL SHENKO
JEFFREY WEINZWEIG

INDICATIONS

Tenosynovitis of extensor compartments 2 through 6 is not as commonly described as tenosynovitis of the first extensor compartment, but it does occur (1–3). A new surgical technique for the management of this problem when conservative methods fail is presented. This technique has the benefits of early mobility, prevention of bowstringing, and reproducibility.

CONTRAINDICATIONS

There are no contraindications to performing a cocompartment release for extensor tenosynovitis.

SURGICAL TECHNIQUE

A transverse incision is made over the dorsum of the wrist near the distal margin of the extensor retinaculum. The symptomatic compartment typically demonstrates a thickened roof. The adjacent compartment (cocompartment) is identified; the third extensor (EPL) compartment is usually excluded. The corresponding tendons are retracted ulnarly and radially as the septum between the compartments is identified (Fig. 76.1). The septum is then incised and partially excised; synovectomy is performed if significant synovial overgrowth is present. The two smaller compartments are thus combined to form one larger compartment. This maintains the integrity of the extensor retinaculum and allows early full mobilization at 2 days.

POSTOPERATIVE MANAGEMENT

The bulky dressing applied at the time of cocompartment release is removed 2 days following surgery and the patient is fully mobilized.

CLINICAL CASE

A 33-year-old male patient sustained a hyperextension injury to his right wrist during a fall. Two months postinjury, he was treated elsewhere for a dorsal wrist ganglion. Postoperatively, the patient had some resolution of pain but, over the subsequent 6 months, developed increasing pain on extension of his digits. He was then seen by one of us (H.K.W.) and treated for extensor tenosynovitis of the fourth compartment with antiinflammatory medication and splinting. Because of persistent symptoms, a partial resection of the extensor retinaculum was performed 12 months following the injury. Postoperatively, the patient still complained of unremitting pain without improvement of his symptoms. He was reexplored 1 year and 5 months postinjury, at which time synovectomy and further resection of the thickened retinaculum was performed. Histologic evaluation of the resected retinaculum indicated a chronic inflammatory response. Significant pain with finger extension postoperatively precluded the patient's return to

---

J. Weinzweig: Department of Plastic Surgery, Brown University School of Medicine, Rhode Island Hospital, and Hasbro Children's Hospital, Providence, Rhode Island 02905.

J. M. Shenko: Department of Plastic Surgery, University of Masssachusetts Memorial Health Care, Worcester, Massachusetts 01605.

H. K. Watson: Connecticut Combined Hand Surgery Fellowship, Hartford Hospital, and Connecticut Children's Medical Center, Hartford, Connecticut 06106; Department of Orthopaedics, University of Connecticut School of Medicine, Farmington, Connecticut 06032; Department of Orthopedics, Rehabilitation, and Plastic Surgery, Yale University School of Medicine, New Haven, Connecticut 06520.

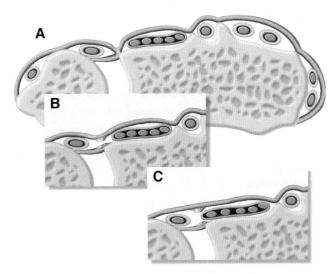

FIGURE 76.1. A: The contents for the fourth dorsal compartment are constricted. Note the septum between the fourth and fifth dorsal compartments. **B:** As the verical septa are transected, the compartments begin to expand, and the contents of the fourth dorsal compartment are free to migrate slightly ulnarward. **C:** With complete resection of the septa, the condition is relieved. There is now a single compartment for the contents of the two cocompartments. The entire extensor retinaculum remains intact.

work. Two years following his initial injury, a cocompartment release was performed, producing immediate, complete relief of his symptoms and return to work status. At follow-up 2 years later, the patient has no symptoms and demonstrates no bowstringing of any tendons with full finger and wrist extension.

COMPLICATIONS

Five patients diagnosed with tenosynovitis of the fourth, fifth, and sixth extensor compartments over a 4-year period have been treated by cocompartment release. The last four patients underwent primary cocompartment release with resolution of their pain symptoms and return to work within a 2- to 4-week period without loss of function. No patient has experienced recurrence of symptoms, and there have been no tendon ruptures. Two of these patients have had follow-up longer than 3 years.

DISCUSSION

Extensor constriction tenosynovitis is typically treated with antiinflammatory medication and immobilization when the extensor compartment roof becomes thickened and fibrotic. Earlier approaches have included either a partial excision of the retinaculum (3) or transection of the extensor retinaculum (4–6). The former approach has limited success in relieving symptoms; the latter allows bowstringing with a concomitant reduction in extension strength. A similar surgical technique was described by Hajj (7): the extensor retinaculum was opened, the septum removed, and the retinaculum repaired. This prevented bowstringing, with resolution of symptoms, but did not allow early mobility.

The cocompartment release technique achieves resolution of symptoms and return to work status within a 2- to 4-week period. This technique addresses the problem of tendon compression in the extensor compartments without sacrificing wrist or finger function.

REFERENCES

1. Burman M. Stenosing tenovaginitis of the dorsal and volar compartments of the wrist. *Arch Surg* 1952;65:752–762.
2. Lapidus PW, Fenton R. Stenosing tenovaginitis at the wrist and fingers. A report of 423 cases in 269 patients with 354 operations. *Arch Surg* 1952;64:475–487.
3. Stern PJ. Tendinitis, overuse syndromes, and tendon injuries. *Hand Clin* 1990;6:467–476.
4. Ambrose J, Goldstone R. Anomalous extensor digiti minimi proprius causing carpal tunnel syndrome in the dorsal compartment. *J Bone Joint Surg Am* 1975;57:706–707.
5. Hooper G, McMaster MJ. Stenosing tenovaginitis affecting the tendon of extensor digiti minimi at the wrist. *Hand* 1979;11:299–301.
6. Ritter MA, Inglis AE. The extensor indicis proprius syndrome. *J Bone Joint Surg Am* 1969;51:1645–1648.
7. Hajj AA, Wood MB. Stenosing tenosynovitis of the extensor carpi ulnaris. *J Hand Surg [Am]* 1986;11:519–520.

SUBJECT INDEX

A

ABC (aneurysmal bone cyst), 709–710
Abduction test, 55
Abductor digiti minimi ligament, 183, 225
Abductor pollicis longus tendon (APL)
    anatomy, 8, 16, 17
    in basal joint resection, 577
    with Bennett's fracture, 256
    de Quervain's disease and, 55
    in distal radius fixation, 317
    intersection syndrome and, 56
    repetitive strain injuries and, 96–97
    with Rolando's fractures, 257
Above-elbow thumb-spica cast, 249, 813
Ace wraps, 778
Acrylic cement, in total wrist prostheses, 662, 668, 676
Activities, everyday. *See* Daily activities
Acute trauma, diagnostic imaging algorithm, 74–75
Adduction test, 54
Adductor pollicis muscle
    with Bennett's fracture, 256
Adhesions
    with articular fracture of the radius, 90
    FCR tendinitis associated with, 99
    lysis, 84
Adjunctive modalities in rehabilitation, 764–765
α-Adrenergic agonists, 696
α-Adrenoceptors, 742, 743, 744
Adson's test, 592
Agee technique, 114
Aging, effects of. *See also* Elderly patients
    carpal tunnel syndrome, 118–119
    Darrach procedure, 803
    ligament mobility, 42
    lunotriquetral ligament, 594
    TFCC perforations, 619
    triangular fibrocartilage complex, 1, 594
Algorithms
    diagnostic imaging, 74–79
    focal bone lesions, 78
    infection, 78–79
    Kienböck's disease, 405–408
    perilunate dislocations, 243
    rotary subluxation of the scaphoid, 529
    scaphoid fractures, 189–190
    subacute and remote trauma, 75–76

Allen's test, 102, 164, 598, 694, 759
Allopurinol, 586
Aluminum, in total wrist prostheses, 660, 661
American Association for Hand Surgery, 742
Amphibians, limb evolution, 1–4
Amputation
    disarticulation for revision, 275
    malignant tumors and, 735, 736, 737
    traumatic. *See* Replantation
ANA. *See* Antinuclear antibodies; Articular-nonarticular junction
Anastomosis
    lunate, patterns of, 396
    microvascular, during replantation, 269, 270, 271, 273
Anatomy, 7–18, 231–232
    arthrology, 11–14
    carpal bones, 231–232, 455–456
    carpal ligament, 107–108
    carpometacarpal joint, 567–568
    column unit concepts, 231
    distal radioulnar joint, 11–12, 369–370
    dorsal extrinsic ligaments, 15
    finger carpometacarpal joint, 260
    hamate, 568, 598
    ligaments, 231–232, 432–435
        intrinsic, 15–16
        palmar extrinsic, 14–15
        of the scapholunate joint, 435–438
    lunate, 8, 458, 504, 508, 525
    lunotriquetral joint, 501–502
    nerves, 9, 945–946
    neutral anatomy positions, 456, 508, 513, 642
    ontogenesis, 7
    osteology, 7–11
    radius, 8, 525
    retinacular system, 16–17
    scaphoid, 187, 434
    trapeziometacarpal joint, 256
    triangular fibrocartilage complex, 8, 11–12, 42–43, 370, 435, 607, 612, 616
Anesthesia
    bone-retinaculum-bone autograft, 916
    carpal tunnel release, 110, 120
    distal radius fractures, 289, 315–316

local, 97
    proximal row carpectomy, 546
    replantation, 270
    triangular fibrocartilage complex tears, 610
Aneurysmal bone cyst (ABC), 709–710
Aneurysms, 692–694
    false, 164, 692, 693
    in the immature wrist, 164–165
    true, 692
Ankylosis, 645, 646, 650
Anlagen, ontogenesis, 7
Antebrachial cutaneous nerves, 946
Antebrachial glenoid, 12
Anterior interosseous nerve, 945–946, 947
Anterior oblique ligament (AOL), 256, 257
Anteroposterior drawer test, 53
Antibiotics, prophylactic, 672, 916
Anticoagulants, 275
Anticonvulsants, 746
Antidepressants, 746
Antiinflammatory medication, 308, 573, 609, 954
Antinuclear antibodies (ANA), 165
Antirheumatic drugs, 667
AO comprehensive classification. *See* Comprehensive Classification of Fractures of Long Bones
AO distracter, 625
AO plate, 680
APL. *See* Abductor pollicis longus tendon
Aponeurotic fibroma, 689
Argon laser, 695
ARIF. *See* Arthroscopic reduction and internal fixation
Arterial repair, 269, 270, 271, 273
Arteriography
    aneurysm, 692
    benign tumors, 696
    hemangioma of the median nerve, 703
Arteriovenous fistula, 692, 693
    acquired, 696–697
    congenital, 695–696
Arthritis. *See also* Osteoarthritis; Rheumatoid arthritis
    arthrodesis of the DRUJ with, 357–358
    basal joint, 572–574
    with carpal dislocation, 246, 251

955

Arthritis (*contd.*)
  complications. *See* Scapholunate
    advanced collapse
  degenerative. *See also* Carpal boss
    with Bennett's fracture, 257
    carpometacarpal, 797–801
    distal radioulnar joint, 351, 852
    pisiform, 602
    and the scaphoid, 197, 525
    with scapholunate dissociation, 491,
      498
    trapeziometacarpal, 572
    and the triscaphe joint, 532–533
  diagnostic imaging, 61, 63, 70
  distal radioulnar joint, 381–385, 391,
    596–597
  FCR tendinitis associated with, 99
  ganglion cysts and, 686
  hamate-lunate joint, 602
  juvenile, 165–167, 168
  with Kienböck's disease, 400, 406
  lunotriquetral joint, 626
  pisiform, 602, 603
  posttraumatic
    carpometacarpal joints, 568–569
    and the Darrach procedure, 803, 805
    with distal radius fractures, 299
    from scaphoid dislocation treament,
      220
    with trapezium dislocation, 223
  proximal row carpectomy and, 551, 552,
    553, 566
  radioscaphoid, 495
  with scaphoid internal fixation, 194,
    196
  thumb carpometacarpal, 770–771
  total wrist arthrodesis and, 556
  tuberculous, 556
  ulnocarpal, 608
Arthrocentesis. *See* Needle aspiration
Arthrodesis
  with arthroplasty, 666
  capitate-lunate, 538
  carpometacarpal, 263, 568, 569, 580. *See
    also* Arthrodesis, total wrist
  distal radioulnar joint, 167, 357–358,
    383, 384–385, 875–877
  fifth metacarpal, 579–580
  "four-corner" or "four-bone," 344, 538,
    552, 921
  of growth cartilage, 64, 68
  intercarpal, 403–404, 666
  limited wrist, 765–767, 777–784
  lunotriquetral, 344, 505–507, 508, 538,
    636, 833–835
  nonunion, 542, 891
  principles of, 521–522
  radiocarpal joint, 216, 217, 652,
    861–865. *See also* Arthrodesis, total
    wrist
  radiolunate joint, 540–542, 652,
    867–874
  radioulnar, 153, 811, 875–877. *See also*
    Sauvé-Kapandji procedure
  in replantation, 271
  rotary subluxation of the scaphoid and,
    523–525, 880
  scaphocapitate, 403, 406, 540, 855,
    895–899
  scapholunate, 539–540
  scapholunatocapitotriquetral, 404
  scaphotrapeziotrapezoid, 249, 403, 521,
    855
    computed tomography, 67
    failed, and total wrist arthrodesis, 555
    for Kienböck's disease, 419, 420,
      423–426
  thumb trapeziometacarpal joint, 577–578
  total wrist, 271, 405, 420, 555–566,
    650–651
  triquetral-hamate joint, 538–539
  triscaphe, 522–523, 931–937
    for carpal instability, 499
    for Kienböck's disease, 403, 406, 415,
      416, 531
    load transmission with, 540
    rehabilitation, 766–767
    for rotary subluxation of the scaphoid,
      487
    with triquetral impingement ligament
      tear surgery, 636
  vs. arthroplasty, 659
Arthrofibrosis with trapezium dislocation,
  223
Arthrography, 69. *See also* Radiography
  carpal dislocation, 237–238
  cinearthrography, 83, 915
  distal radioulnar joint disorders, 373
  lunotriquetral instability, 504
  triangular fibrocartilage complex, 608,
    609, 622
  triple-injection, 342, 593
  ulnar wrist pain, 593–594
Arthrogryopsis, 154
Arthrology, 11–14
Arthroplasty. *See also* Silicone replacement
    arthroplasty
  basal joint resection, 574–577, 580
  carpometacarpal fracture-dislocations,
    267
  carpometacarpal tendon, 797–801
  DRUJ hemiresection-interposition,
    355–356, 837–844
  excision/fascial interposition, 404–405
  hemiresection, with DRUJ arthritis, 383,
    384
  Kienböck's disease, 404–405, 419–420,
    531
  loosening of total wrist implants,
    665–666, 668, 669
  low-friction, 659
  matched hemiresection-interposition,
    355–356, 837–844
  matched ulnar, 847–853, 863
  modified DRUJ, 852
  muscle imbalance with total wrist
    implants, 665, 668–671
  "nonunion." *See* Pseudarthrosis
  prostheses, 275, 404, 430, 653, 659–663,
    664, 728, 870
  proximal row carpectomy, 551
  radiocarpal, 861–865
  soft tissue tumor and, 738
  total carpometacarpal joint, 578
  total wrist
    contraindications, 672
    dislocation of the prosthesis, 671–672,
      679–680
    failure, 556, 659, 663, 665–672, 680
    the future of, 680–681
    historical background, 659
    implants. *See* Arthroplasty, prostheses
    indications, 672
    with rheumatoid arthritis, 652–653
    with triquetral impingement ligament
      tear syndrome, 636
  ulnar, 296, 627, 629, 644, 769, 809,
    847–853, 863
  vs. arthrodesis, 659
Arthroscope, 83, 84, 595
Arthroscopic reduction and internal fixation
  (ARIF), 90
Arthroscopy, 83–93
  carpal instabilities, 448
  distal radioulnar joint disorders,
    373–374, 596
  distal radius fractures, 277
  lunotriquetral instability, 504
  osteoarthritic thumb, 578
  scapholunate interosseous ligament status,
    246
  triangular fibrocartilage complex, 85–90,
    593, 595, 608, 609, 612, 623–624
  ulnar wrist pain, 594–595
Arthrosis, hamate, 599–600
Articular fractures, four basic components,
  299–300
Articular-nonarticular junction (ANA),
  103–104
  physical examination, 49, 58, 528
  rotary subluxation of the scaphoid and,
    526
Asepsis, with total wrist implants, 665
Aseptic necrosis, 126–127
Aspiration. *See* Needle aspiration
Aspirin, 167, 275
Asymptotic wrist, reasons for diagnostic
  imaging, 69
Atherosclerosis, 693
Athletes. *See* Sports

Atlas of Arthroscopy
Australopithecus afarenesis, 4
Avascular necrosis (AVN)
  bone grafts and, 190
  with carpal dislocation, 249–250
  diagnostic imaging, 70, 77–78
  first identification, 396
  lunate. *See* Kienböck's disease
  with perilunate fracture dislocation, 210, 211
  proximal row carpectomy and, 546
  of the scaphoid. *See* Preiser's disease
  with scaphoid fracture or dislocation, 192, 196–197, 220, 222, 223, 413, 904
  with trapezoid dislocation, 220
  vascular implantation for, 401–402
  from venous congestion, 397
AVN. *See* Avascular necrosis
Avulsion
  fractures
    distal radius, 333–335
    ulna, 608
  of ligaments, 173, 174, 178, 179, 181, 492
  of the TFCC, 610–612
Awl, 319, 323, 327
Axial dislocation. *See* Carpal bones, dislocations and instability, axial
Axonal growth, 100
Axonotmesis, 100

B

Backfire fracture. *See* Chauffeur's fracture
Ballottement tests, 52, 55, 474–477, 592, 600, 686
Baltimore Therapeutic Equipment (BTE), 52, 604, 758
Barium impregnation of implants, 660
Barton fracture, reversed, 286
Basistyloid fovea, 8, 11
Basket forceps. *See* Forceps, basket
Benign tumors. *See* Tumors, benign
Bennett retractor, 320, 806
Bennett's fracture, 175, 256–257, 259
Bennett's fracture-dislocation, reverse, 262, 265, 569
Biaxial wrist prosthesis, 661, 670
Biomechanics, 27–43, 232–236
  capitate shortening, 786
  carpal, 464–465
  collagen fiber bundles, 441
  distal ligamentous complex, 439
  distal radioulnar joint, 371, 617
  distal ulna, 616
  extension and flexion, 444, 445
  extrinsic ligaments, 432
  scapholunate interosseous ligament, 439
  triangular fibrocartilage complex, 442, 607
  wrist ligaments, 439, 441–442, 444–446
Biophosphonates, 746
Biopsy of malignant tumors, 724–725, 739
Birth defects. *See* Congenital abnormalities
Blades
  arthroscopy, 609
  banana, 610
  free saw, 625
  hook knife, 109, 114
  retrograde knife, 112, 113
Blatt capsulodesis, 343, 790, 826, 918
Bleeding, persistent, 695
Blood chemistry workup, for replantation, 270
Blood flow
  of the distal radius, 907–908
  reestablishment with replantation, 270–271, 273
  reflex sympathetic dystrophy and, 741, 743–744, 752
Blood pool, in bone scintigraphy, 70
Blount's disease, 151
Bone bruise, 75, 76
Bone cortex, computed tomography of fracture, 66, 73
Bone cysts
  aneurysmal, 709–710
  unicameral, 710–711
Bone death, 412, 414
Bone degradation
  with reflex sympathetic dystrophy, 745
  with rheumatoid arthritis, 645
Bone dysplasias, 143–144
Bone formation, 777. *See also* Bone growth
  effects of ultrasound on, 193
  following osteectomy, 892
  following vascular bundle implantation, 401, 420–421
Bone fragments
  with carpometacarpal fracture-dislocation, 267
  with distal radius fracture, 309, 310, 323, 337
  "healing" time, 337
  with lunate fracture, 872
  osteochondral, with Kienböck's disease, 416
  in total wrist arthrodesis, 558
  ulnar styloid, 602, 603
Bone grafts
  avascular necrosis and, 190
  biconcave, for scaphoid nonunion, 901–905
  bone-retinaculum-bone autograft, 915–919
  "caging" of, 354, 928, 929
  capitate-hamate fusion, 788
  carpal bone fractures, 183
  carpal dislocation, 249

  carpometacarpal fracture-dislocations, 267
  computed tomography of, 67
  distal radius fracture, 287, 317, 323, 326
  donor sites
    contralateral wrist, 927
    distal radius, 427, 428, 815–817, 833, 867, 868, 873, 895, 934
    foot, 918
    iliac crest, 306, 352, 353, 359, 557, 558, 563, 565, 677, 867, 895–896
    Lister's tubercle, 918
    metacarpal bones, 427
    ulna, 427
  extrusion, 904
  free retinacular, 98
  giant cell tumor excision, 728, 729–732
  hook of hamate, 179, 184
  interpositional wedge, 911–912
  for Kienböck's disease, 419, 420, 426–428
  lunotriquetral arthrodesis, 507, 833–834
  "peg," 184, 557
  in radiolunate arthrodesis, 867, 873
  in radioulnar arthrodesis, 875
  radius, 728, 730, 731, 733, 734
  in scaphocapitate arthrodesis, 895–896
  scaphocapitate syndrome, 245
  scaphoid dislocation, 245
  scaphoid fracture, 158, 168, 169, 195, 196, 197, 198, 901–905
  scapholunate advanced collapse reconstruction, 921, 922, 923
  "slot," 557
  solitary enchondroma, 705
  split fibular, 680
  total wrist arthrodesis, 557–559
  with total wrist arthroplasty, 666, 669, 677
  trapezoidal malunion, 353, 364
  "turnabout," 557, 558
  ulna, with giant cell tumor, 729, 731, 732
  vascularized, for scaphoid nonunion, 907–914
  xenografts, 558
Bone growth
  congenital abnormalities and, 123
  diagnostic imaging of turnover, 70
  with distal ulnoradial joint disorders, 388
  overgrowth due to repetitive ulnar loading, 156
  post-fracture arrest, 162
  rate, 161
Bone marrow, magnetic resonance imaging, 73, 74, 75
Bone necrosis. *See* Osteonecrosis
Bone resorption, 189, 193
Bone scan. *See* Bone scintigraphy

958 Subject Index

Bone scintigraphy, 69–71
  algorithms in treatment, 75, 76, 79
  distal radioulnar joint disorders, 373
  fractures, 70, 71, 189, 190
  Kienböck's disease, 398
  osteoid osteoma, 708
  reflex sympathetic dystrophy, 594
  three-phase, 70, 724, 746
  ulnar wrist pain, 594
Bone stock
  deficient, 351, 889
  maintenance with Sauvé-Kapandji procedure, 653
Bone substitutes. See Arthroplasty
Bone tumors, benign, 683, 704–711
Bone turnover, diagnostic imaging, 70
Boss. See Carpal boss
Boutonnière deformity, 641
Boxer's fracture, 260
Bradykinin, 743, 744
Broach, 674, 675, 676
BTE. See Baltimore Therapeutic Equipment
Bunnell's-soaked cotton balls, 274
Bunnell suture techniques, 812
Bunnell test, 640, 654
Burns, 102, 784
Buttress plate, 326, 328, 330, 331, 333. See also L-plate; T-plate

C

Calcification of soft tissue, 695
Calcifying aponeurotic fibroma, 689
Calcinosis, 683, 713–714
Calcitonin, 746
Calcitonin gene-related peptide (CGRP), 743
Calcium channel blockers, 696, 746
Calcium pyrophosphate deposition disease (CPPD), 555, 583, 586–589
Callus, 198
Candida albicans, 679
Cannula, 84, 86. See also Slotted cannula
Cannulated screw. See Screw fixation, cannulated
Capillary hemangioma, 694
Capitate. See also Scaphocapitate fracture syndrome
  computed tomography of fracture, 65
  in development of Kienböck's disease, 411, 412, 413
  dislocation, 225–226
  in flexion-extension, 37
  fractures, 159, 176–177
  motion of the second and third metacarpals, 255
  ontogenesis, 7
  ossification, 149
  osteology, 9–10
  partial resection, 551

  in proximal row carpectomy, 535, 548–549, 551, 553
  with radial deficiency, 131, 132, 134
  shortening, 402, 404, 785–790
  synostosis, 123, 124
Capitate-hamate fusion, 785–790
Capitate-hamate ligament, 14, 15
Capitate-hamate-lunate-triquetrum fusion (CHTL), 344, 538, 552
Capitate-lunate arthrodesis, 538
Capitate-lunate instability pattern (CLIP), 511, 514–515
Capitate metacarpal, 7, 9–10
Capitate-trapezoid joint, 87
Capitate-trapezoid ligament, 14, 15
Capitellar joint, dislocation, 146
Capitohamate interosseous ligament with capitate dislocation, 225
Capitohamate joint (CH)
  anatomy, 232
  fusion, 39, 404
Capitolunate joint, 24. See also Lunocapitate joint
  arthrodesis, 555
  instability, 431, 440–449
Capitotriquetral ligament, anatomy, 432, 435
Capsaicin, 746
Capsular-bone impingement, 633
Capsular contractures, 196
Capsular ligaments, 432
Capsule defects, 69
Capsulodesis, 212–213, 214, 247–249, 495
  Blatt, 343, 790
  in ligamentous repair for scapholunate dissociation, 495, 496, 497, 498
  for rotary subluxation of the scaphoid, 819–827
  vs. bone-retinaculum-bone autograft, 918
Capsulolysis, of the DRUJ, 359
Capsulotomy
  for cerebral palsy wrist contractures, 154
  distal radioulnar joint, 805
  for distal radius fracture, 320, 321, 326
  dorsal radial, for scaphoid nonunion, 910
  for perilunate dislocation, 211, 244
"Caput ulnae" syndrome, 647
Carpal angles, determination of, 236–237, 250
Carpal arch
  anatomy, 232
  flattening, 178
  with Madelung's deformity, 151
  in scapholunate instability, 448
  structural strength, 10
Carpal bones
  congenital synchondrosis, 533–535
  dislocations and instability, 231–251, 446–447
  anatomy, 231–232, 455–458

  axial, 204, 217–219, 231, 241
  biomechanics, 232–234, 455
  definition, 76
  diagnosis, 236–238
  expected outcomes, 249
  in gymnasts, 154
  injury patterns, 234–238
  isolated, 204, 219–226
  longitudinal, 241, 242, 246
  midcarpal, 203, 204
  miscellaneous patterns of, 226
  nomenclature, 477–479
  perilunar, 203–214, 466–469, 546
  posttraumatic, 158–159
  predynamic, 483–489
  proximal row carpectomy and, 546
  radiocarpal, 204, 205, 215–217
  from scaphoid fracture surgery, 196
 distal carpal row. See also Capitate; Trapezium; Trapezoid
  in carpal instability biomechanics, 455
  osteology, 10–11
  "Roman arch," 567
 dysfunction and reconstruction following distal radius fracture, 341–364
 evolution of the, 1–5
 fractures
  in children, 156–157, 159
  excluding scaphoid fractures, 173–184
  with juvenile arthritis, 166–167
 kinematics, 27–28, 36–37, 444–446, 461–465
 with Madelung's deformity, 140
 normal alignment, 190, 455–461, 479
 normal external dimensions, and arthrodesis, 522
 ossification, 7, 149, 533
 pathogenesis of ligament instability, 431, 435–451
 with polydactyly, 138
 with radial deficiency, 123–125, 128, 134
 in radioulnar deviation, 23, 24
 ulnar, nonunion, 602
 ulnar carpal translocation, secondary, 341, 355, 364
 with ulnar deficiency, 135
Carpal boss, 55, 146, 683
  cause of formation, 569, 580, 712
  diagnostic imaging, 62, 63, 712–713, 794
  first use of term, 793
  pediatric, 149–151
  physical examination, 48, 793
  treatment, 63, 150–151, 570, 713, 770, 793–795
"Carpal boss view," 149
"Carpal box" images, 189
Carpal component of total wrist implants, 665–667, 676–677, 679
Carpal condyl, 12

Carpal height, 398, 677, 679, 882
Carpal instability. *See* Carpal bones, dislocations and instability
Carpal instability combined (CIC), 478–479
Carpal instability dissociative (CID), 76, 477, 478, 503, 600, 879, 880. *See also* Rotary subluxation of the scaphoid
Carpal instability nondissociative (CIND), 349, 477–478, 503, 600
Carpal kinematics. *See* Kinematics, carpal
Carpal ligament. *See* Carpal tunnel release; Carpal tunnel syndrome
"Carpal link" concept, 464
Carpal plate, in universal wrist prosthesis, 663, 664, 666
"Carpal ring" concept, 464, 501
Carpal tumors, benign, 693
Carpal tunnel
 anatomy, 100
 approach in perilunate dislocation surgery, 212, 214
 complaints with Kienböck's disease, 415
 computed tomography, 178
Carpal tunnel release
 Agee technique, 114
 alternative Chow technique, 113–114
 Chow technique, 109–114
 distal radius surgery, 321
 dorsal wrist syndrome and, 831
 endoscopic, 101, 109–114, 115, 120
 Japanese technique, 114
 open, 109, 115
 in perilunate dislocation algorithm, 243
 during replantation, 270
 in scaphoid dislocation, 245
Carpal tunnel syndrome (CTS), 100–101, 107–120
 computed tomography, 64
 from distal radius fractures, 336
 with dorsal wrist syndrome, 487
 pathophysiology, 108
 in perilunate dislocation algorithm, 243
 with rotary subluxation of the scaphoid, 527
 secondary to gout, 584
 from total wrist arthrodesis, 562
Carpal volume, 64
Carpectomy
 for giant cell tumor, 709
 for Kienböck's disease, 405, 407
 proximal row. *See* Proximal row carpectomy
 during replantation, 271, 275
 with rheumatoid arthritis, 654
Carpometacarpal column/complex/joints (CMC), 103–104, 567–580. *See also* Trapeziometacarpal joint
 anatomy, 260

 arthrodesis, 263, 568, 569, 580. *See also* Arthrodesis, total wrist
 with capitate dislocation, 225
 with degenerative arthritis, 797–801
 dislocation, 217, 218, 579, 642
 evaluation of motion, 24–25
 fractures and fracture-dislocations, 255–267
 injuries, 258–267, 579
 instability classification, 262
 mechanism of injury, 260–261
 physical examination, 54–55, 758
 with rheumatoid arthritis, 641–642, 649, 653, 654, 770
 in scaphoid fracture fixation, 194
 tendon arthroplasty, 797–801
 total arthroplasty, 578
 with trapezium dislocation, 223
Carpus. *See also* Carpal bones; Soft tissue
 evolution of the, 2–5
 osteology, 7–8
Carrying, in the Dystrophile program, 885, 886, 887
Cartilage
 benign tumors, 704–705
 with carpal dislocation, 251
 compression of, 38–39, 42, 465, 479
 degradation with rheumatoid arthritis, 645
 growth, fusion of, 64, 68
 in the immature wrist, 159
 magnetic resonance imaging, 189
Case studies
 capsulodesis for rotary subluxation of the scaphoid, 825–826
 cocompartment release for tenosynovitis, 953–954
 giant cell tumor, 729–733
 osteosarcoma, 733–736
 Sauvé-Kapandji procedure, 892
 scaphocapitate arthrodesis, 897
 vascularized bone graft, scaphoid nonunion, 913–914
Castaing classification, 279
Cast immobilization
 distal radius fractures, 291–296, 305–306, 311, 343
 five factors which predict instability, 289
 Kienböck's disease, 400
 limited wrist arthrodesis, 777–784
 lunotriquetral instability, 505
 scaphoid fracture, limitations of, 191
 TFCC tears, 770
 total wrist arthrodesis, 557
 vascular bundle implantation, 422
Casts
 above-elbow, 249, 813
 diagnostic imaging and, 64
 effects of extended treatment, 193

 fiberglass, 780–781
 gauntlet, 184, 357, 834, 903
 "Groucho Marx," 198, 777–778, 779, 873, 903, 929, 935
 long arm. *See* Long arm cast; Long arm thumb-spica cast
 molding, 292, 293
 Muenster, 224, 336, 357, 611, 841
 short arm. *See* Short arm cast; Short arm thumb-spica cast
 swelling with, 192
 technique, 779–782, 783
 tightness and reflex sympathetic dystrophy, 744
Catecholamines, 742
Catheterization, 270
Cavernous hemangioma, 694
Cavernous lymphangioma, 697
Celestone, 574
Cell dynamometers, 28, 29
Cement. *See* Acrylic cement
Cenani syndactyly, 137
Center of rotation (COR), 23–24, 670
Centralia, fusion, 7
Centralia intermedium, ontogenesis, 7
Central sensitization, 743
Cephalosporin, 316, 916
Cerebral palsy, 154
CGRP (calcitonin gene-related peptide), 743
CH. *See* Capitohamate joint
"Champagne flute" appearance, 146, 533, 534, 538
Charcot joint, 945, 950
Chauffeur's fracture, 240, 278
Chemotherapy for malignant tumors, 726, 736, 737, 739
Children. *See* Pediatrics
Chirulen, 661
Chloropromazine, 275
Chondroblastoma, 723
Chondrodysplasia, 705
Chondromalacia, 595, 615, 623
Chondrosarcoma, 705
Chow techniques, 109, 110–114
CHTL (capitate-hamate-lunate-triquetrum fusion), 344, 538, 552
CID. *See* Carpal instability dissociative
CIND. *See* Carpal instability nondissociative
Cinearthrography, 83, 469, 871, 915
Clamps
 Kelly, 799
 mosquito, 799
Classifications
 carpal dislocations, 217, 218, 238, 241, 242
 carpal tunnel syndrome, 116
 distal radius fractures, 277–289, 299–304, 309, 314–315

Classifications (contd.)
  DRUJ lesions, 286, 288
  finger carpometacarpal injuries, 262–265, 266
  Galleazzi fracture complex, 163
  instability, 206
  Kienböck's disease, 399–400, 786, 855, 939
  ligament injury following distal radius fracture, 342
  lunate fractures, 179
  malignant tumors, 725
  midcarpal instability, 511, 516–520
  perilunar instability, 206
  radiocarpal dislocation, 215
  reflex sympathetic dystrophy, 742
  rotary subluxation of the scaphoid, 486–487
  scaphoid fractures, 190–191
  scapholunate interosseous ligament ruptures, 486
  trapezial ridge fractures, 175
  triangular fibrocartilage complex injury, 88, 595–596, 608, 616, 619–622
  triquetrum fractures, 181
  ulnar styloid nonunion, 597
  ulnar translation, 216
Clayton-Volz-Ferlic prosthesis, 660–661, 670
Clicking. See Wrist "click"
Clinical assessment
  bone graft, scaphoid nonunion, 903–904
  capitate shortening with capitate-hamate fusion, 788–789
  carpal boss repair, 794
  carpal tunnel release, 114–115
  denervation, 949
  dorsal wrist syndrome, 830–831
  lunotriquetral arthrodesis, 834–835
  matched hemiresection-interposition arthroplasty, 841–843
  matched ulnar arthroplasty, 850
  radiocarpal arthrodesis-arthroplasty, 863, 865
  radiolunate arthrodesis, 868–870
  reflex sympathetic dystrophy, 744–745, 885
  scaphocapitate arthrodesis, 897
  scapholunate advanced collapse reconstruction, 924–925
  trapezoidal osteotomy of the distal radius, 929–930
  triscaphe arthrodesis, 935, 937
  ulnar lengthening, 940–941
  vascularized bone graft, scaphoid nonunion, 913
CLIP (capitate-lunate instability pattern), 511, 514–515
Clonidine, 746
Closed biopsy, 724

Closed reduction
  axial dislocation of carpus, 219
  Bennett's fracture, 256, 257
  capitate dislocation, 225
  distal radius fracture, 277, 287, 289–296, 305–306, 309, 316, 343
  perilunate fracture dislocation, 210, 211
  pisiform dislocation, 225
  radiocarpal dislocation, 215
  scaphoid dislocation, 220
  scaphoid fracture, 190–191, 193
  trapeziometacarpal joint dislocation, 258
  trapezium dislocation, 223
  trapezium fracture, 258
  trapezoid dislocation, 219
Closed wedge osteotomy. See Osteotomy, closed wedge
Club hand, 128, 131, 144
CMC. See Carpometacarpal column/complex/joints
C nociceptors, 743
Cobalt chrome, in prostheses, 660, 663, 668
Coban, 90, 778
Cocompartment release, 639, 654, 953–954
Colchicine, 586
Cold intolerance, 591, 603
Cold stress testing, 746
Collagen
  compression of, 42, 612
  fiber bundle orientation, 439, 441, 617
  production with inflammatory response, 95
  in scapholunate interosseous ligament, 436
Colles' fracture, 25, 91
  classification, 279, 289, 291
  in the elderly, 296–297
  as indicator for Sauvé-Kapandji procedure, 890
  ligament rupture following, 390
  malunion, 37, 930
  matched hemiresection-interposition arthroplasty following, 844
  silver fork deformity, 516
  tendinitis following, 98
  ulnar impaction syndrome and, 615, 628–629
Color changes
  café-au-lait spots, 698
  cyanotic, with benign tumors, 693
  ecchymosis, 591
  hemangiomas, 694, 695, 715
  "port-wine," with benign tumors, 694, 695
Columnar theory of the wrist, 28
Comminution in distal radius fractures, 280, 281, 300, 302, 306
"Communicating defect," 69
Communication during replantation decision, 270

Compartment syndrome, 336, 783
Complex fractures, 335–336
Complex regional pain syndrome. See Reflex sympathetic dystrophy
Complications
  arthrodesis, 542, 835, 871, 937
  arthroplasty, 801, 843, 865
  bone graft, scaphoid nonunion, 904
  bone graft harvest, 815, 817
  capitate shortening with capitate-hamate fusion, 790
  capsulodesis for rotary subluxation of the scaphoid, 824–825
  carpal boss repair, 794
  carpal dislocations, 249–250
  carpal tunnel release, 115
  carpometacarpal fractures, 266–267
  carpometacarpal tendon arthroplasty, 801
  cast immobilization, 783–784
  cocompartment release for tenosynovitis, 953–954
  Darrach procedure, 355, 808
  denervation, 950
  distal radius fractures, 336–337, 341
  dorsal wrist syndrome, 831
  external fixation, 308–309, 336, 771
  ganglion excision, 164, 688
  juvenile arthritis medications, 167
  Kienböck's disease treatment, 790
  lunotriquetral arthrodesis, 835
  matched hemiresection-interposition arthroplasty, 843
  matched ulnar arthroplasty, 850–851
  nonunion of hook of hamate fracture, 179
  osteotomy, 859, 930
  pin fixation, 790
  proximal row carpectomy, 551–552
  radial shortening osteotomy, 859
  radiocarpal arthrodesis-arthroplasty, 865
  radiocarpal dislocation treatment, 216–217
  radiolunate arthrodesis, 871
  Sauvé-Kapandji procedure, 891–892
  scaphoid dislocation treatment, 220
  scaphoid fractures, 196–197
  scaphoid-lunate dislocation, 222
  scapholunate advanced collapse reconstruction, 925
  sling immobilization, 308
  trapezium dislocation, 223
  trapezoidal osteotomy of the distal radius, 930
  triscaphe arthrodesis, 937
  of untreated Madelung's deformity, 151
  of untreated scaphoid fracture in children, 157, 158–159
Comprehensive Classification of Fractures of Long Bones, 280–284, 289, 303, 314–315, 323, 327

Compression jig, 194
Compression neuropathy. See Nerves, entrapment
Compression plate. See Ender compression blade plate; Plate fixation
Compression screws. See Screw fixation, Herbert
Compression test, 52, 54, 189, 686
Compressive forces of everyday activities, 233
Computed tomography (CT), 64–69, 75–79
  capitate fracture, 177
  carpal dislocation, 237
  carpal tunnel, 178
  disadvantages, 69
  distal radioulnar joint disorders, 373, 596
  distal radius fracture, 312, 331
  hamate fracture, 178, 599
  hook of hamate fracture, 178
  Kienböck's disease, 398
  lunate fracture, 180
  malignant tumor, 724
  osteoid osteoma, 707, 708
  perilunar dislocation, 207, 210
  in pisotriquetral joint dysfunction, 598
  prior to arthroscopy, 90
  scaphoid fracture, 189, 198
  spiral, 69
  three-dimensional, 594
  ulnar wrist pain, 594
Concave-Convex rule, 764
"Concertina deformity," 431
Congenital abnormalities, 123–146
  arteriovenous fistula, 695–696
  aseptic necrosis, 126–127
  bipartite scaphoid, 158
  bone dysplasias, 143–144
  carpal synchondrosis, 533–535
  carpal synostosis, 123–125
  distal radioulnar synostosis, 136–137
  hereditary multiple exostoses, 142–143
  ligamentous laxity, 203
  lunotriquetral fusion, 508
  Madelung's deformity. See Madelung's deformity
  mirror hand, 138
  polydactyly, 138
  radial deficiency, 127–134
  synchondrosis, 833
  triquetral-lunate joint, 603
  ulnar, 135–136, 619, 627, 628
Connective tissue disease, 203
Contact area of force distribution, 38–40
Continuous passive motion (CPM), 336, 764
Contraindications
  bone graft, 815, 901
  capsulodesis for rotary subluxation of the scaphoid, 819

carpal boss repair, 793
cocompartment release for tenosynovitis, 953
Darrach procedure, 803, 805
denervation, 945
distal radius malunion surgery, 351, 362
dorsal wrist syndrome, 829
lunotriquetral arthrodesis, 833
matched ulnar arthroplasty, 847
proximal row carpectomy, 545–546
radiocarpal arthrodesis-arthroplasty, 861
replantation, 270
Sauvé-Kapandji procedure, 889
scapholunate advanced collapse reconstruction, 921
total wrist arthrodesis, 556
total wrist arthroplasty, 672
trapezoidal osteotomy of the distal radius, 927
triscaphe arthrodesis, 523, 766, 931
wafer procedure, 624
COR (center of rotation), 23–24, 670
"Coral bone," 337
Cortex. See Bone cortex
Cortical bridge, 797, 798, 801
Cortical wall, "collapsability" of the, 414
Cortical window, in bone graft harvest, 815, 816
Corticocancellous graft, 184, 557–558, 559, 677
Corticosteroids
  for gout, 586
  for reflex sympathetic dystrophy, 746
  for repetitive strain injuries, 97, 98, 99, 100
Cortisone
  carpal tunnel syndrome and, 119
  for distal radioulnar joint arthritis, 597
  for osteoarthritis, 574, 580
  for pisotriquetral joint dysfunction, 598
Corundum, in total wrist prostheses, 661
Cosmesis with de Quervain's disease, 97
Cosmetic aspects of distal radius fracture, 296
Cotton-Loder position, 291
CPM (continuous passive motion), 336, 764
CPPD (calcium pyrophosphate deposition disease), 555, 583, 586–589
Cradle boot, 274
Crossopterygia, 1, 2
Cross-pin fixation, 272
Crush injury, 119, 223, 579
Crystalline arthropathies, 583–589
CT. See Computed tomography
CTS. See Carpal tunnel syndrome
Cuff resection. See Ulna, cuff resection
Cumulative trauma disorder. See Repetitive injury
Curettage, 709, 728, 933

Cyriax evaluation, 758
Cystic lymphangioma, 697
Cystoscope, 83
Cysts. See Bone cysts; Epidermal inclusion cysts; Ganglion cysts

D

Daily activities
  with carpal tunnel syndrome, 117, 120
  compressive force of, 233
  effects of wrist fusion, 659
  fracture immobilization and, 296
  importance of psychological aspects in surgery to, 296
  increase in, Dystrophile program, 886
  modification with TFCC tears, 609
  wrist-fixed, 117
Darrach procedure, 358–359, 803–809
  complications, 355, 808, 943
  distal ulna resection, 653
  with DRUJ disorders, 381, 383, 388, 803
  force and pressure analysis, 34, 38–40
  for Madelung's deformity, 153
  triquetral impingement ligament tear syndrome and, 636
  ulnar impaction syndrome after, 615, 627
DC plate, 328, 337, 357, 405, 857, 939, 940
Debridement
  arthroscopy, 84, 89
  with axial dislocation of carpus, 219
  distal radius fracture, 328, 329
  flexor carpi radialis tendon, 99
  intercarpal ligament tears, 609
  lunotriquetral ligament, 344, 505, 600
  for replantation, 270, 271, 273
  scaphoid fracture, 195
  triangular fibrocartilage complex tears, 609, 610, 611, 623–624
Decompression plate. See DC plate
Decompressive procedures
  for Kienböck's disease, 402–404
  lipofibromatous hamartoma, 702
Deep ligaments, 14–15
Deformities. See Congenital abnormalities; Rheumatoid arthritis, deformities
Degenerative joint disease (DJD), 48, 381
  diagnostic imaging, 70
  scapholunate joint, 486
  subpisiform, 55–56
  trapeziometacarpal joint, 54
Delayed treatment
  carpal dislocation, 246
  perilunate dislocation, 210
Delayed union of scaphoid fracture, 193, 196, 197
"Delta-bones." See Epiphyseal brackets
Demyelination, 100
Denervation, 405, 420, 945–950

de Quervain's disease, 47, 55, 96–97, 103–104, 573, 600, 715, 758
Dermatitis, 784
Dermatofibroma, 689
Desmoplastic fibroma, 689
Devices. *See* Arthroplasty
Dexamethasone, 765
Dextran, 275
DI. *See* Dorsal intercarpal ligament
Diabetes with carpal tunnel syndrome, 100, 119
Diagnosis, reproducability, 277, 281. *See also* Misdiagnosis; Patient history; Physical examination
Diagnostic imaging, 61–79. *See also* Bone scintigraphy; Computed tomography; Diagnostic imaging; Fluoroscopy; Magnetic resonance imaging; Radiography; Three-dimensional carpal motion studies; Tomography
 attenuation coefficients, 64
 for carpal dislocations, 236–238
 for carpometacarpal fracture-dislocations, 265–266
 for Kienböck's disease, 398–399
 metabolic, 70
 selection algorithms, 74–79
 ultrasound, 72
Diaphyseal aclasia, 705
Die-punch fractures
 of the distal radius
  classification, 314, 327
  double, 300, 302
  effects on the radiolunate joint, 872, 873
  first use of term, 278
  lunate, 344, 873
  mechanism of injury, 300, 302
  surgical technique, 321, 327–328
 of the lunate, 344, 871
Diet, post-replantation, 275
Digit. *See also* Metacarpal
 deformities with rheumatoid arthritis, 639–642, 647–648
 evolution of the, 1–3, 5
 joint contractures, 308
 replantation, 269
 rotational malalignment with axial dislocation of carpus, 218
Digitization of data, 21, 34, 40
Dipnoi, 1
Dipyridamole, 275
Disarticulation for revision amputation, 275
DISI. *See* Dorsal intercalated segment instability
Dislocations. *See also specific bones and joints*
 axial, 261
 of the total wrist prosthesis, 671–672, 679–680

 volar-ulnar, 640
 vs. fracture-dislocation, 215
 vs. subluxation, 241
Dissectors, 84
Distal ligamentous complex, 439, 441–442
Distal radial physis
 fracture, 160–161
 injury from gymnastics, 154–155, 156
 ulnar impaction syndrome and, 619
Distal radioulnar joint (DRUJ)
 anatomy, 11–12, 369–370, 595
 with arthritis, 166, 167, 381–385, 596–597, 601, 642, 645, 650
  modified arthroplasty for, 852
  treatment, 653, 654–655. *See also* Darrach procedure
 arthrodesis, 167, 357–358, 383, 384–385, 875–877
 arthroscopy, 90
 biomechanics, 371, 617
 causes of pain, 768
 classification of lesions, 286, 288, 314
 contractures, 838
 deformity after fracture, 162–163
 dislocation
  pain associated with, 48, 603
  stabilization, 811–813
  volar, 374, 375
 in distal radius surgery, 317, 318, 320, 321
 evolution of the, 3, 4, 369, 388
 force and pressure analysis, 39
 injury following distal radius fracture, 343–344, 346–347, 351, 359–362
 with Madelung's deformity, 151, 388
 matched hemiresection-interposition arthroplasty, 355–356, 837–844, 853
 matched resection, 356–357
 in matched ulnar arthroplasty, 847, 849, 850, 852–853
 physical examination, 51–52, 592, 758
 replacement arthroplasty, 662
 resection, 355
 subluxation, 64, 374, 601, 838
 synostosis, 136, 137
 synovectomy, 650, 654
 with TFCC tears, 610
 ulnar shortening and, 625, 627, 629
 vascular anatomy, 595, 617
Distal radioulnar joint capsule, 359, 369–370
Distal radius
 effects of shortening on outcome, 305
 fractures, 327–333
  in children, 160–163
  classification, 277–289, 296, 314–315
  with distal radioulnar joint disorders, 377
  external fixation, 299–309

  in the immature wrist, 160–163
  incidence rate, 341
  initial assessment, 312–314
  malunion. *See* Malunion, distal radius fracture
  principles of management, 305
  reconstruction of secondary carpal problems, 341–364
  reduction and stabilization, 305–306
  reflex sympathetic dystrophy and, 744
  rehabilitation, 308–309
  secondary carpal problems following, 341–364
  surgical technique, 306–308
  treatment, 289–296, 771
 as landmark for arthroscopy, 85
 pedical graft to the lunate, 402
Distal ulnar physis, 162–163
DJD. *See* Degenerative joint disease
Dominant/nondominant aspects of strength, 29
DonJoy wrist splint, 30
Doppler examination, 686, 746
Dorsal approach to internal fixation, 195, 197, 198
Dorsal carpal impingement syndrome, 468
Dorsal intercalated segment instability (DISI), 241, 459, 478
 with Kienböck's disease, 400
 lunate shape and, 513
 pathogenesis, 431
 with perilunate dislocation, 205, 208
 prevention of deformity, 247
 as result of SLIL injury, 915
 with rotary subluxation of the scaphoid, 819, 879–880
 with scaphoid fracture, 189, 193
 in scapholunate advanced collapse reconstruction, 923
 with scapholunate dislocation, 222, 469, 472, 532
 secondary, following distal radius fracture, 341, 343, 349
Dorsal intercarpal ligament (DI), 14, 16
 anatomy, 502
 in capsulodesis, 247–249
Dorsal radiocarpal ligament
 anatomy, 432–434, 502
 in carpal dislocation, 446
 failure location and mode, 433
Dorsal radiolunotriquestral ligament, 8, 12
Dorsal radioulnar ligament (DRUL), 370, 371, 372
Dorsal wrist syndrome (DWS), 49, 58, 436, 483–489, 498
 arthroscopy, 93
 in children, 169
 physical examination, 49, 58, 528
 treatment, 767–768, 829–831

triquetral impingement ligament tear syndrome and, 636
Dorsoradial ligament (DRL), 256
Double-crush syndrome, 119
Double die-punch fracture, 300, 302
Dowel grip, 155
Dressing
   distal radioulnar joint arthritis surgery, 601
   distal radius surgery, 336
   external fixation pins, 308–309
   limited wrist arthrodesis, 777, 779, 780
   matched hemiresection-interposition arthroplasty, 844
   postoperative, technique for, 778–779
   replantation, 274, 275
   scapholunate advanced collapse reconstruction, 924
   skin graft, 274
   total wrist arthrodesis, 562, 563
Drill guide, 316
Drill technique
   biconcave bone graft, scaphoid nonunion, 901–902
   distal radioulnar joint disorders, 812
   dorsal capsulodesis, 822–823
   hook of hamate bone graft, 184
   plate fixation for total wrist arthrodesis, 561
   Sauvé-Kapandji procedure, 889, 890
   universal wrist prosthesis surgery, 674
DRUJ. *See* Distal radioulnar joint
DRUL. *See* Dorsal radioulnar ligament
Drummer boy's palsy, 98
Dupuytren's fibromatosis, 689
DWS. *See* Dorsal wrist syndrome
Dye studies, 904
Dynamic compression plate. *See* DC plate
Dynamic ulnar impaction syndrome, 627
Dynamometer, 592, 758, 870
Dyschondrosteosis, 151
Dysplasias, bone, 143–144, 710
Dystrophile program, 391, 747–751, 801, 835, 885–888

E

Ecchymosis, 591
Echo time (TE), 73
Economic aspects
   of diagnostic imaging, 61, 64, 72, 74
   insurance and carpal tunnel syndrome, 118
   of total wrist arthroplasty, 659
ECRB. *See* Extensor carpi radialis brevis tendon
ECRL. *See* Extensor carpi radialis longus tendon
ECTR. *See* Endoscopic carpal tunnel release
ECU. *See* Extensor carpi ulnaris tendon

EDC. *See* Extensor digitorum comunis tendon
Edema, 757
   with cast immobilization, 784
   diagnostic imaging, 73, 76, 77
   management, 918
   with reflex sympathetic dystrophy and treatment, 745, 885, 887
EDM. *See* Extensor digitis minimi tendon
EDQ. *See* Extensor digiti quinti tendon
Education of the patient
   for juvenile arthritis, 167
   for replantation, 270
EIP. *See* Extensor indicis proprius syndrome; Extensor indicis proprius tendon
Elastic bandage, 90
Elastic fibers, 441
Elastic modulus, 441
Elastin, 441
Elbow
   with hereditary multiple exostoses, 143
   with mirror hand, 138
Elderly patients. *See also* Aging, effects of
   age as a contraindication to surgery, 351
   Colles' fracture in the, 296–297
   fracture immobilization and daily activities, 296
   treatment following distal radius fracture, 351, 355, 357–358
Electrical injuries, 102
Electrical stimulation, 158, 193, 765
Electroacupuncture, 747
Electrogoniometer, 30, 34, 40
Electromyography, with carpal tunnel syndrome, 108
Elephantiasis, 698
Elevator, 318, 327. *See also* Freer elevator
Emboli, 693
Embolization techniques, 696
Embryonic development, 7
   carpal bones, 5, 146
   collagen fiber, 617
   histologic section, 12
   radioscaphoid ligament, 437
   triangular fibrocartilage complex, 12
   triquetral-lunate joint, 146
En bloc resection, 725, 728
Encapsulation process, 660
Enchondromas, 164, 704–705. *See also* Maffucci syndrome
Enchondromatosis, multiple, 151, 705
Ender compression blade plate, 194
Endoscopic carpal tunnel release (ECTR), 101, 109–120
Environment, room temperature after replantation, 275
EPB. *See* Extensor pollicis brevis tendon
EPDQ. *See* Extensor propius digiti quinti
Epidentinous stitch, 274
Epidermal inclusion cysts, 685, 688–689

Epineurotomy, 101
Epiphyseal brackets, 137
Epiphysis
   fracture, 161, 162
   ossification, 149
   premature union, 151, 156
Epithelioid sarcoma, 736–737, 738
EPL. *See* Extensor pollicis longus tendon
Eponyms, use of, 278, 289, 309, 889
Eryops, 1, 2
Esmarch bandage, 856, 858, 916
Esmarch compression, 687
Essex-Lopresti Lesion, 377–378, 595, 619, 627
Ethilon, 120
Etiology
   aneurysms, 693
   carpal tunnel syndrome, 116
   ganglia, 163
   Kienböck's disease, 396–397, 411–415
   rotary subluxation of the scaphoid, 879
   scapholunate advanced collapse, 535–536, 545, 921
Everyday activities. *See* Daily activities
Evolution, 1–5, 42, 154
   digits, 1–3, 5
   distal radioulnar joint, 3, 4, 369, 388
   distal ulna, 616
Ewing's tumor, 723
Examination. *See* Physical examination
Excision
   benign tumors, 696, 700, 702, 706, 708, 709
   carpal boss, 713, 770
   distal ulna, 875
   ganglia, 685, 686, 687–688, 714
   giant cell tumor, 728
   hook of hamate, 179
   lunate, 416, 548
   malignant tumor, 724–726
   pisiform dislocation, 225
   trapezium, 574, 575, 576
   trapezoid dislocation, 219, 220
   triangular fibrocartilage complex, 609, 618, 623
   triquetrum dislocation, 224, 225
   ulnar head, 596, 889
   ulnar styloid, 840
   "unplanned," 724, 736, 737, 739
Exercise. *See* Rehabilitation
Exostoses, hereditary multiple, 142–143
Explosion fracture, 303, 304, 309, 310
Exsanguination, 687
Extension. *See* Flexion-extension
Extensor brevis manis muscle, 104
Extensor carpi radialis brevis tendon (ECRB)
   anatomy, 8, 16, 17
   in carpal boss repair, 793
   in distal radius fracture fixation, 307

Extensor carpi radialis brevis tendon (ECRB) (contd.)
 function, 668
 intersection syndrome and, 97
 in ligamentous repair for scapholunate dissociation, 495
 with rheumatoid arthritis, 645
 in scaphoid internal fixation, 195
 in scapholunate joint reconstruction, 438
 tenodesis with perilunate dislocation, 213
Extensor carpi radialis longus tendon (ECRL)
 anatomy, 16, 17
 biomechanics, 668
 in carpal boss repair, 793
 in distal radius fracture fixation, 307
 intersection syndrome and, 97
 to-ECU transfer, 654, 807–808
 transfer, 670
Extensor carpi radialis tendon
 anatomy, 260
 as landmark for arthroscopy, 85
Extensor carpi ulnaris tendon (ECU)
 anatomy, 8, 11, 16, 17, 370, 391
 arthroscopy, 85, 89
 with Bennett's fracture, 256
 in Darrach procedure, 805, 806–808
 with distal radioulnar joint disorders, 372, 373, 378–379, 382, 391
 with distal radius fracture, 346–347, 356, 358
 in distal radius surgery, 321, 337
 function, 668–669
 in hemiresection arthroplasty, 837, 838–841, 843, 844
 moment arm, 41, 42
 physical examination, 55, 592
 with reverse Rolando's fracture, 263
 with rheumatoid arthritis, 645, 649, 650, 654, 806–808
 in Sauvé-Kapandji procedure, 891
 subluxation, 592, 597–598
 synovitis, 47, 55
 tendinitis, 98, 600
 tenosynovitis, 600, 602
 in total wrist arthroplasty, 671, 672, 677
Extensor compartment arteries, 907–908, 909
Extensor compartment tendinopathies, 96–98, 953
Extensor digiti quinti minimi ligament, 389
Extensor digiti quinti minimi tendon, 8
Extensor digiti quinti tendon (EDQ), 274, 321, 647, 838, 839, 841
Extensor digitis minimi tendon (EDM), 98
Extensor digitorum comunis tendon (EDC), 8, 17, 40, 867
Extensor indicis proprius syndrome (EIP), 98
Extensor indicis proprius tendon (EIP), 17, 274

Extensor pollicis brevis tendon (EPB), 8, 17
 in carpometacarpal tendon arthroplasty, 797
 de Quervain's disease and, 55
 in distal radius fixation, 317
 intersection syndrome and, 56
 moment arm, 42
 repetitive strain injuries and, 96–97
Extensor pollicis longus tendon (EPL)
 anatomy, 8
 in bone-retinaculum-bone autograft, 916, 917
 with distal radius fracture, 359
 in distal radius surgery, 320
 as landmark for arthroscopy, 85
 in ligamentous repair for scapholunate dissociation, 495, 497
 moment arm, 42
 in proximal row carpectomy, 547
 rupture with rheumatoid arthritis, 647, 648
 in scaphoid internal fixation, 195
 tendinitis, 98
 in total wrist arthrodesis, 559, 563
Extensor propius digiti quinti (EPDQ), 17
Extensor retinaculum
 anatomy, 17, 182
 in bone-retinaculum-bone autograft, 915–919
 in capitate shortening, 790
 in Darrach procedure, 805
 in distal radioulnar joint stabilization, 812
 in extensor carpi ulnaris tenosynovitis, 600
 in hemiresection arthroplasty, 839, 840
 in ligamentous repair for scapholunate dissociation, 495, 497
 in lunotriquetral arthrodesis, 507
 in perilunate dislocation surgery, 244
 in proximal row carpectomy, 547, 549
 in radial shortening osteotomy, 859
 in radiocarpal arthrodesis-arthroplasty, 861, 862, 863
 in radioulnar arthrodesis, 875
 in scaphocapitate arthrodesis, 895, 896
 in scaphoid internal fixation, 195
 in universal wrist prosthesis surgery, 672, 673
Extensor tendons
 entrapment, 161
 tenosynovitis, 96
External fixation
 carpal bone fractures, 183
 carpal dislocation, 251
 complications, 308–309, 336, 771
 distal radius fractures, 287, 294, 311, 316–318, 320, 337
  with secondary ligament injury, 343
  surgical technique, 306–308, 309–310

 as intraoperative tool for internal fixation, 317
 Kienböck's disease, 400–401
 pin care, 308–309
 pin removal, 309
Extrinsic ligaments, 501–502
 anatomy, 432
 dorsal, 14, 15
 magnetic resonance imaging, 74
 palmar, 14–15, 456
Eye inflammation with juvenile arthritis, 165–166, 167

F

Failure
 Darrach procedure, 943
 ligamentous, 28, 433, 441–443, 468
 total wrist arthroplasty, 556, 659, 665, 680
False aneurysms, 164
Fascial interposition arthroplasty, 404–405
Fasciotomy, 333
Fat
 replacement of fused physis with, 154
 scaphoid, 157
 subcutaneous, and diagnosis, 157
Fat stripe, 189
Fault plate hypothesis, 411, 414
FCR. See Flexor carpi radialis tendon
FCU. See Flexor carpi ulnaris muscle; Flexor carpi ulnaris tendon
FDP. See Flexor profundae tendon
FDS. See Flexor digitorum sublimis tendon
FE. See Flexion-extension
Fernandez classification
 DRUJ lesions, 286, 288, 315
 fractures, 286–287, 303, 323–336
FET (finger extension test), 48–49, 57, 58, 528
Fetus. See Embryonic development
Fiberglass casting, 780–783
Fiberoptics, 83
Fibroblasts, 420–421
Fibromas, 689–690
Fibromatosis, 689, 690
Fibroosseous tissues, 711
Fibroosseus tunnel, 95, 98, 715
Fibrosis
 immobilization for the prevention of, 95
 pericapsular, 741
 treatment, 749–750, 886
Fibrous histiocytoma, malignant, 736
Fibrous xanthoma, 691–692, 715
Film
 pressure-sensitive, 38, 40, 786
 "spot," 62, 75, 78, 593
 stress, 492
Finger extension test (FET), 48–49, 57, 58, 528
Fingerprint changes, 48

Finger trap traction, 84, 289, 290, 291, 307
Finite element model, 38
Finkelstein's test, 96, 103
Finklestein's test, 55, 573
Fish, limb evolution, 1
Fistula. See Arteriovenous fistula
Fixation. See also External fixation; Internal fixation; Kirschner wires; Percutaneous pinning; Pins; Plate fixation; Screw fixation
  arthroscopically-assisted, 90, 91, 195–196, 612
  hardware failure, 196
  improper implant placement, 196
  intramedullary, 194
  three-point, 191
Flexible hinge silastic implant, 660
Flexible splint. See Mobilization splint
Flexion-extension (FE)
  in activities of daily living, 31
  after proximal row carpectomy, 550
  degrees of freedom, 28
  following scaphocapitate arthrodesis, 895, 897
  kinematics, 21–23
  moment arm and, 40, 42
  muscle imbalance with total wrist arthroplasty, 670
  in scaphoid and lunate rotation, 458–460, 462–464
  in specific activities, 33–34
  strength, 28, 29
  in wrist motion studies, 35, 36
Flexion moment, scaphoid, 9
Flexor carpi radialis tendon (FCR), 104
  anatomy, 9, 16, 17, 260
  in carpometacarpal tendon arthroplasty, 797, 798–799, 801
  function, 669
  ganglion cysts, 688
  as landmark for arthroscopy, 85
  in ligament reconstruction for basal joint resection, 574–577
  moment arm, 40, 41, 42
  in radial shortening osteotomy, 856
  in rotary subluxation of the scaphoid, 879–884
  in scaphoid dislocation surgery, 245
  in scaphoid internal fixation, 194
  tendinitis, 57, 99, 758
  in trapeziometacarpal surgery, 571
Flexor carpi ulnaris muscle (FCU)
  anatomy, 16, 17
  in fifth metacarpal dislocation, 261
  hook of hamate fractures and, 177
  pisiform fractures and, 182, 183
Flexor carpi ulnaris tendon (FCU)
  anatomy, 465
  with distal radioulnar joint disorders, 372, 379, 382–383

  in distal radius surgery, 321, 322
  function, 669, 671
  tendinitis, 99
  in ulnar impingement syndrome, 596
Flexor digitorum, anatomy, 9
Flexor digitorum profundus tendon, 321
Flexor digitorum sublimis tendon (FDS), 17
Flexor digitorum superficialis, 321
Flexor pollicis longus muscle, 856, 857
Flexor pollicis longus tendon (FPL), 104
  anatomy, 17
  Linburg's syndrome, 99
  physical examination, 57
  in radius fracture surgery, 321
  rupture with rheumatoid arthritis, 641, 648
Flexor profundae tendon (FDP), 17
Flexor retinaculum, 182
  anatomy, 9, 17
  in rheumatoid arthritis treatment, 649
  structural strength and, 10
Flexor superficialis muscle, hypertrophied extension of, 96
Flexor tendons
  of the little finger, 179
  during replantation, 274
  transposition as wrist extensors, 138
"Floppy" wrist, 650
Fluid collection, magnetic resonance imaging, 73
Fluidotherapy, 764
Fluoroscopy
  carpal dislocations, 219, 238, 239
  distal radius fracture, 316, 318, 319, 320, 327, 331, 345
  in hemiresection arthroplasty, 839, 840
  ligament injuries, 217
  monitoring of arthrography, 69
  osteoid osteoma, 708
  scaphoid fracture, 190
  "spot" film, 62, 75, 78, 593
"Fluted champagne glass" joint, 146, 533, 534, 538
Force. See also Biomechanics; Kinematics; Load; Restraining forces
  in the Dystrophile program, 886
  to pull out the carpal component of universal wrist prosthesis, 666
  vector analysis of musculotendinous units, 669
Force and pressure transducers, 38
Forceps, basket, 609
Forearm
  orthosis, 357
  radial deficiency, 127–134
  with radioulnar synostosis, 137
  rotation of the, 42, 369, 389
  with ulnar deficiency, 135
Foreign bodies
  diagnostic imaging, 72

  granuloma, 685, 715
  penetration trauma, 206
"Four-corner" or "four-bone" fusion, 344, 538, 552, 921
Four-unit concept, 27, 28, 34–36
Four-view wrist series, 61–63
FPL. See Flexor pollicis longus tendon
Fractures
  articular, four basic components, 299–300
  avulsion, 333–335, 608
  axial, 261
  Barton, reversed, 286
  Bennett's, 256–257, 259
  Bennett's, reverse, 262, 265, 569
  bone scintigraphy of, 70, 71, 189, 190
  boxer's, 260
  capitate, 159, 176–177
  carpal bones
    in children, 156–157, 159
    excluding scaphoid fractures, 173–184
    incidence rate, 173–174
    six features of, 173
  carpmetacarpal, 255–267
  chauffeur's, 278
  chip, 179, 181–182
  Colles'. See Colles' fracture
  complex, 335–336
  compression, 327–333
  computed tomography of, 64–66, 68, 75
  dead bone, 412
  determination of union, 197
  die-punch. See Die-punch fractures
  dislocation vs. fracture-dislocation, 215
  distal radius. See Distal radius, fractures
  distal ulnar physis, 162–163
  explosion, 303, 304, 309, 310
  Galeazzi, 162–163, 377
  Galliazzi, 595
  of gymnasts, 154
  hamate, 179, 261, 265, 598–599
  hand, incidence rate, 173–174
  healing mechanism, 198
  hook of hamate, 177–179, 261
  iliac crest, 565
  implants, 663, 665
  lunate, 179–181
  magnetic resonance imaging, 70, 75
  metacarpal intraarticular displaced fractures, 260
  moment arm and tendon excursion after, 42
  osteochondral, 416
  pediatric. See under Pediatrics
  perilunate, 210, 432
  philosophy and priorities for treatment, 362–364
  pisiform, 55–56, 182–183
  progression of force with, 234–235
  radial head, 377–378

Fractures (contd.)
  radial styloid, 205–206, 212, 240, 342, 345, 446
  radius. See Distal radius, fractures; Radius, fractures
  Rolando's, 257
  Rolando's, reverse, 262, 263
  scaphoid. See Scaphoid, fractures
  shear stress, 159, 173, 174, 175, 179, 323, 325–327, 455
  sigmoid notch, 374–375
  Smith, 289, 291, 294
  spike, 300, 303, 314
  transscaphoid perilunate, 196
  trapezium, 174, 175, 258, 259
  trapezoid, 174, 175
  triquetrum. See Triquetrum, fractures
  ulna. See Ulna, fractures
  ulnar styloid, 346–347, 375–377
  x-ray of, 66, 75
Fragments. See Bone fragments
Free-body diagrams, 38
Freer elevator, 245, 319, 323, 328
Frykman classification, 278–279, 289, 303, 314, 342
Functional capacity evaluation (FCE), 759–760
Fusion. See Arthrodesis

G

Gabapentin, 746
Gadolinium. See Gadopentate dimeglumine
Gadopentate dimeglumine (Gd-DTPA), 73, 78
Galleazzi fracture, 162–163, 377, 595
"Gamekeeper's thumb," 42
Ganglion cysts, 104, 684–688, 699, 714–715
  around the FCR, 99
  in children, 149, 163–164, 714
  complications, 164, 688
  diagnostic imaging, 72, 73, 76, 78
  dorsal wrist, confusion with carpal boss, 149
  etiology, 163
  fluid and pedicle, 685, 686, 687, 688, 714
  metacarpal, 580
  of the nerve sheath, 703–704
  nonoperative treatment, 164
  recurrence, 686, 688, 715
  with rotary subluxation of the scaphoid, 527
  satellite, 685
  scapholunate joint, 829, 830, 831
  scapholunate ligament, 485
  true occult dorsal carpal, 467, 468
  ulnar nerve, 102
Ganglionectomy, open, 92
Ganglionotomy, 84, 92

Gauze. See Dressing
GCT. See Giant cell tumor
Gd-DTPA (gadopentate dimeglumine), 73, 78
Gender aspects
  columnar-type wrists, 27
  juvenile arthritis, 165, 166
  Kienböck's disease, 395
  Madelung's deformity, 138
  osteoid osteoma, 707
  strength, 28, 29
  unicameral bone cyst, 710
Giachinao device, 662
Giant cells, 708
Giant cell tumor (GCT)
  of bone, 708–709, 723, 725, 726–733
  case studies, 729–733
  of tendon sheath, 691–692
  vs. aneurysmal bone cyst, 710
Gigantism, 698, 700
Gilula's lines, 207, 236, 237, 238, 239
Gold, as antirheumatic, 667
Goniometry, 757–758, 885
Gout, 583–586
Granuloma
  foreign bodies, 685, 715
  infectious, 685
Grasper, 84
Greater arc injuries, 203, 205, 207, 212
Grind test, 54, 592, 598
Grip strength
  average maximum, 233
  with carpal tunnel syndrome and release, 115
  evaluation, 592
  following capitate shortening, 789
  following carpometacarpal tendon arthroplasty, 801
  following Darrach procedure, 809
  following dorsal capsulodesis, 825
  following osteotomy, 352
  following perilunate dislocation treatment, 249
  following proximal row carpectomy, 551, 552
  following radiolunate arthrodesis, 870
  following scaphocapitate arthrodesis, 897
  following SLAC reconstruction, 924
  following triscaphe arthrodesis, 935
  gender differences, 28, 29
  with reflex sympathetic dystrophy, 745, 885
  with triquetral impingement ligament tear syndrome, 633
  ulnar variance and, 618
Gross and microscopic findings
  aneurysmal bone cyst, 710
  epidermal inclusion cyst, 689
  fibroma, 690

  fibrous xanthoma, 691–692
  ganglion cyst, 686
  giant cell tumor, 709
  hemangioma of the median nerve, 703
  lipofibromatous hamartoma, 701–702
  lipoma, 691
  neurilemmoma, 699
  neurofibroma, 698
  osteochondroma, 706
  osteoid osteoma, 708
  rheumatoid tenosynovitis, 712
  solitary enchrondroma, 704
  unicameral bone cyst, 711
Ground substances, production with inflammatory response, 95
Growth disturbances. See Bone growth
Guepar wrist prosthesis, 662
Guyon's canal, 178, 179
  fibroma, 690
  ganglion cysts, 686, 688
  release during replantation, 270
  release with hamate fracture, 599
  testing, 758
  ulnar artery thrombosis and, 603
Guyon's syndrome, 101–102
Guyon's tunnel, anatomy, 101
"Gymnast's wrist," 154–156

H

Hamartoma, lipofibromatous, 700–702
Hamate. See also Hook of hamate
  anatomy, 568, 598
  arthrosis, 599–600
  with carpal dislocation, 242
  dislocation, 218, 225, 226
  evolution of the, 3
  in flexion-extension, 37
  fractures, 179, 261, 265, 598–599
  kinematics, 462, 463
  motion of the fourth and fifth metacarpals, 255
  ossification, 7, 149
  osteology, 11
  in radioulnar deviation, 23
  synostosis, 123, 124
Hamate-capitate fusion, 785–790
Hamate-lunate joint, arthritis, 602
Hamulus hamati. See Hook of hamate; Unciform process
Hand
  amputated, proper handling technique, 270
  color changes, 591, 693, 694, 695
  crush injury, 119, 223, 579
  evolution of the, 1–5
Handcuff neuropathy, 103
Hand-forearm unit, with extension injuries, 465–468, 473
Hayes retractor, 673
Heat therapy, 764

Hemangioma, 692, 694–695, 702–703, 715. *See also* Maffucci syndrome
Hematoma, total wrist arthrodesis, 563
Hemiresection arthroplasty, 34, 38–40, 355–356, 837–844
Hemostat, 86, 623
Herbert screw. *See also* Screw fixation, headless
 fracture-dislocation, 194, 195, 267
 scaphoid dislocation, 245
Hereditary patterns. *See also* Congenital abnormalities
 hereditary multiple exostoses, 142–143, 705
 Madelung's deformity, 138
Hibiclens, 270
Histiocytoma, 690, 736
Histology
 giant cell tumor, 728
 ligaments, 436, 439, 441
 neurilemmoma, 699–700
 neurofibroma, 698
 triangular fibrocartilage complex, 617
 triquetral impingement ligament tear syndrome, 637
Historical background
 anatomic description, 7
 arthroscopy, 83, 92
 carpal biomechanics, 464–465
 carpal ligament instability, 431–432
 carpal tunnel syndrome, 107
 distal radius fracture classification, 277–279
 endoscopic carpal tunnel release, 109–110
 gout, 583
 Kienböck's disease, 396, 419–420
 kinematic research, 21
 motion research, 34
 proximal row carpectomy, 545
 replantation, 269
 total wrist arthrodesis, 556–557, 659
 total wrist arthroplasty, 659
History. *See* Historical background; Patient history
"Hockey stick" incision, 797
Hohmann retractor, 320
Hominidae, evolution of the wrist, 4–5
Homo erectus, 5
Homo habilis, 4
Homo sapiens, 5
Hook of hamate, 56
 computed tomography, 68
 excision, 179
 fractures, 177–179, 183, 261
 functional mechanism, 184
 nonunion, 602
 "waist of the hook," 178, 179
Hori procedure, 401–402, 420
House wrist prosthesis, 662

"Humpback deformity," 188, 191, 249, 911
Hurler disease, 143–144, 151
Hygromas, cystic. *See* Cystic lymphangioma
Hyperuricemia, 583
Hypervascularity, 741
Hypoplasia
 of the radius, 128, 129–130, 144–145
 of the thumb, 126, 128, 130, 131, 144
Hypothenar hammer syndrome, 164

I
Ibuprofen, 167
ICSRA. *See* Intercompartmental supraretinacular arteries
Iliac crest, 323
 donor site morbidity, 353
 fracture, 565
 harvest for bone grafts. *See under* Bone grafts, donor sites
Imaging techniques. *See* Bone scintigraphy; Computed tomography; Diagnostic imaging; Fluoroscopy; Magnetic resonance imaging; Radiography; Three-dimensional carpal motion studies; Tomography
Immunohistochemical analysis
 neurilemmoma, 699–700
 neurofibroma, 698
Immunoregulation and juvenile rheumatoid arthritis, 165
Immunosuppressive drugs, 672
Implants. *See* Arthroplasty
Incidence rate
 capitate fractures, 176
 carpal bone fractures, 173–174
 carpometacarpal fractures, 255
 gout, 583
 scaphoid fractures, 174, 187, 255
 scapholunate dissociation, 498
 total wrist arthroplasty failure, 663, 665
 trapezium fractures, 174, 175
 triquetrum fractures, 174
 wrist trauma needing radiography, 255
Inclusion cysts, epidermal, 685, 688–689
"Indiana tome," 101
Indications
 bone graft, 815, 901
 capitate shortening and capitate-hamate fusion, 786
 capsulodesis for rotary subluxation of the scaphoid, 819
 cocompartment release for tenosynovitis, 953
 Darrach procedure, 803
 denervation, 945
 distal radioulnar joint dislocation stabilization, 811
 dorsal wrist syndrome, 829
 lunotriquetral arthrodesis, 833

 matched hemiresection-interposition arthroplasty, 837–838, 844
 matched ulnar arthroplasty, 847
 proximal row carpectomy, 545–546
 radial shortening osteotomy, 855
 radiocarpal arthrodesis-arthroplasty, 861
 radiolunate arthrodesis, 867
 Sauvé-Kapandji procedure, 889, 890
 scaphocapitate arthrodesis, 895, 899
 scapholunate advanced collapse reconstruction, 921
 total wrist arthrodesis, 555–556
 total wrist arthroplasty, 672
 trapezoidal osteotomy of the distal radius, 927
 triscaphe arthrodesis, 766, 931
 ulnar lengthening, 939
 vascularized bone grafts, scaphoid nonunion, 907
Indivis propius, 8
Infantile dermatofibroma, 689
Infection
 as a contradindication to surgery, 351
 diagnostic imaging, 78–79
 following SLAC reconstruction, 925
 from ganglion cyst excision, 688
 with matched hemiresection-interposition arthroplasty, 843
 from scaphoid fracture surgery, 196
 total wrist arthrodesis and, 556, 563, 565, 671–672, 679
 with total wrist implants, 665, 668
Inflammation
 carpal dislocation and instability from, 203
 following capitate shortening, 789
 magnetic resonance imaging, 73
 reflex sympathetic dystrophy and, 743, 752
 shake test for, 592
 stages of inflammatory response, 95
Injury
 crush, 119, 223, 579
 explosion, 303, 304, 309, 310
 lesser arch, 203, 206
 multiple partial, 84
 penetration trauma, 206, 696
 from punching, 188, 599
 repetitive. *See* Repetitive injury
Instability. *See also* Dorsal intercalated segment instability; Midcarpal instability; Volar intercalated segment instability
 anatomic displacement in use of term, 450–451
 capitate-lunate instability pattern, 511, 514–515
 capitolunate joint, 431, 448–449
 carpal. *See* Carpal bones, dislocations and instability

Instability (contd.)
  classifications, 511, 516–520
  dynamic vs. static, 451
  as indicator for Sauvé-Kapandji
    procedure, 890
  from inflammation, 203
  lunotriquetral joint, 449–450, 451,
    501–508, 516
  proximal ulna stump, 891–892
  transcarpal, 262
  trapeziometacarpal joint, 571
  triangular fibrocartilage complex,
    378–380
  triquetrohamate joint, 516
Instantaneous screw axis (ISA), 23–24
Inteq repair kit, 89
Intercalated segment instability. See Dorsal
    intercalated segment instability;
    Volar intercalated segment
    instability
Intercarpal arch, 396, 910
Intercarpal ligaments, definition, 432
Intercompartmental supraretinacular arteries
    (ICSRA), 908–911, 913
Intermetacarpal ligament (IML), 256, 258,
    260
Internal fixation
  of the arthrodesis, 557, 559–563
  arthroscopically-assisted, 195–196
  Bennett's fracture, 257
  capitate dislocation, 225
  carpal bone fracture, 182, 183
  cross-pin, 272
  distal radius fracture, 287, 294, 317
  hook of hamate, 179
  irritation from, 563–564, 891
  lag screw, 182, 183
  ligamentous repair for scapholunate
    dissociation, 491, 494–496
  lunate fracture, 180
  perilunate dislocation, 243–244
  perilunate fracture-dislocation, 210, 212
  pin. See Pin fixation; Pins
  placement to avoid bone growth arrest,
    162
  plate. See Plate fixation
  radiocarpal dislocation, 216, 217
  radiolunate, 870, 873
  scaphoid dislocation, 220, 245
  scaphoid fracture, 157, 158, 193–196,
    771
  trapezium dislocation, 223
  triquetrum dislocation, 224
  ulnar shortening osteotomy, 626
  ulnar styloid fracture, 377
  wire. See Kirschner wires
International Association for the Study of
    Pain, 741
International Federation of Societies of the
    Hand, 451
International Society of Orthopaedic
    Surgery, 280
International Wrist Investigators' Workshop,
    469, 477
Interosseous ligaments. See Lunotriquetral
    interosseous ligament; Scapholunate
    interosseous ligament
Interosseous membrane
  scapholunate, 9
  stabilization of the DRUJ by, 370, 389,
    619
Interphalangeal joint (IP), 801. See also
    Proximal interphalangeal joint
Intersection syndrome, 56, 95, 97, 758
Intraarticular bodies, bone fragments with
    hamate fracture, 179
Intracapsular ligaments, 432, 435
Intracarpal instability with carpal bone
    fractures, 173
Intrascaphoid angulation, measurement,
    193
"Intrasound vibration" pain, 189
Intrinsic ligaments, 502
  anatomy, 14, 15–16
  definition, 432
  diagnostic imaging, 69, 76
  material properties, 28
  palmar, anatomy, 456
Intrinsic release, 641–642
Involuting hemangioma, 694
Iontophoresis, 765
Irrigation technique
  during arthroscopy, 84
  during replantation, 270, 271
ISA. See Instantaneous screw axis
Isolated carpal bone dislocation, 204,
    219 226

J
JA. See Pediatrics, juvenile arthritis
Jansen type chondrodysplasia, 143
Japanese technique, 114
Jebsen test, 843
Jenkins classification, 280, 281
Jigs
  compression, 194
  placement, scaphoid fracture, 195
  radial cutting, 673, 674, 676
Job aspects. See Occupational aspects;
    Occupational health
Joint distraction technique, 83
Joint motion. See Kinematics
Joints, 11–14. See also Arthroplasty; specific
    joints
  incomplete development, 835
  testing in wrist evaluation, 758–759
  therapeutic mobilization, 764
Joint stiffness, 196
"Joysticks," 212, 243, 244, 245, 247, 494,
    548, 917
JRA. See Juvenile rheumatoid arthritis
Jupiter classification. See McMurtry
    classification
Juvenile arthritis. See Pediatrics, juvenile
    arthritis
Juvenile rheumatoid arthritis (JRA), 645,
    646–647

K
Kapandji operation, 140. See also Sauvé-
    Kapandji procedure
Keith needle, 213, 823
Keliod formation, 688
Kessler stitch, 274
Ketanserin, 746
Ketorolac, 746
Kienböck's disease
  diagnostic imaging, 62, 64, 77, 398–399
  etiology, 396–397, 860
  finger extension test, 49
  force and pressure analysis, 39
  gender aspects, 395
  incidence of carpal bone fracture and,
    174
  interosseous ganglia with, 715
  lunate collapes with, 179, 180–181, 529,
    531
  presentation, 414–415, 855
  proximal row carpectomy and, 545–546,
    551, 552, 553
  staging, 399–400, 405–408, 426
  symptoms, 48
  treatment, 400–408, 415–417, 419–429,
    531, 785, 895, 939–943
  ulnar impaction syndrome and, 619,
    627
  vascular anatomy, 395–396
Kinematics, 21–25, 233–236
  carpal, 27–28, 36–37, 233–236,
    444–446, 457, 461–465, 501
  carpal height ratio, 398
  Ståhl index, 398
  triquetrum, 502–503
Kirschner wires, 89, 91. See also "Joysticks";
    Percutaneous pinning
  Bennett's fracture, 257
  biconcave bone graft, scaphoid nonunion,
    901–902, 905
  bone-retinaculum-bone autograft, 917
  capitate-hamate fusion, 788
  capitate osteotomy, 787
  carpal bone fractures, 183
  carpal dislocation, 251
  carpometacarpal fracture-dislocations,
    266–267
  distal radius fractures, 306, 307, 309,
    311, 316, 317–318, 319, 328, 329
  distal radius malunion treatment,
    351–354, 358
  dorsal capsulodesis, 821

ligamentous repair for scapholunate dissociation, 494–496
lunotriquetral joint arthrodesis, 834
lunotriquetral joint instability, 505
perilunate dislocation, 212, 213, 243–244
placement technique to minimize risk of neuropathy, 244
radial club hand treatment, 145
radial shortening osteotomy, 859
radius bone graft with osteosarcoma, 733, 734–735
replantation, 271, 272
Rolando's fractures, 257
in rotary subluxation of the scaphoid correction, 880, 881–882
scaphoid dislocation, 245
scaphoid fracture, 195, 913
scaphoid reduction stabilization, 191, 822
scapholunate joint reconstruction, 438, 923
scaphotrapeziotrapezoid arthrodesis, 426
SLIL injury following distal radius fracture, 346
total wrist arthrodesis, 557
trapezoidal osteotomy of the distal radius, 927, 928, 929
triangular fibrocartilage complex tears, 611, 612
triscaphe arthrodesis, 931, 932, 933
Knowles pin, 548
K-wire. *See* Kirschner wires

L

Laboratory tests
  blood chemistry workup for replantation, 270
  malignant tumor, 723
  of needle aspirate, 594
  for replantation, 270
Lag screws, 182, 183, 328, 877, 891
La maladie des synostoses multiples, 125
Landmarks
  for arthroscopy, 84–86, 88
  capsulodesis for rotary subluxation of the scaphoid, 820
  carpal tunnel syndrome, 111
  in determination of carpal angles, 236–237, 250
  Gilula's lines, 207, 236, 237, 238, 239
  for proximal row carpectomy, 546–547
  for radiography for distal radius fractures, 313
  for scaphocapitate arthrodesis, 895
Langenskiold procedure, 153
Laser treatment. *See* Argon laser
Lateral cutaneous nerve of the thigh (LCNT), 565

Lauenstein's procedure. *See* Sauvé-Kapandji procedure
LCNT. *See* Lateral cutaneous nerve of the thigh
Le Club des Dix classification, 279
Lederhose's fibromatosis, 689
Leri-Weill syndrome, 151
Lesions. *See also* Debridement
  arthroscopy, 89–90
  diagnostic imaging, 73–74, 76, 78
  DRUJ, classification, 286, 288
  fibrotic. *See* Fibromas
Lesser arc injuries, 203, 206
Lidocaine, 97, 289, 593, 600, 746
Ligament of Testut, 232, 472
Ligamentotaxis with distal radius fractures, 291, 305, 306, 309, 311, 327, 337
Ligament repair
  carpal fracture-dislocations, 238–251
    with perilunate dislocation, 212–214
    with radiocarpal dislocation, 216
    with scaphoid dislocation, 220
  distal radioulnar joint disorders, 389–390
  distal radius fractures, 312, 315, 335, 344
  lunotriquetral ligament, 344
  trapeziometacarpal dislocations, 258, 571–572
Ligaments. *See also* Extrinsic ligaments; Intrinsic ligaments; *specific ligaments*
  anatomy, 13–16, 231–232, 432–438
  biomechanics, 439, 441–442, 444–446
  elongation at total failure, 441
  following distal radius fracture, 296
  histology, 436, 439, 441
  as landmarks for arthroscopy, 85, 87
  material properties, 28
  resorption, 362
  tears, 189
  variability in elastic fiber content, 296
Ligation of benign tumors, 696
Limited wrist arthrodesis, 765–767, 777–784
Linburg's syndrome, 99
Lipofibromatous hamartoma, 700–702
Lipoma, 690–691, 699
Liquid crystal thermography, 189
Lister's tubercle
  in distal radius fracture fixation, 320, 321, 330, 352
  osteotomy, 560
  in plate fixation, 330
  in radial shortening osteotomy, 858, 859
  in radiocarpal arthrodesis-arthroplasty, 861, 862
  resection, 895
  in scaphoid fracture fixation, 195
  in wrist arthroscopy, 85
Load, 34, 38–40
  axial, 261, 445, 461–462, 607
  distal radioulnar joint, 370

in the Dystrophile program, 886, 887
from gymnastic events, 155
Kienböck's disease and, 396–397, 402, 411–413, 414–415, 428, 785, 790
midcarpal, 514
under normal anatomy position, 455, 464, 660
progression across the carpals, 234–235, 251, 811
rheumatoid arthritis and, 639, 640, 654
with rotation of scaphoid and lunate, 458–460, 487
scaphocapitate arthrodesis, 898, 899
through the lunate, 785, 790
through the radiolunate, 939
through the radius, 618–619
through the scaphoid, 447–448, 811
through the ulna, 388–389, 462, 618–619, 811
triangular fibrocartilage complex, 607, 612
uneven, 396–397, 402
wrist extension injury, 465–467
Long arm cast
  application technique, 779–782, 783
  distal radius fracture, 291, 294
  pisiform dislocation, 225
  triangular fibrocartilage complex injury, 595
  triquetrum dislocation, 224
Long arm splint, 671, 873
Long arm thumb-spica cast
  perilunate dislocation, 213, 245
  scaphoid fracture, 192
  scaphoid nonunion, 158
  scapholunate advanced collapse reconstruction, 924
  scaphotrapeziotrapezoid arthrodesis, 425
Longitudinal disruptions, 241, 242, 246
Long radiolunate ligament. *See* Radiolunate ligament, long
Longus, 8
Loosening of total wrist implants, 665–666, 668, 669, 679
L-plate, 326, 328, 330, 337
LT. *See* Lunotriquetral interosseous ligament; Lunotriquetral joint
LTq. *See* Lunotriquetral interosseous ligament
Lunate
  anatomy, 8, 458, 504, 508, 525
  in capitate shortening with capitate-hamate fusion, 787, 790
  dislocation, 203, 205, 222, 226, 231, 238–239, 240, 432, 446
  evolution, 3
  fault plates in, 411, 414
  fractures, 70, 179–181
  giant cell tumor, 728
  with Madelung's deformity, 140

Lunate (contd.)
  neutral anatomy position, 513
  in normal carpal alignment, 190
  ontogenesis, 7
  osteology, 9–10
  "pre-Kienböck" condition, 429
  proximal pole collapse, 786
  in radioulnar deviation, 23, 24, 37
  revascularization for Kienböck's disease, 401–404, 419–429
  rotation with the scaphoid, 458–460, 462–464
  sclerosis and collapse. See Kienböck's disease
  shape of, and Kienböck's disease, 414
  silicone replacement arthroplasty, 413, 811
  type D, 412, 414, 459, 513, 518
  type N, 512, 513
  type V, 414, 459, 508, 512, 513
  vascular anatomy, 395–396, 411, 412, 414
Lunate fossa
  anatomy, 8, 463
  in die-punch fractures, 871
  osteotomy, 867
Lunatomalacia, 77
Lunatotriquetral joint, in distal radius fracture, 346
Lunatotriquetral ligament
  with calcium pyrophosphate dihydrate, 588
  dislocation, 205, 213
  in triquetrum dislocation, 224
Lunocapitate joint. See also Capitolunate joint
  carpal kinematics and, 27
  physical examination, 53–54
Lunotriquetral interosseous ligament (LT;LTq)
  anatomy, 14, 15, 16, 232, 435
  dissociation, kinematics, 37, 473–477
  with distal radius fracture, 341, 344–348
  with lunate fracture, 872
  in lunotriquetral instability, 450
  material properties and strain at failure, 28
  tears, 508, 600, 636, 872
  with TILT, 636
Lunotriquetral joint (LT). See also Triquetral-lunate joint
  anatomy, 501–502
  arthrodesis, 344, 505–507, 508, 538, 636, 833–835
  dissociation, vs. midcarpal instability, 515–516
  with distal radius fracture, 344
  instability, 449–450, 451, 501–508, 592, 626
  physical examination, 52–53, 592

Lunotriquetral ligaments
  arthrography, 69, 504
  with distal radioulnar joint disorders, 372, 373
  with lunotriquetral joint dissociation, 516
  with perilunate dislocation, 239, 244
  reconstruction, 505
  total rupture, 603
  in triquetrum dislocation, 224
  with ulnar impaction syndrome, 626
Lymphangioma, 683, 692, 697

M
MA. See Moment arm
Macrodactyly, 700
Madelung's deformity, 138–141, 146
  in children, 151–154, 156, 162, 168–169
  distal radioulnar joint involvement, 151, 388
  gymnast's wrist and, 156
  as indicator for Sauvé-Kapandji procedure, 890
  reverse, 153
  treatment, 151, 153, 168
  twelve criteria for, 151
  ulnar impingement syndrome from, 596, 629
Maffucci syndrome, 164, 705
Magnetic resonance imaging (MRI), 70, 72, 73–74, 75–79
  avascular necrosis, 192
  capitate fracture, 176
  carpal dislocation, 238
  distal radioulnar joint disorders, 373
  extensor carpi ulnaris subluxation, 598
  following dorsal capsulodesis, 826
  ganglion cysts, 686
  giant cell tumor, 732, 733
  hook of hamate fracture, 179, 184
  Kienböck's disease, 398–399, 402, 424, 429
  limitations of, 74, 83
  lipofibromatous hamartoma, 701
  low-field, 74
  lunotriquetral instability, 504, 600
  malignant tumor, 724
  neurofibroma, 698
  osteonecrosis, 189
  scaphoid fracture, 157, 158, 189, 190, 192
  triangular fibrocartilage complex, 608–609
  ulnar wrist pain, 594
Magnetic tracking, 444
Malacia, lunate, 77
Malalignment, fixed carpal, 351
Malformations. See Congenital abnormalities
Malignant tumors. See Tumors, malignant
Malingering, 47, 57, 58

Malunion
  with carpal dislocation, 249
  Colles' fracture, 37, 930
  distal radius fracture, 299, 307, 336, 341, 385, 386, 867
    dorsal, 352–353
    intraarticular, 868
    secondary carpal instability with, 348–351
    treatment, 351–364
  humpback deformity with, 188, 191, 911
  radius shaft, 385, 387
  scaphoid fracture, 192, 196
  total wrist arthrodesis, 564
  trapezoidal, 353, 364
  ulna shaft, 385, 387
Mammals, evolution, 2–5
Management
  aneurysm, 694
  aneurysmal bone cyst, 710
  benign tumors, 687, 689
  calcinosis, 714
  congenital arteriovenous fistula, 696
  epidermal inclusion cysts, 589
  fibrous xanthoma, 692
  giant cell tumor, 709, 728
  hemangioma, 695, 703
  lipofibromatous hamartoma, 702
  lipoma, 691
  nerve sheath ganglion, 703–704
  neurilemmoma, 700
  neurofibroma, 698
  osteochondroma, 706
  osteoid osteoma, 708
  rheumatoid nodules, 712
  rheumatoid tenosynovitis, 712
  solitary enchondroma, 704–705
  unicameral bone cyst, 711
Mannerfelt lesion, 648
Manual reduction, 289, 290, 307
Markers, carpal, 34, 35
Masquelet's test, 52, 53
Massage therapy, 97, 308
Mathoulin, Letrosne, and Saffar classification, 283, 284
Maturation, accelerated. See Pediatrics, juvenile arthritis
Mayo Clinic
  biaxial wrist prosthesis, 661
  classification of fractures, 286, 289, 314
  wrist score, 352
McGill Pain Questionnaire, 745
MCI. See Midcarpal instability
McMurtry classification, 284–285, 289
Mechanism of injury
  Bennett's fracture, 256
  carpal instability, 431–432, 446–448
  dorsal lunate dislocation, 240
  finger carpometacarpal joint fracture, 260–261

in fracture classification, 286
ligament injury following distal radius fracture, 341
palmar perilunate dislocation, 240
perilunar carpal dislocation, 206
radiocarpal dislocation, 215
scaphoid fracture, 188, 431–432
triquetral impingement ligament tear syndrome, 633–634
triquetrum dislocation, 224

Median nerve
anatomy, 9, 107, 945–946
with carpal dislocation, 236, 250
in carpal tunnel release, 101, 120, 758
denervation, 947
hemangioma, 702–703
irritation by a fracture spike, 161
with perilunar dislocation, 206, 211–212
with scaphoid-lunate dislocation, 222
sensory:motor ratio, 100
surgical decompression. See Endoscopic carpal tunnel release
with trapezium dislocation, 223

Medullary compression screws, 210
Megalodactyly, 700
Melone classification, 279–280, 289, 314
Meniscal repair needle, 212
Metabolic imaging, 70

Metacarpal, fifth
anatomy, 260
chronic sprains, 568
dislocation, 259, 261, 262, 265, 579–580, 599
flexor tendons of the, 179
motion of the, 255
posttraumatic degenerative arthritis, 568–569

Metacarpal, first. See also Thumb
anatomy, 260, 568
dislocation, 262, 264
mobility of the, 255
motion of the, 255
non-Rolando's fractures, 257
pollicization, 138, 139
posttraumatic degenerative arthritis, 568–569
Rolando's fractures, 257
with trapezium dislocation, 222–223

Metacarpal, fourth
anatomy, 260, 568
chronic sprains, 568
dislocation, 265, 599
motion of the, 255
posttraumatic degenerative arthritis, 568–569

Metacarpal, second
anatomy, 260, 567–568
chronic sprains, 568
dislocation, 266
Fusi counterrotation, 580

motion of the, 255
pollicization, 130, 131, 134, 137
posttraumatic degenerative arthritis, 568–569
with trapezoid dislocation, 219, 220

Metacarpal, third
anatomy, 260, 567
capitate joint, 21, 24
chronic sprains, 568
dislocation, 266
flexion-extension motion, 21, 24
fracture from total wrist arthrodesis, 564
Fusi counterrotation, 580
motion of the, 255
osteology, 9–10
posttraumatic degenerative arthritis, 568–569
in total wrist implants, 666

Metacarpal arch, 396
Metacarpal bones. See also Carpometacarpal column/complex/joints
dysplasias, 143
harvest for bone graft, 427
intraarticular displaced fractures, 260
as landmarks for arthroscopy, 85
synostoses, 124, 125

Metacarpal vein, Hori procedure of implantation, 401–402
Metacarpophalangeal joints, subluxation of the, 639–641
Metal replacement arthroplasty for Kienböck's disease, 404, 420
Metaphyseal chondrodysplasia, 143
Metastases, 737, 739
Metastatic bone disease, diagnostic imaging, 70, 78
Methotrexate, 667
Methylmethacrylate, 665, 668, 676, 725, 728
Methylprednisilone, 711
Methylprednisolone, 711, 746
Meuli device, 661, 670, 679
Microscopic findings. See Gross and microscopic findings
Midazolam hydrochloride, 110
Midcarpal instability (MCI), 511–520
arthrodesis, 532
arthroscopy, 88
classifications, 511, 516–520
misdiagnoses, 514–516

Midcarpal joint
anatomy, 12
arthrodesis. See Arthrodesis, total wrist
arthrography, 69
arthroscopy, 86, 88
distribution of force, 38
in flexion-extension motion, 22–23, 35
instability, 88
physical examination, 49, 53–54
in radioulnar deviation, 35

Midcarpal space, 85, 87
Minnesota Rate of Manipulation Test, 843
Mirror hand, 138
Misdiagnosis
midcarpal instability, 514–516
nerve sheath ganglion, 703
scapholunate dissociation, 342–343
sprain, 250
triquetrum fractures, 179
Mobilization splint, scaphoid, 192, 193, 195

Models
finite element, 38
motion of a cadaver wrist, 34, 35
rigid-body spring, 38, 39

Moment arm and tendon excursion, 40–43
Moments, 233–234
Monitoring after replantation, 275
Morbidity, iliac crest donor site, 353
Mosquito hemostat, 86
Motion. See Biomechanics; Kinematics; Range-of-motion; Wrist motion
MRI. See Magnetic resonance imaging
Mucopolysaccharidosis, 143, 144, 151
Muenster cast, 336, 841
Multidisciplinary team. See Team approach
Multiple hereditary enchondromatosis, 151
Multiple synostoses syndrome, 125, 129
Munster cast, 224, 357, 611
Muscle belly syndrome, 104, 670
Muscle disorders
imbalance with total wrist implants, 665, 668–671
neuromuscular disease, 546, 556
overactivity with rheumatoid arthritis, 639, 641–642, 670
with radial deficiency, 128
wasting with extended cast treatment, 193

Musculoskeletal Tumor Society, 725
Musculotendinous units, 669
Musicians
carpal tunnel syndrome, 100
range-of-motion of, 33–34, 42

N

Nailbeds, capillary refill, 592
Nail curvature, 48, 885
Naproxen, 167
Naviculocapitate fracture syndrome, 209
Necrosis, aseptic, 126–127. See also Avascular necrosis; Osteonecrosis
Needle aspiration
ganglion cysts, 686–687
ulnar wrist pain, 594
ultrasound, 72
unicameral bone cyst, 711
Needles
Keith, 213, 823
precision microcaliber, 269

Neoplasms. *See* Tumors
Nerve block, 946
Nerve conduction studies, 119
Nerve conduction velocity (NCV), 108, 109
Nerves. *See also* Neuropathy; *specific nerves*
　anatomy, 9, 945–946
　denervation, 405, 420, 945–950
　entrapment, 95, 99–100. *See also* Carpal tunnel syndrome; Guyon's syndrome; Thoracic outlet syndrome; Wartenberg's syndrome
　with ganglion cysts, 685, 688
　graft technique, 274
　growth rate, 100
　regeneration, 950
　repair in replantation, 270, 271, 274
　with schwannoma, 699
　testing in wrist evaluation, 759
Nerve sheath ganglia, 703–704
Neural tissue provocation testing (NTPT), 759
Neurectomy, interosseous, 852
Neurilemmoma, 698–700
Neurofibroma, 697–698
Neurolysis, 101, 702
Neuroma, 563, 688, 843, 850
Neuromuscular disease
　proximal row carpectomy and, 546
　total wrist arthrodesis and, 556
Neuropathic Pain Scale, 745
Neuropathy, 95, 405, 420, 945–950. *See also* Reflex sympathetic dystrophy
　with axial ulnar dislocation, 218
　benign tumors, 102, 683, 697–704
　carpal tunnel syndrome and, 115, 119
　with cast immobilization, 784
　with fibrous xanthoma, 691
　following distal radius fracture, 336, 341
　handcuff, 103
　median, with carpal dislocation, 236, 250
　peripheral nerve tumors, 702
　radial, with perilunate dislocation surgery, 244
　from scaphoid fracture surgery, 196
　from total wrist arthrodesis, 563
　ulnar, 266–267
Neuropeptide Y, 742
Neurotmesis, 100
Nifedipine, 746
Niobium, in total wrist prostheses, 661
Nociceptors, 743, 744
Noninvoluting hemangioma, 694
Nonsteroidal antiinflammatory drugs (NSAIDS)
　carpal tunnel syndrome, 109, 119
　ganglion cysts, 687
　gout, 586, 588
　juvenile arthritis, 167
　osteoarthritis, 574

reflex sympathetic dystrophy, 746
rheumatoid arthritis, 667
triangular fibrocartilage complex injury, 596
ulnar styloid nonunion, 597
Nonunion
　arthrodesis, 542, 891
　capitate fracture, 176
　carpal, 210, 249, 603
　distal radius fracture, 336
　effects of smoking, 777
　following SLAC reconstruction, 925
　hook of hamate fracture, 178, 179, 184, 602
　resorption at the fracture, 189
　scaphoid fracture, 196, 529–531, 771
　　biconcave bone grafting, 901–905
　　in children, 158
　　"humpback" deformation and, 188, 911
　　imaging, 189, 197
　　incidence rate, 187
　　need for surgery, 198
　　proximal row carpectomy, 545
　　treatment, 192, 198, 771
　　vascularized bone grafting, 907–914
　subchondral sclerosis with, 189
　timeframe, 190
　triscaphe arthrodesis, 766, 937
　ulnar styloid, 385, 597, 602
Norepinephrine, 742, 743
Normal parameters
　alignment of carpal bones, 190, 455–461, 479
　anatomy positions, 456, 508, 513, 642, 671
　definition, 456
　load under, 455, 464, 660
　dorsal carpal subluxation, 350
　external dimensions of the carpal bones, 522
　"functional" range-of-motion, 30–32, 521, 760
　strength, 28, 29
　wide variation in, 42, 96
　wrist motion, 557
NSAIDS. *See* Nonsteroidal antiinflammatory drugs

O

Obesity and carpal tunnel syndrome, 100
Oblique osteotomy, 940
Occupational aspects
　constraints on wrist arc of motion, 556
　contraindication for total wrist arthroplasty, 672
　retraining, 151, 835
　return to work, 765
Occupational health
　athletes. *See* Sports

carpal tunnel syndrome, 100
　musicians, 33–34, 42, 100
　range-of-motion disorders, 33–34, 42
　repetitive injury syndrome, 96, 97
　vibration disorders, 78, 102, 164, 413, 568
Ollier's dyschondroplasia, 151, 705
Ontogenesis, 7
Open biopsy, 724, 725
Opening wedge osteotomy. *See* Osteotomy, opening wedge
Open reduction. *See also* Bone grafts
　Bennett's fracture, 257
　carpal dislocation, 239, 241–251
　carpal fracture-dislocations
　　capitate, 225
　　perilunate, 210–211
　　pisiform, 225
　　radiocarpal, 216
　　scaphoid, 220
　　trapezium, 223
　　trapezoid, 219, 220
　　triquetrum, 224
　distal radius fracture, 287, 294, 318–322
　　dorsal approaches, 320–321
　　limited, 318–320, 327
　　volar approaches, 321–322
　ligamentous repair for scapholunate dissociation, 491, 492–498
　limited, 318–320, 327
　perilunate dislocation, 241, 243–245
　Rolando's fracture, 257
　scaphoid dislocation, 245
　scaphoid fracture, 193, 197, 771
　trapezium fracture, 258
　triquetrum fracture, 182
　ulnar styloid fracture, 377
Open wounds, 206
Operating microscope, 269, 270
Operating room. *See* Surgical suite
Opponens digiti minimi muscle, 113, 256
ORIF. *See* Internal fixation; Open reduction
Orthoplast splint, 309
Os capitatum. See Capitate; Carpal bones
Os centrale, 130
Os hamatum. See Hamate
Os lunatum. See Lunate
Os magnum, evolution of the, 3. *See also* Capitate; Carpal bones
Os radius. See Radius
Ossification
　after scaphoid fracture, 157
　confusion with scaphoid fracture in children, 189
　with congenital abnormalities, 123, 127, 128, 533
　with distal radioulnar synostosis, 136
　distal radius, 160
　mechanism of fracture healing, 198
　normal carpus and distal forearm, 149

ontogenesis, 7
  with ulnar deficiency, 135
Os styloideum, 149, 580, 793, 794
Osteoarthritis, 61
  distal radioulnar joint, 385, 837
  distal radius fractures, 312
  as indicator for Sauvé-Kapandji
    procedure, 890
  posttraumatic
    with carpometacarpal fracture-
      dislocations, 267
    and the Darrach procedure, 803, 805
    salvage options, 362, 364
  thumb, 578
  trapeziometacarpal, 572
Osteoblastic activity, 70
Osteochondral fractures, 416
Osteochondromas (multiple exostoses),
  142–143, 164, 705–706
Osteochondrosis, 157
Osteoclastoma. *See* Giant cell tumor
Osteoid osteoma, 706–708
Osteology, 7–11
Osteomyelitis, 78
Osteonecrosis. *See also* Avascular necrosis
  absorption of necrotic bone, 420
  with calcium pyrophosphate deposition
    disease, 587
  diagnostic imaging, 70, 76–78
  removal with Surgi-Airtome, 426–427
Osteopore, 337
Osteoporosis, 70, 193, 585, 889
Osteosarcoma, 710
  age distribution, 723, 733
  case study, 733–736
Osteotome, 194, 547, 787, 927
Osteotomy
  arthroscopy and, 88
  capitate, 404, 785–786, 787
  carpal bones, 673–674
  closed wedge, 351–352
  curved, 363
  distal radius
    dorsal malunion, 353
    palmar malunion of, 353
    trapezoidal, 353–355, 359–361, 364,
      636, 927–930
  in DRUJ resection, 356
  lunate fossa, 867, 873
  oblique, 940
  opening wedge, 352, 353, 361–362, 928
  radial wedge, 39, 403, 790
  radius
    for Kienböck's disease, 402, 405, 406
    for Madelung's deformity, 153
    shortening, 855–860
    with total wrist arthroplasty, 677
  step-cut, 729, 847, 851
  trapezium, 797
  trapezoidal, 927–930

ulna, 357, 769, 840. *See also* Sauvé-
    Kapandji procedure
  for Kienböck's disease, 402
  for Madelung's deformity, 153
  nonunion, 625
  for ulnar impaction syndrome,
    624–626
  for ulnar lengthening, 940
  in universal wrist prosthesis surgery,
    673
  wedge, 39, 153, 403
Os trapezoidium. See Trapezoid
Os triangulare, 7. *See also* Triquetrum
Os triquetrum. See Triquetrum
Os ulna. See Ulna
Overload, chronic, 42
Overprotection, 57
Overuse syndrome. *See* Repetitive injury

P
Paget's disease, 733
Pain
  apprehensive posturing, 592
  arthritis, 572–574
  Bennett's fracture, 257
  carpal boss, 149
  cast immobilization, 784
  denervation for, 405, 420, 945–950
  de Quervain's disease, 96
  in distal radius fracture assessment, 312
  evaluation in children, 169
  extensor carpi ulnaris tendinitis, 98
  extraarticular, 95–104
  following capitate shortening, 789
  iliac crest, 565
  incidence rate in gymnasts, 154
  intersection syndrome, 97
  "intrasound vibration," 189
  midcarpal instability, 513
  osteochondroma, 706
  during physical examination, 50, 52, 55
  postactivity ache, 484
  proximal row carpectomy for relief, 552
  with reflex sympathetic dystrophy and
    treatment, 742, 743, 745, 752, 885,
    887
  repetitive injury syndrome, 96, 97, 98,
    100, 103
  rotary subluxation of the scaphoid, 527
  sympathetic-maintained, 336, 742
  symptoms of, 57–58
  three categories of, 61
  with TILT, 637
  total wrist arthrodesis for, 556
  treatment, 746–747
  ulnar wrist, 591–604, 615
Palmaris brevis muscle, 113
Palmaris longus muscle
  Guyon's syndrome, 102
  hypertrophied extension of, 96

Palmaris longus tendon, coiled
    interposition, 404–405
Palmar radiocarpal ligament (PRCL)
  anatomy, 8, 12
  evolution of the, 4
Palmar radioulnar joint, 371
Palmar radioulnar ligament (PRUL), 370,
    371, 372
Palmar scapholunate ligament (SL), 14, 15
Palmar tilt
  loss of normal, 349–350
  radiographic parameters, 348, 349
  with total wrist prosthesis, 662
Palmar ulnocarpal ligament (PUCL), 3–4
Paraffin therapy, 764
Paresthesia
  with aneurysm, 693
  with carpal tunnel syndrome, 108
  with repetitive injury syndrome, 100, 103
Park-Harris growth arrest lines, 162
Passive fist, 57
Patient history
  aneurysm, 693
  aneurysmal bone cyst, 710
  benign tumors, 685, 689
  calcinosis, 713
  carpal boss, 712
  carpal tunnel syndrome, 116–117
  congenital arteriovenous fistula, 695
  dorsal radioulnar joint disorders, 371
  fibrous xanthoma, 691
  giant cell tumor, 708
  hemangioma, 694
  lipofibromatous hamartoma, 701, 703
  lipoma, 691
  malignant tumors, 723–724
  neurilemmoma, 699
  neurofibroma, 697
  osteochondroma, 705–706
  osteoid osteoma, 707
  rheumatoid nodules, 712
  rheumatoid tenosynovitis, 711
  role in physical examination, 47
  solitary enchondroma, 704
  ulnar wrist pain, 591
  wrist evaluation, 757
Patient selection
  Darrach procedure, 805
  distal ulna resection, 653
  dorsal capsulodesis, 827
  proximal row carpectomy, 546
  replantation, 269
Pauciarticular juvenile arthritis, 165–166
Pediatrics, 149–169
  aponeurotic fibroma, 689
  bone graft harvest, 815
  carpal fracture, 156–157, 159
  distal radius fracture, 160–163
  dorsal wrist syndrome, 169
  fracture classification, 287

Pediatrics (contd.)
  ganglia, 149, 163–164
  hemangioma, 695
  juvenile arthritis, 165–167, 168
  Madelung's deformity, 151–154, 156, 162, 168–169
  ossification vs. fracture, 189
  pain evaluation, 169
  radius fracture, 160–163
  scaphoid fracture, 157, 158–159, 196
  triquetrum fracture, 159
  triquetrum tear, 160
  ulna fracture, 160–163
Pedicle bone graft for Kienböck's disease, 401, 402, 419–420
Penetration trauma, 206, 696
Penicillamine, 667
Percutaneous pinning
  of the arthrodesis, 557
  Bennett's fracture, 257
  capitate dislocation, 225
  carpal dislocation, 219, 226, 239
  carpometacarpal fracture, 264, 265, 266–267
  distal radius fracture, 287, 294, 306, 307, 311, 316–318, 344–345
  perilunate dislocation, 244
  radiocarpal dislocation, 215–216, 217
  Rolando's fracture, 257
  scaphoid dislocation, 220
  scaphoid fracture, 194
  trapezium dislocation, 223
  trapezoid dislocation, 219–220
  triquetrum dislocation, 224–225
Percutaneous screw fixation. See Screw fixation
"Perforation," 69
Perilunar carpal dislocation. See Carpal bones, dislocations and instability, perilunar
Perilunate
  dislocation, 231, 238–240, 241, 243–245, 249, 472
  fracture-dislocations, 432, 446, 447
  injury with scaphoid fracture, 188, 190
  instabilities, 235, 438, 446–450, 466–467
Periosteal artery, 816
Periosteum, 198, 355
Peripheral sensitization, 743
Peritendinitis crepitans, 97
Peyronie's fibromatosis, 689
Phalen's test, 108, 117
Phenoxybenzamine, 746
Phonophoresis, 97
Phylogeny, 1–5, 42
Physical examination, 47–59, 83, 528–529
  aneurysmal bone cyst, 710
  aneurysms, 693–694
  articular-nonarticular junction, 49, 58, 528

benign tumors, 685–686, 689
carpal boss, 712, 793
carpal tunnel syndrome, 108, 117–118
congenital arteriovenous fistula, 695–696
distal radioulnar joint disorders, 371–373, 389, 847
dorsal wrist syndrome, 483, 485, 528
extensor carpi ulnaris subluxation, 598
fibrous xanthoma, 691
giant cell tumor, 708–709
hemangioma, 694–695, 703
lipofibromatous hamartoma, 701
lipoma, 691
lunatotriquetral instability, 474–477
lunotriquetral instability, 503–504
malignant tumor, 723
neurilemmoma, 699
neurofibroma, 697–698
osteochondroma, 706
osteoid osteoma, 707
pain during, 12, 50, 55
radial, 48–51
radiocarpal and midcarpal joints, 53–54
for replantation, 270
rheumatoid nodules, 712
rheumatoid tenosynovitis, 711–712
rotary subluxation of the scaphoid, 49, 528–529, 819
scaphoid fracture, 188–189
scapholunate instability, 469–473
solitary enchrondroma, 704
substitution maneuvers in, 57–58
triscaphe joint, 49, 50, 528
ulna, 51–53, 591–592, 597, 601
wrist evaluation, 757–760
Physical therapy. See Rehabilitation
Physiolysis, 140
Physis. See Distal radial physis; Distal ulnar physis
Physis pins, 162
Piano key test, 592, 843
Pinch strength
  with carpal tunnel syndrome and release, 115
  diminished, with carpometacarpal fracture, 255
  following carpometacarpal tendon arthroplasty, 801
  with reflex sympathetic dystrophy, 885
  therapeutic exercises, 771
Pin fixation. See also Percutaneous pinning
  complications, 790
  cross-, 272
  distal radioulnar joint surgery, 390
  during proximal row carpectomy, 548, 549
  scaphoid fracture, 194
  total wrist prosthesis dislocation, 679–680

Pins
  buttress, 923
  care, 336
  diagnostic imaging and, 64
  distal radius external fixation, 316
  placement to avoid growth arrest, 162
  Rush, 564
  Schanz, 316
  Steinman, 555–556, 564, 651, 812
Pins-and-needles sensation, 100
PIP. See Proximal interphalangeal joint
π-plate, 326, 328, 330, 333
Pisiform
  anatomy, 12–13, 465, 598
  arthritis, 602, 603
  with carpal dislocation, 218, 242
  dislocation, 177, 225
  evolution, 1, 3, 5
  fractures, 55–56, 182–183
  ossification, 149
  osteology, 8
  physical examination, 55–56
  transfer graft for Kienböck's disease, 401, 420
  with ulnar deficiency, 135
Pisiformectomy, 182, 598
Pisihamatum ligament, 182
Pisimetacarpicum ligament, 182
Pisohamate ligament, 225
Pisotriquetral joint (PT)
  anatomy, 12–13
  arthroscopy, 89
  dysfunction, 598
  impaction fracture, 182
  physical examination, 592
  in triquetrum dislocation, 372
"Pivot shift" test, 53–54
Plaquenil, 667
Plaster of Paris for casting, 780–783
Plate fixation
  AO/ASIF, 267, 408
  distal radius fractures, 277, 287, 326–328, 330, 333, 337
  Ender compression blade plate, 194
  in replantation, of radius to metacarpals, 271
  total wrist arthrodesis, 559–563
  total wrist prosthesis failure, 680
  with ulnar shortening osteotomy, 357, 625
PLI. See Perilunate, instabilities
Pollicis longus, 8, 9, 855
Pollicization
  of the index finger, 130, 131, 134, 137
  with mirror hand, 138
  of the thumb, 138, 139
Polyarticular juvenile arthritis, 166
Polydactyly, 138
Polyethylene, in total wrist prosthesis, 661, 662, 663, 668, 676

Portals for arthroscopy, 85–86, 88
"Position of compromise," 659
Position of patient for arthroscopy, 84
Posterior interosseous nerve, 946, 948
Posterior interosseous nerve (PIN)
  in distal radius surgery, 320
  neurectomy with repair for scapholunate dissociation, 492
Posterior oblique ligament (POL), 256
Postoperative management
  bone graft for scaphoid nonunion, 903, 913
  capitate shortening with capitate-hamate fusion, 788
  capsulodesis for rotary subluxation of the scaphoid, 824
  carpal boss repair, 794
  cocompartment release for tenosynovitis, 953
  Darrach procedure, 808
  distal radioulnar joint stabilization, 813
  distal radius fracture, 336
  dorsal wrist syndrome, 830
  lunotriquetral arthrodesis, 834
  matched hemiresection-interposition arthroplasty, 841
  matched ulnar arthroplasty, 850
  proximal row carpectomy, 551
  radiocarpal arthrodesis-arthroplasty, 863
  radiolunate arthrodesis, 868
  radioulnar arthrodesis, 875
  replantation, 274–275
  Sauvé-Kapandji procedure, 889–891
  scaphocapitate arthrodesis, 897
  scapholunate advanced collapse reconstruction, 924
  total wrist arthrodesis, 563
  trapezoidal osteotomy of the distal radius, 929
  triscaphe arthrodesis, 934–935
Posttraumatic arthritis. See Arthritis, posttraumatic; Osteoarthritis, posttraumatic
Posttraumatic carpal instability, 158–159
Potentiometer, 40
PQ transfer. See Pronator quadratus, transfer in distal radioulnar joint disorders
PR. See Pronosupination
PRC. See Proximal row carpectomy
PRCL. See Palmar radiocarpal ligament
Prebend plate, 680
Prednisone, 672
Preiser's disease, 126–127, 413, 555, 921
"Pre-Kienböck" condition, 429
Preoperative planning, dorsal capsulodesis, 824–825
Prepollex, evolution of the, 1
Pressure in the wrist, 38–40
Pressure-sensitive film, 38, 40
Pressure sores, 783–784

Prestyloid recess, evolution of the, 4
Prieser's disease, 157
Primates, evolution of the wrist, 3–4, 369, 616
Procolbus verus, 4
Profundus tendons, 116
Progressive perilunar instability theory, 234, 466
Pronator quadratus muscle
  in distal radius surgery, 321, 322, 856, 857, 858
  entrapment, 161
  in matched ulnar arthroplasty resection salvage, 852
  pedicle graft for Kienböck's disease, 401, 419, 426–428
  in Sauvé-Kapandji procedure, 890
  transfer in distal radioulnar joint disorders, 379–380, 381, 382, 807
Pronosupination (PR), 28, 29, 48
Propofol, 120
Prostheses. See Arthroplasty, prostheses
Protasul, 661
Proton density, 73
Proximal interphalangeal joint (PIP), 57–58, 640, 641
Proximal row carpectomy (PRC), 154, 246, 417, 526, 545–553, 566, 652
PRUL. See Palmar radioulnar ligament
Pseudarthrosis, 563, 615, 643, 654, 861, 862, 889
Pseudoaneurysm. See Aneurysms, false
Pseudogout. See Calcium pyrophosphate deposition disease
Pseudoradiocarpal joint, 729
Psychological aspects
  effects of patient motivation, 308
  of pain, 591
  reflex sympathetic dystrophy, 744, 749, 752
  return to work, 765
  of the surgeon, 296, 579
  worry of tumor malignancy, 683
PT. See Pisotriquetral joint
PUCL. See Palmar ulnocarpal ligament
Pulsed electrical stimulation. See Electrical stimulation
Punching, 188, 599
Purgatorius ceratops, 3
Pyarthrosis, 78

R

Racial aspects
  Kienböck's disease, 397
  lunotriquetral synostosis, 123
Radial artery, 395, 396, 623
  anatomy, 907, 908
  aneurysm, 692, 693, 694
  ganglion cysts, 688
  in radial shortening osteotomy, 855, 856

Radial club hand, 128, 131, 144
Radial collateral ligament, 432, 456
Radial deficiency, 127–134, 136
Radial head
  excision, 385, 387, 388, 391
  fracture, 377–378
Radial inclination
  loss of normal, 350–351
  radiographic parameters, 348, 349
Radial midcarpal portal (RMC), 86, 87
Radial nerve
  anatomy, 946
  denervation, 948, 949
  de Quervain's disease and, 97
  in distal radius fixation, 307, 317
  entrapment, 103
  neuroma from total wrist arthrodesis, 563
  in perilunate dislocation surgery, 244
  in trapeziometacarpal surgery, 571
  in triangular fibrocartilage debridement, 623
Radial recurrent artery, 396
Radial styloid
  absence with radial deficiency, 128
  in distal radius fixation, 317, 318, 319, 325
  with distal radius fractures, 313
  fractures, 205–206, 212, 240, 342, 345, 446
  impaction following triscaphe arthrodesis, 937
  as landmark for arthroscopy, 85
  removal in radiocarpal arthrodesis-arthroplasty, 863
  vascularization, 187
Radial styloidectomy, 91–92, 495, 551, 937
Radial ulnar joint. See Radioulnar joint
Radiation therapy
  hemangioma, 695
  malignant tumor, 726, 736, 737, 739
Radical excision, 725
Radiocapitate ligament (RCL)
  anatomy, 432–434
  biomechanics, 441, 444
  in capitolunate instability, 431, 448–449
  failure location and mode, 442–443
  with scaphoid-lunate dislocation, 222
Radiocarpal arch, 396, 908, 910
Radiocarpal dislocation. See Carpal bones, dislocations and instability, radiocarpal
Radiocarpal joint
  anatomy, 12
  arthrodesis, 216, 217, 650, 861–865. See also Arthrodesis, total wrist
  arthroplasty, 861–865
  dislocation, 277, 333–335
  in distal radius fractures, 299
  flexion-extension motion, 22–23
  ganglia of the, 685, 688

Radiocarpal joint (contd.)
 physical examination, 53–54
 reconstruction, creation of
   pseudoradiocarpal joint, 729
 in scaphoid fracture fixation, 194
 subluxation, 216
 synovectomy, 650
Radiocarpal ligaments
 in distal radius fractures, 312
 dorsal, 432–434, 446, 502
 ganglia of the, 164
 ligamentotaxis, 306
Radiographic agents. See Arthrography;
   Bone scintigraphy
Radiography
 abuse or overuse, 61
 aneurysm, 694
 aneurysmal bone cyst, 710
 axial dislocation of carpus, 219
 "axial loading grip," 461
 benign tumors, 686, 689–690
 Bennett's fracture, 256, 257
 calcinosis, 713–714
 calcium pyrophosphate deposition
   disease, 587–588
 capitate fractures, 176–177
 carpal boss, 62, 63, 712–713
 "carpal box" images, 189
 carpal dislocations, 236–239, 250
 carpal tunnel syndrome, 108–109
 carpometacarpal tendon arthroplasty, 801
 congenital arteriovenous fistula, 696
 conventional, 61–63
 Darrach procedure, 804
 distal radioulnar joint disorders, 373,
   389, 804
 in distal radius external fixation,
   307–308, 316
 in distal radius fracture assessment,
   312–314
 dorsal wrist syndrome, 489
 dynamic ulnar impaction syndrome, 627
 exploded view of wrist in traction, 207
 fibrous xanthoma, 691
 giant cell tumor, 708, 709, 727, 730–733
 gout, 585–586
 gymnast's wrist, 156
 hamate fracture, 599
 hemangioma, 695, 703
 of the immature wrist, 159, 160
 incidence of wrist trauma needing, 255
 juvenile arthritis, 166–167
 Kienböck's disease, 398, 399
 lipoma, 691
 lunate, 250, 251
 lunotriquetral instability, 504
 malignant tumor, 723
 matched hemiresection-interposition
   arthroplasty, 842, 843
 neurofibroma, 698
 osteoarthritis, 572, 573
 osteochondroma, 706
 osteoid osteoma, 707–708
 perilunar dislocation, 207, 208–209, 214,
   240
 radiolunate arthrodesis, 871, 872
 rheumatoid arthritis, 643, 648, 654, 804
 rheumatoid nodules, 712
 rheumatoid tenosynovitis, 712
 rotary subluxation of the scaphoid, 461,
   471, 472, 819, 820
 scaphocapitate arthrodesis, 897, 898
 scaphoid dislocation, 220, 221
 scaphoid fracture, 157, 189–190, 192,
   195
 scapholunate instability, 222, 461,
   469–473
 sclerosis, 250
 solitary enchondroma, 704
 total wrist arthroplasty, pre- and post-,
   667–668
 triangular fibrocartilage complex, 608
 triquetrum dislocation, 224
 ulnar wrist pain, 592–593
 unicameral bone cyst, 711
Radiolunate joint
 angle, following scaphocapitate
   arthrodesis, 897
 arthrodesis, 540–542, 565, 652, 865,
   867–874
Radiolunate ligament (RL)
 anatomy, 14, 434, 456
 long
   anatomy, 231, 232, 501, 502
   with scaphoid dislocation, 236, 241
   in perilunate dislocation surgery, 212
   in scaphoid internal fixation, 194
   with scaphoid-lunate dislocation, 222,
     236, 241
 short, anatomy, 14, 231, 232, 501
Radiolunotriquetral ligament (RLTq), 14,
   15, 456, 501
Radioscaphocapitate ligament (RSC;RSCL),
   8, 12, 14, 187, 432. See also
   Radiocapitate ligament
 anatomy, 231–232, 456, 457, 501–502
 arthroscopy, 87
 in perilunate dislocation surgery, 212
 with scaphoid dislocation, 220
 in scaphoid internal fixation, 194
 with scaphoid subluxation, 241
Radioscaphoid joint
 angle, following scaphocapitate
   arthrodesis, 897
 degenerative arthritis, 525–526
 distribution of force, 39, 525
 in scaphoid dislocation surgery, 245
Radioscaphoid ligament (RSL)
 anatomy, 432, 434, 437–438, 441, 444
 in carpal dislocation, 446
 failure location and mode, 443
 reconstruction, 438, 439
Radioscapholunate ligament (RSL), 14, 15
 anatomy, 456, 501
 arthroscopy, 86–87
 injury with distal radius fracture, 343
 with midcarpal instability, 513
Radiostereophotogrammetric techniques, 34
Radiotherapy. See Radiation therapy
Radiotriquetral ligament (RTL)
 anatomy, 432–434, 456
 biomechanics, 441, 444
 in carpal dislocations, 446, 447, 448
 failure location and mode, 442–443
 with scaphoid-lunate dislocation, 222
 in scapholunate joint reconstruction, 438
 in triquetrum dislocation, 224
Radioulnar deviation (RUD), 23, 24
 in activities of daily living, 31, 32
 degrees of freedom, 28
 kinematics, 469, 471
 moment arm and, 40, 42
 in specific activities, 33, 34
 strength and, 29
 with total wrist arthrodesis, 557
 in wrist motion studies, 35, 36
Radioulnar joint. See also Distal radioulnar
   joint
 in amputation, 275
 arthrodesis, 153, 811, 875–877. See also
   Sauvé-Kapandji procedure
 in distal radius fractures, 299
 distribution of force, 39
 flexion-extension motion, 23, 24
 instability in gymnasts, 154
 physical examination, 51–52
 synostosis, 136–137
Radioulnar ligament, dorsal, 370, 371, 372
Radius
 anatomy, 8, 434, 525
 arthroscopy, 90–91
 closing wedge osteotomy, 403
 computed tomography, 66, 90
 dorsal angulation, with carpal overload,
   514
 duplication of the, 139
 fractures, 39–40
   arthroscopy, 90–91
   in children, 160–163
   with distal radioulnar joint disorders,
     377, 381
   force and pressure analysis, 39–40
   from total wrist arthrodesis, 564
 giant cell tumor and, 728, 730, 731
 harvest for bone graft, 427, 428,
   815–817
 hypoplasia of the, 128, 129–130,
   144–145
 malunion, 385, 387, 867
 force and pressure analysis, 39–40

ulnar impaction syndrome and, 619
migration after radial head excision, 385, 387, 388
osteosarcoma, 733, 734
in proximal row carpectomy, 535, 548, 549, 553, 652
reconstruction, after giant tumor cell excision, 728, 729
reestablishment of the articular surface, 362–364
shortening, 855–860
 effects on outcome, 305
 for Kienböck's disease, 402, 405, 406, 419, 420, 428, 943
 problems associated with, 350–351
total wrist arthrodesis and, 564, 565
with ulnar deficiency, 135
in universal wrist prosthesis surgery, 673
Radius metacarpal
 distal epiphysis of the, 8
 osteology, 9–10
"Railroad track," of carpal ligament, 111
Range-of-motion
 after perilunate dislocation treatment, 249
 after TFCC repair, 770
 carpal synostosis, 123
 exercises in immediate post-operative period, 610
 following bone-retinaculum-bone autograft, 918
 following capitate shortening, 789
 following carpometacarpal tendon arthroplasty, 801
 following distal radius fracture, 315
 following radiolunate arthrodesis, 870
 following SLAC reconstruction, 924
 following triscaphe arthrodesis, 935
 "functional," 30–32, 521, 760
 radiocarpal and midcarpal joints, 22
 in rotary subluxation of the scaphoid correction, 883
 for specific activities, 33–34
 thumb, 570–571
 with total wrist arthroplasty, 659, 660
 with triquetral impingement ligament tear syndrome, 636, 637
 triscaphe arthrodesis, 767
Rapid exchange grip test, 592
Rayhack's classification, 283–284
RCL. See Radiocapitate ligament
Reagan's test, 52
Reconstruction
 after giant cell tumor excision, 728–729
 carpal bones, 341–364
 carpometacarpal joint ligament, 571–572, 574–577, 579
 with the Darrach procedure, 805, 806–808
 with Madelung's deformity, 151

radioscaphoid ligament, 438, 439
scapholunate advanced collapse, 144, 145, 488, 516, 531, 536–538, 766, 767, 921–926
scapholunate joint, 438–439, 440
scapholunate ligament, 915–919
Recreational injuries. See Sports
Recurrence
 congenital arteriovenous fistula, 696
 ganglion cysts, 164, 686, 688
Reduction. See also Closed reduction; Open reduction
 arthroscopy and, 90
 finger trap traction, 289, 290, 291
 manual, 289, 290
Reexploration, post-replantation, 275
Reflex sympathetic dystrophy (RSD), 57, 308, 336, 741–753
 bone scintigraphy, 594
 carpal tunnel release and, 115
 from carpometacarpal tendon arthroplasty, 801
 causes, 564, 742–744, 751, 752, 801
 clinical assessment, 744–745
 diagnosis, 70, 741–742, 744–746
 Dystrophile program for, 391, 835, 885–888
 following SLAC reconstruction, 925
 from total wrist arthrodesis, 564
 treatment, 746–752
Rehabilitation, 757–772
 bone-retinaculum-bone autograft, 918
 carpal tunnel release, 113, 120
 distal radius fractures, 308–309, 345, 771
 juvenile arthritis, 167
 proximal row carpectomy, 551
 reflex sympathetic dystrophy, 746–752, 885–888
 replantation, 274–275
 rheumatoid arthritis, 768
 "six pack" exercises, 296
 total wrist arthrodesis, 565
Remote trauma, 75–76
Renographin, 593
Repetition time (TR), 73
Repetitive injury
 aneurysm, 693
 definition, 95, 765
 from gymnastics, 154, 155
 paresthesia with, 100, 103
Replantation, transcarpal and radiocarpal, 269–275
Reproducibility of diagnosis, 277, 281
Resection
 basal joint, 574–577
 capitate, 794
 carpal bone fracture, 183
 distal radioulnar joint, 837–844
 distal ulna, 355, 358–359, 380, 653, 654, 803, 805, 806, 809

ganglion, 92
 for Kienböck's disease, 419–420
 Lister's tubercle, 895
 malignant tumor, 725–726
 ulna, 89, 806, 841, 849, 851
 ulnar artery, 102
Resisted opposition maneuver, 55
Resorption. See Bone resorption
Restoration
 aneurysm, 164–165
 arthroscopy and, 90
 carpal bone fractures, 183
Restraining forces, 34
Retinacular system, 16–17
Retinaculum. See Extensor retinaculum; Flexor retinaculum
Retractors, 320, 673, 806
Revascularization
 for Kienböck's disease, 419–420
 direct, 401–402
 effects of age, 786
 indirect, 402–404
 lunate, 419–429, 786, 788–789
 in replantation, 269, 270, 271, 273
Reverse Bennet's fracture-dislocation, 262, 265
Reverse Blatt capsulodesis, 918
Rhabdomyosarcoma, 737
Rheumatoid arthritis
 carpal tunnel syndrome and, 100, 116
 in carpometacarpal joints, 570, 580
 deformities, 639–642, 647–648, 654, 670, 679
 distal radioulnar joint, 385, 642, 803, 837–838
 evaluation, 647–649
 fusion secondary to, 679, 680
 as indicator for Sauvé-Kapandji procedure, 890
 juvenile, 165, 168
 medications, 667
 pathomechanics, 645–647
 principles of, 639–644
 proximal row carpectomy and, 552
 radiocarpal arthrodesis-arthroplasty for, 861–865
 radiography, 61
 thumb basal joint, 578
 treatment, 648–655, 768
 ulnar impaction syndrome with, 624, 629
 vs. gout, 585
Rheumatoid nodules, 683, 685, 712
Rheumatoid tenosynovitis, 683, 711–712
Rigid-body spring model, 38, 39
Ringer's lactate solution, 84, 270, 328, 336
"Ring sign," 819, 825
RL. See Radiolunate ligament
RLTq. See Radiolunotriquetral ligament
RMC. See Radial midcarpal portal

Roentgenogram, 660
Rolando's fracture, 257
Rolando's fracture, reverse, 262, 263
Rongeur, use in surgery
  biconcave bone graft, 901
  bone-retinaculum-bone autograft, 917
  carpal boss repair, 793
  carpometacarpal tendon arthroplasty, 797
  dorsal capsulodesis, 825
  DRUJ degenerative arthritis, 601, 852
  proximal row carpectomy, 548
  radiocarpal arthrodesis-arthroplasty, 861, 862, 863
  radiolunate arthrodesis, 873
  scaphoid fracture, 194
  triscaphe arthrodesis, 931, 932
Rotary subluxation of the scaphoid (RSS), 413, 431, 484, 486–487
  carpal kinematics in, 36–37
  classification, 486–487, 526–527
  clinical presentation, 527
  diagnosis, 250, 511, in 49
  dorsal capsulodesis for, 819–827
  fixed or static, 400, 406, 524
  as indicator for triscaphe arthrodesis, 931
  physical examination, 49, 528–529
  progression, 485, 523–526
  radiography, 461, 471, 472
  treatment
    algorithm, 529
    using the flexor carpi radialis, 879–884
  two types, 883–884
  vs. dislocation, 241
Rotation
  with capitate fractures, 176
  center-of, 23–24
  of the forearm, 42, 369, 389, 769, 843
  Fusi counterrotation, 580
  of the scaphoid vs. the lunate, 458–460, 462
  shift with total wrist arthroplasty, 670
  of the total wrist arthrodesis, 564
  of the wrist, 4, 38, 233
Row theory of the wrist, 27
RSC. See Radioscaphocapitate ligament
RSCL. See Radioscaphocapitate ligament
RSD. See Reflex sympathetic dystrophy
RSL. See Radioscaphoid ligament; Radioscapholunate ligament
RSS. See Rotary subluxation of the scaphoid
RTL. See Radiotriquetral ligament
RUD. See Radioulnar deviation

S

Sacroiliac joint, 565
Saddle-shaped configuration, of trapeziometacarpal joint, 256
Salter-Harris II injuries, 160–162
Salter-Harris V injuries, 162
Salvage procedures. See also Sauvé-Kapandji procedure
  for Kienböck's disease, 405
  long-term strategy for, 25
  matched ulnar arthroplasty, 851–852
  for osteoarthritis, 362, 364
  radioulnar arthrodesis, 875–877
  ulnar impaction syndrome, 626–627
  ulnar lengthening, 943
Sarcoma
  degeneration of benign tumor to, 705
  epithelioid, 736–737, 738
  osteosarcoma, 710, 723, 733–736
  rhabdomyosarcoma, 737
  synovial cell, 736, 737
  vs. neurilemmoma, 700
Sarmiento classification, 279
Sauvé-Kapandji procedure, 167, 357–358, 384–385, 388, 811, 889–893
  with rheumatoid arthritis, 643, 653, 809, 837–838
  ulnar impaction syndrome and, 627, 629
Saw, low-speed oscillating, 625
"Scallop sign," 648, 804
Scaphocapitate fracture syndrome, 176, 207, 209
Scaphocapitate joint
  angle, and midcarpal instability, 512
  arthrodesis, 403, 406, 540, 855, 895–899
Scaphocapitate syndrome, 188, 240–241, 245
Scaphocapitate-trapezoid ligament (SCTd), 14, 15
Scaphoid. See also Rotary subluxation of the scaphoid
  anatomy, 70, 187, 434, 458
  articular-nonarticular junction of the, 103–104
  aseptic necrosis, 126–127
  dislocations, 220–222, 235–236, 239, 240, 245
  evolution of the, 3
  fractures, 188–198
    associated with perilunate dislocation, 207, 208
    with carpal instability, 432, 447–448
    in children, 157–158, 167–168
    healing time, 191
    incidence rate, 174, 187, 255
    nonunion. See Nonunion, scaphoid fracture
    stability, 190, 191
    treatment, 192–193, 771
    waist, 190, 191, 192
  horizontalization, 868, 869
  hypermobile, and capitate shortening, 790
  instability. See Rotary subluxation of the scaphoid
  with Madelung's deformity, 140
  as a mnemonic, 25
  in normal carpal alignment, 190, 934
  ontogenesis, 7
  osteology, 8–9
  proximal pole, 821
  with radial deficiency, 127, 128, 130, 131, 134
  in radioulnar deviation, 23, 24, 27, 37, 462–464
  role in wrist biomechanics, 27, 36, 37, 190, 458–460, 462–464
  rotation with Kienböck's disease, 400, 406
  subluxation vs. dislocation, 241
Scaphoideum. See Scaphoid
Scaphoid fossa, 8
Scaphoid impaction syndrome, 467, 468
Scaphoid nonunion advanced collapse (SNAC), 158, 545. See also Nonunion, scaphoid fracture
Scaphoid shift maneuver, 49, 50, 51, 58, 528–529, 686, 915
Scaphoid-trapezium-trapezoid ligament complex (STT)
  anatomy, 14, 16
  fusion and pressure analysis, 39
  fusion and wrist motion, 25, 249
  physical examination, 49, 50, 58
  in rotary subluxation of the scaphoid, 879–880, 883
Scapholunate advanced collapse (SLAC)
  arthritis and, 91, 198, 603
  bone graft for, 815, 816
  with calcium pyrophosphate dihydrate, 588
  etiology, 535–536, 545, 921
  following triscaphe arthrodesis, 937
  physical examination, 47–48
  proximal row carpectomy and, 545, 552, 553
  radial styloidectomy and, 91
  radiography, 489, 530
  reconstruction, 144, 145, 488, 516, 531, 536–538, 766, 767, 921–926
  with scaphoid nonunion or dissociation, 198, 343
  in spectrum of scaphoid instability, 484, 525
Scapholunate interosseous ligament (SLIL)
  anatomy, 232, 434, 435–437, 441, 444, 458
  biomechanics, 439, 441, 458–459
  with carpal dislocation, 235, 236, 239, 446, 448, 449, 450, 459
  failure location and mode, 443, 468
  fibrotic granulation, 821, 822, 825
  kinematics, 36
  with lunate fracture, 872
  reconstruction, 439, 440
  repair, 241, 246–247, 249, 488, 915–919

tear
    classification, 486
    following distal radius fracture, 341, 342–343, 344, 345–346, 362
    and ganglia, 714
    posttraumatic incidence rate, 436
    with scapholunate dissociation, 531, 872

Scapholunate joint (SL)
  arthrodesis, 271, 539–540
  dislocation or dissociation, 491–499, 531, 790, 825. See also Rotary subluxation of the scaphoid
    with Kienböck's disease, 414
    with perilunate dislocation, 205, 207
    with simultaneous scaphoid and lunate dislocation, 222
    and total wrist arthrodesis, 555
  in dorsal wrist syndrome surgery, 829–830, 831
  evaluation for bone-retinaculum-bone autograft, 916
  evaluation for midcarpal instability surgery, 512
  force and pressure analysis, 39, 472
  function with, 42
  ganglia of the, 163–164
  instability, 448
  ligamentous anatomy, 435–438, 444
  with midcarpal instability, 513, 518–519
  normal anatomy position following, 456
  overload. See Dorsal wrist syndrome
  physical examination, 48, 52
  reconstruction, 438–439
  in replantation, 271

Scapholunate ligament (SL)
  anatomy, 456
  arthrography, 69
  arthroscopy, 87
  with calcium pyrophosphate dihydrate, 588
  in dorsal carpal impingement syndrome, 468
  in dorsal wrist syndrome, 485–486, 829, 831
  ennervation, 12, 198
  ganglia of the, 92, 684–685, 687
  material properties, 28
  palmar, 14, 15
  repair, 212, 213, 214, 246–249, 915–919
  in rotary subluxation of the scaphoid, 879
  with scaphoid nonunion bone graft, 904

Scapholunatocapitotriquetral fusion, 404

Scaphotrapezial joint
  ganglia of the, 685, 688
  in ligament reconstruction for basal joint resection, 574
  in scaphoid internal fixation, 194
  in trapezium fractures, 175

Scaphotrapezial ligament, ganglia of the, 164

Scaphotrapeziotrapezoid joint (STT). See also Triscaphe joint
  arthritis, 532–533
  arthrodesis, 249, 403, 419, 420, 423–426, 521, 555, 826, 855, 895
  arthroscopy, 86, 87
  in capitate fractures, 176, 177
  congenital synchondrosis, 535
  in dorsal capsulodesis, 821
  ganglia and, 714
  pinning with Kienböck's disease, 415
  synovitis, 485
  in triscaphe arthrodesis, 933

Scaphotrapezoidal joint, computed tomography, 67

Scaphotrapezoidal ligament
  in trapezium dislocation, 223
  in trapezoid dislocation, 219

Scaphotriquetral ligament
  anatomy, 434, 456
  in perilunate dislocation surgery, 212, 213, 214
  with scaphoid-lunate dislocation, 222
  in triquetrum dislocation, 224

Scar contracture from ganglion cyst excision, 688

Scar tissue
  from hemangioma laser treatment, 695
  hypertrophy, 196
  from reflex sympathetic dystrophy, 741
  soft tissue mobilization of, 763
  in wrist evaluation, 759

Scheffe's analysis of variance, 35
Schwann cells, 697, 699
Schwannoma, 698–700
Scintigraphy. See Bone scintigraphy
Sclerosing hemangioma, 694, 695
Sclerosis, 126, 250, 646, 695, 864

Screw fixation
  alignment guide for, 194
  cannulated, 194, 196, 212, 245
  compression, 245
  of distal radius fractures, 287, 869
  headless, 194, 195
  Herbert, 194, 195, 245, 267, 896, 913
  lag, 182, 183, 259, 328, 877, 891
  medullary compression, 210
  noncannulated, 194
  of scaphoid fracture, 194
  in total wrist prostheses, 662, 663, 664, 666, 667, 675

Scrubbing action, in the Dystrophile program, 885, 886

SCTd. See Scaphocapitate-trapezoid ligament

Secondary gain, 351. See also Malingering
Secondary ulnar impaction syndrome, 627–628

Semmes-Weinstein monofilament testing, 592, 757
Seven University Study Group, 110
Shake test, 592
Shaver, motorized, 609, 610, 611, 623–624

Shear force
  Bennett's fracture, 256
  carpal instability, 455
  lunotriquetral instabiity, 503

Shear fractures, 323, 325–327
Shear tests. See Ballottement tests
Shift test, scaphoid, 189

Short arm cast, 779–782, 783
  capitate-hamate fusion, 788
  distal radius malunion, 355
  pisiform dislocation, 225
  radiolunate arthrodesis, 874
  scaphocapitate arthrodesis, 897
  trapezoid dislocation, 219
  ulnar shortening, 625
  ulnar styloid fracture, 375

Short arm thumb-spica cast
  dorsal capsulodesis, 824
  perilunate dislocation, 245
  scaphoid fracture, 157, 192
  scapholunate advanced collapse reconstruction, 924
  scaphotrapeziotrapezoid arthrodesis, 425

Short radiolunate ligament. See Radiolunate ligament, short

Shoulder abduction, 57
Shoulder pain with carpal tunnel syndrome, 100
Shuck test, 592, 600
Sigmoid notch, 8, 55, 369, 374–375, 616, 648
"Signet ring" sign, 238
Silicone gel sheeting, 765

Silicone replacement arthroplasty
  basal joint resection, 574, 577
  distal ulnar cap, 853
  flexible hinge, 660, 663
  force and pressure analysis, 34, 38–40
  Kienböck's disease, 404, 420
  lunate, 413, 811
  silicone synovitis from, 642, 871, 923

Silver fork deformity, 516
"Six pack" exercises, 296

Skin. See also Scar tissue
  coverage after replantation, 270, 274
  grafts, 274, 563, 695
  inadequate coverage, total wrist arthrodesis for, 556
  with radial club hand treatment, 144–145
  soft tissue mobilization of, 763
  temperature, and arteriovenous fistula, 695
  testing in wrist evaluation, 759

Skin temperature, post-replantation monitoring, 275
SL. See Scapholunate joint; Scapholunate ligament
SLAC. See Scapholunate advanced collapse
SLIL. See Scapholunate interosseous ligament
Sling immobilization, complications, 308
Sling procedure, for tendon grafts, 379, 382
Slotted cannula, 109, 111, 112, 113, 114
Smith's fractures, 91, 289, 291, 294
Smoking, effects on healing, 777, 924
Snuff box
  anatomy, 321, 908
  tenderness with scaphoid fracture, 188
  ulnar, 52, 85, 86
Sodium morrhuate, 695
Soft tissue. See also Scar tissue; Swelling; Triangular fibrocartilage complex; Tumors
  adaptation with carpal tunnel syndrome, 118
  with carpal dislocation, 250
  with complex fracture, 335–336
  in the Darrach procedure, 805, 806–808
  debridement during replantation, 270, 271
  diagnostic imaging, 64, 70, 72, 73, 75
  with distal radioulnar joint disorders, 374, 378–380, 391
  with distal radius fracture, 277, 312
  in distal ulna resection, 653
  post-fracture contractures, 162
  with radial deficiency, 128
  in rheumatoid arthritis treatment, 649–650
  sarcoma, 726, 736–737, 738
  with scaphoid fracture, 188, 191
  testing in wrist evaluation, 758–759
Sonic digitization, 444
Space of Poirer
  anatomy, 434, 444, 457
  biomechanics, 445
  in carpal dislocation, 232, 235, 446
  with distal radius fracture, 344
Spike fracture, 300, 303, 314
"Spilled teacup" sign, 207, 238, 239
Spinal cord stimulation, 747
Spin-echo sequences, 73
Splints, 761–763
  after replantation, 274, 275
  for carpal tunnel syndrome, 109, 119, 120
  circumferential thermoplastic, 761, 763, 769
  cock-up, 309
  flexible (mobilization;dynamic), 192, 193, 195, 750, 888
  Futuro, 824
  for hamate fracture, 599
  for lunotriquetral instability, 505
  Orthoplast, 309
  "pancake," 762
  for proximal row carpectomy, 549
  with repetitive injury syndrome, 97, 98, 99
  for rheumatoid arthritis, 768
  scaphoid, 192, 193, 195
  serial static, 762–763
  silicone rubber, 761
  sugar-tong, 89, 291, 293–294, 336, 357, 671, 677
  TAP, 769
  for TFCC tears, 609
  thumb-spica, 770
  for TILT, 634, 687
  tin, 341
  ulnar gutter, 98
Sports, 635
  bicycling, 176
  de Quervain's disease and, 96
  following distal radius fracture
  gymnastics
    carpal instability, 154
    dorsal carpal impingement syndrome from, 468
    "gymnast's wrist," 100, 154–156
  hook of hamate fractures, 177, 184
  hook of hamate nonunion, 602
  range-of-motion for, 33–34, 42
  repetitive injury syndrome from, 96, 97, 100, 102
  splints worn during, 761
Sprain
  carpometacarpal joints, 568
  misdiagnosis, 250
Spurling's test, 592
Stability of the wrist, 27
Staging
  gymnast's wrist, 156
  Kienböck's disease, 399–400, 405–408, 426
Ståhl index, 398
Staphylococcus aureus, 679
Staples, 194
Steinman pin technique, 555–556, 564, 651, 812
Stereophotography, 444
Steroids. See also Corticosteroids
  for osteoarthritis, 574
  for repetitive injury syndromes, 97, 98, 99, 100, 103
Stiffness
  external fixation frame modification, 309
  from ganglion cyst excision, 688
  with Kienböck's disease, 395
  of ligaments, 441
  proximal row carpectomy for relief, 553
Still's disease, 166
STIR imaging, 77
Strain, maximum, 441
Strain gauges, 38
Strength. See also Grip strength; Pinch strength
  gender aspects, 28, 29
  normal, 28, 29
  structural, 10
Stress-loading Dystrophile program, 391, 747–751, 801, 835
Stress testing, 87, 217, 759–760, 786
STT. See Scaphoid-trapezium-trapezoid ligament complex
Styloidectomy, 84, 91–92, 495, 549, 551, 904, 937
Styloid fractures. See Radial styloid, fractures; Ulnar styloid, fractures
Subacute trauma, 75–76
Subchondral sclerosis, 189
Subluxation. See also Rotary subluxation of the scaphoid
  after basal joint resection, 575
  carpal, 205
  distal radioulnar joint, 64, 374, 601, 838
  dorsal carpal, 343, 349–350, 478
  extensor carpi ulnaris tendon, 592, 597–598, 600, 650
  metacarpophalageal joints, 639–641
  rotary, 241, 250, 431
  tendon, 98
  triscaphe joint, 512
  vs. dislocation, 241
Substitution maneuvers, 57–58
Suction drains, 336
Suction punch, 84, 623
Sudomotor changes, with reflex sympathetic dystrophy, 745, 885
Sugar-tong splint, 89, 291, 293–294, 336, 357, 671, 677
Sulfasalazine, 667
Superficial ligaments, 14, 15
Supernumerary muscle belly syndrome, 104
Supination deformity, 671–672
Supraretinacular arch, 910
Surgeon, psychological aspects, 296, 579
Surgery
  basis for, 92
  as prophylactic or reconstructive, rather than salvage, 667
  time spent on procedures, 93
Surgi-Airtome, 426–427
Surgical assistant, role in arthroscopy, 84
Surgical suite for arthroscopy, 84
Surgical technique. See also Excision; Resection; Sutures
  arthritis of the distal radioulnar joint, 601
  arthroscopy, 84, 86, 87
  bone graft, biconcave, 901–903
  bone graft, vascularized, 910–912
  bone harvest, 815, 816

capitate shortening with capitate-hamate fusion, 786–788
capsulodesis for rotary subluxation of the scaphoid, 820–824
carpal boss repair, 793–794
carpal tunnel release, 101, 110–114, 120
carpometacarpal joint ligament reconstruction, 571–572, 574–577, 579
carpometacarpal tendon arthroplasty, 797–800
cocompartment release for tenosynovitis, 953, 954
Darrach procedure, 805–808
de Quervain's disease, 97
distal radioulnar joint dislocation stabilization, 812–813
distal radius fractures, 315
   approaches, 320–322
   external fixation, 316–318, 323–336
   Fernandez Type I bending fractures, 323, 324
   Fernandez Type II shearing fractures, 323, 325–327
   Fernandez Type III compression fractures, 327–333, 337
   Fernandez Type IV avulsion fractures, 333–335
   Fernandez Type V complex fractures, 335–336
   fixation, 306–308, 309–310
distal radius malunion, 351–364
dorsal intercarpal ligament in capsulodesis, 247–249
dorsal wrist syndrome, 485–486, 829–830
drilling, 184
endoscopic-assisted, 101
ganglia, 164
hereditary multiple exostoses, 143
incision placement, 17
ligamentous repair for scapholunate dissociation, 492–498
lunotriquetral arthrodesis, 833–834
Madelung's deformity, 140
malignant tumor biopsy, 724–725
malignant tumor excision, 725–726
matched ulnar arthroplasty, 847–850
perilunate dislocation, 211–214, 243–245
proximal row carpectomy, 546–551
radial club hand treatment, 145–146
radial shortening osteotomy, 855–859
radiocarpal arthrodesis-arthroplasty, 861–863, 864
radiolunate arthrodesis, 867–868, 869
radioulnar arthrodesis, 875, 876–877
replantation, 269, 270–274
rheumatoid arthritis, 649
Sauvé-Kapandji procedure, 889–891

scaphocapitate arthrodesis, 895–897, 898
scaphoid fractures, 193–196, 901–903
scapholunate advanced collapse reconstruction, 921–924, 925
scapholunate ligament repair, 246–249
"short-incision," 101
total wrist arthrodesis, 558–563, 651
trapezoidal osteotomy of the distal radius, 927–929
triangular fibrocartilage complex tears, 609–612
triquetral impingement ligament tear syndrome, 633–634
triscaphe arthrodesis, 931–934, 936
ulnar lengthening, 939–940, 941, 942
ulnar shortening osteotomy, 625
universal wrist prosthesis, 672–679
vascular implantation, 401–402, 405, 406, 421–424
Survival rate for replantation, 275
Sutures
   anchor, 89, 823–824
   Dacron, 924
   Dexon, 799, 863
   Ethibond, 577
   mini-Mitek-anchor, 577
   monofilament nonabsorbable, for replantation, 274
   prolene pullout, 822, 823
   3-0 silk retraction, 672
   Tycron, 577
   ultrafine nonreactive, 269
   used to transect a tendon, 799
   Vicryl, 577, 799, 812
Swan-neck deformity, 641, 645, 801
Swanson silastic wrist implant, 660, 663, 870
Swelling. See also Epidermal inclusion cysts; Ganglion cysts
   carpal dislocation, 218, 236, 250
   carpometacarpal fracture-dislocation, 265
   with a cast, 192, 783
   computed tomography, 68
   distal radius fracture, 336
   "double hump" configuration, 647
   Kienböck's disease, 395
   perilunate instability, 206–207, 211
   pisiform dislocation, 225
   scaphoid-lunate dislocation, 222
   from total wrist arthrodesis, 564
   trapezoid dislocation, 219
   triquetral impingement ligament tear syndrome, 633
   triquetrum dislocation, 224
Swiss Association for the Study of Problems of Internal Fixation, 280
Symbrachydactyly, 124, 125, 136
Sympathectomy, 746
Sympathetically maintained pain, 742
Sympathetic nervous system, 742–743, 744

Synchondrosis, 533–535, 833
Syndactyly, 131, 137
Synostoses
   associated with radial deficiency, 131
   capitate, 123, 124
   carpal, 123–125, 479
   distal radioulnar, 136–137
   hamate, 123, 124
   lunotriquetral, 123
   metacarpal, 124, 125
   multiple synostoses syndrome, 125, 129
   radioulnar, 136–137
Synovectomy, 101, 167
   distal radioulnar joint, 650, 654, 803
   intercarpal ligament tears, 609
   with rheumatoid arthritis, 639, 642, 650, 654, 803, 861
   in universal wrist prosthesis surgery, 673
Synovial cell sarcoma, 736, 737
Synovial compartment, 69
Synovial cyst, 76. See also Ganglion cysts
Synovitis. See also Tenosynovitis
   after reconstruction of the scapholunate joint, 439
   carpal tunnel, 118
   diagnostic imaging, 70, 74, 76, 78
   distal radioulnar joint, 601
   extensor carpi ulnaris, 47, 55
   with juvenile arthritis, 166
   mechanism of injury, 451
   scapholunate, 483, 484
   shake test for, 592
   with shearing of hyaline cartilage, 465
   silicone, 871, 923
   with total wrist implants, 665
Synovium, 639, 654
Systemic lupus erythematosis, 672

T

Tagging, importance during replantation, 270, 271
Tajima stitch, 274
TCL. See Transverse carpal ligament
TE. See Echo time
Team approach
   cerebral palsy, 154
   juvenile arthritis, 167
   replantation, 270
Technetium-99. See Bone scintigraphy
Technetium-99-methylene diphosphate. See Bone scintigraphy
Teeth suck, 57
Temperature
   of casting material during application, 782
   post-replantation monitoring, 275
   of skin, 695, 885
Tendinitis
   calcified, 371, 615
   diagnostic imaging, 74

Tendinitis (contd.)
  extensor carpi ulnaris, 55, 600
  flexor carpi radialis, 57, 99, 758
  flexor carpi ulnaris, 99
  neural disorders which mimic, 95
  with radial shortening osteotomy, 859
  with total wrist arthrodesis, 564
Tendon excursion and moment arms, 40–43
Tendonitis
  calcific, diagnostic imaging, 70
  extensor carpi ulnaris tendon, 47
Tendon roll replacement, 420
Tendons
  adherence. See Tenosynovitis
  arthroplasty, 797
  effects of distal radius fracture and surgery, 336–337
  graft technique, 378–379, 382
  implantation in amputation, 275
  as landmarks for arthroscopy, 85
  outpouching from sheath. See Ganglion cysts
  repair during replantation, 270, 271, 274
  repair with rheumatoid arthritis, 649
  rupture from Darrach procedure, 809
  rupture from pin track irritation, 790
  rupture from rheumatoid arthritis, 640–642, 647–648
  rupture from scaphoid fracture surgery, 196
  subluxation, 98
  testing in wrist evaluation, 759
Tendon sheath xanthoma, 691–692
Tendon slips, 99
Tenodesis
  in amputation, 275
  extensor carpi radialis brevis, 213
  rheumatoid arthritis, 650
  total wrist arthrodesis for, 556
Tenosynovectomy, 649
Tenosynovitis, 95–96. See also Carpal tunnel syndrome
  accelerated. See Pediatrics, juvenile arthritis
  cocompartment release for, 639, 654, 953–954
  diagnosis, 74, 758, 759
  from distal radius surgery, 337
  extensor carpi ulnaris, 600, 602
  extensor compartment, 47, 95–96, 98
  of the first dorsal compartment, 47, 55, 573
  fluoroquinolone-induced, 96
  of the fourth dorsal compartment, 954
  with gout, 584
  infection and, 78
  with intersection syndrome, 56
  nonspecific, 99
  rheumatoid, 647, 648, 649, 683, 711–712

  from total wrist arthrodesis, 564
Tensile forces in fractures, 173
Tensile properties of ligaments, 441
Tension-band technique, 377
Tension wiring for distal radius fractures, 287
"Terry Thomas" sign, 239, 819, 820
TFCC. See Triangular fibrocartilage complex
TH. See Triquetrohamate joint; Triquetrohamate ligaments
Thalidomide, 127
Thenar muscle, 113, 117, 119
Thermography, liquid crystal, 189
Thermometers, 275
Thoracic outlet syndrome (TOS), 95, 103, 592
Three-dimensional carpal motion studies, 34–36
3M Corporation, 114
Three-phase bone scan, 70, 724, 746
Three-point fixation method, 191
Thrombosis
  with Guyon's syndrome, 102
  of the ulnar artery, 598, 603
Thumb. See also Metacarpal, first; Trapeziometacarpal joint
  absence of, 129, 138, 146
  anatomy, 568
  in carpal tunnel syndrome diagnosis, 117–118
  hypoplasia, 126, 128, 130, 131, 144
  osteoarthritis, 578
  positioning during trapeziometacarpal joint arthrodesis, 578
  range-of-motion, 570–571
  replantation, 269
  rheumatoid arthritis, 578
  substitute. See Pollicization
  suspensionplasty, 183
  triphalangeal, 131, 132, 133
  triplication of, 138, 139
  zed, 641–642, 654
Thumb-spica cast
  basal joint resection, 577
  scaphoid dislocation, 220
  scaphoid-lunate dislocation, 222
  scapholunate joint reconstruction, 438
  trapezium dislocation, 223
Thyroid disease with carpal tunnel syndrome, 100
Tibia vara, 151
TILT. See Triquetral impaction ligament tear syndrome
Timeframe
  for external fixation removal, 337
  for replantation, 269
Tinel's sign, 103, 108, 686, 699
Titanium plates, 326
Titanium replacement arthroplasty, 404, 430, 660, 661, 663, 666–667

TL. See Triquetral-lunate joint
TMC. See Trapeziometacarpal joint
"Toe of the boot" osteophyte, 798, 799
Tolmetin for juvenile arthritis, 167
Tomography
  carpal dislocation, 237
  carpometacarpal fracture-dislocations, 265–266
  computed. See Computed tomography
  conventional, 63–64
  distal radius fracture, 312, 318, 332
  Kienböck's disease, 398
  perilunar dislocation, 207, 210
  vascularized bone graft, 913, 914
T1-weighted images, 73, 190
Tophi. See Gout
TOS. See Thoracic outlet syndrome
Total wrist arthrodesis. See Arthrodesis, total wrist
Tourniquet control
  bone-retinaculum-bone autograft, 916
  distal radius fracture, 316
  pneumatic, for arthroscopy, 84
  in replantation, 271, 273
  total wrist arthroplasty, 672
  tumors, 695
T-plate
  for distal radius fracture, 326, 328, 330, 337, 352, 353
  in radial shortening osteotomy, 857, 859
TqHC. See Triquetrum-hamate-capitate ligament complex
TR. See Repetition time
Traction
  for arthroscopy, 84
  during distal radius fixation, 307, 309–310
  finger trap, 84, 211, 241, 289, 290, 291, 307
  to the thumb, for Bennett's fracture reduction, 257
Traction Tower, 84, 90, 595
"Trampoline effect," 610
Transcarpal instability classification, 262
Transcutaneous nerve stimulation (TENS), 747. See also Electrical stimulation
Transmetacarpal instability classification, 262
Transradial styloid perilunate dislocation, 240, 245
Transscaphoid perilunate, fracture-dislocations, 196
Transtriquetral fracture-dislocations, 241
Transverse carpal ligament (TCL). See also Surgical technique, carpal tunnel release
  anatomy, 17, 434
  first surgical release, 107
  in perilunate dislocation surgery, 212
  with pisiform dislocation, 225

trapezium, 175
Trapezial ridge, 175
Trapeziolunate external fixator, 194
Trapeziometacarpal joint (TMC)
  anatomy, 256
  arthrodesis, 577–578
  dislocations, 258
  ganglia of the, 685, 688
  injuries, 255–258
  instability, 571
  ligament repair, 574–577
  osteoarthritis, 572
  physical examination, 53
  in trapezium fractures, 175
Trapeziotrapezoidal joint, computed tomography, 67
Trapezium
  with Bennett's fracture, 257
  with carpal dislocation, 242
  computed tomography, 68
  dislocation, 222–223, 226
  displacement with axial dislocation of carpus, 218
  evolution of the, 3
  excision, 574, 575, 576
  fractures, 174, 175, 579
  motion of the first metacarpal, 255
  ontogenesis, 7
  ossification, 149
  osteology, 9, 10
  osteotomy, 797
  with radial deficiency, 128–129, 130, 131, 132
  in radioulnar deviation, 24, 463–464
  unstable fractures, 258, 259
Trapezoid
  with carpal dislocation, 242
  dislocation, 218, 219–220, 226, 261
  evolution of the, 3
  fractures, 174, 175
  fusion, 219
  motion of the second and third metacarpals, 255
  ontogenesis, 7
  osteology, 9, 10
  in radioulnar deviation, 24
Trapezoidal osteotomy, 927–930
Trapezoid-trapezium ligament, 14, 15
Trauma
  acute, diagnostic imaging algorithm, 74–75
  as cause of reflex sympathetic dystrophy, 741, 743, 744
  explosion, 303, 304, 309, 310
  Kienböck's disease and, 397
  penetration, 206, 696
  remote, 75–76
  subacute, 75–76
  twisting, 98
Trebeculae, 413, 414

Triangular fibrocartilage complex (TFCC)
  in amputation, 275
  anatomy, 8, 11–12, 42–43, 232, 370, 435, 607, 612, 616
  arthroscopy, 85–86, 87, 88–90, 593, 595
  biomechanics, 442, 607
  calcium pyrophosphate deposition disease in, 587
  changes in thickness, 351
  chronic instability, 378–380
  classification system, 88, 595–596, 608
  debridement and reattachment, 378–379, 380
  diagnostic imaging, 69, 74, 75, 76
  differential diagnosis, 595–596
  with distal radioulnar joint disorders, 374, 377–378, 812
  in distal radius surgery, 321
  distribution of force, 38
  evolution of the, 3, 4
  following distal radius fracture, 341, 342, 343–344, 346–347, 350, 356
  with lunotriquetral joint instability, 450, 505, 835
  ontogenesis, 7
  physical examination, 52, 592
  tears, 88, 89, 93, 284
    age-related, 343
    arthroscopy, 84, 608
    classification, 88, 595–596, 608, 616, 619–622
    diagnosis, 48, 52
    with distal radioulnar joint disorders, 374
    in gymnasts, 154
    with TILT, 636, 637
    treatment, 609–610, 769–770. See also under Debridement
  ulnar detachment of the, 610–611
  vascular anatomy, 607
Triphalangeal thumb, 131, 132, 133
Triquetral capitate ligament, 224
Triquetral impaction ligament tear syndrome (TILT), 604, 613, 633–638
  clinical examination, 389, 601
  following ulnar arthroplasty, 851
  physical examination, 48, 53
  treatment, 768
  with ulnar wrist pain, 601, 604
Triquetral-lunate joint (TL). See also Lunotriquetral joint
  congenital abnormalities, 534, 603
  dissociation, 511, 601
  embryonic development, 146
Triquetrocapitate ligament, 502
Triquetrohamate joint (TH)
  arthrodesis, 538–539
  arthroscopy, 86, 88
  in capitate fractures, 176

  dissociation, 511
  instability, 516
  Kienböck's disease load transfer and, 790
  kinematics, 462, 501, 508
Triquetrohamate ligaments (TH)
  anatomy, 502
  with capitate dislocation, 225
  with triquetrohamate joint dissociation, 516
  in triquetrum dislocation, 224
Triquetrolunate ligaments. See Lunotriquetral ligaments
Triquetrum
  displacement and dislocation, 218, 224–225, 238, 472
  fracture-dislocations, 241
  fractures, 181–182, 184, 446, 447
    differential diagnosis, 599
    in the immature wrist, 159
    incidence rate, 174
    misdiagnosis, 179
  with Kienböck's disease, 400
  kinematics, 502–503
  ossification, 149
  osteology, 10
  tears in children, 160
  in triquetral impingement ligament tear syndrome, 633–634
Triquetrum-hamate-capitate ligament complex (TqHC), 14, 15, 16
Triscaphe joint
  arthrodesis, 522–523, 540, 931–937
    with dorsal wrist syndrome, 487
    indications, 406
    outcomes, 403, 766–767
    with scapholunate dissociation, 531
    and triquetral impingement ligament tear syndrome, 636
    wrist motion following, 249
  with carpal dislocation, 226
  degenerative arthritis, 532–533
  dislocation, 531–532
  fusion, 403, 406, 499
  physical examination, 49, 50, 528
  subluxation, 512
Trispherical total wrist prosthesis, 661–662, 670
Trocar, 86, 113
Trophic changes, 48, 745, 885
T2-weighted images, 73, 594
Tubercle, 9. See also Lister's tubercle
Tumors
  benign
    bone, 683, 704–711
    carpal, 693
    nerve, 102, 683, 697–704
    subcutaneous tissue, 683, 684–692
    vascular, 683, 692–697
  diagnostic imaging, 73, 74

Tumors (contd.)
  distal radius, and total wrist arthrodesis, 556
  in the immature wrist, 164
  magnetic resonance imaging, 73
  malignant. See also Giant cell tumor; Histiocytoma; Sarcoma
    biopsy of, 724–725
    metastatic, 737, 739
    patient evaluation, 723–724
  multiple hereditary exostoses, 142–143
Turner's syndrome, 151
Two-point substitution, 58

U

UL. See Ulnocapitate ligament; Ulnolunate ligament
Ulcers, in the fingers, 696
Ulna
  allograft replacement and giant cell tumor, 729, 731, 732
  anatomy, 8, 434, 847
  arthroplasty, 296, 629, 644, 769, 809, 847–853, 863
  congenital deficiencies, 134, 135–136
  cuff resection, 357, 615, 635, 638
  deficiency, 135–136
  distal
    epiphysis of the, 8
    excision after arthrodesis, 564
    fractures, 162–163
    impingement after arthrodesis, 564
    resection, 355, 358–359, 653, 654
    shaping, 844
    stabilization in Darrach procedure, 806–807
  duplication of. See Mirror hand
  evolution of the, 3, 4, 5
  fractures, 284
    in children, 160–163
    with distal radioulnar joint disorders, 377
    in the immature wrist, 160–163
  harvest for bone graft, 427
  lengthening, 402, 939–943
    for distal radioulnar joint disorders, 391
    for Kienböck's disease, 419, 420, 428, 769
    and triquetral impingement ligament tear syndrome, 636
  with Madelung's deformity, 151
  ontogenesis, 7
  osteotomy. See Osteotomy, ulna
  overgrowth due to repetitive loading, 156
  pain associated with the, 591–604, 615
  in replantation, 272
  resection, 89, 806, 841, 849, 851
  with rheumatoid arthritis, 642–643, 803.
    See also Darrach procedure
  rotatory displacement, 263
  shaft, malunion, 385, 387
  shortening, 160, 357
    with distal radioulnar joint disorders, 380–381, 391
    formal, for ulnar impaction syndrome, 624–625
    with hereditary multiple exostoses, 143
    stabilization with, 625
    with triquetral impingement ligament tear syndrome, 638
  stabilization, 11, 809
  translocation, 809
  variance. See Ulnar variance
Ulnar artery
  anatomy, 395, 396
  aneurysms, 692
  thrombosis, 598, 603
Ulnar collateral ligament, 432, 435
Ulnar deficiency, 135–136
Ulnar detachment of the TFCC, 610–611
Ulnar deviation deformity, 670–671, 675, 679
Ulnar drift, 639–641
Ulnar head
  anatomy, 369
  cross-section, 839
  excision, 596, 889
  fracture with distal radioulnar joint disorders, 374–375
  with Madelung's deformity, 151
  resection, 89, 806, 839, 841
  shortening, "wafer procedure," 610, 624, 626, 628
Ulnar impaction syndrome, 350–351, 602–603, 615–629, 633
  diagnostic imaging, 62, 63, 74
  with distal radioulnar joint disorders, 380
  dynamic, 627
  force and pressure, 40, 388–389
  physical examination, 592
  secondary, 627–628
  treatment, 622–627
  vs. ulnar impingement syndrome, 615–616
Ulnar impingement syndrome (UIS), 633
  differential diagnosis, 596, 615
  matched ulnar resection for, 851
  vs. ulnar impaction syndrome, 615–616
Ulnar midcarpal portal (UMC), 86
Ulnar nerve
  anatomy, 946
  with carpal tunnel syndrome, 119
  complications from total wrist arthrodesis, 563, 564
  compression, 102
  denervation, 948–949
  in distal radioulnar joint surgery, 390
  injury with Sauvé-Kapandji procedure, 891
  lipofibromatous hamartoma, 702
  neuroma, 843, 850
  in perilunate dislocation surgery, 244
  in pisotriquetral joint dysfunction, 598
Ulnar physis, 154–155, 156
Ulnar recurrent artery, 396
Ulnar sling mechanism
  anatomy, 613, 633
  with distal ulna resection, 809, 844
  in matched ulnar arthroplasty, 849, 850
  TILT and, 633, 638
  ulnar lengthening and, 769
"Ulnar snuff box," 52, 85, 86
Ulnar stump instability, 809
Ulnar styloid
  anatomy, 8
  with carpal fracture, 159
  in distal radius surgery, 320, 804
  excision, 840
  fractures, 212, 284, 346–347, 375–377
  with matched hemiresection-interposition arthroplasty, 844
  nonunion, 385, 597, 602, 603
  ontogenesis, 7
  with TFCC tears, 160, 611
Ulnar translation
  definition, 456
  with radiocarpal dislocation, 205, 216–217
  with scaphoid-lunate dislocation, 222
Ulnar variance
  determination, 617
  with distal radius fractures, 313
  force and pressure with, 37, 39, 42, 234–235, 388–389, 462
  with Kienböck's disease, 396–397, 405, 412, 419, 420, 428, 785, 939, 941, 942
  progression of force with, 234–235, 350
  radiographic parameters, 348, 349
  with triquetral impingement ligament tear syndrome, 635
Ulnocapitate ligament (UL), 14, 502
Ulnocarpal abutment syndrome, 608, 615
Ulnocarpal impaction/impingement, 843, 844
Ulnocarpal ligament, 224, 456
Ulnolunate joint, distribution of force, 39
Ulnolunate ligament, anatomy, 14, 50, 232, 370, 389, 432, 434, 435, 456
Ulnotriquetral ligament (UTL;UTq), 444
  anatomy, 14–15, 232, 370, 389, 432, 435, 502
  in carpal dislocations, 448, 450
Ultrasound, 72
  ganglion cysts, 486, 686
  for heat therapy, 764
  scaphoid fractures, 189, 193
  ulnar wrist pain, 594
UMC. See Ulnar midcarpal portal
Unciform bone. See Hamate

Unciform process, 11. *See also* Hook of hamate
Unicameral bone cyst, 710–711
Union, delayed
  resorption at the fracture, 189
  subchondral sclerosis, 189
  timeframe, 190
Universal Classification, 314
Universal wrist prosthesis, 663, 664, 666–667, 672–679
Uric acid. *See* Gout
Uricosuric drugs, 586
U.S. Department of Labor, 765
UTL. *See* Ulnotriquetral ligament
UTq. *See* Ulnotriquetral ligament

V
Vanadium, in total wrist prostheses, 660
Vascular anatomy
  in bone scintigraphy, 70
  distal radioulnar joint, 595, 617
  distal radius, 907–910
  distal ulna, 617
  in the fracture healing process, 198
  hamate, 178
  injury from scaphoid fracture surgery, 196
  lunate, 395–396, 411, 412, 414, 786
  scaphoid, 158, 187, 198, 220
  scapholunate interosseous ligament, 437
  scapholunate ligament, 904
  testing in wrist evaluation, 759
  transverse carpal ligament, 107–108
  trapezoid, 219, 220
  triangular fibrocartilage complex, 607
Vascular bundle implantation, 405
  historical background, 401
  Hori procedure, 401–402
  for Kienböck's disease, 420–426
Vascular component of reflex sympathetic dystrophy, 743–744
Vascular examination, 592
Vascularized bone grafts, 907–914
Vascular tumors, benign, 683, 692–697
Vasomotor changes, with reflex sympathetic dystrophy, 745, 885
Vaughan-Jackson lesion, 647, 803
Vein grafts, 273, 274
Vein repair, 269, 270, 271, 273–274
Venous congestion and Kienböck's disease, 397
Venous hemangioma, 694
Viability. *See* Survival rate for replantation
Vibration disorders
  fatigue, 413
  focal bone lesions from, 78
  hypothenar hammer syndrome, 164
  trauma, 102
Vibration sense, 592
Video technique, 83, 84, 110, 469, 871, 915, 916
Viral infections and juvenile rheumatoid arthritis, 165
VISI. *See* Volar intercalated segment instability
Visual analog scale, 949
Vitamin E, 120
Volar approach to internal fixation, 194–195
Volar intercalated segment instability (VISI), 478
  collapse pattern, 238
  with Kienböck's disease, 400
  lunate shape and, 513
  with lunotriquetral instability, 503
  midcarpal instability and, 512, 517, 518
  neutral anatomy position and, 508
  with perilunate dislocation, 205, 208
  progression of force and pathogenesis, 235, 431, 473–474
  radiography, 250–251
  with scaphoid-lunate dislocation, 222
  secondary, following distal radius fracture, 341, 346
Volar plate test, 57–58, 745, 887
Volar radiolunotriquetral ligament. *See* Radiolunate ligament, long
Volar tilt, 350
Volar-ulnar dislocation, 640
Volar wrist crease, 144
Volz prosthesis, 653, 660, 666, 670, 679
von Recklinghausen's disease, 697
"V sign," 250

W
"Wafer procedure," 88–89, 610, 624, 626, 628
Waist fractures of the scaphoid, 190, 191, 192
Wartenberg's syndrome, 96, 103, 758
"Washboard," of carpal ligament, 111
Wedge. *See* Bone grafts, interpositional wedge; Osteotomy
Wire fixation. *See* Kirschner wires
Wire suture passer, 212
Work aspects. *See* Occupational aspects; Occupational health
Wounds, open, 206, 783
Wright's test, 592
Wrist "click"
  ganglion cysts, 686
  with lunotriquetral instability, 503, 504–505
  with scapholunate instability, 469, 471
  with scapholunate interosseous ligament injury, 343
  with triangular fibrocartilage complex tears, 160, 610
  with ulnar impaction syndrome, 622
  with ulnar wrist pain, 591, 595, 600, 892
Wrist "clunk"
  with carpal instability nondissociative, 477, 478
  with dynamic scapholunate instability, 469, 471
  with Kienböck's disease, 400
  with midcarpal instability, 511, 514, 517
  with rotary subluxation of the scaphoid, 819, 825
  with scaphoid wrist maneuver, 5229
Wrist fusion. *See* Arthrodesis, total wrist
Wrist motion
  advantages of wrist arthroplasty, 659
  continuous passive motion, 764
  effects of arthrodesis, 521, 542, 659
  following proximal row carpectomy, 551, 552
  functional assessment, 759–760
  general, 28–32
  normal arc, 557
  occupational demands, and total wrist arthrodesis, 556
  in physical examination, 51
  physiologic, 32–33
  rotation, 38, 233
Wrist preparation for arthroscopy, 84
Wrist simulators, dynamic, 36. *See also* Models
Wrist "snap," 349

X
Xanthine oxidase inhibitors, 586
Xanthoma, fibrous, 691–692, 715
Xeroform gauze, 274, 275
X-ray. *See also* Radiography
  in conventional diagnostics, 61–63
  early studies, 21, 34
  four routine exposures, 61–63, 75, 77
  limitations of, 63
  radiolunate arthrodesis, 871, 874
  of scaphoid shift, 51
Xylocaine, 111

Y
Young's modulus, 441, 444
Yttrium-90, 588

Z
Zed thumb deformity, 641–642, 654